EIGENTUM DER
LANDESKRANKENANSTALTEN
SALZBURG

CARDIAC ARRHYTHMIAS: Where To Go From Here?

edited by

PEDRO BRUGADA, M.D.

Associate Professor, University of Limburg
Director, Clinical Electrophysiology Laboratory
Department of Cardiology, Academic Hospital
Maastricht, The Netherlands

and

HEIN J.J. WELLENS, M.D.

Professor of Cardiology, University of Limburg
Chairman, Department of Cardiology
Academic Hospital
Maastricht, The Netherlands

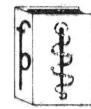

FUTURA PUBLISHING COMPANY, INC.
Mount Kisco, New York
1987

Library of Congress Cataloging-in-Publication Data

Cardiac arryhythmias.

   Include bibliographies and index.
   1. Arrhythmia. I. Brugada, Pedro. II. Wellens,
H. J. J. [DNLM: 1. Arrhythmia—diagnosis. 2. Arrhythmia
—therapy. WG 330 C2688]
RC685.A65C284   1987   616.1′28   87-9005
ISBN 0-87993-306-2

Copyright 1987
Futura Publishing Company, Inc.

Published by
Futura Publishing Company, Inc.
295 Main Street
Mount Kisco, New York

L.C. No.: 87-9005
ISBN No.: 87993-306-2

All rights reserved.
No part of this book may translated or reproduced in any form
without the written permission of the Publisher.

Dedication

This book is in appreciation of all the investigators who inspired us and showed us the way to study and treat our patients suffering from cardiac arrhythmias. It is dedicated to all human beings who hold our future in their hands. Among them, our children Isabel, Floor, Willemijn, Maarten en Jooske.

Contributors

Masood Akhtar, MD
University of Wisconsin, Milwaukee Clinical Campus, Mount Sinai Medical Center, Milwaukee, Wisconsin, USA

Maurits A. Allessie, MD, PhD
Department of Physiology, University of Limburg, Maastricht, The Netherlands

H. Dieter Ambos, MD
Cardiovascular Division, Washington University School of Medicine, St. Louis, Missouri, USA

Angel Arenal, MD
Department of Medicine, Montreal Heart Institute, Montreal, Quebec, Canada

Anirban Banerjee, PhD
Department of Surgery, University of Colorado, Denver, Colorado, USA

M. Baraka, MD
Service de Rythmologie et de Stimulation Cardiaque, Hôpital Jean Rostand, Ivry, France

Anton E. Becker, MD
Department of Pathology, University of Amsterdam, Academic Medical Center, Amsterdam, The Netherlands

Felix I.M. Bonke, MD, PhD
Department of Physiology, University of Limburg, Maastricht, The Netherlands

Ivan M.G.P. Bourgeois, Ir, MBA
Int. Research and Science Center B.V. Medtronic, Maastricht, The Netherlands

Josep Brugada, MD
Service de Cardiologie B, Clinique St. Eloi, Montpellier, France

Pedro Brugada, MD
Department of Cardiology, University of Limburg, Maastricht, The Netherlands

Alfred E. Buxton, MD
Cardiovascular Section, Department of Medicine, University of Pennsylvania, Philadelphia, Pennsylvania, USA

Michael E. Cain, MD
Cardiovascular Division, Washington University School of Medicine, St. Louis, Missouri, USA

CONTRIBUTORS

Dennis Cassidy, MD
Department of Medicine, Montreal Heart Institute, Montreal, Quebec, Canada

Agustin Castellanos, MD
Division of Cardiology, Department of Medicine, University of Miami School of Medicine, Miami, Florida, USA

Mark J. Cooper, FRACP
Cardiology Unit, Westmead Hospital, Westmead, Australia

Angelika Costard, MD
Department of Cardiology, University Hospital Eppendorf, Hamburg, Fed. Rep. of Germany

Philippe Coumel, MD
Hôpital Lariboisière, Paris, France

James L. Cox, MD
Division of Cardiothoracic Surgery, Barnes Hospital, St. Louis, Missouri, USA

Elizabeth Darling, RN
Krannert Institute of Cardiology, Indiana University School of Medicine, Indianapolis, Indiana, USA

Willem Dassen, PhD
Department of Cardiology, University of Limburg, Maastricht, The Netherlands

Paolo Della Bella, MD
Department of Cardiology, University of Limburg, Maastricht, The Netherlands

A. Robert Denniss, MD
Department of Medicine, Westmead Hospital, Westmead, Australia

Stephen Dillon, PhD
Department of Pharmacology, Columbia University, New York, New York, USA

Thierry Dugernier, MD
Department of Cardiology, University of Limburg, Maastricht, The Netherlands

Karel den Dulk, MD
Department of Cardiology, University of Limburg, Maastricht, The Netherlands

G. Thomas Evans, Jr., MD
Department of Medicine and Cardiovascular Research Institute, University of California, San Francisco, California, USA

Paul Fahey BSc, Dip Med Stat
Department of Community Medicine, Westmead Hospital, Westmead, Australia

G. Farenq, MD
Service de Rythmologie et de Stimulation Cardiaque, Hôpital Jean Rostand, Ivry, France

Jerónimo Farré, MD
Department of Cardiology, Fundacion Jimenez Diaz, Universidad Autonoma, Madrid, Spain

Pedro Fernandez, MD
Division of Cardiology, Department of Medicine, Univeristy of Miami School of Medicine, Miami, Florida, USA

Naomi Fineberg, PhD
Krannert Institute of Cardiology, Indiana University School of Medicine, Indianapolis, Indiana, USA

Charles Fisch, MD
Krannert Institute of Cardiology, Indiana University School of Medicine, Indianapolis, Indiana, USA

John D. Fisher, MD
Montefiore Medical Center, Albert Einstein College of Medicine, Bronx NY, New York, USA

Guy Fontaine, MD
Service de Rythmologie et de Stimulation Cardiaque, Hopital Jean Rostand, Ivry, France

Julián Fraile, MD
Department of Cardiovascular Surgery, Fundacion Jimenez Diaz, Universidad Autonoma, Madrid, Spain

Robert Frank, MD
Service de Rythmologie et de Stimulation Cardiaque, Hôpital Jean Rostand, Ivry, France

Jean-Louis Funck-Brentano, MD
Hôpital Lariboisière, Paris, France

Y. Gallais, MD
Service d'Anesthesiologie, Hôpital Jean Rostand, Ivry, France

Annette Geibel, MD
Innere Medizin III, Universitaetsklinik Freiburg, Freiburg, West Germany

Manfred Geiger, MD
Department of Cardiology, University Hospital Eppendorf, Hamburg, Fed. Rep. of Germany

Daniel Godin, MD
Department of Medicine, Montreal Heart Institute, Montreal, Quebec, Canada

CONTRIBUTORS

Anton P. Gorgels, MD
Department of Cardiology, University of Limburg, Maastricht, The Netherlands

Charles Gottlieb, MD
Cardiovascular Section, Department of Medicine, University of Pennsylvania, Philadelphia, Pennsylvania, USA

Angel Grande, MD
Department of Cardiology, Fundacion Jimenez Diaz, Universidad Autonoma, Madrid, Spain

Y. Grosgogeat, MD
Service de Rythmologie et de Stimulation Cardiaque, Hopital Jean Rostand, Ivry, France

Gerard M. Guiraudon, MD
University Hospital, London, Ontario, Canada

Alden H. Harken, MD
Department of Surgery, University of Colorado, Denver, Colorado, USA

Michael G. Havenith, MD
Department of Pathology, University of Limburg, Maastricht, The Netherlands

James J. Heger, MD
Krannert Institute of Cardiology, Indiana University School of Medicine, Indianapolis, Indiana, USA

Richard W. Henthorn, MD
Department of Medicine, Case Western Reserve University, Cleveland, Ohio, USA

Joseph A. Hill Jr., PhD
Departments of Medicine and Pharmacology, Duke University Medical Center, Durham, North Carolina, USA

Brian F. Hoffman, MD
Departments of Pharmacology and Pediatrics, Columbia University College of Physicians & Surgeons, New York, New York, USA

Stefan Hohnloser, MD
Innere Medizin III Universitaetsklinik Freiburg, Freiburg, Fed. Rep. of Germany

Hiroshi Inoue, MD
Krannert Institute of Cardiology, Department of Medicine, Indiana University School of Medicine, Indianapolis, Indiana, USA

Les Irwig, FFCM
School of Public Health and Tropical Medicine, University of Sydney, Sydney, Australia

Michiel J. Janse, MD
Department of Clinical and Experimental Cardiology, University of Amsterdam, Amsterdam, The Netherlands

Mohammad Jazayeri, MD
University of Wisconsin, Milwaukee Clinical Campus, Mount Sinai Medical School, Milwaukee, Wisconsin, USA

David C. Johnson, FRACS
Cardiothoracic Surgical Units, Westmead Hospital, Westmead, Australia

Nancy J. Johnson, MD
Departments of Pharmacology and Pediatrics, Columbia University College of Physicians & Surgeons, New York, New York, USA

Mark E. Josephson, MD
Cardiovascular Section, Department of Medicine, University of Pennsylvania, Philadelphia, Pennsylvania, USA

Hansjoerg Just, MD
Innere Medizin III, Universitaetsklinik Freiburg, Freiburg, Fed. Rep. of Germany

Kenneth M. Kessler, MD
Division of Cardiology, Department of Medicine, University of Miami School of Medicine, Miami, Florida, USA

Hosen Kiat, FRACP
Cardiology Unit, Westmead Hospital, Westmead, Australia

Soo G. Kim, MD
Montefiore Medical Center, Division of Cardiology, Bronx, New York, USA

Elizabeth Kindwall, MD
Cardiovascular Section, Department of Medicine, University of Pennsylvania, Philadelphia, Pennsylvania, USA

Charles J.H.J. Kirchhof, MD
Department of Physiology, University of Limburg, Maastricht, The Netherlands

George J. Klein, MD
University Hospital, London, Ontario, Canada

Chee Choong Koo, MRCP
Cardiology Unit, Westmead Hospital, Westmead, Australia

S. Kounde, MD
Service de Rythmologie et de Stimulation Cardiaque, Hôpital Jean Rostand, Ivry, France

CONTRIBUTORS

Karl-Heinz Kuck, MD
Department of Cardiology, University Hospital Eppendorf, Hamburg, Fed. Rep. of Germany

Henri E. Kulbertus, MD
Department of Cardiology, University of Liège Medical School, Liege, Belgium

Klaus-Peter Kunze, MD
Department of Cardiology, University Hospital Eppendorf, Hamburg, Fed. Rep. of Germany

Wim J.E.P. Lammers, MD
Department of Physiology, University of Limburg, Maastricht, The Netherlands

Richard Langendorf, MD
The Michael Reese Hospital, Chicago, Illinois, USA

Ralph Lazzara, MD
Department of Medicine, University of Oklahoma Health Sciences Center, Oklahoma City, Oklahoma, USA

Jean François Leclercq, MD
Clinique Cardiologique, Lariboisiere Hospital, Paris, France

Antoine Leenhardt, MD
Clinique Cardiologique, Lariboisiere Hospital, Paris, France

Robert Lemery, MD
Department of Cardiology University of Limburg, Maastricht, The Netherlands

Bruce D. Lindsay, MD
Cardiovascular Division, Washington University School of Medicine, St. Louis, Missouri, USA

Gerard C.M. Linssen, BA
Department of Cardiology, University of Limburg, Maastricht, The Netherlands

Elwyn A. Lloyd, MD
Krannert Institute of Cardiology, Indiana University School of Medicine, Indianapolis, Indiana, USA

Etienne Marchand, MD
Department of Medicine, Montreal Heart Institute, Montreal, Quebec, Canada

Jorge Martinell, MD
Department of Cardiovascular Surgery, Fundacion Jimenez Diaz, Universidad Autonoma, Madrid, Spain

William J. McKenna, MD
Cardiovascular Disease Unit, Royal Postgraduate Medical School, London, United Kingom

Contributors • xi

Thomas Meinertz, MD
Innere Medizin III, Universitaetsklinik Freiburg, Freiburg, Fed. Rep. of Germany

Anthony Mercando, MD
Division of Cardiology, Montefiore Medical Center, Bronx, New York, USA

Michel Mirowski, MD
Department of Medicine, Sinai Hospital of Baltimore, Baltimore, Maryland, USA

Peter Mortensen, MD
Cardiothoracic Surgical Units, Westmead Hospital, Westmead, Australia

Morton M. Mower, MD
Department of Medicine, Sinai Hospital of Baltimore, Baltimore, Maryland, USA

Robert J. Myerburg, MD
Division of Cardiology, Department of Medicine, University of Miami School of Medicine, Miami, Florida, USA

Seah Nisam
Cardiac Pacemakers Inc., St. Paul, Minnesota, USA

Ken Okumura, MD
Department of Medicine, Case Western Reserve University, Cleveland, Ohio, USA

Brian Olsahnsky, MD
Department of Medicine, Case Western Reserve University, Cleveland, Ohio, USA

Olaf C. Penn, MD
Department of Cardiothoracic Surgery, University of Limburg, Maastricht, The Netherlands

Eric N. Prystowsky, MD
Krannert Institute of Cardiology, Indiana University School of Medicine, Indianapolis, Indiana, USA

Paul Puech, MD
Service de Cardiologie B, Clinique St. Eloi, Montpellier, France

Gregorio Rábago, MD
Department of Cardiology, Fundacion Jimenez Diaz, Universidad Autonoma, Madrid, Spain

Shahbudin H. Rahimtoola, MB
Section of Cardiology, Department of Medicine, LAC-USC Medical Center, University of Southern California School of Medicine, Los Angeles, California, USA

José A. Ramirez, MD
Department of Cardiovascular Surgery, Fundacion Jimenez Diaz, Universidad Autonoma, Madrid, Spain

CONTRIBUTORS

Pieter L. Rensma, MD
Department of Physiology, University of Limburg, Maastricht, The Netherlands

David A. Richards, MD, FRACP
Cardiology Unit, Westmead Hospital, Westmead, Australia

Michael R. Rosen, MD
Departments of Pharmacology and Pediatrics, Columbia University College of Physicians & Surgeons, New York, New York, USA

David L. Ross, MD, FRACP
Cardiology Unit, Westmead Hospital, Westmead, Australia

Denis Roy, MD
Department of Medicine, Montreal Heart Institute, Montreal, Quebec, Canada

Sanjeev Saksena, MD, FACC
Division of Cardiology, Newark Beth Israel Medical Center, Newark, New Jersey, USA

Masayuki Sakurai, MD
Department of Medicine, University of Oklahoma Health Sciences Center, Oklahoma City, Oklahoma, USA

Melvin M. Scheinman, MD
Department of Medicine and Cardiovascular Research Institute, University of California, San Francisco, California, USA

Benjamin J. Scherlag, MD
Department of Medicine, University of Oklahoma Health Sciences Center, Oklahoma City, Oklahoma, USA

Michael Schlüter, PhD
Department of Cardiology, University Hospital Eppendorf, Hamburg, Fed. Rep. of Germany

Peter J. Schwartz, MD
Ist. Clinca Medica Generale, Ospedale Maggiore e Universita di Milano, Milano, Italy

Arjun D. Sharma, MD, FRCP(C), FACC
University Hospital, London, Ontario, Canada

Mohammad Shenasa, MD, PhD
Centre de Recherche, Hôpital du Sacre-Coeur, University of Montreal, Montreal, Quebec, Canada

Michael B. Simson, MD
Cardiovascular Section, Department of Medicine, University of Pennsylvania, Philadelphia, Pennsylvania, USA

Michael Skinner, MBBS
Cardiology Unit, Westmead Hospital, Westmead, Australia

Contributors • xiii

Robert Slama, MD
Clinique Cardiologique, Lariboisière Hospital, Paris, France

William G. Stevenson, MD
Department of Cardiology, University of Limburg, Maastricht, The Netherlands

Harold C. Strauss, MD
Departments of Medicine and Pharmacology, Duke University Medical Center, Durham, North Carolina, USA

John Sun, MD
Department of Surgery, University of Columbia, Denver, Colorado, USA

Raed Sweiden, MD
Department of Medicine, University of Oklahoma Health Sciences Center, Oklahoma City, Oklahoma, USA

Mario Talajic, MD
Department of Cardiology, University of Limburg, Maastricht, The Netherlands

Amanda Taylor, BSc
Cardiology Unit, Westmead Hospital, Westmead, Australia

Patrick J. Tchou, MD
University of Wisconsin, Milwaukee Clinical Campus, Sinai Medical Center, Milwaukee, Wisconsin, USA

Pierre Theroux, MD
Department of Medicine, Montreal Heart Institute, Montreal, Quebec, Canada

Andrea Thomas, RN
Cardiac Pacemakers Inc., St. Paul, Minnesota, USA

J.L. Tonet, MD
Service de Rythmologie et de Stimulation Cardiaque, Hôpital Jean Rostand, Ivry, France

I. Touzet, MD
Service de Rythmologie et de Stimulation Cardiaque, Hôpital Jean Rostand, Ivry, France

Richard G. Trohman, MD
Division of Cardiology, Department of Medicine, University of Miami School of Medicine, Miami, Florida, USA

Philip C. Ursell, MD
Department of Pathology, Columbia University, New York, New York, USA

John B. Uther, MD, FRACP
Cardiology Unit, Westmead Hospital, Westmead, Australia

CONTRIBUTORS

Marc A. Vos, MS
Department of Cardiology, University of Limburg, Maastricht, The Netherlands

Albert L. Waldo, MD
Department of Medicine, Case Western Reserve University, Cleveland, Ohio, USA

David D. Waters, MD
Department of Medicine, Montreal Heart Institute, Montreal, Quebec, Canada

James N. Weiss, MD
Division of Cardiology, UCLA School of Medicine, Los Angeles, California, USA

Hein J.J. Wellens, MD
Department of Cardiology, University of Limburg, Maastricht, The Netherlands

Glenn J. R. Whitman, MD
Department of Surgery, University of Colorado, Denver, Colorado, USA

Isaac Wiener, MD
Cardiovascular Consultants Medical Group, Van Nuys, California, USA

Roger A. Winkle, MD
Cardiovascular Medicine Coronary Interventions and Cardiac Arrhythmias, Paolo Alto, California, USA

Andrew L. Wit, PhD
Department of Pharmacology, Columbia University, New York, New York, USA

Raymond Yee, MD FRCP(C)
University Hospital, London, Ontario, Canada

Liaqat Zaman, MD
Division of Cardiology, Department of Medicine, University of Miami School of Medicine, Miami, Florida, USA

Manfred Zehender, MD
Innere Medizin III, Universitaetsklinik Freiburg, Freiburg, West Germany

Marc Zimmerman, MD
Hôpital Lariboisière, Paris, France

Douglas P. Zipes, MD
Krannert Institute of Cardiology, Department of Medicine, Indiana University School of Medicine, Indianapolis, Indiana, USA

Preface

Diagnosis, prognostic significance, and treatment of cardiac arrhythmias continue to be a common and frequently puzzling problem in our daily cardiology practice.

In recent years, several new techniques such as 24-hour ECG recordings, programmed electrical stimulation of the heart, measurement of the left ventricular ejection fraction, and the recording of signal averaged cardiac potentials have been advanced as new methods to help us in making diagnostic, prognostic, and therapeutic decisions. Apart from these techniques, several new treatment modalities including new antiarrhythmic drugs, pacing, surgery, and fulguration have become available.

Nineteen eighty-seven marks the twentieth anniversary of the introduction of programmed electrical stimulation of the heart. In 1967, independently from one another, Durrer and co-workers in Amsterdam and Coumel and associates in Paris started to use this technique to investigate the mechanism of arrhythmias in the intact human heart. By doing so, they opened a new era in arrhythmology. It took 10 years before programmed electrical stimulation of the heart became applied world-wide, the major breakthrough being the demonstration that the technique could be used safely in patients suffering from ventricular arrhythmias.

After 20 years of programmed electrical stimulation of the heart, we felt it was appropriate to evaluate what we have learned—not only about the value of programmed electrical stimulation of the heart, but also about the place of the other techniques. More important, however, than reflecting on the past or evaluating our present state of the art is a careful exploration of the future; i.e., what we can expect from the presently available diagnostic and therapeutic possibilities and what information or new techniques are required to improve our treatment of patients with cardiac arrhythmias.

That discussion by the leading experts in the field of cardiac electrophysiology and arrhythmias was held in Maastricht, the Netherlands, in June 1987 and is presented in this book. We are indebted to the contributors, not only because of their timely evaluation of the state of the art, but also, and probably more so, because they were willing to indicate to us which new roads should be explored. It is obvious that we still have a long way to go before the problems of cardiac arrhythmias are solved. The purpose of this book is to stimulate the investigator to go on!

PEDRO BRUGADA, M.D., and HEIN J. J. WELLENS, M.D.

Acknowledgments

This book could not be written without contributors. This book is the result of their work and not of the editors. Our task was easy. We simply had to read the manuscripts and make them more uniform. Peer review was limited. We were interested as much in facts as in ideas, even when ideas were not always supported by hard data. We wanted to know "where to go from here."

The contributors presented their data and ideas during a Congress organized in Maastricht, The Netherlands, June 1987.

In finalizing the book, some hands and brains were invaluable such as those of our secretarial staff, which included Mrs. Miep Hinskens, Miss Carla Wetzels, Miss Anna Lemmens, and Mrs. Janine Weymarshausen, expertly led by Miss Patricia Krekels. Much help was also provided by Mr. Ivan Bourgeois, Mrs. Françoise Regnier, and Mr. Jean-François Gaulis.

Ms. Linda Shaw, editor, and Mr. Jacques Strauss from Futura Publishing Company performed the incredible task of getting this book ready in time for the Congress. They managed to offer the reader a pleasantly designed, high-quality book. The result speaks for itself.

To all our sincere thanks.

Contents

Contributors v
Preface *Pedro Brugada, MD, and Hein J.J. Wellens* xv
Acknowledgments xvi

I. PATHOLOGIC SUBSTRATES OF ARRHYTHMIAS

1. Morphologic Characteristics of Arrhythmias
   Anton E. Becker, MD 3
2. Influences of Anisotropic Tissue Structure on Reentrant Ventricular Tachycardia
   Andrew L. Wit, PhD, Stephen Dillon, PhD, and Philip C. Ursell, MD 27

II. MECHANISMS OF ARRHYTHMIAS

3. Sinus Node Reentry: Fact or Fiction?
   Charles J.H.J. Kirchhof, MD, Felix I.M. Bonke, MD, PhD, and Maurits A. Allessie, MD, PhD 53
4. Flutter and Fibrillation in Experimental Models: What Has Been Learned that Can Be Applied to Humans?
   Maurits A. Allessie, MD, Wim J.E.P. Lammers, MD, Pieter L. Rensma, MD, and Felix I.M. Bonke, MD 67
5. Metabolic Effects of Ischemia: What are the Implications for Arrhythmogenesis and the Treatment of Arrhythmias?
   James N. Weiss, MD 83
6. Arrhythmias during Acute Ischemia in Experimental Models
   Michiel J. Janse, MD 105
7. The Distinction between Triggered Activity and other Cardiac Arrhythmias
   Nancy J. Johnson, MD, and Michael R. Rosen, MD 129
8. The Clinical Relevance of Abnormal Automaticity and Triggered Activity
   Anton P.M. Gorgels, MD, Marc A. Vos, MS, Pedro Brugada, MD, and Hein J.J. Wellens, MD 147
9. Current Perspective on Entrainment of Tachyarrhythmias
   Albert L. Waldo, MD, Brian Olshansky, MD, Ken Okumura, MD, and Richard W. Henthorn, MD 171

10. Localization of the Area of Slow Conduction during Ventricular Tachycardia
    R. Frank, MD, J.L. Tonet, MD, S. Kounde, MD, G. Farenq, MD, and G. Fontaine, MD 191

11. Effects of Simultaneous Vagal and Sympathetic Stimulation on Spontaneous Sinus Cycle Length, Atrial and Ventricular Refractoriness, and Atrioventricular Nodal Conduction
    Hiroshi Inoue, MD, and Douglas P. Zipes, MD 209

12. Modification of the Electrophysiologic Matrix by Antiarrhythmic Drugs
    Brian F. Hoffman, MD 219

III. SUPRAVENTRICULAR ARRHYTHMIAS

13. Role of Electrophysiologic Studies in Supraventricular Tachycardia
    Masood Akhtar, MD, Mohammad Shenasa, MD, PhD, Patrick J. Tchou, MD, and Mohammad Jazayeri, MD 233

14. Atrial Unipolar Waveform Analysis during Retrograde Conduction over Left-Sided Accessory Atrioventricular Pathways
    Jerónimo Farré, MD, Angel Grande, MD, Jorge Martinell, MD, Julián Fraile, MD, José A. Ramirez, MD, and Gregorio Rábago, MD 243

15. Is Understanding the Mechanism of a Supraventricular Arrhythmia Necessary for Correct Treatment?
    Jean Francois Leclercq, MD, Antoine Leenhardt, MD, and Robert Slama, MD 271

16. Antitachycardia Pacing: Is There a Universal Pacing Mode to Terminate Supraventricular Tachycardia?
    Karel den Dulk, MD, Paolo Della Bella, MD, Willem Dassen, PhD, Thierry Dugernier, MD, Pedro Brugada, MD, and Hein J.J. Wellens, MD 285

IV. VENTRICULAR TACHYCARDIA AND SUDDEN DEATH

17. Signal Averaging of the ECG in the Management of Patients with Ventricular Tachycardia: Prediction of Antiarrhythmic Drug Efficacy
    Michael B. Simson, MD, Elizabeth Kindwall, MD, Alfred E. Buxton, MD, and Mark E. Josephson, MD 299

18. Fast Fourier Transform Analysis of the Signal-Averaged Electrocardiogram in the Management of Patients with or Prone to Ventricular Tachycardia or Fibrillation
    Michael E. Cain, MD, H. Dieter Ambos, MD, and Bruce D. Lindsay, MD 311

19. Identification of Patients at Risk of Sudden Death after Myocardial Infarction: The Continued Australian Experience
    David Richards, FRACP, Amanda Taylor, BSc, Paul Fahey, BSc, Dip Med Stat, Les Irwig, FFCM,

Contents • xix

   Chee Choong Koo, MRCP, David Ross, FRACP,
   Mark Cooper, FRACP, Hosen Kiat, FRACP,
   Michael Skinner, MBBS, and John Uther, FRACP 329
20. The Canadian Experience on the Identification of Candidates
  for Sudden Cardiac Death After Myocardial Infarction
   Denis Roy, MD, Angel Arenal, MD, Daniel Godin, MD,
   Etienne Marchand, MD, Dennis Cassidy, MD,
   Pierre Théroux, MD, and David D. Waters, MD 343
21. Sudden Death in Hypertrophic Cardiomyopathy: Identification
  of the "High Risk" Patient
   William J. McKenna, MD 353
22. Programmed Electrical Stimulation in Patients with Hypertrophic
  Cardiomyopathy: Results in Patients with and without Cardiac
  Arrest or Syncope
   Karl-Heinz Kuck, MD, Klaus-Peter Kunze, MD,
   Manfred Geiger, MD, Angelika Costard, MD, and
   Michael Schlüter, PhD 367
23. Late Death After Myocardial Infarction: Mechanisms, Etiologies, and
  Implications for Prevention of Sudden Death
   William G. Stevenson, MD, Gerard C.M. Linssen, BA,
   Michael G. Havenith, MD Pedro Brugada, MD, and
   Hein J.J. Wellens, MD 377
24. Sudden Cardiac Death: A Multifactorial Problem
   Hein J.J. Wellens, MD, and Pedro Brugada, MD 391

V. STRATEGIES OF TREATMENT OF VENTRICULAR ARRHYTHMIAS

25. Antiarrhythmic Therapy: Noninvasive Guided Stategy Versus
  Empirical or Invasive Strategies
   Philippe Coumel, MD, Jean-François Leclercq, MD,
   Marc Zimmerman, MD, and Jean-Louis Funck-Brentano, MD 403
26. The Preference of Programmed Stimulation-Guided Therapy for
  Sustained Ventricular Arrhythmias
   Charles Gottlieb, MD, and Mark E. Josephson, MD 421
27. Standardization of Noninvasive and Invasive Studies in the
  Assessment of Patients with Ventricular Arrhythmias
   Manfred Zehender, MD, Annette Geibel, MD,
   Stefan Hohnloser, MD, Thomas Meinertz, MD, and
   Hanjoerg Just, MD 435
28. Treatment of Patients with Ventricular Tachycardia or Ventricular
  Fibrillation: First Lessons from the "Parallel Study"
   Pedro Brugada, MD, Robert Lemery, MD,
   Mario Talajic, MD, Paolo Della Bella, MD, and
   Hein J.J. Wellens, MD 457
29. Prospective Criteria for the Selection of Therapy for Ventricular
  Tachycardia and Ventricular Fibrillation
   John D. Fisher, MD, Anthony D. Mercando, MD,
   Soo G. Kim, MD 471

VI. ANTIARRHYTHMIC DRUGS

30. A Clinical Classification of Antiarrhythmic Drugs
    Paul Puech, MD, and Josep Brugada, MD 485
31. A Comparison of Electrophysiologic Effects of Antiarrhythmic Agents in Humans
    Eric N. Prystowsky, MD, Elwyn A. Lloyd, MD,
    Naomi Fineberg, PhD, Douglas P. Zipes MD,
    Elizabeth Darling, RN, and James J. Heger, MD 495
32. Factors Leading to Decreasing Mortality among Patients Resuscitated from Out-of-Hospital Cardiac Arrest
    Robert J. Myerburg, MD, Kenneth M. Kessler, MD,
    Liaqat Zaman, MD, Richard G. Trohman, MD,
    Pedro Fernandez, MD, and Agustin Castellanos, MD 505

VII. PERCUTANEOUS ABLATION

33. Catheter Electrical Ablation of Cardiac Arrhythmias: A Summary Report of the Percutaneous Cardiac Mapping and Ablation Registry
    Melvin M. Scheinman, MD, and G. Thomas Evans, MD 529
34. Electrode Catheter Ablation of Resistant Ventricular Tachycardia by Endocavitary Fulguration Associated with Antiarrhythmic Therapy: Experience of 38 Patients with a Mean Follow-Up of 23 Months
    G. Fontaine, MD, J.L. Tonet, MD, R. Frank, MD,
    Y. Gallais, MD, I. Touzet, MD, S. Kounde, MD, G. Farenq, MD,
    M. Baraka, MD, and Y. Grosgogeat, MD 539

VIII. SURGICAL TREATMENT OF ARRHYTHMIAS

35. Surgical Treatment of the Wolff-Parkinson-White Syndrome: Current Indications, Techniques, and Results
    Olaf C. Penn, MD 573
36. Surgical Treatment of Supraventricular Tachycardia without the WPW Syndrome: Current Indications, Techniques, and Results
    David L. Ross, FRACP, David C. Johnson, FRACS,
    Chee Choong Koo, MRCP, Peter Mortensen, MD,
    Mark J. Cooper, FRACP, A. Robert Denniss, MD,
    David A. Richards, MD, and John B. Uther, MD 591
37. Preoperative and Intraoperative Mapping of Ventricular Tachycardia: Is it Necessary for the Success of Surgical Treatment?
    Isaac Wiener, MD 605
38. Intraoperative Computerized Mapping Techniques: Do They Help Us to Treat Our Patients Better Surgically?
    James L. Cox, MD 613
39. Use of Old and New Anatomic, Electrophysiologic, and

Technical Knowledge to Develop Operative Approaches to Tachycardia
Gerard M. Guiraudon, MD, George J. Klein, MD, Arjun D. Sharma, MD, and Raymond Yee, MD 639

IX. THE IMPLANTABLE DEFIBRILLATOR

40. The Automatic Implantable Defibrillator: Some Historical Notes
M. Mirowski, MD, and Morton M. Mower, MD 655
41. The Automatic Implantable Cardioverter Defibrillator: U.S. Experience
Roger A. Winkle, MD, and Andrea Thomas, RN 663
42. The Implantable Defibrillator AICD: European Clinical Experience
Henri E. Kulbertus, MD, and Seah Nisam 681

X. SCIENTIFIC RESEARCH

43. Control of Scientific Research
Shahbudin H. Rahimtoola, MB 689
44. The Electrocardiogram as a Marker for Future Cardiovascular Events
Charles Fisch, MD 699
45. Relations Between University and Industry
Ivan M.G.P. Bourgeois, Jr., MBA 707
46. How Everything Started in Clinical Electrophysiology
Richard Langendorf, MD 715

XI. NEW PROSPECTS IN DIAGNOSIS AND TREATMENT OF ARRHYTHMIAS

47. New Forms of Anomalous Conduction in the AV Junction
Benjamin J. Scherlag, MD, Masayuki Sakurai, MD, Raed Sweidan, MD, and Ralph Lazzara, MD 725
48. Manipulation of the Autonomic Nervous System in the Prevention of Sudden Cardiac Death
Peter J. Schwartz, MD 741
49. Quantitation of Myocardial Ischemic Surface and Volume by NADH and Magnetic Resonance Imaging with Correlation to Ventricular Arrhythmias
Alden H. Harken, MD, Anirban Banerjee, PhD, John Sun, MD, and Glenn J.R. Whitman, MD 767
50. Characterizing Cardiac Ion Channels Using the Bilayer Reconstitution Technique
Joseph A. Hill, Jr., PhD, and Harold C. Strauss, MD 779
51. Laser Ablation for Tachyarrhythmia Control: Current Status and Future Development
Sanjeev Saksena, MD 803

INDEX 819

PATHOLOGIC SUBSTRATES OF ARRHYTHMIAS

1

Morphologic Characteristics of Arrhythmias

Anton E. Becker

Introduction

Cardiac arrhythmia is defined as any condition in which the normal rhythm of the heart is disturbed and, hence, includes a wide variety of pathologic conditions that may range from congenital to acquired and may affect almost any part of the heart. It is beyond the scope of this chapter to attempt to encompass all these abnormalities. Some of the pathological states, such as those that relate to sinus node dysfunction and arrhythmias conditioned by ischemia, are discussed in other chapters. This contribution, therefore, will be devoted solely to the pathology of supraventricular tachycardias and, in particular, to the Wolff-Parkinson-White syndrome.

Ventricular Preexcitation

The term preexcitation was first introduced by Öhnell in 1944.[1] It is defined as the condition in which "the whole or some part of the ventricular muscle is activated earlier by the impulse originating from the atrium than would be expected if the impulse reached the ventricles by way of the normal specific conduction system only."[2] The incidence of the electrocardiographic pattern of preexcitation has been estimated to occur in approximately 1 to 3 per 1000 individuals.[3] In other words, a rather esoteric condition, particularly since it includes individuals with an abnormal electrocardiogram as the sole manifesta-

From: Brugada P, Wellens HJJ. CARDIAC ARRHYTHMIAS: Where To Go From Here? Mount Kisco, NY, Futura Publishing Company, Inc., © 1987.

tion as well as patients with potentially life-threatening arrhythmias, usually due to atrial fibrillation with a rapid ventricular response. Basically, however, the common denominator in all individuals with this syndrome is some kind of anomalous connection between atrial and ventricular myocardium so that the usual delay-producing area of the atrioventricular conduction system is short-circuited. It is in this particular arena that many eponyms have been introduced, all related to a particular morphology considered to underlie preexcitation. On historical ground, the name "Kent" has been linked to the atrioventricular connection that commonly occurs in the Wolff-Parkinson-White syndrome. The fact that Kent's description of an atrioventricular muscular bridge seems unrelated to the bundle presently held responsible for preexcitation has led to lively discussions in the literature.[4-7] A scholastic historical overview of ventricular preexcitation, which considers the background of these divergent viewpoints in detail has recently been provided by Burchell.[8]

In this chapter, the descriptive nomenclature proposed on behalf of the European Study Group of Preexcitation will be used,[9] but to quote Burchell, "the interested physician should remain facile in his cognition of Kent's, Mahaim's, Öhnell's, James', and Brechenmacher's fibers."

Basic Pathology in Preexcitation

As outlined previously, preexcitation is a rare condition and, hence direct morphologic correlations between electrocardiographically proven cases of preexcitation and cardiac pathology are limited. The first histological demonstration of an accessory connection between the atrium and ventricle in a patient with the Wolff-Parkinson-White syndrome was reported in 1943 by Wood et al.[10] Shortly thereafter a pathway was reconstructed in exemplary fashion by Öhnell[1] (Fig. 1). Subsequent studies showed that preexcitation could occur because of abnormal connections between atrial and ventricular myocardium or in the setting of abnormal connections between the conduction axis and the ventricular musculature (see for review[11]).

Once the morphological basis for the Wolff-Parkinson-White syndrome was firmly established, the first surgical and, at the time, most daring procedure to interrupt the bundle was performed in 1968.[12] It is because of the pioneering efforts of Dr. Sealy that surgical intervention has now become an established mode of treatment in patients whose arrhythmias prove resistant to medication.[13,14] Recently catheter ablation for ventricular preexcitation has been introduced as a new option in treating patients who do not respond well to medication, although the technique is presently still considered experimental and should be considered only in patients with life-threatening or disabling arrhythmias not responding to drug therapy and in whom surgery is contraindicated.[15]

Ironically, the successes obtained with both conventional drug therapy and other forms of treatment have hampered further progress in the understanding of the underlying pathologic substrates. For instance, it remains a puzzling phenomenon why retrograde (ventriculoatrial) conduction occurs commonly in case of an accessory atrioventricular connection, while conduction in antegrade fash-

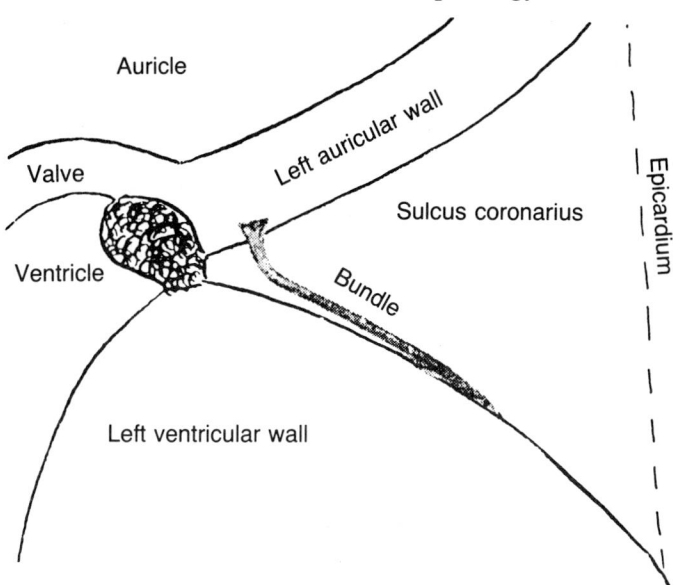

Figure 1: Original drawing by Öhnell of a reconstructed atrioventricular connection.

ion appears to be rare. To answer such detailed questions from a morphologic viewpoint, the material available for study is extremely limited, particularly since a precise correlation between morphologic and electrophysiologic data is mandatory. Nevertheless, with a few heart specimens and proper electrophysiologic back-up, much can be achieved. Quality definitely outweighs quantity in this respect.

There are other questions, however, that probably will never be answered with any degree of certainty. For instance, one may wonder what the frequency will be of abnormal connections in hearts of individuals who never presented electrocardiographic evidence of preexcitation. At present, it is well established from clinical experiences that "concealed" accessory connections occur, but the incidence in the population remains pure speculation. An attempt can be made to study normal hearts in order to verify whether or not such connections can be found, but one must then be sure that the individual whose heart is studied has had proper electrocardiographic evaluation during life, which is not always the case. Moreover, how many hearts should be studied in order to come up with a reliable answer? Taking into consideration that the incidence of connections that lead to a manifest delta wave is approximately 1 to 3 per 1000 individuals, it is likely that a vast number of hearts should be studied in order to meet the statistical challenge of encountering one such "concealed" connection. The very fact that thousands of histologic sections per heart have to be studied most meticulously in order to rule out that a connection exists—negative findings are always difficult to defend—makes this study extremely time-consuming, costly, and hardly justifiable.

On the other hand, some morphologic questions to which the pathologist was exposed in the early days may presently better be answered by clinicians and surgeons. The question as to the multiplicity of connections may serve as an example, since this feature can be studied clinically and during perioperative mapping procedures. Some questions may nevertheless remain, such as the incidence of the combined occurrence of accessory atrioventricular connections and abnormalities of the atrioventricular conduction axis.

The following sections will deal in detail with the material that over the years has become available for morphologic study in an attempt to unravel some of the mysteries that still remain.

Morphologic Basis of Preexcitation

Currently ventricular activation can occur when the usual delay-producing area of the atrioventricular node is short-circuited. There are several potential means by which this may occur (Fig. 2). Basically, two main conditions can be distinguished: (1) accessory atrioventricular connections that occur outside the area of the specialized atrioventricular junctional tissues, and (2) pathways intimately related to the conduction axis. The latter consists of accessory nodoventricular connections and accessory fasciculoventricular connections, both connecting node and penetrating bundle, respectively, to the crest of the underlying ventricular septum. In addition, fibers can occur from the atrium penetrating the nodal bundle axis distal to the delay-producing area, so-called accessory atriofascicular connections. Finally, atrial fibers may penetrate the atrioventricular node forming an intranodal bypass tract, circumventing part of the delay-producing area within the junctional region.

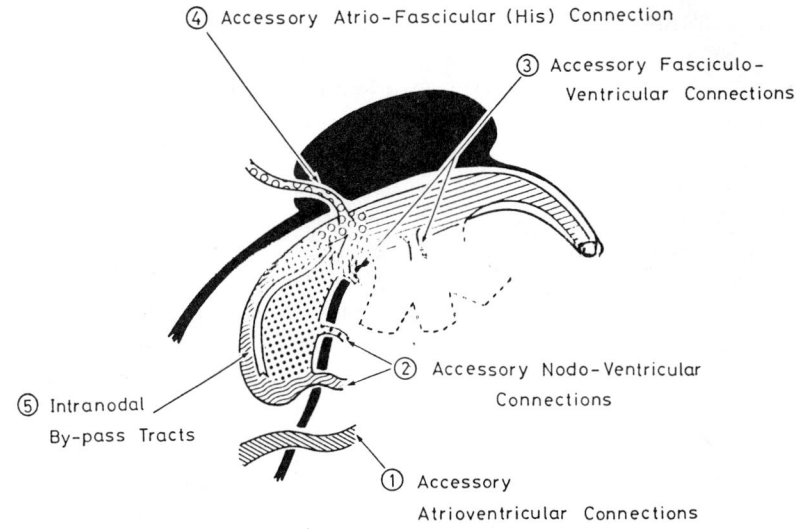

Figure 2: Scheme of the morphologic basis of preexcitation.

Accessory Atrioventricular Connections

It is presently well acknowledged, both from pathological studies[16] and from surgical series,[17] that accessory atrioventricular connections outside the area of the atrioventricular node and bundle underlie the classic Wolff-Parkinson-White syndrome. The connection can be present at any site along either atrioventricular junction, including the area of aortic–mitral fibrous continuity.[18]

Initial classifications of the Wolff-Parkinson-White syndrome separated the electrocardiographic patterns into types A and B.[19] In this classification, type A represented a left-sided connection, whereas type B was due to a right-sided connection. This classification, however, does not take into account septal connections and for these reasons it is preferable to distinguish left-sided, right-sided, and septal atrioventricular connections rather than types A and B.[20] It is important, in this respect, to be aware of the fact that septal connections have been divided into posterior and anterior ones.[21] According to the diagram provided, however, it is our impression that the anterior area is not truly septal, but rather anterior to the region of the central fibrous body (Fig. 3). Accessory connections in that area, therefore, should connect the right atrium to the musculature of the right ventriculo-infundibular fold and no longer to the septum. The posterior septal connections are truly septal. Such posterior septal connections may cause preexcitation of ventricular myocardium which, according to surface

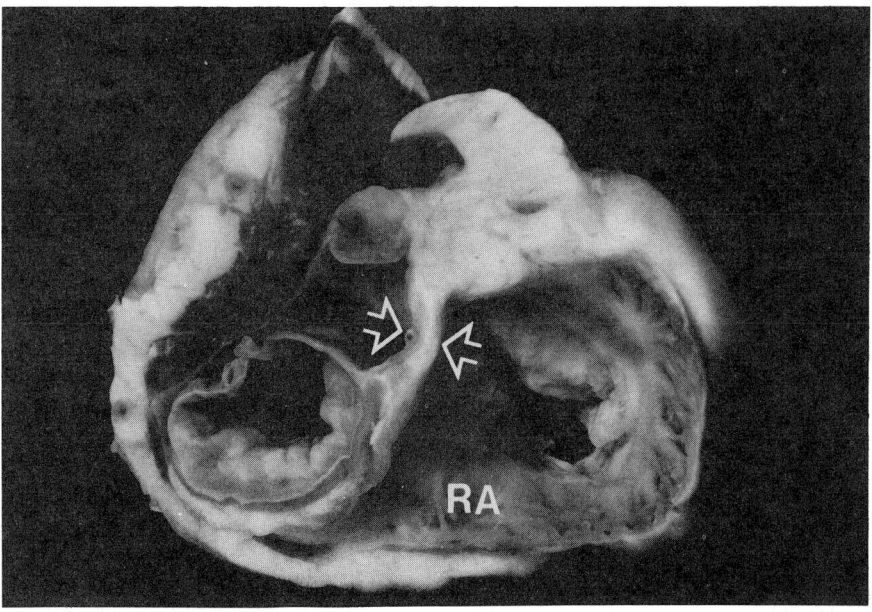

Figure 3: Superior view of heart following removal of the atria. The septal area is relatively small and relates to the zone where the so-called posterior septal connections can occur. The area where so-called anterior septal connections can occur (arrows) is not a septal structure, but a mural wall separating the right atrium (RA) from the left ventricular outflow tract.

mapping studies, produce early activation either to the left or the right side of the crux of the heart and may mask the anatomical side of the connection within the septum.

The accessory atrioventricular connection is almost always composed of common "working" myocardial fibers (Fig. 4). The bundle connects the atrial musculature to the ventricular myocardium and, hence, facilitates spread of activation from atrial to ventricular musculature outside the delay-producing zone. Within this basic framework, however, a wide variety exists with respect to the precise morphology of the connection.

The anomalous bundle may skirt the annulus fibrosus, which separates atrial from ventricular myocardium and gives rise to the fibrous core of the atrioventricular valve involved. In other instances, the bundle may run within the epicardial fat remote from the atrioventricular junction. As a rule, the bundle ramifies before merging with ventricular myocardial fibers. In other words, the bundle usually originates from atrial myocardium as a common trunk, but soon diverges into several much smaller bundles that taper out before rooting into the ventricle (Fig. 5). This could be an important morphologic feature responsible for the clinical observation that retrograde conduction over an accessory atrioventricular connection is common, whereas antegrade conduction is rare. One may envision that in case of retrograde spread of activation, there is a massive input from many ventricular myocardial cells into almost single cells that contribute the distal ramifications of the connection. This situation, with converging small bundles, may then easily lead to spread of activation towards the main trunk and, hence, toward atrial cells. With antegrade conduction over the bundle, small patches of ventricular myocardial cells may become activated potentially, but because of the minute input may not necessarily be effective in activating the surrounding ventricular myocardium.

Another variable is the length of the total bundle. From the reconstruction of histologic sections, the length of the bundle could be calculated as approximating between 5 to 10 mm.[16] The diameter, moreover, may likewise vary, although the bundle is usually tiny with diameters of approximately 1 to 2 mm. Due to ramifications as alluded to above, the diameter may become even less and eventually single cell strands may hook up to myocardial fibers.

From a functional viewpoint, it may be important also that the composition of the bundle may vary considerably. Although basically composed of working myocardial cells, it is common to find extensive fibrosis within the bundle (Fig. 6) and at the sites of continuity with ventricular myocardium. One can only speculate on the pathophysiologic consequences of this phenomenon, but in general terms, one may expect a negative effect.

Nodoventricular and Fasciculo-Ventricular Connections

These are connections present between the nodal and fascicular components of the nodal bundle axis and the crest of the ventricular septum. The anatomical substrates implicated in this form of preexcitation were first described by Mahaim and Winston in 1941[22] and in a further communication by Mahaim in 1947.[23]

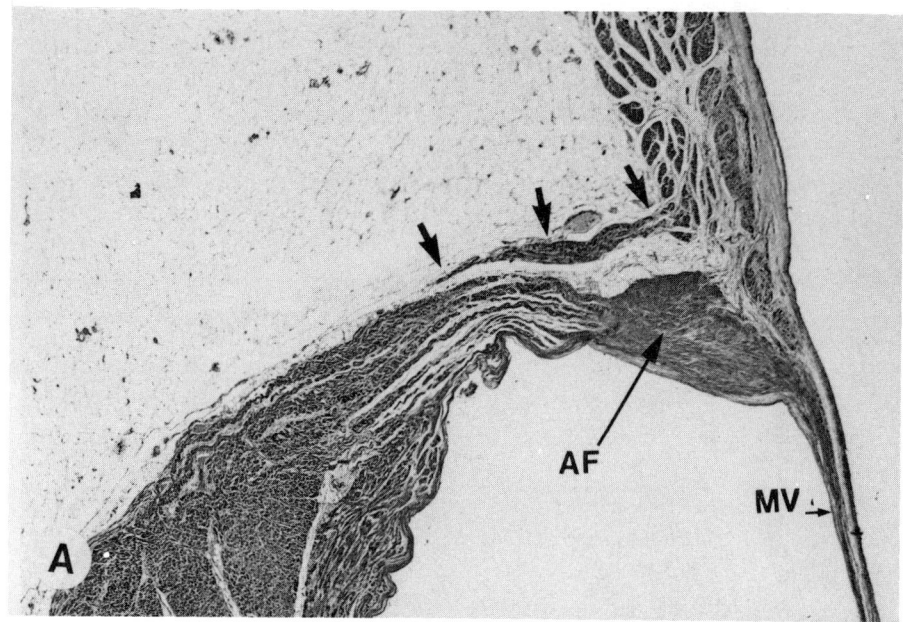

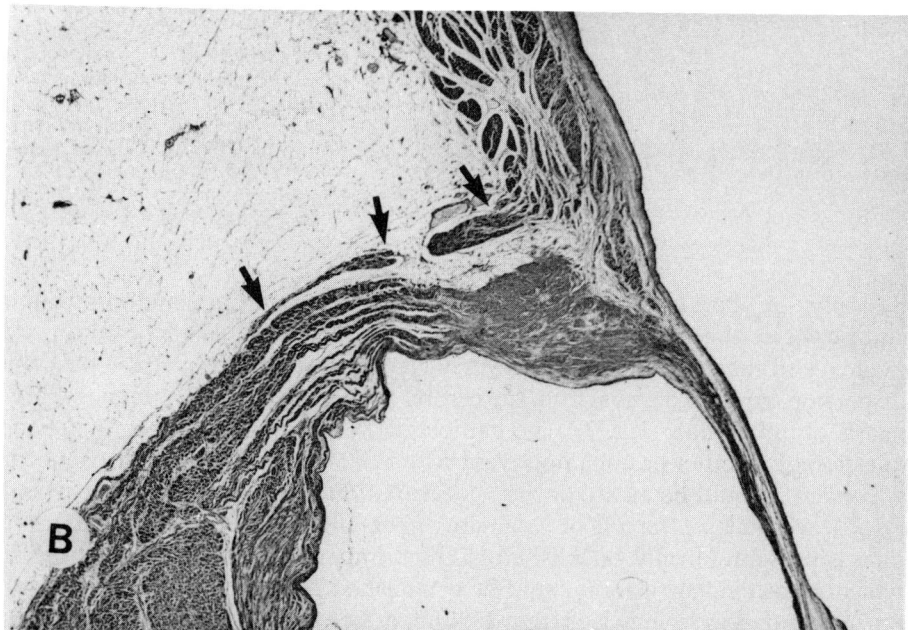

Figure 4: Accessory atrioventricular connection (arrows), skirting the annulus fibrosus (AF) supporting the mitral valve (MV). A and B show sections 0.3 mm apart. The bundle originates from atrial myocardium and divides into smaller bundles prior to its ventricular insertion. Elastic tissue stain; ×20.

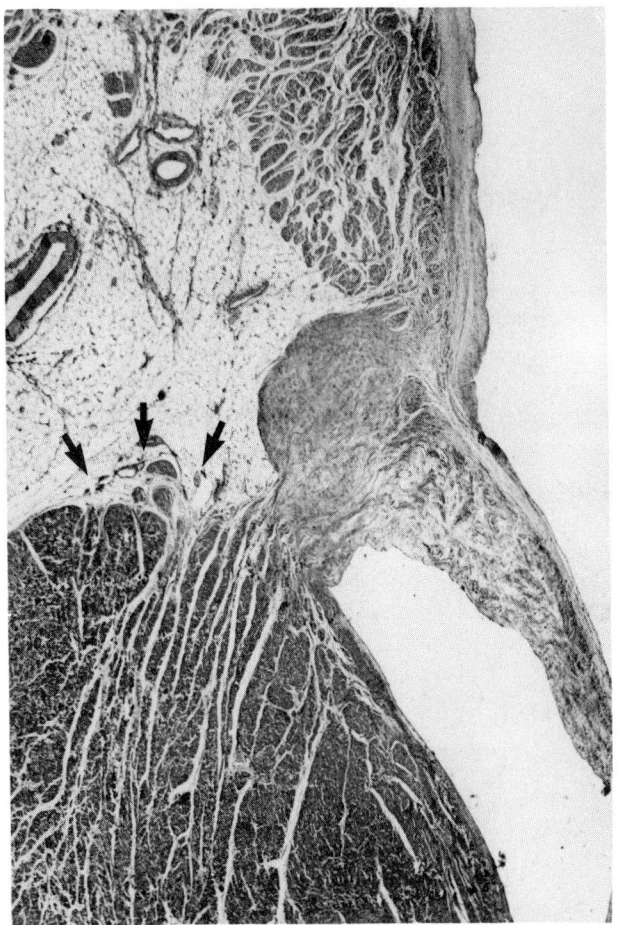

Figure 5: Atrioventricular connection immediately prior to its ventricular insertion. The common trunk has divided into several small bundles (arrows). Elastic tissue stain; ×16.

Basically, the fibers originate from the atrioventricular node or penetrating bundle and perforate the central fibrous body to contact ventricular myocardium. The existence of these connections, however, has been debated over the past since dispersion of nodal tissue within the central fibrous body is a common finding in hearts of individuals (Fig. 7). The pathologist, examining hearts with a specific question of whether or not a nodoventricular or fasciculo-ventricular connection is present, should be aware of the wide variation in histology in this particular area. Nevertheless, the role of "Mahaim" fibers in the genesis of cardiac arrhythmias is presently firmly established.[24] The number of well-documented cases in which a positive correlation could be established between electrocardiographic tracings and morphology is extremely limited. Lev and associates[25] were the first to report such a correlation. Recently a unique case has been documented by Gmeiner and co-workers.[26] They recorded paroxysmal tachycardia with widened QRS complexes in an 11-year-old boy who had suffered brain damage, which had

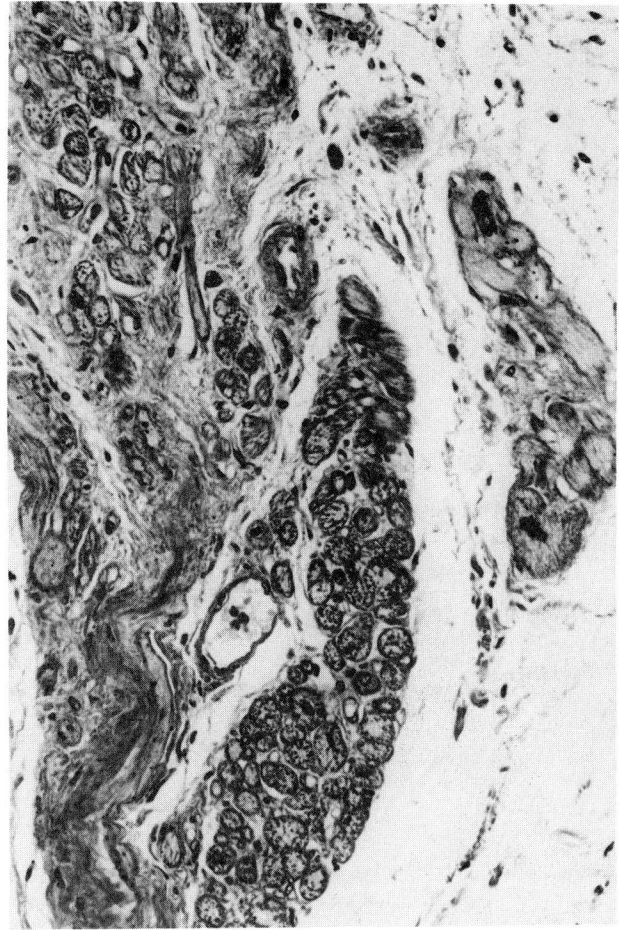

Figure 6: Detail of accessory atrioventricular connection. The bundle shows extensive fibrosis and hydropic cell swelling. Masson trichrome stain; ×230.

resulted from an episode of ventricular fibrillation. Atrial stimulation produced an increased atrioventricular conduction, sudden disappearance of the His bundle deflection, and a complete left bundle branch block pattern. Tachycardias of this morphology were initiated by early atrial and ventricular premature beats. The findings suggested the presence of a macro-reentry circuit, utilizing a slow nodoventricular connection as the anterograde limb and the nodal bundle axis as the retrograde limb. Serial sectioning of the atrioventricular specialized junctional area revealed a nodoventricular tract originating from the posterior extension of the compact part of the atrioventricular node inserting into the crest of the ventricular septum (Fig. 8). It is interesting that the same heart specimen showed extensive dispersion of conduction fibers, derived from the atrioventricular node and penetrating bundle, within the central fibrous body. The fragmentation often suggested additional connections, but careful observations never substantiated this particular viewpoint.

12 • CARDIAC ARRHYTHMIAS

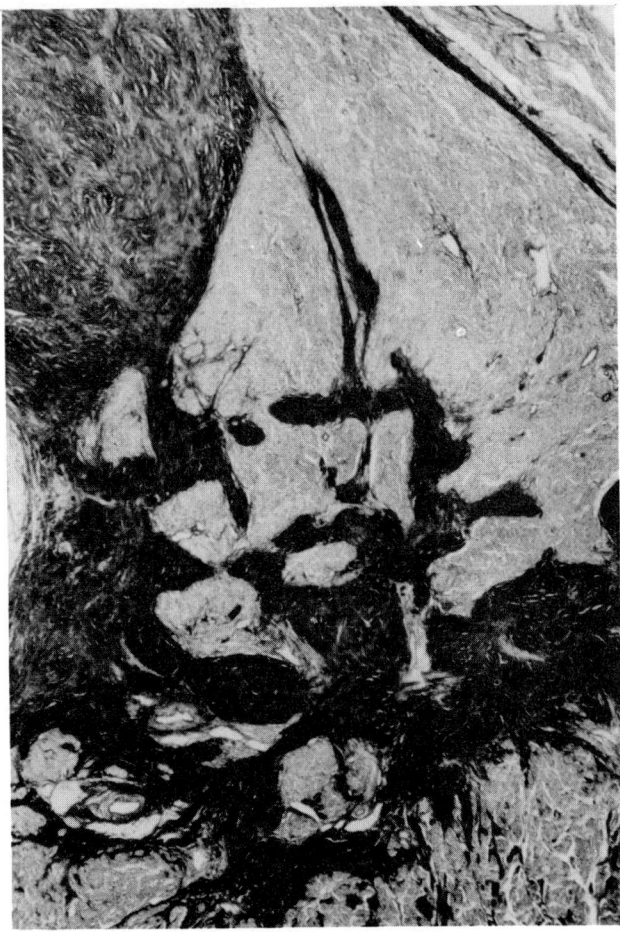

Figure 7: Dispersion of nodal tissue within the central fibrous body. Elastic tissue stain; ×35.

Atrio-Fascicular and Intranodal Bypass Tracts

The hallmark of these anatomical options is that although the area of conduction delay is "bypassed," the impulse is still conducted into the ventricles along the usual conduction axis. The atrio-fascicular tract consists of a bundle of atrial fibers which contacts the penetrating or branching bundle beyond the point of differentiation between node and bundle. For the pathologist, this may pose a problem, since recognition of the tract is heavily influenced by the criterion used for the distinction between node and bundle. The penetrating bundle is considered that part of the nodal bundle axis which becomes completely encased by collegenous tissue of the central fibrous body and, hence, is thereby insulated from atrial inputs.[27] This implies that an atrio-fascicular tract can be identified with certainty only when the fibers actually penetrate the insulating fibrous tissue before contacting the nodal bundle axis (Fig. 9). This becomes of paramount significance since the study of series of hearts, without indications for preexcita-

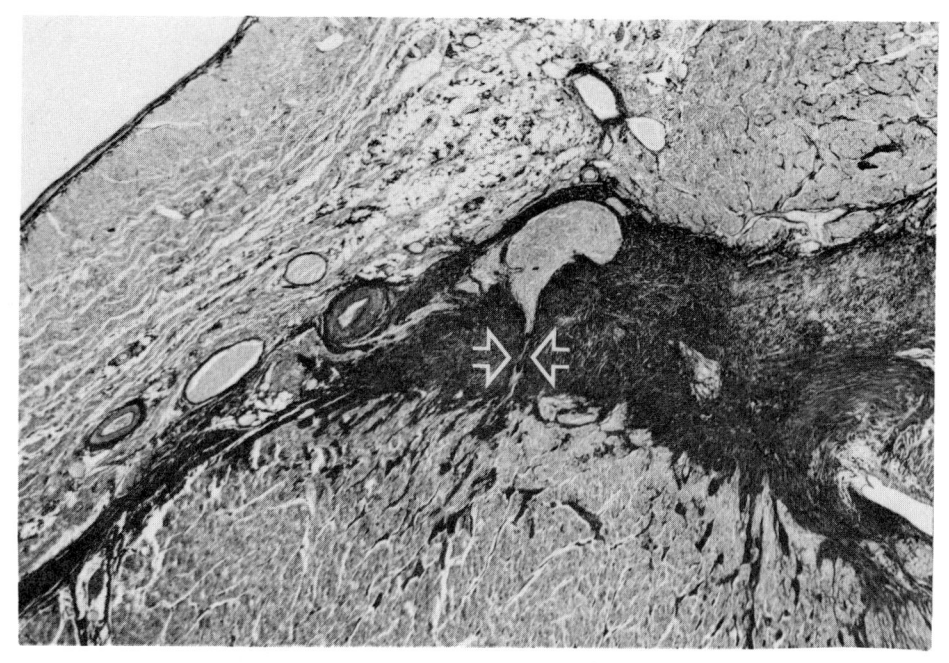

Figure 8: Example of a nodoventricular connection (between arrows). The accessory connection originates from the posterior extent of the node, itself fully embedded within the connective tissue of the central fibrous body. Elastic tissue stain; ×17.5. (Used with permission of the Eur Heart J 1984; 5:233–242.)

tion, has shown that the degree of development of the central fibrous body varies considerably from one case to the other. The precise architecture of the nodal-bundle axis and its relationship with the atrial input fibers, therefore, also shows variation. It is extremely difficult from a purely morphologic viewpoint to be sure whether the "last" input fiber from atrial musculature is still within the delay-producing area of the node or whether it is so far distally that one may expect considerable shortening of the PR interval. Moreover, it should be clearly understood that the central fibrous body with aging is much influenced by degenerative changes that mold the area considerably. In fact, so-called Lev's disease is attributed to such rearrangements of the central fibrous body which by necessity affect the conduction tissues.[28]

Atrio-fascicular tracts should not be confused with the so-called "James fibers."[29] The latter constitute atrial fibers, which he considered to be derived from the "posterior internodal tract," which ran anteriorly to make contact with the node more distally than the bulk of the common posterior input fibers (Fig. 9). It should be emphasized, in this context, that James's description was based on the study of normal hearts, so that any functional significance to be attributed to this finding remains pure speculation. Nevertheless, the eponym "James fiber" is often used to indicate any atrial fiber which bypasses the area of delay in the atrioventricular junctional area. It is our belief that this is an inappropriate use of the eponym and for those who want to use eponyms, the term "Brechenmacher fiber" seems much more adequate.[30]

14 • CARDIAC ARRHYTHMIAS

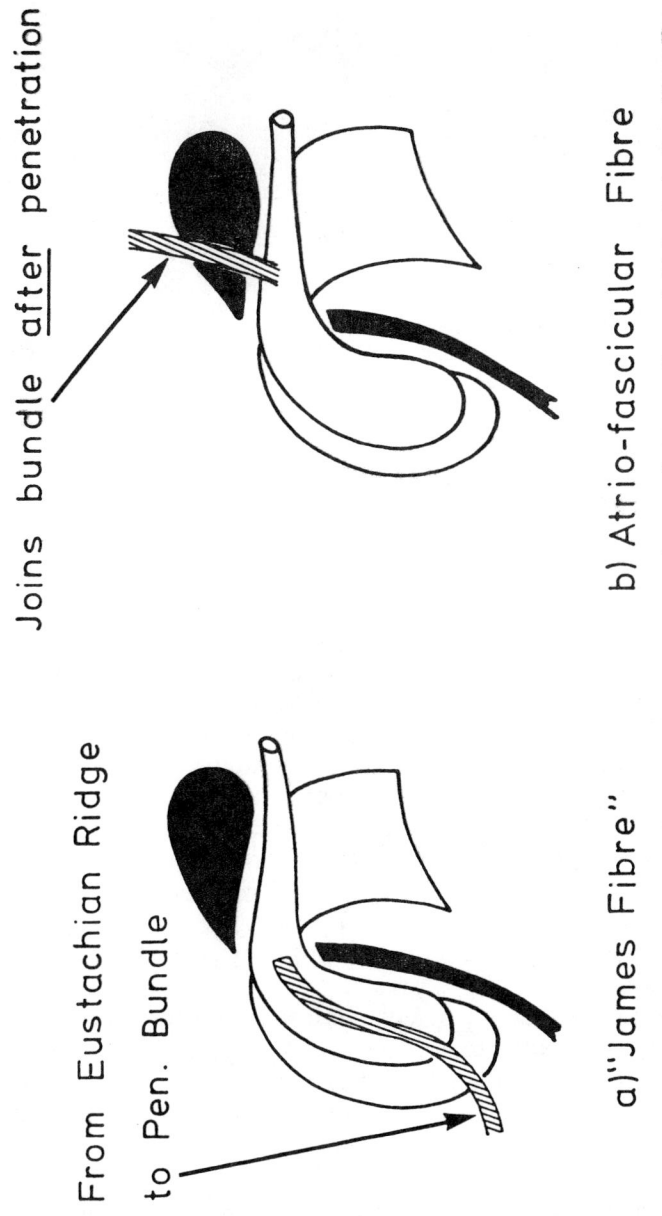

a) "James Fibre"
From Eustachian Ridge to Pen. Bundle

b) Atrio-fascicular Fibre
Joins bundle *after* penetration

Figure 9: Schematic drawing indicating the basic difference between the so-called James fiber and atriofascicular fiber. (From The Conduction System of the Heart: Davies MJ, et al. With permission of Butterworths.)

The existence of intranodal bypass tracts, although suggestive from electrophysiological data, remains difficult to establish by the morphologist. Nevertheless, careful examination of the fragmented conduction tissue elements, within the central fibrous body, often reveals that such isolated cells may veer back towards the main nodal bundle axis, thus forming loops within the specialized junctional zone. One may hypothesize that this is an underlying substrate for rapid conduction through the node. Thus far, no conclusive data are available.

Specific Questions to the Morphologist

What is the Incidence of "Concealed" Atrioventricular Connections?

A "concealed accessory atrioventricular connection" is defined as an accessory pathway capable of conduction in only the retrograde (ventriculoatrial) direction, in other words, exhibiting an anterograde unidirectional block. Nevertheless, such patients can develop paroxysmal supraventricular tachycardia, often referred to as the "concealed WPW syndrome."[31] Programmed ventricular stimulation in such instances has revealed that the characteristics of retrograde atrial activation and the retrograde atrioventricular conduction properties are those of accessory atrioventricular connections.[32]

The mechanisms underlying unidirectional block under these circumstances remain unsolved. It has been suggested that "impedence mismatch" could be the mechanism involved,[33] but it is fair to state that the pathophysiology still remains speculative. Since the "concealed" accessory atrioventricular connection under normal circumstances does not show the characteristic electrocardiographic pattern of the Wolff-Parkinson-White syndrome, the question remains as to what extent such connections may occur in "normal" individuals. For this particular reason, a small series of 10 hearts has been studied. None of the patients whose hearts were used for this particular study had presented evidence of the preexcitation syndrome during life. The total circumference of both atrioventricular rings, including the septum, were blocked, according to the technique previously outlined.[11,16]

An accessory atrioventricular connection was not recognized. The most important aspect that was revealed by this study related to the morphology of the left (mitral) atrioventricular annulus fibrosus. In a previous communication on the architecture of the annulus fibrosus,[34] it is stated that in the left-sided atrioventricular junction, the annulus is composed usually of a firm band of collagen which, only in its most parietal parts, shows a tendency to fade out. This contrasts sharply with the right-sided annulus which, despite its greater circumference, is poorly formed and largely composed of adipose tissue. In the present series of 10 hearts, these findings were endorsed, but in addition, the variability of the mitral annulus along the oblique margin of the heart was most striking (Fig. 10). At many sites, the fibrous core of the annulus fibrosus had faded or was represented by tiny collagenous strands only. Moreover, atrial and ventricular musculature was

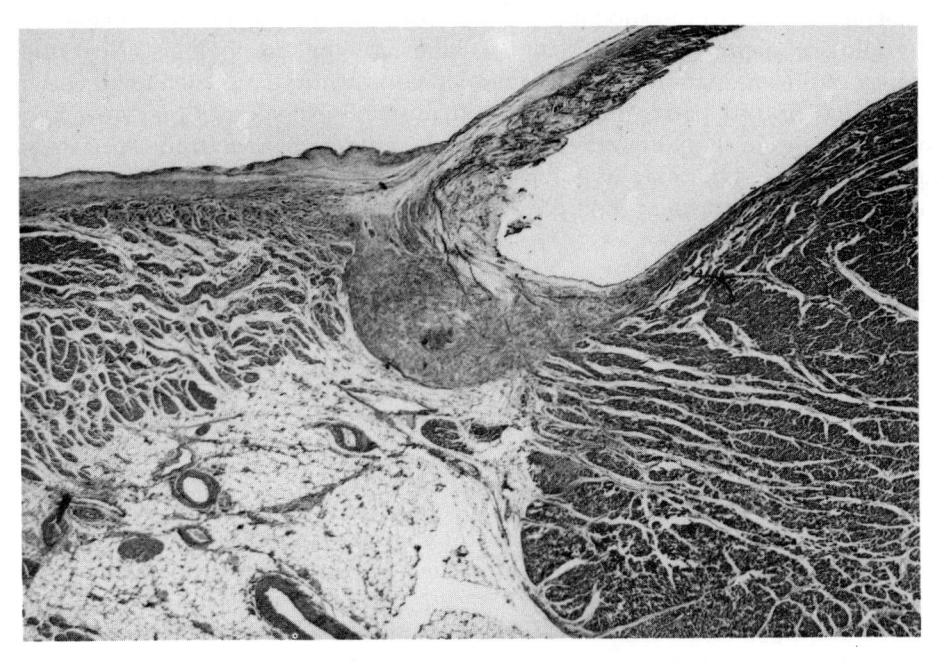

Figure 10: Cross-section through the oblique margin of the mitral orifice. The case illustrates a well-formed fibrous annulus. The connective tissue extends into the mitral valve leaflet and forms the fibrosa. Elastic tissue stain; ×16.

often widely separated by adipose tissue and the site of origin of the mitral valve leaflet varied accordingly. In some instances, the valve leaflet took off at the basal aspect of the atrial musculature, whereas at other sites, the leaflet attachment was intimately related to the crest of mural ventricular myocardium. The area with a deficient mitral annulus was much larger than initially thought. This brings back to memory the clinical observations that the majority of left-sided accessory atrioventricular connections occur along the obtuse margin of the left atrioventricular groove. It remains speculative whether or not these two observations are related (see below).

The present study, therefore, does not provide a clue as to the incidence of accessory atrioventricular connections in individuals without an electrocardiographic pattern of preexcitation. As outlined previously, it seems highly unlikely that this particular question will ever be solved by morphologists.

What is the Incidence of Multiple Accessory Atrioventricular Connections?

The occurrence of multiple accessory atrioventricular connections is presently well established,[35] but atrioventricular reciprocating tachycardia incorporating two or more accessory atrioventricular connections is considered exceedingly rare.[36] Nevertheless, clinical studies reveal that approximately 10% of patients with the preexcitation syndrome have more than one accessory atrioventricular connection.[35]

The number of anatomically documented cases of multiple accessory connections is extremely limited. Indeed, almost all instances reported are case reports. A particularly well-documented case was reported by Dreifus and associates in 1976.[37] The late Dr. Truex showed three left-sided atrioventricular connections histologically. One connected the posterior wall of the left atrium to the posterior aspect of the ventricular septum, while the remaining two atrioventricular connections occurred in the left lateral wall. Both were closely adjacent, but one skirted the annulus fibrosus, while the other was more superficial within the epicardial fat.

At present, this author had the opportunity to study the hearts of 10 patients with proven preexcitation. In only one of these hearts was a dual connection encountered which was, as it appears, a most remarkable case in many aspects. In this particular patient (case 1; Becker et al.[16]), autopsy revealed Ebstein's anomaly of the tricuspid valve and an accessory atrioventricular connection in the posterior wall of the left atrium. The same heart also contained an accessory atrioventricular connection originating from a node-like structure in the anterior margin of the tricuspid orifice (Fig. 11). From this node, a bundle, composed of slender "specialized" cells, bridged the atrioventricular groove and connected to the right ventricular myocardial fibers present in the dysplastic anterior leaflet of the tricuspid valve. The presence of a node-like structure in this particular location is fascinating, since this is precisely the area in which Kent described his node.[38] It is also the area from which the penetrating atrioventricular bundle may originate in hearts with congenital malformations with gross malalignment of the atrial and ventricular septa, such as congenitally corrected transposition and double inlet ventricles.

To the best of our knowledge, only two previous reports of an accessory connection document a histologic composition of a specialized nature, rather than "ordinary" working myocardium usually found in these connections. The first case was reported by Verduyn-Lunel,[39] who described the bundle as composed of "Purkinje cells." The second case was reported by James and Puech[40] who described a left lateral connection as composed of "p cells," thus suggesting a relation with pacemaker cells. Whether the "specialized" connection encountered in the present series was functionally significant remains speculative.

In view of these collected data, it seems once more that the clinician is better equipped to answer the question of multiplicity than is the morphologist.

Are Accessory Atrioventricular Connections in Epicardial or Subendocardial Position?

This has been a topic of some interest in the past, but at the same time has led to major confusion regarding the precise topography of the accessory connections in relation to the annulus fibrosus. Morphologic experience dictates that almost all accessory atrioventricular connections traverse through the epicardial fat in bridging atrial and ventricular musculature. In this sense, the connection is epicardial,

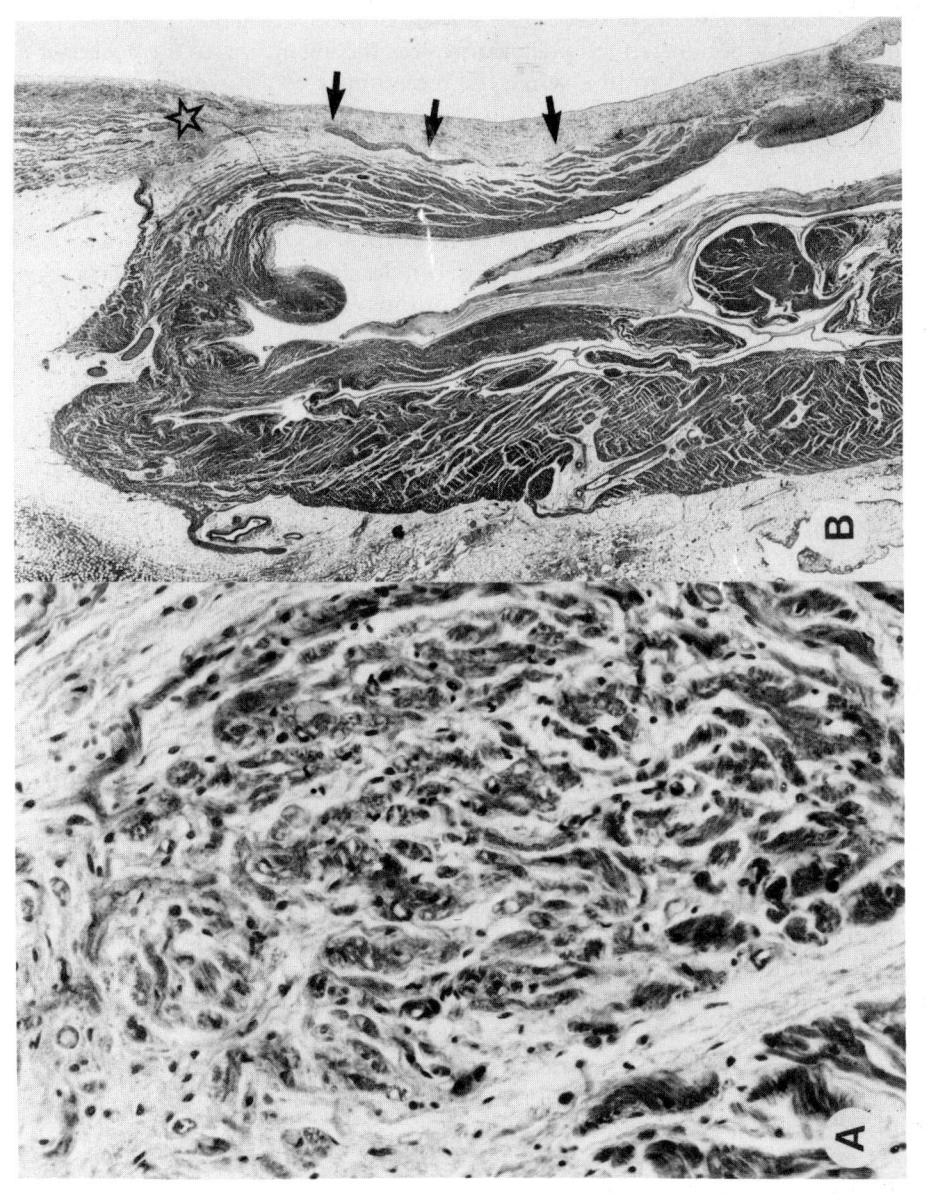

Figure 11: Accessory atrioventricular connection composed of specialized cells, derived from a node-like structure. A: detail of the node. B: overview of the bundle (arrows) inserting into right ventricular myocardium extending into a dysplastic anterior tricuspid valve leaflet in a case of Ebstein's anomaly. The site of the node is indicated by an asterisk. Masson trichrome stain; A, ×230; B, ×7.

since it is located on the epicardial aspect of the annulus fibrosus. As outlined previously, however, the annulus is often deficient, particularly along the tricuspid orifice but to a large extent also along the obtuse margin of the left atrioventricular annulus. Hence, it is not always feasible to relate the accessory connection to the presence of a fibrous annulus. Moreover, despite its position in the epicardial fat, the bundle may be more closely related to the inner aspect of the heart than to the epicardial surface. Therefore, a distinction between subendocardial and epicardial seems irrelevant. The bundle or bundles may be present in positions almost skirting the atrioventricular junction and much more superficial almost directly underneath the epicardium. There is no guideline to predict beforehand what the precise course of the connection will be.

The truly subendocardial connections present in the series of hearts studied were encountered in septal position and in hearts only with Ebstein's malformation of the tricuspid valve (Fig. 12). In these instances, atrial and ventricular septal musculature was no longer separated by a fibrous annulus and a bundle bridged the gap in the immediate subendocardial location. It is important, in this context, to be aware of the fact that in hearts without any indication for preexcitation, the annulus in the posterior septal area in particular is often deficient. The downward cascading atrial fibers, known also as Paladino's tract, thus are closely adjacent to ventricular myocardial cells through gaps in the annulus. In some instances, there may be no fibrous tissue whatsoever and contiguity of muscle cells of atrial and ventricular origin is often the case. These histologic pictures can easily be mistaken for continuity and, hence, an accessory atrioventricular connection (Fig. 13).

What is the Incidence of "Mahaim" Connections in Normal Individuals?

Following the initial descriptions,[22,23] the potential of connections at the level of the atrioventricular node or penetrating bundle has been a matter of much dispute. Presently, it is firmly acknowledged that "Mahaim" connections may play a role in the genesis of cardiac arrhythmias, although their incidence remains unsolved. This issue is clouded particularly by the morphology of the specialized tissues of the nodal-bundle axis in relation to the central fibrous body. Histologic sections of the specialized atrioventricular junctional area will often reveal dispersion or fragmentation of small groups of cells, derived from either the node or the bundle, within the dense connective tissue of the central fibrous body. Indeed, dispersion may be so extensive that the presence of a connection is highly suggestive (Fig. 14). Nevertheless, careful reconstruction of serial histologic sections under these circumstances usually reveals that no true continuity between specialized cells of the nodal-bundle axis and the crest of the ventricular septum occur. The groups of cells separate from the main axis and further branch within the fibrous tissue, often to confluence and veer back towards the main bundle, although at a more distal end. In other words, it seems that loops of specialized cells are formed within the central fibrous body. The question thus arises of whether this peculiar architecture may play a role in intranodal conduction, rather

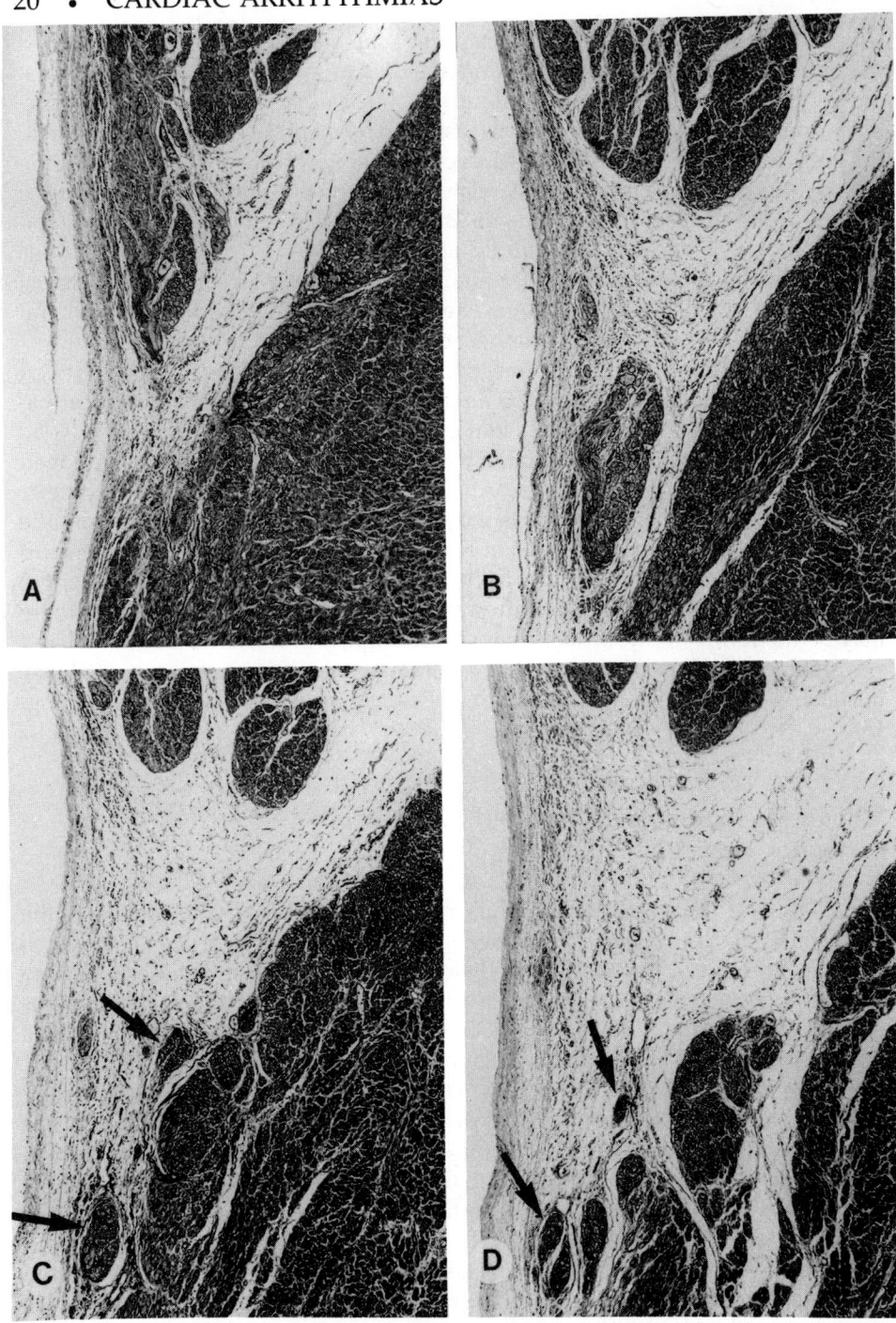

Figure 12: Accessory atrioventricular connection in subendocardial right septal position, in a patient with Ebstein's malformation of the tricuspid valve. A: the atrial take off of the bundle. B: the bundle between atrial and ventricular musculature. C: the bundle, already divided (arrows), approximates the ventricular myocardium. D: the area of ventricular insertion characterized by multiple bundles (arrows). Masson trichrome stains; A-D, ×55.

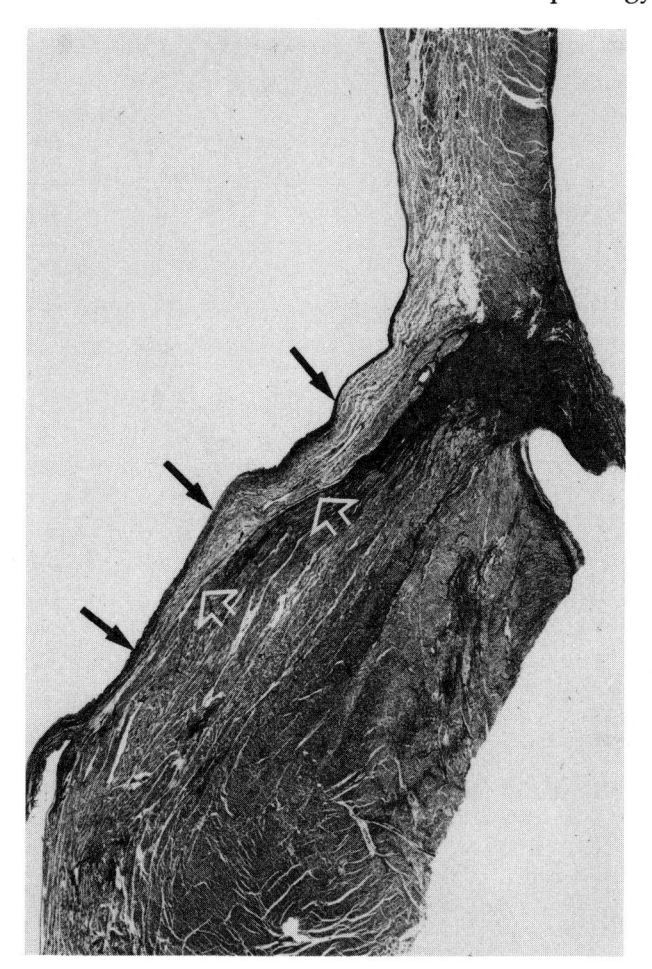

Figure 13: Cross-section through the junction of the atrial and ventricular septa. The mitral valve originates from a well-formed central fibrous body. The atrial musculature cascades down on the right side of the ventricular septum (solid black arrows) and is contiguous with the ventricular myocardium, separated only by a small rim of fibro-fatty tissue (open white arrows). There is no atrioventricular connection. Elastic tissue stain; ×6

than in connecting the node to the ventricular myocardium. It is in this arena, which needs further investigation, that the pathologist may well play a major role in unraveling the functional morphology.

Our experiences suggest that hesitation on histologic grounds, whether or not a nodoventricular or fasciculo-ventricular connection is present, almost always dictates that such a connection is not there. When present, it is usually obvious as encountered in the few cases personally observed. One of these has previously been alluded to.[26] In that particular instance, a distinct bundle connected the posterior extent of the node to the crest of the ventricular septum. The architecture in no way resembled dispersion as encountered so commonly. The second case was that of a 19-year-old-male who suddenly and unexpectedly died during exercise. Histologic examination of the specialized atrioventricular junctional zone disclosed a tract connecting the main mass of the compact atrioventricular node to the underlying ventricular myocardium (Fig. 15). In this particular instance, the bundle took a zig-zag course, somewhat resembling the situation encountered in fragmented nodes, but still obviously different (compare Figs. 14 and 15).

22 • CARDIAC ARRHYTHMIAS

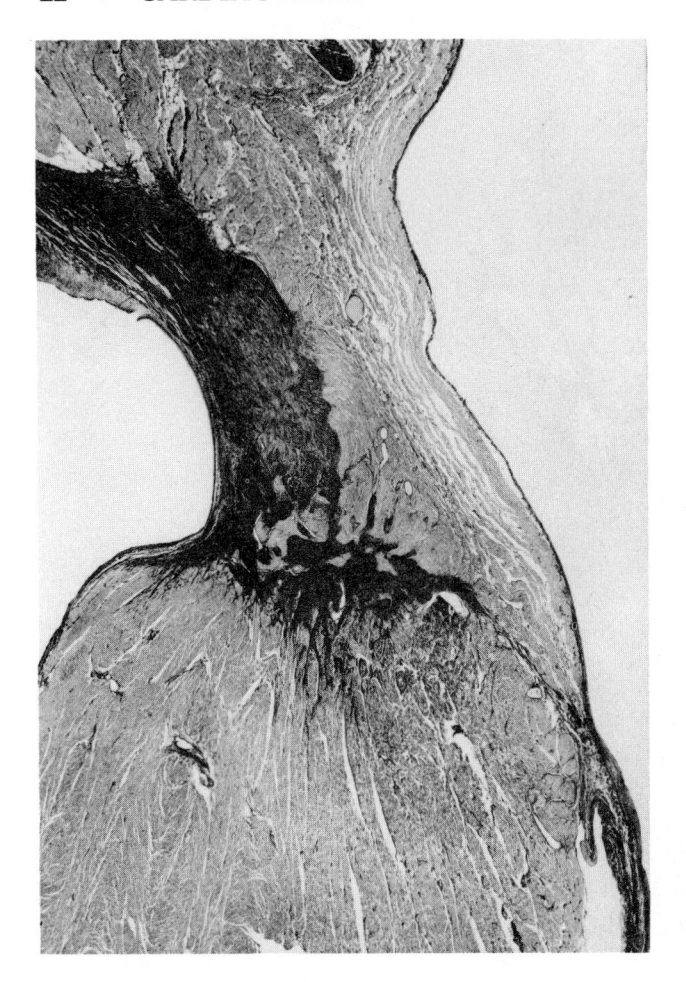

Figure 14: Dispersion of the atrioventricular node within the central fibrous body, suggesting a connection. Serial sectioning reveals that direct continuity is not present. Elastic tissue stain; ×12.

How Often do Accessory Atrioventricular Connections Occur in Addition to Nodoventricular and Fasciculo-Ventricular Connections?

In order to answer this question with any degree of certainty, the problem of solving the true nature of nodal and bundle dispersion within the central fibrous body should be solved. At this stage there is little morphologic evidence that the combined occurrence of nodoventricular and fasciculo-ventricular connections, with accessory atrioventricular connections outside the specialized atrioventricular junctional area are frequent. Nevertheless, there is definite clinical evidence that dual connections in which both anatomic substrates take part do occur and, most probably, not at all infrequently.

In the series presently studied, one heart specimen was encountered in which nodoventricular dispersion with a possible connection was encountered (case 5; Becker et al.[16]). The electrocardiogram in this particular patient suggested a right lateral accessory connection, which on extensive histologic serial sectioning could not be documented. This particular case further illustrates that the

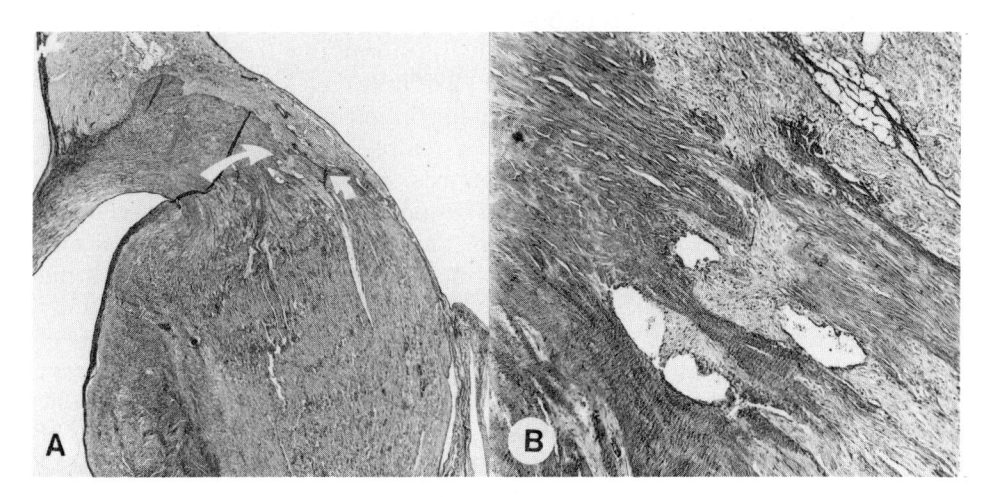

Figure 15: Nodoventricular connection in a patient with sudden death. A: low power view of the atrioventricular node and dispersion of nodal tissue within the central fibrous body (arrows). B: detailed view of the zone with specialized cells connecting the node (upper part) to the crest of the ventricular septum. Elastic tissue stain; A, ×7; B, ×55.

problem can be solved by the morphologist only when extensive and advanced electrophysiological studies are available to relate to the anatomic findings. Thus far, such cases have, to the best of my knowledge, not been produced.

Should Ventricular Preexcitation be Considered as a Form of Congenital Heart Disease?

The answer to this question is *yes*. One has to accept that accessory atrioventricular connections bridging the gap between atrial and ventricular musculature are remnants of an early developmental state in which direct physical continuity between atrial and ventricular anlagen is still present. The fibrous annulus, as we know it in the mature heart, is formed by ingrowth of atrioventricular sulcus tissue, thus creating discontinuity between atrial and ventricular musculature. The anatomical studies of the right- and left-sided fibrous annulus in normal hearts previously alluded to,[34] clearly show that discontinuity between both compartments is established although not necessarily by a fibrous annulus. In other words, there is much variation which has to be considered at least in part as developmental in origin. In this setting, one may easily envision the situation that occasional remnants of the original cardiac tube remain and eventually may develop into working myocardial cells forming bridges between atrial and ventricular musculature. The concept does not imply that a deficiency of the annulus fibrosus is the hallmark of the presence of an accessory atrioventricular connection, but rather that the whole developmental process at the level of the atrioventricular junction is variable as far as details are concerned and that the occasional presence of bridging muscle fibers may well fit within this spectrum.

Similarly, it has previously been pointed out that the specialized atrioventricular junctional area is highly variable in its detailed architecture.[9,11] Once more, the formation of the central fibrous body is relevant in this context. In the classical fashion, the atrioventricular node gradually transforms into the penetrating bundle, defined as that part of the nodal-bundle axis fully enveloped by fibrous tissue of the central fibrous body and, hence, no longer in contact with atrial fibers. A poorly developed central fibrous body, therefore, may markedly change the morphology of this part of the conduction axis. The functional significance remains speculative, although the clinical significance of atrio-fascicular connections directly relate to this phenomenon. Similarly, dispersion of nodal and bundle tissues within the central fibrous body may be considered along the same lines. Indeed, there is evidence that at birth the central fibrous body is not yet fully completed and, hence, may still have an effect upon the definitive architecture of the atrioventricular conduction axis. For instance, the composition changes from a tissue with a high content of glycosaminoglycans into a densely packed sclerotic tissue at older ages. However, at present, it remains pure speculation whether these changes within the central fibrous body may lead to a disappearance of connections between the node and bundle with the musculature of the ventricular crest with increasing maturation. Indeed, the developmental aspects of nodoventricular and fasciculoventricular connections remain as yet unsolved.

Some of the questions that relate to developmental aspects can be solved only by studying large numbers of hearts of different age groups. Ideally, one would like to be able to follow the various transformations in one and the same heart, but this of course is a practical impossibility. Since the variability from one heart to the other is enormous, by definition, it implies that a study as suggested above will have to encompass an enormous number of cases in order to come up with a reliable answer.

Conclusions

At the present stage, it is well established that ventricular preexcitation is due to connections that bypass the normal delay-producing area of the atrioventricular node. The most common condition is the accessory atrioventricular connection, bridging the gap between atrial and ventricular musculature. Within this framework, however, a marked variation can occur. The bundle may be short and directly related to a well-formed fibrous annulus and it may be long and slender and located superficially in the epicardial fat. Moreover, the bundle may ramify, and it appears that, as a rule, the ventricular insertion of an accessory atrioventricular connection is by way of multiple smaller branches sometimes represented by single cell strands. This particular architecture may have electrophysiological significance in facilitating retrograde spread of activation rather than antegrade conduction. Furthermore, the accessory connection and the ventricular musculature at the site of insertion usually show marked fibrotic changes. This may also affect the possibility for spread of activation. Specific questions, such as the incidence of multiple connections and the incidence of combined occurrence of accessory atrioventricular connections with nodoventricular and fasciculoventricular connections, remain unanswered from a morphologic point of view.

In this context, the dispersion of specialized cells derived from the atrioventricular node and bundle needs further evaluation. Here, progress may be expected from the morphologist although the work will be tedious and possibly will never be definitive since electrophysiologic correlates are necessary to prove that a morphologic substrate can be held responsible for electrical phenomena in the heart.

From a morphologic stance, a plea should be made to concentrate all heart specimens of patients with well-documented ventricular preexcitation in a few centers where pathologists have a keen interest in this particular syndrome. Only through such an effort progress in this particular field may be expected from morphologists.

References

1. Öhnell RF. Pre-excitation, a cardiac abnormality, pathophysiological, pathoanatomical and clinical studies of excitatory spread phenomenon bearing upon the problem of the WPW (Wolff-Parkinson-White) electrocardiogram and paroxysmal tachycardia. Acta Med Scand Suppl 1944;152:79–81.
2. Durrer D, Schuilenburg RM, Wellens HJJ. Preexcitation revisited. Am J Cardiol 1970; 25:690–697.
3. Chung, KY, Walsh TJ, Massie E. Wolff-Parkinson-White syndrome. Am Heart J 1965;69:116–133.
4. Anderson RH, Becker AE. Accessory atrioventricular connections. J Thorac Cardiovasc Surg 1979;78:310–311.
5. Sealy WC. Reply to accessory atrioventricular connections. J Thorac Cardiovasc Surg 1980;79:637–638.
6. Burchell HB. In support of Kent. J Thorac Cardiovasc Surg 1980;79:637–638.
7. Anderson RH, Becker AE. Stanley Kent and accessory atrioventricular connections. J Thorac Cardiovasc Surg 1981;81:649–658.
8. Burchell HB. Ventricular preexcitation: historical overview. In: Benditt DG, Benson DW Jr, eds. Cardiac Preexcitation: Origins, Evaluation and Treatment. Boston, Martinus Nijhoff Publishing, 1986;3–19.
9. Anderson RH, Becker AE, Brechenmacher C, Davies MJ, Rossi L. Ventricular preexcitation: A proposed nomenclature for its substrates. Eur J Cardiol 1975;3:27–36.
10. Wood FC, Wolferth GK, Geckeler GD. Histologic demonstration of accessory muscular connections between auricle and ventricle in a case of short P-R interval and prolonged QRS complex. Am Heart J 1943;25:454–462.
11. Davies MJ, Anderson RH, Becker AE. The Conduction System of the Heart. London, Butterworths, 1983;181–202.
12. Cobb FR, Blumenschein SD, Sealy WC, Boineau JP, Wagner GS, Wallace AG. Successful surgical interruption of the bundle of Kent in a patient with Wolff-Parkinson-White syndrome. Circulation 1968;38:1018–1029.
13. Cox JL, Cain ME. Surgery for preexcitation syndromes. In: Benditt DG, Benson DW Jr, eds. Cardiac Preexcitation: Origins, Evaluation and Treatment. Boston, Martinus Nijhoff Publishing, 1986;527–534.
14. Guiraudon GM, Klein GJ, Sharma AD, Jones DL. Surgical treatment of Wolff-Parkinson-White syndrome: the epicardial approach. In: Benditt DG, Benson DW Jr, eds. Cardiac Preexcitation: Origins, Evaluation and Treatment. Boston, Martinus Nijhoff Publishing 1986;535–541.
15. Scheinman MM. Catheter ablation for patients with ventricular preexcitation. In: Benditt DG, Benson DW Jr, eds. Cardiac Preexcitation: Origins, Evalution and Treatment. Boston, Martinus Nijhoff Publishing, 1986;493–506.
16. Becker AE, Anderson RH, Durrer DR, Wellens HJJ. The anatomical substrates of Wolff-Parkinson-White syndrome: A clinicopathologic correlation in seven patients. Circulation 1978;57:870–879.
17. Gallagher JJ, Sealy WC, Cox JL, German LD, Kasell JH, Bardy GH, Backer DL. Results of surgery for preexcitation caused by accessory atrioventricular pathways in 267

consecutive cases. In: Josephson PH, Josephson ME, Wellens HJJ, eds. Tachycardias: Mechanisms, Diagnosis and Treatment. Philadelphia, Lea & Febiger, 1984:259–269.
18. Gotlieb AI, Chan M, Palmer WH, Huang SN. Ventricular preexcitation syndrome. Accessory left atrioventricular connection and rhabdomyomatous myocardial fibers. Arch Pathol Lab Med 1977;101:486–489.
19. Rosenbaum FF, Hecht HH, Wilson FH, Johnston FD. Potential variations of thorax and the oesophagus in anomalous atrioventricular excitation (Wolff-Parkinson-White syndrome). Am Heart J 1945;29:281–326.
20. Gallagher JJ, Svenson RH, Sealy WC, Wallace AG. The Wolff-Parkinson-White syndrome and the pre-excitation dysrhythmias: Medical and surgical management. Med Clin N Am 1976;60:101–123.
21. Sealy WC, Gallagher JJ. The surgical approach to the septal area of the heart based on experience with 45 patients with Kent bundles. J Thorac Cardiovasc Surg 1980; 79:542–551.
22. Mahaim I, Winston MR. Recherches d'anatomie comparée et de pathologie expérimentale sur les connexions hautes de His-Tawara. Cardiologia 1941;5:189–260.
23. Mahaim I. Kent's fibers and the A-V paraspecific conduction through the upper connections of the bundle of His-Tawara. Am Heart J 1947;33:651–653.
24. Gallagher JJ, Smith WM, Kasell JH, Benson DW Jr, Sterba R, Grant AO. Role of Mahaim fibers in cardiac arrhythmias in man. Circulation 1981;64:176–189.
25. Lev M, Fox SM, Bharati S, Rosen KM, Langendorf R, Pick A. Mahaim and James fibers as a basis for a unique variety of preexcitation. Am J Cardiol 1975;36:880–888.
26. Gmeiner R, Ng CK, Hammer I, Becker AE. Tachycardia caused by an accessory nodoventricular tract: A clinico-pathologic correlation. Eur Heart J 1984;5:233–242.
27. Anderson RH, Becker AE. Morphology of the normal conduction system. In: Van Mierop LHS, Oppenheimer-Dekker A, Bruins CLDCh, eds. Embryology and Teratology of the Heart and the Great Arteries. The Hague, Martinus Nijhoff Medical Division, 1978;25–33.
28. Lev M. The pathology of complete atrioventricular block. Prog Cardiovasc Dis 1964; 6:317–326.
29. James TN. Anatomy of the human atrioventricular node with remarks pertinent to its electrophysiology. Am Heart J 1961;62:756–771.
30. Brechenmacher C, Atrio-His bundle tracts. Br Heart J 1975;37:853–855.
31. Sung RJ, Gelband H, Castellanos A, Aranda JM, Myerburg RJ. Clinical and electrophysiologic observations in patients with concealed accessory atrioventricular bypass tracts. Am J Cardiol 1977;40:839–847.
32. Wellens HJ, Durrer D. Patterns of ventriculo-atrial conduction in the Wolff-Parkinson-White syndrome. Circulation 1974;49:22–31.
33. De la Fuente D, Sasyniuk B, Moe GM. Conduction through a narrow isthmus in isolated canine atrial tissue: A model for the WPW-syndrome. Circulation 1971; 44:803–809.
34. Anderson RH, Davies MJ, Becker AE. Atrioventricular ring specialized tissue in the normal heart. Eur J Cardiol 1974;2:219–230.
35. Gallagher JJ, Sealy WC, Kasell J, Wallace AG. Multiple accessory pathways in patients with the preexcitation syndrome. Circulation 1976;54:571–591.
36. Brady GH, Packer DL, German LD, Gallagher JJ. Preexcited reciprocating tachycardia in patients with Wolff-Parkinson-White syndrome: Incidence and mechanisms. Circulation 1984;70:377–391.
37. Dreifus LS, Wellens HJ, Watanabe Y, Kimbiris D, Truex R. Sinus bradycardia and atrial fibrillation with the Wolff-Parkinson-White syndrome. Am J Cardiol 1976;38:149–156.
38. Kent AFS. The right lateral auriculo-ventricular junction of the heart. J Physiol 1914; 48:22–24.
39. Verduyn-Lunel AA. Significance of annulus fibrosus of heart in relation to AV conduction and ventricular activation in cases of Wolff-Parkinson-White syndrome. Br Heart J 1972;34:1263–1271.
40. James TN, Puech P. De subitaneis mortibus IX. Type A Wolff-Parkinson-White syndrome. Circulation 1974;50:1264–1280.

2

Influences of Anisotropic Tissue Structure on Reentrant Ventricular Tachycardia

Andrew L. Wit
Stephen Dillon
Philip C. Ursell

Introduction

Reentrant excitation is an important cause of both experimental and clinical ventricular arrhythmias accompanying myocardial infarction. In discussing the mechanisms for reentry in this situation, it has been assumed that alterations in transmembrane action potentials of myocardial cells are usually the primary cause of the slow conduction and block necessary for reentry to occur.[1-4] For example, in acute ischemia, membrane depolarization of ventricular muscle fibers leads to a reduced action potential amplitude and upstroke velocity, inhomogeneous recovery of excitability, slow conduction, and reentry that causes tachycardia and fibrillation.[5,6] Purkinje fibers in subacute infarcts (1–3 days old) have a reduced maximum diastolic potential, spontaneous diastolic depolarization, and delayed afterdepolarizations that cause ventricular premature beats and tachycardia.[7-9] Muscle cells surviving in chronic infarcts may have abnormal and inhomogeneous repolarization so that premature impulses may block in some regions and not in others, leading to the formation of reentrant circuits.[10] However, in this chapter we present evidence that altered or depressed transmembrane potentials

---

From: Brugada P, Wellens HJJ. CARDIAC ARRHYTHMIAS: Where To Go From Here? Mount Kisco, NY, Futura Publishing Company, Inc., © 1987.

may not always be necessary for reentry in infarcts and that reentry might occur primarily from the influences of infarct structure on conduction.

Influences of Structure on Conduction: Anisotropy

The factors governing conduction in cardiac muscle are complex.[11] The velocity at which the impulse propagates is dependent on the characteristics of the transmembrane action potentials as well as the passive electrical properties (Fig. 1). An action potential occurring at a particular site (A) is accompanied by an inward current (I_{Na}). Part of this current flows along the fiber towards another site (B) which has not yet been excited. This intracellular flow is called axial current. The current exits at the distal site through the membrane as capacitive current (I_C) which depolarizes the membrane potential or as membrane current (I_i) flowing through ionic channels. If the depolarization caused by the capacitive current is large enough to reach threshold, an action potential will occur at site B and thus the impulse propagates from site A to B. Hence, a reduction in the upstroke of an action potential (I_{Na}) leading to a decrease in axial current can slow conduction. There are also intracellular resistances to axial current flow which

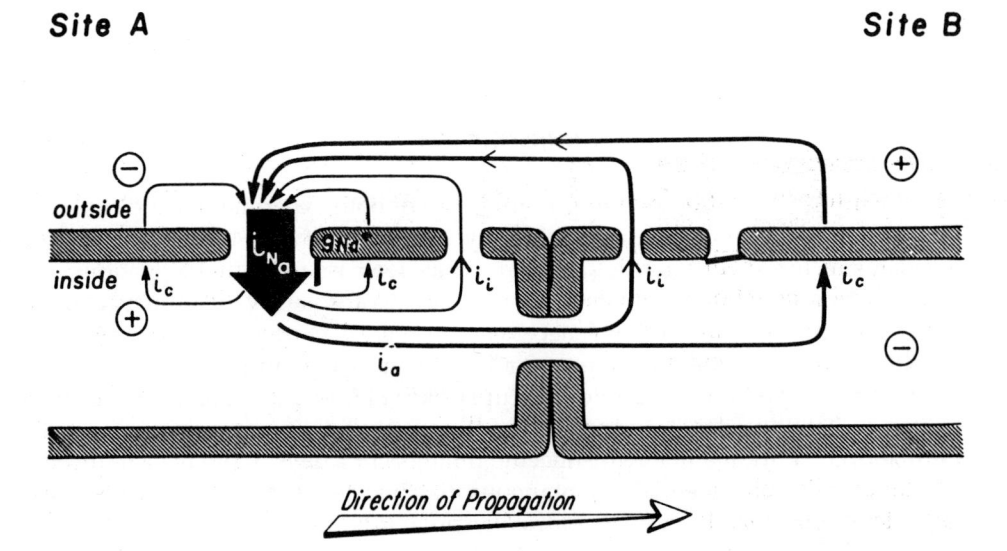

Figure 1: Diagram of current flow resulting in conduction of the cardiac impulse. Site A is excited by a stimulus and an action potential occurs. The large black arrow labeled ^{i}Na depicts the fast inward Na current flowing through the Na channels (g Na) during the action potential upstroke. This inward membrane current, in turn, results in intracellular axial current flow, along the myocardial fiber away from the stimulus' site (horizontal arrows) and extracellular current flow back toward the stimulus site. Axial current is composed of capacitive current (^{i}c) and membrane current (^{i}i) (see text). Capacitive current causes depolarization at site B to threshold potential and the occurrence of an action potential. (Reproduced from Frame LH, Hoffman, BF: Mechanisms of Tachycardia In Tachycardias, Surawicz B, Pratrap Reddy C, Prystowsky EN, eds. Martinus Nijhoff, The Hague, pp 7–36, 1984.)

determine how far the current spreads and its effectiveness in depolarizing membranes at a distance. An increase in intracellular resistance may decrease axial current spread and slow conduction. The cytoplasm offers minimal resistance to the spread of axial current. A larger portion of the intracellular resistance is normally located at the intercellular connections between myocardial fibers—the gap junctions of the intercalated discs. During conduction, axial current flows from one myocardial cell to the adjacent cell through the gap junctions of the disc (which normally have a relatively low resistance) and therefore the resistance, size, and distribution of these junctions have a profound influence on conduction. The resistance of the discs is influenced by changes in intracellular Ca^{++} concentration and pH and may increase substantially when Ca is elevated and pH is low during ischemia.[12] This, in turn, may slow or block conduction.[13] The size and distribution of these junctions influence conduction even in normal myocardium and may be further modified by pathology.

Cardiac muscle is anisotropic; its anatomic and biophysical properties vary according to the direction in the cardiac syncytium in which they are measured. In regions where the cardiac muscle fibers are closely packed together and arranged parallel to each other in a uniform manner, conduction in the direction parallel to the myocardial fiber orientation (along the long axis of the myocardial fibers) is much more rapid than in the direction perpendicular to the long axis.[14–17] Conduction perpendicular to the long axis of atrial or ventricular muscle fibers can be as slow as 0.1 m/sec even when resting and action potentials of the fibers are normal. The slow conduction is caused by an effective axial resistance ($\bar{R}a$: resistance to current flow in the direction of propagation dependent to a large extent on intracellular resistivity) which is higher in the direction perpendicular to fiber orientation than parallel to fiber orientation.[15] This higher axial resistivity results in part from fewer and shorter intercalated discs in a side-to-side direction than in the end-to-end direction. These characteristics have been called uniform anisotropy.[15]

In addition, although it may seem paradoxical, in spite of more rapid conduction down the long axis of the myocardial fibers than perpendicular to the long axis, Spach et al. have proposed that premature impulses block more readily when propagating along the long axis than perpendicular to it and have provided supporting evidence for this hypothesis.[16] Spach calculated the relationship between maximum axial current (Ia_{max}) and effective axial resistance ($\bar{R}a$), using data obtained from action potential measurements during transverse and longitudinal propagation in uniformly anisotropic muscle. In the idealized situation where $\dot{V}_{max}$ does not change with $\bar{R}a$, the maximum axial current is inversely proportional to the square root of $\bar{R}a$. Therefore, it is predicted that conduction block will occur when $\bar{R}a$ increases to such an extent that the decreased axial current is no longer effective in depolarizing the membrane to the threshold potential. However, this does not apply to uniformly anisotropic muscle, where $\dot{V}_{max}$ *increases* when $\bar{R}a$ increases during slowing of conduction in the transverse direction. In anisotropic tissue, axial current increases as $\bar{R}a$ decreases but reaches a peak at low values of $\bar{R}a$ and decreases sharply when $\bar{R}a$ decreases further. The maximum propagation velocity occurs at the peak of the Ia_{max} curve (in the direction of the long fiber axis). Propagation fails first in the direction of a low $\bar{R}a$

as the ability of the membrane to supply depolarizing current is reduced (a decrease in $\dot{V}_{max}$). In the direction of low $\bar{R}a$ (longitudinal), a decrease of depolarizing current fails to depolarize the membrane to threshold causing block, whereas in the direction of higher $\bar{R}a$ (transverse), the membrane may still be depolarized to threshold, and conduction occurs. This hypothesis does not preclude the possibility that conduction block will also occur at a very high $\bar{R}a$. Others do not agree with this proposal,[18,19] and therefore, additional studies are necessary. However, if the site of block of premature impulses is determined to some extent by the orientation of the myocardial fibers, this influence of structure on conduction may be important for the initiation of reentrant tachycardias. We discuss this possibility in a later section.

When myocardial fiber bundles are separated by nonmuscular tissue, such as connective tissue, the conduction properties may be altered because of the effects on axial resistivity. For example, fibrosis in the heart separates myocardial fibers reducing the number of disc connections and possibly decreasing the extent or area of connections that remain. An example is provided by the effects of fibrosis on the structure and conduction properties of aging atrial myocardium.[20] We will discuss later the influences of the fibrosis that occurs during infarct healing on conduction.

Severe changes in fiber orientation in the direction of propagation which results from branching of muscle bundles also slows conduction and can cause block, even in the absence of changes in transmembrane potentials. Slowing of conduction and block may occur because of the sudden increase in axial resistivity associated with the change in orientation.[16] For example, an impulse conducting along a muscle bundle in a direction parallel to fiber orientation (low effective axial resistivity) may conduct into a branch of that bundle; at the branching point, the orientation of the myocardial fibers may be perpendicular to the original direction of conduction, and therefore, the effective axial resistivity suddenly becomes high. Conduction may therefore block because of the sudden increase in axial resistivity. The separation of fibers by connective tissue and the branching of bundles results in a nonuniform anisotropic structure. We will describe how both uniform and nonuniform anisotropy might cause reentry in hearts with healing or healed infarcts.

Mechanisms for Reentry Caused by Anisotropic Structure of Cardiac Fibers Surviving in Subacute Infarcts

Experimental Model

Our experimental studies, which have suggested to us that anisotropy is an important cause of reentry, have been done on the canine heart with myocardial infarction caused by complete occlusion of the left anterior descending coronary artery (LAD) near its origin.[21-23] After occlusion, a transmural infarct of the anterolateral left ventricular wall often occurs, but epicardial muscle bundles survive probably because they have an additional blood supply from epicardial branches of the circumflex. These surviving muscle fibers comprise the epicardial border zone of the infarct which is a thin sheet of muscle on the epicardial surface (Fig. 2).[21-23]

When complete transmural necrosis occurs, there is no underlying muscular connections to this surviving epicardial muscle; the epicardial border zone is connected to normal muscle only around the margins of the infarct.[21-22] Im-

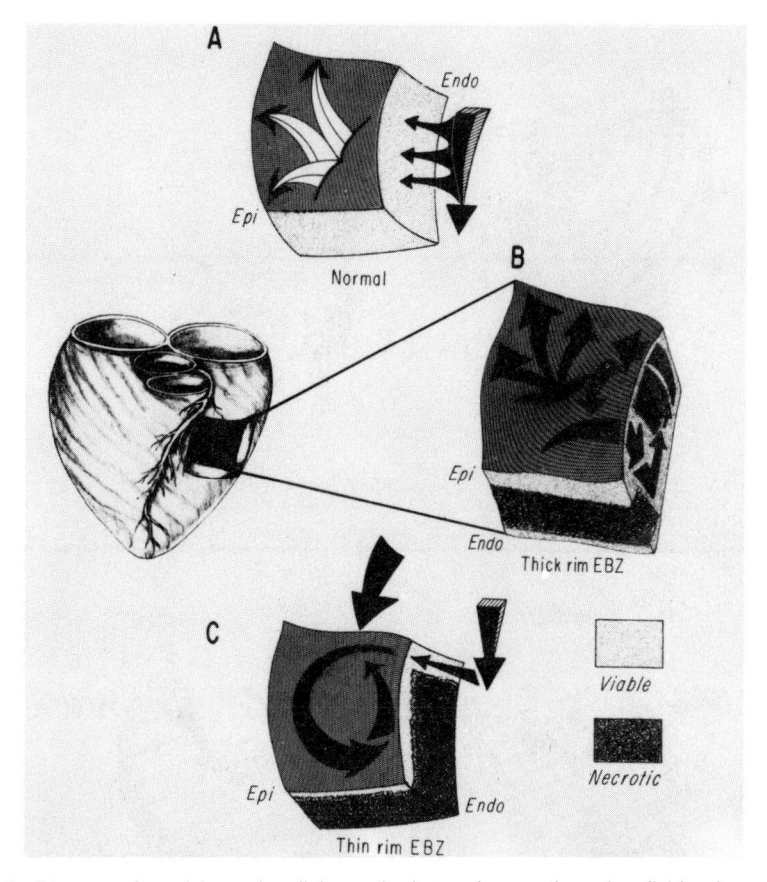

Figure 2: Diagram of surviving epicardial muscle that makes up the epicardial border zone after a transmural infarction caused by LAD occlusion, and possible activation patterns. Panel A shows a section of the anterior wall from a noninfarcted ventricle. The epicardial surface is indicated by the striped shading; the thickness of the wall by the light stipples. The black arrows at the right indicate that activation normally occurs along the endocardial surface and transmurally toward the epicardial surface. Epicardial breakthrough is indicated by the white arrows. B and C indicate possible location of surviving muscle fibers and reentrant circuits after occlusion of the LAD. Necrotic regions are indicated by dark shading, viable regions by the light stippling. In B, a large amount of muscle survived in the infarct region and a thick border zone of muscle is on the epicardial surface. The arrows show that reentrant circuits may be comprised of epicardial, intramural, and endocardial muscle. In C only a thin rim of epicardial muscle survived the coronary occlusion and there are no intramural muscle bundles connecting epicardial and endocardial regions as often occurs after complete and permanent occlusion of the LAD. Reentry in this type of infarct may be confined to the epicardial surface. (Reproduced from Gardner PI, Ursell PC, Pham TD, Fenoglio JJ, Wit AL: Experimental chronic ventricular tachycardia: Anatomic and electrophysiologic substrates, In: Tachycardias: Mechanisms, Diagnosis, Treatment, ME Josephson and HJ Wellens, eds. Philadelphia, Lea and Febiger, pp 29-60, 1984.)

pulses conduct over the surface of the infarct in the surviving muscle and the muscle cannot be activated from intramural regions as it is prior to coronary occlusion (Fig. 2). Reentrant excitation occurs in this region to cause tachycardia.[21,24-27] Many of the anatomic features of the epicardial border zone are similar to the subendocardial regions of human infarcts where tachycardias originate[28] and the results of electrophysiologic studies on conduction in the epicardial border zone of canine infarcts may provide information relevant to properties of conduction in human infarcts.

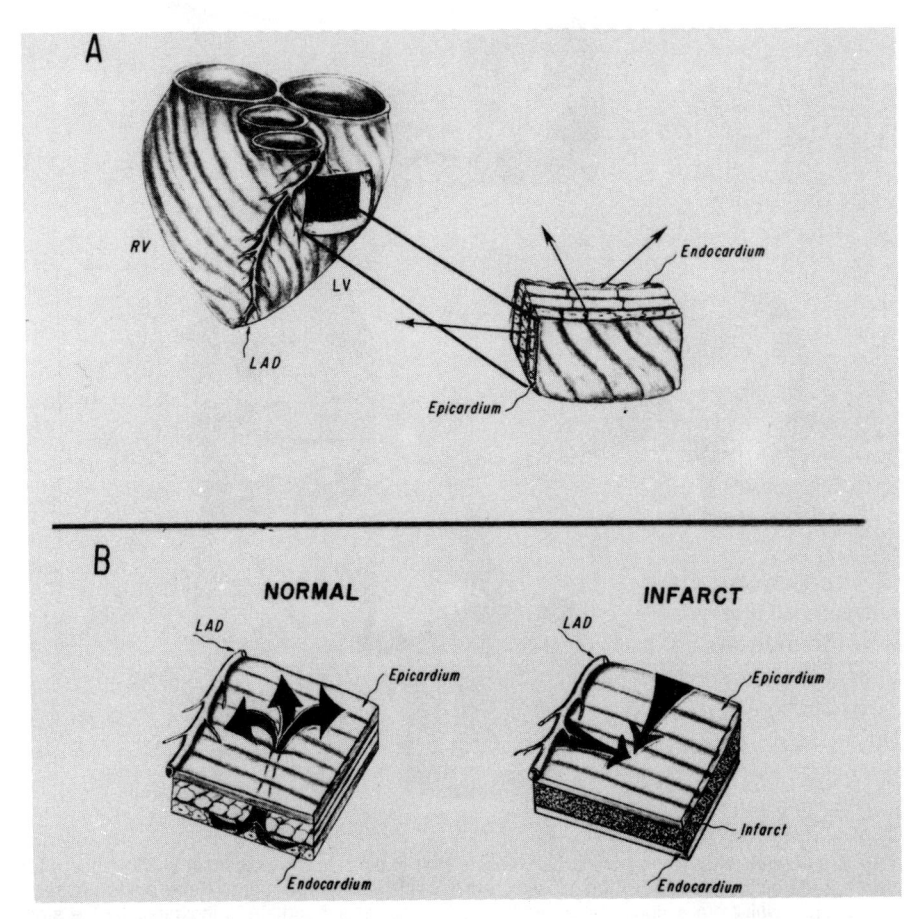

Figure 3: Epicardial border zone of transmural canine infarcts and orientation of the muscle fibers that comprise it. Panel A shows an anterior view of the heart. LAD = left anterior descending coronary artery, LV = left ventricle, and RV = right ventricle. In the section of the anterior wall at the right, the orientation of the muscle fiber on the epicardial surface is shown by the arrows. The epicardial fibers course at right angles to the LAD toward the apex and lateral left ventricular wall. Panel B diagrammatically shows the influence of fiber orientation on conduction. In the normal noninfarcted left ventricle at the left, activation occurs from below as indicated by the arrows; hence the orientation of the epicardial muscle fibers does not significantly influence conduction. In the narrow epicardial border zone of a transmural infarct (right), the impulse conducts horizontally across the epicardial surface as indicated by the arrow and the orientation of the muscle fibers significantly influences conduction. (Reproduced from Gardner PI, Ursell PC, Pham TD, Fenoglio JJ, Wit AL: Experimental chronic ventricular tachycardia: Anatomic and electrophysiologic substrates In: Tachycardias, Mechanisms, Diagnosis, Treatment, ME Josephson and HJ Wellens, eds., Philadelphia, Lea and Febiger, pp 29-60, 1984.)

During the first several weeks after occlusion, the muscle fibers in the epicardial border zone are arranged in parallel with their long axis extending from the anterior descending coronary artery toward the lateral left ventricle and apex (Fig. 3). Little connective tissue separates individual fiber bundles at this time but the bundles are separated by variable amounts of edema. Intercalated discs connecting myocardial cells end to end are more numerous than discs connecting fibers side to side. Thus, the border zone at this time is an anisotropic structure which is relatively uniform in terms of fiber orientation but which may have some nonuniform properties because of the separation of the fibers by edema.[22]

Effects of Anisotropy on Conduction

The canine epicardial border zone can be used as a model to test the hypothesis that the anatomical arrangement of cardiac fibers surviving in an infarcted region affects conduction properties in a way that may cause reentrant excitation. The influence of the myocardial fiber orientation on conduction in the epicardial border zone is shown by the activation map in Figure 4. In this experiment, an array of 190 bipolar electrodes embedded in a 4×5 cm, thin rubber sheet was placed on the epicardial surface of the anterolateral ventricle of a canine heart with a 4-day-old infarct. The ventricles were then stimulated through electrodes at the center of this electrode array. In the figure, each small number is an activation time at each of the bipolar electrodes and the "SS" shows the site of stimulation. Isochrones are drawn at 10 ms intervals and identified by the dark black numbers. During stimulation, excitation spread rapidly toward the left margin of the electrode array which is aligned along the left anterior descending coronary artery (LAD) and toward the right margin on the lateral left ventricle (LL). Activation reached these margins within 30 to 40 ms. This is the general direction of the long axis of the myocardial fibers. On the other hand, activation upward toward the base and downward toward the apex—perpendicular to the long axis—occurred much more slowly as indicated by the decreased spacing between isochrones. The basal and apical margins of the electrode array were activated after 80 to 110 ms. In general, the ratio of fast to slow conduction is 2.5–3 to 1.

The slow conduction in the direction toward the base and apex (in Fig. 4) is not caused by depressed action potentials but is a result of high axial resistivity[16] in the direction transverse to the myocardial fibers. This is shown from experiments on isolated blocks of tissue from the epicardial border zone, superfused in a tissue chamber with Tyrode's solution.[22] In the experiment illustrated in Figure 5, the isolated preparation was stimulated at a regular cycle length through bipolar electrodes in the upper left corner. Conduction velocity was determined by recording action potentials at 1 mm intervals from the stimulus site both parallel to fiber orientation (longitudinal axis) (LAD towards lateral ventricle) and perpendicular to fiber orientation (transverse axis) (towards the apex). The upstroke velocities ($\dot{V}_{max}$) of the action potentials were also measured. In general, maximum diastolic potential of muscle fibers 4–5 days after coronary occlusion are depolarized by approximately 10 mV and upstroke velocity is decreased by 10–20% compared to muscle in normal regions.[22] Conduction velocity in the

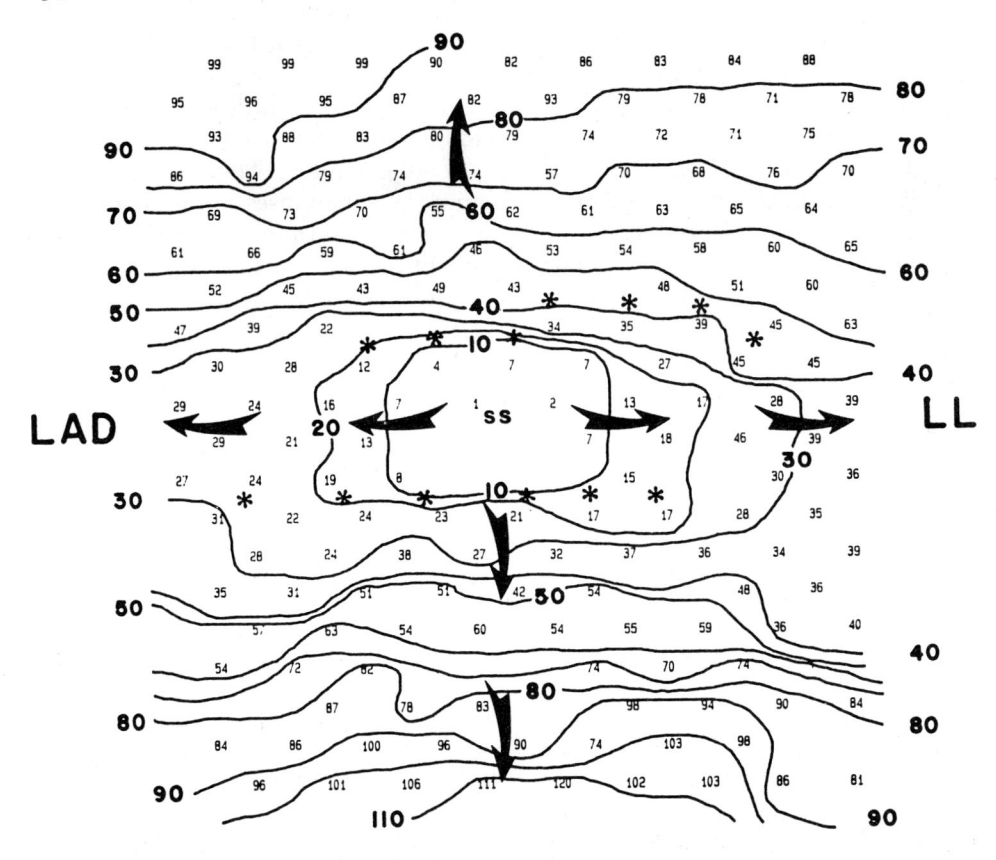

Figure 4: Activation map of impulse propagation in the epicardial border zone demonstrating the influence of anisotropy. An array of 190 bipolar electrodes were placed on the anterior left ventricle; one margin of the array adjacent to the left anterior descending coronary artery (LAD) and the opposite margin on the lateral left ventricle. The ventricles were stimulated through electrodes in the center of this array (SS). Each small number indicates an activation time. Isochrones are drawn at 10 ms intervals and are labeled with dark black numbers. Arrows show spread of activation away from central stimulus site. Note rapid activation in the horizontal direction (widely spaced isochrones) and slow activation in the vertical direction (narrow spaced isochrones).

longitudinal direction in this experiment was 0.50 m/sec while it was 0.12 m/sec in the transverse direction. Despite this marked difference, the $\dot{V}_{max}$ of the action potentials in each direction were not significantly different—80 ± 9 v/sec in the longitudinal direction and 84 ± 9 v/sec in the transverse direction. Thus, slower conduction in the direction from base to apex (transverse to fiber orientation) is not the result of a lower $\dot{V}_{max}$ of the myocardial fibers.

In addition to this prominent influence of myocardial fiber orientation on conduction velocity in the epicardial border zone, there may sometimes be additional factors resulting in slow conduction that are superimposed on the anisotropic effects. Although maximum diastolic potential and $\dot{V}_{max}$ of the muscle action potentials are usually only moderately depressed, in some regions a more

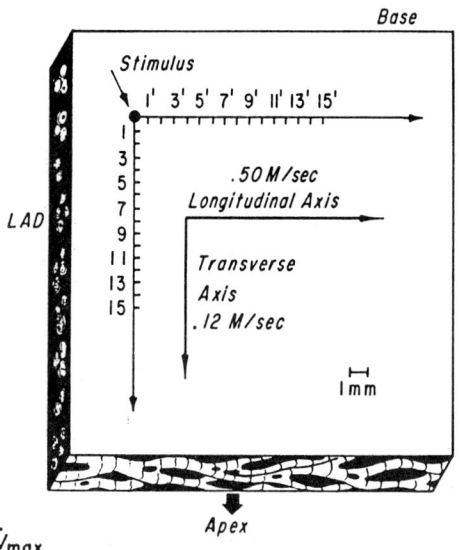

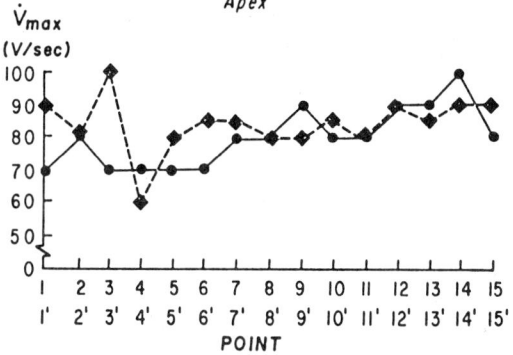

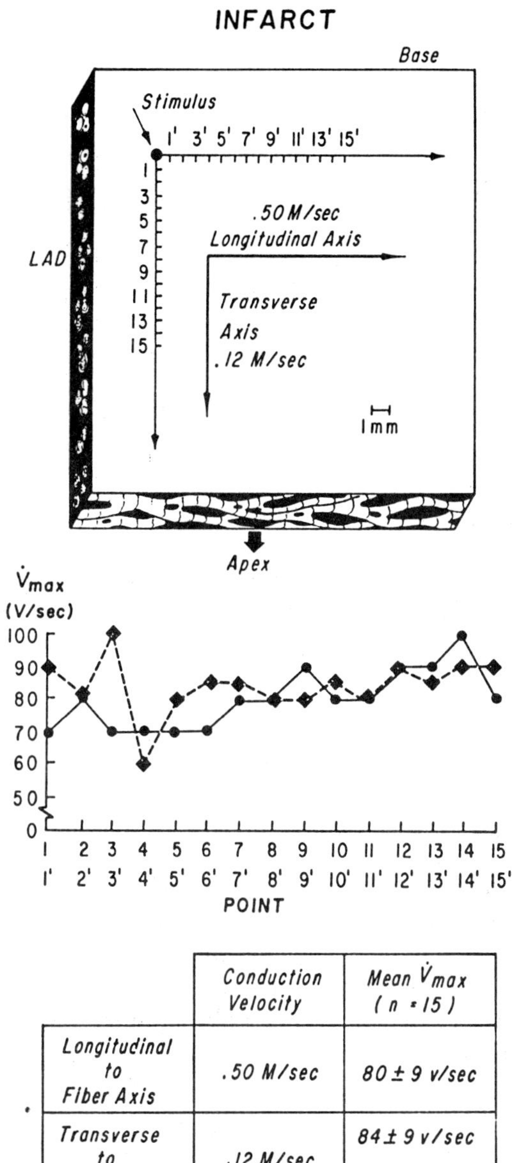

Figure 5: At the top is a diagram of a block of tissue removed from the epicardial surface of a canine infarct 5 days after LAD occlusion. The preparation was stimulated from the upper left corner and action potentials recorded at 1 mm intervals along the base and LAD margins (parallel and transverse to the longitudinal axis of myocardial fiber orientation). V_{max} of action potentials at each recording site are plotted below the diagram (circles are in longitudinal direction and diamonds in transverse direction). In the table conduction velocity and mean V_{max} are given. (Records kindly provided by Dr. Phyllis Gardner.)

	Conduction Velocity	Mean $\dot{V}_{max}$ (n = 15)
Longitudinal to Fiber Axis	.50 M/sec	80 ± 9 v/sec
Transverse to Fiber Axis	.12 M/sec	84 ± 9 v/sec (p > 0.05)

severe depression may occur because of the prior period of ischemia. Also, the infarcted myocardium may sometimes extend all the way to the epicardial surface resulting in regions of "anatomical" conduction block. This occurred in the experiment illustrated in Figure 6 in which activation was mapped in an isolated superfused preparation from the epicardial border zone of a 5-day-old myocardial infarct. Stimuli were applied at the left margin (LAD margin). In general, activation is more rapid from left to right (parallel to myocardial fiber orientation) than

36 • CARDIAC ARRHYTHMIAS

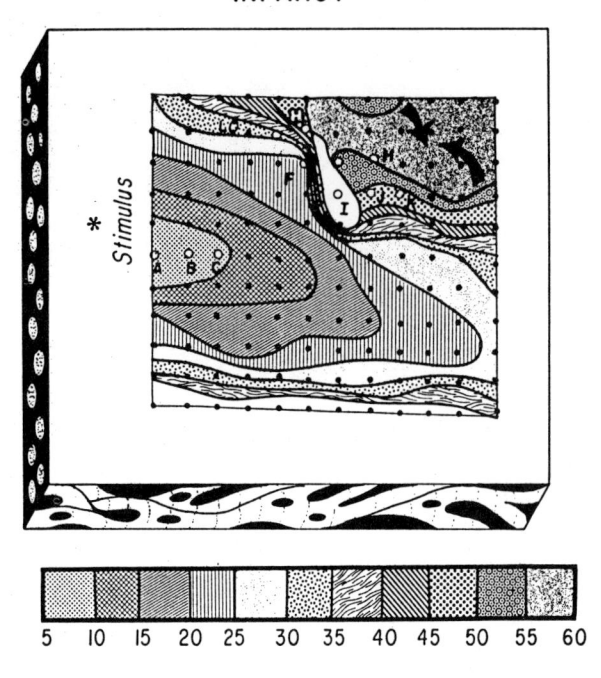

Figure 6: Diagram of activation of an isolated preparation of epicardial border zone from a 5-day-old infarct caused by LAD occlusion. The left border was adjacent to the LAD and the long axis of the parallel myocardial fibers are in the left to right direction. Isochrones are drawn at 10 ms intervals according to the scale below. Recording sites are indicated by black dots. The preparation was stimulated at the asterisk and the isochrones show rapid spread in the left to right direction except between recording sites F and I. Here there is slow activation and block. (Records kindly provided by Dr. Phyllis Gardner.)

towards the top or bottom (transverse to fiber orientation) except between sites labeled F and I. Here there is a bunching together of isochrones indicating very slow activation in the parallel direction, and finally conduction block in the white area (I). At site I, there were no surviving myocardial fibers. Whereas during slow conduction caused by anisotropy of parallel oriented fibers, "bunched" isochrones are oriented parallel to the long axis of the myocardial fibers (see Fig. 4), isochrones during slow conduction caused by depressed transmembrane potentials or anatomical obstacles may be oriented transverse to the long axis of the fibers as shown in Figure 6. The importance of the direction of the isochrones for distinguishing possible mechanisms for slow conduction and block during reentrant tachycardias is discussed in the following sections.

Is Anisotropy Important for Initiation of Reentry?

Despite the slower conduction perpendicular to myocardial fiber orientation than parallel to fiber orientation, Spach et al. showed that conduction block of premature impulses might occur more readily in the parallel direction then in the perpendicular direction in a uniformly anisotropic structure as was described earlier.[15] If this occurs in the epicardial border zone, it might contribute to the initiation of reentry by premature impulses.[21]

Figure 7 shows activation maps during initiation of reentrant tachycardia by programmed premature stimulation from electrodes on the right ventricle adjacent to the LAD coronary artery. The activation map during basic drive at a cycle

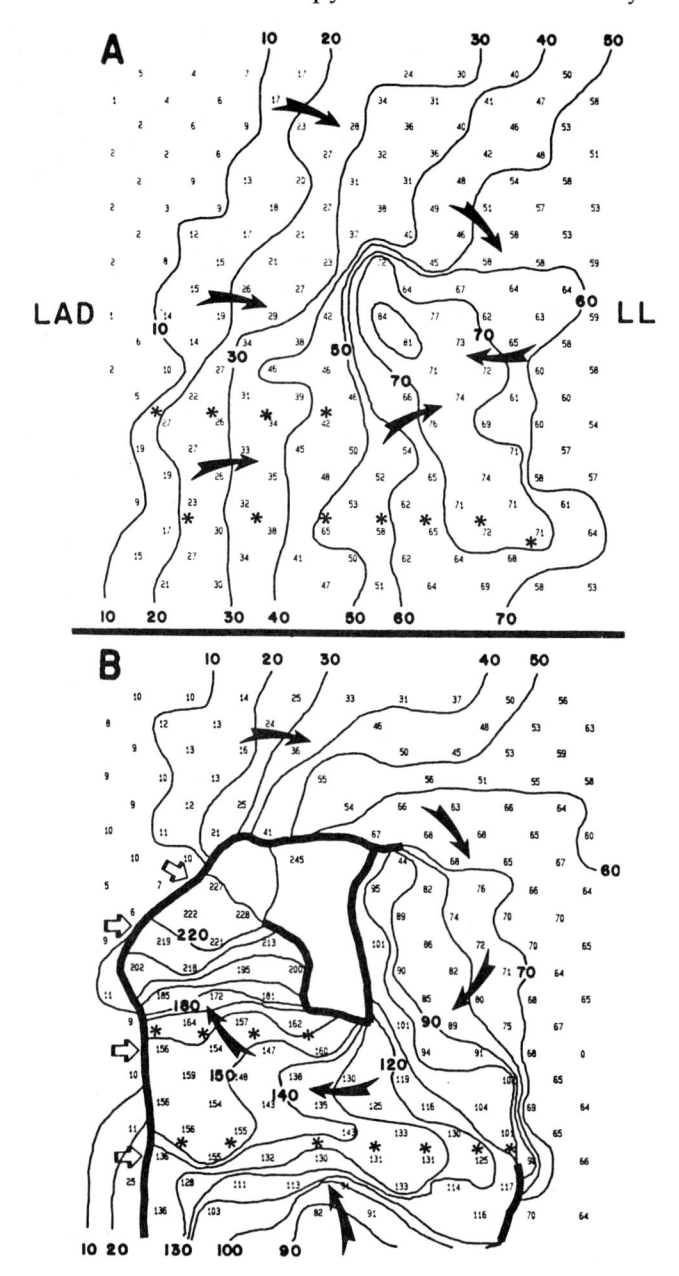

Figure 7: Activation maps of the epicardial border zone during initiation of reentrant ventricular tachycardia. The orientation of the electrode array on the anterior left ventricle is shown in Figure 10. LAD is the margin of the array adjacent to the left anterior descending coronary artery and LL is the margin on the lateral left ventricle. The stimuli during the programmed stimulation protocol were applied to the right ventricle adjacent to the LAD. Each small number is an activation time at one of the recording sites. Isochrones are drawn at 10 ms intervals and labeled with dark black numbers. Arrows indicate direction of activation.

length of 300 ms is shown in A. A broad wavefront sweeps across the left side of the epicardial border zone (from the 10 to the 50 ms isochrones). The pattern then becomes more heterogeneous because of a small region of slow activation indicated by the bunched isochrones (note that the orientation of these isochrones perpendicular to fiber orientation means that slow activation in this region is not caused by anisotropy). An activation wave also comes eventually from the lateral margin (right side of the map) as well. Panel B shows the activation pattern of the stimulated premature impulse (coupling interval of 180 ms) which initiated tachycardia. This wavefront blocked along the LAD margin at the 10–30 ms isochrones. The blocked wavefront is denoted by the unfilled arrows and the thick black line at the left of the figure. Conduction block is indicated by (1) the markedly different activation time at sites to the left and to the right of the region designated as block—the thick black line, and (2) activation is occurring in nearly the opposite direction on either side of the region of block. Above, the line of block also extends toward the right. Activation during the premature impulse circulates around this block along the basal margin above (isochrones 10–60) and the lateral margin at the right (isochrones 60–90) and then proceeds back to the LAD margin (isochrones 90–230). This sequence of activation is pointed out by the black arrows. Activation during the premature impulse also seems to conduct around the line of block towards the apex (below), out of the field of the recording electrodes. The activation wave appears from the apical margin at the 90 ms isochrone and then proceeds toward the LAD margin while merging with the activation wave from the base and lateral margin. The circulating activation wave returned to the site of conduction block long after the block occurred (isochrones 180–220). It was, therefore, able to continue propagating through this region toward the LAD and basal margins of the electrode array (map not shown) causing the first reentrant tachycardia beat. Reentry then continued during the tachycardia.

The conduction block of the premature impulse initiating tachycardia occurred toward the LAD margin in a region where the wavefront propagated in partially refractory tissue parallel to the long axis of the myocardial fibers (the fibers are oriented from left to right in Fig. 7). The safety factor for conduction of early premature impulses in this direction should be low according to Spach's[15] hypothesis and, therefore, conduction block may be caused by this parallel arrangement of the myocardial fibers. The returning impulse is presumably conducting in tissue that is nearly fully excitable so the low safety factor in the parallel direction now has little significant influence on conduction velocity. However, although premature impulses readily block in the direction parallel to fiber orientation in the epicardial border zone, other factors may also contribute to the occurrence of the block. In Figure 7, the line of conduction block of the premature impulse does bend in the left-to-right direction at its upper extremity and, therefore, in this region it cannot be caused by the supposed low safety factor parallel to fiber orientation. The effective refractory period of the muscle fibers increases from the margin of the epicardial border zone with normal myocardium toward the center of the border zone and the site of conduction block has been correlated with regions of long refractory periods.[29] Therfore both long refractory periods and anisotropy might contribute to the occurrence of block or one of these mechanisms may be more important than the other. More experiments are required to elucidate the relative contributions of each mechanism.

The Role of Anisotropy in Sustained Reentry

Not only might anisotropy be important for initiation of reentrant tachycardia but it also may be a major factor that causes the slow conduction necessary for continued reentry during sustained tachycardia in the epicardial border zone. Figure 8 shows the activation sequence of the epicardial border zone of a 4-day-old infarct in situ during two cycles of sustained tachycardia induced by a premature impulse. This tachycardia persisted for 15 minutes and these activation patterns were repeated in a nearly identical manner during each beat. In the time frame represented by each map, activation begins at the asterisk (10 ms isochrone) and ends at the 150 ms isochrone—the tachycardia cycle length was a consistent 146–150 ms. In panel A, activation proceeds initially from the 10 ms isochrone towards the lateral left ventricular margin of the electrode array (LL) (from the left to right as indicated by the solid black arrows) which it reaches between 60–70 ms. The sequence of isochrones then shows the activation wave splitting into two wavefronts. One moves upward toward the base and back toward the LAD margin which it reaches after 150 ms, completing a reentrant circuit (indicated by arrows). The other wave of excitation moves downward toward the apex and then back toward the LAD margin which it also reaches after 150 ms, completing a second reentrant circuit. These two wavefronts (one from the base and one from the apex), merge into the single activation wave that moves from the LAD to the LL margin. Panel B shows essentially the same pattern of activation during another time frame. Activation at the beginning of this time frame (10 ms isochrones indicated by asterisks) is toward the lateral margin at the right of the figure where the common activation wave splits into the upper (basal) and lower (apical) wavefronts. These two wavefronts move toward the LAD margin (as shown by the arrows) which they reach after 90–100 ms and again merge into the common activation wave that moves back to the LL margin.

During continuous reentry in the epicardial border zone, as exemplified in Figure 8, the circuitous activation patterns are roughly in the shape of ovals. The long axis of each oval extends in the general direction from the LAD margin to the left lateral margin of the electrode array. Activation is rotating around narrow long lines (indicated by the thick black lines in each panel) extending in the direction of the long axis of the oval. Activation proceeds in one direction on one side of the line and in the opposite direction on the other side of the line. The extent and location of these lines are defined by the marked differences in activation times on either side of them. According to convention, interpolation of the large number of isochrones between these markedly disparate activation times results in the thick black lines which are actually formed by closely bunched isochrones. Such marked differences in activation times are traditionally interpreted as indicating areas of conduction block. However, a large number of isochrones bunched closely together to form the thick black lines might also result from slow activation across a narrow region.

40 • CARDIAC ARRHYTHMIAS

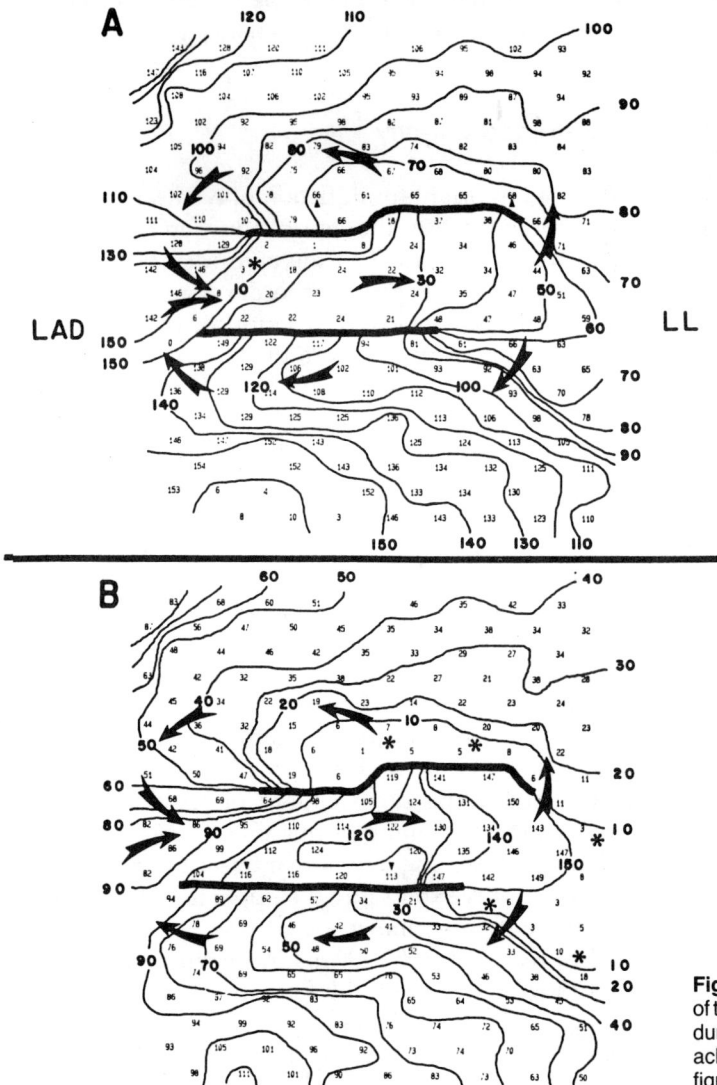

Figure 8: Activation maps of the epicardial border zone during reentrant ventricular achycardia. Format of the figure is the same as Figure 7.

We have reason to propose that much of the lines of block around which activation appears to be circulating during tachycardia are actually regions of very slow conduction caused by anisotropy and that anisotropic slow conduction is one important factor that enables reentry to occur. This proposal is based on consideration of the following observations.

1. The lines of block are often functional. In most cases they are not evident during sinus rhythm but only appear during ventricular tachycardia. However, there are exceptions; sometimes areas or lines of permanent anatomical block do occur that are always evident no matter what the rhythm. We are not discussing the tachycardias associated with this anatomical block.

2. Lines of functional block are oriented parallel to the long axis of the muscle fibers as they should be if they are formed by slow conduction transverse to the long axis of the myocardial fibers. In Figure 9, the location of the recording electrode array on the heart is shown at the left. The long axis of the myocardial fibers runs from the LAD margin of the array to the margin on the lateral left ventricle. At the right are diagrams of the orientation of lines of block in three different experiments. In the top panel, only a single reentrant circuit was mapped. In the middle and bottom panels, two reentrant circuits occurred as was also shown in Figure 8. In general, the lines of block are parallel to the long axis of the fibers except for a vertical component of the upper line of block in the third diagram. Vertical lines of block such as this are anatomical and not functional.

3. Isochrones adjacent to the lines of block are often parallel to the line of

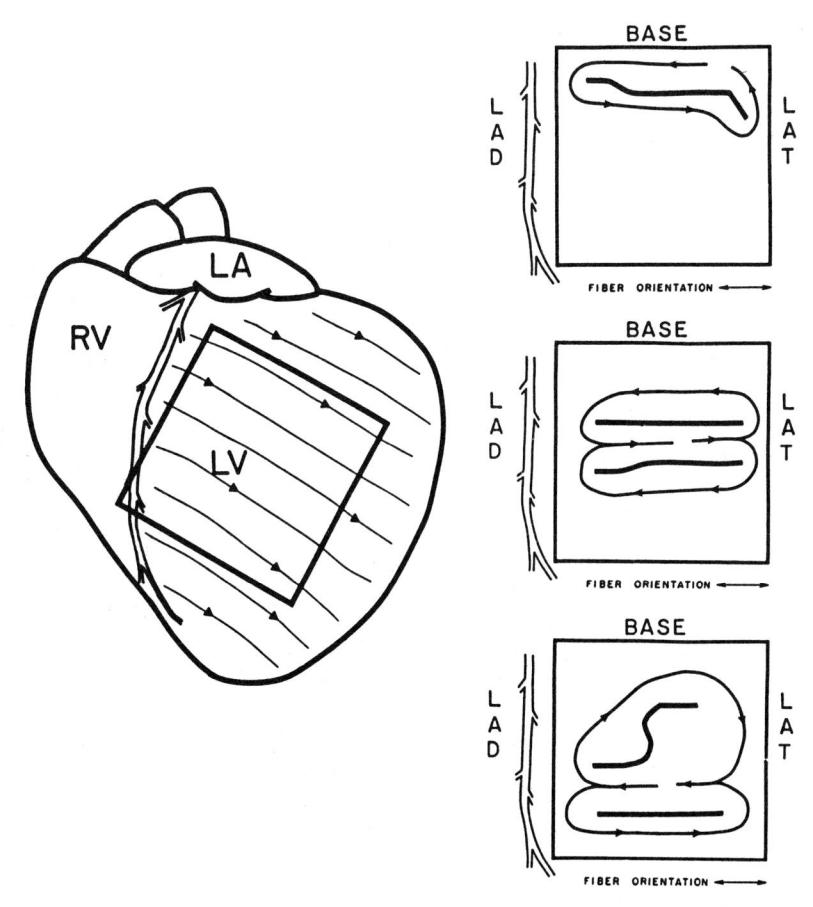

Figure 9: Location of the array of 190 bipolar electrodes used to map activation of the epicardial border zone is shown in the diagram at the left. The relationship of the electrode array position relative to the long axis of the myocardial fibers is also diagrammed. The long axis of the fibers run from the left (LAD) to the right margin (on the lateral left ventricle of the electrode array). At the right, three diagrams of the electrode array in position adjacent to the LAD are shown during three different tachycardias. Location of the lines of apparent conduction block are shown and the reentrant circuit indicated by arrowheads. In general, lines of apparent conduction block during sustained tachycardia are oriented parallel to the long axis of the myocardial fibers.

block. This is evident in Figure 8. In panel A, isochrones 70 and 80 above the top line of block are parallel to this line of block. In panel B, a large region of isochrone 120 also is parallel to the lower line of block. The occurrence of these parallel isochrones strongly suggests that activation occurs across the line. For example, in panel A, activation along the upper line of block within the 70 ms isochrone occurs within 2 ms (66–68 ms) over a distance of about 20 mm. This could not occur if the impulse conducted only around the line and then in a right to left direction. In panel B, activation along the lower line of block occurs within 7 ms (activation times ranging from 113 to 120 ms), also much too rapid to be explained only by conduction around the line and then in the left to right direction.

4. The electrograms at the lines of block have multiple components whereas several millimeters away from the lines of block they usually have only a single component. An important question pertains to the meaning of multicomponent electrograms. In a previous study it was shown that activity persists within a region where multicomponent electrograms are recorded with bipolar electrodes, for the duration of the electrogram.[23] Fractionated, multicomponent electrograms may represent slow activation proceeding from one fiber bundle to the next across high resistance connections. For the same reason, multicomponent electrograms also occur in anisotropic cardiac muscle when activation occurs transverse to myocardial fiber orientation.[16,20]

In constructing the activation maps shown in Figure 8, only one activation time was assigned to multicomponent electrograms at the fastest, largest amplitude component. Figures 10 and 11 show how the data can be reinterpreted if each component of a fractionated electrogram is given a separate activation time (a different tachycardia beat is illustrated). Electrodes a–j in Figure 10 are located along the line of apparent conduction block (upper line of block in Fig. 8). Activation times at electrodes above and below these electrodes have a difference in their activation times of 40–80 ms and thus might suggest block. However, electrograms a–e and g–j have two components while f has at least three components. The multiple component electrogram recorded at site f is shown below (it did not have multiple components in the absence of tachycardia such as during ventricular drive). Each component of multiple-component electrograms was assigned an activation time. The single line of conduction block (in Fig. 8) is resolved into its components, consisting of closely bunched isochrones indicating slow conduction. The reinterpretation of the activation pattern is also shown by the diagrams in Figure 11. At the top, a single line of block is shown, with activation for the most part rotating around it (large arrows) although the possibility of activation progressing through the line, as suggested by parallel isochrones, is also indicated by the small wavy arrows. In the bottom diagram, the line of apparent block has been subdivided into a number of isochrones from the analysis of the fractionated electrograms. According to this interpretation, there is a small center region of functional block (F) (rather than a long line of block) with activation circulating around it. Activation is rapid in the part of the circuit in which it occurs parallel to myocardial fiber orientation and very slow in the part of the circuit in which it occurs perpendicular to fiber orientation.

In summary, the consequences of the anisotropy are the following. (1) It provides the basis for the slow conduction that enables reentry to occur, since in

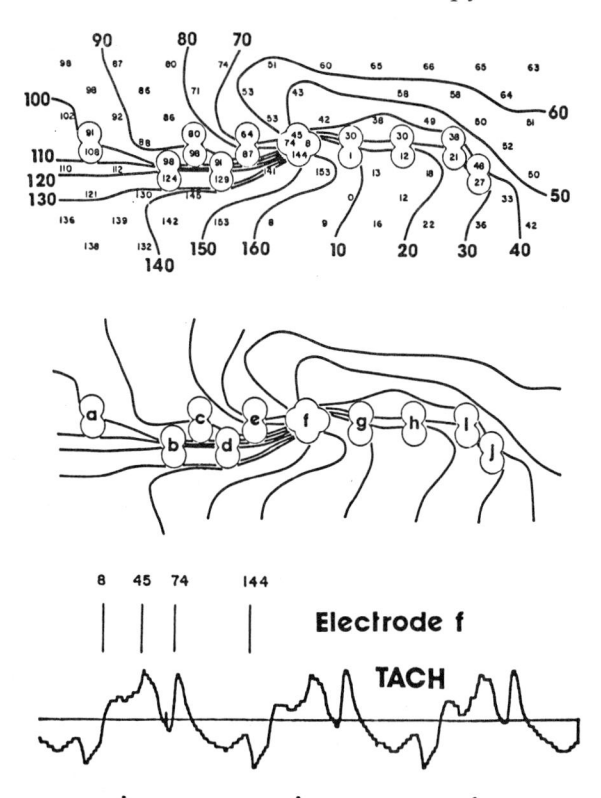

Figure 10: Activation in the region of the upper line of apparent conduction block during the tachycardia shown in Figure 8. In the middle diagram the location of recording electrodes along the line are labeled a–j. The electrogram recorded from electrode f during tachycardia (Tach) and stimulation of the ventricles (drive) is shown below. At the top is the activation map when all components of the fractionated electrodes along the line of block are given activation times.

all likelihood, action potentials are not depressed sufficiently to account for the slow conduction alone (see ref. 22). (2) It imparts certain properties to the functional reentrant circuit that may be different from the leading circle mechanism. The marked changes in conduction velocity as activation progresses around the circuit may result in the occurrence of an excitable gap.[30] (3) The effects of antiarrhythmic drugs on conduction in the circuit may be dependent on the effects of drugs on anisotropy.

Mechanisms for Reentry Caused by Anisotropic Structure of Cardiac Fibers Surviving in Chronic Infarcts

The structure of a myocardial infarct changes with time as the infarct heals. These changes also influence the electrophysiological properties. We have studied these changes in the epicardial border zone of the canine infarct model described in the preceding section. Fibrosis occurs in this region during healing and by 8 weeks after coronary occlusion the muscle bundles are widely separated,

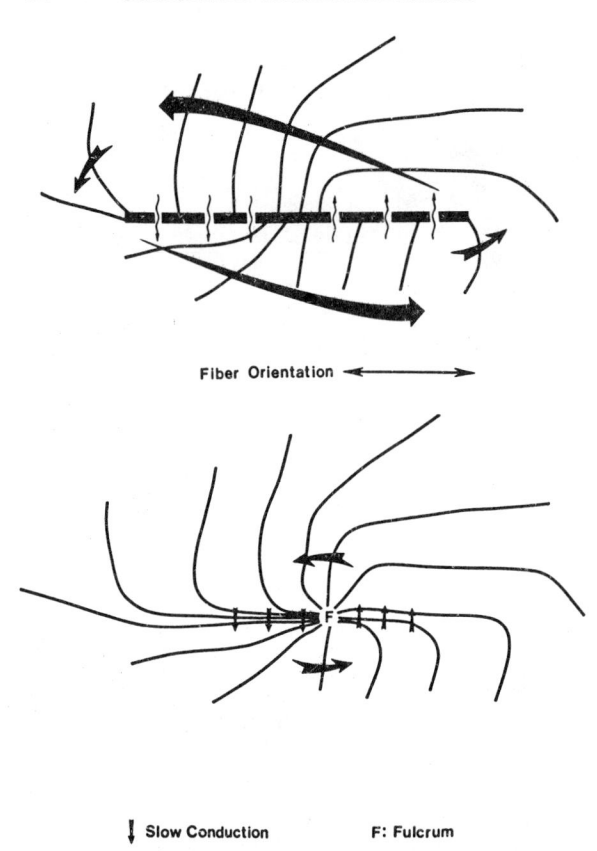

Figure 11: Diagram of reentrant circuit in the anisotropic epicardial border zone. The diagram at the top shows the line of apparent conduction block (horizontal thick line) as previously shown in Figure 8. Activation is shown to be occurring, for the most part, around this line (large arrows) but some activation also occurs through it (small vertical arrows). Below, the activation map is redrawn showing the individual bunched isochrones which comprise the line of apparent block, based on assigning activation times to each component of multiple component electrograms.

leaving fewer side to side connections (Fig. 12). The development of connective tissue further impedes transverse conduction, leading to additional slowing despite the normal resting potential and, upstroke velocities of the muscle action potentials.[22] After several months, in addition to the separation of the muscle fibers by connective tissue, the fibers in some regions are no longer oriented in parallel. Orientation is distorted by the large amounts of connective tissue with the long axis of fiber bundles coursing in all directions. Muscle fibers are connected to each other only by short segments of intercalated discs. The broad wide discs which occur at the longitudinal ends of normal cells are no longer present because of the deformation of the cells by connective tissue. The changes in the size and distribution of the discs are expected to cause a marked increase in effective axial resistivity in all directions and, therefore, to slow conduction. This slowing of conduction occurs even though the transmembrane potentials of the muscle fibers in healed infarcts may be normal. The effects of the structural changes on conduction are illustrated in Figure 13. Activation of an isolated epicardial border zone preparation from an 8-week-old infarct superfused in normal Tyrode's solution is shown during stimulation from the left margin at a basic cycle length of 800 ms. The spread of the impulse was mapped by using

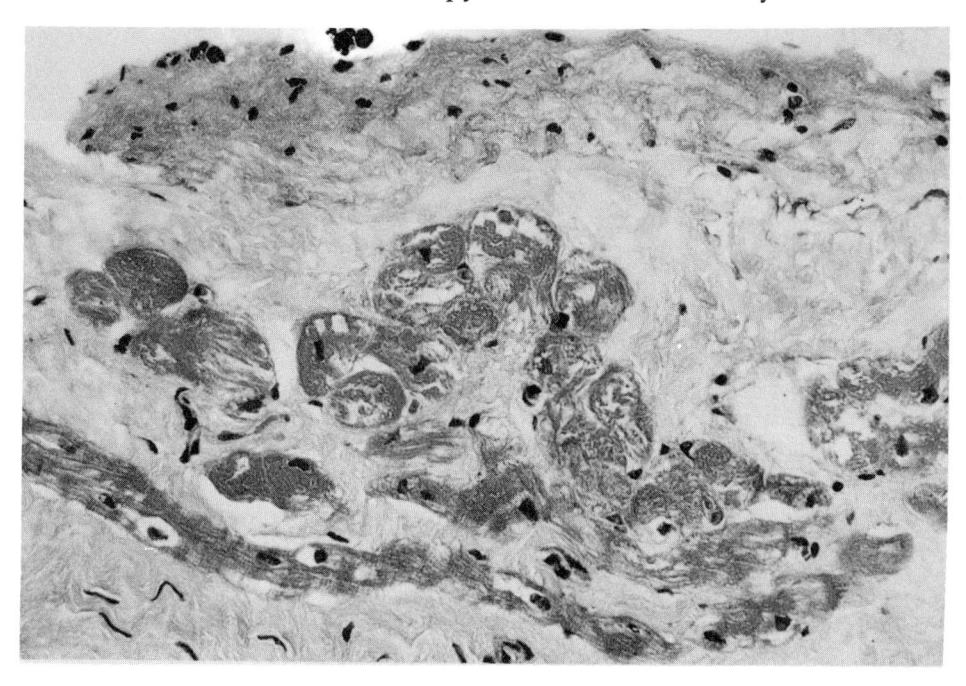

Figure 12: Muscle fibers trapped in connective tissue in the epicardial border zone of a 2-month infarct are shown. The fibers are widely separated by the connective tissue and are no longer oriented in a parallel manner.

intracellular recordings from a microelectrode that was moved sequentially from site to site on the surface of the preparation. Action potentials and relative activation times were recorded from the ventricular muscle fibers at each site. It is apparent from the spacing of the isochrones that activation in some regions is very slow (compare with spacing of isochrones during activation of normal epicardial muscle below) and this slow activation is not dependent on the direction of propagation. For example, between isochromes 40 and 55 ms the apparent conduction velocity is 0.02 ms in a direction perpendicular to the isochrones. Conduction is more rapid between isochrones 55 and 60 (0.1 m/sec). Between isochrones 60 and 85 ms, apparent conduction velocity is 0.01 m/sec. Normal resting and action potentials were recorded from fibers in this region of very slow activation as well as fractionated electrograms, as shown in the insets at the top of the figure.

The marked slowing of conduction in muscle fibers surviving in healed infarcts probably results from the poor connections between the fibers. Since the effective axial resistance depends to a large extent on the intracellular resistivity which in turn is influenced by the resistance, extent, and distribution of cell-to-cell couplings, a decrease in intercellular connections might increase resistance to current flow and thereby slow conduction. A reduced space constant has been found in regions of chronically infarcted canine myocardium to support this suggestion.[31] It is possible that slow electrotonic transmission across high-resistance or inexcitable gaps sometimes cause the marked conduction delays.

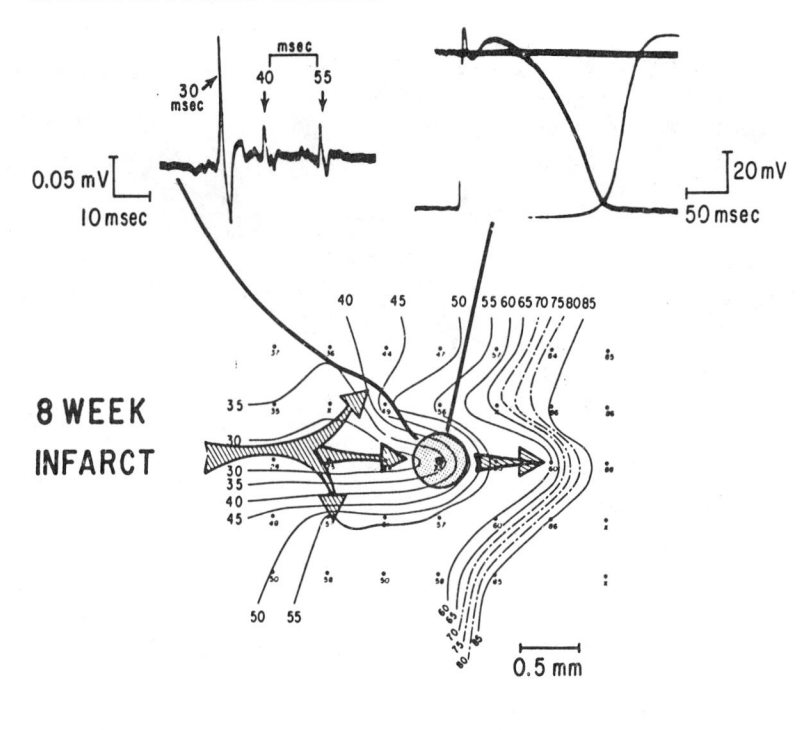

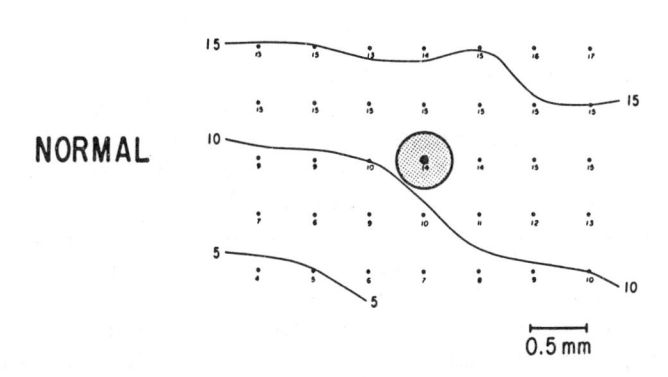

Figure 13: Activation map of an isolated preparation of epicardial border zone from an 8-week-old infarct (top) and of epicardial muscle from the same region of a noninfarcted heart. In the top panel the preparation was stimulated from the left margin (which was adjacent to the LAD in situ). Arrows show direction of activation. Activation times from microelectrode recordings are indicated by small numbers. Isochrones are drawn at 5 ms intervals and labeled with large numbers. A fractionated electrogram recorded from the site indicated by the large circle on the map is in the top left section and a representative action potential is showin in the top right section. The normal preparation in the bottom panel was stimulated from the lower margin. Note the much more rapid activation as indicated by the wider spacing of the isochrones.

Action potentials in regions where there is slowed conduction sometimes show prepotentials before the upstroke, similar to the prepotentials recorded from regions just distal to an area of block in other experiments in which slow, electrotonic transmission has been demonstrated (Fig. 14).[32-35] On occasion we have also seen two distinct components during the depolarization phase of the action potentials, which has previously been associated with electrotonic transmission.[35]

It is predicted that the slow activation which occurs in healed infarcts should

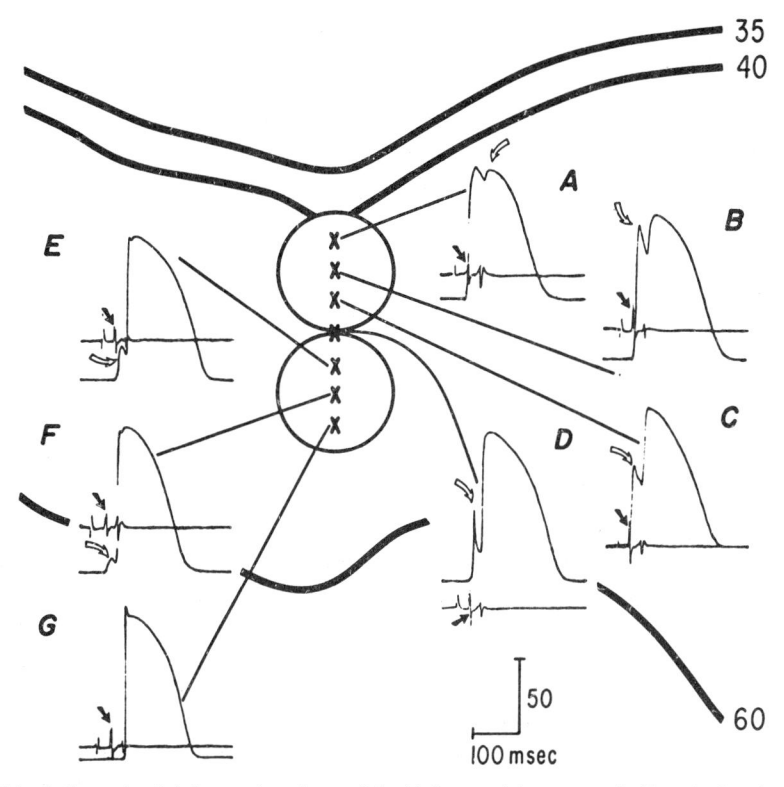

Figure 14: Action potentials in a region where a "double" potential was recorded in an isolated epicardial border zone preparation from a 2-month-old infarct. The two circles in the middle of the figure indicate the bipolar electrode. The x's show where action potentials were recorded. (The microelectrode was actually adjacent to the bipoles and not beneath them.) The thick dark lines are isochrones indicating activation times and the direction of propagation at this recording site. Panels A to G show simultaneous recordings of the action potentials and the extracellular electrogram. The solid arrows in each panel indicate the first component of the "double" potential. This component is preceded by a stimulus artifact. The upstroke of the action potentials in A and B occur simultaneously with the first electrogram deflection. The unfilled arrows indicate possible electrotonic influences on the plateau phase. The upstrokes of the action potentials in C and D have two components, one corresponding to the first electrogram deflection (unfilled arrow) and one corresponding to the second electrogram deflection. The upstrokes of the action potentials in E and F are simultaneous with the second electrogram deflection but are preceded by an electrotonic prepotential (unfilled arrows) that begins with the first electrogram deflection and spans the isoelectric segment between the two deflections. The upstroke of the action potential in G occurs just after the second electrogram deflection and is not preceded by a prepotential. Voltage calibration is for the transmembrane potential recording. (Reproduced from Gardner PI, Ursell PC, Fenoglio JJ Jr, Wit AL: Electrophysiologic and anatomic basis for fractionated electrograms recorded from healed myocardial infarcts. Circulation 1985;72:596–611.)

lead to reentrant excitation. However, no activation maps have yet been published from experiments on such hearts showing reentry.

Anisotropy and Antiarrhythmic Drug Action

One means by which antiarrhythmic drugs terminate reentrant ventricular tachycardia is by causing conduction block of the circulating impulse in the reentrant circuit. In some instances, drugs may bring about this effect by depressing the inward Na current that flows during the upstroke of the action potential (type 1 drugs). Other drugs may prolong the time course of action potential repolarization, thereby lengthening the effective refractory period.[37]

In order for the type 1 drugs to cause condition block in reentrant circuits by depressing the Na current, it is likely that the inward Na current must already be quite depressed by the cardiac pathology.[38] Such depressed fast responses might not always exist in reentrant circuits, especially where the slow conduction necessary for reentry is a result of the anisotropic tissue properties. However, it is conceivable that antiarrhythmic drugs might also influence the axial current flow by effecting intracellular resistivity, particularly at the intercalated disk. The effects of drugs on anisotropic conduction is, surprisingly, unknown. The level of intracellular Ca plays an important role in the control of the resistance of gap junctions of intercalated disks. Spach et al. have shown that ouabain increases the ratio of fast axis to slow axis conduction velocity by preferentially slowing conduction in the direction transverse to the long axis of the myocardial fibers.[39] It may do this by elevating intracellular Ca. Drugs that decrease inward Na current may also have an effect. It has been shown with ion selective electrodes that intracellular [Na] may decrease during the course of exposure of cardiac fibers to lidocaine because of the decrease in fast Na current.[40] This in turn may lead to a decrease in intracellular Ca by means of the Na-Ca exchange mechanisms. What would be the effect on conduction in regions of lines of block in the reentrant circuits we described in the previous sections of this chapter? If slow conduction in the region of lines of apparent block are crucial for reentry to occur, either improving or further depressing activation in this region might terminate reentry. Decreasing intracellular Ca might improve activation while increasing Ca might depress it and cause block. The influence of drugs on anisotropic conduction properties is currently under investigation.

Acknowledgment: This research was supported by Program Project Grant HL30557 from the National Heart, Lung and Blood Institute.

References

1. Wit AL, Bigger JT Jr. Possible electrophysiological mechanisms for lethal arrhythmias accompanying ischemia and infarction. Circulation 1975;51, 52 (Suppl II):96–115.
2. Lazzara R, El-Sherif N, Hope RR, Scherlag BJ. Ventricular arrhythmias and electrophysiological consequences of myocardial ischemia and infarction. Circ Res 1978;42: 740–749.
3. Janse MJ, Kleber AG. Electrophysiological changes and ventricular arrhythmias in the early phase of regional myocardial ischemia. Circ Res 1981;49:1069–1081.

4. Gettes LS. Effects of ischemia on cardiac electrophysiology. In: Fozzard HA, Jennings RB, Haber E, Katz AM, eds. The Heart and Cardiovascular System: Scientific Foundations. New York, Raven Press, 1986;1317–1342.
5. Downar E, Janse MJ, Durrer D. The effects of acute coronary occlusion on subepicardial transmembrane potentials in the intact porcine heart. Circulation 1977;56:217–224.
6. Janse MJ, van Capelle FJL, Morsink H, Kleber AG, Wilms-Schopman E, Cardinal R, Naumann d'Alvoncout C, Durrer D. Flow of "injury current" and patterns of excitation during early ventricular arrhythmias in acute regional myocardial ischemia in isolated porcine and canine hearts: evidence for 2 different arrrhythmogenic mechanisms. Circ Res 1980;47:151–165.
7. Friedman PL, Steward JR, Fenoglio JJ Jr, Wit AL. Survival of subendocardial Purkinje fibers after extensive myocardial infarction in dogs: In vitro and in vivo correlations. Circ Res 1973;33:597–611.
8. Lazzara R, El-Sherif N, Scherlag BJ. Electrophysiological properties of canine Purkinje cells in 1-day-old myocardial infarction. Circ Res 1973;33:722–734.
9. El-Sherif N, Gough WB, Zeiler RH, Mekra R. Triggered ventricular arrhythmias in 1-day-old myocardial infarction in the dog. Circ Res 1983;52:566–579.
10. Myerburg RJ, Gelband H, Nilsson K, Sung RJ, Thurer RJ, Morales AR, Bassett AL. Long term electrophysiological abnormalities resulting from experimental myocardial infarction in cats. Circ Res 1977;41:73–84.
11. Fozzard HA. Conduction of the action potential. In: Berne RM, ed. Handbook of Physiology Section 2: The Cardiovascular System, Vol. 1, The Heart Amer Physiol Soc, Baltimore, 1979;335–356.
12. Page E, Shibata Y. Permeable junctions between cardiac cells. Am Rev Physiol 1981;43: 431–441.
13. Kléber AG, Rugger CB, Janse MJ. Electrical uncoupling and increase of extracellular resistance after induction of ischemia in isolated, arterially perfused rabbit papillary muscle. Circ Res (In Press).
14. Clerc L. Directional differences of impulse spread in trabecular muscle from mammalian heart. J Physiol (London) 1976;255:335–346.
15. Spach M, Miller WT, Geselowitz DB, Barr RC, Kootsey JM, Johnson EA. The discontinuous nature of propagation in normal canine cardiac muscle: Evidence for recurrent discontinuities of intracellular resistance that effect the membrane currents. Circ Res 1981;48:39–54.
16. Spach MS, Miller WT, Dolber PC, Kootsey JM, Summer JR, Moscher CE. The functional role of structural complexities in the propagation of depolarization in the atrium of the dog: Cardiac conduction disturbances due to discontinuities of effective axial resistivity. Circ Res 1982;50:175–191.
17. Spach MS, Kootsey JM. The nature of electrical propagation in cardiac muscle. Am J Physiol: Heart and Circ Physiol 1983;13:3–22.
18. van Capelle F. Slow conduction and cardiac arrhythmias. Academisch Proefschrift, Universiteit van Amsterdam, 1983.
19. Delmar M, Michaels DC, Jalife J. Effects of increasing intercellular resistance on transverse and longitudinal propagation in sheep epicardial muscle. Circ Res (In Press).
20. Spach MS, Dolber PC. Relating extracellular potentials and their derivatives to anisotropic propagation at a microscopic level in human cardiac muscle: Evidence for electrical uncoupling of side to side fiber connections with increasing age. Circ Res 1986;56:356–371.
21. Wit AL, Allessie MA, Bonke FIM, Lammers W, Smeets J, Fenoglio JJ Jr. Electrophysiologic mapping to determine the mechanism of experimental ventricular tachycardia initiated by premature impulses: Experimental approach and initial results demonstrating reentrant excitation. Am J Cardiol 1982;49:166–185.
22. Ursell PC, Gardner PI, Albala A, Fenoglio JJ Jr, Wit AL. Structural and electrophysiological changes in the epicardial border zone of canine myocardial infarcts during infarct healing. Circ Res 1985;56:436–451.

23. Gardner PI, Ursell PC, Fenoglio JJ Jr, Wit AL. Electrophysiologic and anatomic basis for fractionated electrograms recorded from healed myocardial infarcts. Circulation 1985; 72:596–611.
24. El-Sherif N, Smith A, Evans K. Canine ventricular arrhythmias in the late myocardial infarction period: Epicardial mapping of reentrant circuits. Circ Res 1981;49:255–265.
25. Mehra R, Zieler RH, Gough WB, El-Sherif N. Reentrant ventricular arrhythmias in the late myocardial infarction period: Electrophysiologic-anatomic correlation of reentrant circuits. Circulation 1983;67:11–23.
26. Cardinal R, Savard P, Carson DL, Pagé P. Mapping of ventricular tachycardia induced by programmed stimulation in canine preparation of myocardial infarction. Circulation 1984;70:136–148.
27. Kramer JB, Saffitz JE, Witkowski FX, Corr PB. Intermural reentry as a mechanism of ventricular tachycardia during evolving myocardial infarction. Circ Res 1985;56: 736–748.
28. Fenoglio JJ Jr, Pham TD, Harken AH, Horowitz LN, Josephson ME, Wit AL. Recurrent sustained ventricular tachycardia: Structure and ultrastructure of subendocardial regions where tachycardia originates. Circulation 1983;68:518–533.
29. Gough WB, Mehra R, Restivo M, Zuler RH, El-Sherif N. Reentrant ventricular arrhythmias in the late MI period in the dog: Correlation of activation and refractory maps. Circ Res 1985;57:432–442.
30. Lammers WJEP, Wit AL, Allessie MA. Effects of anisotropy on functional reentrant circuits: Preliminary results of computer simulation studies. In: Sideman S, Beyar R, eds. Electromechanical Activation, Metabolism and Perfusion of the Heart—Simulation and Experimental Models. Dordrecht/Boston/Lancaster, Martinus Nijhoff Publishers, (In Press).
31. Spear JF, Michelson EL, Moore EN. Reduced space constant in slowly conducting regions of chronically infarcted canine myocardium. Circ Res 1983;176–185.
32. Joyner RW. Effects of the discrete pattern of electrical coupling on propagation through an electrical syncytium. Circ Res 1982;50:192–200.
33. Joyner RW, Veenstra R, Rawling D, Chorro A. Propagation through electrically coupled cells; effects of a resistive barrier. Biophys J 1984;45:1017–1025.
34. Bandura JP. The role of electrotonics in slow potential development and conduction in canine Purkinje tissue. In Zipes DP, Bailey JC, Elharrer V (editors) The Slow Inward Current and Cardiac Arrhythmias. The Hague, Martinus Nijhoff Publishing Co, 1980; 327–355.
35. Antzelevitch C, Jalife J, Moe GK. Characteristics of reflection as a mechanism of reentrant arrhythmias and its relationship to parasystole. Circulation 1980;61:182–191.
36. Wennemark JR, Ruesta VJ, Brody DA. Microelectrode study of delayed conduction in the canine right bundle branch. Circ Res 1968;23:753–769.
37. Boyden PA, Wit AL. Pharmacology of antiarrhythmic drugs. In: Rosen MR, Hoffman BF, eds. Cardiac Therapy, The Hague, Martinus Nijhoff Publishing Co, 1983;171–235.
38. Brennan FJ, Cranefield PF, Wit AL. Effects of lidocaine on slow response and depressed fast response action potentials of canine cardiac Purkinje fibers. J Pharmacol Exp Ther 1978;204:312–324.
39. Spach MS, Kootsey JM, Sloan JD. Active modulation of electrical coupling between cardiac cells of the dog. A mechanism for transient and steady state variations in conduction velocity. Circ Res 1982;51:347–362.
40. Sheu SS, Lederer WJ. Lidocaine's negative inotropic and antiarrhythmic actions: Dependence of shortening of action potential duration and reduction of intracellular sodium activity. Circ Res 1985;57:578–590.

MECHANISMS OF ARRHYTHMIAS

II

3

Sinus Node Reentry: Fact or Fiction?

Charles J.H.J. Kirchhof
Felix I.M. Bonke
Maurits A. Allessie

Introduction

Cardiac arrhythmias can be based on disturbed impulse formation or on disturbed conduction of the impulse. A reentry circuit is often the underlying mechanism in case of disturbed impulse conduction. In case of a reentry circuit, the impulse is captured in an "endless" loop of reexitation whereby the circulation frequency of this impulse is higher than sinus rhythm. Therefore such a reentry circuit will function as pacemaker and will control heart rhythm.

A (unidirectional) conduction block is the prerequisite for the occurrence of the reentry phenomenon: when the impulse is blocked somewhere in the myocardium, it will turn around this area of blockade and activate the tissue behind the conduction block in a retrograde direction. Then if the area of block is reexcitable again, the impulse can be entrapped in a loop of reexcitation or reentry circuit.

In case of supraventricular arrhythmias, three reentrant circuits are possible: (1) a circuit completely situated in the atrial myocardium; (2) a circuit completely located in one or both nodal structures, the AV node or the sinus node; (3) a heterogeneous circuit with a pathway partially composed of atrial tissue and partially of nodal tissue.

If we focus on the possible involvement of the sinus node in such a circuit—

From: Brugada P, Wellens HJJ. CARDIAC ARRHYTHMIAS: Where To Go From Here? Mount Kisco, NY, Futura Publishing Company, Inc., © 1987.

54 • CARDIAC ARRHYTHMIAS

thus the theoretical possibilities mentioned before as second or third—there are several clinical observations suggesting the occurrence of sinus node reentrant arrhythmias: Barker and co-workers[1] were the first to consider the involvement of the sinus node in auricular paroxysmal tachycardias, but could not give any actual evidence; later, other investigators suggested a crucial role of the sinus node in clinical as well as experimental observations of high right atrial tachycardias.[2-8]

Nevertheless, all these investigators speculated and could only suggest a role of the sinus node as explanation for the observed atrial arrhythmias.

The Possible Role of the Sinus Node in a Reentrant Arrhythmia

In all mammalian hearts, the cardiac pacemaker is normally found in the sinus node. In principle there are no basic differences between the sinus nodes of the species investigated: in the sinus node of the mouse, rat, guinea pig, rabbit, cat, mole, dog, pig, cow, monkey, and man, two distinct regions can be distinguished morphologically as well as electrophysiologically:[9-14] the nodal center or compact zone and the border zone or zone of perinodal fibers.[9] In the isolated sinus node impulse formation occurs in the center, whereas the border zone, which circumferences this nodal center, serves as the conduction pathway for the impulse towards the atrium.

Theoretically the sinus node can be involved in a reentry circuit in several ways whereby the nodal center, border zone, or both can play an essential role. Figure 1 depicts schematically three different models of sinus node involvement in a reentrant circuit. In case of an early atrial premature beat, the impulse might arrive at the border of the sinus node and finds itself blocked; however, if this entrance block is not complete, the impulse might enter the sinus node at one side

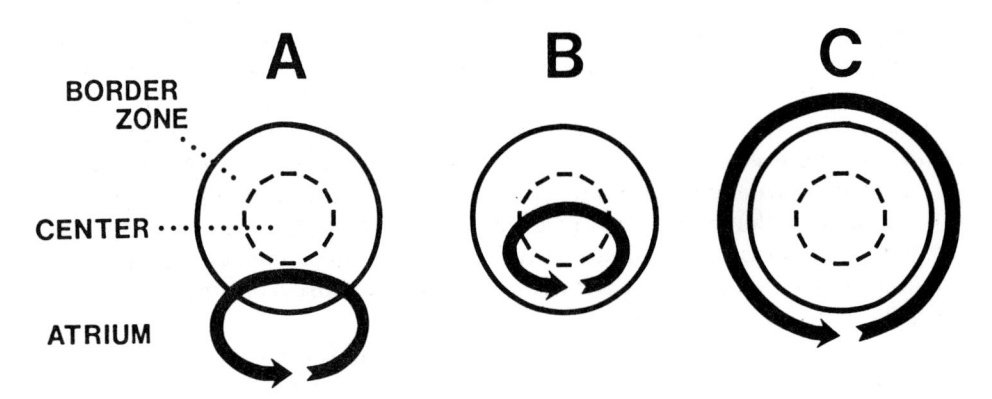

Figure 1: The role of the sinus node in a reentry circuit. The closed circle represents the atrio-sinus border; the dotted circle represents the transition between border zone and center of the sinus node. A: The sinus node as a part of an atrial reentry circuit. Both the border zone and the center of the node can be involved. B: The reentry circuit is completely located within the sinus node. C: An atrial reentry circuit around the sinus node. The circulating wavefront will depolarize the sinus node continuously but will not use it as a consequent part of the circuit.

and travel through the border zone or nodal center and finally might find an exit at the other side of the sinus node where the area of previous entrance block has become excitable again. Then the atrium is reactivated and the impulse might enter the sinus node again at the previous entrance side. This situation is depicted in panel A of Figure 1. In panel B, the whole reentrant pathway is located in the sinus node, using both the border zone and nodal center as part of the circuit. This situation can occur during a transient intranodal conduction block and can be indicated as an "intranodal reentry." In that case also an atrio-sinus entrance block must exist since otherwise conduction of the impulse through the border zone is shortcutted by the atrial myocardium. In panel C, the sinus node functions as a center around which the impulse is circulating, probably activating the nodal fibers from several sides, but without using these as part of the reentrant pathway. For the initiation of such a circuit, it is necessary that the impulse of an early premature atrial beat is split into two activation fronts around the sinus node, one of which is blocked.

Is There Any Evidence for a Role of the Sinus Node in a Reentry Circuit?

Several experimental studies using the isolated rabbit sinus node as preparation were performed to obtain direct evidence for the occurrence of sinus node reentry.[15-18] In this preparation, it is possible to reconstruct the intranodal activation pattern by using microelectrode recordings. In whole animal studies, mostly the canine was used;[19-20] however, the sinus node of the canine heart is, as in the human heart, very difficult to approach since it is covered by atrial tissue. Therefore in these experiments, the activation pattern within the sinus node could not be determined.

Besides experimental studies, clinical studies with respect to the occurrence of sinus node reentry are also available.[4,6-8,21-25] However, in humans, it is not possible to study the sinus node by any direct method necessary to demonstrate the reality of a sinus node reentry. Consequently, clinical studies of sinus node reentry in fact only report patient cases in which the existence of sinus node reentry is suggested. However, these suggestions are based solely on indirect criteria and are therefore purely speculative.

The first experimental in vitro study dealing with the phenomenon of sinus node reentry was performed by Han and co-workers.[15] In the isolated rabbit right atrium, these investigators described the phenomenon of so-called echo beats. After induction of an early atrial premature beat, an atrial return response was observed which came markedly earlier than expected in case of a spontaneous sinus beat. By using multiple atrial electrograms as well as intracellular recordings, they gave evidence suggesting that this early atrial premature impulse was blocked at one side of the sinus node while entering it from another side; thus there was a local sinus entrance block. Because the impulse was conducted slowly through the sinus node, it reached the site of entrance block antegradely. This region of conduction block had become excitable again, and via this route, the impulse reactivated the atrium giving rise to the early atrial return response. The mechanism supposed to underly these echo beats is depicted in the ladder diagram of Figure 2. During sinus rhythm (A1), an early premature impulse (A2) induced in the atrium is followed by an atrial response (A3) which comes much earlier than expected on basis of the known A1-A1 interval. Based on these findings, it was stated that an early atrial premature impulse followed by an earlier than expected atrial response represents a sinus echo or sinus node reentry if A1-A2 + A2-A3 << A1-A1. In studies of Bonke and co-workers,[26,27] it was found that the difference between the A1-A3 and the A1-A1 interval must be marked since early atrial premature beats can cause changes in the A1-A1 interval by electrotonic modulation of the pacemaker.

In further experimental studies, also using the isolated rabbit sinus node as preparations, the behavior of early atrial premature beats and the occurrence of echo beats was investigated more intensively by Bonke et al.;[27] nevertheless, these studies did not bring more actual evidence for the existence of sinus node reentry than the attempts by Han et al.[15] since the pathway of the supposed reentry was still not demonstrated. It was Allessie and Bonke[17] who finally succeeded in an attempt to produce an activation map of the sinus node during an echo beat. In one experiment, these investigators were able to evoke an echo beat many times while performing a large number of intracellular recordings in the sinus node area. In this way, the pathway of the echo beat could be reconstructed (Fig. 3). The suggestions of Han and co-workers[15] in fact were proven to be real: the occurrence of a local entrance block at one side of the sinus node and entrance of the impulse via another side was followed by a slow conduction of the impulse through the sinus node and reactivation of the atrium. However, in Figure 3, it can be seen that the impulse enters the sinus node and even describes an intranodal loop before leaving the sinus node to reactivate the atrium. The results of this study as well as those of Han et al.[15] represent the only direct evidence for the occurrence of a sinus node reentrant pathway as depicted in Figure 1 (A and B).

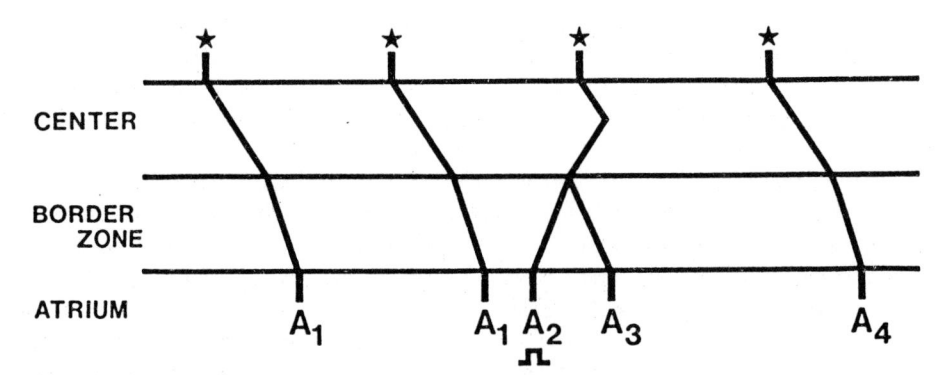

Figure 2: Ladder-diagram indicating the mechanism underlying an echo beat. The upper line represents the nodal center, the level of pacemaking; the middle line represents the transition between nodal center and border zone; the lower line represents the level of the atrium (crista terminalis). The star represents a spontaneous sinus beat, the pulse sign, an early stimulated atrial depolarization. The premature atrial impulse (A_2) enters the sinus node from one side and finds an exit at another side, thereby reactivating the atrium (A_3) before it would be activated by a normal sinus beat.

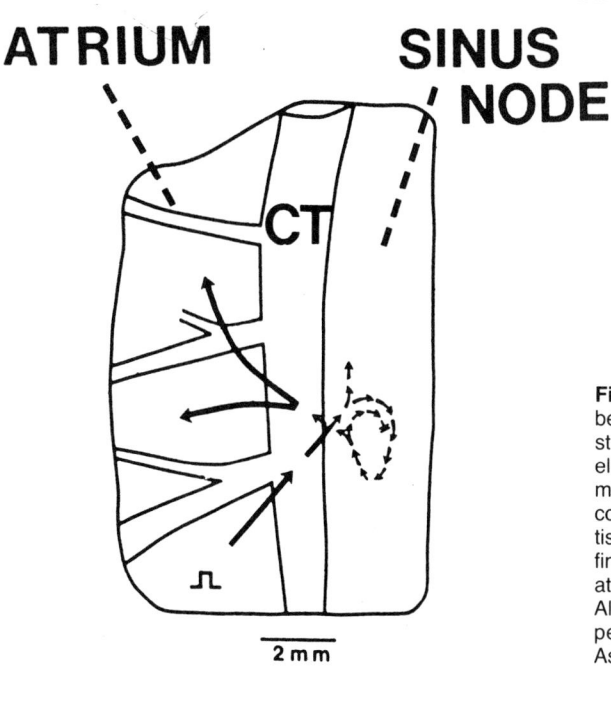

Figure 3: The pathway of an echo beat through the sinus node as reconstructed by means of multiple microelectrode implements. The atrial premature impulse enters the node, is conducted slowly through the nodal tissue (note the intranodal loop), and finally finds an exit to reactivate the atrium. CT = crista terminalis. (From Allessie and Bonke, 1979; used with permission of the American Heart Association.)

Several experimental in vivo studies[3,19,20] as well as clinical studies reported the existence of echo beats and even short trains of echo beats or sinus reentrant tachycardias.[1,3,4,6–8,18,22–25,28] In all of these studies, the diagnosis of sinus node reentry was based on indirect evidence obtained from the atrial activation pattern. In all cases, a high right atrial tachycardia or premature atrial response was found and indicated as sinus node reentry when fitting to the following indirect criteria: (1) initiation of the supposed echo beat or sinus node reentry by a properly timed premature atrial beat, reproducible from different stimulation sites; (2) the A1-A3 interval must be remarkably shorter than spontaneous cycle length (A1-A2 + A2-A3 << A1-A1); (3) P-wave morphology must be identical to that of sinus beats; (4) The A3-A4 cycle must be longer than the A1-A1 interval, since this excludes a sinus entrance block (sinus reset); (5) exclusion of a right-sided accessory bypass tract which can mimic a high-to-low activation pattern of the right atrium.[29]

However, it should be emphasized that these indirect criteria are definitely insufficient to diagnose sinus node reentry with certainty.[30] The occurrence of a sinus node reentry is still completely speculative with respect to the in vivo situation, whereas with respect to the in vitro situation, some important remarks must be made to assure that the significance of the presented findings is not overestimated. The isolated rabbit sinus node cannot be compared to the in vivo situation in canine or man. In vivo, the influence of autonomic transmitters might play an important role, but in vitro a denervated preparation was studied. Furthermore, it must be realized that the demonstration of the intranodal pathway of an echo beat by Allessie and Bonke[17] is still a single fortunate attempt which might not be reproducible; the preparation in this experiment might have been extraordinary or even pathologic, since the occurrence of a sinus nodal entrance block over such a long part of the atrio-sinus border is not a common finding.

Finally, for the reality of a reentrant loop as illustrated in Figure 1C, no clinical or experimental evidence, directly or indirectly, exists. Nevertheless, every high right atrial reentrant tachycardia is a candidate: an atrial premature beat will not only depolarize the sinus node but also the tissue around the sinus node, thereby splitting the impulse into two activation fronts which will collide somewhere behind the sinus node. In case of blockade of one or both activation fronts in the neighborhood of the sinus node, the latter might activate this area of block sufficiently later and in the opposite direction to be engaged in a reentry circuit around the sinus node.

How Can the Reality of the Sinus Node Reentry be Investigated More Basically?

Reentrant circuits in which the sinus node can play a role will be of the functional type as described by Allessie and co-workers.[31-33] In such a circuit, the front of the activation wave will always activate tissue that has just restored its excitability enough to be activated again. The length of a functional circuit is given by the wavelength[34] or the product of conduction velocity and refractory period. Therefore we investigated both conduction velocity and refractoriness in the isolated rabbit sinus node; this preparation was used because it is easy to approach with invasive techniques and different regions of the node can be investigated separately.

In the upper part of Figure 4, the method used is depicted schematically. The atrial part of the preparation was divided into two halves by an incision perpendicular to the crista terminalis. This incision was continued through the crista terminalis into the border zone of the sinus node. Thus a preparation was obtained in which both atrial halves were connected only by a bridge of sinus nodal tissue. In this way, an impulse induced in one atrial half could be conducted towards the other atrial half only through the bridge of sinus nodal tissue. The conduction time of the impulse through this bridge was monitored by two surface electrodes placed on top of the crista terminalis at the "entrance" and "exit" of the sinus nodal bridge (Fig. 4). Since the length of the pathway of the impulse through the sinus node was known and the impulse was always conducted via the shortest route (i.e., just around the tip of the incision), conduction velocity could be calculated. Conduction time was measured at different pacing frequencies starting with 3 Hz, which is faster than sinus rhythm, and continued until the maximal pacing frequency (F_{max}) was reached whereby conduction in a 1:1 manner through the sinus node was still present. Thereafter, the conduction time of premature atrial beats was calculated. While pacing with a frequency of 3 Hz, the coupling interval of the premature stimulus was shortened repetitively until the coupling interval of the earliest premature impulse which was still conducted through the sinus node was reached; this was the effective refractory period

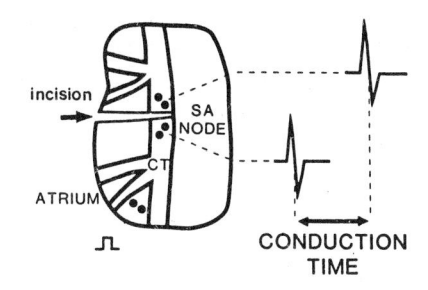

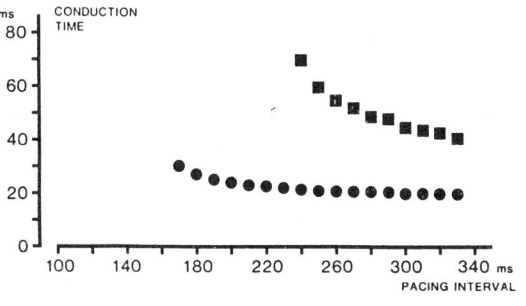

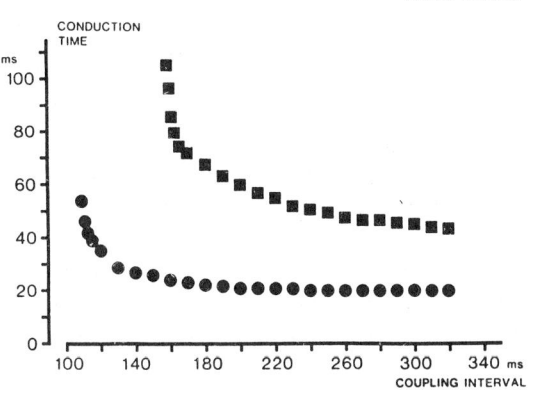

Figure 4: Conduction in the sinus node. A schematic representation of the preparation used: isolated right atrium of the rabbit, placed in a tissue bath and superfused with modified Tyrode solution containing in mM: NaCl 130, KCl 5.6, $CaCl_2$ 2.2, $MgCl_2$ 0.6, $NaHCO_3$ 24.2, Na_2PO_4 1.2, glucose 11 and sucrose 13. Oxygenated by 95% O_2 and 5% CO_2; temperature: 38°C. The two diagrams depict the conduction time measured at different pacing intervals (upper diagram) and the conduction time of a premature beat with different coupling intervals (lower diagram; a premature beat was induced after 15 basic beats paced at a rate of 3 Hz). The lower curves (circles) in both diagrams represent conduction in the border zone, the upper curves (squares), conduction in the nodal center. The left end of both curves in the upper diagram represent the maximal pacing frequency (F_{max}); the left end of both curves in the lower diagram represent the effective refractory period, measured with an accuracy of 1 ms. Note that a premature beat can be conducted with more prematurity and lower conduction velocity than a train of stimuli during regular pacing. CT = crista terminalis.

(ERP). To investigate conduction properties through the nodal center, the incision had to be lengthened by at least 600 micron into the sinus node.

The diagrams in Figure 4 illustrate conduction times during different pacing frequencies (upper diagram) and of premature atrial impulses (lower diagram). In each diagram, the lower curve (circles) represent conduction through the border zone whereas the upper curve (squares) represent conduction through the nodal center. The presented data are obtained from one representative experiment. During regular pacing with a frequency of 3 Hz (333 ms interval), conduction time through the border zone is 20 ms; when increasing the pacing frequency (decreasing the pacing interval), initially no significant change in conduction time was observed. However, at a frequency of about 4.5 Hz (220 ms pacing interval) conduction time starts to increase and at the maximal pacing frequency of almost 6 Hz (170 ms pacing interval) conduction time is 30 ms. Obviously, in the border zone, rate-dependent conduction delay occurs only at relatively high pacing frequencies. In the lower diagram, the conduction times of single premature beats are depicted. In the border zone (circles), the conduction time of a late premature beat is not different from a normal paced beat and amounts to 20 ms. While shortening the coupling interval, initially no increase in conduction time is observed. In case of relative early premature stimuli, starting at about 150 ms coupling interval, conduction time starts to increase markedly while shortening the coupling interval further. The earliest premature beat—representing the effective refractory period of the sinus nodal tissue bridge—can be delivered with a coupling interval of 109 ms and is conducted through the border zone in 54 ms. Thus premature beats can be conducted with greater prematurity and a slower conduction velocity through the nodal border zone than a train of stimuli.

In the center of the sinus node, the situation is different in comparison to the border zone. Conduction time during 3 Hz pacing (squares; upper diagram) is markedly longer than in the border zone, namely 43 ms. Furthermore, when increasing the pacing frequency, conduction time is immediately prolonged. This rate-dependent prolongation of conduction time progresses while the pacing frequency is increased. The maximal pacing frequency through the center was slightly above 4 Hz (240 ms pacing interval) whereas the conduction time was prolonged to 70 ms. In case of premature beats, in fact the same situation was found (squares; lower diagram): the conduction time prolonged immediately when shortening the coupling interval, but most pronounced in case of early premature stimuli. The shortest coupling interval (effective refractory period) in the center was 159 ms accompanied by a conduction time of 105 ms. A series of experiments was performed in which conduction properties of border zone and nodal center was investigated. The data obtained are given in Table I.

An interesting phenomenon was observed in some experiments while investigating conduction through the border zone (Fig. 5). Premature stimuli were applied and conduction time was measured according to the described protocol. The course of the curve was as expected until early premature stimuli were given: when decreasing the coupling interval from 150 to 145 ms, conduction time

Table I
Conduction Properties of the Rabbit Sinus Node (mean ± SD)

	Border Zone (n = 41)	Center (n = 39)
Conduction time during pacing 3 Hz (ms)	17 ± 6	42 ± 24
Conduction time during maximal pacing (ms)	33 ± 12	73 ± 37
Conduction time of earliest premature beat (ms)	53 ± 30	125 ± 61
Effective refractory period (ms)	110 ± 16	165 ± 29
Maximal pacing rate (interval in ms)	165 ± 25	240 ± 38

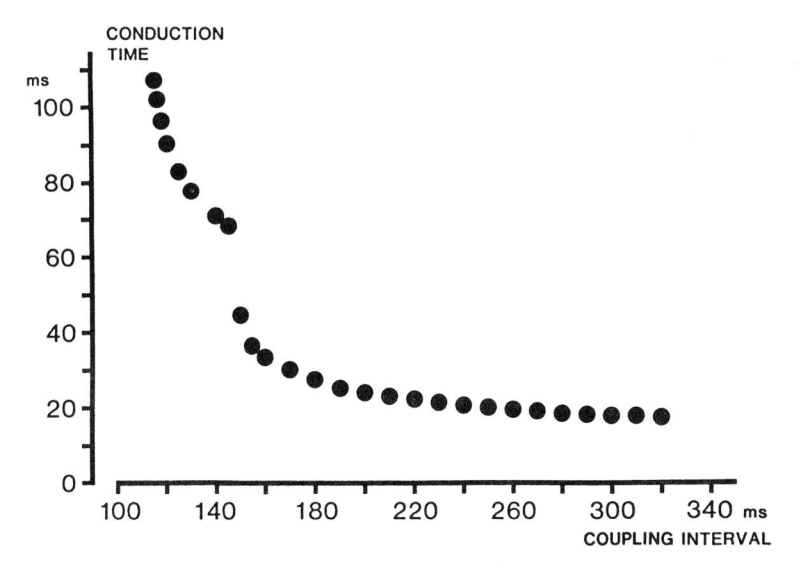

Figure 5: Curve depicting conduction time at different coupling intervals in case of conduction through the border zone. A sudden increase in conduction time is observed with relative early premature beats suggesting alteration of the conduction pathway after local intranodal conduction block.

suddenly increased from 45 to 67 ms. Further shortening of the coupling interval caused a further increase in conduction time but in the same proportion as before the abrupt increase. This disproportionate increase in conduction time during a very small range of coupling intervals occurred often but was observed only in case of conduction through the border zone. The most reasonable explanation for this event is an alteration of the conduction pathway of the impulse through the sinus node. This sudden change of the pathway during early premature stimuli strongly suggests local conduction blockade in the border zone of the sinus node, a condition suggested to be favorable for the development of sinus node reentry.[15]

In order to compare conduction velocity and refractoriness in atrium, border zone, and nodal center, we have summarized these properties, for the rabbit atrium, in Table II. A very marked decrease of conduction velocity is observed when going from the atrium (50–60 cm/sec) towards the border zone (7–11 cm/sec) of the sinus node; it decreases further when entering the nodal center (2–5 cm/sec). This reveals that the sinus node is, in comparison to the atrium, indeed a slow-conducting structure. In all three types of tissue, conduction velocity decreases by about 50% while pacing with the maximal frequency, and decreases by about 70% in case of the earliest premature beat. Refractoriness, which determines the circulating frequency of a functional reentrant circuit, is markedly longer in the sinus node than in the atrium. Furthermore, it should be noted that in the nodal center, maximal pacing frequency hardly exceeds the normal range of sinus rate.

From the present results, it was concluded that conduction in the border zone of the sinus node is markedly slower and refractory period longer than in the atrium, whereas conduction and refractory period in the nodal center are even

Table II
Comparison of Ranges of Conduction Properties in Atrium and Sinus Node

	Atrium	Border Zone	Center
Conduction velocity during 3 Hz pacing (cm/sec)	50–60	7–11	2–5
Conduction velocity during maximal pacing (cm/sec)	25–30	3–5	1–2.5
Conduction velocity of earliest premature beat (cm/sec)	15–20	2–3.5	0.7–1.5
Maximal pacing frequency (Hz)	9–12	5–7	3.5–5
Effective refractory period (ms)	60–70	95–125	135–195

markedly slower and shorter than in the border zone. Furthermore, a single premature beat can be conducted both through the border zone and through the nodal center at far greater prematurity and with a lower conduction velocity than a train of regular impulses. From these data, it can be concluded that the wavelength (product of conduction velocity and refractory period) in atrial tissue will be much larger than in sinus nodal tissue (in the center, the wavelength will be about half of that in the border zone).

Significance of the Present Results for the Reality of the Sinus Node Reentry

The clarification of conduction properties within the rabbit sinus node implicates several important prerequisites for both the occurrence and diagnosis of a sinus node reentry. From the described findings, it can be concluded that a reentry circuit with the rabbit sinus node as part of the pathway cannot have a circulation frequency higher than about 6 Hz in case of a pathway through the border zone and about 4 Hz in case of a pathway through the nodal center. This is markedly slower than pure atrial reentry circuits having frequencies between 10 and 12 Hz.[31–33] However, this does not implicate an easy diagnosis of the sinus node reentry in the rabbit since in case of a pathway through the nodal center, it will have a rate hardly faster than accelerated sinus rhythm.

As explained earlier, the dimensions of a functional reentry circuit are in principle determined by the refractory period and the impulse conduction velocity (wavelength) of the tissue including the pathway. In case of a reentry (Fig. 2) with a pathway through the sinus node, more types of tissue are involved. This makes it very difficult to determine the wavelength of such a circuit. However, some important features must be considered. As suggested and revealed by several investigators,[15,17] an echo beat can only be initiated by an early atrial depolarization in the presence of a transient sinus nodal entrance block. However, this entrance block must have some specific features. First, the refractory period of the atrium ranges between 60 and 70 ms whereas the conduction velocity of an early impulse through the border zone ranges between 2 and 3.5 cm/sec. This means that the premature impulse, after activating the atrium and entering the sinus node, must have a pathway through the border zone of about 2 mm (taking 65 ms and 3 cm/sec as representative values) before the atrium can be activated again. This implicates that the entrance block must also be at least 2 mm in length along the atrio-sinus border zone. Second, the block area must be located in such a way that the early atrial depolarization finds only one entrance into the sinus node; otherwise it will travel around the block area at two sides and collide in the sinus node. Such an entrance block is not a common finding in the normal heart.

If we speculate about the possibility of an echo beat reentering the sinus node, it should be emphasized that the reentry of the impulse cannot occur before the original entrance site of the premature atrial beat into the sinus node has become excitable again; therefore, the impulse has to make a detour through the atrium of at least 1 cm (taking 115 as refractory period of the border zone and also taking into account that the entrance site of the sinus node was activated 65 ms before the impulse leaves the border zone and starts to reexcite the atrium; furthermore, for conduction velocity through the atrium, a value of 20 cm/sec is taken arbitrarily). Such a long detour is hardly probable in the right rabbit atrium.

If we consider the possibility of reentrant tachycardias in which the border zone of the sinus node is included in the pathway, we can calculate that in case of a frequency of 6 Hz (F_{max} border zone) and an atrial part of the circuit of about 1 cm, the part of the pathway through the border zone has to have a length of about 5 mm, which is in a healthy rabbit sinus node an unrealistic supposition. Therefore, in the rabbit the occurrence of sustained sinus nodal reentrant tachycardias is even less probable than a reentering echo beat.

Summary

The sinus node reentry is today, despite all of the clinical and experimental, indirect and direct evidence, still very speculative. Only in the isolated rabbit, right atrium direct evidence for a pathway through the sinus node in case of an echo beat was found, but this seemed to be an extraordinary situation. Investigation of the basic conduction properties of the rabbit sinus node revealed that the occurrence of a stable sinus node reentry in the right atrium of the rabbit is almost impossible under normal conditions. However, in the described studies, an isolated preparation was used that is not equal to the human situation. Nevertheless, although in case of a "sick" human heart the conditions might be more favorable, sinus node reentry as a basis of supraventricular tachycardia will probably remain a fiction.

References

1. Barker PS, Wilson RJ, Johnston FD. The mechanism of auricular paroxysmal tachycardia. Am Heart J 1943;26:435–445.

2. Wallace AG, Daggett WM. Reexcitation of the atrium. "The echo phenomenon." Am Heart J 1964;68:661–666.
3. Childers RW, Arnsdorf MF, Fuente DJ, Gambetta M, Svenson R. Sinus nodal echoes. Am J Cardiol 1973;31:220–231.
4. Narula OS. Sinus node reentry: A mechanism for supraventricular tachycardia. Circulation 1974;50:1114–1128.
5. Paritzky, Z, Obayashi K, Mandel WJ. Atrial tachycardia secondary to sino-atrial node reentry. Chest 1974;66:526.
6. Wu D. Demonstration of sustained sinus and atrial reentry as a mechanism of paroxysmal supraventricular tachycardia. Circulation 1975;51:234–243.
7. Pahlajani DB, Miller RA, Serratto M. Sinus node reentry and sinus node tachycardia. Am Heart J 1975;90:305–311.
8. Castellanos A, Aranda J, Moleiro F, Mallon SM, Befeler B. Effects of the pacing site in sinus node reentrant tachycardia. J Electrocardiol 1976;2:165–169.
9. Strauss HC, Bigger JT. Electrophysiological properties of the rabbit perinodal fibers. Circ Res 1972;31:490–506.
10. Tranum-Jensen J. The fine structure of the sinus node: A survey. In Bonke FIM, ed. The Sinus Node: Structure, Function and Clinical Relevance. The Hague, Martinus Nijhoff Medical Division, 1978;149–165.
11. Bleeker WK, Mackaay AJC, Masson-Pevet M, Bouman LN, Becker AE. Functional and morphological organization of the rabbit sinus node. Circ Res 1980;46:11–22.
12. Opthof T, De Jonge B, Mackaay AJC, Bleeker WK, Masson-Pevet M, Jongsma HJ, Bouman LN. Functional and morphological organization of the guinea-pig sinoatrial node compared with the rabbit sinoatrial node. J Mol Cell Cardiol 1985;17:549–564.
13. Opthof T, De Jonge B, Masson-Pevet M, Jongsma HJ, Bouman LN. Functional and morphological organization of the cat sinoatrial node. In Opthof T. The Mammalian Sinus Node: A Comparative Morphological and Electrophysiological Study (thesis). University of Amsterdam, 1986;105–121.
14. Opthof T, De Jonge B, Jongsma HJ, Bouman LN. Functional morphology of the pig sinoatrial node. In Opthof T. The Mammalian Sinus Node: A Comparative Morphological and Electrophysiological Study (thesis). University of Amsterdam, 1986;123–144.
15. Han J, Malozzi AM, Moe GK. Sino-atrial reciprocation in the isolated rabbit heart. Circ Res 1968;22:355–362.
16. Miller HC, Strauss HC. Measurement of sino-atrial conduction time by premature atrial stimulation in the rabbit. Circ Res 1974;35:935–947.
17. Allessie MA, Bonke FIM. Direct demonstration of sinus node reentry in the rabbit heart. Circ Res 1979;44:557–568.
18. Matsuo H, Takayanagi K, Ueda K. Sinoatrial responses to premature atrial stimulation: Clinical observations and experimental study. Jap Circ J 1980;44:551–560.
19. Paulay KL, Varghese PJ, Damato AN. Sinus node reentry: An in vivo demonstration in the dog. Circ Res 1973;32:455–463.
20. Ogawa S, Dreifus LS, Osmick MJ. Induction of sinus node reentry: Its relation to inhomogeneous atrial conduction. J Electrocardiol 1978;11:109–116.
21. Breithart G, Seipel L. Further evidence for the site of reentry in so-called sinus node reentrant tachycardia in man. Eur J Cardiol 1980;11:105–113.
22. Paulay KL, Ruskin JN, Damato AN. Sinus and atrioventricular nodal reentrant tachycardia in the same patient. Am J Cardiol 1975;36:810–816.
23. Curry PVL, Evans TR, Krikler DM. Paroxysmal reciprocating sinus tachycardia. Eur J Cardiol 1977;6/3:199–228.
24. Garson A, Gillette PC. electrophysiological studies of supraventricular tachycardia in children. I. Clinical-electrophysiologic correlations. Am Heart J 1981;102:233–250.
25. Reiffel JA, Bigger JT, Ferrick K, Livelli FD, Gliklich J, Wang P, Bosner R. Sinus node echoes and concealed conduction: Additional sinus node phenomena confirmed in man by direct sinus node electrography. J Electrocardiol 1985;18:259–266.
26. Bonke FIM, Bouman LN, Van Rijn HE. Change of cardiac rhythm in the rabbit after an atrial premature beat. Circ Res 1969;24:533–544.

27. Bonke FIM, Bouman LN, Schopman FJG. Effect of an early atrial premature beat. Circ Res 1971;29:704–715.
28. Dhingra RC, Wyndham C, Amat-y-Leon F, Denes P, Wu D, Rosen KM. Sinus nodal responses to atrial extra stimuli in patients without apparent sinus node disease. Am J Cardiol 1975;36:445–452.
29. Breithart G, Seipel L. Role of sinus node reentry in the genesis of supraventricular arrhythmias. In Masoni A, Alboni P, ed. Cardiac Electrophysiology Today. London/New York, Academic Press, 1982;99–122.
30. Waldo AL. Need for additional criteria for the diagnosis of sinus node reentrant tachycardias. J Electrocardiol 1977;10:103–104.
31. Allessie MA, Bonke FIM, Schopman FJG. Circus movement in rabbit atrial muscle as a mechanism of tachycardia. Circ Res 1973;33:54–62.
32. Allessie MA, Bonke FIM, Schopman FJG. Circus movement in rabbit atrial muscle as a mechanism of tachycardia II: The role of nonuniform recovery of excitability in the occurrence of unidirectional block, as studied with multiple microelectrodes. Circ Res 1976;39:168–177.
33. Allessie MA, Bonke FIM, Schopman FJG. Circus movement in rabbit atrial muscle as a mechanism of tachycardia III. The "leading circle" concept: A new model of circus movement in cardiac tissue without the involvement of an anatomical obstacle. Circ Res 1977;41:9–18.
34. Smeets JLRM, Allessie MA, Lammers WJEP, Bonke FIM, Hollen SJ. The wavelength of the cardiac impulse and reentrant arrhythmias in the isolated rabbit atrium. Circ Res 1986;58:96–108.

4

Flutter and Fibrillation in Experimental Models: What Has Been Learned that Can Be Applied to Humans?

Maurits A. Allessie
Wim J.E.P. Lammers
Pieter L. Rensma
Felix I.M. Bonke

Introduction

Although several possible mechanisms of cardiac arrhythmias have been identified in animal experiments, the exact mechanisms underlying atrial flutter and fibrillation in man are still unknown. Clinical studies with intracavitary and intraesophageal leads and programmed electrical stimulation sometimes point to an ectopic focus of abnormal impulse formation,[1-5] whereas other studies conclude that continuous circus movement of the impulse in a smaller or larger area of the atria is responsible for atrial tachyarrhythmias.[3,5-11] Detailed epicardial and endocardial mapping of the atria in patients with atrial flutter or fibrillation who are subjected to cardiac surgery could be an excellent and direct way to visualize the abnormalities in atrial excitation in these patients. This would also give the

---

From: Brugada P, Wellens HJJ. CARDIAC ARRHYTHMIAS: Where To Go From Here? Mount Kisco, NY, Futura Publishing Company, Inc., © 1987.

opportunity to establish the (ultra)structural and electrophysiological "background" of the myocardium which creates favorable circumstances for the occurrence of flutter and fibrillation. Intraoperative mapping is presently being carried out in several specialized cardiosurgical centers. It is to be expected that in the near future this will lead to a great increase in our knowledge of mechanisms of arrhythmias in man.

Up to now most of our understanding of atrial flutter and fibrillation has been derived from animal experiments. In one model, atrial flutter is induced by topical application of aconitine on the exposed atrial surface.[12] At the site of application, aconitine induces early afterpotentials and rapid abnormal automaticity.[13] Perpetuation of the arrhythmia is dependent on this single focus of abnormal impulse formation, and isolating the aconitine spot from the rest of the heart by a forceps immediately terminates the arrhythmia.[14] The majority of animal models of atrial flutter are based on a reentrant mechanism. After Mines and Garrey had introduced the classical concept of continuous circus movement around a gross anatomic obstacle,[15,16] Lewis studied atrial flutter induced by rapid pacing in open chest dogs.[6,17] Using a double string galvanometer, he measured the local moments of activation during an episode of flutter at multiple sites of the right and left atrium and concluded that common atrial flutter was based on a continuous circus movement of the impulse around the orifices of the great veins. Rosenblueth and Garcia Ramos modified this model by crushing the intercaval auricular bridge, thus converting the two orifices into a single but larger obstacle.[18] More recently Frame et al.[19] described a canine model of atrial flutter in which they forced the circulating impulse around the tricuspid valve orifice by making a Y-shaped right atrial incision. Boineau et al.[20] produced atrial flutter by focal suture ligation of the crista terminalis. Their maps suggest that an area of the tuberculum intervenosum was the pathological substrate for atrial flutter.

Opposed to these different varieties of "obstacle flutter," a number of models have been developed based on the "leading circle" mechanism in which no anatomic obstacle is involved.[21-23] Boyden and Hoffman[24] described leading circle flutter in dogs in which right atrial enlargement was produced by surgically induced partial tricuspid insufficiency and graded pulmonary artery stenosis. Allessie et al.[25] mapped episodes of rapid atrial flutter in isolated canine hearts under the influence of a low dosage of acetylcholine. Induction of sterile pericarditis also proved to be a way to induce "leading circle" flutter.[26] The two different types of reentry (with and without a gross anatomic central obstacle) have different properties and can be expected to react differently to changes in basic electrophysiological parameters. In Figure 1, the differences in "anatomical" and "functional" circus movement have been summarized. These two types of reentry should be considered as extreme representatives of a wide variety of reentrant circuits of various sizes and different degrees of excitable gaps. Models of reentry can be more complex if the circuit is comprised of tissue with different electrophysiological properties. The presence of diseased myocardium or uniform or nonuniform anisotropy[27-30] may further add to the complexity of reentrant circuits in patients.

CIRCUS MOVEMENT

Anatomically determined
(Mines, 1913)

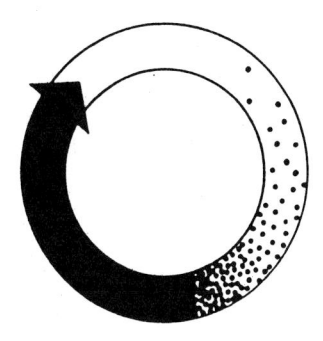

Functionally determined
(Allessie et al. 1977)

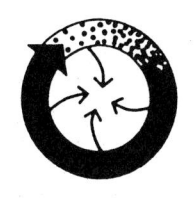

1. Fixed length and localization of circuit.

2. Circuit length equal to anatomical pathway.

3. Excitable gap between head and tail of impulse.

4. Rate proportional to conduction velocity and length of pathway.

1. Variable size and localization of circuit.

2. Circuit length equal to the length of the excitation wave.

3. No gap of full excitability.

4. Rate proportional to refractory period.

Figure 1: Comparison of characteristics of anatomically and functionally determined circus movement.

Atrial Flutter and Fibrillation in the Normal Heart

In Figures 2, 3, and 4, color maps of atrial flutter and fibrillation are given from experiments in isolated canine hearts.[25,31] Atrial flutter and fibrillation were induced by the combination of acetylcholine infusion and rapid pacing. The activation maps were constructed on the basis of local electrograms recorded with a right and a left multiple endocardial electrode, containing 960 leads (spatial resolution 2–3 mm).[25] Figure 2 shows the excitation of the atria during an episode of flutter with a cycle length of 145 ms (flutter rate 410/min). For comparison, the map during normal sinus rhythm before the induction of flutter is given at the left.

During sinus rhythm, there was a normal sequence of atrial activation. The impulse originating in the sinus node excited the atrium along the lateral border of the superior vena cava. From here, the right atrium was activated in less than 50 ms. Electrical activity in the left atrium was noted 15 ms after the impulse emerged from the sinus node. In this example, the area of earliest endocardial activation was located somewhat posteriorly from which the left atrium was activated in a regular manner, resulting in a total atrial conduction time during sinus rhythm of 70 ms. No areas of conduction block or depressed conduction were noted.

During the episode of atrial flutter, which lasted for more than half an hour, the excitation of the atria was completely different compared to sinus rhythm. First, it is evident that the source of the arrhythmia was located in the left atrium, the right atrium now being activated from the left. The light green area of first right atrial activation corresponds with the insertion of Bachmann's bundle. Apart from this shift in origin of the atrial impulse, the right atrium was activated quite normally, with the impulse spreading more or less radially from its point of entrance in the right atrium. In contrast, the left atrium showed a completely different way of excitation. During flutter, the radial conduction pattern was lost and replaced by a continuous circus movement in the free lateral wall. The length of this intra-atrial circuit was about 10 cm. It should be emphasized that with less extensive mapping techniques, the identification of such a circuit can be easily missed. About half the length of the circuit the impulse was propagating in a rather narrow pathway along the inferior margin of the atrium. If this limb of the circuit, in which conduction was somewhat depressed, had remained unrecognized, the flutter could have been erroneously attributed to a focus of rapid impulse formation in the low left atrium.

In Figure 3, some other examples of rapid atrial flutter are shown. In all cases the flutter was based on continuous circus movement of the impulse in the atrial myocardium. However, the localization of the intra-atrial circuits differed from case to case even in the same heart. Apart from the free lateral wall of the left atrium, circuits were identified in the left atrial appendage, the posterior left atrium, the right atrial appendage, and the posterior right atrium. Both the size of the circuits and the cycle length of the flutter varied from case to case. In the examples given, the cycle length ranged from 65 to 145 ms and the length of the circuits between 5 and 10 cm. These differences may in part have been due to different effective dosages of acetylcholine leading to a different degree of shortening of the atrial refractory period in the different experiments.

Figure 4 gives the excitation of the right (upper part) and the left (lower part) atrium during atrial fibrillation. Each series of activation maps covers a time window of less than half a second. Although the right and left atrium were mapped consecutively and cannot be directly time-aligned, it seems justified to consider the two different episodes as part of one and the same process. In panel A of the right atrium, which starts at an arbitrary moment during sustained atrial fibrillation, we encounter three independent wavelets. One wavelet (smallest arrow) is traveling down the septum and is extinguished at time 30 at the AV junction. The other two waves originally propagated in opposite directions, the middle one traveling along the medial wall of the atrium in a posterior direction

Sinus Rhythm

Atrial Flutter

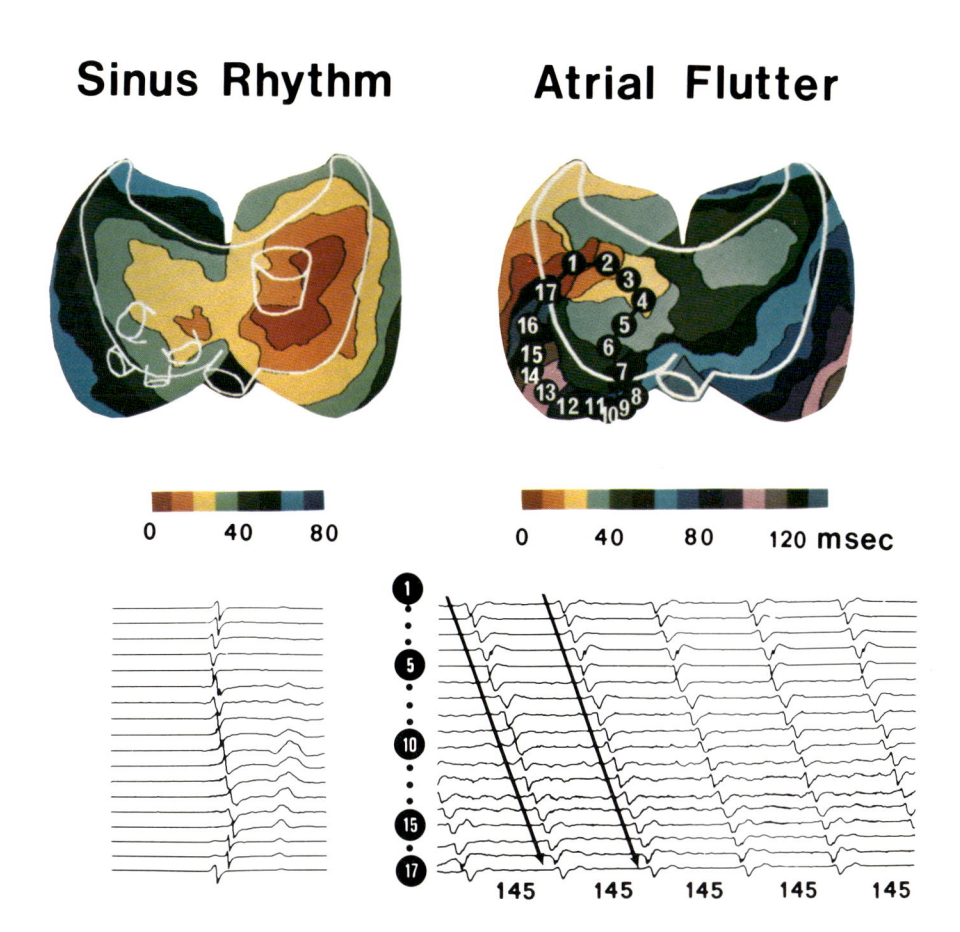

Figure 2: Maps of total endocardial activation during sinus rhythm (left) and an episode of atrial flutter (right). The maps are based on the recording of 960 unipolar endocardial electrograms resulting in a spatial resolution of the maps of 3 mm. Each color represents an isochrone of 10 ms. During sinus rhythm, there is normal spread of the impulse from the sinus node to both the right and the left atria. During atrial flutter, the source of the rapid repetitive impulses is located in the left atrium and consists of an intra-atrial circuit located in the lateral wall. At the bottom of the figure, 18 electrograms from 17 different sites in the left lateral wall are shown. The recording sites of these electrograms were identical during sinus rhythm and atrial flutter and are indicated on the flutter map. From these electrograms, the continuous circulating excitation during atrial flutter can be seen. During sinus rhythm, the area of the future circuit was excited almost synchronously and did not show any abnormalities in conduction or configuration of the electrograms.

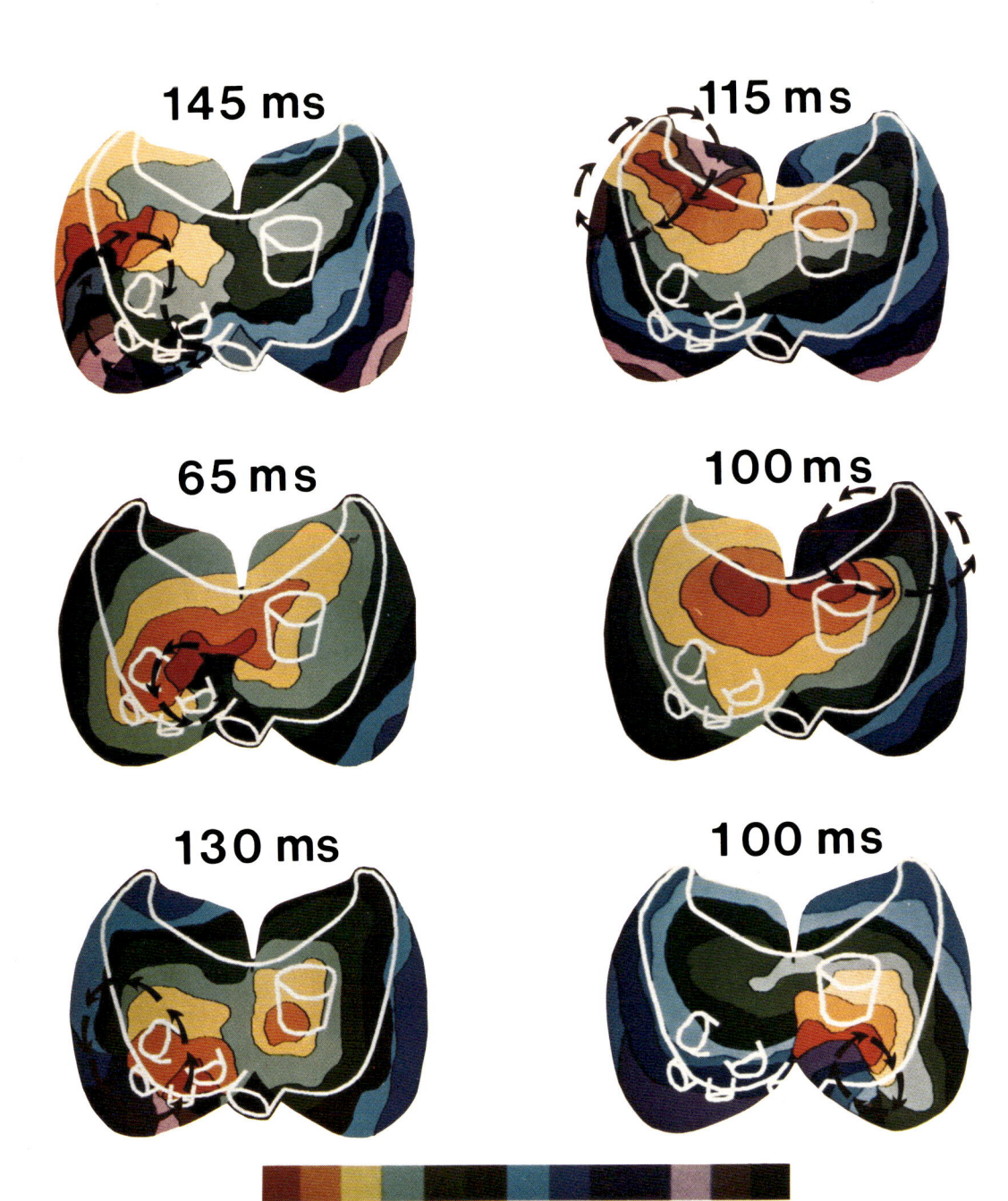

Figure 3: Atrial excitation maps of six different cases of rapid atrial flutter are shown. Maps at top left and middle right are taken from the same heart. In all cases atrial flutter was based on intra-atrial reentry. There was marked variation both in the rate of the flutter and in the localization of the circuits. Top left: The circuit (cycle length 145 ms) was found in the lateral wall of the left atrium. Top right: The impulse circulated around the left atrial appendage with a revolution time of 115 ms. Middle left: This extremely rapid flutter (cycle length 65 ms) was based on a circuit in the posterior wall of the left atrium. The episodes of the other three cases of atrial flutter were caused by an intra-atrial circuit located around the right atrial appendage (middle right panel), in the left lateral wall (bottom left), and the posterior right atrium (bottom right). The estimated size of the circuits varied between 5 and 10 cm. Each color represents an isochrone of 10 ms.

RIGHT ATRIUM

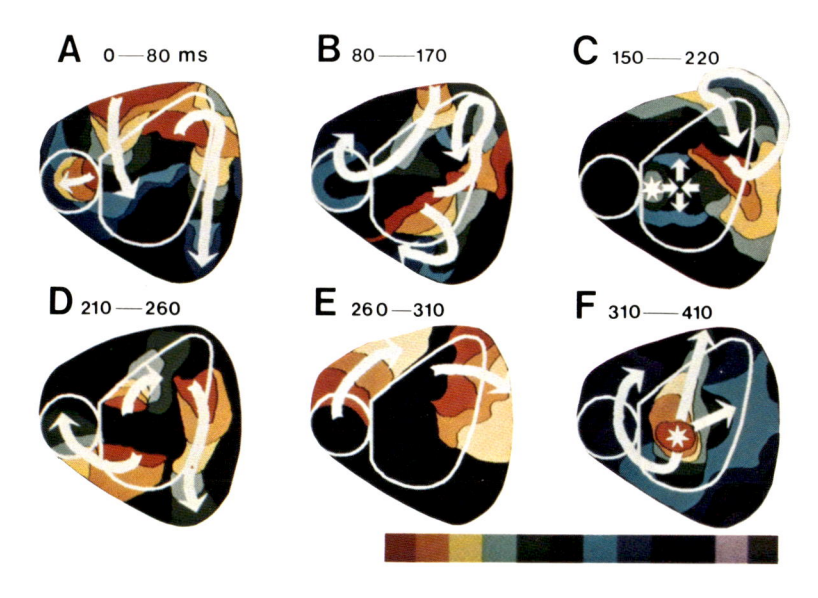

A 0—80 ms   **B** 80—170   **C** 150—220

D 210—260   **E** 260—310   **F** 310—410

LEFT ATRIUM

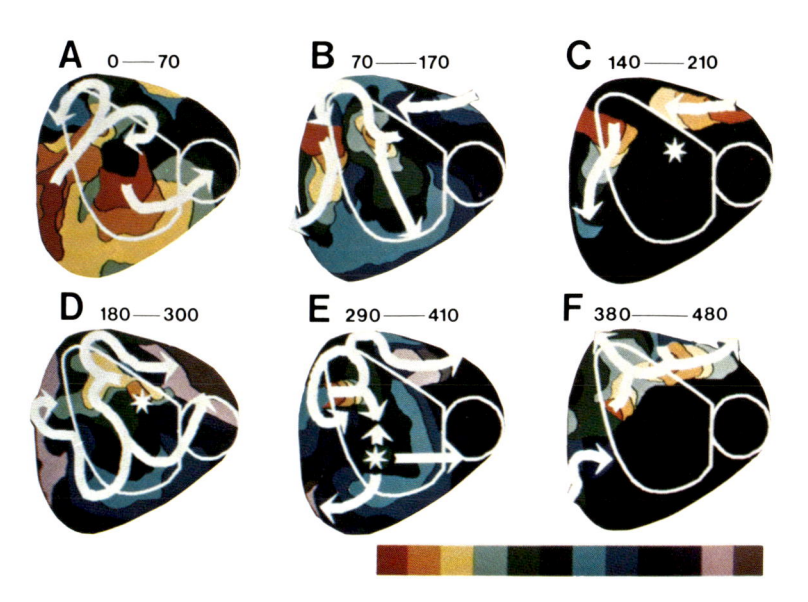

A 0—70   **B** 70—170   **C** 140—210

D 180—300   **E** 290—410   **F** 380—480

Figure 4: A series of consecutive activation maps covering the spread of excitation in the right (upper part of figure) and left atrium (lower part) during half a second of stable self-perpetuating atrial fibrillation. The recordings from the right and left atrium are not recorded simultaneously and therefore cannot be time-aligned. Each color represents an isochrone of 10 ms. The propagation of the various wavelets is indicated by white arrows. Asterisks indicate sites of origin of "new" impulses, entering the atrium from the other side. See text for description.

(downwards in the map) and the right wave upwards to the tip of the appendage. At time 20, the two waves collide, resulting in a sudden narrowing of the middle wave. The right wave, finding its way to the appendage suddenly blocked, changes its direction of propagation by 180° and continues its course as a narrow wavelet in the lateral wall until, at time 80, it dies out at the AV ring. In panel B, the large activation wave at the end of panel A is split into smaller wavelets. One wavelet (lower arrow in panel B) encounters an area in the posterior wall of the right atrium which obviously has not yet restored its excitability, resulting in a 180° clockwise turn. At time 170, this turning wavelet extinguished at the atrial border. A second wave (counterclockwise arrow in panel B) entered the lateral wall of the appendage and made a full 360° turn in the anterior part of the lateral wall. As can be seen from panel C, this wavelet created a closed local circuit which continued for/another revolution although the size and location of the circuit changed (compare counterclockwise arrows in panels B and C).

Panel C shows two other interesting phenomena. First, at time 180, a new impulse appears at the site indicated by the asterisk. The origin of this impulse cannot be explained from the propagation of wavelets in the right atrium and most probably is the continuation of a wavelet in the left atrium. The second noteworthy phenomenon is the event indicated by the four little arrows. Here we can see what can happen if two narrow wavelets collide. Instead of mutual extinction, we see something which we have called the "clash and go" phenomenon. The two narrow impulses approaching each other collide, and after the collision diverge again in opposite directions with a 90° change in direction. The phenomena in panel C led to the presence of three clearly separated and narrow wavelets in panel D. The right one is an offspring of the circuit around the appendage which has ceased to exist. The other two are the result of the "clash and go" phenomenon. After the right wavelet has died out at time 260 at the AV ring, in panel E only two wavefronts are left. At time 290, these two remaining wavelets are simultaneously extinced by the coincidental combination of reaching the AV ring and conduction block at refractory tissue. This sudden disappearance of multiple wandering wavelets in the right atrium did *not* result in termination of atrial fibrillation. About 20 ms after the right atrium has become electrically silent, a new impulse penetrated the right atrium from the left (asterisk in panel F). The activation map in panel F further illustrates that the impulse entering the right atrium at time 310 is immediately broken up into three separate depolarization waves. Obviously the short time that the right atrium has been electrically silent has not been long enough to bring the fibers in the same phase of excitability. The new impulse therefore encounters islands of refractoriness and the process of fragmented multiple wandering wavelets is restarted.

The lower part of Figure 4 shows the fibrillatory process in the left atrium. In general, the left atrium exhibited the same pattern of excitation as described for the right atrium. During sustained fibrillation, each atrium contained an average of about three wandering wavelets. Also in the left atrium, frequent entries of "new" impulses from the right atrium were seen (asterisks in panels C, D, and E). Once more, the ever-changing pathways of the various wavelets become evident, giving the impression of looking through a kaleidoscope.

The Role of the Wavelength in Atrial Reentrant Arrhythmias

In any model of reentry, the length of the excitation wave plays a crucial role both in the initiation and the perpetuation of circuitous excitation. When the wavelength—defined by the product of refractory period and conduction velocity—is long, a large area of unidirectional conduction block is required to make the impulse reenter itself. On the other hand, when the impulse is short—either by depressed conduction or by a short refractory period—small areas of conduction block may already set up reentrant circuits. Since conduction block is more likely to occur in small areas than in a large portion of the myocardium, the *inducibility* of reentrant arrhythmias must to be directly related to the length of the cardiac impulse.

Also, for the perpetuation of reentrant rhythms, the wavelength is important. Interventions that prolong the wavelength will increase the minimal size of intramyocardial circuits. If an excitable gap is present in the reentrant loop, prolongation of the wavelength will first reduce and finally close the excitable gap, leading to instability and a high chance of block of the circulating impulse. In the case of *multiple* reentering wavelets as during fibrillation,[32] a prolongation of the wavelength will result in an increase in average circuit size. Since the tissue mass in a given heart is constant, this will diminish the total number of wandering impulses and thus increase the likelihood of simultaneous dying out of the wavelets and spontaneous termination of the arrhythmia. On the other hand, interventions that shorten the wavelength will either stabilize the reentrant process by creating or enlarging an excitable gap or it may lead to degeneration into multiple randomly reentering circuits (fibrillation).

These considerations led us to develop a chronic conscious dog model in which the wavelength of the atrial impulse could be measured and directly correlated with the induction of arrhythmias.[33] Figure 5 shows the set of double row electrodes for measurement of the wavelength in the bundle of Bachmann and the free wall of the right and left atrium. The lower part of the figure shows a superimposition of unipolar electrograms recorded from neighboring electrodes. The principle of the wavelength measurement is the simultaneous determination of conduction velocity and refractory period.[34] If the corresponding electrodes of the double row are activated simultaneously, the impulse propagates parallel to the electrode and conduction times can be used to calculate the actual conduction velocity. To measure the refractory period, the heart was driven at a certain basic rate and after every 15th beat a premature stimulus ($4 \times$ threshold) was given at progressively shorter intervals in steps of 2–5 ms. The shortest possible A_1-A_2 interval, measured at the recording electrode closest to the stimulus site, was taken as the functional refractory period. By applying a second premature stimulus, the refractory period of the first premature impulse could be measured from the shortest A_2-A_3 interval. The wavelength of the basic rhythm is given by the product of the conduction velocity of A_1 and the A_1-A_2 interval. The premature wavelength is the product of conduction velocity of the A_2 impulse and the A_2-A_3 interval.

In all dogs (n=19), atrial arrhythmias (n=549) could be induced with single

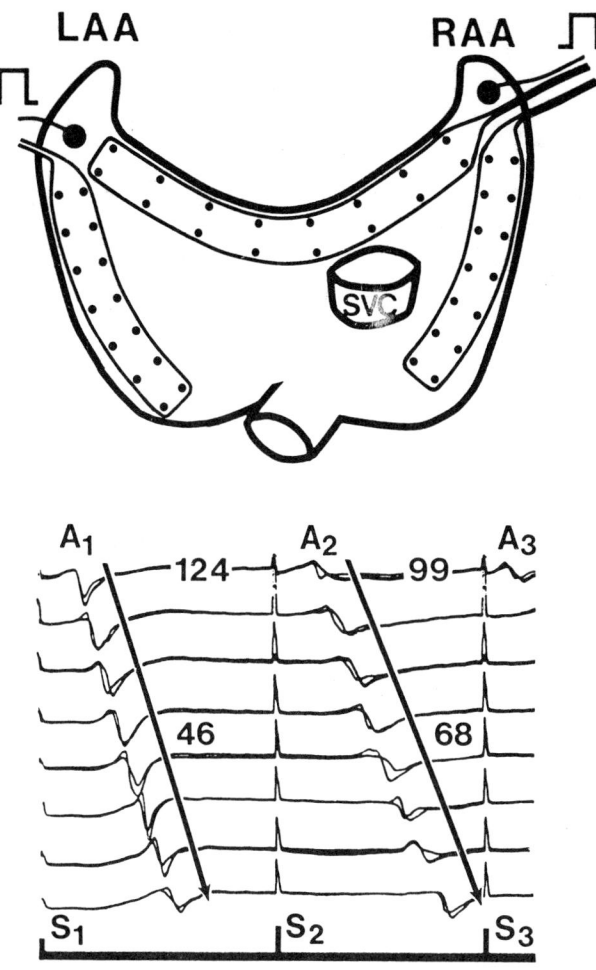

Figure 5: Upper panel: Schematic representation of the position of the implanted electrodes. The long electrode is positioned on Bachmann's bundle from the right to the left atrial appendage (RAA and LAA). The other electrodes are attached to the free wall of the right or left atrium parallel to the AV ring. Two pairs of stimulating electrodes (black dots) are fixed to the atrial appendages (SVC = superior vena cava). Lower panel: Superimposed unipolar electrograms recorded from neighboring electrodes along a row of double electrodes (interelectrode distance 8 mm). The electrograms recorded at the pairs of electrodes are almost simultaneous, and thus the impulse is propagating parallel to the long axis of the electrode. Conduction under the electrode was uniform as can be seen from the constant conduction times between the electrodes. Total conduction time for the basic impulse (A_1) was 46 ms and for the premature impulse (A_2) 68 ms. The shortest A_1-A_2 interval was 124 ms. Thus the wavelength of the basic impulse can be calculated to be 56 mm/46 ms * 124 ms = 15.0 cm. The wavelength of the premature impulse was 8.2 cm.

premature stimuli. Figure 6 shows the different types of arrhythmias that were induced by extrasystoles with varying prematurity. Premature stimuli with long coupling intervals (tracing A) elicited only single premature responses (A_2), after which sinus rhythm resumed. Moderately premature stimuli (tracing B) were followed by short series of rapid repetitive responses (RRR) (n=223). Early premature stimuli (tracing C) sometimes resulted in a longer or shorter paroxysm of atrial flutter (n=118). Premature stimuli given immediately after the end of the

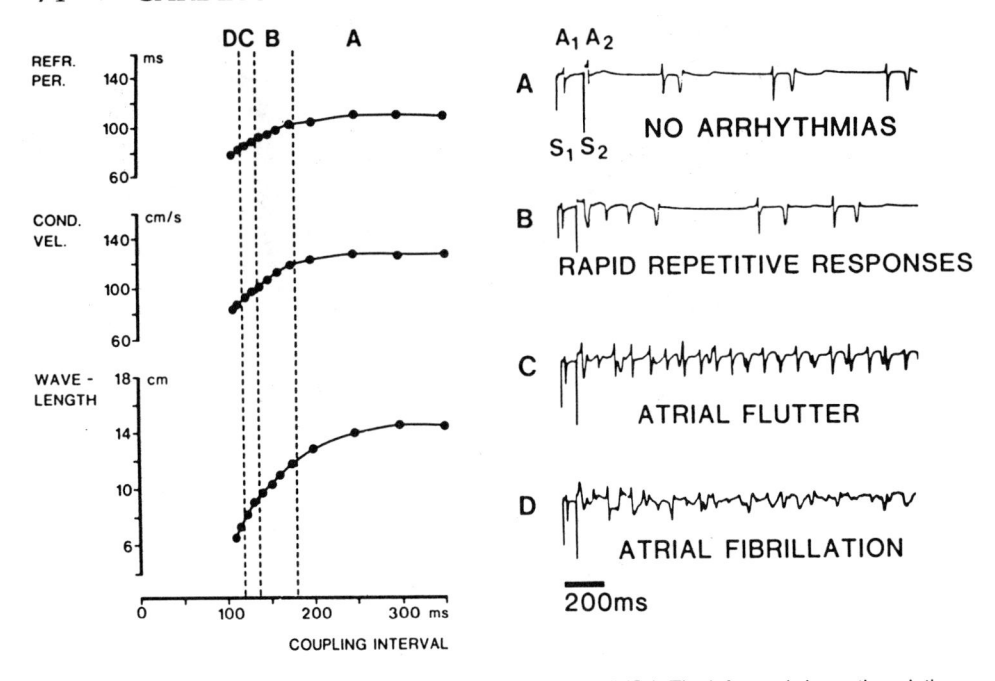

Figure 6: Atrial arrhythmias induced by single premature stimuli (S_2). The left panel shows the relationship among the coupling interval of premature impulses and refractory period, conduction velocity, and wavelength. The prematurity zones in the left panel correspond to the tracings in the right panels. Premature stimuli with a long coupling interval (zone A) elicited only single premature responses (A_2). Moderately premature stimuli (B) were followed by a short run of rapid repetitive reponses (RRR). Still earlier extrasystoles (zone C) resulted in a paroxysm of atrial flutter. Premature stimuli given immediately after the refractory period (zone D) induced episodes of atrial fibrillation.

refractory period frequently induced atrial fibrillation (n=208) (tracing D). Comparison with the curves in the left panel shows that the observed atrial response to progressively shorter coupled extrasystoles coincided with a progressive decrease in both refractory period, conduction velocity, and wavelength. To find out how these different parameters affected the induction of arrhythmias, we manipulated the electrophysiological properties of the atrium by administration of a variety of drugs (acetylcholine, propafenone, lidocaine, ouabain, quinidine, and d-sotalol). Under all these different circumstances, the values of the refractory period, conduction velocity and wavelength of the premature impulse were correlated with the induction of atrial arrhythmias. To get the best separation between the different subpopulations, linear discriminant analysis was used and the predictive power, sensitivity, and specificity of each variable for the occurrence of arrhythmias was calculated. In Table I, the results of this analysis are given. It clearly shows that the wavelength of the atrial impulse is the best parameter to predict the inducibility of reentrant arrhythmias (predictive power 75%). Both conduction velocity and refractory period had a rather poor predictive value, the overall correct prediction of occurrence of arrhythmias being 38% and 48%, respectively. In addition, the sensitivity and specificity of the wavelength were better than the sensitivity and specificity of either conduction velocity or refrac-

Table I
Predictive Power, Sensitivity, and Specificity of Refractory Period, Conduction Velocity, and Wavelength for the Induction of Atrial Arrhythmias

		Refractory Period	Conduction Velocity	Wavelength
Predictive power (% correct classification)	n = 750	48%	38%	75%
Fibrillation versus	Sens:	84%	71%	100%
No Arrhythmias	Spec:	89%	72%	96%
Flutter versus	Sens:	65%	75%	100%
No Arrhythmias	Spec:	72%	70%	89%
Repetitive Responses versus	Sens:	67%	66%	88%
No Arrhythmias	Spec:	68%	57%	80%
All Arrhythmias versus	Sens:	69%	68%	88%
No Arrhythmias	Spec:	76%	70%	89%

tory period alone. The *critical wavelengths* for induction of atrial arrhythmias were: (1) for rapid repetitive responses, 12.3 cm; (2) for atrial flutter, 9.7 cm; and (3) for atrial fibrillation, 7.8 cm.

In Figure 7, the correlation among the induction of atrial fibrillation and refractory period, conduction velocity, and wavelength of the provoking premature impulse is plotted graphically. The refractory period is plotted on the abscissa, the conduction velocity is plotted on the ordinate, and the value of the wavelength is given by the curved "isowave"-lines (product of refractory period and conduction velocity). The critical wavelength where atrial arrhythmias started to occur (12 cm) and the critical wavelength for atrial fibrillation (8 cm) are indicated by thick curves. The values of premature beats which did not induce an arrhythmia are plotted with open symbols, whereas premature impulses which provoked atrial fibrillation are plotted as filled symbols. Because of the use of a variety of drugs, the values for refractory period and conduction velocity varied widely. From this graph, one can see that the duration of the refractory period alone is not a reliable parameter for the prediction of atrial fibrillation. The same holds true for the conduction velocity. For each of the two parameters, there is considerable overlap between the population of "no arrhythmias" and "fibrillation." However, if one uses the wavelength as a criterion, a clear separation between the two populations becomes evident. Three wavelength-bands can be distinguished: a band of "no arrhythmias" (wavelength >12 cm), a "fibrillation band" (wavelength < 8 cm), and an intermediate band (wavelength between 8 and 12 cm) in which rapid repetitive responses or atrial flutter occurred.

The concept of a critical wavelength for reentrant arrhythmias suggests that it might be useful to describe part of the antiarrhythmic properties of cardiac drugs in terms of changes in the wavelength. Drugs that shorten the wavelength must

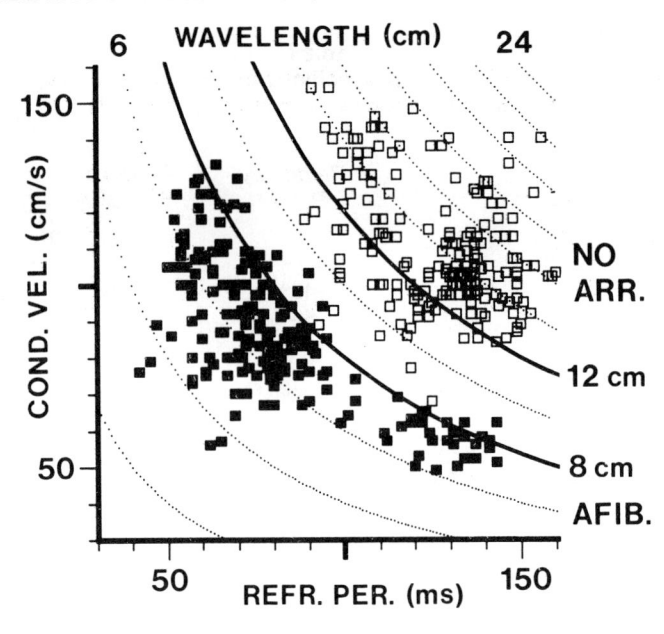

Figure 7: Relationship among the induction of atrial fibrillation and the refractory period, conduction velocity, and wavelength of the initiating premature beat. The refractory period is plotted on the abscissa and the conduction velocity on the ordinate. Because the wavelength is the product of refractory period and conduction velocity also, "iso-wavelength" curves can be drawn. Open squares are premature beats that did not result in an atrial arrhythmia. Filled squares indicate premature impulses which initiated atrial fibrillation. If the wavelength was longer than 12 cm, no arrhythmias occurred. At a critical wavelength below 8 cm, atrial fibrillation was often induced, whereas in the intermediate wavelength band between 8 and 12 cm, atrial flutter or repetitive responses occurred.

be regarded as arrhythmogenic, whereas agents that prolong the wavelength can be expected to possess antiarrhythmic properties. An increase in wavelength is most effectively accomplished by a combined increase in refractory period and conduction velocity. Compounds whose action on one variable is totally or partially counteracted by an opposite effect on the other variable are less effective. The correlation between the length of the impulse and the occurrence of arrhythmias as found in this animal study seems to be applicable to the human heart. Pharmacological prolongation of the wavelength might offer a rational basis for therapy of clinical arrhythmias. In our study in dogs, class III drugs were the most powerful wavelength-prolonging agents. This may explain the effectiveness of these drugs in treating atrial flutter and fibrillation.

Different Models of Reentry

In Figure 8, a variety of different models of reentry are summarized. Panel A shows the earliest model of circus movement as introduced by Mines in 1913.[15] It is the simplest model of reentry, in which the impulse continuously encircles a large anatomic obstacle. Implicit to this model is the existence of a fully excitable

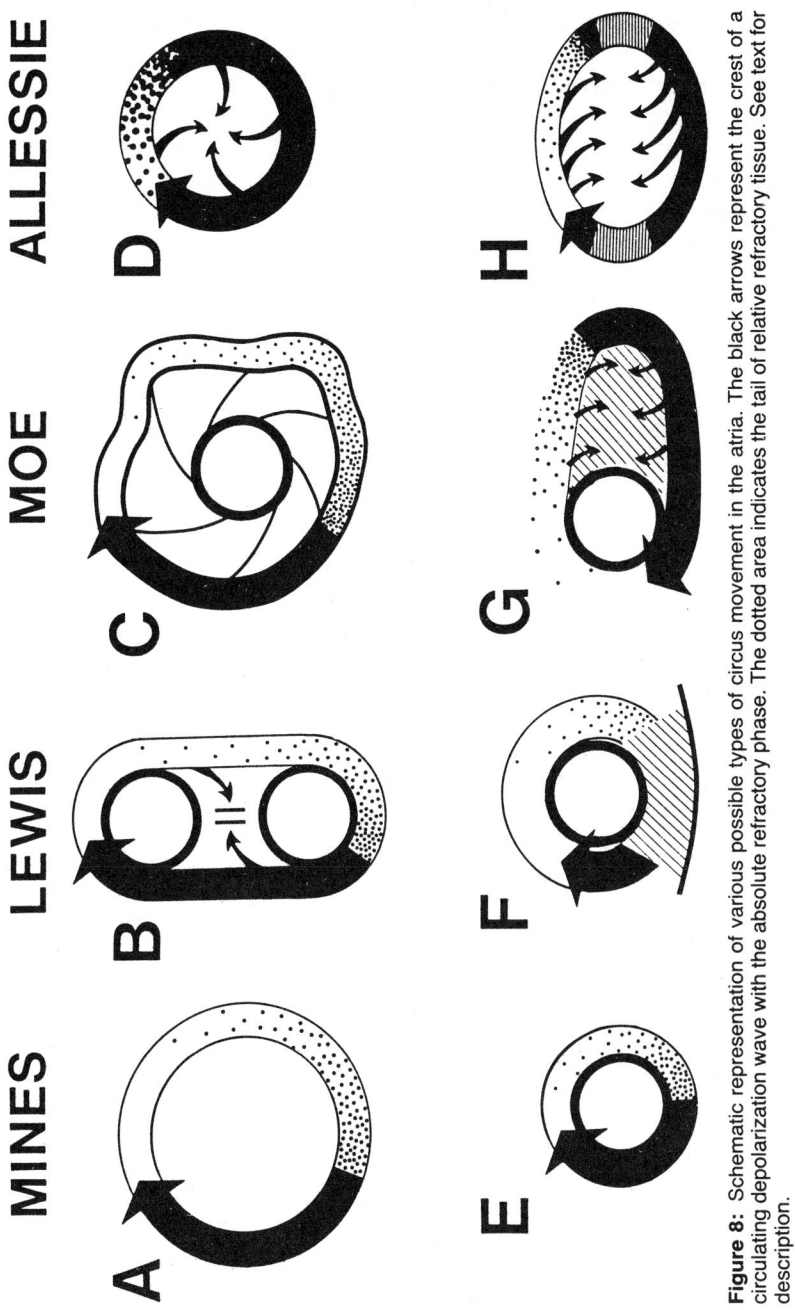

Atrial Flutter and Fibrillation • 77

Figure 8: Schematic representation of various possible types of circus movement in the atria. The black arrows represent the crest of a circulating depolarization wave with the absolute refractory phase. The dotted area indicates the tail of relative refractory tissue. See text for description.

gap (white part of the circuit) between the crest of the excitation wave and its tail of relative refractoriness (dotted area). The presence of such a fully excitable gap explains the high degree of regularity and stability of this kind of rhythm. Since the studies of Rosenblueth and Garcia Ramos,[18] there is little doubt that by the creation of a large obstacle in the atria, atrial flutter can be produced that is based on this mechanism. The problem, however, is that in patients suffering from atrial flutter, such large anatomic obstacles have never been actually demonstrated.

In panel B, circus movement around two obstacles (like the venae cavae) as popularized by Lewis[6,17] is shown. A functional conduction block is assumed in the isthmus between the two obstacles. As long as the excitable gap remains shorter than the circumference of the smallest of the two obstacles, short-circuit of the circulating impulse through the interobstacle band is prevented and the flutter rate is determined by the revolution time around both obstacles. The behavior of this type of reentry is identical to the Mines model with one exception. As soon as the excitable gap gets larger than the perimeter of the smallest of the two obstacles, the impulse can shortcut the circuit. This may result either in sudden termination of flutter, or when the impulse continues to circulate around the larger obstacle, in abrupt acceleration of the flutter. In this case, when other parts of the atria cannot follow the higher rate, degeneration into atrial fibrillation may occur.

In another attempt to overcome the problem that natural obstacles in the atria under normal circumstances do not seem to be large enough to allow for sustained circus movement, Moe et al.[35,36] took differences in conduction velocity into account. In Moe's model (panel C), the rapidly conducting muscle bundles, such as the internodal bands and the bundle of Bachmann, form closed loops which serve as preferential circuits through which flutter waves may circulate.

In panel D, the leading circle type of reentry[23] is given schematically. When there is no anatomic obstacle that defines the length of a circular pathway, the circuit in which the impulse circulates is completely defined by the electrophysiological properties of the fibers composing the circuit. Under these circumstances, the smallest possible pathway in which the impulse can circulate is the circuit in which the "stimulating efficacy" of the circulating impulse is just enough to excite the tissue ahead which is still in its relative refractory phase. In other words, in this smallest circuit possible, the leading edge of the circulating wavefront is continuously biting in its own tail of refractoriness. Because of this tight fit, the length of the leading circuit is equal to the wavelength of the circulating impulse. In the center of the leading circle, dimensions are too small for a sustained circus movement. Instead, the area within the leading circle is activated by centripetal wavelets that collide in the middle of the circuit.

In the lower row of Figure 8, we propose some additional variants of intramyocardial circuits that may be responsible for atrial arrhythmias. In panel E, intra-atrial reentry is facilitated by shortening of the wavelength of the impulse. The wavelength defined as the distance traveled by the impulse during the functional refractory period is determined by the product of conduction velocity and refractory period. For instance, under the influence of acetylcholine, the refractory period of the atrial myocardium shortens while the speed of conduction remains essentially unaltered.[33,34] When this occurs, small natural openings in the atria may suffice as central anatomic obstacles for stable reentry. Conditions that shorten the wavelength will also favor leading circle reentry. A small arc of functional conduction block that may occur during the propagation of a premature beat then may be sufficient to initiate reentrant excitation within the myocardium.

In panel F, an area of depressed conduction is assumed in the inferior atrium between an internal obstacle (such as the inferior vena cava or a pulmonary vein) and the atrioventricular ring. The presence of such an isthmus of depressed conduction would not only bring the rate of a reentrant rhythm down to the range of common atrial flutter, but it will also stabilize the reentrant process because it produces an excitable gap at least in the healthy segment of the circuit. In panel G, an area of prolonged refractoriness neighbors an anatomic obstacle. The revolution time in such a circular pathway may be long enough to create an excitable gap in the normal atrial myocardium. There is a tight fit between the circulating depolarization wave and its tail of refractoriness only at the free end of the arc of functional conduction block in the area with prolonged refractoriness. This functionally determined turning point then is the only unstable part of the circuit. During subsequent cycles, the impulse may pivot at slightly different points, resulting in only minor variations in size and cycle length of the circuit. However, the localization of the circuit will be fixed and the resulting flutter could last for a long time.

Finally, the diagram in panel H introduces anisotropy in a reentrant process. Conduction of the cardiac impulse (including circulating excitation) is strongly influenced by the structural interrelationships of the myocardial fiber bundles. One of the fundamental characteristics is that impulse propagation is more rapid parallel to the fiber orientation than perpendicular to it. This anisotropic property has been subdivided by Spach et al.[27-30] According to their definitions, *uniform anisotropy* occurs in cardiac muscle in which the fibers are all arranged parallel to each other. *Nonuniform anisotropy* occurs when nonconductile barriers such as those formed by connective tissue influence conduction or when myocardial fibers are not arranged in parallel. Such anisotropic properties of cardiac muscle may play an important role in the genesis of reentrant arrhythmias. Spach et al.[27-30] proposed that it may cause conduction block of premature impulses that may initiate reentry because of a low safety factor for conduction in the longitudinal direction. Conduction perpendicular to fiber orientation can also be slow enough even in normal tissue to cause reentry. Slowed conduction caused by anisotropy in the epicardial border zone of canine infarcts may be an important factor in the genesis of ventricular tachycardia.[37] Recently, a simple experimental model of anisotropic reentry has been developed.[38] The properties of anisotropic reentry are: (1) The central arc of conduction block where the impulse is turning around is oriented parallel to the orientation of the muscle fibers. (2) The circuit is ellipsoid in shape. (3) Conduction velocity along the circuit is not constant, being fast along the long axis of the circuit and slowing down at the two pivoting points. (4) The slowing in conduction at the pivoting points—because the impulse is forced to travel perpendicular to the fiber orientation—creates an excitable gap.

Summary

The above-reviewed experimental studies have greatly increased our knowledge and understanding of cardiac arrhythmias. It has become clear that there is not a *single* mechanism but a variety of arrhythmogenic mechanisms. Not only does one have to distinguish between abnormal impulse formation and circus movement, but each of the two groups again have to be subdivided into different mechanisms. Experimentally, several different models of reentry have been described. Until now, it was not clear what the *clinical significance* of these different mechanisms is. Experimental models are useful to provide insight in *possible* mechanisms. However, the obvious limitations of animal studies is that they are always to some extent artificial and cannot be regarded identical to human hearts, especially not to diseased human hearts. Mapping of electrophysiological properties in humans during cardiac surgery seems to be the only way to answer this question. From experimental models of arrhythmias, we have learned what we have to look for and use adequate recording tools. Application of this knowledge and techniques in cardiac surgery is required to extend our understanding of mechanisms of atrial flutter and fibrillation to the human heart.

References

1. Prinzmetal M, Corday E, Brill IC, Oblath RW, Kruger HE. The auricular arrhythmias. Springfield, IL, Charles C Thomas, 1952.
2. Scherf D, Schott A. Extrasystoles and allied arrhythmias. London, Heinemann Medical Books, 1973.
3. Kishon Y, Smith RE. Studies in human atrial flutter with the use of proximity electrodes. Circulation 1969;40:513–525.
4. Rosen KM, Lau SH, Damato AN. Simulation of atrial flutter by rapid coronary sinus pacing. Am Heart J 1969;78:635–642.
5. Wellens HJJ. Value and limitations of programmed electrical stimulation of the heart in the study and treatment of tachycardias. Circulation 1978;57:845–853.
6. Lewis T. The Mechanism and Graphic Registration of the Heart Beat. ed. 3. London, Shaw & Sons, 1925.
7. Puech P, Latour H, Grolleau R. Le flutter et ses limites. Arch Mal Coeur 1970;61:116–120.
8. Waldo AL, MacLean WAH, Karp RB, Kouchoukos NT, James TN. Entrainment and interruption of atrial flutter with atrial pacing: studies in man following open heart surgery. Circulation 1977;56:737–745.
9. Watson RT, Josephson ME. Atrial flutter. I. Electrophysiologic substrates and modes of initiation and termination. Am J Cardiol 1980;45:732–741.
10. Inoue H, Matsuo H, Takayanagi K, Murao S. Clinical and experimental studies of the effects of atrial extrastimulation and rapid pacing on atrial flutter cycle. Am J Cardiol 1981;48:623–631.
11. Disertori M, Inama G, Vergara G, Guarnerio M, Del Favero A, Furlanello F. Evidence of a reentry circuit in the common type of atrial flutter in man. Circulation 1983;67:434–440.
12. Scherf D. Studies on auricular tachycardia caused by aconitine administration. Proc Soc Exp Biol Med NY 1947;64:233–239.
13. Cranefield PF. The conduction of the cardiac impulse. The slow response and cardiac arrhythmia. Mt. Kisco, NY, Futura Publishing Co., 1975.

14. Moe GK, Abildskov JA. Atrial fibrillation as a self-sustaining arrhythmia independent of focal discharge. Am Heart J 1959;58:59–70.
15. Mines GR. On dynamic equilibrium in the heart. J Physiol 1913;46:349–383.
16. Garrey WE. The nature of fibrillary contraction of the heart: Its relation to tissue mass and form. Am J Physiol 1914;33:397–414.
17. Lewis T, Feil S, Stroud WD. Observations upon flutter and fibrillation. II. The nature of auricular flutter. Heart 1920;7:191–246.
18. Rosenblueth A, Garcia Ramos J. Studies on flutter and fibrillation: the influence of artificial obstacles on experimental auricular flutter. Am Heart J 1947;33:677–684.
19. Frame LH, Page RL, Hoffman BF. Atrial reentry around an anatomic barrier with a partially refractory excitable gap. Circ Res 1986;58:495–511.
20. Boineau JP, Schuessler RB, Mooney CR, Miller CB, Wylds AC, Hudson RD, Borremans JM, Brockus CW. Natural and evoked atrial flutter due to circus movement in dogs. Am J Cardiol 1980;45:1167–1181.
21. Allessie MA, Bonke FIM, Schopman FJG. Circus movement in rabbit atrial muscle as a mechanism of tachycardia. Circ Res 1973;32:54–62.
22. Allessie MA, Bonke FIM, Schopman FJG. Circus movement in rabbit atrial muscle as a mechanism of tachycardia. II. The role of nonuniform recovery of excitability in the occurrence of unidirectional block as studied with multiple microelectrodes. Circ Res 1976;39:168–177.
23. Allessie MA, Bonke FIM, Schopman FJG. Circus movement in rabbit atrial muscle as a mechanism of tachycardia. III. The "leading circle" concept: a new model of circus movement in cardiac tissue without the involvement of an antomic obstacle. Circ Res 1977;41:9–18.
24. Boyden PA, Hoffman BF. The effects on atrial electrophysiology and structure of surgically induced right atrial enlargement in dogs. Circ Res 1981;49:1319–1331.
25. Allessie MA, Lammers WJEP, Bonke FIM, Hollen J. Intra-atrial reentry as a mechanism for atrial flutter by acetylcholine and rapid pacing in the dog. Circulation 1984;70: 123–135.
26. Page P, Plumb VJ, Waldo AL. Total epicardial mapping of atrial flutter in a new animal model (abstr). J Am Coll Cardiol 1983;1:716.
27. Leier CV, Schaal SF. Biatrial electrograms during coarse atrial fibrillation and flutter-fibrillation. Am Heart J 1980;99:331–341.
28. Cosio FG, Palacios J, Vidal J, Cocina EG, Gomez-Sanchez MA, Tamargo L. Electrophysiologic studies in atrial fibrillation. Slow conduction of premature impulses: a possible manifestation of the background for reentry. Am J Cardiol 1983;51:122–130.
29. Spach MS, Miller WT, Dolber PC, Kootsey M, Sommer JR, Mosher CE. The functional role of structural complexities in the propagation of depolarization in the atrium of the dog: Cardiac conduction disturbances due to discontinuities of effective axial resistivity. Circ Res 1982;50:175–191.
30. Spach MS, Dolber PC. Relating extracellular potentials and their derivatives to anisotropic propagation at a microscopic level in human cardiac muscle. Circ Res 1986;58: 356–371.
31. Allessie MA, Lammers WJEP, Bonke FIM, Hollen J. Experimental evaluation of Moe's multiple wavelet hypothesis of atrial fibrillation. In Zipes DP, Jalife J, eds. Cardiac Arrhythmias. New York, Grune & Stratton, 1985;265–276.
32. Moe GK. On the multiple wavelet hypothesis of atrial fibrillation. Arch Int Pharmacodyn Ther 1962;140:183–188.
33. Rensma PL, Allessie MA, Lammers WJEP, Bonke FIM, Schalij MJ. The length of the excitation wave as an index for the susceptibility to reentrant atrial arrhythmias. 1987 (in press).
34. Smeets JLRM, Allessie MA, Lammers WJEP, Bonke FIM, Hollen J. The wavelength of the cardiac impulse and reentrant arrhythmias in isolated rabbit atrium. Circ Res 1986;58:96–108.
35. Moe GK, Pastelin G, Mendez R. Circus movement excitation of the atria. In Little RC, ed. Physiology of Atrial Pacemakers and Conductive Tissue. New York, Futura Publishing Co., 1980;207–220.

36. Pastelin G, Mendez R, Moe GK. Participation of atrial specialized conduction pathways in atrial flutter. Circ Res 1978;42:386–393.
37. Wit AL, Allessie MA, Bonke FIM, Lammers WJEP, Smeets J, Fenoglio JJ Jr. Electrophysiologic mapping to determine the mechanism of experimental ventricular tachycardia initiated by premature impulses. Am J Cardiol 1982;49:166–185.
38. Allessie MA, Schalij MJ, Wit AL, Lammers WJEP, Augustijn CH. Does anisotropy play a role in the creation of an excitable gap in reentrant ventricular tachycardia? In Breithardt G, ed. Non-Pharmacological Therapy of Tachyarrhythmias. Mt. Kisco, NY, Futura Publishing Company, 1987.

5

Metabolic Effects of Ischemia: What are the Implications for Arrhythmogenesis and the Treatment of Arrhythmias?

James N. Weiss

Introduction

Ventricular arrhythmias during acute myocardial ischemia are the major cause of mortality from coronary artery disease in the world today. Of the more than one million cases of myocardial infarction each year in the United States alone, approximately 60% die before reaching a hospital, the majority succumbing to lethal arrhythmias.[1] If the electrical instability leading to arrhythmias could be prevented in this group of individuals, the majority would probably survive since the size of the infarction is not generally large enough to cause intractable pump failure. Although modern cardiac care units have had a significant impact on the in-hospital mortality from ischemic arrhythmias, they obviously do not prevent arrhythmic deaths in the majority of patients whose arrhythmias develop before they can reach a hospital. To date, the most effective strategies for preventing life-threatening arrhythmias in the setting of coronary disease have been devised for the minority of patients who develop chronic ventricular arrhythmias. Although prevention of acute myocardial ischemia and infarction by early recognition and treatment of coronary artery disease may be the most effective strategy for preventing arrhythmic deaths, unravelling the pathophysiology of arrhythmo-

---

From: Brugada P, Wellens HJJ. CARDIAC ARRHYTHMIAS: Where To Go From Here? Mount Kisco, NY, Futura Publishing Company, Inc., © 1987.

genesis during acute ischemia has contributed significantly to the management of this critically important clinical problem.

Basal Cardiac Metabolism

Under normal conditions, the heart derives over 90% of its energy requirements from aerobic metabolism, with anaerobic glycolysis accounting for less than 10% of total cardiac adenosine triphosphate (ATP) production when adequate oxygen is present.[2] Fatty acids are the preferred substrate (60% or greater) for aerobic metabolism with the remainder being supplied largely by carbohydrates. The degradation of a molecule of glucose to two pyruvate or lactate molecules anaerobically through the glycolytic pathway yields a net production of two ATP molecules, whereas 34 ATP molecules result from the subsequent aerobic metabolism of the two pyruvate molecules to CO_2 and H_2O by the mitochondria. Thus the aerobic pathway is by far a more efficient pathway for converting substrate into ATP. During ischemia, the aerobic pathway is shut down and the only pathway for ATP generation is glycolysis. Although the rate of glycolysis initially accelerates many-fold in response to ischemia, glycolytic ATP production, even when maximal, cannot fully meet myocardial energy requirements. Furthermore, as lactate (the end-product of anaerobic glycolysis) and hydrogen ions accumulate due to lack of washout by normal blood flow, glycolysis is progressively inhibited by feedback mechanisms. By 10 minutes of ischemia, ATP production through this pathway is also markedly impaired.

Despite its critical dependence on aerobic metabolism, the heart extracts virtually the maximal amount of oxygen possible (about 75%) from the coronary blood flow. In contrast, most other tissues extract 20–25% of delivered oxygen. It is clear that an increased oxygen demand by the heart muscle must be met by a proportional increase in coronary flow. With a normally responsive coronary vasculature, a sensitive feedback mechanism matches coronary flow to the metabolic requirements of the heart.[3] As ATP utilization increases (or production decreases), levels of adenosine diphosphate (ADP) and adenosine monophosphate (AMP) rise. AMP is dephosphorylated to adenosine by 5'-nucleotidase in the cardiac cell. Adenosine is an extremely potent arteriolar vasodilator which increases coronary flow, providing more substrate and oxygen for ATP replenishment.

At rest ventricular oxygen consumption is about 9 ml/100 g/min.[4] At a heart rate of 80 beats/min about 20% of oxygen consumption is utilized by processes unrelated to electrical and mechanical activity directly but necessary for maintaining basal cellular integrity, e.g., protein synthesis and replacement of structural components. Electrical activity consumes less than 5% of myocardial energy, primarily to supply ATP to the Na^+-K^+ pump in order to maintain steady-state levels of sodium and potassium within the cell. The maintenance of these ionic gradients is crucial for the generation of normal action potentials which result from membrane voltage- and time-dependent changes in sarcolemmal ionic currents. Fifteen percent of oxygen consumption is required to pump calcium into the intracellular vesicular system, the sarcoplasmic reticulum, in order to maintain intracellular calcium concentration at low levels at which the myofilaments are relaxed. The remaining 60% of oxygen consumed is utilized for tension development, with 40% required to develop force within the cell ("internal tension"), which never appears as external work. These internal forces are applied to elastic and viscous structures in the cell. The other 20% of oxygen consumption is used to accomplish external work, i.e., to pump blood. With a component lost to heat, the overall mechanical efficiency of the heart as a pump is less than 20%.

Priorities of Energy Utilization during Myocardial Ischemia

In time, all aspects of cardiac function described above are impaired by myocardial ischemia. However, these functions do not fail with the same time course nor do they fail in an order predicted by the proportion of energy they consume. In isolated preparations, the two most rapid events, occurring within seconds of the onset of severe ischemia, are a slowing of the rate of relaxation before the force of contraction actually declines,[5] and a loss of cellular potassium.[6-11] Both events occur long before there is a significant decrease in total cellular ATP content. The defect in relaxation is probably related to a failure of intracellular Ca^{++} sequestration by the sarcoplasmic reticulum. The sarcoplasmic reticulum absorbs Ca^{++} against a marked concentration gradient using ATP as the source of energy. The Ca^{++} pumping ability of the sarcoplasmic reticulum may be more sensitive to the quantity of free energy released when a molecule of ATP is hydrolyzed than to the concentration of ATP per se.[12] The free energy of ATP hydrolysis is proportional to the log ([ATP]/[ADP]×[P_i]) and falls more rapidly than [ATP] during ischemia due to the accumulation of ADP and inorganic phosphate (P_i) as ATP is degraded. Cellular K^+ loss during ischemia is caused by an increased rate of K^+ efflux rather than decreased influx from suppression of the Na^+-K^+ pump.[6,8,10] The mechanisms responsible for the increased K^+ efflux will be discussed in detail later. In isolated cardiac preparations such as the rabbit interventricular septum, the development of active tension is the next function to deteriorate after 60 to 90 seconds of ischemia.[5] By contrast, in situ hearts may develop apparent systolic dysfunction (paradoxical systolic bulging) within seconds after coronary occlusion because of passive distension of the ischemic area by adjacent nonischemic and reflexively hypercontractile myocardium. Active tension development ceases completely by 5 minutes, at which time ATP levels are only modestly decreased, although creatine phosphate levels are significantly depressed by this time. The cause of the total loss of contractile force has not been conclusively determined, but a number of potential explanations have been proposed, some better supported by experimental evidence than others. These include: (1) the negative inotropic effect of intracellular acidosis, (2) reduction in intracellular Ca^{++} due to the rapid accumulation of P_i which exceeds the solubility product of $CaHPO_4$, (3) depletion of a critical compartmentalized pool of ATP at the myofilaments or at sites regulating Ca^{++} influx, (4) a decrease in the amount of Ca^{++} released from the sarcoplasmic reticulum as a result of the reduced Ca^{++} sequestration of the sarcoplasmic reticulum, (5) a decrease in transsarcolemmal Ca^{++} influx, and (6) collapse of the vascular space, which reduces myocardial stretch and shifts the heart to a lower position on the Starling curve.

Loss of systolic force development is followed by an increase in diastolic or rest tension, occurring at 7–10 minutes of ischemia in isolated hearts with development of full contracture after 20 minutes or greater.[13] It is controversial as to whether the early rise of rest tension is due to diastolic Ca^{++} overload or rigor from ATP depletion. The late contracture, however, is probably a direct result of depletion of ATP at the myofilaments, which prevents crossbridges between actin and myosin from detaching once formed. Total cellular levels of ATP are less than 50% of normal at this point.[13]

The final system to fail during ischemia is the Na^+-K^+ pump. Despite the marked cellular K^+ loss, intracellular $[Na^+]$ measured directly with ion selective electrodes does not increase for at least 15 minutes of global ischemia.[10] It is perhaps not surprising that the Na^+-K^+ pump is the last function to deteriorate, since from the standpoint of the cell's survival, the maintenance of ionic gradients is the cornerstone on which all electrical and contractile functions ultimately depend.

Electrophysiological Alterations during Acute Myocardial Ischemia

Figure 1 illustrates the time course of the changes in action potential configuration, extracellular $[K^+]$, and tension during global ischemia in an isolated arterially perfused rabbit interventricular septum. Electrophysiological alterations develop even more rapidly in the in situ heart, and include cellular depolarization, decreased excitability, depression of the action potential upstroke velocity (V_{max}), shortening of action potential duration, and altered refractoriness. These abnormalities cause marked slowing of conduction and eventually conduction block within the ischemic zone. During global ischemia, these changes are fairly homogenous and reentrant arrhythmias are infrequent. However, during regional ischemia, e.g., following coronary occlusion, the marked inhomogeneity in the electrophysiological properties between the ischemic and adjacent perfused tissue provides the ideal substrate for the development of reentrant arrhythmias. Injury currents arising from slowly conducting impulses in the ischemic zone may excite adjacent normal tissue, producing extrasystoles which then commonly act as the trigger for initiating reentrant ventricular tachycardia and fibrillation.[14] During the initial 20 minutes of ischemia, there is a high incidence of ventricular arrhythmias due to reentry.[15] As the ischemic zone becomes inexcitable, the frequency of arrhythmias decreases transiently for several hours after which ventricular extrasystoles reappear as a result of enhanced automaticity in damaged subendocardial Purkinje fibers overlying the area of infarct.[16]

Figure 2 shows the activation map of a three-beat run of ventricular tachycardia which occurred 7 minutes after the onset of regional ischemia in an isolated rabbit ventricle. The electrical activity at 128 sites over the surface of the left ventricle (flayed open along the posterior interventricular grove and pinned down as a sheet) was measured with a membrane potential sensitive optical dye

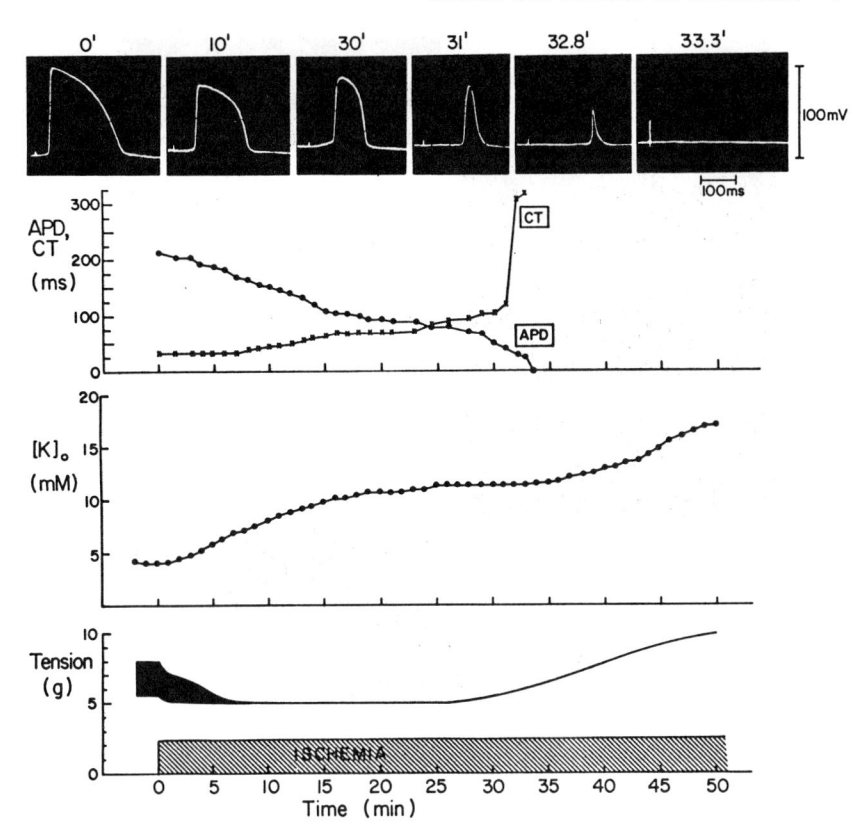

Figure 1: Changes in action potential duration, conduction time, [K$^+$]$_o$, and tension during a 50-minute period of global ischemia in an isolated rabbit interventricular septum. Upper panel shows representative action potentials recorded at various times after the onset of ischemia, from which action potential duration and conduction time from the site of stimulation to recording site have been measured and plotted in the graph below. The third panel shows the change in [K$^+$]$_o$ measured with an intramyocardial K$^+$ sensitive electrode, showing the triphasic pattern of [K$^+$]$_o$ accumulation. The lower panel shows changes in the peak systolic and diastolic tension during the ischemic period. The development of contracture coincides with the secondary rise in [K$^+$]$_o$. APD = action potential duration; CT = conduction time.

(WW 781) using a laser scanning system.[17] Representative optical signals from the surface of the preparation during the arrhythmia are shown in Figure 2A. Although the action potential configuration is distorted by mechanical artifacts, the upstroke can be readily identified. The activation maps constructed from the timing of the action potential upstroke at each point for the three beats are shown in Figure 2B-D. The first extrasystole arose in the normal myocardium, possibly induced by injury currents from the ischemic zone.[14] Conduction block occurred as this impulse spread across the border zone into the ischemic region at the base of the left ventricle, but the impulse was able to conduct slowly around the apex. As a result of the slow conduction in this region, the base recovered excitability and the impulse reentered the normal zone to initiate the second beat. The reentry circuit persisted for one more beat before bidirectional block occurred, extinguish-

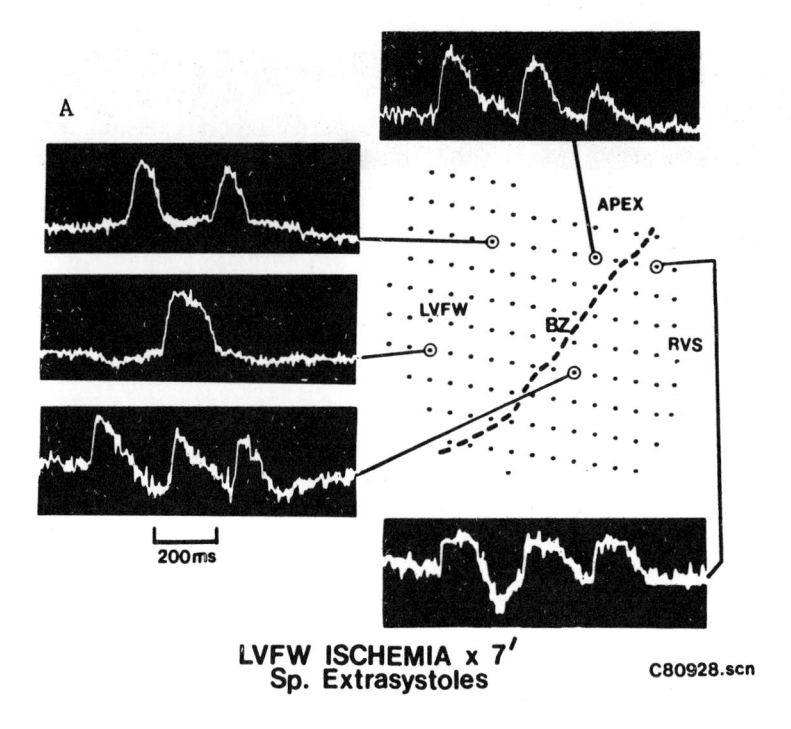

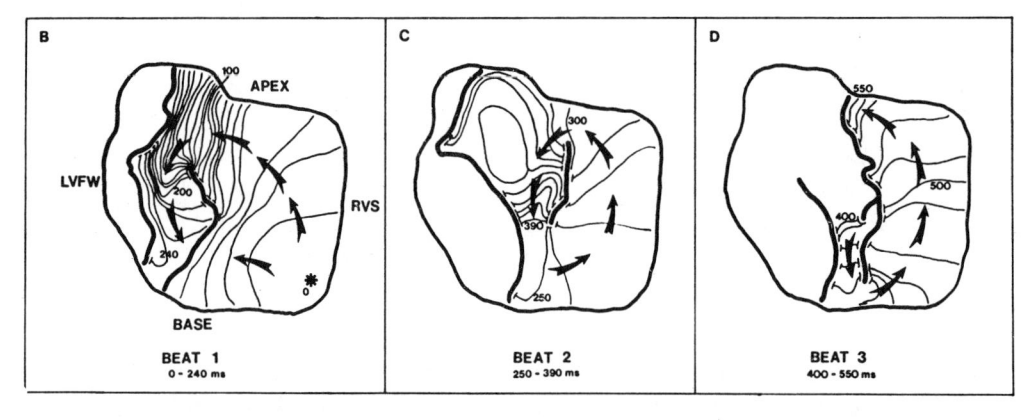

Figure 2: Activation mapping of a three-beat run of reentrant ventricular tachycardia during regional ischemia in an isolated rabbit ventricle. **A:** Electrical activity was measured over the surface of an arterially perfused isolated rabbit ventricle with the membrane potential sensitive dye WW 781, using a computer-controlled acousto-optical device directed laser beam to scan 128 sites (indicated by dots) every 4 ms. Optically measured action potentials from representative sites are shown during a three-beat run of ventricular tachycardia which occurred 7 minutes after coronary flow to the left ventricular free wall (LVFW) was stopped. Flow to the interventricular septum (RVS) was maintained. The border zone (BZ) between the two vascular beds is indicated by the dashed line.

Figure 2B–D: Activation maps of each of the three ventricular tachycardia beats reconstructed from the timing of the action potential upstroke at all 128 sites. Isochrome lines are 10 ms apart. Asterisk indicates the earliest site of activation of the first beat (time zero). Arrows show the direction of impulse spread for the beat 1 (0–240 ms), beat 2 (250–390 ms) and beat 3 (400–550 ms). Zones of block are indicated by the heavy lines.

ing the arrhythmia. Figure 3 shows the activation map for an arrhythmia due to enhanced automaticity, using the same laser scanning system. Although the arrhythmia in this case was induced by exposure to a toxic concentration of acetylstrophanthidin, a similar activation pattern might be expected in the setting of the late ischemic arrhythmias due to enhanced automaticity in damaged Purkinje fibers overlying the area of infarct. Note that the optically measured action potential configuration was more uniform over the surface of the preparation, and earliest activation occurred at the same site for each beat. Unlike the example of reentry in Figure 2, there was a long gap (approximately 250 ms) between the latest activation time of the first beat and the earliest activation time of the second beat.

Table I lists the major factors which contribute to the electrophysiological abnormalities causing arrhythmias during acute myocardial ischemia. Extracellular K^+ accumulation plays an important role in causing slowing of conduction and altered refractoriness leading to reentrant arrhythmias during the early phase of acute ischemia.[18-20] Studies in in vivo pig and dog hearts have documented increases in extracellular K^+ concentration ($[K^+]_o$) of up to 12 meq/l in the central ischemic zone within 10 minutes after coronary occlusion.[7-11] $[K^+]_o$ rises in a triphasic pattern characterized by an initial rapid increase leading to a plateau phase after about 10 minutes, followed by a secondary rise after about 25 minutes (Fig. 1). The latter phase probably reflects loss of sarcolemmal integrity and is associated with irreversible cellular damage on reperfusion.[7,8] Acidosis significantly exacerbates the electrophysiologic alterations produced by elevated $[K^+]_o$.[20] Lactate has electrophysiologic effects independent of its effects on pH.[21] Catecholamine release and its extracellular accumulation due to lack of washout is significant during ischemia and has frankly arrhythmogenic influences. By increasing intracellular cyclic AMP levels, catecholamines augment the slow Ca^{++} channel and facilitate slowly conducting action potentials and triggered and nontriggered automaticity in depressed myocardium. Activation of intracellular phospholipases during early ischemia results in the generation of lysophospholipids, such as lysophosphatidyl choline, which contribute to cyclic AMP elevation and also have marked electrophysiologic effects of their own.[22] These compounds cause a reduction in K^+ conductance leading to cellular depolarization,[23] and can produce changes in excitability, V_{max}, and refractoriness resembling ischemia. Their effects are potentiated by acidosis. Derangements in fatty acid metabolism during ischemia lead to the intracellular accumulation of fatty acid esters, particularly long chain acyl carnitines, which have been shown to cause electrophysiological alterations mimicking ischemia.[22] Fatty acid esters may interfere with the Na^+-K^+ pump and intracellular membrane-mediated function as well. Both lysophospholipids and fatty acid esters are thought to act in low concentrations by inserting into membranes and modifying their functions, and in higher concentrations via a detergent-like effect. Whether they accumulate rapidly enough and in sufficient quantity to account for the earliest electrophysiological changes during ischemia remains controversial, however. Elevated free fatty acids may also have direct arrhythmogenic effects in ischemic tissue.[22] Finally, the generation of the free radicals during ischemia and reperfusion has recently received a great deal of attention as a potential mediator of membrane

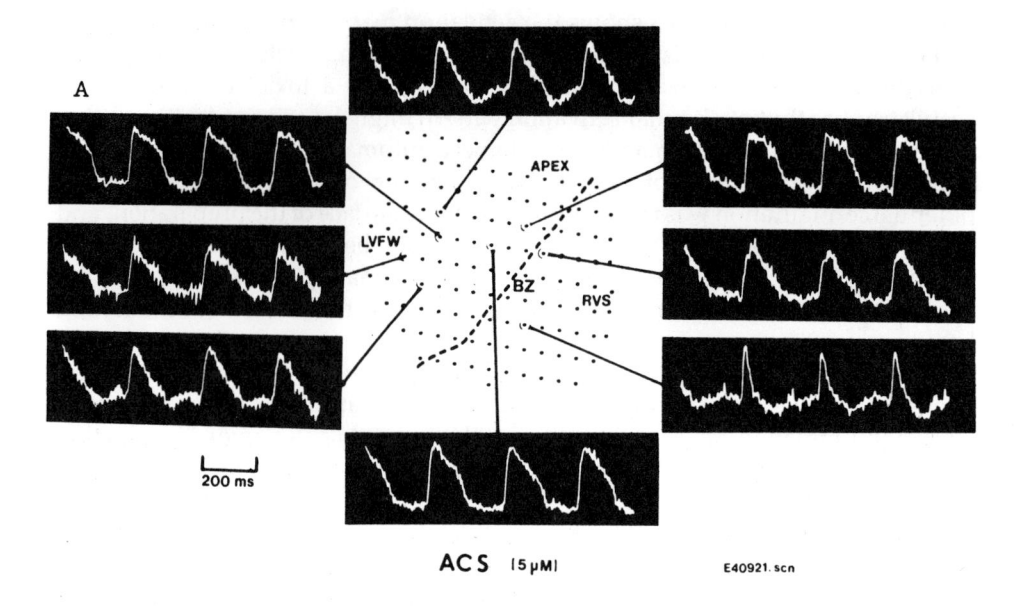

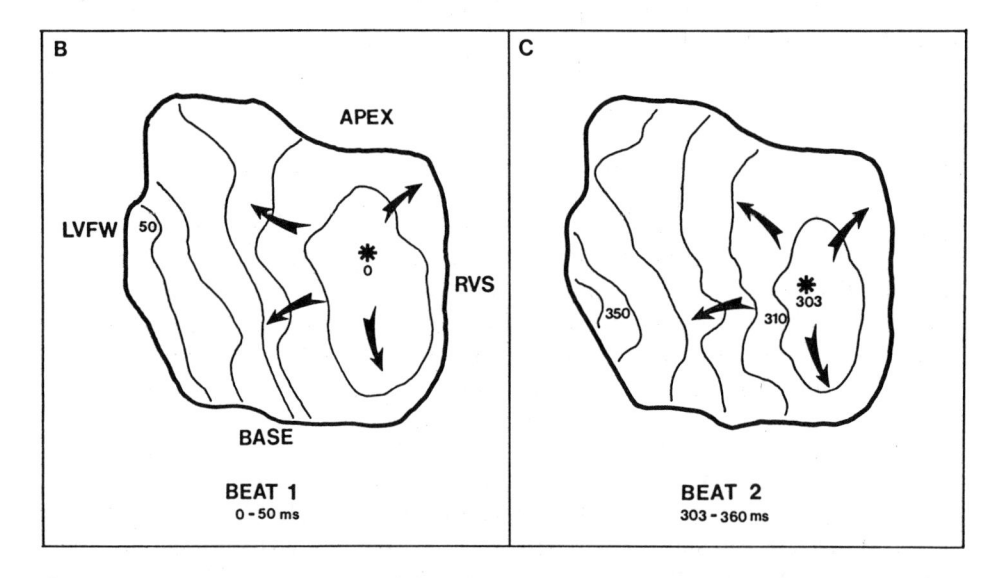

Figure 3: Activation mapping of automatic ventricular tachycardia in an isolated arterially perfused rabbit ventricle. **A:** Optically detected action potentials from representative points on the surface of the ventricle were recorded during automatic ventricular tachycardia using the laser scanning system described in Figure 2. The tachycardia occurred after exposure to a toxic concentration (5 μM) of the cardiac glycoside acetylstrophanthidin (ACS).
Figure 3B,C: Activation maps of two beats of tachycardia. Earliest detected electrical activity for both beats (indicated by an asterisk) began in the same region and fully activated the ventricle in 50–60 ms. The second beat began after an electrically silent gap of approximately 250 ms. Isochrome lines are 10 ms apart. LVFW = left ventricular free wall, RVS = interventricular septum.

Table I
Factors Contributing to Electrophysiologic Abnormalities during Acute Ischemia

Elevated extracellular [K^+]
Intracellular acidosis
Lactate accumulation
Catecholamine release
Elevated intracellular cyclic adenosine monophosphate
Lysophospholipid accumulation
Fatty acid ester accumulation
Free fatty acid accumulation
Free radicals

---

dysfunction.[24] Free radicals may produce marked electrophysiological changes in isolated preparations,[25] and free radical scavengers reduce the incidence of reperfusion arrhythmias.[26] However, their precise role in ischemic arrhythmogenesis is unestablished.

The individual importance of each of the various factors listed above in ischemic arrhythmogenesis has been difficult to quantify because ischemia is a non-steady-state condition in which both the impairment of metabolism and the accumulation of toxic metabolic byproducts due to lack of washout contribute to cardiac dysfunction. However, considerable information about how these factors interact to produce the marked electrophysiological alterations has been gained from studies in cardiac preparations in which the arterial perfusate has been modified to simulate various components of the ischemic environment. Without diminishing the importance of the other factors, I would now like to describe some of the recent experimental findings relating to the mechanism of the marked cellular K^+ loss which occurs in response to metabolic inhibition in heart.

Mechanisms of Cellular K^+ Loss during Myocardial Ischemia and Hypoxia

It is now well established that cellular K^+ loss during early acute ischemia results from an increase in K^+ efflux rather than a decrease in K^+ influx.[6,8,10] Several mechanisms may contribute to the increase in K^+ efflux during ischemia: (1) an increase in $[K^+]_o$ due to movement of free water from the extracellular to intracellular space as osmotically active metabolic byproducts, e.g., lactate and inorganic phosphate (P_i), accumulate intracellularly,[27] (2) K^+ efflux linked to the efflux of intracellularly-generated anions such as lactate and P_i in order to maintain neutral net charge movement across the sarcolemma,[28,29] (3) an increase in sarcolemmal [K^+] conductance.[30–32] The first mechanism cannot account for the increased K^+ efflux observed during other metabolic insults such as hypoxia in which flow is maintained, and is clearly not the sole mechanism operating during ischemia. This factor could significantly augment the magnitude of $[K^+]_o$ accumulation during ischemia, however. Support for the second mechanism comes from the observation that on a mole-per-mole basis, the quantity of anion loss (lactate + P_i) during ischemia exceeds K^+ loss by a factor of 2 to 3[28] (Fig. 4). Other evidence, however, indicates that anion and K^+ loss during ischemia are not closely coupled.[33]

Figure 5 compares the magnitude of K^+, lactate, P_i, and pyruvate loss during successive 10 minute periods of ischemia in eight isolated arterially perfused rabbit septa. One period of ischemia was preceded by 10 minutes of exposure to glucose-free perfusate in order to diminish the ability of the preparation to produce lactate during the ischemic period. The other period of ischemia served as the control, and the order was reversed in half the preparations. As expected, pre-exposure to the substrate-free perfusate reduced lactate loss during ischemia by 20 ± 3% ($p < 0.005$). P_i loss was not significantly changed, and total anion loss decreased by 16 ± 4% ($p < 0.02$). K^+ loss, however, increased by 29 ± 12% ($p < 0.05$). Similarly, during hypoxia with maintained flow, omission of glucose from the hypoxic perfusate resulted in reduced lactate loss (and no change in P_i loss) but increased K^+ loss.[33] These findings indicate that although anion efflux during ischemia and hypoxia must be accompanied by the equal and opposite charge movement of some ionic specie(s), K^+ is not the predominant ion which serves this function. H^+ is a more likely candidate since in the case of lactate, the lactic acid molecule is much more membrane-permeable than the lactate ion. These results do not exclude the possibility that a portion of the increased K^+ efflux during ischemia and hypoxia is coupled to anion efflux.

The third potential mechanism of K^+ loss during ischemia is a change in the membrane conductance to K^+ ions. Unfortunately, it is not currently possible to voltage-clamp truly ischemic cardiac muscle in order to analyze the time course of

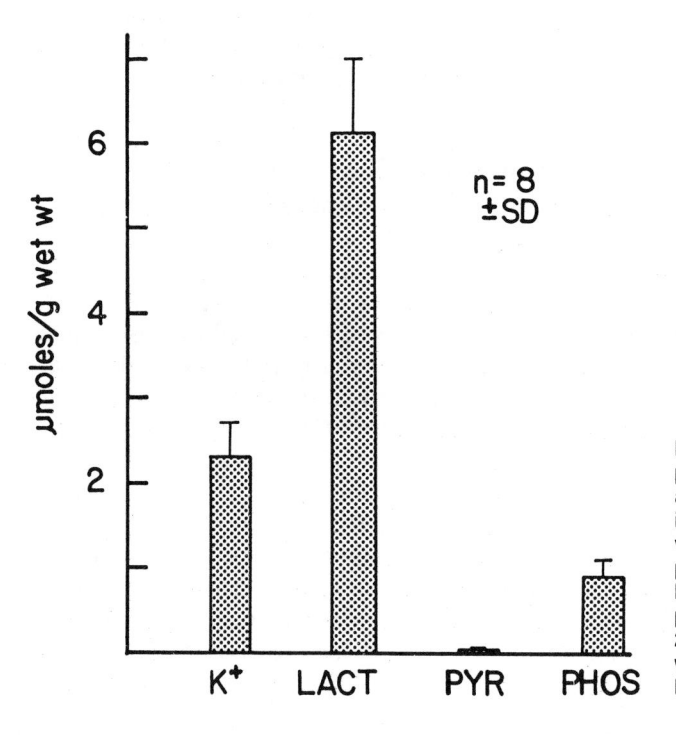

Figure 4: Quantitative comparison of magnitudes of K^+ vs anion loss during 10 minutes of ischemia in isolated rabbit interventricular septa. On a mole-per-mole basis, the ratio of K^+ : lactate (LACT) : inorganic phosphate (PHOS) loss was 1.0 : 2.7 : 0.4. Pyruvate (PYR) loss was insignificant compared to K^+ loss.

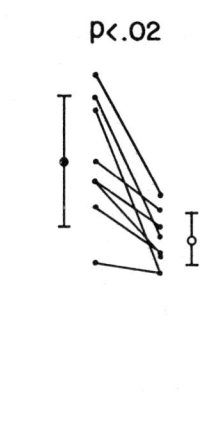

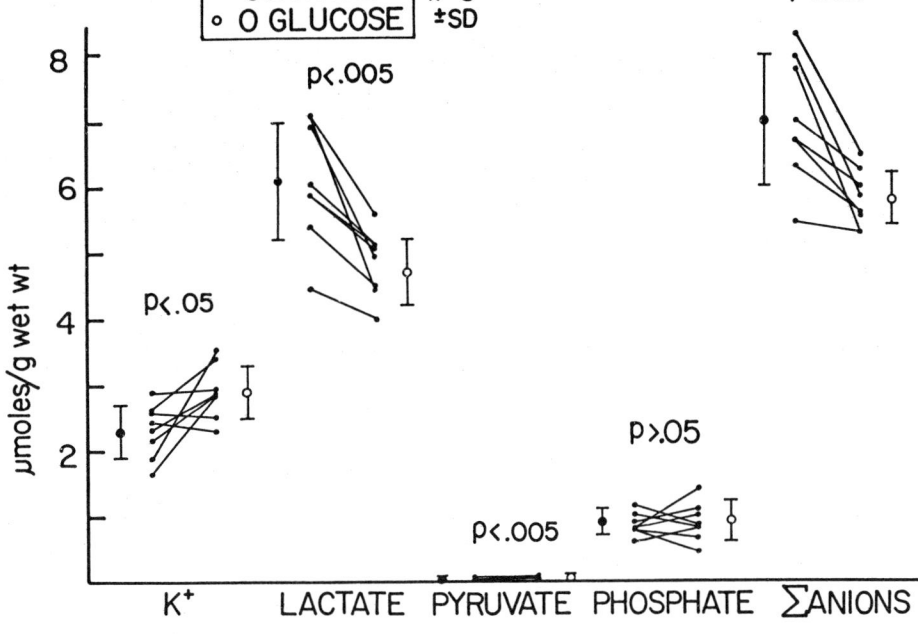

Figure 5: The effect of preexposure to substrate-free perfusate on K$^+$ vs anion loss during ischemia. Net loss of K$^+$, lactate, pyruvate, inorganic phosphate, and the sum of the latter three anions are compared during two sequential 10 minute periods of ischemia in eight isolated rabbit septa. One period of ischemia (O GLU) was preceded by a 10 minute exposure to glucose-free perfusate immediately prior to ischemia; the other ischemic period (CONTROL) served as the control. The order was reversed in half of the experiments. Lines connect the values obtained from individual preparations, with the mean and standard deviation of each group shown alongside. Paired t-tests were used to assess statistical significance.

changes in ionic currents. However, voltage-clamp studies in both multicellular and single cell cardiac preparations during exposure to hypoxia and metabolic inhibitors have demonstrated abnormalities in K$^+$ currents.[30–32] Voltage-clamped papillary muscles develop an increase in background K$^+$ currents when subjected to hypoxia.[30,31] In enzymatically isolated single ventricular cells, exposure to either hypoxia or metabolic inhibitors produces a marked increase in K$^+$ conductance which can be completely prevented by dialyzing the interior of the cell with ATP[35] (Fig. 7). Figure 6 shows records from a guinea pig ventricular cell which has been exposed to metabolic inhibitors. During the 50 ms voltage-clamp pulse, a progressive increase in outward current can be seen with each beat. The current voltage relation indicates that the large outward current reverses near the K$^+$ equilibrium potential E_K. Because the outward current is so large at membrane potentials in the range of the action potential plateau, marked action potential shortening results[32] (Fig. 11), similar to that during ischemia in multicellular preparations (Fig. 1). The relevance of these findings to ischemia in the intact heart, however, is uncertain. In particular, it is unclear whether these abnormal K$^+$ currents could be activated early enough to account for the rapidity of onset of

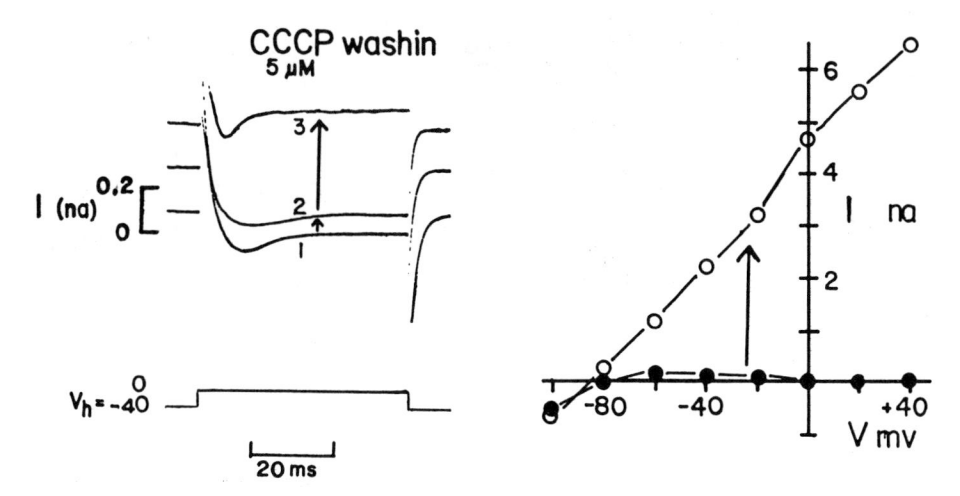

Figure 6: Effects of metabolic inhibition on ionic currents in a voltage-clamped single guinea pig ventricular myocyte. The tracing to the left shows superimposed 50 ms voltage clamps applied every 5 sec from a holding membrane potential of −40 mv to 0 mv. About 5 minutes after the mitochondrial inhibitor CCCP (5 μm) + the glycolytic inhibitor 2-deoxyglucose (20 mM) were washed in, the current became progressively more outward (upward direction) with each successive clamp (labeled 1−3). The current-voltage relations under control conditions (filled circles) and after 5 minutes' exposure to the metabolic inhibitors (open circles) are shown on the right. Note that the direction of the latter current reverses near E_K, and is very large (outward) at positive membrane potentials compared to control.

ischemic K^+ loss. Indirect evidence suggesting that increased K^+ conductance may occur quite early has been derived from studies of the effects of heart rate on $[K^+]_o$ accumulation during ischemia.[34] At faster rates, the heart spends a greater portion of time in the depolarized state, where the driving force for K^+ to leave the cell is very large in comparison to the diastolic driving force. If an increase in K^+ conductance underlies the increase in K^+ efflux during ischemia, then one might expect the cumulative time spent in the depolarized (systolic) state to be a more important determinant of the magnitude of $[K^+]_o$ accumulation than the total duration (systolic + diastolic) of ischemia. Figure 7 shows that this was the case in the arterially perfused rabbit septum paced at 75 or 150 beats per minute. For example, at 75 bpm the cumulative time depolarized after a total of 5 minutes of ischemia was 1 minute, at which time $[K^+]_o$ was approximately 8 mM. At 150 bpm, the same cumulative time depolarized was achieved after only 2.5 minutes of ischemia, and K^+ was also approximately 8 mM at this point (Fig. 7A). However, after the same total duration of ischemia (5 minutes) at 150 bpm, $[K^+]_o$ was approximately 10.5 mM (Fig. 7B).

The ATP-Sensitive K^+ Channel

The ability to record current passing through single ionic channels with the gigaseal patch-clamp technique[36] has contributed greatly to our understanding of the metabolically sensitive K^+ currents described above. The patch-clamp tech-

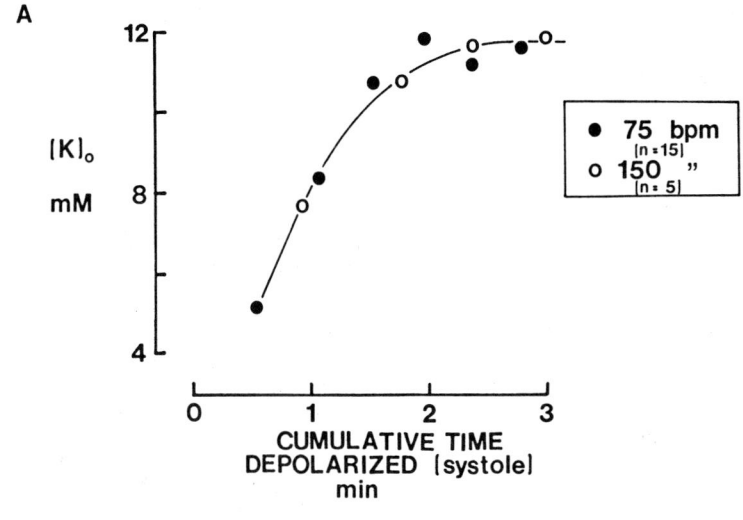

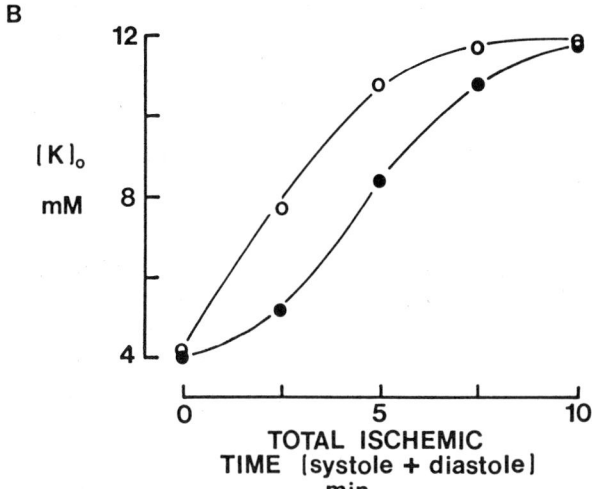

Figure 7: The level of $[K^+]_o$ accumulation plotted as a function of either the cumulative time spent depolarized during ischemia (**A**) or the total duration of ischemia (**B**) at two different heart rates, 75 bpm (closed circles) and 150 bpm (open circles) in isolated rabbit interventricular septa. At each heart rate the action potential duration was measured during ischemia and summed over time to estimate the total time spent depolarized (systole) after various total durations (systole + diastole) of ischemia. Intracellular potential was recorded with floating glass microelectrodes and $[K^+]_o$ with extracellular valinomycin K^+ selective electrodes.

nique is schematically illustrated in Figure 8. Briefly, a glass microelectrode with a tip diameter of 1–2 µ is brought into contact with the surface membrane of the cell. Gentle suction is applied to form a very high resistance ($>10^{10}$ ohms) seal between the glass rim of the electrode and the membrane. With a very high seal resistance, if a voltage difference is imposed between the electrode and the bath (grounded), the only pathway for current flow is through the membrane patch in the tip of the electrode. This membrane patch also has a very high resistance unless an ionic channel is present and happens to open. When a channel does open, the resistance of the patch suddenly decreases and the amount of current necessary to hold the voltage at the same level increases proportionately according to Ohm's law. Openings and closings of individual ionic channels are thus detected as stepwise jumps in current necessary to clamp the voltage to a constant

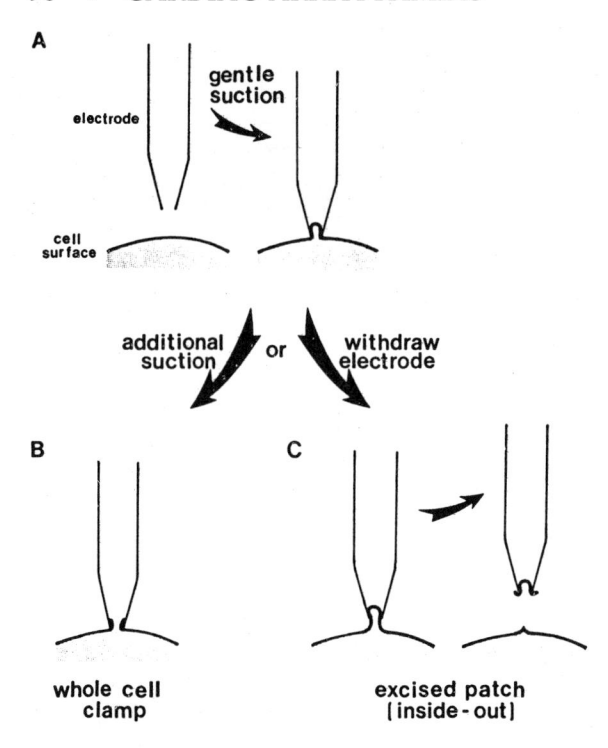

Figure 8: The tight gigaseal patch clamp technique. **A:** The patch electrode (tip diameter 1–2 μ) is brought into contact with the surface membrane of the cell and light suction applied to form a high resistance seal (>10^{10} ohms) between the bath and the electrode. **B:** Additional suction can be applied after the initial seal to rupture the membrane patch in the tip of the electrode in order to voltage-clamp the whole cell or record the action potential. **C:** Alternatively, after the initial seal is formed the electrode can be withdrawn from the cell, excising a patch of membrane in the tip of the electrode. In this configuration (inside-out patch) the surface of the membrane previously facing the cytoplasm now faces the bath.

predetermined level (Fig. 9). After a high resistance seal has been formed with the electrode, additional suction can be applied to rupture the patch (Fig. 8B) in order to voltage-clamp the whole cell, as in Figure 6. Alternatively, the electrode can be withdrawn after the seal is formed, excising altogether the patch of membrane from the cell to create an inside-out patch. The latter configuration allows complete control over the environment of both the cytoplasmic and extracellular surface of the membrane patch by manipulating the contents of the solutions in the electrode and the bath. If an inside-out patch is excised from a mammalian ventricular cell, the normal cardiac K$^+$ channels which pass current only in an inward direction are observed as long as ATP is present in the solution bathing the cytoplasmic surface of the membrane patch. If the ATP is removed, however, a much larger K$^+$ current appears which passes current in both the inward and outward direction[35,37,38] (Fig. 9). This ATP-sensitive K$^+$ channel is the same channel that causes the large outward current in response to metabolic inhibition (Figs. 6,11).

A major difficulty in attributing K$^+$ loss during ischemia to activation of the ATP-sensitive K$^+$ channel is that the threshold concentration of ATP which completely suppresses the channel is very low (approximately 0.2 mM).[35] Normal ATP levels in the cytoplasm are 3–5 mM, and after 10 minutes of ischemia, ATP has generally fallen by only one-third. There is some evidence that in the intact cell, a higher concentration of ATP (approximately 2 mM) may be necessary to suppress activity of the ATP-sensitive K$^+$ channel,[38] but even at this threshold it is unlikely that the channel would be activated during the early minutes of

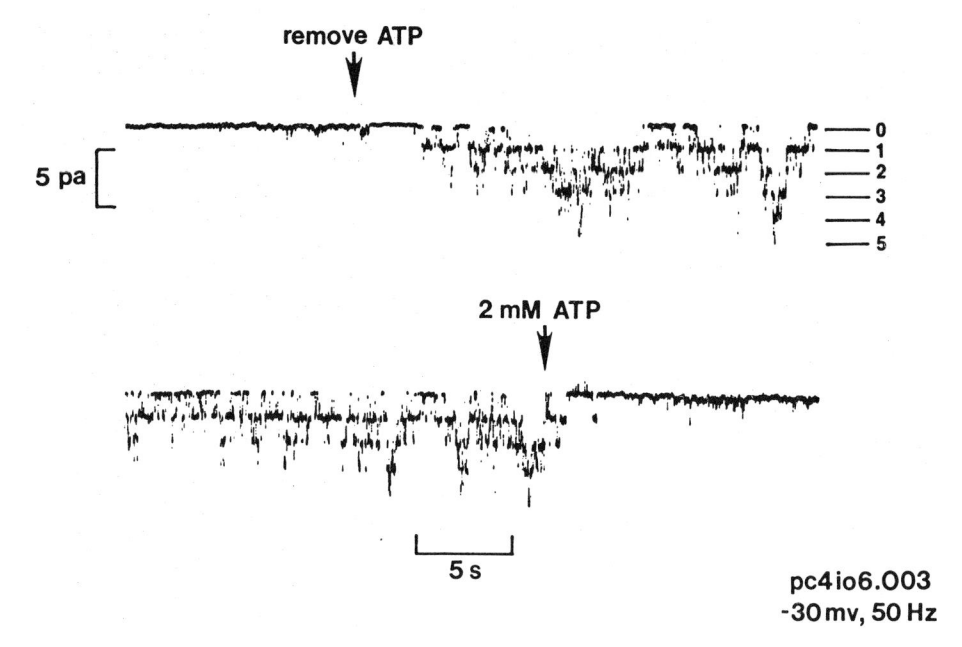

Figure 9: Single channel current recording of the ATP-sensitive K$^+$ channel. An inside-out membrane patch was excised from a guinea pig ventricular myocyte (see Fig. 8) and voltage-clamped to a potential of -30 mv (bath relative to inside of electrode). With 2 mM ATP in the bath (facing the cytoplasmic surface of the membrane patch), no channel openings were detected, i.e., the current required to clamp the potential difference across the membrane at -30 mv was constant. When ATP was removed from the bath, however, five levels of current steps (right upper tracing) were observed, indicating openings of at least five separate ionic channels. Replacing ATP (at arrow) promptly suppressed openings of these channels. The electrode and bath solutions contained respectively (in mM): 150 KCl, 5 HEPES, pH 7.3; and 150 KCl, 5 HEPES, 2 EGTA, 0.5 CaCl$_2$, 2 MgCl$_2$, with or without 2 MgATP, pH 7.1. Current tracings were filtered at 50 Hz. Inward current is downward.

ischemia. One possibility is that the sensitivity of the ATP-sensitive K$^+$ channel to ATP is altered by factors such as metabolic byproducts accumulating during early ischemia (Table I). We have found that exposure of the rabbit septal preparation to hydrogen peroxide, which is both a product and a source of free radicals during ischemia, resulted in an almost immediate increase in K$^+$ efflux at concentrations as low as 10 μM (Fig. 10). In single rat or guinea pig ventricular myocytes, 1 mM hydrogen peroxide caused activation of a large outward K$^+$ current indistinguishable from that induced by metabolic inhibitors (Fig. 11). Dialyzing the interior of the cell with 5 mM ATP, however, prevented activation of this current by metabolic inhibitors, but not by hydrogen peroxide. Thus hydrogen peroxide, either by a direct effect or through the generation of free radicals, appears to interfere with the ability of ATP to suppress ATP-sensitive K$^+$ channel. Other components of ischemia (see Table I) could also potentially affect the ATP sensitivity of this channel, but they have not yet been investigated in this context.

Alternatively, compartmentation of ATP in the heart might also explain why the ATP-sensitive K$^+$ channel would be activated earlier during ischemia than predicted from total cellular levels of ATP. According to this hypothesis, a com-

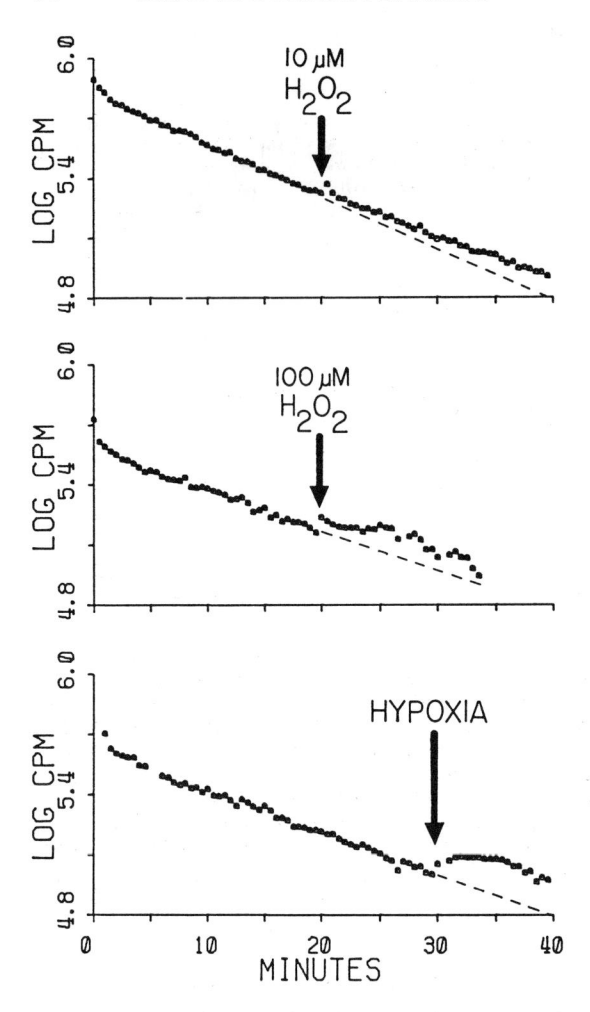

Figure 10: Effects of hydrogen peroxide (H_2O_2) vs hypoxia on the rate of $^{42}K^+$ washout in isolated rabbit septa. After loading preparations with $^{42}K^+$ for approximately 50 minutes, washout with "cold" perfusate (no $^{42}K^+$) was begun and timed venous effluent samples were collected and their $^{42}K^+$ activity measured. After establishing the control rate of $^{42}K^+$ washout, the preparations were exposed either to hydrogen peroxide or hypoxia at the arrow. An immediate increase in the effluent $^{42}K^+$ activity was seen in both cases.

partmentalized pool of ATP preferentially supplying ATP to the ATP-sensitive K^+ channel might be depleted more rapidly during ischemia than is reflected by measurements of total cellular ATP content. Although compartmentation of metabolic energy in heart remains a highly controversial topic, there is evidence in support of this hypothesis. Based on the observation that creatine phosphate levels fall much more rapidly than ATP levels during ischemia despite the rapid kinetics of the creatine kinase reaction, Gudbjarnason and co-workers[39] postulated that ATP becomes effectively trapped in mitochondria during ischemia, unable to be used in the cytoplasm by energy-consuming processes. Recently ^{31}P-nuclear magnetic resonance studies have supported the existence of the creatine phosphate energy shuttle, in which creatine phosphate acts as a preferential shuttle mechanism for transporting ATP from the mitochondria to the contractile apparatus.[40] Other evidence suggests that high energy phosphates generated via mitochondrial metabolism are used preferentially for tension development, whereas glycolytically generated high energy phosphates are used pref-

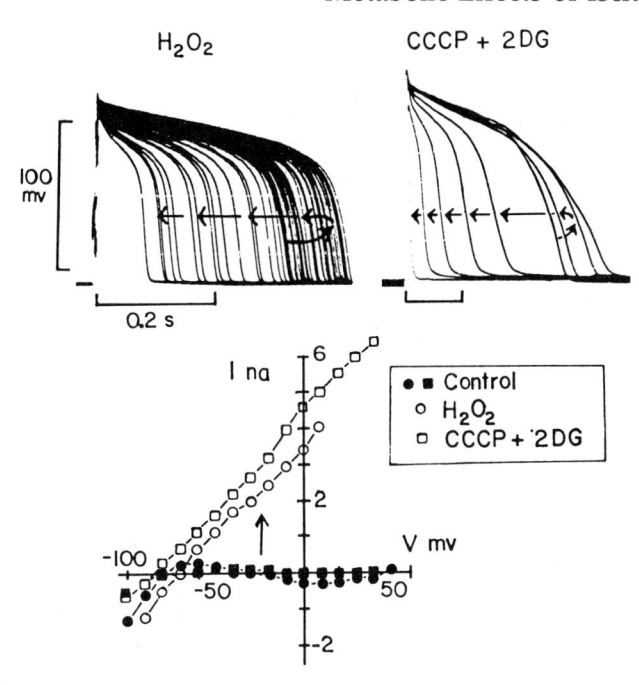

Figure 11: Comparison of the efffects of hydrogen peroxide vs metabolic inhibitors on the action potential and current-voltage relations in single guinea pig ventricular myocytes, using the patch-clamp technique (whole cell clamp configuration shown in Fig. 8B). Upper left tracing of superimposed action potentials shows that in response to 1 mM hydrogen peroxide (H_2O_2), the action potential duration transiently prolonged and then shortened progressively until the cell became inexcitable. This effect was almost identical to that produced by exposure to the combination of the mitochondrial inhibitor CCCP (5 μM) and glycolytic inhibitor 2-deoxyglucose (20 mM). The current-voltage relations under both conditions are shown in the graph below (50 ms clamp duration, holding potential −40 mv). The patch electrode solution dialyzing the interior of the cell contained 5 mM MgATP during exposure to hydrogen peroxide, but no ATP during exposure to the metabolic inhibitors.

erentially to support sarcolemmal function.[41–46] For example, during low flow ischemia in the isolated Langendorff rat heart, concomitant inhibition of glycolysis resulted in much greater enzyme loss and contracture development on reperfusion (reflecting more severe membrane damage) than concomitant inhibition of oxidative metabolism. Total cellular levels of high energy phosphates were nearly identical in the two cases, however.[42,46] This finding was interpreted to indicate that glycolytically generated ATP was more effective in protecting membrane function during ischemia than oxidatively generated ATP. With regard to K^+ loss, in the isolated arterially perfused rabbit septum, selective inhibition of oxidative metabolism caused marked loss of developed tension, but only modest $[K^+]_o$ accumulation measured with intramyocardial K^+ sensitive electrodes.[45] In contrast, selective inhibition of glycolysis had little effect on developed tension but caused marked $[K^+]_o$ accumulation (Fig. 12). The dosages of the metabolic inhibitors (iodoacetate [IAA], dinitrophenol [DNP], and sodium azide) were adjusted so that total cellular levels of high energy phosphates were not significantly different from control despite causing marked abnormalities in cardiac

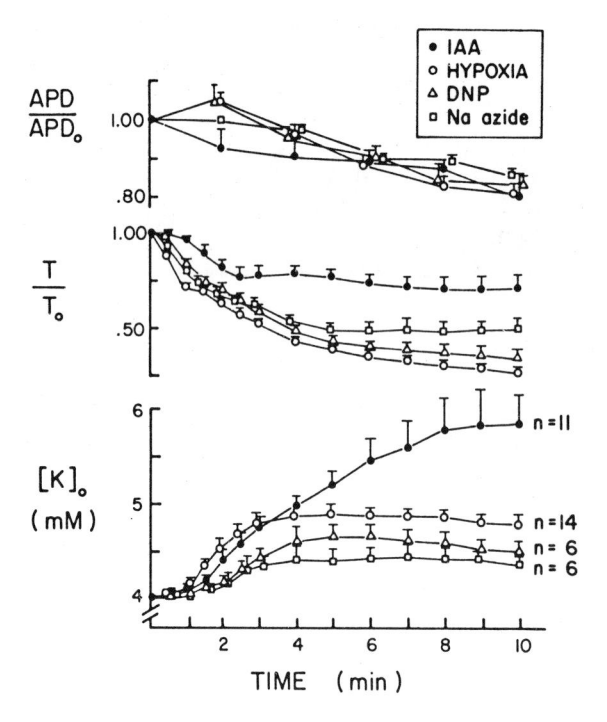

Figure 12: Comparison of the effects of selective inhibition of glycolytic versus oxidative metabolism on action potential duration (APD/APD$_o$), tension (T/T$_o$) and [K$^+$]$_o$ accumulation in isolated arterially perfused rabbit interventricular septa. Glycolysis was inhibited by adding 1 mM iodoacetate (IAA) to glucose-free perfusate containing pyruvate as substrate for oxidative metabolism (filled circles). Oxidative metabolism was inhibited with either hypoxia (open circles), 0.01 mM dinitrophenol (DNP) (triangles), or 1 mM Na azide (squares) with glucose present as substrate for glycolysis. Values are mean ± SE.

function. The interpretation of these findings was that during selective partial inhibition of oxidative metabolism, glycolysis accelerated to maintain normal total cellular levels of high energy phosphates, but the glycolytically generated high energy phosphates could not be effectively used by the contractile apparatus to maintain normal tension. Conversely, during selective inhibition of glycolysis, oxidatively generated high energy phosphates could not be effectively used by the sarcolemma to prevent cellular K$^+$ loss. If it exists in heart, compartmentation of metabolic energy is only partial because combined inhibition of glycolytic and oxidative metabolism had much more severe effects on cellular K$^+$ loss and force development than selective inhibition of either pathway alone.[45] One mechanism by which glycolysis could potentially provide a preferential supply of ATP to ATP-sensitive K$^+$ channels is if glycolytic enzymes were bound to the sarcolemma in the immediate vicinity of the channels. Sarcolemmal-bound glycolytic enzymes appear to act as a preferential source of ATP for sarcolemmal functions in other tissue.[47,48] To test this hypothesis in heart we studied the effects of glycolytic substrates on activity of the ATP-sensitive K$^+$ channel in excised inside-out membrane patches from guinea pig ventricular myocytes. If glycolytic enzymes were bound to the sarcolemma and remained functional when a membrane patch was excised, then when provided with the appropriate substrates they might be capable of generating sufficient ATP locally to prevent ATP-sensitive K$^+$ channels from opening when exogenous ATP was removed. In one excised inside-out patch, the combination of 2 mM phosphoenolpyruvate (PEP) and 0.5 mM ADP, which are converted to pyruvate and ATP by the glycolytic enzyme pyruvate kinase, was effective in preventing the ATP-sensitive K$^+$ channels from opening when exogenous ATP was removed (Fig. 13). In the same

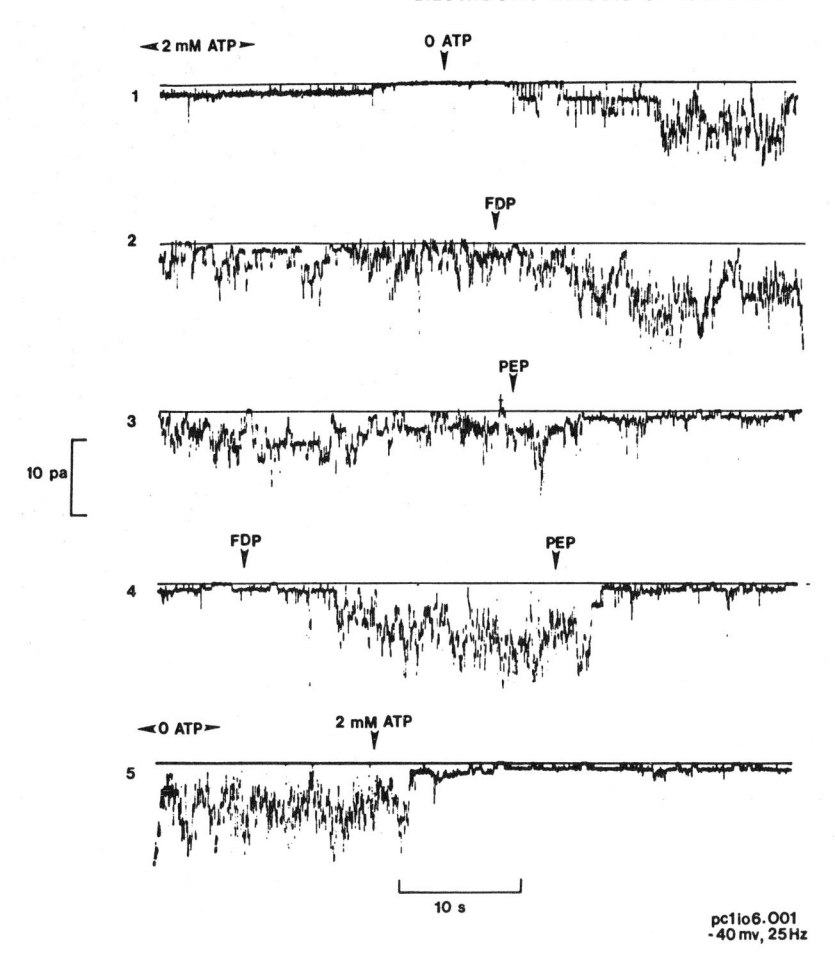

Figure 13: Effects of glycolytic substrates on the ATP-sensitive K$^+$ channel. Tracings show single channel current recordings from an inside-out patch excised from a guinea pig ventricular myocyte and voltage-clamped to a potential of −40 mv (bath with respect to inside of the electrode). In tracing 1, with 2 mM ATP present in the bath solution (facing the cytoplasmic surface of the membrane patch) a long opening of an inwardly rectifying (normal) K$^+$ channel occurred at beginning of the record. The magnitude of the current step for this single channel was 2−3 times smaller than the magnitude of single ATP-sensitive K$^+$ channels, which began to open as soon as ATP was removed from the bath solution (arrow). Tracing 2 shows that adding the combination of glycolytic substrates labelled FDP which included 2 mM fructose 1,6-diphsophate, 1 mM NAD, 1 mM P$_i$, and 0.5 mM ADP did not suppress openings of the ATP-sensitive K$^+$ channels. However, in tracing 3, the combination labelled PEP (2 mM phosphoenolpyruvate + 0.5 mM ADP), substrates for an ATP-producing step further in the glycolytic sequence, did reversibly suppress the ATP-sensitive K$^+$ channel. The smaller inwardly-rectifying K$^+$ channel remained active in the presence of PEP. In tracing 4, replacement of PEP with the FDP substrates again caused the ATP-sensitive K$^+$ channels to open reversibly in this patch. Tracing 5 shows that the ATP-sensitive K$^+$ channels were again active after all the glycolytic substrates were removed (0 ATP), and were completely suppressed by 2 mM ATP, leaving only the normal inwardly rectifying K$^+$ channel actively opening and closing. The electrode and bath solutions were the same as in Figure 9 with various substrates added as described above. Tracings 1−3 are continuous. The zero current level is indicated by the thin narrow line in each tracing, with inward current downward. Tracings were filtered at 25 Hz. Some artifacts are present due to the rapid perfusion rate during the recordings.

patch, a combination of substrates more proximal in the glycolytic sequence including 2 mM fructose 1,6-diphosphate, 1 mM NAD, 1 mM P_i, and 0.5 mM ADP did not suppress activity of the channels. In nine subsequent inside-out patches, however, the above substrates were ineffective in suppressing the ATP-sensitive K^+ channel. Although it is possible that the glycolytic enzymes may have become nonfunctional or dislodged in the process of excising the patch, these experimental findings do not convincingly support the hypothesis that glycolytic enzymes bound to the sarcolemma act as a preferential source of ATP for the ATP-sensitive $[K^+]$ channel.

Conclusions

It is apparent from the discussion of cellular K^+ loss during ischemia in the preceding sections that many questions remain as to both the fundamental mechanisms involved and the quantitative contribution of this factor to ischemic arrhythmias. Although they have not been discussed in detail, a similar situation applies to most of the other factors listed in Table I which have been implicated in ischemic arrhythmogenesis. Arrhythmias during acute ischemia remain the single most common cause of mortality from coronary artery disease, and account for the majority of nontraumatic sudden deaths in our society. Despite the great amount of effort that has gone into unravelling the pathophysiology of this problem, the impact on the clinical management of acute ischemic arrhythmias is severely limited by the fact that most events occur outside of a controlled setting such as the coronary care unit. Because of this limitation, the prevention of atherosclerosis and aggressive early detection and treatment of coronary artery disease before myocardial infarction occurs will have the greatest impact on cardiovascular mortality. Nevertheless, elucidation of the basic mechanisms relating cardiac metabolism and function will continue to play a crucial role in improving methods for implementing the above strategies (e.g., enhancing myocardial preservation during cardiopulmonary bypass) and improving the in-hospital and paramedic-assisted management of myocardial ischemia. Understanding the mechanisms of ischemic arrhythmogenesis in greater detail may also suggest strategies for reducing the risk of sudden death from myocardial infarction in the out-of-hospital setting.

Acknowledgments: This work was supported by USPHS grants HL27846, HL36729, and Research Career Development Award HL01890; by American Heart Association Grants-in-Aid 83-626 and 736 G2 (Greater Los Angeles Affiliate); and by the Laubisch Cardiovascular Research Endowment. For their generous help, advice, and collaborative efforts in parts of this work, I would like to express my appreciation to Kenneth Shine, Glenn Langer, Richard Weiss, Martin Morad, Steven Dillon, Raman Mitra, Richard Horn, Scott Lamp, Joshua Goldhaber, and Bradley Hiltbrand. The experiments using the laser scanning technique (Figs. 2 & 3) were performed at the University of Pennsylvania in collaboration with Drs. Dillon and Morad.

References

1. Goldman L, Cook F, Hashimoto B, Stone P, Muller J, Loscalzo A. Evidence that hospital care for acute myocardial infarction has not contributed to the decline in coronary mortality between 1973–1974 and 1978–1979. Circulation 1982;65:936–42.

2. Kobayashi K, Neely JR. Control of maximum rates of glycolysis in rat cardiac muscle. Circ Res. 1979;44:166−75.
3. Berne RM, Knabb RM, Ely SW, Rubio R. Adenosine in the regulation of blood flow; a brief overview. Fed Proc. 1983;42:3136−42.
4. Gibbs CL, Chapman JB. Cardiac energetics. In Berne RM, Sperelakis N, Geiger S, eds. *Handbook of Physiology, The Cardiovascular System.* Bethesda, MD. American Physiological Society, 1979;775−804.
5. Shine KI, Douglas AM, Ricchiuti NV. Ischemia in isolated ventricular septa: Mechanical events. Am J Physiol 1976;231:1225−32.
6. Shine KI, Douglas AM, Ricchiuti NV. ^{42}K exchange during myocardial ischemia. Am J Physiol 1977;232:H564−70.
7. Hill JL, Gettes LS. Effect of acute coronary artery occlusion on local myocardial extracellular K^+ activity in swine. Circulation 1980;61:768−78.
8. Weiss J, Shine KI. Extracellular K^+ accumulation during myocardial ischemia in isolated rabbit heart. Am J Physiol 1982;242:H619−28.
9. Hirche HJ, Franz CHR, Bos L, Bissig R, Lang R, Schramm, M. Myocardial extracellular K^+ and H^+ increase and noradrenaline release as possible cause of early arrhythmias following acute coronary artery occlusion in pigs. J Mol Cell Cardiol 1980;12:579−93.
10. Kleber A. Resting membrane potential, extracellular K^+ activity, and intracellular Na^+ activity during global ischemia in isolated perfused guinea pig hearts. Circ Res 1983;52:442−50.
11. Wiegand V, Guggi M, Meesmann W, Kessler M, Greitschus F. Extracellular potassium activity changes in the canine myocardium after acute coronary occlusion and the influence of beta-blockade. Cardiovasc Res 1979;13:297−302.
12. Kammermeier H, Schmidt P, Jüngling E. Free energy change of ATP-hydrolysis: A causal factor of early hypoxic failure of the myocardium? J Mol Cell Cardiol 1982;14: 267−77.
13. Hearse DJ, Garlick PB, Humphrey SM. Ischemic contracture of the myocardium: Mechanisms and prevention. Am J Cardiol 1977;39:986−93.
14. Janse MJ, van Capelle FJL, Morsink H, et al. Flow of "injury" current and patterns of excitation during early ventricular arrhythmias in acute regional myocardial ischemia in isolated porcine and canine hearts. Circ Res 1980;47:151−65.
15. El-Sherif N, Scherlag BJ, Lazzara R. Electrode catheter recordings during malignant ventricular arrhythmia following experimental acute myocardial ischemia. Circulation 1975:51:1003−14.
16. Witt AL, Bigger, JT Jr. Possible electrophysiological mechanisms for lethal arrhythmias accompanying myocardial ischemia and infarction. Circulation. 1975;51,52(Suppl III): III−96−III−115.
17. Morad M, Dillon S, Weiss J. An acousto-optical steered laser scanning system for the measurement of action potential spread in intact heart. In Deweer P, Salzburg BM, eds. *Optical Methods in Cellular Physiology.* New York, John Wiley and Sons, 1986; 211−226.
18. Harris AS, Bisteni A, Russell RA, Brigham JC, Firestone, JE. Excitatory factors in ventricular tachycardia resulting from myocardial ischemia: Potassium a major excitant. Science 1954;119:200−3.
19. Morena H, Janse MJ, Fiolet JWT, Krieger WJG, Crijins H, Durrer D. Comparison of the effects of regional ischemia, hypoxia, hyperkalemia, and acidosis on intracellular and extracellular potentials and metabolism in the isolated porcine heart. Circ Res 1980;46: 634−46.
20. Weiss J, Shine KI. $[K^+]_o$ accumulation and electrophysiological alterations during early myocardial ischemia. Am J Physiol 1982;243:H318−27.
21. Saman S, Opie LH. Mechanism of reduction of action potential duration of ventricular myocardium by exogenous lactate. J Mol Cell Cardiol 1984;16:659−62.
22. Corr PB, Gross RW, Sobel BE. Amphipathic metabolites and membrane dysfunction in ischemic myocardium. Circ Res 1984;55:135−54.
23. Clarkson CW, Ten Eick RE. On the mechanism of lysophosphatidyl choline-induced depolarization of cat ventricular myocardium. Circ Res 1983;52:543−56.

24. Hess ML, Manson NH. Molecular oxygen: Friend and foe. J Mol Cell Cardiol 1984;16: 969–85.
25. Barrington PL, Meier CF, Dickens BF, Weglicki WB. Free radical scavengers protect canine myocytes from free radical-induced changes in the action potential (abstract). Circulation 1985;72(Suppl III):III–228.
26. Bernier M, Hearse DJ, Manning AS. Reperfusion-induced arrhythmias and oxygen-derived free radicals. Circ Res 1986;58:331–40.
27. Jennings RB, Steenbergen C. Nucleotide metabolism and cellular damage in myocardial ischemia. Ann Rev Physiol 1985;47:727–749.
28. Mathur PP, Case RB. Phosphate loss during reversible myocardial ischemia. J Mol Cell Cardiol 1973;5:375–393.
29. Kleber AG. Extracellular potassium accumulation in acute myocardial ischemia. J Mol Cell Cardiol 1984;16:389–94.
30. Vleugels A, Vereecke J, Carmeliet E. Ionic currents during hypoxia in voltage-clamped cat ventricular muscle. Circ Res 1980;47:501–508.
31. Conrad CH, Mark RG, Bing OL. Outward current and repolarization in hypoxic rat myocardium. Am J Physiol 1983;244:H341–H350.
32. Isenberg G, Vereecke J, van der Heyden G, Carmeliet E. The shortening of the action potential by DNP in guinea-pig ventricular myocytes is mediated by an increase of a time-independent K conductance. Pflügers Arch 1983;397:251–59.
33. Weiss J, Hiltbrand B, Shine KI. On the mechanism of cellular K^+ loss during acute myocardial ischemia. Circulation 1983;68(Suppl III):66.
34. Weiss J, Shine KI. The effect of heart rate on $[K^+]_o$ accumulation during myocardial ischemia. Am J Physiol 1986;250:H982–H991.
35. Noma A. ATP regulated K^+ channels in cardiac muscle. Nature 1983;305:147–8.
36. Hamill OP, Marty A, Neher E, Sakmann B, Sigworth FJ. Improved patch clamp for high resolution recording from cells and cell-free membrane patches. Pflügers Arch 1981;391:85–100.
37. Trube G, Hescheler J. Inward-rectifying channels in isolated patches of heart cell membrane: ATP dependence and comparison with cell-attached patches. Pflügers Arch 1984;401:178–84.
38. Kakei M, Noma A, Shibasaki T. Properties of adenosine triphosphate-regulated K^+ channels in guinea pig ventricular cells. J Physiol 1985;363:441–62.
39. Gudbjarnason S, Mathes P, Ravens KG. Functional compartmentation of ATP and creatine phosphate in heart muscle. J Mol Cell Cardiol 1970;1:325–39.
40. Jacobus WE. Respiratory control and the integration of heart high-energy phosphate metabolism by mitochondrial creatine kinase. Ann Rev Physiol 1985;47:707–25.
41. McDonald TF, MacLeod DP. Metabolism and the electrical activity of anoxic ventricular muscle. J Physiol 1973;229;559–82.
42. Bricknell OL, Opie LH. Effects of substrates on tissue metabolic changes in the isolated rat heart during underperfusion and on release of lactate dehydrogenase and arrhythmias during reperfusion. Circ Res 1978;43:102–15.
43. Higgins TJC, Bailey PJ, Allsopp D. Interrelationship between cellular metabolic status and susceptibility of heart cells to attach by phospholipase. J Mol Cell Cardiol 1982;14: 645–54.
44. Hasin Y, Barry WH. Myocardial metabolic inhibition and membrane potential, contraction, and potassium uptake. Am J Physiol 1984;247:H322–9.
45. Weiss J, Hiltbrand B. Functional compartmentation of glycolytic vs. oxidative metabolism in isolated rabbit heart. J Clin Invest 1985;75:436–47.
46. Bricknell OL, Daries PS, Opie LH. A relationship between adenosine triphosphate, glycolysis and ischemic contracture in the isolated rat heart. J Mol Cell Cardiol 1981;13: 941–5.
47. Parker JC, Hoffman JF. The role of membrane phosphoglycerate kinase in the control of glycolytic rate by active cation transport in human red blood cells. J Gen Physiol 1967;50:893–916.
48. Paul RJ. Functional compartmentalization of oxidative and glycolytic metabolism in vascular smooth muscle. Am J Physiol 1983;244:C399–C409.

6

Arrhythmias During Acute Ischemia in Experimental Models

Michiel J. Janse

Introduction

It has been known for more than 100 years that in the experimental animal, both occlusion of a coronary artery and reperfusion after a brief ischemic episode can lead to ventricular fibrillation.[1] There is no doubt that persistent coronary artery occlusion (because of occlusive thrombi or long-lasting coronary spasm) in man can lead to ventricular arrhythmias, although the incidence of ventricular fibrillation in the acute phase of myocardial infarction varies in the different reports from 4% to 36%.[2] These differences are probably related to variability in the time elapsed between onset of symptoms and the moment the patient was examined. The evidence that transient episodes of myocardial ischemia in man are the main causes of sudden cardiac death is far from complete. The following arguments, supporting the concept that myocardial ischemia is an important factor for the genesis of lethal ventricular arrhythmias, may be presented.

Sudden cardiac death occurs almost exclusively in patients with coronary artery disease.[3,4] Only a minority of patients who are successfully resuscitated from ventricular fibrillation outside the hospital subsequently develop a myocardial infarction,[4,5] suggesting that when indeed myocardial ischemia was involved, it was transient. In patients with coronary artery spasm, severe ventricular arrhythmias including ventricular fibrillation can occur within minutes after

---

From: Brugada P, Wellens HJJ. CARDIAC ARRHYTHMIAS: Where To Go From Here? Mount Kisco, NY, Futura Publishing Company, Inc., © 1987.

the beginning of electrocardiographic signs of ischemia.[6] Most often, arrhythmias develop when segment elevation is growing or has reached maximal levels, but it has also been reported that arrhythmias occur at the time when ST changes return to normal,[6-9] indicating that arrhythmias can result from both ischemia and reperfusion. Ventricular tachycardia and fibrillation occur in about one-fifth of patients with coronary artery spasm, but in only 3.6% of the ischemic episodes.[6] This suggests that other factors besides transient ischemia determine whether lethal arrhythmias will occur or not. Independent risk factors for the occurrence of sudden death include the presence of complex forms of ventricular premature depolarization[10-12] and left ventricular dysfunction.[13] Other factors could be changes in the activity of the autonomic nervous system, changes in ionic composition of plasma, use of antiarrhythmic drugs, or presence of supraventricular arrhythmias. It may even be questioned whether myocardial ischemia always is present when ventricular fibrillation suddenly develops. Analysis of ambulatory electrocardiographic recordings prior to the occurrence of ventricular fibrillation has shown that in a substantial number of cases, no signs of acute ischemia could be detected.[14-16] At this time, it is difficult enough to identify and quantify the different factors that may play a role in the sudden death syndrome, let alone to understand their electrophysiological arrhythmogenic effect.

Since in the past decade, a great deal has become known about the electrophysiological changes occurring in the first minutes following occulsion of a coronary artery and the way in which these changes result in lethal arrhythmias, it seems justified to review these experimental studies, and to attempt to indicate which interventions could possibly be of benefit in the prevention of sudden death. Some preliminary experiments on the nature of ischemia-induced ventricular fibrillation will be described as well.

Experimental Models for the Study of Ischemia-Induced Arrhythmias: Factors Influencing Incidence of Arrhythmias

There is a great variety in the models designed for the study of arrhythmias caused by myocardial ischemia, although all of them involve occlusion of a coronary artery. For this reason it is difficult to give precise figures about the incidence of the different types of arrhythmias during the various phases of ischemia and to compare them with the figures available for man. Many factors determine whether arrhythmias occur, and when and how often they occur.

The Size of the Ischemic Area

It has been known for quite some time that the level at which a coronary artery is occluded influences the incidence of ventricular fibrillation, and the general rule is that the larger the ischemic area, the more frequent the arrhythmias.[17,18] Still, even when in dogs the circumflex branch is occluded at the point of origin, the incidence of ventricular filbrillation may vary in different reports from 58% to 75%.[17,19] Among the factors that could explain such differences the following seem very important.

The Presence of Preexisting Collaterals

When the circumflex branch is occluded at its origin in dogs that have no preexisting collateral connections, ventricular fibrillation occurs in 100% of the animals, whereas its incidence is reduced to 3.7% in animals with collaterals.[20,21] This indicates that both the size of the ischemic area and the severity of ischemic changes are important determinants for arrhythmogenesis. This latter factor is also influenced by the degree of coronary stenosis and the way coronary occlusion is produced.

The Mode of Coronary Artery Occlusion

To avoid the occurrence of ventricular fibrillation, Harris[22] developed a method by which complete coronary artery occlusion is achieved in two stages. Initially, the artery is constricted but not occluded, and only after 30 minutes is the vessel completely occluded. This largely prevents ventricular fibrillation. The reasons for the protective effect of a period of coronary stenosis are unclear.[23]

In pigs, a stenosis that reduced flow in the left anterior descending coronary artery to 40% of baseline level did not result in ventricular fibrillation, but a flow reduction of 25% of control value led to ventricular fibrillation in about one-third of the animals.[24,25]

Gradual occlusion of a coronary artery by an ameroid constrictor implanted around a coronary artery can produce lethal arrhythmias, which occur, however, at unpredictable times, most often within 3 weeks following implantation.[26] A similar unpredictability in timing of lethal arrhythmias is present in the experimental model of Lee et al.[27] where pigs are fed a high cholesterol diet and irradiated precordially by X-ray. Several of the animals die within a few months from ventricular fibrillation or asystole. They have an advanced degree of coronary atherosclerosis and even myocardial infarcts are found.

Presence of a Previous Infarct

In man, the presence of a healed infarct is associated with a higher incidence of sudden death.[28] Several animal models have been developed to study the effect of an acute ischemic episode in hearts with a chronic infarct. Patterson and co-workers[29] produced an anteroseptal infarct in dogs by occluding the left anterior descending artery for 90 minutes and then reperfusing the ischemic area. During reperfusion, an area of stenosis was maintained to reduce flow. At the same time, a wire was inserted into the lumen of the circumflex branch. After several days, when the dogs were conscious, current was applied through this wire, which led to platelet aggregation and transient reduction of flow through the circumflex artery. Application of current produced venticular fibrillation more often in animals with a previous infarction than in dogs without an infarct.

In the presence of multiple stenotic lesions, sudden occlusion of another coronary artery can cause a decrease in flow in the areas supplied by the stenotic vessels, thus creating "ischemia at a distance."[30,31] Thus, the size of the ischemic area will be larger than in the case of a single occlusion without stenoses elsewhere, and hence the chance for arrhythmias will be greater.

Another factor that could, in part, explain why an acute ischemic episode superimposed upon a healed infarct is more arrhythomogenic than acute coronary occlusion alone is the greater degree of dispersion of actionpotential duration.[32]

A model, combining acute ischemia, a healed infarct, and exercise, was developed by Schwartz and co-workers.[33,34] Conscious dogs with a chronic anteroseptal infarct were exercised, and beginning with the last minute of exercise, a balloon occluder around the circumflex branch was inflated for 2 minutes. This brief occlusion did not produce arrhythmias in resting animals but resulted in frequent ventricular fibrillation when coupled with exercise, especially after cessation of exercise. This finding emphasizes the role of changes in the activity of the autonomic nervous system, a factor that also may account for the differences in the incidence of ischemia-induced arrhythmias in anesthetized and conscious animals.

Anesthetized Versus Conscious Animals

Anesthesia may decrease the incidence of severe arrhythmias,[35] and both the depth[36] and the type of anesthesia play a role.[37] It cannot be excluded that changes in heart rate contribute to these differences.[20]

In conscious animals, the occurrence of ischemia-induced arrhythmias depends on the level of stress. Pigs adapted to the laboratory environment develop severe arrhythmias much less frequently after coronary occlusion than do stressed animals.[38] Reperfusion arrhythmias occur less often in conscious trained dogs than in open-chested anesthetized dogs.[39]

The way in which the activity of the autonomic nervous system may interact with acute ischemia to enhance or reduce the chances for arrhythmias may be manyfold, but one important parameter is undoubtedly heart rate.

Heart Rate

There is some controversy regarding the arrhythmogenic effects of changes in heart rate in the setting of acute ischemia since both sinus bradycardia and sinus tachycardia have been reported to increase the incidence of arrhythmias. In the early phase of myocardial infarction, changes in the activity of the autonomic nerves can cause both bradycardia (often together with hypotension) and tachycardia.

Bradycardia usually occurs in inferior wall infarction, and was seen in 48% of patients observed within 30 minutes after the onset of symptoms. Sinus tachycardia, as a sign of enhanced sympathetic activity is most often associated with anterior wall infarction, and was found in 35% of patients seen in the first half hour.[40,41] It must be emphasized that an unchanged heart rate does not necessarily indicate absence of elevated sympathetic tone, since normal sinus rhythm may be present with both sympathetic and vagal tone being enhanced.[42] The sudden occurrence of severe bradycardia and hypotension has been reported as precipitating ventricular fibrillation,[43] but it is uncertain whether the lower heart rate or the hypotension is the main arrhythmogenic factor. The experimental evidence that bradycardia would be arrhythmogenic stems from the work of Han et al.[44] but in this study ventricular tachycardia and fibrillation are not mentioned, and only the number of ventricular premature depolarizations occurring after 5 minutes of ischemia was greater at low than at rapid heart rates.

In an experimental study on isolated Purkinje fibers in which a segment was exposed to a milieu containing high K+ and epinephrine, premature depolarizations based on reentry occurred only at very low and very rapid rates of stimulation. In an intermediate range of cycle lengths, reentry was not observed.[45] This concept of an optional heart rate was later also formulated for arrhythmias occurring in the first 3 hours following coronary occlusion.[46] In these experiments, ventricular premature depolarization and fibrillation occurred predominantly at rates between 60 and 90 beats/min and at rates between 180 and 200/min. The drawback of this study is that the time at which the arrhythmias occurred is not specified. The effects of bradycardia are different in the early phase of ischemia from those several hours later. Vagal stimulation during the first 30 minutes following coronary occlusion does not precipitate ventricular fibrillation, but after 4 to 5 hours it induced ventricular tachycardia in all dogs studied.[47] In other studies, slow heart rates even protected against arrhythmias in the acute phase of ischemia, while after 3 hours slow heart rates facilitated the occurrence of ectopic rhythms.[48-50] These effects can be explained on the basis of arrhythmia mechanisms. In the early phase of ischemia, idioventricular automaticity is unchanged, whereas several hours later it is enhanced.[50-52] Slowing of the sinus rate several hours after coronary occlusion may therefore unmask the enhanced automaticity and lead to ectopic activity. In the early phase of ischemia, reentry is the dominant mechanism for lethal arrhythmias. As will be discussed later, low heart rates protect against reentry.

The sudden introduction of a long cycle, however, may be very arrhythmogenic. The extrasystole which initiates ventricular fibrillation is often preceded by a long pause, most often a post-extrasystolic pause.[53] This has been observed in patients with acute myocardial infarction[43] and in patients dying suddenly during ambulatory electrocardiographic recording.[14,15]

The evidence that rapid heart rates are arrhythmogenic in acute ischemia is strong. Patients developing ventricular fibrillation in the very early phase of myocardial infarction show a significant increase in sinus rate immediately prior to the arrhythmias.[54] Acceleration of sinus rate in the hour preceding ventricular fibrillation was also noted in patients who underwent ambulatory electrocardiographic recording.[14-16] Increase in heart rate exacerbates arrhythmias in dogs following coronary occlusion.[52] The arrhythmogenic effects of sinustachycardia may be both direct and indirect. Direct effects are related to the delayed recovery of excitabililty of ischemic cells, and will be discussed later. Indirect effects include an increase in the size of the ischemic area.[55]

Activity of the Sympathetic Nervous System

It is generally believed that enhanced activity of the cardiac sympathetic nerves is a factor increasing the incidence of ischemia-induced arrhythmias. There is a vast literature of both clinical and experimental studies on the relationship between sympathetic activity and arrhythmogenesis, and many different approaches have been followed: correlation between plasma catecholamine levels and occurrence of arrhythmias; efforts to document increased catecholamine release in the heart at the time arrhythmias are most frequent; attempts to demonstrate a reduction in incidence and severity of arrhythmias following cardiac denervation, unilateral or bilateral stellectomy, adrenergic blockade, or cardiac catecholamine depletion; correlation between arrhythmias and emotional stress; and attempts to show that increased sympathetic activity induces arrhythmias. It is beyond the scope of this paper to review the whole literature, but a few remarks can be made. There is great variability in results, and many studies have conflicting results. For example, some authors report on increased catecholamine release in the first 10 minutes of ischemia,[56] while others were unable to confirm this.[57] Some authors found a correlation between circulating catecholamines and arrhythmias[58] while others did not.[59] Some authors found that left stellectomy reduced the number of ischemia-induced arrhythmias;[60] others found no effect.[61] In some experimental studies, beta-adrenergic blocking agents had an antiarrhythmic effect;[62] in others they precipitated arrhythmias.[38] In some studies, stress was found to be arrhythmogenic,[38,63] but in others stress had no effect.[64] These differences may to a large extent be due to the variability in animal models. In the various studies, many of which used too small a number of animals to reach statistically significant results, no standardization was attempted regarding animal species, heart size, size of the ischemic area, number of collaterals, heart rate, blood pressure, whether or not the animals were conscious, depth of anesthesia, mode of coronary occlusion, time of occurrence of arrhythmias, or type of arrhythmias.

When considering in which way enhanced sympathetic activity could be arrhythmogenic, it must be recognized that this could occur by indirect effects, such as sinus tachycardia, hypokalemia,[65] or an increase in the size of the ischemic area. Not enough data are available to evaluate the possible direct electrophysiological effects of noradrenaline on ischemic myocardial cells.

Two Phases of Early Arrhythmias

In all animal species studied (rat, guinea pig, dog, sheep, and pig) there is a bimodal distribution of arrhythmias during the first half hour following complete occlusion of a coronary artery. The first phase (phase 1a, or "immediate ventricular arrhythmias") occurs between 2 and 10 minutes, with the highest incidence at 5 to 6 minutes. The second phase (phase 1b, or "delayed early ventricular arrhythmias") extends approximately from 12 to 30 minutes, with a peak between 15 and 20 minutes.[66-71] Individual animals may exhibit only 1a or only 1b arrhythmias, but both types may occur in the same animal. It is not known whether in man with acute ischemia a similar distinction between 1a and 1b arrhythmias can be made.

There are several findings suggesting that the mechanims underlying 1a and 1b arrhythmias may be different. Phase 1a arrhythmias are correlated to the degree of conduction delay and fragmentation of extracellular electrograms recorded from the ischemic subepicardium. Often, continuous fragmented activity extends from the QRS complex of a normally propagated sinus impulse to the beginning of a premature ventricular depolarization.[70] This so-called "diastolic bridging" was not observed in 1b arrhythmias, which also were not related to epicardial conduction delay.[68,70] During the 1b phase, both the mean activation delay and their variance were significantly less than during the 1a phase, indicating less spatial inhomogeneity.[72] These findings have been interpreted as indicating that 1a arrhythmias are reentrant in nature, whereas mechanisms such as abnormal automaticity would cause 1b arrhythmias.

There is some evidence that 1b arrhythmias are related to release of endogenous catecholamines, which occurs between 15 and 20 minutes of ischemia.[57] Thus, 1b arrhythmias in isolated guinea pig hearts were always preceded by improvement of action potential upstroke characteristics of ischemic cells.[71] This improvement was absent in hearts from animals that were depleted of catecholamines by pretreatment with 6-hydroxydopamine, which also resulted in a reduction in 1b arrhythmias.[71] Regional sympathectomy in dogs had no effect on 1a arrhythmias, but abolished 1b arrhythmias.[73]

Some Conclusions Based on the Review of Animal Models

Several conclusions can be drawn from this brief review on animal models. When evaluating experimental studies, especially those that are designed to test interventions meant to reduce incidence and severity of ischemia-induced arrhythmias, it is of vital importance to know about the following: type of arrhythmias, time of occurrence, size of the ischemic area, degree of collateralization, and heart rate. Since both the underlying mechanism (and thus the effect of an eventual pharmacological intervention) and the influence of the sympathetic nervous system may be different for 1a and 1b arrhythmias, it is obviously of importance to know the interval betwen onset of ischemia and manifestation of ectopic activity. Important factors that increase the incidence of arrhythmias are a large ischemia area, a small degree of collateralization and sinus tachycardia. There are very few studies in which these parameters are known, let alone standardized. Most studies on the effects of antiarrhythmic drugs, or other interventions, are performed on so-called "mongrel dogs" and usually a small number of animals are used. Since these animals have widely varying coronary artery systems, even a standardized coronary artery occlusion (for example: "just distal to the first diagonal branch") may result in ischemic areas of varying sizes, in which the degree of ischemic changes may vary as well. Extrapolation of antiarrhythmic interventions in animal studies to man with coronary artery disease must therefore be made with extreme caution. While it is difficult to design prophylactic measures that could influence the size of an ischemic area, or the degree of collateralilzation, it is quite feasible to reduce heart rate. It is possible that the success of beta-adrenergic blockade in reducing the incidence of sudden death in post-infarction patients is related to this effect.

Electrophysiological Changes During Acute Ischemia

In understanding arrhythmia mechanisms during the different phases of acute ischemia, we have to consider the time course and nature of changes in both the passive and active electrical properties of ischemic myocardium. In the following, the changes in intra- and extracellular longitudinal resistance, in transmembrane potential characteristics, and in excitabillity will be briefly reviewed, as will be the resulting effects on conduction velocity and the occurrence of conduction block.

Changes in Longitudinal Extra- and Intracellular Resistance

In arterially perfused papillary muscles, the arrest of coronary flow, combined with a change in the surrounding gaseous atmosphere to 94% N_2 and 6% CO_2, led to the following changes in passive electrical properties: an immediate, but small increase in logitudinal extracellular resistance caused by the decrease in vascular volume, and a subsequent gradual increase by about 80% of control value after 20 minutes, most likely due to a reduction in extracellular volume consequent to osmotic cell swelling. Intracellular resistance remained constant during the first 12 to 18 minutes, but thereafter the ischemic cells rapidly uncoupled, with intracellular resistance increasing to 200 to 400% within a few minutes. This cellular uncoupling was associated with irreversible cell damage.[74] The consequences of these changes are a mild reduction in conduction velocity during the initial 12 to 18 minutes (due to the increase in extracellular resistance), and inhomogeneous conduction and conduction block during the later phase of cellular uncoupling. The initial changes are too small to have significance for 1a arrhythmias, but the increase in coupling resistance could play an important role in the genesis of 1b arrhythmias. Agents that could prevent or postpone cellular uncoupling, such as calcium entry blockers, might have a beneficial effect on 1b arrhythmias. This possibility, however, is purely hypothetical, and at the present time untested.

Changes in Transmembrane Potential

Within minutes following coronary occlusion, resting membrane potential depolarizes until at levels of about -60 mV ischemic cells become inexcitable. This occurs at times varying from 5 to 10 minutes in tissue where coronary flow is reduced to zero. Concomitant with depolarization of resting membrane potential, actionpotential amplitude and upstroke velocity decrease. Actionpotentials often alternate with respect to amplitude and duration, and 2:1 responses may precede the phase of unresponsiveness. With maintained ischemia, actionpotentials may return for a brief period in previously inexcitable cells after 15 to 20 minutes. These changes are depicted in Figure 1. The 1a arrhythmias occur during the phase when actionpotentials become markedly depressed: the phase of in-

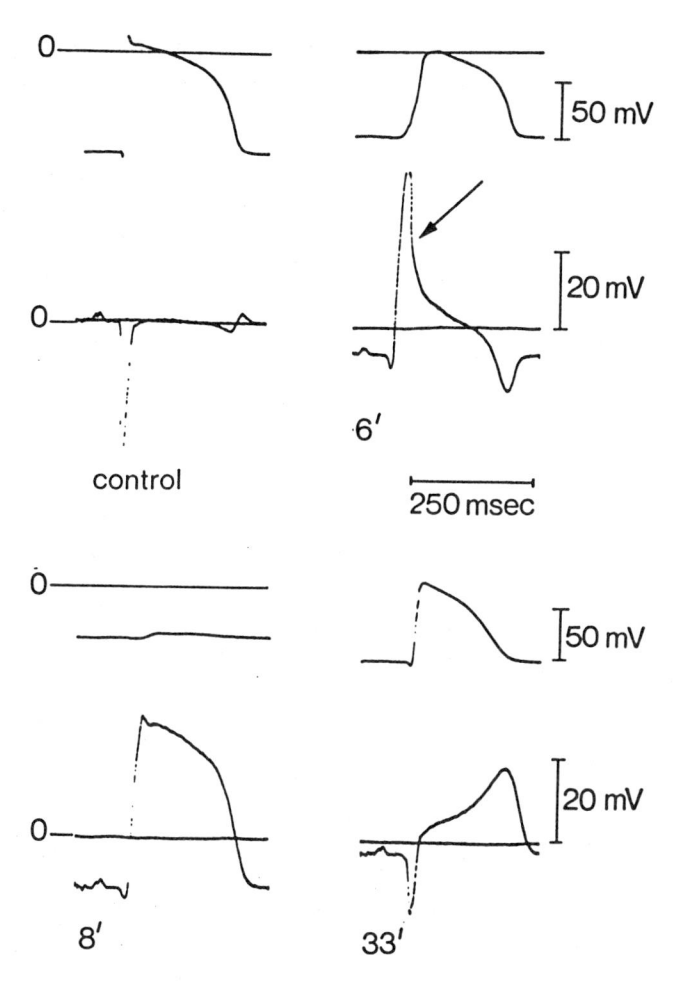

Figure 1: Electrophysiological changes in the isolated perfused pig heart after coronary artery occlusion. Top trace: transmembrane potentials; lower trace: local extracellular DC electrograms. Zero potentials in the extracellular recordings is the potential of the aortic root. After coronary occlusion, resting membrane potential decreases, resulting in a TQ depression in the extracellular signal. The decrease in plateau voltage is reflected by ST elevation. Note decrease in upstroke velocity and delayed activation (arrow points to intrinsic deflection in upper right panel). After 8 min of ischemia, the actionpotential has disappeared and the extracellular complex is monophasic. A transient recovery in electrical activity is seen after 33 minutes. (Reproduced with permission from Janse JM, Durrer D: Ned Tijdschr Geneesk 122:1964–1968, 1978.)

excitability is associated with the period during which sinus rhythm is the predominant rhythm; the transient recovery of electrical activity coincides with the phase of 1b arrhythmias.

For many years, it was believed that the actionpotential of acutely ischemic cells would be a so-called slow response, in which inward current is carried through the slow channels, predominantly by calcium ions. This possibility was suggested because conditions in which slow responses can be elicited in vitro (high extracellular K^+, and catecholamines) also are present in ischemic myocardium. Recently obtained evidence, however, indicates that the actionpotential during the 1a phase of arrhythmias is not a slow response, but a "depressed fast response," with inward current flowing through partially inactivated fast sodium channels. Briefly, the evidence is as follows. When ischemic cells are depolarized beyond the level at which fast channels are inactivated, and at which slow channels become activated, the cells remain inexcitable. Resting membrane potentials at which inexcitability occurs during ischemia is on the average -61 mV, resting membrane potentials at which slow responses could be induced in the same hearts by elevating extracellular potassium and adding catecholamines in control conditions was on the average -47 mV. Conduction velocity of the slow response is much lower than the lowest values observed during ischemia. The refractory period of the slow response is much longer (i.e., 1.5 sec) than that of ischemic cells. Lidocaine, which does not affect slow channels but inactivates fast channels in partially depolarized cells, abolishes action potentials of ischemic cells.[75,76]

Changes in Conduction Velocity

The increase in extra- and intracellular resistance, and the decrease in actionpotential upstroke velocity and amplitude lead to a reduction in conduction velocity. Experiments in which spread of activation in the globally ischemic left ventricle of the pig heart was measured by recording simultaneously from 100 electrodes, spaced at 1.5 mm distances around a central stimulus electrode, gave the following results: conduction velocity in the direction parallel to the long axis of the myocardial fibers decreased from a control value of about 50 to about 30 cm/sec after 4 to 5 minutes of ischemia, just before the fibers became inexcitable. For conduction in the direction perpendicular to the long fiber axis, velocity decreased from 21 to 13 cm/sec.[75] Thus, during the 1a phase of arrhythmias, conduction velocity is reduced by approximately 50%.

As shown in Figure 2, at a certain point in time, asymmetrical conduction block occurs. In this experiment, the area to the left of the stimulating electrode was not directly excited, and two semicircular wavefronts from the right part make an unsuccessful attempt to invade the area of block. The conduction block is cycle length-dependent since a sudden increase in cycle length (panel B) results in restoration of elliptical spread of excitation. Apparently, slight differences in recovery of excitability of the myocardium to the right and left of the stimulus electrode accounted for the conduction block in panel A.

Effect of Stimulus Interval on Epicardial Activation

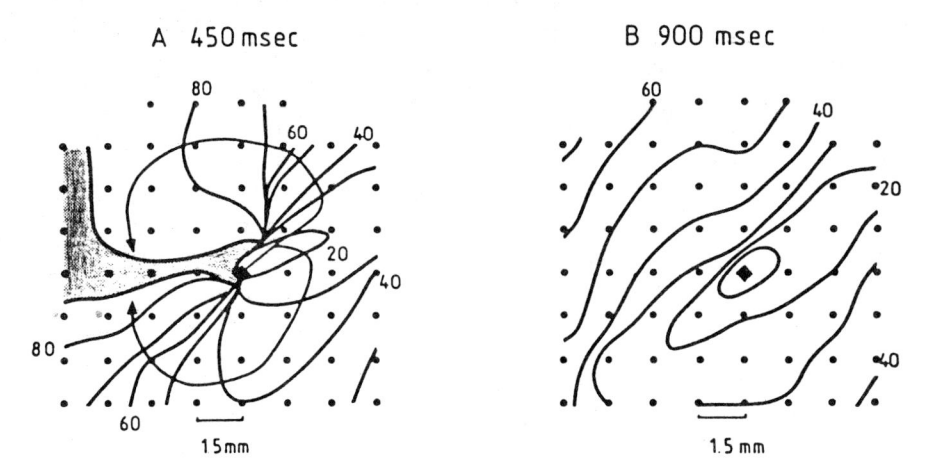

A 450 msec

B 900 msec

Figure 2: Effects of an abrupt change in stimulus interval on epicardial activation 6 minutes after interruption of coronary flow. Position of the central stimulus electrode is indicated by a quadrangle. Dots indicate individual recording electrodes. Activation on isochronal maps is given in increments of 10 ms. A: stimulus interval 450 ms. Block occurs on the left and upper parts of the map (shaded area). Electrode sites adjacent to shaded area are activated with delay by circulating excitation (arrows). B: activation during the beat after A, when the stimulus interval was suddenly increased to 900 ms. This causes immediate restoration of elliptic spread of activation. (Reproduced with permission.[75])

Changes in Excitability

Changes in refractory period duration in acutely ischemic myocardium are difficult to measure for a number of reasons. The classical method to determine local refractoriness is in essence to pace the ventricle regularly and to apply an extrastimulus of, for example twice diastolic threshold strength, after every eighth regular stimulus. The shortest coupling interval at which a propagated premature beat is elicited is then equal to the local refractory period. If the refractory period is to be determined with a millisecond precision, this is a time-consuming procedure which, in view of the rapidity at which ischemic myocardium changes its electrophysiologic characteristics, presents with considerable problems. In particular, since diastolic current requirements for threshold excitation gradually increase during ischemia, it becomes very difficult to set the intensity of the premature stimulus at twice diastolic threshold strength. When stimulation currents increase, fibers with shorter refractory periods and lower thresholds may be excited at considerable distance from the stimulating electrode, and this may lead to erroneous values for local refractory period duration.[77] Furthermore, when actionpotentials alternate in duration, refractory periods alternate as well, and it depends on the number of beats preceding the test stimulus whether one finds a short or a long refractory period.[78] Finally, in partially depolarized cells, recovery of excitability lags behind repolarization, and stimuli delivered well after repolarization is complete elicit so-called "graded responses": actionpotential with reduced amplitudes and upstroke velocities, which gradually become larger and with faster upstrokes when evoked later in diastole.[79] For these reasons, it is difficult to speak of *the* refractory period of acutely ischemic myocardium.

In general, recovery of excitability in the central ischemic zone, where cells are partially depolarized, is prolonged. Cells close to the border, with unchanged, or minimally depolarized resting membrane potentials, may have refractory periods that are shorter than those of normal myocardium (see Fig. 3). This results in an increase in the spatial dispersion of refractory periods within the ischemic area, which may be one of the most important reasons for the occurrence of reentry.

In vitro studies, in which ischemic conditions were simulated by exposing isolated papillary muscles to elevated concentrations of potassium, low pO_2, and low pH, have shown that the time-dependent recovery of excitability is very sensitive to small changes in resting membrane potential.[80] Therefore, small local gradients in resting membrane potential caused by small gradients in extracellular potassium[81] within the ischemic zone explain the spatial dispersion in refractori-

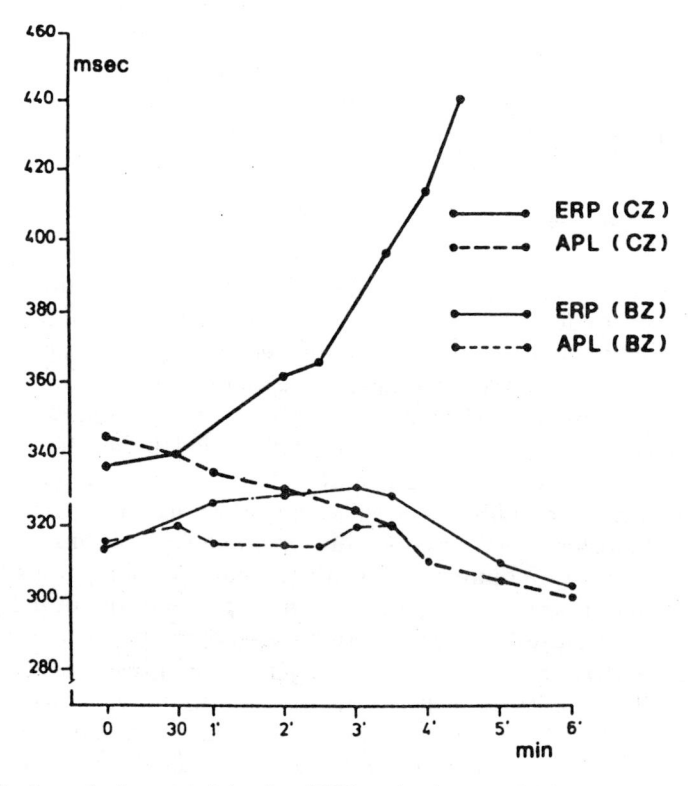

Figure 3: Effective refractory period duration (ERP) and actionpotential duration (APL) of the central ischemic zone (CZ) and border zone (BZ) in an isolated porcine heart following coronary occlusion. In both the central ischemic and the border zone, actionpotential duration decreases (dotted line). In contrast, the effective refractory period in the central ischemic zone lengthens considerably from 338 to 444 ms, whereas in the border zone, refractory period shortens slightly. (Reproduced with permission from Capucci et al: New Frontiers of Arrhythmias, OIC Medical Press, 1984; 7–17.)

ness. An important consequence is that ischemic cells that generate actionpotentials of similar configuration at low heart rates may not do so as heart rate increases. Those cells with the longest recovery times will show alternation or 2:1 responses; those with shorter recovery times will still be able to respond in a 1:1 fashion. Thus, increases in heart rate may unmask electrical inhomogeneity, create zones of unidirectional block, and set the stage for reentry (see Fig. 4).

Mechanisms of Ventricular Fibrillation

Our experiments, in which spread of activation during spontaneously developing ventricular fibrillation in the first 10 min following coronary artery occlusion was mapped, led to the conclusion that two different arrhythmogenic mechanisms are operative during this phase. Spontaneous ventricular premature depolarizations could, in our experiments, not be attributed to macro-reentry. Instead, such ectopic beats originated at the ischemic border, often in the subendocardium, and appeared to be of "focal" origin. Although the exact mechanism remains to be elucidated, the following possibilities can be considered: reexcitation of nonischemic myocardium or Purkinje fibers at the normal side of the border by currents of injury: triggered activity in such fibers induced by flow of injury current; and micro-reentry or reflection across the ischemic border.[82,83] Premature ventricular depolarizations can induce macro-reentry in much the same way as an increase in heart rate, namely by unmasking inhomogeneities and creating areas of unidirectional block. Macro-reentry can result in short bouts of ventricular tachycardia, or degenerate into ventricular fibrillation. In the following, we will concentrate on this mechanism.

Figure 5 shows 12 selected electrograms out of 125 simultaneously recorded

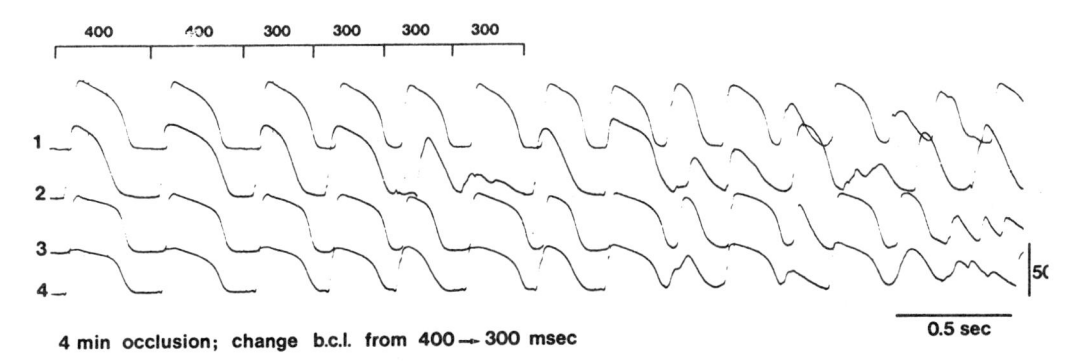

Figure 4: Effect of an increase in heart rate on acutely ischemic myocardium. Four transmembrane potentials were simultaneously recorded from the ischemic part of the left ventricle of a pig heart, 4 minutes after occlusion of the left anterior descending artery. The atrium was paced at a cycle length of 400 ms. The actionpotentials of the four ischemic cells had a similar configuration, and activation was more or less synchronous. Shortening the pacing cycle to 300 ms unmasked inhomogeneity: cell 2 became activated with delay, and shows block (6th response), and within 2 seconds after increasing pacing rate, the chaotic pattern of ventricular fibrillation is seen. (Reproduced with permission from Janse et al: Ann Cardiol Angeiol 26:551–554, 1977.)

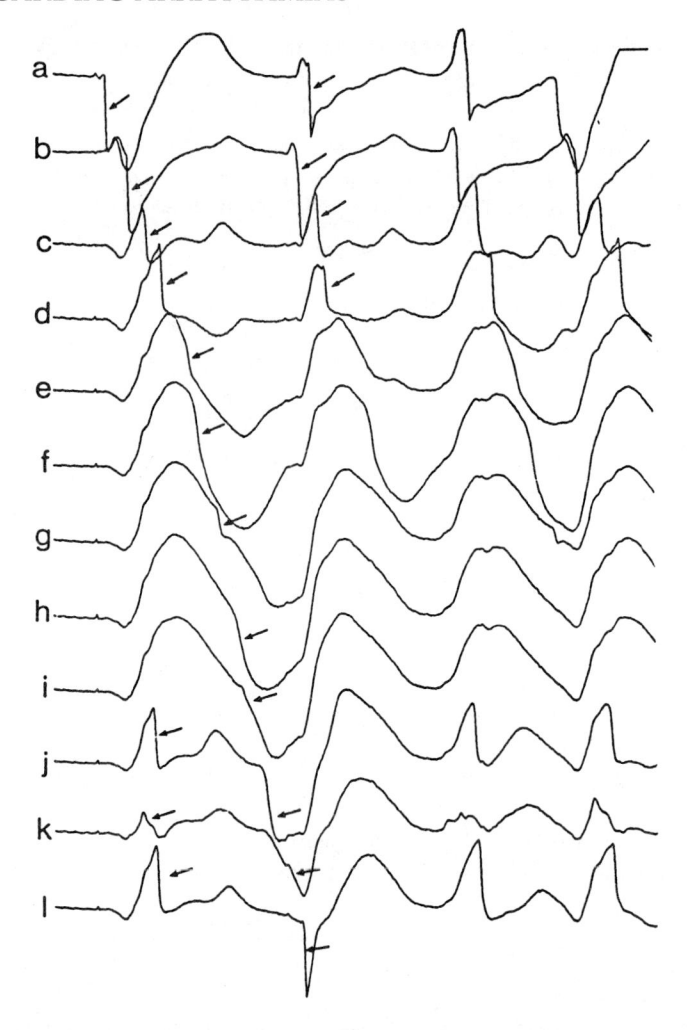

Figure 5: Selected unipolar electrograms from an isolated perfused dog heart, 7 minutes after occlusion of the left anterior descending and circumflex branch. The position of sites a to l is indicated in Figure 6. The first beat is the last paced beat (the stimulus electrode was on the posterior right ventricle), the second beat is an ectopic beat leading to ventricular fibrillation. Arrows point to intrinsic deflections, indicating local activation. See text for discussion. (Reproduced with permission.[85])

signals from the epicardial surface of the left ventricle of an isolated, Langendorff-perfused canine heart, 7 minutes after occlusion of both the left anterior descending coronary artery and the circumflex branch. Ventricular fibrillation was induced by pacing the right ventricle. The first complex is the last paced beat, the following are ectopic beats leading to fibrillation. Sites a to l, from which these potentials were recorded are indicated in Figure 6, where the configuration of the multipolar electrode, wrapped around both ventricles, is shown. Arrows in Figure 5 point to intrinsic deflections resulting from local depolarization. The activation patterns of first (paced) and second (ectopic) beat are shown in iso-

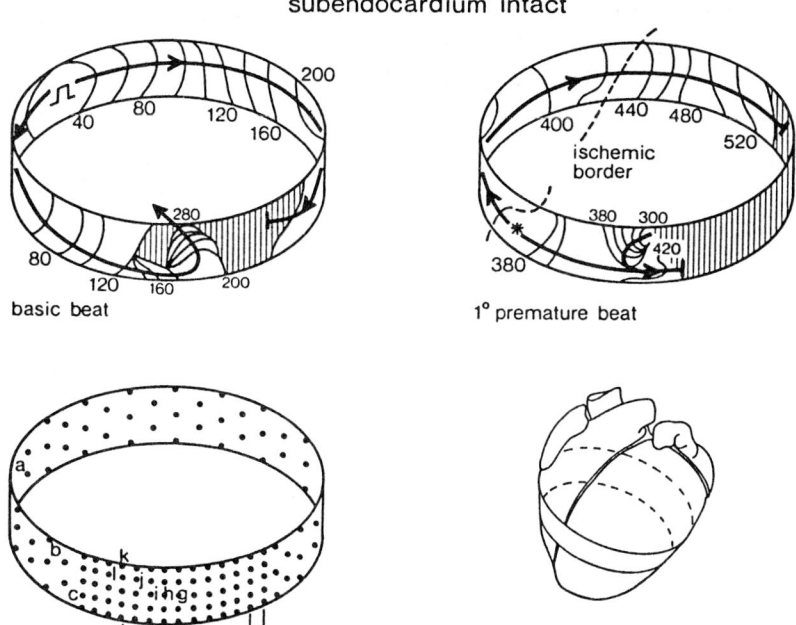

Figure 6: Circus movement reentry between first and second beat of Figure 5. The multipolar electrode was a 2 cm wide band, containing 125 electrodes, wrapped around both ventricles, as schematically shown in the lower right panel. In the lower left panel, each dot is an individual electrode; sites a to l of Figure 5 are indicated. In the upper panels, spread of activation is indicated by isochrones. The site of the stimulus electrode is indicated by a square wave. Time zero is the stimulus artifact, numbers are in milliseconds; shaded areas are zones of block. Note unidirectional block, and circus movement on the anterior aspect of the left ventricle, resulting in reexcitation of the area proximal to the zone of block after 300 ms (upper right panel). In addition, a second ectopic wavefront emerged after 380 ms (asterisk) close to the ischemic border (indicated by the dotted line). See text for discussion. (Reproduced with permission.[85])

chronic maps in Figure 6. From the stimulus site, activity spreads in two directions. After having excited site joules at 110 ms, the wave on the anterior surface meets a region of block around the 120 ms isochrone. The impulse propagates around the zone of block via sites d, e, and f, turns back via sites g, h, and i to reexcite site j after 355 ms. The length of this reentrant circuit was on the order of 8 cm. After reexciting the tissue around site c, another attempt is made to follow the same circular pathway, but now, the wavefront blocks at site g at 420 ms. Another ectopic wavefront emerges at about 380 ms close to the ischemic border (indicated by the asterisk), which is responsible for premature excitation of sites b and a. In other words, two different sources of ectopic activity are present: classical circus movement reentry, and an unknown mechanism located close to the border.

If we want to predict the length of a possible reentrant circuit of the "leading circle" type,[84] we must multiply conduction velocity with refractory period duration. For acutely ischemic myocardium, reasonable figures are 20 cm/sec and 350 ms, respectively, which gives us a wavelength of 7 cm, which agrees well with the pathway length of about 8 cm found in this and in other experiments.[82,85] It must be emphasized that reentrant circuits in ischemic myocardium are large, and that revolution times (because of the prolonged recovery of excitability) are long: on the order of 350 ms. This implies that the rate of a ventricular arrhythmia which is solely dependent on circus movement reentry within the ischemic myocardium would be on the order of 170/min, and that this rate would become slower and slower with the progression of ischemia, concomitant with further prolongation of recovery of excitability, until the rhythm would stop when the ischemic myocardium becomes inexcitable. How then, is it possible that regional myocardial ischemia can cause ventricular fibrillation, where intervals between successive activation in the normal myocardium are on the order of 180 ms, equivalent to rates of about 550/min? Clearly, if we think of fibrillation in terms of multiple wavelet reentry, one must assume that the reentrant process, beginning in the ischemic zone, is somehow transferred to the normal myocardium, where refractory periods are much shorter. Normal canine ventricles can be made to fibrillate by pacing the ventricles at increasingly faster rates.[86] At rapid rates, spatial dispersion of refractory periods in the normal canine ventricle is on the order of 40 ms,[87] and we know that much smaller local differences in refractory period duration are sufficient to create areas of unidirectional block, one of the prerequisites for reentry.[88] In very general terms, the following hypothesis can be formulated: Centrifugal wavefronts, as offshoots from the main reentrant circuit within the ischemic zone, utilizing various "exits" towards normal myocardium, excite the latter at a fairly rapid rate (about 170 to 200/min), but, more importantly, out of phase. As a result, conduction within the normal myocardium becomes inhomogeneous, with colliding wavefronts, areas of block, and areas of normal and reduced conduction velocity when cells are excited in their relative refractory period. This inhomogeneity will lead to multiple wavelet reentry, with many independent wavefronts traveling around many islets of temporary conduction block, reexciting every cell group that has recovered its excitability. Because of the rapid rate of excitation, refractory periods will shorten[87] and, combined with a reduced conduction velocity in partially refractory tissue, wavelengths will become very short. The resulting fibrillation will have become independent from whatever reentrant phenomena may be present in the ischemic myocardium. There are basically three different exit routes from the ischemic area: (1) conduction through ischemic myocardium towards normal myocardium, (2) conduction through the Purkinje system from ischemic to normal myocardium, and (3) conduction through the ischemic subendocardial border zone (where ischemic changes are much less marked than in midmyocardial zones[89]) towards the normal subendocardium.

We have conducted experiments in which the whole subendocardium, including the Purkinje system, was destroyed by intracavitary application of phenol[85] or liquid nitrogen (unpublished results). Ectopic ventricular rhythms developed spontaneously after coronary occlusion following the destruction of the subendocardium, or could be induced by premature stimulation. These ectopic rhythms were regular, and had slow rates (cycle lengths varied from 300 to 350 ms, corresponding to the revolution times of reentrant circuits within the ischemic zone) (see Fig. 7). These rhythms generally terminated spontaneously as

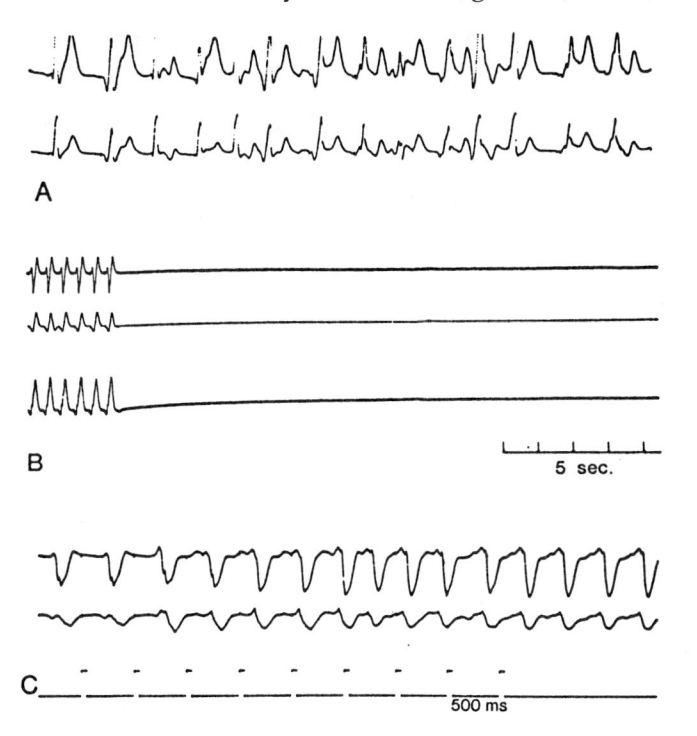

Figure 7: A: Two electrograms recorded 7 minutes after coronary occlusion in an isolated perfused dog heart. The third complex is a spontaneous premature ventricular beat which initiates ventricular fibrillation. B: Three different electrograms recorded from the same heart after intracavitary application of phenol. Destruction of the Purkinje system is evident from the fact that after stopping pacing the ventricles, no escape rhythm developed. C: Ectopic rhythm occurring during regional ischemia in the same heart after destruction of the subendocardium by phenol. The lowest trace is a coded output of the stimulator (actual stimuli had a much shorter duration of 2 ms). Note regular rhythm after stopping pacing. (Reproduced with permission.[85])

excitability in the ischemic zone decreased. They did not degenerate into ventricular fibrillation. Apparently, the daughter waves of the reentrant circuit, which could reach the normal myocardium only via muscle conduction, excited the normal myocardium in a regular, orderly fashion, preventing asynchronous conduction that could result in multiple wavelet reentry. Since destruction of the subendocardium is hardly a suitable way to prevent ischemia-induced ventricular fibrillation in man, we started experiments in an attempt to prolong the refractory period of the Purkinje system, in order to create a "barrier" in one of the exit routes from the ischemic myocardium. Although at this stage these experiments are in too preliminary a phase to draw conclusions, the results thus far have been encouraging. Drugs that prolong the refractory period of the Purkinje system, in doses that do not affect the myocardial refractory period at rapid rates, such as 4-aminopyridine and D-Sotalol, were in a number of cases effective in preventing ischemia-induced ventricular fibrillation in Langendorff-perfused dog hearts, despite the occurrence of circus movement within the ischemic zone.

How Can Sudden Death be Prevented?

One may agree with epidemiologists that "the prevention of sudden death means the prevention of coronary attacks,"[90] but it is not within the scope of this paper to discuss epidemiological studies, or to consider whether changes in smoking habits, diet, or general life style have succeeded in reducing mortality due to ischemic heart disease, even though one should rejoice in the encouraging reports that the incidence of fatal events is on the decline.[91,92]

In discussing mechanisms for sudden death, it may be helpful to emphasize that ventricular fibrillation results from the interplay between three major determinants: the substrate for reentry, triggers, and modulating factors.

The substrate for the fatal arrhythmia may be, for example, an anatomically defined reentry circuit such as may exist within a healed infarct, consisting of surviving muscle and Purkinje fibers. It can also be a functional reentrant circuit in acutely ischemic myocardium, and here local differences in excitability are the major determinants. Finally, the substrate may be a combination of a healed infarct and an acutely ischemic region. Prevention of a substrate for reentry to occur seems to be achieved more easily by anti-ischemic measures (for example, drugs preventing coronary artery spasm, or platelet aggregation; thrombolysis; coronary bypass surgery; percutaneous transluminal angioplasty, etc.) than by conventional antiarryhthmic therapy. Ablation of (part of) the reentrant circuit in patients with sustained ventricular tachycardia in the chronic phase of myocardial infarction, by endocardial resection, cryosurgery, laser ablation, or catheter ablation can be a rationalistic and successful intervention to prevent sudden death in a subgroup of patients.

Theoretically, one could prevent reentry either by abolishing electrical activity within an ischemic region, or by improving conduction. In both cases, the wavelength (the product of conduction velocity and refractory period) would increase, and if the ratio wavelength/size of the ischemic area would be sufficiently large, reentry could no longer occur. An example of the first possibility is provided by experiments in which lidocaine was given prior to coronary occlusion. This resulted in a rapid abolishment of actionpotentials within the ischemic region, and indeed, reentry leading to ventricular fibrillation was only rarely seen.[76] Lidocaine, given in large doses intravenously, has been reported to prevent primary ventricular fibrillation in patients with acute myocardial infarction in the coronary care unit, [93] and intramuscular lidocaine, given outside the hospital to patients suspected of developing a myocardial infarction, reduced the incidence of ventricular fibrillation.[94] However, lidocaine may be a two-edged sword: in myocardium that is not (yet) severely ischemic, it may slow conduction and actually enhance the chances for reentry. It comes as no surprise that in several animal studies, lidocaine was found to have a pro-fibrillatory effect.[95,96] A similar caveat may be made concerning measures that improve conduction: both reperfusion and sympathetic stimulation improve conduction in (previously) ischemic myocardium,[61,79] yet both interventions are capable of inducing ventricular fibrillation. Clearly, there is no simple, safe way in which a drug can prevent reentry by altering the electrophysiological properties of acutely ischemic myocardium. The possibility that drugs which alter the properties of nonischemic

Purkinje fibers and/or myocardium may be effective in protecting the heart against ventricular fibrillation, even in the presence of reentry within the ischemic zone, could be considered. Destruction of the endocardium, including the Purkinje system, prevents ischemia-induced ventricular fibrillation, as described in this paper. Initial results, using drugs that prolong the refractory period of nonischemic Purkinje fibers, showed that the reentrant events could be restricted to the ischemic zone and that the normal part of the ventricles did not become involved in the pattern of multiple wavelet reentry. In other words, the Purkinje system with a prolonged refractory period might act as a filter, more or less in a similar way as the atrioventricular node during atrial fibrillation. It goes without saying that this hypothesis needs thorough testing before it can be considered as a practical approach to prevent ischemia-induced ventricular fibrillation.

Ventricular premature depolarizations, sudden pauses, and increases in heart rate are triggers that can induce reentry. The suppression of premature depolarizations, and the prevention of sinus tachycardia may, even in the presence of a substrate for reentry, be very effective in reducing the incidence of fatal arrhythmias. As said earlier, an important effect of beta-adrenergic blockade may be the reduction in sinus rate. Complete abolition of premature ventricular depolarizations by antiarrhythmic therapy could be important in preventing ventricular fibrillation, but in practice, classical antiarrhythmic therapy has been not very effective.[97-99]

Finally, there are several factors which can be thought of as modulators, such as poor left ventricular function, enhanced sympathetic tone, and electrolyte disturbances (hypokalemia), which enhance the chance for reentry. The precise mechanisms of action of such modulating factors is poorly understood, and some are not easily amenable to treatment.

In conclusion, it must be stated that despite a considerable advancement in our understanding of the genesis of arrhythmias caused by acute ischemia, this has not yet resulted in a simple and safe procedure that effectively prevents these life-threatening arrhythmias.

References

1. Cohnheim J, Von Schulthess-Rechtberg AV. Ueber die Folgen der Kranzarterienverschliessung fuer das Herz. Virchows Arch 1881;85:503–537.
2. Bigger JT, Dresdale RJ, Heissenbuttel, RH, Weld FM, Wit AL. Ventricular arrhythmias in ischemic heart disease: mechanism, prevalence, significance and management. Progr Cardiovasc Dis 1977;19:255–300.
3. Davies MJ. Pathological view of sudden cardiac death. Br Heart J 1981;45:88–96.
4. Goldstein S, Landis JR, Leighton R, Ritter G, Vasu CM, Lantis A, Serokman R. Characteristics of the resuscitated out-of-hospital cardiac arrest victim with coronary heart disease. Circulation 1981;64:977–984.
5. Cobb LA, Werner JA, Trobaugh GB. Sudden cardiac death. I. A decade's experience with out-of-hospital resuscitation. Mod Concepts Cardiovasc Dis 1980;49:31–36.
6. Maseri A, Severi S, Marzullo P. Role of coronary arterial spasm in sudden coronary ischemic death. Ann NY Acad Sci 382:204–212, 1982.
7. Araki H, Koiwaya Y, Nakagaki O, Nakamura M. Diurnal distribution of ST-segment elevation and related arrhythmias in patients with variant angina: a study by ambulatory ECG monitoring. Circulation 1983;67:995–1000.

8. Previtali M, Klersy C, Salerno JA, Chimienti M, Panciroli C, Marangoni E, et al. Ventricular tachyarrhythmias in Prinzmetal's variant angina: clinical significance and relation to the degree and time course of S-T segment elevation. Am J Cardiol 1983;52: 19–25.
9. Tzivoni D, Keren A, Granot H, Gottlieb S, Benhorin J, Stern S. Ventricular fibrillation caused by myocardial reperfusion in Prinzmetal's angina. Am Heart J 1983;105: 323–325.
10. Bigger JT, Weld FM, Rolnitzky LM. Which postinfarction ventricular arrhythmias should be treated? Am Heart J 1982;103:660–664.
11. Moss AJ, Davis HT, De Camilla J, Bayer LW. Ventricular ectopic beats and their relation to sudden cardiac death after myocardial infarction. Circulation 1979;60:998–1003.
12. Ruberman W, Weinblatt E, Goldberg JD, Frank CW, Shapiro S. Ventricular premature beats and mortality after myocardial infarction. N Engl J Med 1977;297:750–757.
13. Myerburg RJ, Conde CA, Sung RJ, Mayorga-Cortes A, Mallon S, Sheps DS, Appel RA, Castellanos A. Clinical, electrophysiologic and hemodynamic profile of patients resuscitated from prehospital cardiac arrest. Am J Med 1980;68:568–576.
14. LeClercq JF, Coumel P, Maison-Blanche P, Couchemez B, Zimmermann M, Chouty F, Slama R. Mise en evidence des mecanismes determinants de la mort subite. Enquete cooperative portant sur 69 cas enregistres par la methode de Holter. Arch Mal Coeur 1986;79:1024–1033.
15. Roelandt J, Klootwijk P, Lubsen J, Janse MJ. Sudden death during long term ambulatory monitoring. Europ Heart J 1984, in press.
16. Pratt CM, Francis MJ, Luck JC, Wyndham CR, Miller RR, Quinomes MA. Analysis of ambulatory electrocardiograms in 15 patients during spontaneous ventricular fibrillation with special reference to preceding arrhythmic events. J Am Coll Cardiol 1983;2: 789–797.
17. Allen JB, Laadt JR. The effect of the level of the ligature on mortality following ligation of the circumflex coronary artery in the dog. Am Heart J 1950;39:273–278.
18. Skelton RBT, Gergely NF, Manning GW, Coles JC. Mortality studies in experimental coronary occlusion. J Thorac Cardiovasc Surg 1962;44:90–96.
19. McEachern CG, Manning GW, Hall GE. Sudden occlusion of coronary arteries following removal of cardiosensory pathways. Arch Intern Med 1940;65:661–670.
20. Meesman W. Early arrhythmias and primary ventricular fibrillation after acute myocardial ischaemia in relation to pre-existing coronary collaterals. In Parratt JR, ed. Early Ventricular Arrhythmias Resulting from Myocardial Ischaemia. London and Basingstoke, Macmillan Press, 1982.
21. Meesmann, W, Schulz FW, Schley G, Adolphsen P. Ueberlebensquote nach akutem experimentellen Koronarverschlusz in Abhaengigkeit von Spontankollateralen des Herzens. Z Ges Exp Med 1970;153:246–264.
22. Harris AS. Delayed development of ventricular ectopic rhythms following experimental coronary occlusion. Circulation 1950;1:1318–1328.
23. Kabell G, Scherlag BJ, Hope RR, Lazzara R. Regional myocardial blood flow and ventricular arrhythmias following one-stage and two-stage coronary artery occlusion in anaesthesized dogs. Am Heart J 1982;104:537–545.
24. Verdouw PD, Remme WJ, De Jong JW, Breeman WAP. Myocardial substrate utilization and hemodynamics following repeated coronary flow reduction in pigs. Basic Res Cardiol 1979;74:477–485.
25. Verdouw PJ, Deckers JW, Rutteman AM, Van Bremen RH, Schefter MG. Efficacy and cardiovascular effects of antiarrhythmic drugs. Progr Pharmacol 1979;24:99–107.
26. Schaper W. The Collateral Circulation of the Heart. Amsterdam, North-Holland Publishing Company, 1971.
27. Lee KT, Lee WM, Han J, Jarmolych J, Bishop MB, Goel BG. Experimental model for study of "sudden death" from ventricular fibrillation or asystole. Am J Cardiol 1973;32: 62–73.
28. Kannel WB, Thomas HE. Sudden coronary death: The Framingham study. Ann NY Acad Sci 1982;382:3–21.

29. Patterson E, Holland K, Eller BT, Lucchesi BR. Ventricular fibrillation resulting from ischemia at a site remote from previous myocardial infarction—a conscious canine model of sudden coronary death. Am J Cardiol 1982;50:1414–1423.
30. Blumgart HL, Schlesinger MJ, Davis D. Studies on the relation of the clinical manifestations of angina pectoris. coronary thrombosis and myocardial infarction to the pathologic findings. Am Heart J 1940;19:1–91.
31. Schwartz JS, Cohn JN, Bache RJ. Effects of coronary occlusion on flow in the distribution of a neighboring stenotic coronary artery in the dog. Am J Cardiol 1983;52:189–195.
32. Myerburg RJ, Epstein K, Gaide MS, Wong SS, Castellanos A, Gelband H, Bassett AL. Electrophysiologic consequences of experimental acute ischemia superimposed on healed myocardial infarction in cats. Am J Cardiol 1982;49:323–330.
33. Schwartz PJ, Stone HL. The role of the autonomic nervous system in sudden coronary death. Ann NY Acad Sci 1982;382:162–180.
34. Billman GS, Schwartz, Stone HL. Baroceptor reflex control of heart rate: a predictor of sudden cardiac death. Circulation 1982;66:874–880.
35. Manning GW, McEachern CG, Hall GE. Reflex coronary artery spasm following sudden occlusion of other coronary branches. Arch Intern Med 1939;64:661–674.
36. Chai CY, Huang TF, Wang SC. Mechanisms of cardiac arrhythmias induced by baroceptor reflexes in cats. Am J Physiol 1968;215:1316–1323.
37. Wenger TL, Harrell FE Jr, Brown KK, Lederman S, Strauss HC. Ventricular fibrillation following canine coronary artery reperfusion: different outcome with pentobarbitol and alpha-chloralose. Can J Physiol Pharmacol 1983;62:224–228.
38. Skinner JE, Lie JT, Entman ML. Modification of ventricular fibrillation latency following coronary artery occlusion in the conscious pig: The effects of psychological stress and beta adrenergic blockade. Circulation 1975;51:656–667.
39. Bolli R, Myers ML, Wei-Xi Zhu, Roberts R. Disparity of reperfusion arrhythmias after reversible myocardial ischemia in open chest and conscious dogs. J Am Coll Cardiol 1986;7:1047–1056.
40. Pantridge FJ, Webb SW, Adgey AAJ, Geddes JS. The first hour after the onset of acute myocardial infarction. In Yu PN, Goodwin JF, eds. Progress in Cardiology (vol. III). Philadelphia, Lea and Febiger, 1974.
41. Webb SW, Adgey AAJ, Pantridge JF. Autonomic disturbance of onset of acute myocardial infarction. Br Med J 1972;3:89–92.
42. Inoue H, Zipes DP. Sinus cycle length may not indicate autonomic tone to the rest of the heart. Circulation 74 (suppl) 1986;11:II–431.
43. Pantridge JF, Webb SW, Adgey AAJ. Arrhythmias in the first hours of acute myocardial infarction. Progr Cardiovasc Dis 1981;23:265–278.
44. Han J, De Traglia J, Millet D, Moe GK. Incidence of ectopic beats as a function of heart rate in the ventricle. Am Heart J 1966;72:632–639.
45. Wit AL, Hoffman BF, Cranefield PF. Slow conduction and reentry in the ventricular conducting system. I. Return extrasystole in canine Purkinje fibers. Circ Res 1972;30:1–10.
46. Chadda KD, Banka VS, Helfant RH. Rate dependent ventricular ectopia following acute coronary occlusion. The concept of an optimal antiarrhythmic heart rate. Circulation 1974;49:654–658.
47. Kerzner J, Wolf M, Kosowsky BD, Lown B. Ventricular ectopic rhythms following vagal stimulation in dogs with acute myocardial infarction. Circulation 1973;47:44–50.
48. Scherlag BJ, Kabell G, Harrison L, Lazzara R. Mechanism of bradycardia-induced ventricular arrhythmias in myocardial ischemia and infarction. Circulation 1982;65:1429–1434.
49. Scherlag BJ, Helfant RH, Robinson MJ, Samet P. Electrophysiology underlying ventricular arrhythmias due to coronary ligation. Am J Physiol 1970;219:1665–1671.
50. Scherlag BJ, Hope RR, Williams DO, El-Sherif N, Lazzara R. Mechanisms of ectopic rhythm formation due to myocardial ischemia: effects of heart rate and ventricular

premature beats. In The Conduction System of the Heart. Wellens HJJ, Lie KI, Janse MJ, eds. The Hague, Martinus Nijhoff, 1976.
51. Kaplinsky E, Horowitz A, Neufeld HN. Ventricular reentry and automaticity in myocardial infarction. Effect of size of injury. Chest 1978;74:66–71.
52. Scherlag BJ, El-Sherif N, Hope RR, Lazzara R. Characterization and localisation of ventricular arrhythmias resulting from myocardial ischemia and infarction. Circ Res 1974;35:372–383.
53. Pick A, Langendorf R. Interpretation of Complex Arrhythmias. Lea & Febiger, Philadelphia 1979.
54. Adgey AAJ. Initiation of ventricular firbillation outside the hospital. In: Acute Phase of Ischemic Heart Disease and Myocardial Infarction. Edited by Adgey AJJ. Martinus Nijhoff, The Hague, Boston, London, 1982.
55. Shell WE, Sobel BE. Deleterious effects of increased heart rate on infarct size in the conscious dog. Am J Cardiol 1973;31:474–479.
56. Shabab L, Wollenberger A, Haase M, Schiller U. Noradrenalinabgabe aus dem Hundeherzen nach voruebergehender Okklusion einer Koronararterie. Acta Biol Med Germ 1969;22:135–143.
57. Schomig A, Dart AM, Dietz R, Mayer E, Kubler W. Release of endogenous catecholamines in the ischemic myocardium of the cat. Part A: Locally mediated release. Circ Res 1984;55:689–701.
58. Ceremuzynski L, Staszewska-Barczak J, Herbaczynska-Cedo K. Cardiac rhythm disturbances and the release of catecholamines after acute coronary occlusion in dogs. Cardiovasc Res 1969;3:190–197.
59. Richardson JA, Woods EF, Bagwell EE. Circulating epinephrine and norepinephrine in coronary occlusion. Am J Cardiol 1960;5:613–618.
60. Schwartz PJ, Stone HL. Left stellectomy in the prevention of ventricular fibrillation caused by acute myocardial ischemia in conscious dogs with anterior myocardial infarction. Circulation 1980;62:1256–1265.
61. Janse MJ, Schwartz PJ, Wilms-Schopman F, Peters RJG, Durrer D. Effects of unilateral stellate ganglion stimulation and ablation on electrophysiologic changes induced by acute myocardial ischemia in dogs. Circulation 1985;72:585–595.
62. Pearle DL, Williford D, Gillis RA. Superiority of practolol versus propranolol in protection against ventricular fibrillation induced by coronary occlusion. Am J Cardiol 1978;42:960–964.
63. Skinner JE, Reed JC. Blockade of frontocortical-brain stem pathway prevents ventricular fibrillation of ischemic heart. Am J Physiol 1981;240:H136–H163.
64. Randall DC, Hasson DM. Cardiac arrhythmias in the monkey during classically conditioned fear and excitement. Pavlov J Biol Sci 1981;16:97–107.
65. Nordrehaug JE, Von Der Lippe G. Hypokalaemia and ventricular fibrillation in acute myocardial infarction. Br Heart J 1983; 50:525–529.
66. Haase M, Schiller U. Zur zeitlichen Parallelitaet zwischen der Aktivitaet ectopischer Schrittmacher und dem Eintritt von Kammerflimmern nach Ligatur eines haupt Koronarastes beim Hund. Acta Biol Med Germ 1969;23:413–422.
67. Hirche HR, Friedrich R, Kebbel U, McDonald F, Zylka V. Early arrhythmias, myocardial extracellular potassium and pH. In Early Arrhythmias Resulting from Myocardial Ischaemia, edited by Parratt JR. London, Basingstoke, Macmillan, 1982.
68. Euler DE, Spear JF, Moore EN. Effect of coronary occlusion on arrhythmias and conduction in the ovine heart. Am J Physiol 1983;245:H82–H89.
69. Parratt JR. Inhibitors of the slow calcium current and early ventricular arrhythmias. In Early Arrhythmias Resulting from Myocardial Ischemia, edited by Parratt JR. London and Basingstoke, Macmillan, 1982.
70. Kaplinsky E, Ogawa S, Balke CW, Dreifus LS. Two periods of early ventricular arrhythmias in the canine acute infarction model. Circulation 1979;60:397–403.
71. Penny WJ. The deleterious effects of myocardial catecholamines on cellular electrophysiology and arrhythmias during ischemia and reperfusion. Eur Heart J 1984;5:960–973.

72. Russell DJ, Lawrie JS, Riemersma RA, Oliver MF. Mechanism of phase 1a and 1b early ventricular arrhythmias during acute myocardial ischemia in the dog. Am J Cardiol 1984;53:307–312.
73. Martin C, Meesman W. Antiarrhythmic effect of regional myocardial chemical sympathectomy in the early phase of coronary artery occlusion in dogs. J Cardiovasc Pharmacol 1985;7:(suppl)5:S76–S80.
74. Kleber AG, Riegger C, Janse MJ. Electrical uncoupling in acute ischemia of rabbit ventricular myocardium. Circulation 1986;74(suppl II);II–116.
75. Kleber AG, Janse MJ, Wilms-Schopman FGJ, Wilde AAM, Coronel R. Changes in conduction velocity during aute ischemia in ventricular myocardium of the isolated porcine heart. Circulation 1986;73:189–198.
76. Cardinal R, Janse MJ, van Eeden I, Werner G, Naumann d'Alnoncourt C, Durrer D. The effects of lidocaine on intracellular and extracellular potentials, activation and ventricular arrhythmias during acute regional ischemia in the isolated porcine heart. Circ Res 1981;49:792–806.
77. Janse MJ, Capucci A, Coronel R, Fabius MAW. Variablity of recovery of excitability in the normal canine and ischemic porcine heart. Eur Heart J 1985;6:(suppl D):41–52.
78. Janse MJ, Downar E. The effect of acute ischemia on transmembrane potentials in the intact heart. The relation to re-entrant arrhythmias. In Re-entrant Arrhythmias, edited by Kulbertus HE. Lancaster, M.T.P. Press, 1977.
79. Downar E, Janse MJ, Durrer D. The effect of acute coronary artery occlusion on subepicardial transmembrane potentials in the intact porcine heart. Circulation 1977;56:217–224.
80. Kodama I, Wilde A, Janse MJ, Durrer D, Yamada K. Combined effects of hypoxia, hyperkalemia, and acidosis on membrane action potential and excitability of guinea pig ventricular muscle. J Mol Cell Cardiol 1984;16:247–259.
81. Hill JL, Gettes LS. Effect of acute coronary artery occlusion on local myocardial extracellular K+ activity in swine. Circulation 1980;61:768–778.
82. Janse MJ, van Capelle FJL, Morsink H, Kleber AG, Wilms-Schopman FJG, Cardinal R, Naumann d'Alnoncourt C, Durrer D. Flow of "injury" current and patterns of excitation during early ventricular arrhythmias in acute regional ischemia in isolated porcine and canine hearts. Evidence for 2 different arrhythmogenic mechanisms. Circ Res 1980;47:151–165.
83. Janse MJ, van Cappelle FJL. Electrotonic interactions across an inexcitable region as a cause of ectopic activity in acute regional ischemia. A study in intact porcine and canine hearts and computer models. Circ Res 1982;50:403–414.
84. Allessie MA, Bonke FIM, Schopman FJG. Circus movement in rabbit atrial muscle as a mechanism of tachycardia. III. The "leading circle" concept: a new model of circus movement in cardiac tissue without the involvement of an anatomical obstacle. Circ Res 1977;41:9–18.
85. Janse MJ, Kleber AG, Capucci A, Coronel R, Wilms-Schopman F. Electrophysiological basis for arrhythmias caused by acute ischemia. Role of the subendocardium. J Mol Cell Cardiol 1986;18:339.
86. Brooks, CMcC, Gilbert JL, Janse MJ. Failure of integrated cardiac action at supernormal heart rates. Proc Soc Exp Biol Med 1964;117:630–634.
87. Janse MJ. The effect of changes in heart rate on the refractory period of the heart. Thesis, University of Amsterdam. Mondeel Offset Drukkerij, 1971.
88. Allessie MA, Bonke FIM, Schopman FJG. Circus movement in rabbit atrial muscle as a mechanism for tachycardia II. The role of non-uniform recovery of excitability in the occurrence of unidirectional block as studied with multiple microelectrodes. Circ Res 1976;39:168–177.
89. Wilensky RL, Tranum-Jensen J, Coronel R, Wilde AAM, Fiolet JWT, Janse MJ. The subendocardial "border" zone during acute ischemia of the rabbit heart: an electrophysiological, metabolic and morphological correlation. Circulation 1986;74:1137–1146.
90. Kannel WB, Doyle JT, McNamara PM, Quickenton P, Gordon T. Precursors of sudden coronary death: factors related to the incidence of sudden death. Circulation 1975;51:606–613.

91. Epstein TH, Pisa Z. International comparison in ischaemic heart disease mortality. Proceedings of the "conference on the decline in coronary heart mortality." National Heart, Lung and Blood Institute, N.I.H., Bethesda, Md, October 24–25, 1978.
92. Stern MP. The recent decline in ischemic heart disease mortality. Ann Int Med 1979;91: 630–640.
93. Lie KI, Wellens HJJ, van Capelle FJL, Durrer D. Lidocaine in the prevention of primary ventricular fibrillation. A double-blind, randomized study of 212 consecutive patients. N Engl J Med 1974;291:1324–1329.
94. Koster RW, Dunning AJ. Intramuscular lidocaine for prevention of lethal arrhythmias in the prehospitalization phase of myocardial infarction. N Engl J Med 1985;313: 1105–1112.
95. Carson DL, Cardinal R, Savarol P, Vasseur C, Nattel S, Lambert C, Nadeau R. Relationship between an arrhythmogenic action of lidocaine and its effects on excitation patterns in acutely ischemic porcine myocardium. J Cardiovasc Pharmacol 1986;8: 126–136.
96. Bergey JL, Nocella K, McCallum JD. Acute coronary artery occlusion-reperfusion arrhythmias in rats, dogs and pigs: antiarrhythmic evaluation of quinidine, procainamide and lidocaine. Eur J Pharmacol 1982;81:205–216.
97. Chamberton DR, Julian DG, Boyle DM, Jewitt DE, Campbell RWF, and Shanks RG. Oral mexiletine in high risk patients after myocardial infarction. Lancet 1980;2: 1324–1327.
98. Peter T, Ross D, Duffield A, Luxton M, Harper R, Hunt D, Sloman G. Effect on survival on long-term treatment with phenytoin. Br Heart J 1978;40:1356–1360.
99. Ryden L, Arnman K, Conradson TB, Hhofvendahl S, Mortensen O, Smedgard P. Prophylaxis of ventricular tachyarrhythmias with intravenous and oral tocainide in patients with and recovering from myocardial infarction. Am Heart J 1980;100: 1006–1012.

7

The Distinction Between Triggered Activity and Other Cardiac Arrhythmias

Nancy J. Johnson
Michael R. Rosen

Introduction

The traditional method for identifying the mechanisms responsible for cardiac arrhythmias has been based on observing their responses to interventions such as overdrive pacing and premature stimulation. These same interventions have been applied to the characterization of arrhythmias induced in experimental animals and in isolated tissues. In this review, we will consider one specific arrhythmogenic mechanism: triggered activity induced by delayed afterdepolarizations, and will address two questions: (1) Given that many types of tissue preparations and diverse experimental conditions produce delayed afterdepolarizations and triggered activity, and that most of the "rules" describing the phenomenology of triggered activity are based on studies of digitalis-toxic Purkinje fibers, to what extent are such rules applicable to triggered arrhythmias induced by other means? (2) Are the characteristics of triggered activity described in isolated tissue preparations sufficiently specific to allow the discrimination of triggered activity from other mechanisms of arrhythmia generation?

To help answer the first question, we will compare the behavior of two experimental tissue preparations: the digitalis-toxic canine Purkinje fiber and the catecholamine-superfused coronary sinus. To consider the second question, we will systematically compare the responses to pacing of triggered rhythms to those of other mechanisms of arrhythmia induction. In so doing, there will be no attempt at an extensive review of the literature relating to arrhythmia induction by each mechanism; rather, we will review such characteristics in summary form.

The Comparison of Delayed Afterdepolarizations and Triggered Activity in Purkinje Fibers with Those Occurring in Coronary Sinus

Delayed afterdepolarizations are oscillations in membrane potential that are induced by and are strongly influenced by the preceding cardiac rhythm.[1-10] Such oscillations may occur singly or as sequences of two or more. Figure 1A is an analog record of delayed afterdepolarizations occurring in a ouabain-toxic Purkinje fiber after the cessation of drive. The two prominent oscillations in the tracing are typical of the multiple delayed afterdepolarizations seen in this type of preparation. The relationship between the basic drive cycle length and the coupling interval between the action potential and the first two delayed afterdepolarizations succeeding it is shown in Figure 1C. Note that the relationship between basic drive and coupling interval is nearly linear for each delayed afterdepolarization, but that the slope for the second afterdepolarization is far steeper than that for the first.

The relationship of delayed afterdepolarization amplitude to basic cycle length is more complex than that of the coupling interval (Fig. 1B), as first one and then the other afterdepolarization predominates. The overall tendency is for the amplitude of the first afterdepolarization to increase and then decrease as drive cycle length decreases. The second afterdepolarization continues to increase in amplitude. Depending on the relationship of afterdepolarization amplitude to threshold potential, either one or the other depolarization may attain threshold and initiate a triggered beat. Hence, either the first or the second delayed afterdepolarization in a sequence can give rise to a triggered rhythm. The coupling interval of the first triggered beat will approximate that of the delayed afterdepolarization. It should be apparent from the record in Figure 1C that if only the first or only the second afterdepolarization attains threshold and induces a triggered rhythm, then the relationship of the coupling interval of the first triggered beat to a sequence of drive cycle lengths will be that of a single line (either the filled or unfilled circles in Figure 1C). However, if at some cycle lengths the first delayed afterdepolarization attains threshold, and at others, the second attains threshold, a discontinuous line will relate coupling interval to drive cycle length.

In contrast to digitalis-toxic fibers, the catecholamine-superfused coronary sinus usually produces only one delayed afterdepolarization.[11-13] (Fig. 2A). The amplitude of the afterdepolarization increases with decreasing drive cycle length (Fig. 2B) and its coupling interval is related to the basic drive cycle length by the single curve shown in Figure 2C. In many ways, the relationship between delayed afterdepolarization amplitude (Fig. 2B) and coupling interval to basic drive (Fig. 2C) in the coronary sinus is similar to that of the *second* delayed afterdepolarization in the digitalis-toxic fiber in Figure 1B and C.

In coronary sinus, action potentials triggered by delayed afterdepolarizations

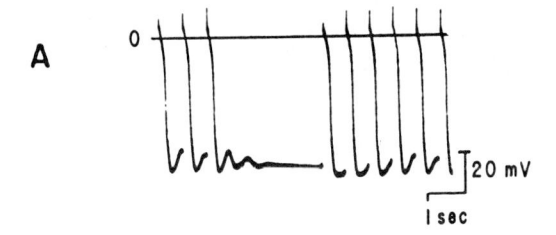

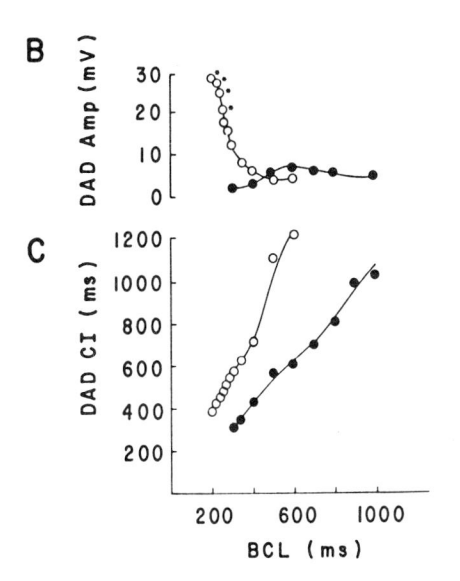

Figure 1: Panel A shows a Purkinje fiber following exposure to ouabain. The first three cycles are driven, after which the drive is discontinued. Two delayed afterdepolarizations are seen, followed by a period of quiescence, until the drive is reinitiated. Several cycles are then required for the afterdepolarizations to attain their peak amplitude. Panels B and C show, respectively, the relationship to the basic drive cycle length of the amplitude and coupling interval of the first (black circles) and the second (white circles) delayed afterdepolarizations in a sequence. Asterisks indicate those afterdepolarizations that attained threshold potential and initiated triggered action potentials. See text for discussion. (Modified after Rosen, et al.[13])

will tend to show a similar relationship between their coupling interval and the basic drive to that demonstrated by the afterdepolarization in Figure 2C. There usually is not the type of complication brought on by the occurrence of more than one afterdepolarization, as in Figure 1. Hence, the similarity between the preparations in Figures 1 and 2 lies in the fact that the coupling interval of the first triggered beat in both settings will tend to decrease as the initiating drive cycle length decreases. The dissimilarity is that for reasons mentioned above, the curve relating coupling interval to basic cycle length is the ouabain-toxic fiber will often be discontinuous; that in coronary sinus will be continuous.

As shown above, at sufficiently rapid drive rates, the afterdepolarization amplitude in digitalis-superfused Purkinje fibers and in catecholamine-treated coronary sinus will attain threshold potential. The result will be a single triggered beat or a series of triggered beats. Several factors can complicate the relationship between the basic drive cycle and the delayed afterdepolarization beyond those already mentioned, thereby influencing whether or not threshold is reached and an arrhythmia occurs.

The first of these factors is membrane potential.[11,13–15] Figure 3 shows the relationship of the membrane potential of a coronary sinus preparation to delayed afterdepolarization amplitude. There is an important effect of membrane poten-

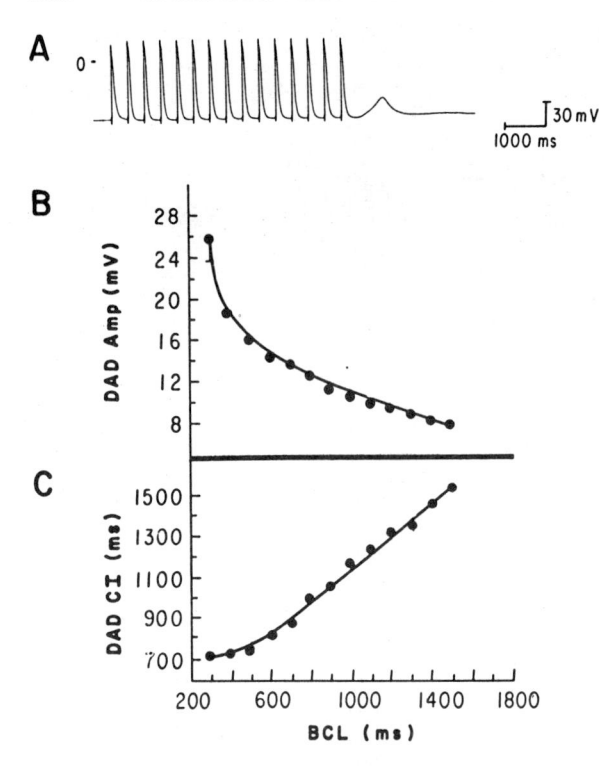

Figure 2: Panel A shows an atrial fiber in the canine coronary sinus during exposure to epinephrine. There are 15 driven cycles and the drive is then discontinued. A single delayed afterdepolarization is seen, followed by quiescence. Panels B and C relate delayed afterdepolarization amplitude and coupling interval to basic drive cycle length. Results are the mean of nine experiments. See text for discussion. (Modified after Johnson, et al.[13])

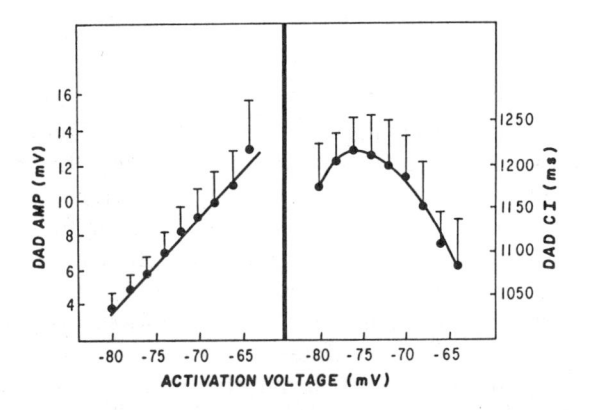

Figure 3: Relationship of the amplitude (left panel) and coupling interval (right panel) of catecholamine-induced delayed afterdepolarizations in coronary sinus to the membrane potential of the preparation (activation voltage). Results expressed as mean ± SE of five preparations. See text for discussion (Modified after Johnson et al.[13])

tial here, such that if drive is occurring at a constant cycle length and membrane potential changes, there is a profound change in the afterdepolarization amplitude and, with this, in the likelihood of triggered activity. The coupling interval of the afterdepolarization also is influenced by changes in membrane potential, as is seen on the right panel of Figure 3. Similar membrane potential dependence has been shown for digitalis-induced delayed afterdepolarizations as well.[16,17]

A second factor to be considered is periods of quiescence (which may occur locally when a site in the conducting system is protected by some degree of entry block from frequent excitation by the primary cardiac pacemaker).[13,14] During quiescence, catecholamine-superfused coronary sinus preparations gradually depolarize to a membrane potential of approximately −60 mV, as demonstrated in Figure 4A. If short bursts of pacing are induced at various intervals during quiescence, the resulting delayed afterdepolarizations will show an increase in amplitude and a decrease in coupling interval as the duration of quiescence preceding pacing increases. As expected, based on the increase in afterdepolarization amplitude, triggering is seen more readily after the longer periods of quiescence. When triggered activity occurs, its peak rate varies inversely with the duration of preceding quiescence (Fig. 4B). These relationships undoubtedly reflect, in part, the change in membrane potential that accompanies quiescence in this preparation, but there may be other contributing factors as well. For example, during quiescence following rapid electrical activity, there is a decay of outward current due to the gradual decline of sodium/potassium pump activity. As outward current decays, delayed afterdepolarizations, which are a manifestation of a transient inward current, should become more prominent. Because the potential for entrance block leading to local areas of quiescence is very real in the intact heart, and because periods of quiescence in their own right or in association with

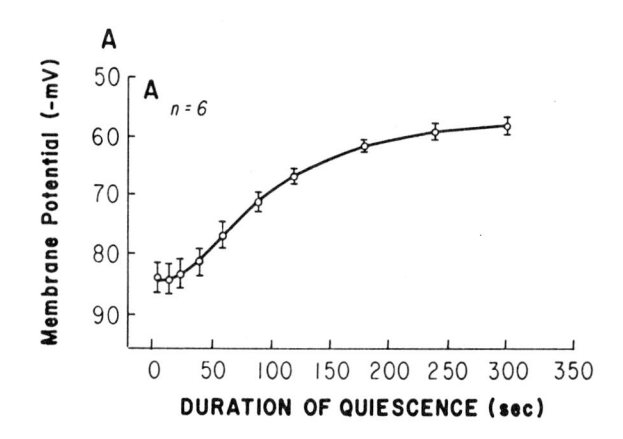

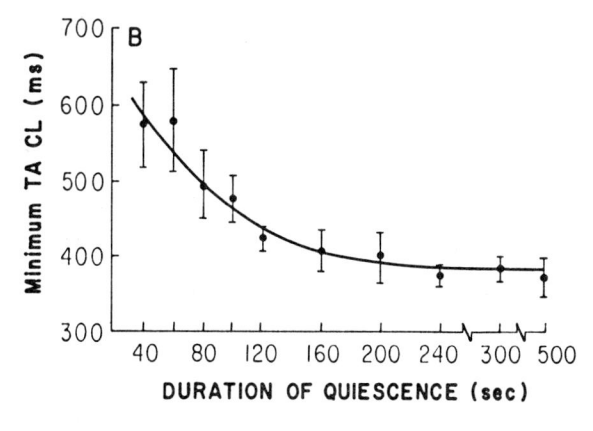

Figure 4: A: Relationship of membrane potential of six canine coronary sinus preparations to the duration of quiescence. B: The relationship of the minimum cycle length of a series of triggered rhythms to the duration of preceding quiescence. As the duration of quiescence increases, the membrane potential depolarizes and the minimum cycle length attained by the subsequent triggered rhythm becomes shorter. Results expressed as mean ± SE. See text for discussion. TA = triggered activity.

changes in membrane potential can induce changes in amplitude of afterdepolarizations, the occurrence of block or quiescence is likely to complicate the behavior of triggered rhythms.

Other factors that can influence delayed afterdepolarization amplitude will be mentioned only briefly. For example, beta-adrenergic catecholamines will increase the amplitude and shorten the coupling interval of delayed afterdepolarizations in coronary sinus,[11-15] in digitalis toxicity[18] and in myocardial infarction;[19,20] acetylcholine has the opposite effect.[21] Alpha-adrenergic catecholamines also can increase afterdepolarization amplitude in the presence of high $[Ca^{2+}]_o$.[22] Interventions that prolong repolarization increase afterdepolarization amplitude, presumably by increasing inward current.[23] Elevating $[K^+]_o$ will change membrane potential and, thereby, can change afterdepolarization amplitude.[24,25] Since all of these variables are important in the clinical setting, the clinical expression of delayed afterdepolarizations and triggered rhythms can be anticipated to show a great deal of variation among individuals.

Initiation of Triggered Activity[13,26]

In ouabain-toxic Purkinje fibers, triggered activity is more readily induced by sustained drive or burst pacing at short cycle lengths than at longer cycle lengths.[26] A similar relationship exists for catecholamine-superfused coronary sinus, as shown in Figure 5, top.[13] Reproducibility of induction differs in the two types of preparations. Induction of triggering is reproducible at the same drive cycle length in only 38% of Purkinje fibers, whereas reproducibility tends to increase with the frequency of triggering in coronary sinus.

The triggered activity induced by basic drive plus a single premature stimulus (S_2) in ouabain-toxic Purkinje fibers shows a variable relationship to the initiating drive. That is, the coupling interval of the first triggered beat either increases or decreases as the S_2 becomes more premature. In contrast, the first triggered beat in catecholamine-treated coronary sinus shows no relationship to the coupling interval of the premature impulse that induces it. Regardless of the S_1-S_2 interval, the coupling interval of the first premature beat remains constant. In both types of tissue, the frequency of triggering increases as the S_2 coupling interval decreases (e.g., Fig. 5, bottom), and in coronary sinus, the reproducibility of triggering at any one cycle length increases along with the frequency.

Sustained episodes of triggered activity in Purkinje fibers often show "warm-up" (an increasing rate) at the outset, and a slowing trend prior to termination. Sustained triggered rhythms in coronary sinus follow one of the four characteristic patterns shown in Figure 6. Whereas the rate of triggered rhythms in Purkinje fibers often is directly related to the cycle length of the initiating drive, both the maximum rate and the equilibrium rate of coronary sinus rhythms are constant within each preparation, independent of the initiating drive cycle length. However, as stated above, the first beat of the triggered rhythm in coronary sinus does show a linear relationship to the preceding drive over a wide range of drive cycle lengths, regardless of the behavior of the subsequent rhythm. In fact, it is the coupling interval relationship of the first beat after cessation of pacing to the basic

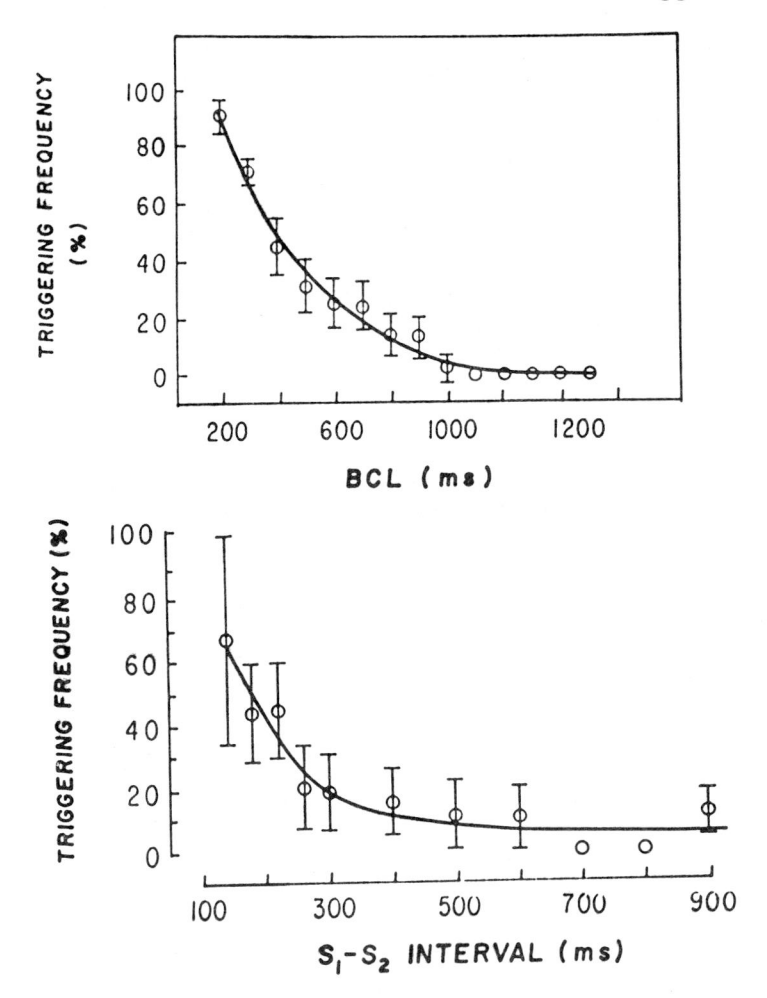

Figure 5: Top: The frequency of triggered activity in 14 canine coronary sinus preparations increases as basic drive cycle length is reduced. Bottom: The frequency of triggered activity in five preparations increases as the S_1-S_2 coupling interval for premature stimulation is reduced. Results are mean ± SE. See text for discussion. (Modified after Johnson et al.[13])

drive cycle length that is the consistent finding regardless of the type of triggered activity.

Response of Sustained Triggered Rhythms to Overdrive Pacing[13,26]

Eighty-nine percent of all episodes of sustained triggered activity in ouabain-toxic Purkinje fibers can be terminated by 15–60 seconds of overdrive pacing at a cycle length of 300 ms. This result is reproducible in 92% of fibers. Seventy-four percent of these terminations are preceded by 1–10 terminal beats on cessation of overdrive. Seventy-five percent of episodes in coronary sinus can be terminated by overdrive pacing at 50% of the intrinsic cycle length for durations of up to 120

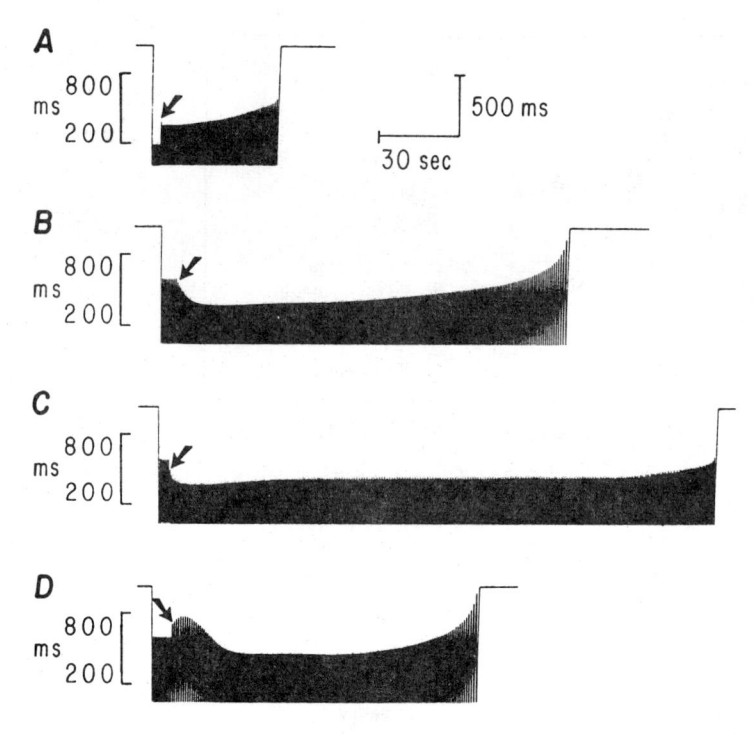

Figure 6: A series of tachometer recordings of the spontaneous rhythms occurring in coronary sinus preparations following periods of drive. In each panel, the cessation of drive is marked with an arrow. Note that the rhythms either slowed gradually until they ceased (A); sped up and then gradually slowed (B); sped up, attained a steady state, and then slowed (C); or slowed down, sped up, and then gradually slowed again (D). The slowing before cessation was a constant in all experiments. See text for discussion. (Reprinted from Johnson et al.[13] by permission of the American Heart Association.)

beats, and this result can be reproduced in 90% of preparations. Similarly, approximately 55% of these terminations are preceded by up to 25 terminal beats, on cessation of the drive. There terminal beats gradually increase in cycle length until the rhythm ceases.

In both types of preparation, short overdrive cycle lengths are more effective in terminating triggered rhythms than are long cycle lengths. When the rhythm persists following overdrive pacing, the coupling interval of the first beat following the cessation of pacing is directly related to the cycle length of the overdrive, in effect duplicating the relationship of these two variables shown in Figures 1 and 2.

In contrast to overdrive pacing, premature stimulation infrequently terminates triggered activity in both Purkinje fibers (14% of rhythms) and coronary sinus preparations (21%). Termination is reproducible in 33% of Purkinje fibers and in approximately 50% of coronary sinus preparations. In the remaining Purkinje fibers, the first triggered beat following the premature stimulus tends to reset the preceding triggered cycle length, whereas in coronary sinus only 21% of preparations show reset in response to S_2. The remaining 79% show a slightly positive slope of the return cycle length in relation to the S_2 coupling interval.

In summary, there are some distinct differences between the triggered activity produced in ouabain-toxic Purkinje fibers and that occurring in catecholamine-superfused coronary sinus. There are, however, many similarities as well. An outline of these characteristics is presented in Table I.

Do the Responses of Triggered Rhythms to Pacing Differ Significantly from Those of Other Arrhythmogenic Mechanisms?

In Table II we have summarized the responses to pacing that occur in various types of arrhythmias. The underscored entries represent those responses which differ from those of delayed afterdepolarization-induced triggered activity.

Table I
Comparison of Triggered Activity in Ouabain-Superfused Purkinje Fibers and Catecholamine Superfused Coronary Sinus[13,26]

	Purkinje Fiber	Coronary Sinus
Initiation by Basic Drive	Freq. of trig. ↑ as BCL ↓ 38% reproducible at critical CL No increase in reproducibility at shorter CL 1st trig. CI ↓ as BCL ↓ Discontinuous curve (because usually have 2 or more DAD)	Freq. of trig. ↑ at BCL ↓ 55% reproducible at critical CL Reproducibility ↑ as BCL ↓ 1st trig. CI ↓ as BCL ↓ Continuous curve (because usually have 1 DAD)
Initiation by Basic Drive + S_2	Freq. of trig. ↑ as S_2CI ↓ 57% reproducible at critical CI 1st trig. CI ↓ or ↑ as S_2CI ↓	Freq. of trig. ↑ as S_2CI ↓ 25% reproducible at critical CI Reproducibility ↑ as S_2CI ↓ 1st trig. CI unchanged as S_2CI ↓
Sustained Triggered Activity	Initital "warm-up" Occasional terminal "slow-down"	Initial "warm-up" Typical terminal "slow-down" 4 characteristic rate patterns
Response of Sustained TA to OD	89% termination with OD Abrupt or delayed termination Freq. of term. ↑ as OD CL ↓ Freq. of term. unchanged as OD dur. ↑ 1st escape CI ↓ as OD CL ↓	75% termination with OD Abrupt or delayed termination Freq. of term. ↑ as OD CL ↓ Freq. of term. ↑ as OD dur. ↓ 1st escape CI ↓ as OD CL ↓
Response of Sustained TA to S_2	14% termination at short S_2CI 33% reproducible at critical CI Abrupt and delayed term. Return CL resets as S_2CI ↓	21% termination at short S_2CI 50% reproducible at critical CI Abrupt and delayed term. Return CL resets or ↓ as S_2CI ↓

BCL = basic cycle length, S_2 = premature stimulus, CI = coupling interval, OD = overdrive, dur = duration, ↑ = increases, ↓ = decreases, TA = triggered activity.

Table II
Comparison of the Characteristics of Triggered Activity Induced by Delayed Afterdepolarizations (see Table I) with Some Other Mechanisms of Arrhythmia Generation

	TA (EADs) (27)	Normal Automaticity (7,8,28,29)	Abnormal Automaticity (7,8,28-31)	Reentry (34-48)
Initiation by Basic Drive	Freq. of trig. ↓ as BCL ↓ 1st trig. CI ↑ as BCL ↓	Spontaneous, not initiated by pacing More manifest at slow heart rates	Spontaneous, not initiated by pacing More manifest at slow heart rate	High reproducibility 1st CI tends to be unchanged or ↓ as BCL ↓
Initiation by Basic Drive & S₂	No trig. with S₂	Spontaneous not initiated by pacing	Spontaneous, not initiated by pacing	Narrow range of critical S₂ CI High reproducibility 1st CI tends to be unchanged or ↑ as S₂ CI ↓
Sustained Rhythm		May show "warm-up" May show "annihilation"	May show "warm-up" May show "annihilation"	Initial stable rate or oscillation of rate, or may "slow-down" Terminal oscillation or abrupt cessation
Response to OD Pacing	No term. with OD 1st escape CI resets or shows OD suppression	No term. with OD 1st escape CI shows OD suppression 1st escape CI ↑ as OD CL ↓	No term. with OD 1st escape CI shows reset, accel., or suppression after OD 1st escape CI ↓ or ↑ as OD CL ↓	High freq. of term. with OD abrupt and delayed term. Narrow range of critical OD CL 1st escape CI resets or ↑ as OD CL ↓
Response to S₂ Pacing	10-75% term. with S₂ Abrupt term. only Return CL resets	No term. with S₂ Return CL resets or ↑ as S₂ CI ↓	No term. with S₂ Return CL resets, ↑ or ↓ as S₂ CI ↓	High freq. of term. with S₂ Narrow range of critical S₂ High reproducibility Abrupt and delayed term. Return CL resets or ↑ as S₂ CI ↓

Abbreviations: TA = triggered activity, DAD = delayed afterpolarization, CI = coupling interval, S₂ = premature stimulus, OD = overdrive, EAD = early afterdepolarization, BCL = basic cycle length, CL = cycle length, ↑ = increases, ↓ = decreases.

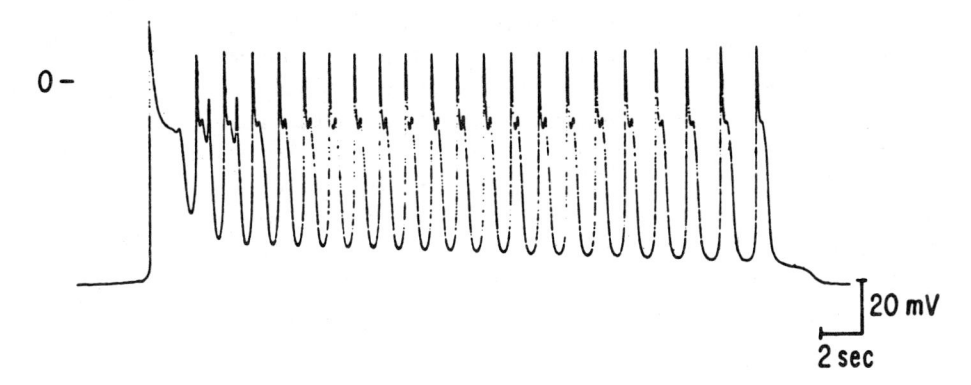

Figure 7: Cesium-induced delayed afterdepolarizations and triggered activity in a canine Purkinje fiber. The initial action potential is driven. An oscillation appears near the termination of the plateau and triggered activity commences during phase 3 repolarization. Early afterdepolarizations persist during the plateau of the first few triggered beats. There is gradual spontaneous hyperpolarization of the membrane and slowing of the rhythm until it stops abruptly and the membrane returns to a high level of membrane potential. See text for discussion. (Reprinted from Damiano and Rosen[27] by permission of the American Heart Association.)

Triggered Activity Induced by Early Afterdepolarizations

Early afterdepolarizations are oscillations in membrane potential that precede the termination of repolarization[7,8] (Fig. 7). They tend to increase in amplitude as drive rate is slowed and/or repolarization is delayed. Moreover, the rate of the triggered activity they induce increases as the basic drive rate is slowed.[27] Hence, rhythms induced by early afterdepolarizations are "bradycardia-dependent tachycardias." This is in clear contrast to triggered rhythms induced by delayed afterdepolarizations. Furthermore, since rhythms generated by early afterdepolarizations are bradycardia-dependent, they tend not to occur following premature stimulation. Once initiated, these rhythms may be suppressed by overdrive pacing, depending on their membrane potential, and, unlike delayed afterdepolarization-induced triggered rhythms, tend not to exhibit terminal beats prior to cessation. Their spontaneous termination (as shown in Fig. 7) is usually associated with hyperpolarization of the membrane to a level at which the inward current responsible for the early afterdepolarization no longer occurs. When these rhythms are subjected to overdrive pacing, their behavior is like that of automatic rhythms (see below); i.e. those rhythms occurring at higher membrane potentials are more readily suppressed.

Automatic Rhythms

Automatic rhythms are those which can be initiated de novo as a result of phase 4 depolarization in the Purkinje system.[7,8] It is obvious that in the beating heart it would be difficult to identify with certainty whether a rhythm that was occurring did, in fact, arise de novo. Hence, this initial descriptor of automatic rhythms, while serving as an excellent means for identifying them in isolated tissues, is of only limited value in vivo. Moreover, automatic rhythms may, at times, be subject to "annihilation."[28] In this case, perhaps as a result of subthreshold depolarizations propagating from another site and modifying the membrane potential of the automatic pacemaker, termination of the rhythm is seen.

Automatic rhythms have been divided arbitrarily into two types.[29-31] The first is referred to as normal automaticity, is initiated in preparations whose membrane potentials are normal (for that tissue type), and tends to be suppressed by overdrive pacing. The second type, abnormal automaticity, occurs in depolarized tissues and is not readily overdrive suppressible. In fact, there is a continuum between the two types of automaticity, and their ability to be overdrive-suppressed is related directly to the level of membrane potential. At higher membrane potentials, more Na^+ is carried into the cell by the action potential upstroke, thereby providing a greater stimulus for the electrogenic Na^+, K^+ pumping that is responsible for overdrive suppression.[32,33] At lower membrane potentials, there is less of a stimulus for Na^+, K^+ pumping (as the action potential may be largely Ca^{2+}-dependent) and overdrive suppression is less readily induced.

Arrhythmias resulting from automaticity at high membrane potentials have marked differences from those induced by triggered activity. The automatic rhythms are not inducible by drive or premature stimuli, but are spontaneous in origin. In contrast to triggered activity, such automatic rhythms show no increase in rate nor are they terminated by overdrive pacing; rather, the coupling interval of the first escape beat following overdrive increases as the cycle length of the overdrive decreases, showing consistent overdrive suppression. In response to premature stimuli, the return cycle length of a normally automatic rhythm is either fully compensatory (if the automatic focus is protected) or resets the preceding rate (if the focus is depolarized by the S_2). Theoretically, a focus of triggered activity might be similarly protected from invasion by pacing, and might be expected to show a compensatory pause in that event. However, this type of pause has never actually been reported in triggered rhythms.

So-called "abnormal automaticity" is a spontaneously occurring rhythm originating from specialized conducting or myocardial fibers at low (usually < -70 mV) membrane potentials.[29-31] Rhythms resulting from abnormal automaticity do not depend on pacing, premature stimuli, or even a preceding action potential for their initiation. As the name implies, they are automatic and spontaneous in origin.

Unlike the usual response of triggered rhythms to overdrive pacing, abnormally automatic rhythms tend not to terminate. The reason for this is the low membrane potentials at which such abnormal automatic rhythms tend to occur. The action potentials here tend to be more Ca^{2+}-dependent than Na^+-dependent. Since Na^+ entry is a potent stimulus for electrogenic Na^+, K^+ pumping and provides the basis for overdrive suppression in fibers having automatic rhythms at normal membrane potentials, one would not expect Na^+, K^+ pumping and overdrive suppression in depolarized fibers having Ca^{2+}-dependent action potentials.[32,33] The extent to which this (or any) automatic rhythm will be overdrive-suppressed, then, depends on its initial membrane potential, and the likelihood of suppression will be a variable, depending on the membrane potential and the duration and rate of overdrive pacing. Moreover, the studies of Dangman and

Hoffman[29] suggest that at low membrane potentials, abnormal automatic rhythms may even increase in rate following a period of overdrive pacing. Hence, the cycle length following pacing can either decrease or increase as the overdrive cycle length is decreased.

This means that some abnormal automatic rhythms will be distinguishable from delayed afterdepolarization-induced triggered activity on the basis of their response to overdrive pacing while others will not. Following premature stimulation, abnormally automatic rhythms tend not to terminate. The return cycle length after premature stimulation can increase, decrease, or simply show reset as the S_2 becomes more premature. Only in the first case will this response aid in the differentiation of this type of rhythm from triggered activity. In summary, it is likely that only a subset of abnormally automatic rhythms is distinguishable from triggered activity on the basis of the response to pacing.

Reentrant Rhythms

In comparing the characteristics of reentrant rhythms to those of triggered activity, there are several distinctions which may be useful. Unlike triggered activity, reentry may be initiated at long or short drive cycle lengths,[34,35] but in any one individual its initiation tends to be highly reproducible over a critical range of cycle lengths. Furthermore, the coupling interval of the first reentrant beat is a function of the circuit that is traversed and can be relatively independent of the cycle length of the initiating drive. When these rhythms are initiated by premature stimuli, there is usually a narrow range of effective S_2 coupling intervals and reproducibility is high. Again, the coupling interval of the first reentrant beat may appear unrelated to the coupling interval of the S_2 that initiated it. Reentrant rhythms tend to have consistent rates, with only one or two oscillations of cycle length preceding the development of a stable rate,[36,38] or they may slow or speed up for as many as 50–100 beats before stabilizing.[39] The former pattern is clearly different from that seen in triggered activity.

Reentry can be terminated by overdrive pacing, but in any individual there usually is a specific and narrow range of cycle lengths which terminate the rhythm. When reentry is not terminated by overdrive pacing, the coupling interval of the first escape beat can reset the succeeding reentrant cycle length independent of the rate of the overdrive. A major difference between triggered activity and reentry lies in the behavior of the return cycle length following the S_2 in response to premature stimulation. In reentry, the return cycle length tends to increase as the S_2 becomes more premature, a phenomenon usually not seen with delayed afterdepolarization-induced triggered activity (although it can be mimicked, as discussed with reference to Figure 1C).

Recently, Waldo and associates[40-43] have studied presumably reentrant arrhythmias in the intact heart, and have considered in detail the response of these rhythms to a specific pacing protocol. They have described a series of rules for the behavior of rhythms that demonstrate "transient entrainment," the rationale being that the occurrence of transient entrainment will definitively identify a rhythm as reentrant. Of particular note as descriptors are the following: (1) one can entrain such a rhythm by pacing and demonstrate fusion at progressively more rapid pacing rates; (2) one can demonstrate differing degrees of fusion at different pacing rates (so-called progressive fusion); (3) once fusion has occurred, it will be constant at any cycle length except for the last entrained beat; (4) on abrupt cessation or gradual slowing of pacing there may be the immediate resumption of the original tachycardia; this will occur at the original tachycardia cycle length. In considering whether a triggered arrhythmia induced by delayed afterdepolarizations might be expected to show a similar, and therefore, confounding, pattern, the following appears to hold: observations 1 and 2 might reasonably be expected with some triggered rhythms: that is, both entrainment and fusion as well as progressive fusion might occur. However, observations 3 and 4 are less likely with triggered activity, especially observation 4: we would expect a triggered rhythm to show, for at least the first beat after cessation of pacing, a coupling interval that approximated that of the overdrive or entraining rhythm or, alternatively, gradual or sudden cessation of the triggered rhythm. Hence, it appears that some real distinctions might be made between triggered and reentrant rhythms in the intact heart based on this particular descriptor. Nonetheless, triggered rhythms have not yet been tested using the rules of transient entrainment, and so no definitive statement can be made.

Summary

The typical responses to pacing that characterize the various mechanisms of arrhythmia generation in isolated experimental preparations are sufficiently different to allow the distinction of triggered activity from other types of arrhythmias in most instances. However, because of overlapping responses to pacing interventions, distinction becomes more difficult in considering the cause of rhythms in the intact heart[49,50] and may be impossible in individual instances of arrhythmias. Hence, whereas pacing may be useful in classifying populations of arrhythmias, it is not presently a sufficient discriminator to permit its use as an identifier of mechanism in individuals with any certainty.[51,52] Nonetheless, only triggered activity and some instances of abnormal automaticity show a nearly linear relationship between basic drive and the initiating beat of a tachycardia. This specific relationship (i.e., a decrease in the cycle length of the first impulse following pacing as drive cycle length decreases) can be used to discriminate triggered and some abnormal automatic rhythms from other mechanisms. More specific differentiation requires additional technology, such as the use of selective cardioactive drugs, monophasic action potential recording techniques, and cardiac mapping.

Acknowledgment: Certain of the studies referred to were supported by USPHS-NHLBI Grant HL-28223.

References

1. Rosen MR, Gelband HB, Merker C. Mechanics of digitalis toxicity. Effects of ouabain on phase 4 of canine Purkinje fiber transmembrane potentials. Circulation 1973;47: 681–689.
2. Rosen MR, Gelband HB, Hoffman BF. Correlation between effects of ouabain on the

canine electrocardiogram and transmembrane potentials of isolated Purkinje fibers. Circulation 1973;47:65–72.
3. Ferrier GR. The effects of tension on acetylstrophanthidin-induced transient depolarizations and aftercontractions in canine myocardial and Purkinje tissue. Circ Res 1976;38:156–162.
4. Ferrier GR. Digitalis arrhythmias: Role of oscillatory afterpotentials. Prog Cardiovasc Dis 1977;19:459–474.
5. Davis LD. Effects of changes in cycle length on diastolic depolarization produced by oaubain in canine Purkinje fibers. Circ Res 1973;32:206–21.
6. Hogan PM, Wittenberg SM, Klocke FJ. Relationship of stimulation frequency to automaticity in the canine Purkinje fiber during ouabain administration. Circ Res 1973;32:377–383.
7. Cranefield PF. The Conduction of the Cardiac Impulse: The Slow Response and Cardiac Arrhythmias. Futura Publishing, Mt. Kisco, NY, 1975.
8. Cranefield PF. Action potentials, afterpotentials and arrhythmias. Circ Res 1972;41:415–423.
9. Cranefield PF. Does spontaneous activity arise from phase 4 depolarization or from triggering? In Bonke FIM, ed. The Sinus Node: Structure, Function and Clinical Relevance, Martinus Nijhoff, The Hague, 1978;348–356.
10. Cranefield PF, Aronson RS. Initiation of sustained rhythmic activity by single propagated action potentials in canine cardiac Purkinje fibers exposed to sodium free solution or to ouabain. Circ Res 1974;34:477–481.
11. Wit AL, Cranefield PF. Triggered and automatic activity in the canine coronary sinus. Circ Res 1977;41:435–445.
12. Wit AL, Cranefield PF, Gadsby DC. Electrogenic sodium extrusion can stop triggered activity in the canine coronary sinus. Circ Res 1981;49:1029–1042.
13. Johnson N, Danilo P, Wit AL, Rosen MR. Characteristics of initiation and termination of catecholamine-induced triggered activity in atrial fibers of the coronary sinus. Circulation 1986;74:1168–1179.
14. Boyden PA, Cranefield PF, Gadsby DC, Wit AL. The basis for the membrane potential of quiescent cells of the canine coronary sinus. J Physiol (Lond) 1983;339:161–183.
15. Boyden PA, Cranefield PF, Gadsby DC. Noradrenalin hyperpolarises cells of the canine coronary sinus by increasing their permeability to potassium ions. J Physiol (Lond) 1983;339:185–206.
16. Ferrier GR. Effects of transmembrane potential on oscillatory afterpotentials induced by acetylstrophanthidin in canine ventricular tissues. J Pharmacol Exp Ther 215:332–341.
17. Wasserstrom JA, Ferrier GR. Voltage dependence of digitalis afterpotentials, aftercontractions, and inotropy. Am J Physiol 1981;241:H646–H653.
18. Hewett KW, Rosen MR. Alpha and beta adrenergic interactions with ouabain-induced delayed afterdepolarizations. J Pharmacol Exp Ther 1984;229:188–192.
19. El-Sherif N, Gough WB, Zeiler RH, Mehra R. Triggered ventricular rhythms in one-day-old myocardial infarction in the dog. Circ Res 1983;52:566–579.
20. LeMarec H, Dangman KH, Danilo P, Rosen MR. An evaluation of automaticity and triggered activity in the canine heart one to 4 days after myocardial infarction. Circulation 1985;71:1224–1236.
21. Hashimoto K, Moe GK. Transient depolarizations induced by acetylstrophanthidin in specialized tissue of dog atrium and ventricle. Circ Res 1973;32:618–624.
22. Kimura S, Cameron JS, Kozlovsky PL, Bassett AL, Myerberg RJ. Delayed afterdepolarizations and triggered activity induced in feline Purkinje fibers by alpha-adrenergic stimulation in the presence of elevated calcium levels. Circulation 1984;70:1074–1082.
23. Henning B, Wit AL. The time course of action potential repolarization affects delayed afterdepolarization amplitude in atrial fibers of the canine coronary sinus. Circ Res 1984;55:110–115.
24. Vassalle M, Mugelli A. An oscillatory current in sheep cardiac Purkinje fibers. Circ Res 1981;48:618–631.

25. Wit AL, Rosen MR. Afterdepolarizations and triggered activity. In Fozzard HA, et al., eds. The Heart and Cardiovascular System, Raven Press, New York, 1986;1449.
26. Moak JP, Rosen MR. Induction and termination of triggered activity by pacing in isolated canine Purkinje fibers. Circulation 1984;69:149–162.
27. Damiano BP, Rosen MR. Effects of pacing on triggered activity induced by early afterdepolarizations. Circulation 1984;69:1013–1025.
28. Jalife J, Antzelevitch, C. Pacemaker annihilation: Diagnostic and therapeutic implications. Am Heart J 1980;100:128.
29. Dangman KH, Hoffman BF. Studies on overdrive stimulation of canine cardiac Purkinje fibers: Maximal diastolic potential as a determinant of the response. JACC 1983;2:1183–1190.
30. Katzung BO, Morgenstern JA. Effects of extracellular potassium on ventricular automaticity and evidence for a pacemaker current in mammalian ventricular myocardium. Circ Res 1977;40:105–111.
31. Imanishi S, McAllister RG Jr., Surawicz B. The effects of verapamil and lidocaine on the automatic depolarizations in guinea-pig ventricular myocardium. J Pharmacol Exp Ther 1978;207:294–303.
32. Vassalle M. Electrogenic suppression of automaticity in sheep and dog Purkinje fibers. Circ Res 1970;27:361–377.
33. Vassalle M. The relationship among cardiac pacemakers: Overdrive suppression. Circ Res 1977;41:268–277.
34. Wit AL, Goldreyer BN, Damato AN. An in vitro model of paroxysmal supraventricular tachycardia. Circulation 1971;43:862–875.
35. Wit AL, Hoffman BF, Cranefield PF. Slow conduction and re-entry in the ventricular conducting system. I. Return extrasystole in canine Purkinje fibers. Circ Res 1972;30:1–10.
36. Frame LH. Mechanisms of termination of re-entry by single premature stimuli: Oscillations, propagated and non-propagated responses. Circulation 1986;74:(Suppl)2:II–350.
37. Bernstein RC, Frame LH. Response to programmed electrical stimulation in reentrant ventricular tachycarida around the canine mitral and aortic valves: An in vitro model. JACC (1987, in press).
38. Frame LH, Page RL, Hoffman BF. Atrial reentry around an anatomic barrier with a partially refractory excitable gap. Circ Res 1986;58:495–511.
39. Allessie MA, Bonke FIM, Schopman FJG. Circus movement in rabbit atrial muscle as a mechanism of tachycardia. Circ Res 1973;33:54–62.
40. Waldo AL, Henthorn RW, Plumb VJ, MacLean WA. Demonstration of the mechanism of transient entrainment and interruption of ventricular tachycardia with rapid atrial pacing. JACC 1984;3:422–430.
41. Waldo AL, MacLean WA, Karp RB, Kouchoukos NT, James TN. Entrainment and interruption of atrial flutter with atrial pacing. Circulation 1977;56:737–745.
42. Okumura K, Henthorn RW, Epstein AE, Plumb VJ, Waldo AL. Further observations on transient entrainment: importance of pacing site and properties of the components of the reentry circuit. Circulation 1985;72:1293–1307.
43. Waldo AL, Plumb VJ, Arciniegas JG, MacLean WA, Cooper TB, Priest MF, James TN. Transient entrainment and interruption of the atrioventricular bypass pathway type of paroxysmal atrial tachycardia. Circulation 1983;67:73–83.
44. Mines GR. On circulating excitations in heart muscles and their possible relation to tachycardia and fibrulation. Trans Roy Soc Can (Section IV) 1914;8:43.
45. Wellens HJ. Value and limitations of programmed electrical stimulation of the heart in the study and treatment of tachycardias. Circulation 1978;57:845–853.
46. Rosenblueth A, Garcia Ramos J. Studies on flutter and fibrillation. II. The influence of artificial obstacles on experimental auricular flutter. Am Heart J 1947;33:677–684.
47. Hayden WG, Hurley EJ, Rytand DA. The mechanism of canine atrial flutter. Circ Res 1967;20:496–505.
48. Durrer D, Schoo L, Schuilenburg RM, Wellens HJJ. The role of premature beats in the initiation and the termination of supraventricular tachycardia in the Wolff-Parkinson-White Syndrome. Circulation 1967;36:644.

49. Gorgels APM, Beekman HDM, Brugada P, Dassen WRM, Richards DAB, Wellens HJJ. Extrastimulus related shortening of the first postpacing interval in digitalis induced ventricular tachycardia. JACC 1983;1:840–857.
50. Zipes DP, Arbel E, Knope RF, Moe GK. Accelerated cardiac escape rhythms caused by ouabain intoxication. Am J Cardiol 1974;33:248–253.
51. Rosen MR, Fisch C, Hoffman BF, Danilo P, Lovelace DE, Knoebel SB. Can accelerated AV junctional escape rhythms be explained by delayed afterdepolarizations? Am J Cardiol 1980;45:1272–1282.
52. Rosen MR, Reder RF. Does triggered activity have a role in the genesis of cardiac arrhythmias? Ann Intern Med 1981;94:794–801.

8

The Clinical Relevance of Abnormal Automaticity and Triggered Activity

Anton P.M. Gorgels
Marc A. Vos
Pedro Brugada
Hein J.J. Wellens

Introduction

According to the classification of Hoffman and Rosen,[1] cardiac arrhythmias are based on three mechanisms (Table I): (1) abnormal impulse generation, including normal and abnormal automaticity and triggered activity, (2) abnormal impulse conduction, including reentry, and (3) simultaneous abnormalities of impulse generation and conduction, including parasystole. Most of our knowledge on abnormal automaticity and triggered activity has been derived from isolated tissue and animal studies. Reentry has also been studied extensively in the human heart. The reason for this is that many reentrant arrhythmias can be reproducibly initiated and terminated by timed electrical stimuli allowing a systematic study.[2] It has been hypothesized that reentry may be the most frequent mechanism of paroxysmal clinical arrhythmias. However, this may be incorrect if one realizes that triggered activity and abnormal automaticity have been demonstrated experimentally in a number of different pathophysiological conditions, which frequently occur clinically. Therefore, it is possible that many clinical arrhythmias are caused by mechanisms different from reentry but are not recog-

From: Brugada P, Wellens HJJ. CARDIAC ARRHYTHMIAS: Where To Go From Here? Mount Kisco, NY, Futura Publishing Company, Inc., © 1987.

148 • CARDIAC ARRHYTHMIAS

Table I
Mechanisms of Arrhythmias

Impulse Formation	
automaticity	• high
	• intermediate
	• low potential
triggered activity:	
early afterdepolarizations	• low membrane
	• high membrane potential
delayed afterdepolarizations	• inhibition sodium-potassium pump
	• calcium
	• beta-receptor stimulation
Impulse Conduction	
reentry	
Abnormal Impulse Formation and Conductance	
parasystole	

Modified from Hoffman and Rosen[1].

nized as such. Knowledge about the mechanism of arrhythmias is of importance to our understanding of its pathophysiology and relation to the etiology but also to open new ways to a more rational treatment. The aim of this chapter will be to review our present knowledge on the clinical relevance of triggered activity and abnormal automaticity.

Techniques for the Study of Mechanisms of Arrhythmias

From a theoretical point of view, mechanisms of arrhythmias can be studied by direct or by indirect means (Table II). To demonstrate abnormal automaticity and triggered activity, intracellular recordings of the electrical activity of the heart are needed. Mapping of a reentry circuit is necessary to identify reentry as the underlying arrhythmia mechanism. At present, it is not possible to record intracellular potentials in the human heart. Direct recordings from the multiple pathways of a reentry circuit can be obtained only in the case of circus movement tachycardia in the Wolff-Parkinson-White syndrome.[3]

For most human arrhythmias, therefore, study of their mechanism can be done only in an indirect way. Techniques to achieve that goal are recording of monophasic action potentials,[4] body surface signal averaging techniques to identify potentials of the bundle of His,[5] late potentials,[6] and possibly also afterdepolarizations causing triggered activity.

Promising results[7,8] have been obtained using monophasic action potentials. Nevertheless, this technique has some inherent limitations: it is an invasive technique, the site of impulse formation where the arrhythmia initiates has to be localized, and one has to prove that the action potentials registered are indeed causing the clinical arrhythmia. Other problems are related to the calibration of the signal, stable positioning of the catheter, and motion artifacts.

Signal averaging techniques from the body surface need a sufficient mass of

Table II
Methods for Studying Mechanisms of Arrhythmias

Direct	• Intracellular recordings of diastolic membrane potential and afterdepolarization.
	• Mapping of reentry circuit.
Indirect	• Recordings of monophasic action potentials.
	• Body surface signal averaging techniques.
	• Programmed electrical stimulation.
	• Surface electrocardiogram.
	• Drugs specifically affecting arrhythmogenic mechanisms.

cardial tissue and a sufficient amount of arrhythmia complexes to show specific abnormalities. Other indirect techniques are programmed electrical stimulation,[2,9-16] analysis of the spontaneous behavior of the arrhythmia on the surface electrocardiogram,[17-19] and the use of drugs specifically affecting arrhythmia mechanisms.

The value of programmed electrical stimulation to identify arrhythmogenic mechanisms is discussed elsewhere in this book.[20] Although useful, this technique cannot be applied in all clinically occurring arrhythmias. The technique is invasive and the arrhythmia has to be sufficiently long and has to be tolerated by the patient to allow a systematic study. In addition, when the arrhythmia does not start spontaneously, it has to be reproducibly initiated which is not always the case. A number of arrhythmias caused by abnormal automaticity and triggered activity are strongly influenced by the pathophysiologic condition facilitating their occurrence and by changes in the autonomic balance.[21-23] These problems interfere with a systematic stimulation study and the acquisition of interpretable data.

Another limitation when using programmed stimulation to identify the mechanism of an arrhythmia is that criteria that have been found to be useful in isolated tissues are less reliable in the intact heart. For instance, the criterium of initiation of a tachycardia "de novo," characteristic of abnormal automaticity and excluding triggered activity, which always requires a preceding rhythm, does not hold in a continuously beating intact heart. Competition between the arrhythmia and the sinus node rhythm may make it difficult to demonstrate in the intact heart phenomena of arrhythmias such as a discontinuous curve,[10,15,24] warming up, overdrive suppression, spontaneous initiation, or delayed termination.

Studies using programmed stimulation in isolated tissues have led to formulations[17-19] about how arrhythmias are expected to behave spontaneously on the surface electrocardiogram depending upon their underlying mechanism. This technique has the advantage of being cheap, noninvasive, and easy to apply and has resulted in a number of interesting observations. Unfortunately, the specificity of this approach is not sufficiently high for general application.

Drugs suppressing specifically a particular arrhythmia mechanism could be of great advantage for both theoretical and practical reasons. They could be easily administered, inform the clinician about the arrhythmogenic mechanism, and suppress the arrhythmia. No such drugs are presently available, however. Most antiarrhythmic drugs affect more than one arrhythmogenic mechanism (see Table III). Recently, however, some steps forward have been made, such as with doxorubicin to suppress ouabain-induced triggered activity[25] and with adenosine to suppress catecholamine-dependent triggered activity.[23] Also, progress is to be expected in the group of calcium entry antagonists.[26] For instance, a drug such as flunarizine does not influence the action potential of Purkinje fibers[26] but strongly inhibits digitalis-induced arrhythmias in the guinea pig heart.[27]

Automaticity

Normal automaticity is a characteristic of the sinus node and AV node at a low diastolic potential and of atrial specialized fibers and Purkinje fibers at a high diastolic potential. Automaticity resulting from a reduced diastolic potential of Purkinje fibers and working myocardium is called abnormal automaticity.[1]

As far as the ionic mechanism for phase 4 depolarization in abnormal automaticity is concerned, it has been suggested that an increase in sodium and/or a decrease in repolarizing potassium current plays a role.[28] Also an inward calcium current has been held responsible for the diastolic depolarization.[29] Diastolic depolarization leading to abnormal automaticity can be achieved by application of intracellular currents[30] or exposure to barium salts,[31] and can occur in the 24 hours of an infarct in Purkinje fibers,[12,32] and possibly in digitalized Purkinje fibers.[33]

The rate of arrhythmias due to abnormal automaticity is related to the maximal diastolic potential. A lower maximal diastolic potential is usually associated with a more rapid rate.[12,34] Also the effect of overdrive stimulation depends on the diastolic membrane potential and the duration and rate of overdrive,[12] i.e., the higher the diastolic membrane potential the easier overdrive suppression of the rhythm can be obtained. These findings are presumably related to the fact that at low membrane potentials, the upstroke of the action potential is primarily calcium-dependent and as a result less sodium enters the cell to prime the pump.[12]

Premature impulses have not been found to influence the length of the return

Table III
Antiarrhythmic Drug Effects

	NA	AA	DAD
verapamil	↑ or ↓	↓ or ↑	↓
lidocaine	↓	—	↓
ethmozin	—	↓	↓
ouabain (toxic)	↓	↑	↑
isoprenaline	↑	↑	↑

NA = normal automaticity; AA = abnormal automaticity; DAD = delayed afterdepolarization.
Modified from refs. 35 and 79.

cycle during spontaneous activity due to abnormal automaticity,[34] but they show reset of the tachycardia focus. High potential or normal automaticity is suppressed by class I antiarrhythmics. Low potential automaticity can be blocked by drugs such as acetylcholine, verapamil, nifedipine, and ethmozin.[34] In contrast, experimentally, lidocaine in therapeutic concentrations does not exert any significant effect on the slope of phase 4 depolarization or rate of impulse generation.

Clinical Relevance

Figure 1 shows an example of high potential automaticity in a patient with complete AV block and an idioventricular rhythm with a cycle length of 1400 ms. This rhythm is overdriven with 50 stimuli and interstimulus intervals of 360 ms. Note the following: (1) the original rhythm is overdrive-suppressed, suggesting that automaticity originates from a high diastolic potential, and (2) a different QRS-complex with a short coupling interval occurs (1100 ms). This accelerated response is probably caused by triggered activity.[35] (3) Following a pause (4360 ms), ventricular activity is resumed out of a different focus.

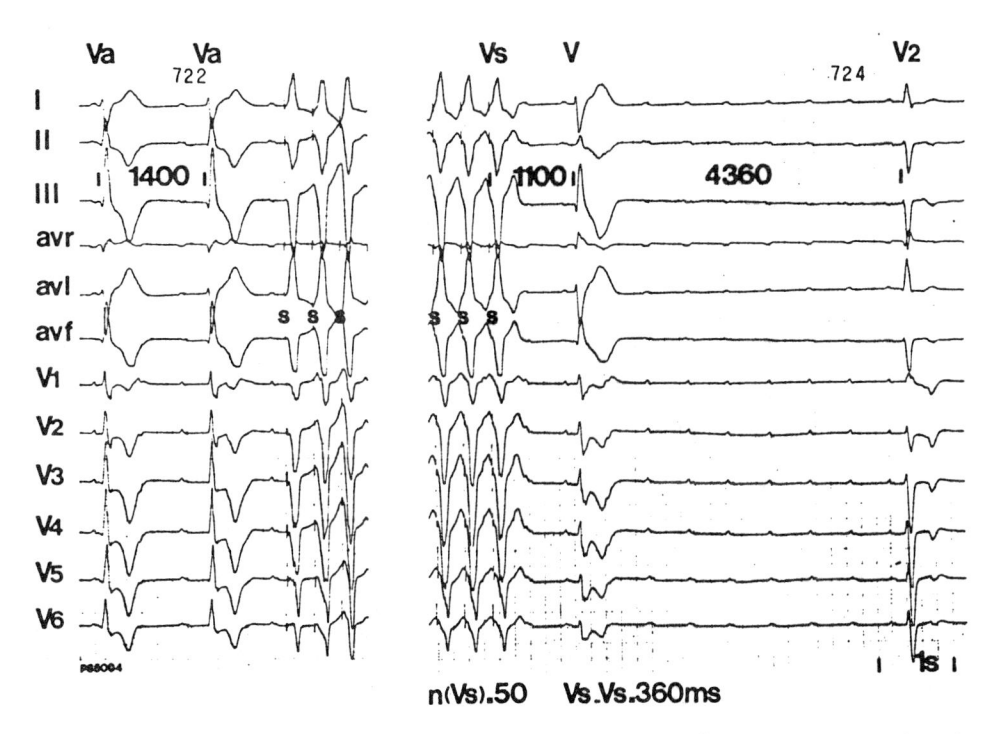

Figure 1: High potential automaticity: Suppression of overdrive stimulation. Simultaneous recording of 12 leads of the electrocardiogram. Chronic complete AV block is present with an idioventricular rhythm (Va) showing a left bundle branch block-like configuration and right axis deviation. The cycle length (Va-Va) equals 1400 ms. This rhythm is overdriven by giving 50 stimuli (nVs = 50) with interstimulus intervals (Vs-Vs) of 360 ms. Following pacing, an accelerated escape beat is observed after 1100 ms. This QRS complex is likely to be due to triggered activity. Thereafter the original rhythm is suppressed and a different focus emerges after another 4360 ms.

152 • CARDIAC ARRHYTHMIAS

There are only a few reports on the occurrence of abnormal automacitity in clinical arrhythmias. An example of an arrhythmia compatible with abnormal automaticity is shown in Figures 2 and 3. These tracings were obtained from a patient with an old myocardial infarction admitted with severe heart failure. An accelerated junctional rhythm was continuously present but was frequently interrupted by sinus node captures which were conducted exclusively over the left bundle. The cycle length of the accelerated junctional rhythm had a duration of about 840 ms. Overdrive stimulation resulted in slight lengthening of only the first coupling interval following pacing (Fig. 3), after which the arrhythmia resumed its original rate. The lack of response to overdrive stimulation and the occurrence of overdrive acceleration at faster rates (Fig. 4) is compatible with reduced potential automaticity.[12] Abnormal automaticity was further supported by the fact that intravenous lidocaine (100 mg) did not result in suppression of the arrhythmia (mean cycle length 870 ms ± 15 before and 890 ± 35 ms after lidocaine administration). The same mechanism has been suggested in five out of 22 patients with spontaneous AV junctional escape rhythms by Tenczer et al.[37]

Ruder et al.[38] have described five adult patients with automatic AV junctional tachycardia, an arrhythmia previously only known in children.[39] These tachycardias were irregular, their rate varied between 110 and 250 beats/min, and the QRS-complex had the same morphology as during sinus rhythm. The inci-

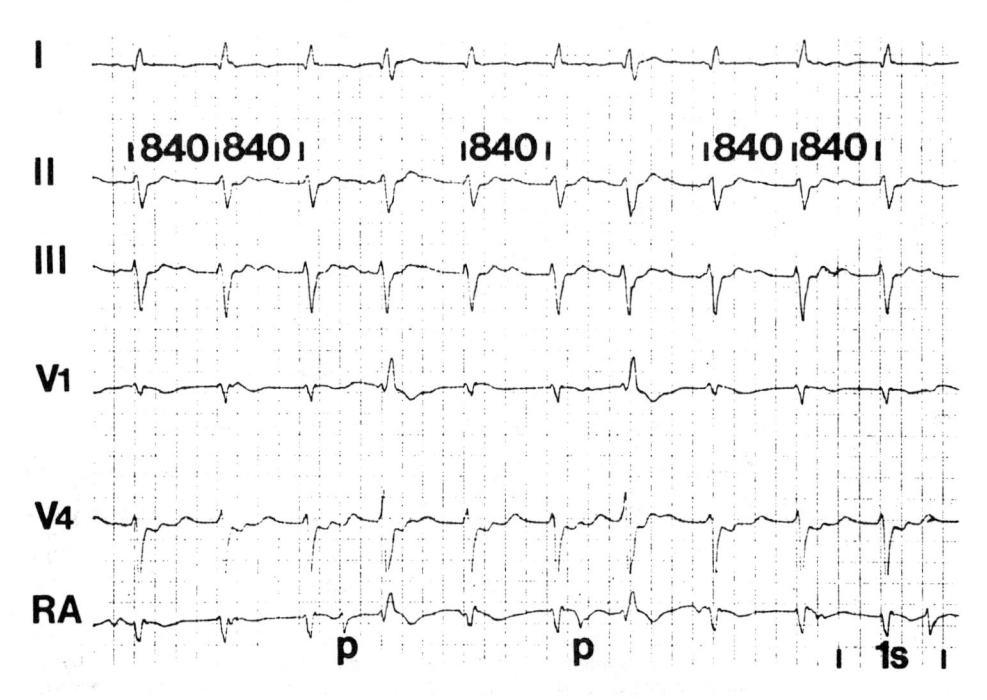

Figure 2: Accelerated junctional rhythm. Simultaneous recording of five surface leads and an intra-atrial lead (RA = right atrium). An accelerated junctional escape rhythm is shown with an interectopic interval of 840 ms. This arrhythmia is interrupted by sinus captures which are conducted exclusively over the posterior fascicle of the left bundle. Note the atrial deflections (p) in the right atrial lead.

Abnormal Automaticity and Triggered Activity • 153

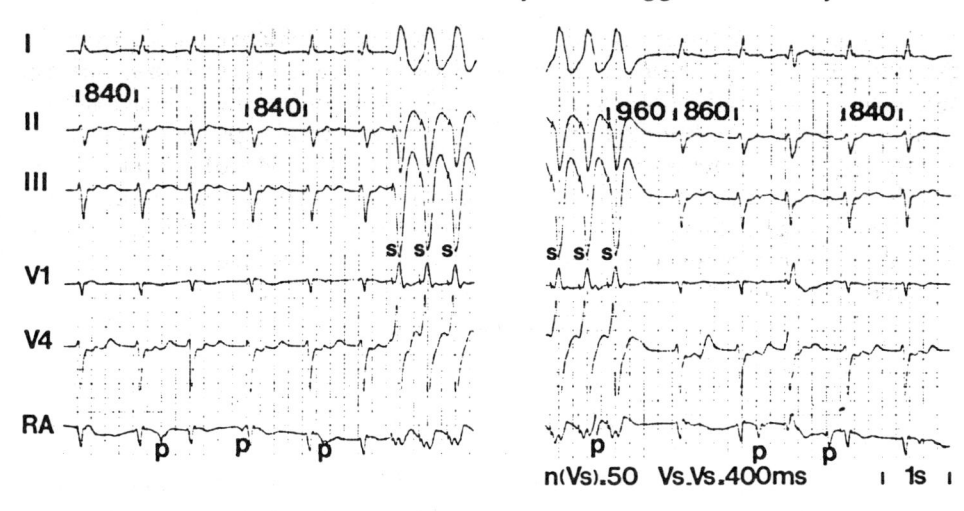

Figure 3: The effect of overdrive stimulation on the accelerated junctional rhythm. The arrhythmia of Figure 2 is overpaced with 50 stimuli (nVs = 50) with interstimulus intervals (Vs-Vs) of 400 ms. Following stimulation, only the first post-pacing interval shows slight overdrive suppression (960 ms).

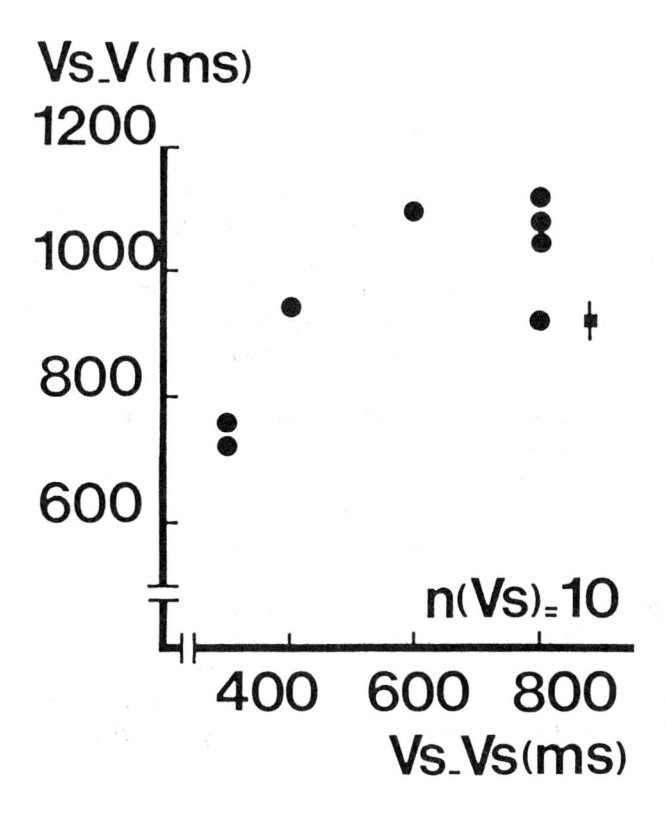

Figure 4: Response of the first post-pacing interval (Vs-V) of the same arrhythmia to overdrive stimulation with 10 stimuli (nVs = 10) and different interstimulus intervals (Vs-Vs). Note that pacing at shorter cycle length does not result in more overdrive suppression, but in overdrive acceleration. Black square = mean of interectopic intervals before stimulation.

dence of episodes of junctional tachycardia varied from relatively infrequent to many times daily, and the duration varied from several seconds to hours, causing significant symptoms in all patients, including syncope. Ventricular activation was preceded by a His bundle deflection, AV dissociation was present, onset and termination of the tachycardia was spontaneous and could not be induced or terminated using atrial or ventricular overdrive pacing. These observations suggested abnormal automaticity as the arrhythmogenic mechanism. Sung et al.[40] described seven patients with spontaneous symptomatic ventricular tachycardia, which could not be induced by electrical stimulation, but isoproterenol infusion readily resulted in ventricular tachycardia.

Triggered Activity

The term "triggered activity," initially introduced by Cranefield and Aronson,[41] is used for arrhythmias that are caused by afterdepolarizations. These are transient depolarizations of the membrane potential during or after an action potential and are caused by this action potential.[41] When the amplitude of an afterdepolarization is sufficiently high, threshold can be attained and an action potential develops.[44] This action potential can again induce an afterpotential, resulting in self-sustaining rhythmic activity.[41] Afterdepolarizations are divided into early and delayed afterdepolarizations (Table I).

Early Afterdepolarizations

Early afterdepolarizations are depolarizing potentials occurring during phase 2 (low membrane potential) or phase 3 (high membrane potential) of repolarization. During phase 2, no triggered activity is inducible, in contrast to phase 3. Early afterdepolarizations occur from action potentials with a normal diastolic potential.[42] They have been induced in isolated cardiac tissues under a variety of conditions that increase inward current or reduce repolarizing current (catecholamines, reduced potassium concentrations, acidosis, low calcium concentrations, hypoxia, aconitine, N-acetyl procainamide, sotalol, and cesium chloride).[13]

Damiano and Rosen have reported on the response of early afterdepolarizations to programmed electrical stimulation.[13] It was found that the induction of high membrane potential early afterdepolarizations are bradycardia-dependent. Sustained rhythms induced by these afterdepolarizations are reset or terminated by premature stimuli, depending upon the maximal diastolic potential. Longer periods of overdrive stimulation influenced the sustained rhythmic activity also in relation to the maximal diastolic potential: the more negative this potential, the longer the period of overdrive suppression.[13] Triggered rhythms induced by early afterdepolarizations behave similarly to abnormal automatic mechanisms in their response to overdrive pacing and extrastimuli.[13] As pointed out by Rosen, abnormal automaticity and early afterdepolarization-induced triggered rhythms at a comparable membrane potential are probably dependent on the same mechanism for their maintenance.[43]

Clinical Relevance

In relation to the possible clinical relevance of high membrane potential early afterdepolarizations, it has been suggested that they may play a role in tachycardias of the QT prolongation syndrome (torsades de pointes),[8,44] and in other bradycardia-related arrhythmias.[45] An example is given in Figure 5 which illustrates recordings obtained from a 65-year-old woman admitted because of polymorphic ventricular tachycardias. During angiography of the left coronary artery,

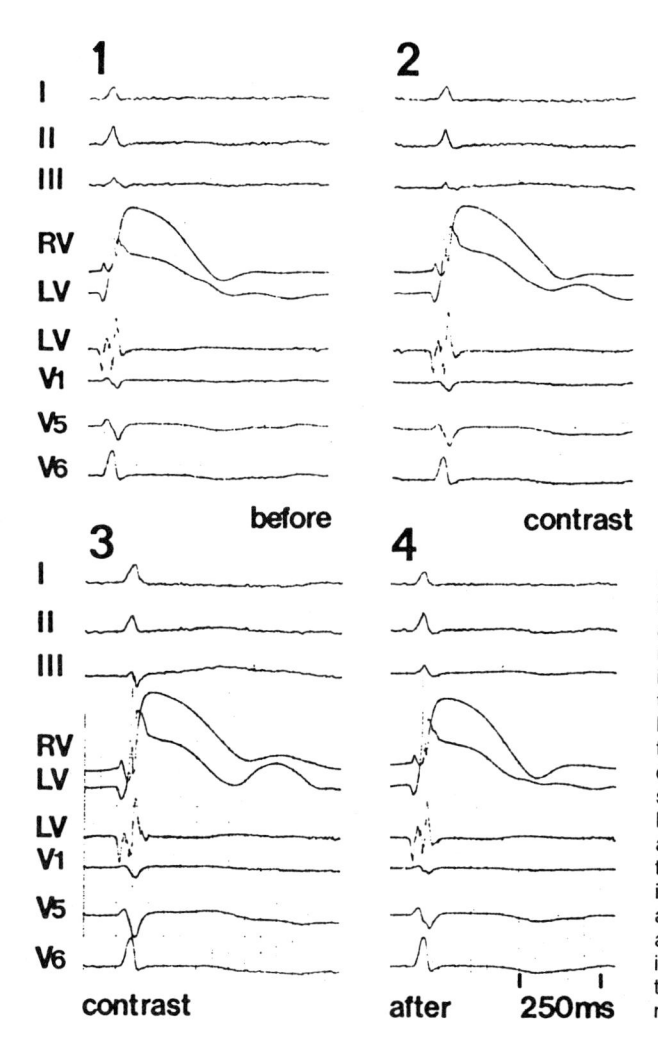

Figure 5: Early afterdepolarizations? Recording by monophasic action potentials. The response of monophasic action potentials to dye injection into the left coronary artery. Six simultaneous surface ECG leads, monophasic action potentials from the right and left ventricle, and a left ventricular lead are simultaneously recorded. Panel 1: Before contrast injection. Panels 2 and 3: During contrast injection; note the marked depolarization especially in the left ventricular monophasic action potential. This deflection is accompanied by a positive U wave in lead 3. Panel 4: Following injection; the high deflection during the repolarization phase disappears.

monophasic action potentials in the base of the left ventricle showed a marked depolarization during phase 3 with the same timing as the occurrence of a U-wave in the surface electrocardiogram. This depolarization, which was less clear in the right ventricular monophasic action potential, possibly reflected the occurrence of a high membrane potential early afterdepolarization. This was further supported by the observation shown in Figure 6.

Following the dye injection, again a depolarization was induced followed by a polymorphic ventricular tachycardia starting with an onset late in the sinus cycle. The concomitant occurrence of phenomena like early afterdepolarizations and polymorphic ventricular tachycardia suggests a causal relationship, although this is difficult to prove definitely.

The clinical relevance of low membrane potential early afterdepolarizations is not yet defined. Although they do not induce full action potentials,[13] they may be arrhythmogenic by causing local prolongation of the repolarization phase in the myocardium. A voltage gradient between continuous structures in the heart can

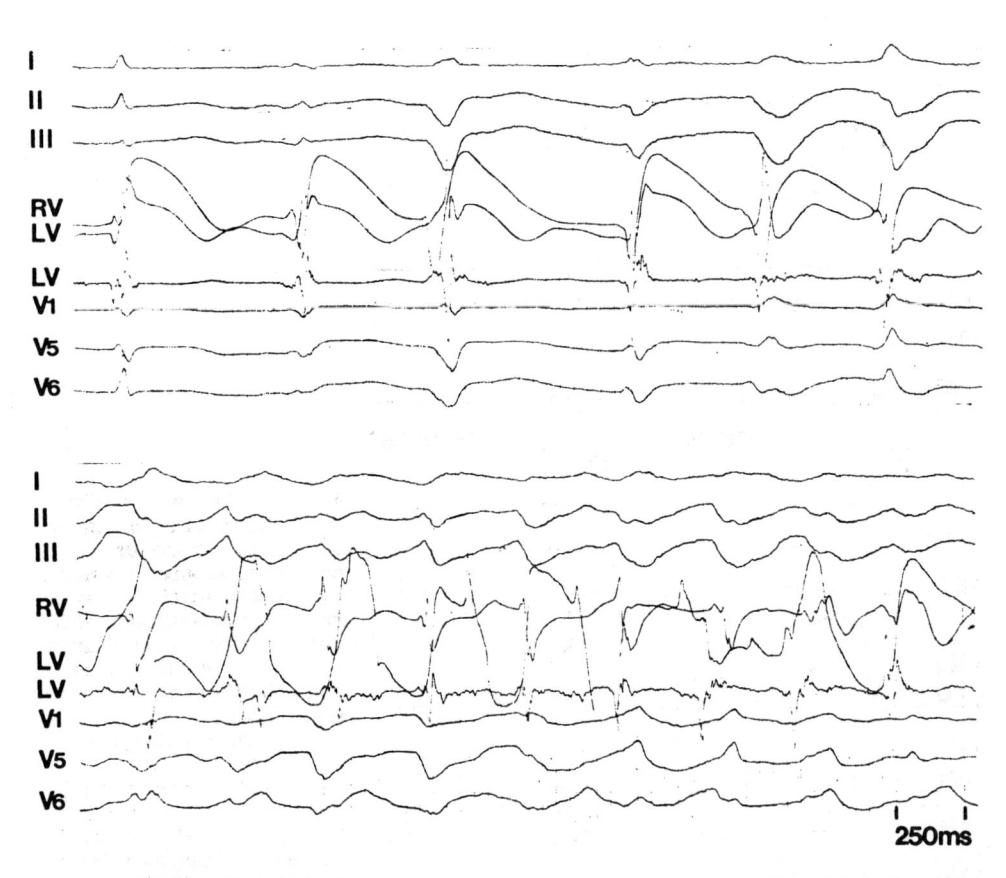

Figure 6: Same patient as in Figure 5. Two panels of a continuous recording of induction of a polymorphic ventricular tachycardia during a subsequent contrast injection. Again, a deflection during the repolarization phase of the sinus beat is observed, which is followed by a rapid polymorphic ventricular tachycardia requiring cardioversion.

be created in this way leading to reexcitation.[46] This hypothesis from our group,[45] which we have termed "prolonged repolarization dependent reexcitation," awaits both experimental and clinical confirmation.

Delayed Afterdepolarizations

Delayed afterdepolarizations are oscillations of the membrane potential, occurring after complete repolarization of the preceding action potential.[41] These transient depolarizations have been demonstrated in normal cardiac tissues such as the canine coronary sinus,[47] the simian mitral valve,[48] and also in atrial tissues from diseased human hearts and in ventricular specialized conducting[49,50] and myocardial tissues[51] from normal and diseased hearts exposed to toxic concentrations of digitalis. Apart from digitalis toxicity, delayed afterdepolarizations have been shown during catecholamine administration,[21,22,52-54] myocardial infarction,[12,32,56] and in sodium-free, calcium-rich solutions.[57]

Mechanism Inducing Delayed Afterdepolarizations

The important feature in the occurrence of delayed afterdepolarizations is an increase of the calcium concentration intracellularly, especially in the sarcoplasmic reticulum.[58] When this structure becomes overloaded with calcium, it releases this electrolyte in an oscillatory fashion.[59,60] This increases monovalent cation conductance, inducing a transient inward sodium current, which is thought to be responsible for the delayed afterdepolarizations. There are three mechanisms through which intracellular calcium overload can occur (Fig. 7): (1) inhibition of the sodium-potassium pump, (2) an increased supply of calcium, and (3) catecholamines.

Inhibition of the Sodium Potassium Pump

When sodium-potassium ATP-ase is inhibited, sodium accumulates within the cell. Through the sodium-calcium exchange mechanism also the intracellular calcium content increases, which results in intracellular calcium overload. The classical inhibitors of the sodium-potassium pump are digitalis glycosides.[61] Clinically, arrhythmias due to digitalis intoxication occur and have been extensively described and studied.[62,63] The sodium-potassium pump is also inhibited in vitro by administration of low potassium solutions.[64] The potentiating effect of hypopotassemia on digitalis intoxication is well known clinically.[65,66]

Increased Supply of Calcium

Delayed afterdepolarizations have been induced in isolated Purkinje fibers superfused with calcium-rich solutions.[57,67-69] Calcium overload of the myo-

158 • CARDIAC ARRHYTHMIAS

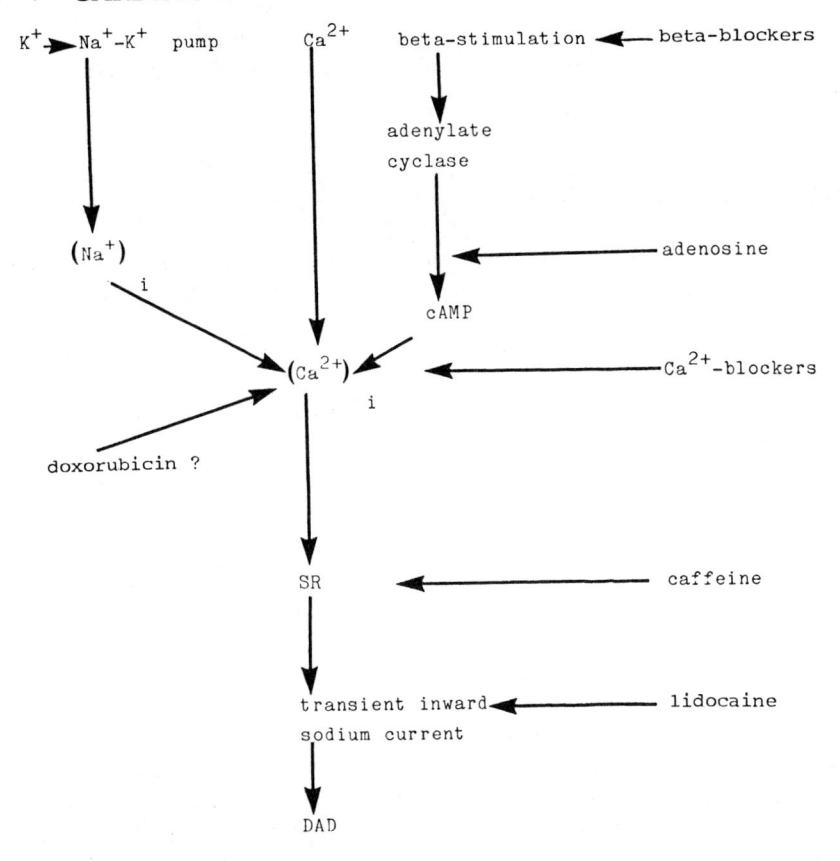

Figure 7: Different mechanisms of induction of delayed afterdepolarizations and the different sites of action of pharmacological intraventions (modified from Lerman et al.[23]). SR = sarcoplasmic reticulum; DAD = delayed afterdepolarizations.

cardium also occurs during the reperfusion phase after coronary artery occlusion.[70] Delayed afterdepolarizations have been demonstrated in isolated Purkinje fibers during reperfusion.[55] The accelerated idioventricular rhythms occurring during the reperfusion phase of acute myocardial infarction in patients receiving thrombolytic therapy are probably based on delayed afterdepolarizations (see below). A third example of an increased calcium supply into the myocardial cells is the one caused by electrical stimulation.[71] By this method, triggered activity has been induced in conscious dogs with AV block.[35]

Catecholamine-Induced Triggered Activity

Calcium overload can also be induced by beta-receptor stimulation.[54,68,69] This mechanism acts through activation of the adenylate-cyclase, c-AMP system. This mechanism may have important clinical implications because it is likely to be related to catecholamine-dependent tachycardias in the human heart.[23]

The three described mechanisms can influence each other in a potentiating but also in an inhibiting manner. For instance, an arrhythmia induced by digitalis intoxication may be facilitated by beta-receptor stimulation.[22,53] However, an increase in rate may activate the sodium-potassium pump enough to suppress delayed afterdepolarizations, resulting in slowing down or termination of the arrhythmia.[54]

Pharmacological Suppression of Arrhythmias Based on Delayed Afterdepolarizations

The mechanisms inducing triggered activity as discussed before allow pharmacological suppression at different sites at the cell membrane and intracellularly (Fig. 7). Triggered activity induced by inhibition of the sodium-potassium pump can be suppressed in several ways: (1) suppletion of potassium, which accelerates the sodium-potassium pump.[72] Also magnesium suppletion suppresses digitalis-induced triggered activity although its action is probably not related to a reactivation of Na-K$^+$ ATP-ase.[73] (2) Cholinomimetic drugs which cause hyperpolarization of the cell membrane.[74] (3) Doxorubicin which has recently been shown to selectively suppress triggered activity in ouabain-treated Purkinje fibers and in the ouabain-treated intact dog heart.[25] Although the exact mechanism of action is not clear, it has been suggested that this drug depresses the Na$^+$–Ca^{++} exchange mechanism in sarcolemmal vesicles.[25]

Calcium overload of the cell can be inhibited by calcium entry blockers. These drugs have indeed been shown to be effective in triggered activity.[33,75,76] Calcium entry blockers differ in respect to their site of action in the heart and throughout the body. For instance, verapamil acts not only at different sites in the working myocardium and the conduction system of the heart, but also causes arteriolar dilatation. The latter leads to hypotension and a reflex catecholamine release, counteracting the initial effect. Also, verapamil is not specific in suppressing triggered activity, but is also active in arrhythmias due to abnormal automaticity.[77] Therefore, it is of importance to look for more specifically acting calcium antagonists. As pointed out before, calcium overload blockers such as flunarizine may be promising because they have no influence on calcium entrance through the slow calcium channel[26] and have been shown to strongly suppress digitalis-induced arrhythmias.[27] Because no additional cardiac effects are to be expected in drugs with this pharmacological profile, they may be useful tools for the study and treatment of clinical arrhythmias due to triggered activity.

Beta-receptor stimulation as a cause of triggered activity can be inhibited by beta-sympathicolytic drugs and are clinically useful in the treatment of exercise-induced arrhythmias. Also, adenosine has recently been shown to be effective in some forms of ventricular tachycardia.[23] Caffeine inhibits the release of calcium from the sarcoplasmic reticulum and in this way suppresses triggered activity.[78,79] The transient sodium inward current is blocked by lidocaine.[81] The suppression of arrhythmias by aprindine[82] is possibly also related to this way of action. Finally, also diphenylhydantoin has been shown clinically to be effective in suppressing digitalis-induced arrhythmias.

Clinical Relevance

During the last few years, an increasing number of reports have appeared on the possible role of triggered activity in clinical cardiology.[9,23,37,38,40,82-84] In most studies, programmed electrical stimulation was used, frequently in combination with an antiarrhythmic drug. Our group has pointed to the lack of specificity of present criteria from programmed stimulation to identify triggered activity. From a retrospective analysis of a large group of patients, we also concluded that triggered activity is only rarely the probable underlying mechanism of recurrent ventricular tachycardia which can be reproducibly initiated and terminated by programmed stimulation.[9] It is more likely that the role of delayed afterdepolarizations has to be sought in arrhythmias occurring in the setting of similar disease states as described in vitro or in animal models.

A number of such clinical conditions is listed in Table IV. They include electrolyte disturbances such as hypokalemia, hypercalcemia, and hypomagnesemia. Hypokalemia inhibits sodium-potassium pumping, as well as hypomagnesemia. Their potential for arrhythmias is also related to their ability to induce QT prolongation and torsades de pointes.[85] Whether these electrolytes clinically induce triggered activity all or not in combination with digitalis or sympathetic stimulation has yet to be defined.

In our experience, the prevalence of arrhythmias due to *digitalis intoxication* is declining in the recent years. This is probably due to the standardization of the bioavailability of the orally ingested digitalis glycosides[86] and because tablets with different strength have allowed more refined dosage regimes. Digitalis intoxication can still occur and should be considered in any patient using digitalis and presenting with an arrhythmia. One should especially be careful about that possibility during intercurrent illness, a gradual or sudden decrease in kidney function, or changes in medication in patients receiving digitalis since a number of drugs have been shown to increase plasma levels and the chance of toxicity.[87,88]

Table IV
Clinical Conditions Possibly Related to Delayed Afterdepolarization-Induced Triggered Activity

1. electrolyte disturbances
    hypokalemia
    hypercalcemia
    hypomagnesemia
2. digitalis glycosides
    diuretics
3. ischemia
    reperfusion
4. increased sympathethic tone
5. increased wall tension
    heart failure

The clinical presentation of digitalis intoxication is related to (1) effects of digitalis on the whole heart, (2) enhancement of impulse formation which is likely to be due to delayed afterdepolarizations, and (3) the vagomimetic effect leading to impairment of impulse conduction.[62,63] These features lead to (1) arrhythmias from different sites in the heart, (2) onset of the arrhythmia late in the cycle, and (3) different degrees of SA and AV block. An example is given in Figure 8.

The fact that digitalis-induced arrhythmias are probably based on delayed afterdepolarizations has the following implications for their management: beta-

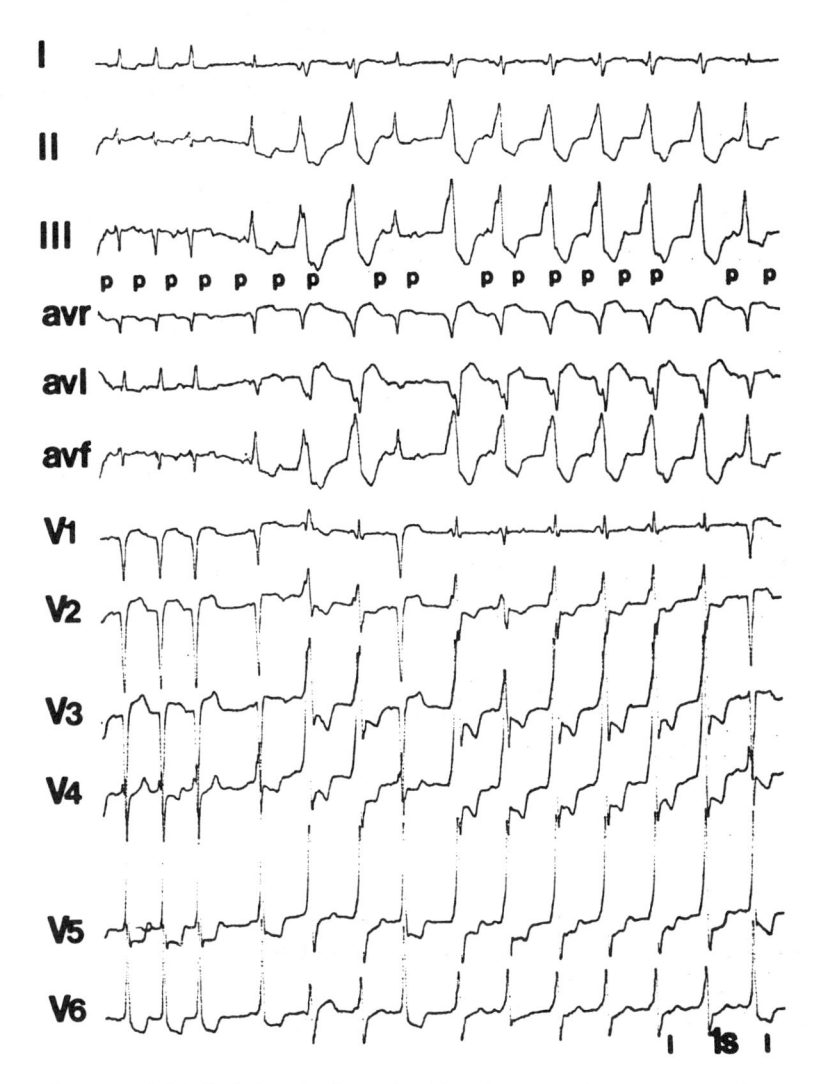

Figure 8: Example of digitalis-induced arrhythmias. Note the concomitant presence of (1) atrial tachycardia, (2) high degree AV block inducing pauses by which a (3) ventricular tachycardia can occur, (4) which starts late in the cycle, and (5) originates in the region of the anterior fascicle of the left bundle.

stimulation, including anxiety, exercise, and the use of sympathicomimetic drugs, should be avoided as well as the administration of cholinolytic drugs such as atropine. When an antiarrhythmic drug is given, a pacemaker lead should be inserted to prevent bradycardia and cardiac arrest.

During the reperfusion phase of acute myocardial infarction, accelerated idioventricular rhythms (AIVR) are observed frequently[89] and characterized by a mostly regular rate between 50 and 120 beats/min. When an idioventricular rhythm occurs during the acute ischemic episode of myocardial infarction, this is a sign (1) of blood flow being restored in the ischemic area, or (2) that damage to the myocardium has already taken place.[90]

Characteristically, an AIVR starts late in the cycle (Fig. 9). This results in a linear relation between the last preceding sinus beat interval and the interval to the first arrhythmia beat (Fig. 10). An AIVR does not behave as a modulated or nonmodulated parasystolic focus, but rather is reset by interrupting ventricular or

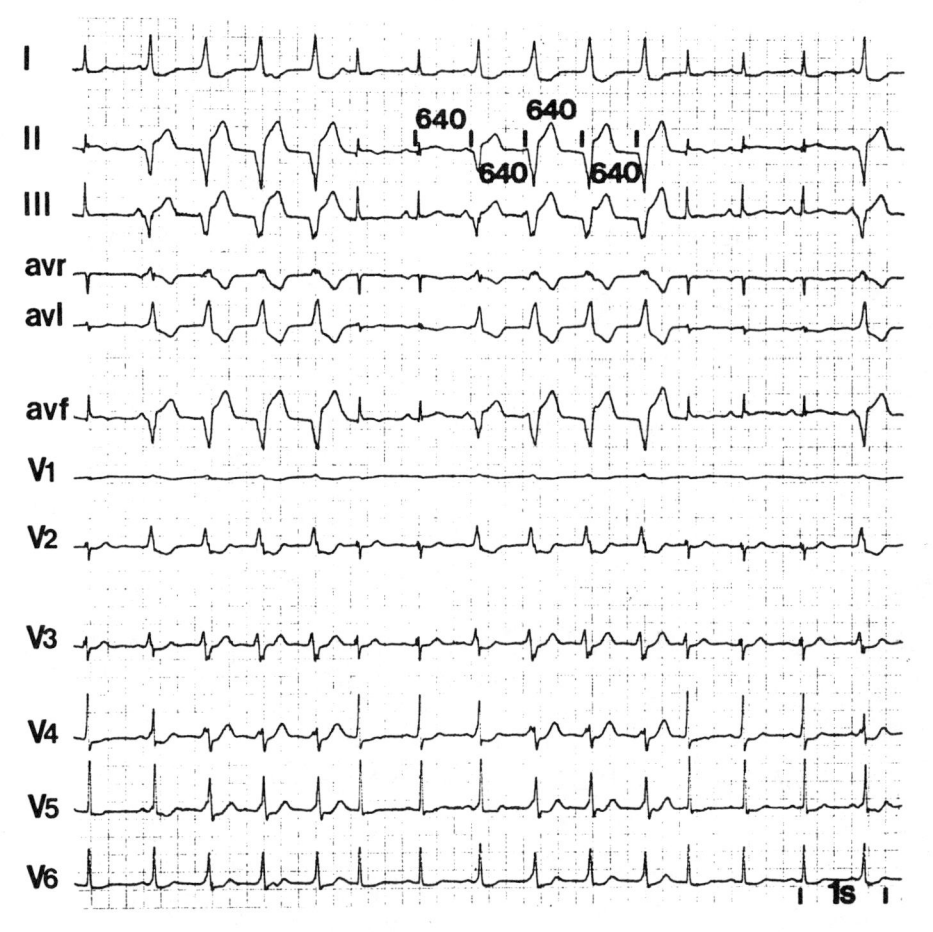

Figure 9: Example of an accelerated idioventricular rhythm. The arrhythmia occurred during the reperfusion phase of an acute inferior wall infarction. The ectopic impulse formation originates from inferiorly. Note that the arrhythmia starts late in the cycle and is reset by capturing sinus complexes.

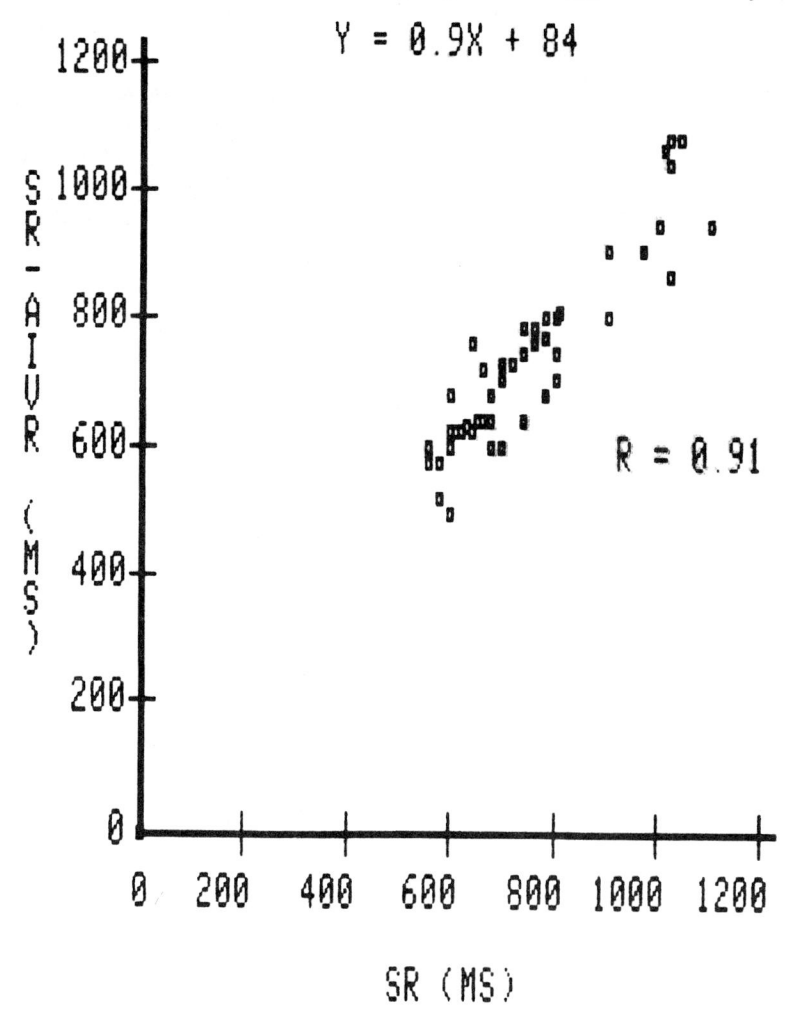

[Figure: scatter plot with Y = 0.9X + 84, R = 0.91, axes SR-AIVR (MS) vs SR (MS)]

Figure 10: Diagram showing the linear relation between the sinus beat interval (SR) before the onset of an accelerated idioventricular rhythm (AIVR) and the interval to the first AIVR-complex (SR-AIVR) from 45 episodes of AIVR in 22 patients.

supraventricular beats. Ferrier et al. have recently studied the effect of ischemia and reperfusion in isolated ventricular tissues.[55] During superfusion with normal oxygen-containing solution, short-lasting hyperpolarization followed by depolarization and finally repolarization to control values were seen. The depolarization phase was accompanied by delayed afterdepolarizations and extrasystoles. Abnormal automaticity was observed during the final repolarization phase. The arrhythmias due to this mechanism had a parasystolic behavior.

Considering the underlying mechanism of the accelerated ventricular rhythm, we think that triggered activity is the more likely mechanism because of the late onset in the cycle and the nonparasystolic behavior. During our recent studies on AIVRs during reperfusion on myocardial infarction, we have observed episodes of ventricular bigeminy (Fig. 11), an arrhythmia recently described to be caused by triggered activity.[91]

Other arrhythmias are possibly related to situations where the sympathetic tone increases.[47,48,68,70] Beta stimulation-dependent triggered activity has been shown in a small number of ventricular tachycardias with the following characteristics:[23] they could be initiated and terminated by timed electrical stimuli, were inducible by exercise and isoproterenol, and responded to adenosine, a drug specifically suppressing CAMP-dependent triggered activity. In the setting of heart failure, triggered activity may occur because of increased tension on the Purkinje fiber tissue, a phenomenon which has been shown to increase the amplitude of delayed afterdepolarizations, induced by acetylstrophantidin.[51]

Conclusions

Abnormal automaticity and early and delayed afterdepolarizations are observed in different species and pathophysiologic conditions. Therefore it is likely that they are also important in human arrhythmias. The recognition of arrhythmo-

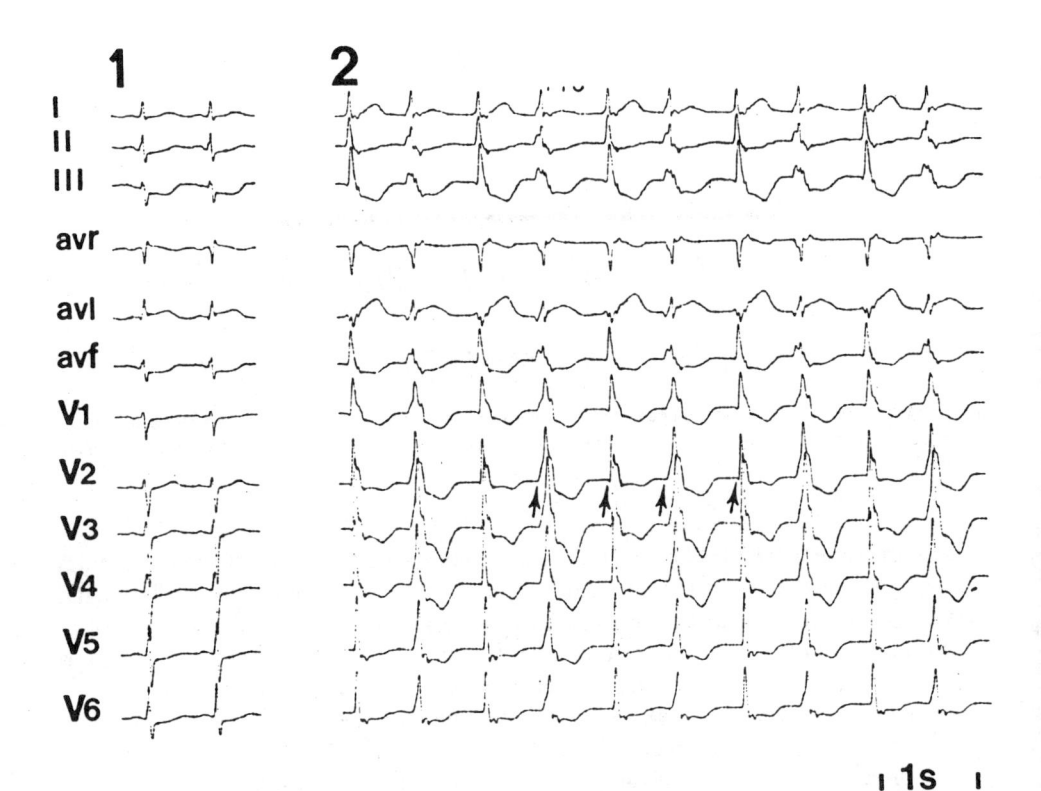

Figure 11: AIVR occurring during reperfusion by way of streptokinase of an obtuse marginal branch. Panel 1 shows an acute lateral infarction. Panel 2 shows the AIVR as a ventricular bigeminy originating from the postero-basal part of the left ventricle. Note the alternation in configuration and cycle length.

genic mechanisms is important for a rational approach to the arrhythmia and the underlying disease state. Present indirect methods to differentiate between arrhythmogenic mechanisms lack sufficient specificity and direct methods are not yet clinically available. More progress can be made by using programmed electrical stimulation together with drugs specifically suppressing particular arrhythmia mechanisms. Those drugs are not yet available, however.

An important step to consider is the application of our present knowledge to arrhythmias which, because of their etiology, presentation, or behavior are likely to be caused by a specific mechanism. Because of possible therapeutic implications, such an approach is far more important than simply being of academic interest. Although we have at our disposal a large number of antiarrhythmic drugs to treat cardiac arrhythmias, we are far from having the ideal antiarrhythmic drug. As with antibiotic therapy, it would be much better if we could use specific antiarrhythmic drugs for specific arrhythmia problems. Digitalis antibodies are an example of that possibility.[92] Obtaining these specific drugs requires first understanding of the pathophysiologic mechanism of the arrhythmia.

References

1. Hoffman BF, Rosen MR. Cellular mechanisms for cardiac arrhythmias. Circ Res 1981;49:1–15.
2. Wellens HJJ. Value and limitations of programmed electrical stimulation of the heart in the study and treatment of tachycardias. Circulation 1978;57:845–853.
3. Durrer D, Schoo L, Schuilenburg RM, Wellens HJJ. The role of premature beats in the initiation and termination of supraventricular tachycardia in the Wolff-Parkinson-White syndrome. Circulation 1967;34:644–662.
4. Hoffman BF, Cranefield PF, Lepeschkin E, Surawicz B, Herlich HC. Comparison of cardiac monophasic potentials recorded by intracellular and suction electrodes. Am J Physiol 1959;196:1297–1301.
5. Flowers N, Hand R, Orander P, Miller C, Walden M, Horan L. Surface recording of electrical activity from the region of the bundle of His. Am J Cardiol 1974;33:384–386.
6. Vasallo J, Cassidy D, Simson M, Marchlinski F, Buxton A, Waxman H, Dresden C, Falcone R, Josephson M. Relationship of signal averaged late potentials, endocardial late activity, and origin of ventricular tachycardia. Circulation 1983;68:(III)174.
7. Levine JH, Spear JF, Guarnieri T, Weisfeldt ML, de Langen CDJ, Becker LC, Moore EN. Cesium chloride-induced long QT syndrome: demonstration of afterdepolarizations and triggered activity in vivo. Circulation 1985;72:1093–1103.
8. Franz MR. Long-term recording of monophasic action potentials from human endocardium. Am J Cardiology, 1983;51:1629–1634.
9. Brugada P, Wellens HJJ. The role of triggered activity in clinical ventricular arrhythmias. PACE 1984;7:260–271.
10. Moak JP, Rosen MR. Induction and termination of triggered activity by pacing in isolated canine Purkinje fibers. Circulation 1984;69:149–162.
11. Johnson N, Danilo P, Wit AL, Rosen MR. Characteristics of initiation and termination of catecholamine-induced triggered activity in atrial fibers of the coronary sinus. Circulation 1986;74:1168–1179.
12. Dangman KH, Hoffman BF. Studies on overdrive stimulation of canine cardiac Purkinje fibers: Maximal diastolic potential as a determinant of the response. JACC 1983;2:1183–1190.
13. Damiano BP, Rosen M. Effects of pacing on triggered activity induced by early afterdepolarizations. Circulation 1984;69:1013–1025.

14. Gorgels APM, de Wit B, Beekman HDM, Dassen WRM, Wellens HJJ. Triggered activity induced by pacing during digitalis intoxication. PACE 1987 (in press).
15. Gorgels APM, de Wit B, Beekman HDM, Dassen WRM, Wellens HJJ. Effect of different modes of stimulation on the morphology of the first QRS-complex following pacing during digitalis induced ventricular tachycardia. PACE 1986;9:842−859.
16. Waldo AL, Plumb VJ, Arciniegas JG, MacLean WA, Cooper TB, Priest MF, James TN. Transient entrainment and interruption of AV bypass pathway type of paroxysmal atrial tachycardia. A model for understanding and identifying reentrant arrhythmias. Circulation 1983;67:73.
17. Rosen MR, Fisch C, Hoffman BF, Danilo P, Lovelace DE, Knoebel SB. Can accelerated atrioventricular junctional escape rhythms be explained by delayed after depolarizations. Am J Cardiol 1980;45:1272−1284.
18. Swenne CA. Interpretation of ventricular arrhythmias. Doctoral thesis, University of Utrecht, The Netherlands, 1984.
19. Van Hemel NM. Identification of mechanisms of ventricular arrhythmias from the surface ECG. Doctoral thesis, University of Utrecht, The Netherlands, 1984.
20. Johnson NJ, Rosen MR. The distinction between triggered activity and other cardiac arrhythmias.
21. Muguelli A, Amerini S, Piazzesi G, Cerbai E, Giotti A. Enhancement by norepinephrine of automaticity in sheep cardiac Purkinje fibers exposed to hypoxic glucose-free Tyrode's solution: a role for alpha-adrenoceptors. Circulation 1986;73:180−188.
22. Hewett KW, Rosen MR. Alpha and beta adrenergic interactions with ouabain-induced delayed afterdepolarizations. Pharmacol Exp Ther 1984;229:188−192.
23. Lerman BB, Belardinelli L, West A, Berne RM, Dimarco JP. Adenosine-sensitive ventricular tachycardia: evidence suggesting cyclic AMP-mediated triggered activity. Circulation 1986;74:270−280.
24. Rosen MR, Reder RF. Does triggered activity have a role in the genesis of cardiac arrhythmias? Ann Int Med 1981;94:794−801.
25. Le Marec H, Spinelli W, Rosen MR. The effects of doxorubycine on ventricular tachycardia. Circulation 1986;74:881−889.
26. Borgers M, de Clerck F, van Reempts J, Xhonneux R, van Nueten J. Selective blockade of cellular Ca^{2+}-overload by flunarizine. Int J Angiol 1984;25−31.
27. Jonkman FAM, Boddeke HWGM, van Zwieten PA. Protective activity of calcium entry blockers against ouabain intoxication in anaesthetized guinea pigs. Cardiovasc Pharmacol 1986;8.
28. Isenberg J. Cardiac Purkinje fibers: (Ca^{2+}) controls the potassium permeability via the conductance components gK_1 and gK_2. Pfluegers Arch 1977;371:77−85.
29. Dangman KM, Hoffman BF. Effects of nifedipine on electrical activity of cardiac cells. Am J Cardiol 1980;46:1059−1067.
30. Imanishi S, Surawicz B. Automatic activity in depolarized guinea pig ventricular myocardium. Cir Res 1976;39:751−759.
31. Toda N. Barium-induced automaticity in relation to calcium ions and norepinephrine in the rabbit left atrium. Circ Res 1970;27:45−57.
32. Le Marec H, Dangman KH, Danilo P, Rosen MR. An evaluation of automaticity and triggered activity in the canine heart one to four days after myocardial infarction. Circulation 1985;71:1226−1236.
33. Rosen M, Danilo P. Effects of tetrodotoxin, lidocaine, verapamil and AHR-2666 on ouabain induced delayed afterdepolarizations in canine Purkinje fibers. Circ Res 1980;46:117−124.
34. Hoffman BF. Disturbances of cardiac electrogenesis. In: Rosenbaum MB, Elizari MV, eds. Frontiers of Cardiac Electrophysiology, Development in Cardiovascular Medicine. Boston, Martinus Nijhoff Publishers, 1983;1−12.
35. Gorgels APM. Ventricular impulse formation and the influence of digitalis intoxication. Doctoral thesis, University of Limburg, Maastricht, The Netherlands; Schrijen-Lippertz bv., Voerendaal, 1985.
36. Vasalle M. The relationship among cardiac pacemakers. Circ Res 1977;41:269−277.

37. Tenczer J, Littmann Z, Rohla M, Fenyvesi T. The effects of overdrive pacing and lidocaine on atrioventricular junctional rhythm in man: the role of abnormal automaticity. Circulation 1985;72:480–486.
38. Ruder MA, Davis JC, Eldar M, Abbott JA, Griffin JC, Seger JJ, Scheinman MM. Clinical and electrophysiological characterization of automatic junctional tachycardia in adults. Circulation 1986;73:930–937.
39. Garson A, Gillette PC. Junctional ectopic tachycardia in children: electrocardiography, electrophysiology and pharmacologic response. Am J Cardiol 1979;44:298–304.
40. Sung RJ, Shapiro WA, Shen EN, Morady F. Effects of verapamil on ventricular tachycardias possibly caused by reentry, automaticity and triggered activity. J Clin Invest 1983;72:350–360.
41. Cranefield PF. Action potentials, afterpotentials and arrhythmias. Circ Res 1977;41:415–423.
42. Frame LH, Hoffman BF. Mechanisms of tachycardia. In: Surawicz B, Reddy CP, Prystowsky EN, eds. Tachycardias. Boston, Martinus Nijhoff Publishers, 1984;2–35.
43. Rosen MR. Is the response to programmed electrical stimulation diagnostic of mechanisms for arrhythmias? Circulation 1986;73(Suppl II):19–27.
44. Brachmann J, Scherlag BJ, Rosenstraukh LV, Lazzara R. Bradycardia dependent triggered activity: Relevance to drug induced multiform ventricular tachycardia. Circulation 1983;68:846–856.
45. Brugada P, Wellens HJJ. Early afterdepolarizations: role in conduction block, prolonged repolarization dependent reexcitation, and tachyarrhythmias in the human heart. PACE 1985;8:889–896.
46. Janse M, van Capelle FJL. Electrotonic interactions across an inexcitable region as a cause of ectopic activity in acute regional myocardial ischemia. Circ Res 1982;50:527.
47. Wit AL, Cranefield PT. Triggered and automatic activity in the canine coronary sinus. Circ Res 1977;44:435–445.
48. Wit AL, Cranefield PF. Triggered activity in cardiac muscle fibers of the simian mitral valve. Circ Res 1976;38:85–98.
49. Ferrier GR. Digitalis arrhythmias: role of oscillatory afterpotentials. Prog Cardiovasc Dis 1977;19:459–474.
50. Rosen MR, Wit AL, Hoffman BF. Electrophysiology and pharmacology of cardiac arrhythmias. IV. Cardiac antiarrhythmic and toxic effects of digitalis. Am Heart J 1975;89:391–399.
51. Ferrier GR. The effects of tension on acetylstrophantidin induced transient depolarizations and aftercontractions in canine myocardial and Purkinje tissue. Circ Res 1976;38:156–162.
52. Wald RW, Waxman MB. Pacing induced automaticity in sheep Purkinje fibers. Circ Res 1981;48:531–538.
53. Kimura S, Cameron JS, Kozlovsky PL, Bassett AL, Meyerburg RJ. Delayed afterdepolarizations and triggered activity induced in feline Purkinje fibers by alpha-adrenergic stimulation in the presence of elevated calcium levels. Circulation 1984;70:1074–1082.
54. Wit AL, Cranefield PF, Gadsby DC. Electrogenic sodium extrusion can stop triggered activity in the canine coronary sinus. Circ Res 1981;49:1029–1042.
55. Ferrier GR, Moffat MP, Lukas A. Possible mechanisms of ventricular arrhythmias elicited by ischemia followed by reperfusion. Circ Res 1985;56:184–194.
56. El-Sherif, Gough WB, Zeiler RH, Mehra R. Triggered ventricular rhythms in 1-day old myocardial infarction in the dog. Circ Res 1983;52:566–579.
57. Cranefield PF, Aronson RS. Initiation of sustained rhythmic activity by single propagated action potentials in canine Purkinje fibers exposed to sodium free solution or to ouabain. Circ Res 1974;34:477–484.
58. Fabiato A, Fabiato F. Calcium release from the sarcoplasmatic reticulum. Circ Res 1977;40:119–129.
59. Orchard CH, Eisner DA, Allen DG. Oscillations of intracellular Ca^{2+} in mammalian cardiac muscle. Nature 1983;304:735–737.
60. Kass RS, Lederer WJ, Tsien RW, Weingart R. Role of calcium ions in transient inward

currents and aftercontractions induced by strophantidin in cardiac Purkinje fibers. J Physiol 1978;281:187–208.
61. Schatzmann HJ. Herzglycoside als Hemmstoff für den aktiven Kalium und Natriumtransport durch die Erythrocyten membran. Helv Physiol Pharmacol Acta 1953;11:346–354.
62. Wellens HJJ. The electrocardiogram in digitalis intoxication. In: Yu PN, Goodwin JF, eds. Progress in Cardiology 5. Philadelphia, Lea and Febiger, 1976;271–290.
63. Vanagt EJ, Wellens HJJ. The electrocardiogram in digitalis intoxication. In: Wellens HJJ, Kulbertus ME, eds. What's New in Electrocardiography? The Hague, Martinus Nijhoff Publishers, 1981;315–343.
64. Eisner DA, Lederer WJ. Inotropic and arrhythmogenic effects of potassium-depleted solutions on mammalian cardiac muscle. J Physiol (London) 1979;294:255–277.
65. Gilman AG, Goodman LS, et al. The Pharmacological Basis of Therapeutics, 6th edition. London, Macmillan, 1980.
66. Mason DT, Foerster JM. Side effects and intoxication of cardiac glycosides: manifestations and treatment. In: Greeff K, ed. Handbook of Experimental Pharmacology, vol. 56/II. Berlin, Heidelberg, New York, Springer-Verlag, 1981;275–292.
67. Hiraoka M, Okamoto Y, Sano T. Oscillatory afterpotentials in dog ventricular muscle fibers. Circ Res 1981;48:510–518.
68. Valenzuela F, Vasalle M. Interaction between overdrive excitation and overdrive suppression in canine Purkinje fibers. Cardiovasc Res 1983;17:608–619.
69. Vasalle M, Knob RE, Lara GA, et al. The effect of adrenergic enhancement on overdrive excitation. J Electrocardiol 1976;9:335–343.
70. Whalen DA, Hamilton DG, Ganote CE, Jennings RB. Effect of a transient period of ischemia on myocardial cells. 1. Effects on cell volume regulation. Am J Pathol 1974;74:381–398.
71. Lado MG, Sheu SS, Fozzard HA. Changes in intracellular Ca^{2+} activity with stimulation in sheep cardiac Purkinje strands. Am J Physiol 1982;243:133–137.
72. Wallick DW, Valencic F, Fratiazze RB, Levy MN. Effects of ouabain and vagal stimulation on heart rate in dog. Cardiovasc Res 1984;18:75–79.
73. Specter MJ, Schweizer E, Goldman RH. Studies on magnesium's mechanism of action in digitalis induced arrhytymias. Circulation 1975;52:1001–1005.
74. Cranefield P. Triggered arrhythmias. In: Rosenbaum MB, Elizari MV, eds. Frontiers of Cardiac Electrophysiology. Boston, Martinus Nijhoff Publishers, pp. 182–194.
75. Gough WB, Zeiler RH, El-Sherif N. Effects of Nifedipine on triggered activity in 1-day-old myocardial infarction in dogs. Am J Cardiol 1983;53:303–306.
76. Klevans LR, Kelly RJ. Effect of autonomic neural blockade on verapamil-induced suppression of the accelerated ventricular escape beat in ouabain-treated dogs. J Pharmacol Exp Ther 1978;206:259–267.
77. Ilvento JP, Provet J, Danilo P, Rosen MR. Fast and slow idioventricular rhythms in the canine heart; a study of their mechanism using antiarrhythmic drugs and electrophysiologic testing. Am J Cardiol 1982;49:1909–1916.
78. Di Gennaro M, Valle R, Pahor M, Carbonin R. Abolition of digitalis tachyarrhythmias by caffeine. Am J Physiol 1983;244:H215–221.
79. Di Gennaro M, Carbonin P, Vassalle M. On the mechanism by which caffeine abolishes the fast rhythms induced by cardiotonic steriods. J Moll Cell Cardiol 1984;16:851–862.
80. Eisner DA, Lederer WJ. A cellular basis for lidocaine antiarrhythmic action. J Physiol 1979;295:25–26.
81. Foster PR, King RM, Nicoll AD, Zipes DP. Suppression of ouabain-induced ventricular rhythms with aprindine HCL: a comparison with other antiarrhythmic agents. Circulation 1976;53(2):315–321.
82. Wellens HJJ, Brugada P, Vanagt EJDM, Ross DL, Bär FWHM. New studies on triggered activity. In: Harrison DC, ed. Cardiac Arrhythmias: A Decade of Progress. Boston, GK Hall Medical Publishers, 1981;601–610.
83. Zipes DP, Foster PR, Troup PJ, Pedersen DH. Atrial induction of ventricular tachycardia: reentry versus triggered automaticity. Am J Cardiol 1981;44(1):1–8.

84. Wu D, Kuo HC, Hung JS. Exercise triggered paroxysmal ventricular tachycardia: A repetitive rhythmic activity possibly related to afterdepolarization. Ann Intern Med 1981;95:410–444.
85. Coumel P, Leclercq JF, Dessertenne F. Torsades de pointes. In: Josephson ME, Wellens HJJ, eds. Tachycardias, Mechanisms, Diagnosis, Treatment. Philadelphia, Lea and Febiger, 1984;325–351.
86. Smith TW, Antman EM, Friedman PL, Blatt CM, Marsh JD. Digitalis glycosides: mechanisms and manifestations of toxicity. Prog Cardiovasc Dis 1984;26:413–458.
87. Bigger JT. the quinidine-digoxin interaction. Int J Cardiol 1981;1:109–116.
88. Lessem J, Bellinetto A. Interaction between digoxin and calcium antagonists. Am J Cardiol 1982;49:1025–1029.
89. Goldberg S, Greenspan AJ, Urban PL, Muza B, Berger B, Walinsky P, Maroko PR. Reperfusion arrhythmia: A marker of restoration of antegrade flow during intracoronary thrombolysis for acute myocardial infarction. Am Heart J 1983;105:26–32.
90. Gorgels APM, Letsch IS, Bär FWHM, Janssen JH, Wellens HJJ. Accelerated idioventricular rhythm in persistent ischemic chest pain indicates necrosis and reperfusion (abstr). Circulation 1986;74:II–11.
91. Kieval RS, Johnson NJ, Rosen MR. Triggered activity as a cause of bigeminy. JACC 1986;8(3):644–647.
92. Smith TW, Butler VP Jr, Haber E, et al. Treatment of life-threatening digitalis intoxication with digoxin-specific Fab antibody fragments: Experience in 26 cases. N Engl J Med 1982;307:1357–1366.

9

Current Perspective on Entrainment of Tachyarrhythmias

Albert L. Waldo
Brian Olshansky
Ken Okumura
Richard W. Henthorn

Introduction

Transient entrainment of a tachycardia is an increase in the rate of all tissue responsible for sustaining the tachycardia to the faster pacing rate, with resumption of the intrinsic rate of the tachycardia upon either abrupt cessation of pacing or slowing of the pacing rate below the intrinsic rate of the tachycardia.[1] Transient entrainment was first recognized one decade ago during rapid pacing of atrial flutter,[2] but, at that time, its explanation was unclear. Subsequent studies during atrioventricular (AV) reentrant tachycardia involving an AV bypass pathway[1] and ventricular tachycardia[3] provided an explanation for its mechanism. On the basis of those studies, we suggested that during transient entrainment of a tachycardia, each wavefront from the pacing impulse enters into the excitable gap of the reentrant circuit and travels in two directions, antidromically, i.e., in the opposite direction of the circulating wavefront of the spontaneous tachycardia, where it collides with the orthodromic wavefront of the preceding beat, and orthodromically, i.e., in the same direction as the circulating wavefront of the spontaneous tachycardia. The latter wavefront continues the tachycardia, resetting it to the pacing rate (Fig. 1).

On the basis of those and subsequent studies,[1,3–12] we suggested that the

From: Brugada P, Wellens HJJ. CARDIAC ARRHYTHMIAS: Where To Go From Here? Mount Kisco, NY, Futura Publishing Company, Inc., © 1987.

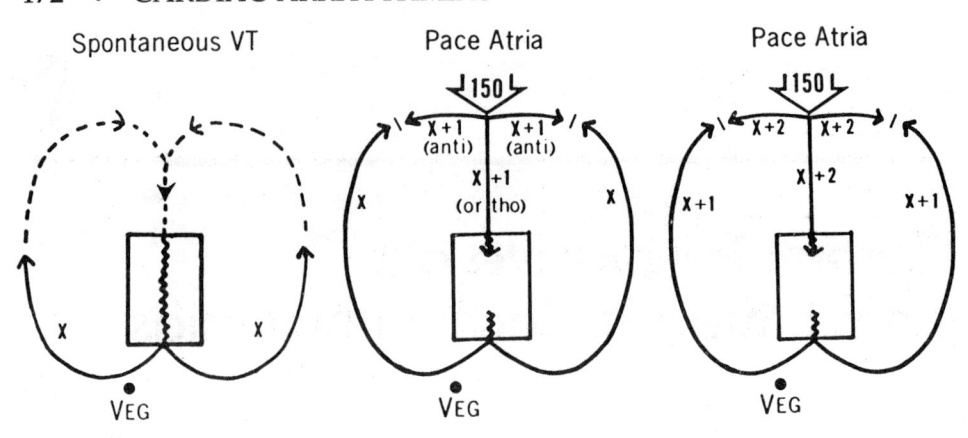

Figure 1: Left Panel: Diagrammatic representation of transient entrainment, in the is case of a ventricular tachycardia by atrial pacing. Diagrammatic representation of the reentry circuit using the figure of eight loop model during spontaneous ventricular tachycardia (VT) at a rate of 141 bpm. The X represents the orthodromic wavefronts of the reentrant rhythm. In this and subsequent diagrams, the arrows indicate the direction of spread of the impulse, the box represents an area of slow conduction, the serpentine line indicates slow conduction of the impulse, the dashed lines indicate the excitable gap in the reentry circuit, the dot represents a right ventricular electrogram (VEG) recording site, and the large arrow (middle and right panels) indicates the wavefront from the pacing impulse entering into the excitable gap of the ventricular tachycardia reentrant circuit, where it is conducted orthodromically (ORTHO) and antidromically (ANTI). Middle Panel: Diagrammatic representation of the introduction of the first pacing impulse (X + 1) during atrial pacing at a rate of 150 bpm during spontaneous ventricular tachycardia. The antidromic wavefronts from the pacing impulse (X + 1) collide with the orthodromic wavefronts from the previous spontaneous beats (X), resulting in fusion of ventricular activation which, in effect, interrupts the tachycardia. However, the orthodromic wavefront from the pacing impulse (X + 1) continues the ventricular tachycardia, resetting it to the pacing rate. Right Panel: Diagrammatic representation of the introduction of the second pacing impulse (X + 2) during atrial pacing at a rate of 150 bpm during the spontaneous ventricular tachycardia. The antidromic wavefronts (X + 2) collide with the orthodromic wave fronts from the previous paced beat (X + 1), again resulting in ventricular fusion, which, in effect interrupts the ventricular tachycardia. However, once again, the orthodromic wavefront (X + 2) from the pacing impulse continues the ventricular tachycardia, resetting it to the pacing rate. Note that during the spontaneous rhythm and during the period of pacing, the right ventricular electrogram (VEG) recording site is always activated by an orthodromic wavefront. From Waldo et al.[3]

ability to demonstrate transient entrainment of a tachycardia indicates that the tachycardia is due to a reentrant mechanism, with an excitable gap being present in the reentrant circuit. Many additional studies have now been performed, expanding our understanding and appreciation of the entrainment phenomena.[13-26] In this paper, we present a perspective on the role of transient entrainment in understanding the nature and mechanisms of tachyarrhythmias and on the use of transient entrainment as a basis for providing more effective treatment.

Establishing the Presence of a Reentrant Rhythm

As recently summarized,[27] until a relatively short time ago, it was generally thought that normal and abnormal rhythms resulted either from an automatic mechanism or a reentrant mechanism. Surprising though it may seem, apart from the early and classic experiments of Mayer[28] on reentry in the Medusa ring, and subsequent studies by Mines[29] on ring preparations cut from dogfish auricles or from canine right ventricles, it was not until the 1972 publications of the in vitro studies of depressed bundles and loops of canine Purkinje fibers by Wit, Hoffman, and Cranefield[30,31] that the occurrence of reentry actually was documented. Prior to the latter studies, there had been an enormous amount of work in which reentrant mechanisms had been postulated as being present, primarily based on indirect evidence. In fact, for in vivo rhythms, it had been thought that one could recognize a reentrant tachycardia by a few key characteristics that distinguished it from an automatic rhythm. Stated simply, these characteristics were that if the rhythm could be either initiated or terminated by premature beats or rapid pacing, it was due to a reentry mechanism.[32]

Of course, it has always been appreciated that the best proof of reentry would be to map the sequence of activation of the heart during the tachycardia, and thereby demonstrate the reentrant circuit. Even so, we must remember Mines' admonition[29] that ". . . the chief error to be guarded against is that of mistaking a series of automatic beats originating in one point of a ring [substitute apparent reentry circuit] and travelling around it in one direction only owing to a complete block close to the point of origin of the rhythm on one side of this point." The point, of course, is that even mapping is not proof of reentry per se. Mines suggested severing the ring (again, substitute reentry circuit) or the like and then demonstrate that no further reentrant excitation could occur was required as proof for reentry. In any event, mapping has now become possible to do in vivo, but only with the use of recording techniques with the chest open and the heart exposed. Since the indirect pacing techniques were far easier to apply, in virtually all clinical studies and most animal studies, investigators had been relying on the above simple responses to cardiac pacing to establish the presence of reentry.

Then, a little more than one decade ago came the recognition that triggered rhythms could be initiated and terminated with premature beats or rapid pacing.[27] This, of course, made it necessary to rethink the criteria which could distinguish reentrant tachyarrhythmias from other arrhythmias, in particular, triggered rhythms.[27,33] In some ways, this may be tilting windmills, because triggered activity has yet to be identified as an important mechanism of clinical arrhythmias.[34,35] However, as summarized recently,[36] largely based on results of studies performed in animal models or deductive reasoning for several patient arrhythmias, it seems possible that some ventricular arrhythmias which follow an acute myocardial infarction, torsade de pointes, some digitalis toxic rhythms, some AV junctional rhythms, and perhaps right ventricular outflow tract tachycardias are due to triggered activity.

In sum, electrophysiologic mapping is technically difficult and, as per Mines, not foolproof for the identification of reentry. And rhythms due to triggered activity can be initiated and terminated by cardiac pacing techniques, making this old technique no longer indicative per se of reentry. It is in this context that we suggested that the demonstration of transient entrainment of a tachycardia with or without its subsequent interruption was an easy and reliable way to identify reentry as the mechanism of the tachyarrhythmia.

Criteria to Establish the Presence of Transient Entrainment

We have proposed four criteria (Table I), any one of which, if demonstrated, establishes the presence of transient entrainment, and thereby the presence of reentry with an excitable gap. Figures 1–7 demonstrate the first three criteria in a single case of ventricular tachycardia. Figures 8–10 demonstrate the fourth criterion, recently described by Henthorn et al.,[9] the example shown being a case of AV reentrant tachycardia involving an AV bypass pathway. These four criteria, to one degree or another, have been demonstrated during five putative reentrant rhythms: classical (type I) atrail flutter,[2,5,12,18,21] ventricular tachycardia,[3,8,10,13,14,16,17] AV reentrant tachycardia involving an AV bypass pathway,[1,4] AV nodal reentrant tachycardia,[7,15] and ectopic atrial tachycardia.[6] In addition, several in vivo studies using mapping techniques to document the presence of reentrant rhythms during ventricular tachycardia[22–24] and atrial flutter[11,25,26] have also demonstrated that the phenomena postulated to occur during transient entrainment and used as part of the entrainment criteria indeed do occur.

Limitations of Transient Entrainment in Identifying a Reentrant Mechanism

Are the Observations during Transient Entrainment Only Explained by the Presence of Reentry?

Altought the phenomena associated with transient entrainment of a tachycardia with or without its subsequent interruption are best explained by reentry, it still must be asked whether any or all of the criteria for the demonstration of transient entrainment can be explained by another mechanism. Present understanding of the response of automatic rhythms to rapid pacing is completely inconsistent with the phenomena (constant fusion beats in the ECG, progressive

Table I
Criteria to Establish the Presence of Transient Entrainment

1) The demonstration of constant fusion beats in the ECG during the period of rapid pacing at a constant rate except for the last captured beat, which is entrained but not fused (i.e., the last entrained beat demonstrates the ECG morphology of the spontaneous tachycardia).

2) The demonstration of progressive fusion, i.e., constant fusion beats in the ECG during rapid pacing at any constant rate, but different degrees of constant fusion at different rapid rates.

3) Interruption of the tachycardia associated with localized conduction block to a site(s) for one beat, followed by subsequent activation of that site(s) from a different direction, manifest by a change in morphology of the electrogram at the blocked site(s), and with a shorter conduction time.

4) A change in conduction time and electrogram morphology at one recording site when pacing from another site at two different constant pacing rates, each of which is faster than the spontaneous rate of the tachycardia but fails to interrupt it.

fusion beats in the ECG) observed during transient entrainment, and observations consistent with overdrive suppression and subsequent warm-up of a pacemaker[37] or observations consistent with entrance block into an automatic focus are not seen during transient entrainment. Also, although it has been demonstrated in the canine heart[37] that automatic foci tend to accelerate and compete with imposed drives which exceed the spontaneous rate by a relatively small percentage, (10–15%) this still seems most unlikely to explain the phenomena observed during transient entrainment, as the automatic pacemaker tends to keep its accelerated rate for a period following termination or slowing of the pacing rate. And finally, automatic rhythms should not be interrupted by pacing.

Whether rapid pacing in the presence of a triggered rhythm can produce any of the entrainment criteria is, to our knowledge, unknown, as this question has yet to be systematically studied. As recently summarized,[36] relevant data such as are published are not consistent with the observations made during entrainment.

Finally, while we believe that entrainment of a tachycardia is best explained by the presence of an underlying reentrant mechanism, we recognize that, as with almost all complex phenomena, it is possible to invent alternative explanations, in this case explanations which have a basis other than reentry, regardless of how convoluted the explanations. Therefore, we submit that presently available data support our hypothesis, but that continued systematic investigation of the hypothesis is in order.

Concealed Entrainment

One additional limitation concerning transient entrainment as a marker of reentry has been recognized. We have shown that a tachycardia may be transiently entrained and even interrupted without being able to demonstrate any of the entrainment criteria, i.e., there may be concealed entrainment.[4] This can result, we have shown, when pacing is performed from a site which is orthodromically distal to the area of slow conduction in the reentry circuit.[4] Thus, it is clear that unless one is able to pace from an appropriate site, a reentry circuit with an excitable gap may be present, but entrainment, though present, will not be demonstrable.

This becomes of particular importance in at least two ways. First, it is obvious that the failure to demonstrate transient entrainment does not per se mean that a reentrant mechanism is not present. And second, it naturally follows that studies which attempt to quantitate the incidence of being able to demonstrate transient entrainment during various putative reentrant rhythms will not be meaningful unless pacing from an adequate number of sites is performed.

Demonstration and Localization of an Area of Slow Conduction in the Reentry Circuit

It is generally assumed that slow conduction is a necessary part of most reentry circuits.[27] However, the original studies of Mayer[28] and subsequent studies by Mines[29] indicated that reentry could occur around a fixed anatomical circuit without the presence of an area of slow conduction as long as the circuit was long enough to allow complete recovery of excitability, and that, at least with the initiation of the reentrant rhythm, there was unidirectional block around the circuit. And, most recently, a reentrant circuit sustaining atrial flutter in a dog model was found not to have a localized area of slow conduction, but rather to have uniformly slow conduction around the reentrant circuit.[25] Thus, there is no question that reentry without a discrete area of slow conduction can occur.

In this context, it is noteworthy that transient entrainment can be used not only to demonstrate the presence of reentry, but also to demonstrate and subsequently localize the area of slow conduction in the reentrant circuit of reentrant tachycardias. As indicated above, if one can demonstrate transient entrainment from one pacing site, but cannot demonstrate it from another (concealed entrainment), one would then know that the former pacing was performed from a site proximal to an area of slow conduction in the reentry circuit, whereas the latter pacing was performed from a site distal to the area of slow conduction.[4,10-12] Thus, this not only would demonstrate the presence of an area of slow conduction, but, also, by pacing from different sites, would localize the area of slow conduction. Furthermore, since one can entrain a reentrant tachycardia in which conduction around the anatomic circuit is uniformly slow,[25] one could identify reentrant rhythms in which there is no localized area of slow conduction because one presumably would be unable to demonstrate concealed entrainment. And finally, as we have shown for ventricular tachycardia in man, one can also localize a recording site as being within or just distal to the area of slow conduction.[10] Thus, we submit that the use of transient entrainment provides a useful technique to demonstrate and localize an area of slow conduction in a reentrant circuit. The usefulness in demonstrating and localizing an area of slow conduction may be theoretical or it may be practical, as in localizing such an area for ablative procedures either during catheter fulguration or during surgery, or to study effects of various interventions, including pharmacologic interventions.

Use of Transient Entrainment in Understanding Antitachycardia Pacemaker Treatment of Tachyarrhythmias

As we have already indicated, rapid pacing techniques can be used to interrupt reentrant tachyarrhythmias in which the reentry circuit includes an excitable gap. These rhythms include classic (type I) atrial flutter, ectopic atrial tachycardia, AV nodal reentrant tachycardia, AV reentrant tachycardia involving an AV bypass pathway, ventricular tachycardia, and probably sinus node reentrant tachycardia. As summarized recently,[38] when utilizing rapid pacing techniques to interrupt any of these arrhythmias, it is necessary to pace at a critically rapid rate (Figs. 2, 4, 8), and then for a critical duration of time at that rapid rate (Fig. 6), or else the tachycardia will not be successfully interrupted. Pacing at rates short of the critically rapid rate or short of the critical time duration will simply transiently entrain the tachycardia to the pacing rate without interrupting it. Therefore, when

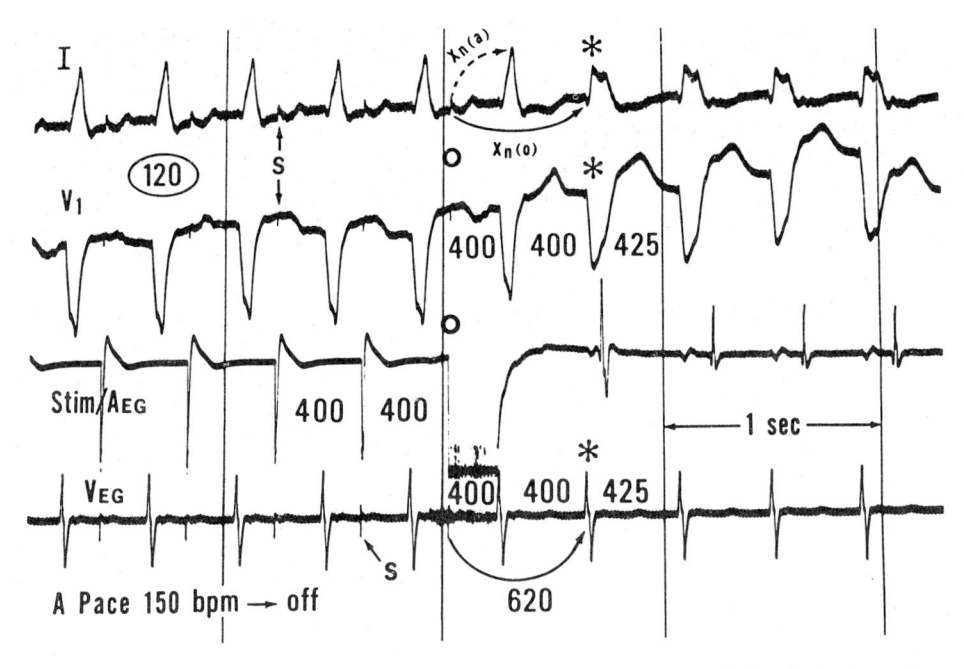

Figure 2: ECG leads I and VI recorded simultaneously with the atrial pacing (A Pace) stimulus artifact (Stim) or atrial electrogram (AEG) and the unipolar ventricular electrogram (VEG) at the termination of atrial pacing at a rate of 150 bpm (400 ms). In this and subsequent figures, the open circle denotes the last stimulus artifact (S), the asterisk denotes the last entrained beat, the arrow from the stimulus artifact in the ventricular electrogram points to the resulting ventricular electrogram (with the stimulus-to-ventricular electrogram interval being indicated in milliseconds), the dashed arrow in lead I represents the last antidromic wavefront ($X_n[a]$), the solid arrow the last orthodromic wavefronts ($X_n[o]$), from the last pacing impulse, and the circled number represents the duration of the QRS complex in the ECG. This figure illustrates the first criterion for transient entrainment (see Table I). From Waldo et al.[3]

such pacing is terminated, the tachycardia will resume promptly at its previous spontaneous rate. Furthermore, for some arrhythmias, pacing may be achieved at an appropriately rapid rate to interrupt the tachycardia and the pacing may be maintained for an appropriate period of time. However, in the latter instances, the phenomenon of termination and reinitiation of the arrhythmia sometimes may occur, in which case cessation of pacing is not associated with interruption of the arrhythmia, but rather with its continuation (Figs. 11-14).[38-41] All these phenomena associated with pacing interruption of tachyarrhythmias are understood by applying the principles of transient entrainment.[38,39]

Insights gained from understanding transient entrainment and interruption of tachyarrhythmias help explain some of the difficulties previously encountered with the use of antitachycardia pacemakers, and should help assist in the more effective use of antitachycardia pacemakers. In this regard, the recent appearance of miltiprogrammable antitachycardia pacemakers with the ability to program coupling intervals and the duration of pacing should make application of these devices to the treatment of tachycardias more effective. Of course, the problem of acceleration of tachycardias by rapid pacing clearly recognized in the

178 • CARDIAC ARRHYTHMIAS

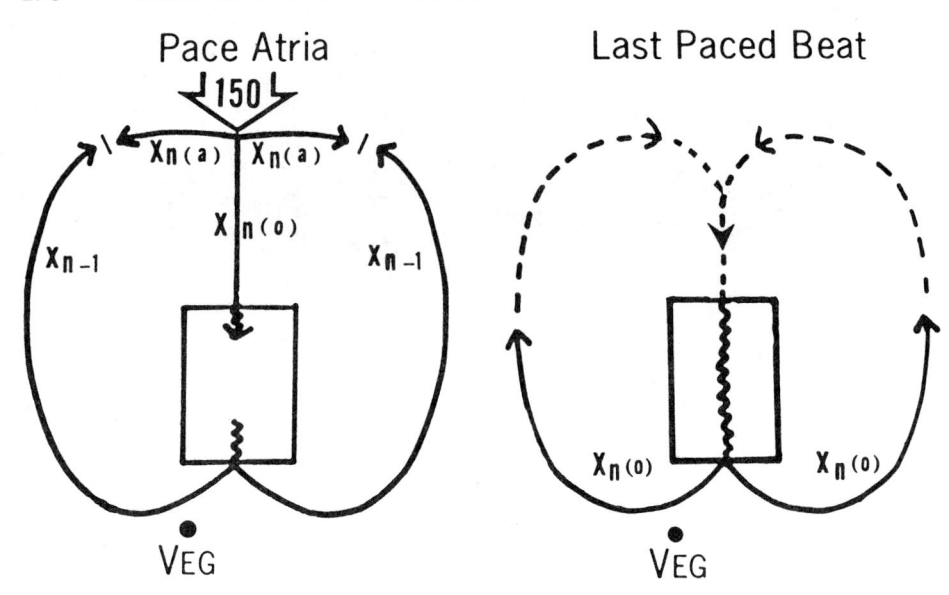

Figure 3: Diagrammatic representation of the termination of atrial pacing illustrated in Figure 2. Left Panel: The large arrow indicates the wavefront from the last pacing impulse delivered at a rate of 150 bpm entering into the excitable gap of the reentrant circuit of the ventricular tachycardia, where it is conducted orthodromically and antidromically. The antidromic wavefronts ($X_n[a]$) collide with the orthodromic wavefronts ($X_n[o]$) of the previous beat ($X_{n}-1$) resulting in fusion of ventricular activation, which, in effect, interrupts the tachycardia, but the orthodromic wavefront from the last pacing impulse continues the tachycardia, resetting it to the pacing rate. Right Panel: The orthodromic wavefronts from the last pacing impulse are now unopposed by antidromic wavefronts from a subsequent pacing impulse, so that no fusion of ventricular activation occurs despite the presence of transient entrainment. This last entrained beat continues the tachycardia (dashed lines), which then resumes at its previous spontaneous rate. This diagrammatically illustrates the first criterion of entrainment (see Table I). From Waldo et al.[3]

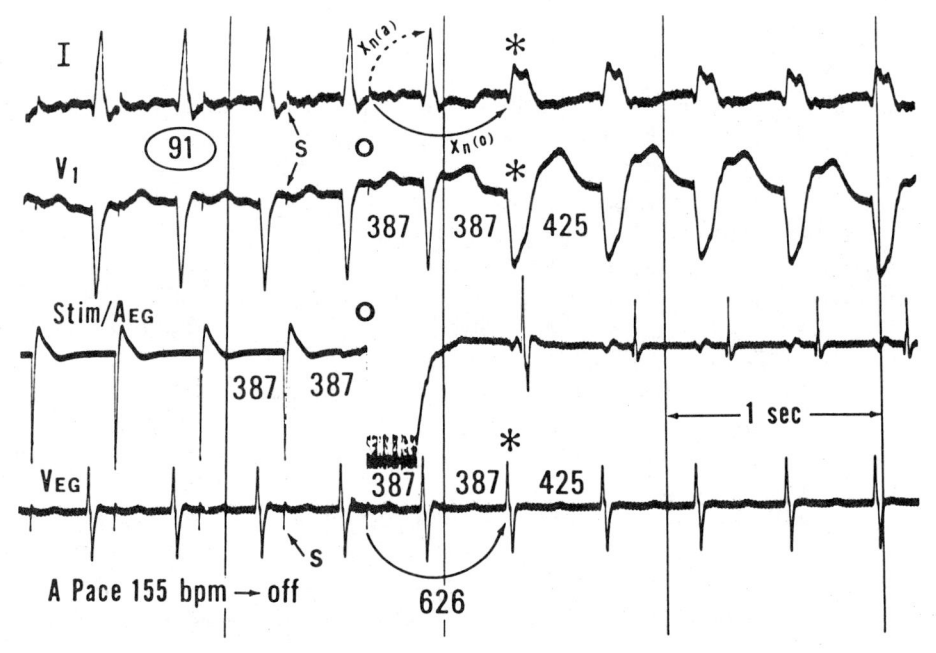

Figure 4: Legend on p. 179.

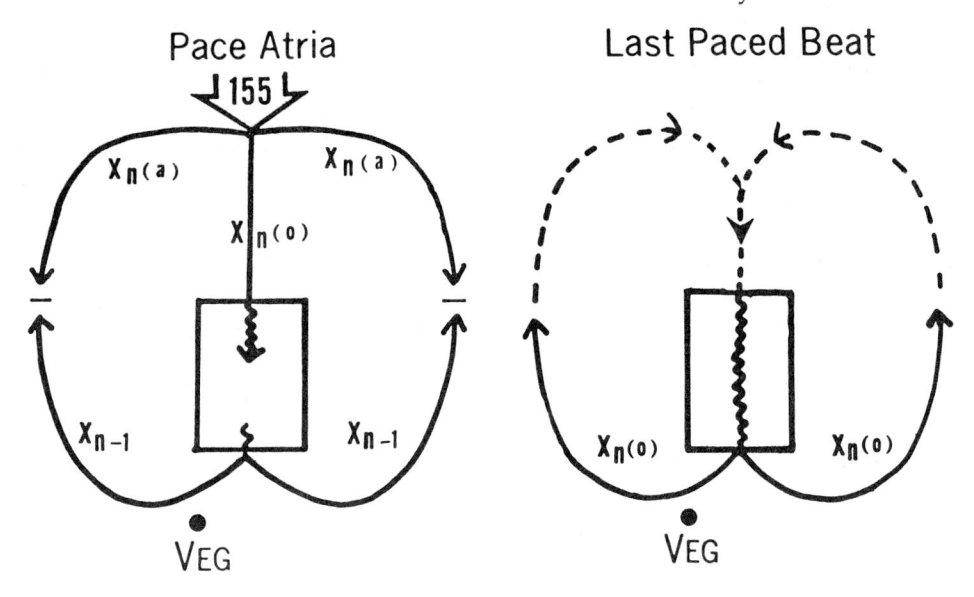

Figure 5: Diagrammatic representation of the termination of atrial pacing illustrated in Figure 4. Left Panel: Identical to the description of the left panel in Figure 3, except that the pacing impulse was delivered at a rate of 155 bpm. Note also that the greater penetration by the antidromic wavefront from the pacing impulse ($X_n(a)$) at this pacing rate when compared to pacing at 150 bpm explains the progressive fusion in the electrocardiogram. Atrial pacing at a rate of 160 bpm once again entrained the ventricular tachycardia, producing still a different degree of fusion beats in the ECG (not shown) because of the still greater penetration of the reentrant circuit by the antidromic wavefront from the pacing impulse. Right Panel: Identical to the description of the right panel in Figure 3. Note that the right ventricular electrogram (VEG) recording site is activated only by an orthodromic wavefront from the pacing impulse. From Waldo et al.[3]

treatment of ventricular tachycardia and atrial flutter remains one of the important present limitations of the use of this mode of treatment.

Understanding Components and Characteristics of the Reentry Circuit

There is much about the reentry circuit that we do not understand very well. We suggest that use of the principles of transient entrainment can help to understand better the various components and characteristics of the reentry circuit. For instance, we have recently noted the presence of double potentials during atrial flutter and ventricular tachycardia, and, using the principles of entrainment, have

Figure 4: ECG leads I and VI recorded simultaneously with either the atrial pacing stimulus (S) artifact (Stim) or atrial electrogram (AEG) and unipolar ventricular electrogram (VEG) at the termination of atrial pacing at a rate of 155 bpm (387 ms). All intervals are in milliseconds. Note the difference in the QRS complexes in the ECG leads during pacing at this rate compared with pacing at 150 bpm (Fig. 2). This figure demonstrates the second criterion of transient entrainment, namely progressive fusion in the ECG leads (see Table I). From Waldo et al.[3]

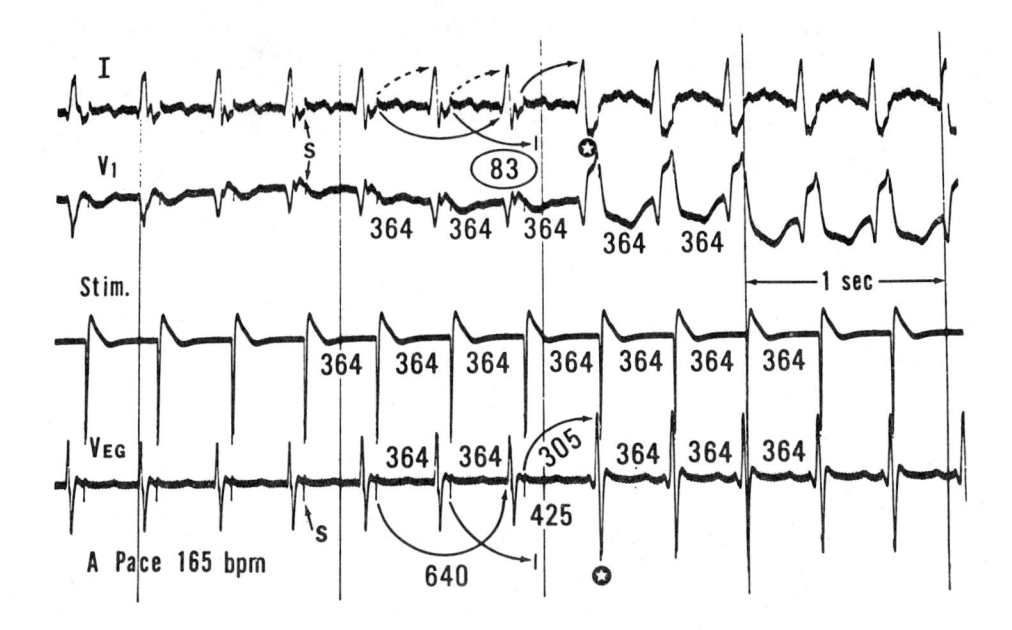

Figure 6: ECG leads I and VI recorded simultaneously with the atrial pacing stimulus (S) artifact (Stim) or atrial electrogram (AEG) and the unipolar ventricular electrogram (VEG) during atrial pacing at a rate of 165 bpm (364 ms cycle length). Note the further progressive fusion of the QRS complexes in the ECG leads when compared with Figures 2 and 4. Then, denoted by the circled stars, there is an abrupt change in configuration of the recorded QRS complexes in both ECG leads and in the unipolar ventricular electrogram complex. In the ventricular electrogram tracing, each arrow points to the resulting ventricular electrogram. Before the change in configuration of the QRS complexes and ventricular electrogram, the stimulus-to-ventricular electrogram interval is 640 ms. Then, after the localized conduction block to the ventricular electrogram recording site, the stimulus-to-ventricular electrogram interval becomes 305 ms. Note that this localized conduction block is associated with a 1 cycle increase in the beat-to-beat cycle length localized to the ventricular electrogram recording site (from 364 ms to 425 ms and then back to 364 ms). In the ECG lead I tracing, the dashed arrows represent the antidromic wavefronts and the associated solid arrows represent the orthodromic wavefronts from the 5th and 6th pacing impulses shown in the Figure. After the block of both the antidromic and orthodromic wavefronts of the 6th pacing impulse in the reentrant circuit of the ventricular tachycardia, the ventricles are activated by the 7th pacing impulse as expected during overdrive atrial pacing of a sinus rhythm because the ventricular tachycardia has been interrupted. Finally, had the pacing been terminated prior to achieving block of both the antidromic and orthodromic wavefronts of the pacing impulse, the tachycardia would not have been interrupted, emphasizing the critical duration of pacing at the critical pacing rate required for interruption of the tachycardia. All intervals are in milliseconds. From Waldo et al.[3]

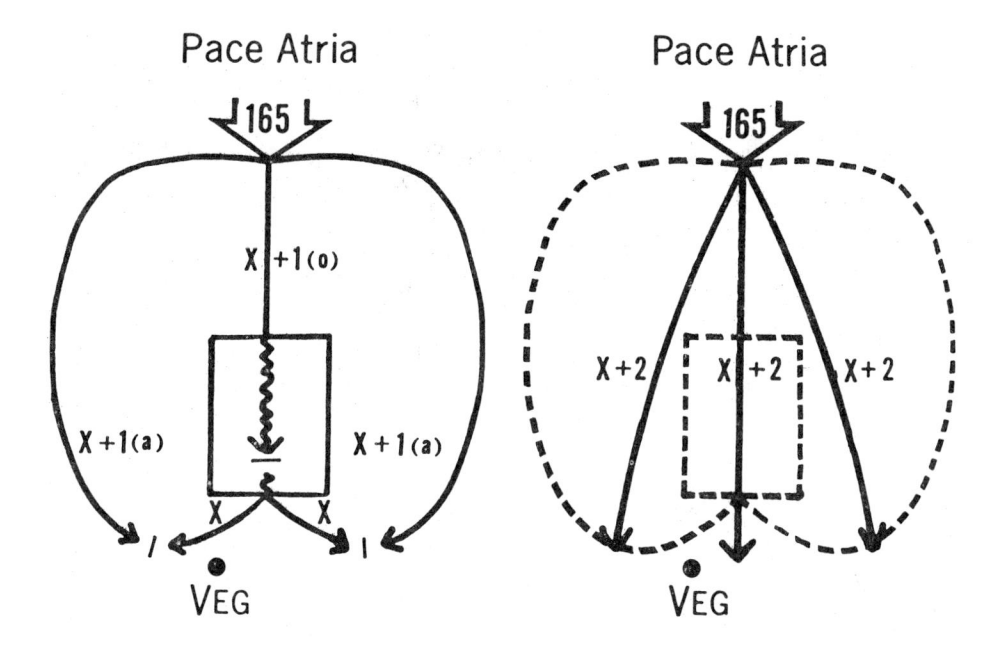

Figure 7: Diagrammatic representation of the events in Figure 6. Left Panel: The large arrow indicates the wavefront from the pacing impulse delivered at a rate of 165 bpm entering into the reentrant circuit of the ventricular tachycardia, where it is conducted orthodromically (X + 1[o]) and antidromically (X + 1[a]). The antidromic wavefronts collide with the orthodromic wavefronts from the previous beat (X) resulting in fusion of ventricular activation. Note the still greater antidromic penetration of the reentry circuit by the wavefront from the pacing impulse, explaining the initial appearance of still more progressive fusion of the QRS complexes in the ECG leads. This time, however, the orthodromic wavefront is also blocked (presumably in the area of slow conduction) during the same beat. Note that the right ventricular electrogram (VEG) recording site is still activated by the orthodromic wavefront of the previous beat (X), but is not activated either by the antidromic or orthodromic wavefront of the X + 1 beat, i.e., there is localized conduction block to that site. Right Panel: The large arrows indicate the next pacing impulse (X + 2) delivered at the same pacing rate (165 bpm) from the same atrial pacing site as in the left diagram. The dashed lines indicate the reentrant circuit present during the previous periods of spontaneous ventricular tachycardia and transient entrainment of the ventricular tachycardia. Because the ventricular tachycardia has been interrupted by the previous pacing impulse (X + 1), the sequence of ventricular activation of the next pacing impulse (X + 2) is as one would expect during overdrive pacing of a sinus rhythm. Therefore, the right ventricular electrogram (VEG) recording site is activated from a different direction than during previous periods of transient entrainment from the same pacing site. In addition, because the presumed area of slow conduction is no longer functionally present, the stimulus-to-right ventricular electrogram conduction time will be shorter. This fulfills and explains the third criterion for transient entrainment (see Table I). From Waldo et al.[3]

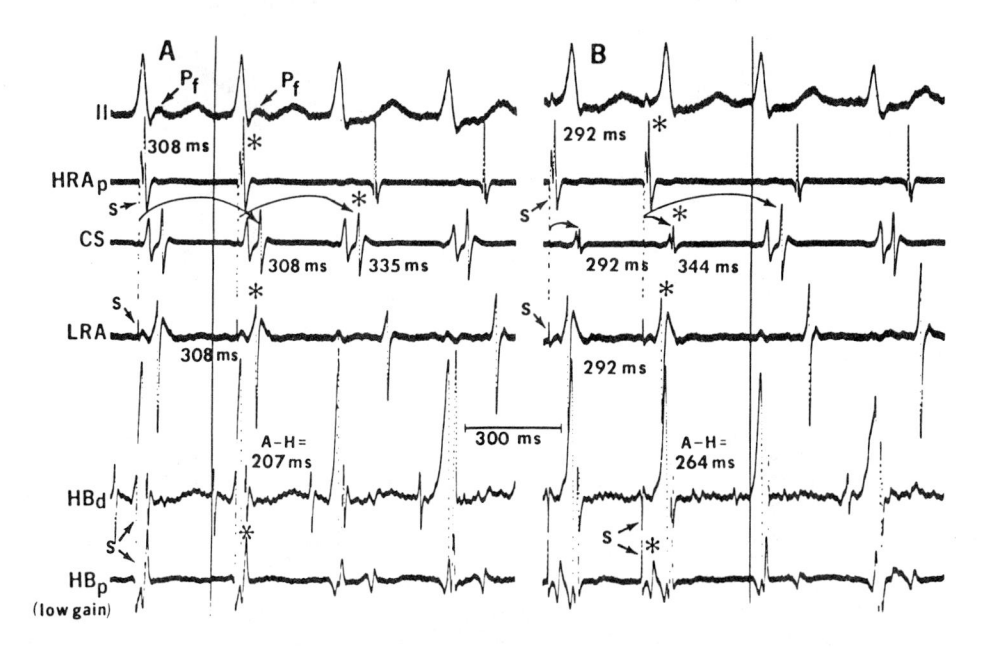

Figure 8: Illustration of the fourth criterion for the demonstration of the transient entrainment (see Table I) during atrial pacing from the high right atrium (HRA) during AV junctional reentrant tachycardia (spontaneous cycle length 339 ms). In both panels, ECG lead II is recorded simultaneously with bipolar electrograms from the proximal pair of electrodes from a catheter electrode placed in the high right atrium (HRA_p), the coronary sinus (CS), the low right atrium (LRA), and the distal pair (HB_d) and proximal pair (HB_p) of electrodes of a tripolar catheter in the His bundle position during termination of pacing at a cycle length of 308 ms (Panel A) and 292 ms (Panel B). In the recordings from the coronary sinus site, the arrows from each stimulus artifact indicate the atrial complexes which result from that stimulus. The asterisk indicates the last transiently entrained beat at each recording site. S = stimulus artifact. P_f = fusion P wave. Note that the atrial electrogram at the coronary sinus site in Panel A is identical to that during the spontaneous rhythm, and that, as indicated by the arrow from the stimulus artifact to the atrial complex at the coronary sinus recording site, conduction time during pacing is long. However, with pacing at the shorter cycle length in Panel B, the atrial electrogram morphology changes at the coronary sinus site and the stimulus-to-atrial electrogram conduction time becomes much shorter. Note also that the tachycardia is not interrupted by pacing in either instance. This fulfills the fourth criterion for the demonstration of transient entrainment (see Table I). From Waldo et al.[1]

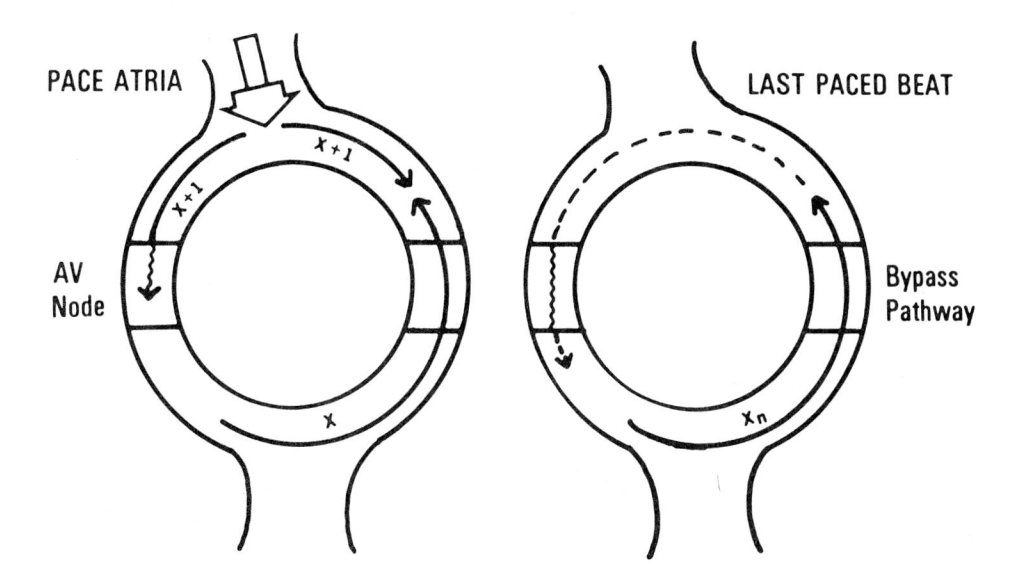

Figure 9: Diagrammatic representation of the events recorded in Panel A of Figure 8. Left Panel: The large arrow indicates the pacing impulse from the high right atrium entering into the reentry circuit, whereupon it is conducted orthodromically (X + 1) and antidromically (X + 1). The antidromic wavefront collides with the orthdromic wavefront of the previous beat (X) resulting in intra-atrial fusion, which, in effect, terminates the tachycardia, but the orthodromic wavefront from the pacing impulse continues and, in fact, resets it. Right Panel: The orthodromic wavefront of the last paced beat (X_n) is unopposed by an antidromic wavefront, so that no atrial fusion occurs despite the presence of transient entrainment, and the tachycardia (dashed lines) then continues spontaneously. The serpentine line indicates slow conduction. Note that the coronary sinus recording site, that is, the area just on the atrial side of the AV bypass pathway, is activated orthodromically during pacing (left panel) and during the spontaneous tachycardia, so that the electrogram recorded at that site is the same during pacing as during the spontaneous rhythm. Also, conduction time from the stimulus artifiact to the coronary sinus recording site is long (left panel) because the impulse must traverse the specialized AV conduction system and the ventricles before reaching that recording site. From Waldo et al.[1]

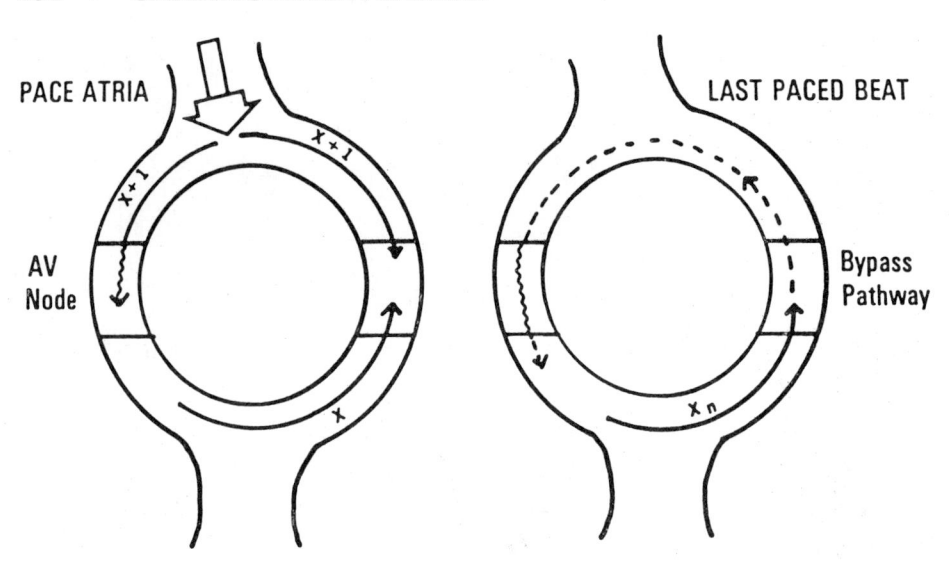

Figure 10: Diagrammatic representation of the events recorded in Panel B of Figure 8. Left Panel: The large arrow indicates the pacing impulse from the high right atrium entering into the reentry circuit, whereupon it is conducted orthodromically (X + 1) and antidromically (X + 1). Antegrade block of the antidromic wavefront from the pacing impulse and retrograde block of the orthodromic wavefront of the previous beat (X) occur in the AV bypass pathway, resulting in the absence of atrial fusion beats in the ECG, and apparent termination of the tachycardia. However, the tachycardia is continued and reset by the orthodromic wavefront of the pacing impulse (X + 1). Note that the coronary sinus recording site, diagrammatically represented as just on the atrial side of the AV bypass pathway, is now activated by the antidromic wavefront from the pacing impulse, so that the morphology of the atrial electrogram recorded at that site is different, and conduction time from the pacing stimulus to the atrial electrogram is now shorter. This fulfills and explains the fourth criterion for the demonstration of transient entrainment (see Table I). Right Panel: The orthodromic wavefront of the last paced beat (X_n) is unopposed by an antidromic wavefront, so that it is now conducted in the retrograde direction over the AV bypass pathway to the atria, so that the tachycardia (dashed lines) continues spontaneously. The serpentine line indicates an area of slow conduction. Note that with resumption of the spontaneous tachycardia, the coronary sinus recording site will again be activated orthodromically. From Waldo et al.[1]

demonstrated that the double potentials really represent two different wavefronts which temporally occur during one beat, but in actual fact are really related to different beats.[42,43] In addition, there are many portions of the reentry loop about which there is much to learn. We have already discussed the opportunity to localize an area of slow conduction in the reentry circuit using the principles of transient entrainment. By the same token, one can begin to examine the nature of the excitable gap and the way that antiarrhythmic drugs act on the different components of the reentry circuit. Likewise, one can look at the effects of other interventions on the reentry circuit, and finally, one can even use entrainment to understand better the nature of the functional center of some reentry circuits.

Summary and Conclusion

It is clear that transient entrainment is a useful tool to use for understanding and better treating cardiac arrhythmias. Its ease of application, particularly for studies in man, makes it particularly useful to apply. As we begin to understand

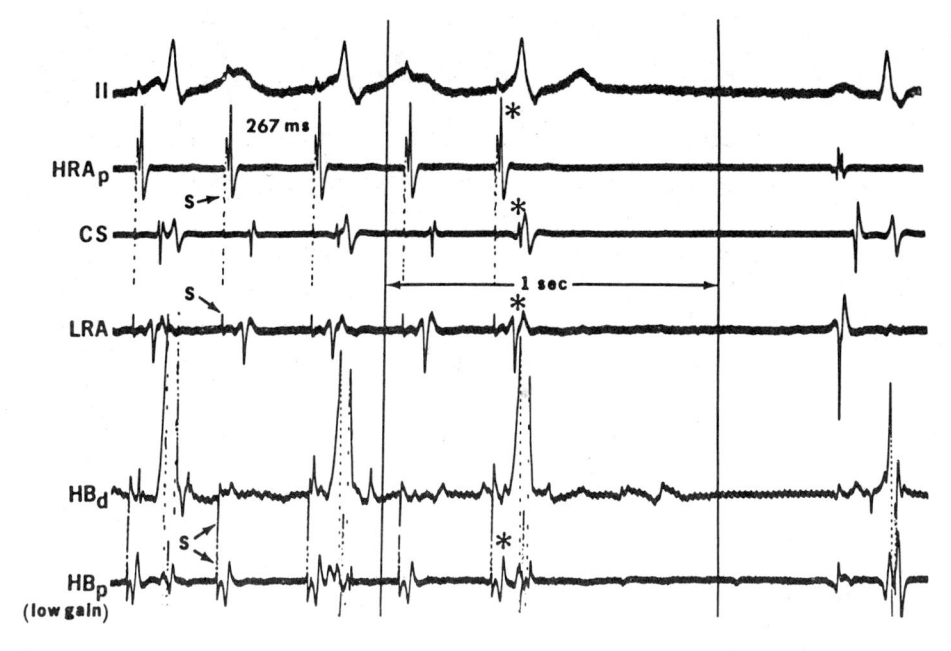

Figure 11: Records from the same patient shown in Figure 8 at the termination of rapid pacing (cycle length 267 ms). The asterisk indicates the last captured beat at each atrial recording site. Upon termination of pacing, the tachycardia was interrupted because both the antidromic and orthodromic wavefronts from the same pacing impulse were blocked during the same beat. Had pacing been terminated following an AV nodally conducted beat, the tachycardia would have been reinitiated (see Fig. 13). S = stimulus artifact. Time lines are at one-second intervals. From Waldo et al.[1]

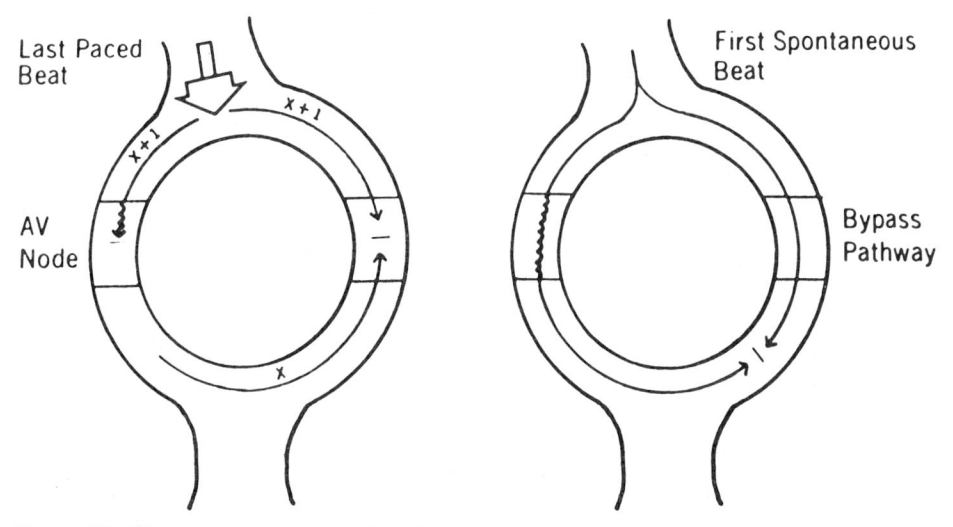

Figure 12: Diagrammatic representation of events recorded in Figure 11. Left Panel: Large arrow indicates pacing impulse from the high right atrium entering into the reentry circuit, whereupon it is conducted orthodromically (X + 1) and antidromically (X + 1). The antidromic wavefront collides with the orthodromic wavefront of the previous beat (X), and the ortodromic wavefront from the same pacing impulse blocks in the AV node. Thus, the AV reentrant tachycardia is interrupted. Right Panel: Since there are no further paced beats, nor any more circulating reentrant wavefronts, the first beat is a spontaneous sinus beat which activates the ventricles simultaneously via a wavefront conducted over the AV node and a wavefront conducted over the AV bypass pathway. From Waldo et al.[38]

186 • CARDIAC ARRHYTHMIAS

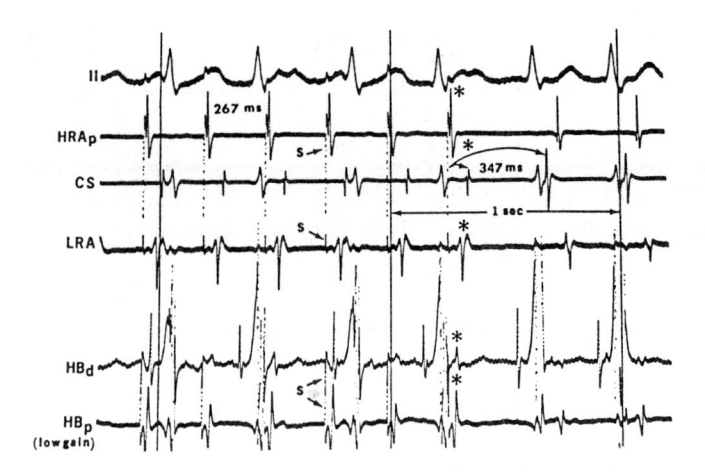

Figure 13: This figure demonstrates termination with reinitiation of a tachycardia during rapid pacing. EG lead II recorded simultaneously with electrograms from the same recording sites as in Figures 8 and 11 at the termination of rapid atrial pacing from the high right atrium of the same AV reentrant tachycardia at the same pacing cycle length as in Figure 11. Although second degree AV block occurred during pacing, because the last paced atrial beat was conducted orthodromically through the specialized AV conduction system with sufficient delay, the tachycardia was reinitiated, and, therefore, continued after the termination of pacing. In the recordings from the coronary sinus site, the arrows point from the last stimulus to the resulting atrial complexes. The asterisk indicates the last captured beat at each recording site. S = stimulus artifact. Time lines are at one-second intervals. From Waldo et al.[1]

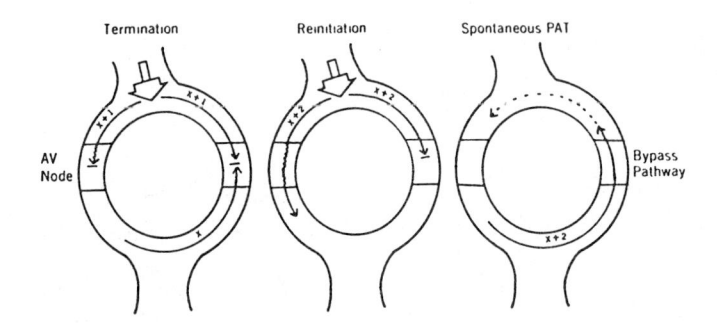

Figure 14: Diagrammatic representation of the events recorded in Figure 13. Left Panel: The large arrow indicates the pacing impulse (X + 1) entering into the reentrant circuit, whereupon it is conducted orthodromically and antidromically. The antidromic wavefront from the same pacing impulse blocks in the AV bypass pathway with the orthodromic wavefront of the previous beat (X), as always happens during transient entrainment. However, the orthodromic wavefront of the same beat (X + 1) blocks in the AV node. Therefore, since the antidromic and orthodromic wavefronts of the same pacing impulse are blocked during the same beat, the tachycardia has been interrupted. Middle Panel: In this example, rapid atrial pacing is continued after the interruption of the tachycardia. The large arrow indicates the next pacing impulse (X + 2) entering into the reentry circuit, whereupon it is conducted antidromically and orthodromically. The antidromic wavefront blocks in the AV bypass pathway, not because it collides with the orthodromic wavefront of the previous beat (there is none because the previous orthodromic wavefront had been blocked in the AV node), but because the impulse arrives during the effective refractory period in the AV bypass pathway. However, the orthodromic wavefront from the pacing impulse (X + 2) is conducted through AV node. Right Panel: Now, rapid atrial pacing is terminated. Therefore, the orthodromic wavefront of the last paced beat (X + 2) is unopposed by an antidromic wavefront from a subsequent pacing impulse. This last wavefront (X + 2) conducts retrogradely through the AV bypass pathway to reexcite the atria and reinitiate the spontaneous AV reentrant tachycardia. Thus, termination with reinitiation is explained by this diagram. From Waldo et al.[38]

more about transient entrainment itself and as we can apply it in vivo to different cardiac arrhythmias, this tool should continue to provide a useful means not only to establish the presence of reentry, but also to understand it better and to apply treatment more effectively.

Acknowledgement: This research was supported in part by Grant R01HL29381 from the U.S. Public Health Service, National Institutes of Health, National Heart, Lung and Blood Institute Bethesda, Maryland.

References

1. Waldo AL, Plumb VJ, Arciniegas JG, MacLean WAH, Cooper TB, Priest MF, James TN. Transient entrainment and interruption of A-V bypass pathway type paroxysmal atrial tachycardia: A model for understanding and identifying reentrant arrhythmias in man. Circulation 1982;67:73.
2. Waldo AL, MacLean WAH, Karp RB, Kouchoukos NT, James TN. Entrainment and interruption of atrial flutter with atrial pacing: Studies in man following open heart surgery. Circulation 1977;56:737.
3. Waldo AL, Henthorn RW, Plumb VJ, MacLean WAH. Demonstration of the mechanism of transient entrainment and interruption of ventricular tachycardia with rapid atrial pacing. J Am Coll Cardiol 1984;3:422.
4. Okumura K, Henthorn RW, Epstein AE, Plumb VJ, Waldo AL. Further observations of transient entrainment: Importance of pacing site and properties of the components of the reentry circuit. Circulation 1985;72:1293
5. Waldo AL, Plumb VJ, Henthorn RW. Observations on the mechanism of atrial flutter. In Surawicz B, ed. Tachycardias. The Hague, Martinus Nijhoff, 1984;213.
6. Henthorn RW, Plumb VJ, Arciniegas JG, Waldo AL. Entrainment of "ectopic atrial tachycardia:" Evidence for re-entry (abstr). Am J Cardiol 1982;49:920.
7. Brugada P, Waldo AL, Wellens HJJ. Transient entrainment and interruption of atrioventricular nodal tachycardia. J Am Coll Cardiol (In press).
8. Plumb VJ, Henthorn RW, Waldo AL. Characteristics of the transient entrainment of ventricular tachycardia by ventricular pacing (abstr). PACE 1984;7:463.
9. Henthorn RW, Plumb VJ, Olshansky B, Okumura K, Hess PG, Epstein AE, Waldo AL. A new criterion for entrainment: More evidence for reentry (abstr). Circulation 1985;72:III-30.
10. Okumura K, Olshansky B, Henthorn RW, Epstein RE, Plumb VJ, Waldo AL. Demonstration of the presence of slow conduction during sustained ventricular tachycardia in man. Circulation (In press).
11. Okumura K, Plumb VJ, Waldo AL. Entrainment of experimental atrial flutter and its use to localize the slow conduction area in the reentry loop (abstr). Circulation 1985;72:III-382.
12. Olshansky B, Okumura K, Henthorn RW, Epstein AE, Plumb VJ, Waldo AL. Entrainment of human atrial flutter localizes the area of slow conduction in the inferior right atrium (abstr). J Am Coll Cardiol 1986;7:128A.
13. MacLean WAH, Plumb VJ, Waldo AL. Transient entrainment and interruption of ventricular tachycardia. PACE 1981;4:358.
14. Anderson KP, Swerdlow CD, Mason JW. Entrainment of ventricular tachycardia. Am J Cardiol 1984;53:335.
15. Portillo B, Mejias J, Leon-Portillo N, Zaman L, Myerburg RJ, Castellanos A. Entrainment of atrioventricular nodal reentrant tachycardias during overdrive pacing from high right atrium and coronary sinus: With special reference to atrioventricular dissociation and 2:1 retrograde block during tachycardias. Am J Cardiol 1984;53:1750.
16. Mann DE, Lawrie GM, Luck JC, Magro SA, Wyndham CRC. Importance of pacing site in entrainment of ventricular tachycardia. J Am Coll Cardiol 1985;5:781.

17. Almendral JM, Gottlieb C, Marchlinski FE, Buxton AE, Doherty JU, Josephson ME. Entrainment of ventricular tachycardia by atrial depolarizations. Am J Cardiol 1985; 56:298.
18. Inoue H, Matsuo H, Takayanag K, Murao S. Clinical and experimental studies of the effects of atrial extrastimulation in rapid pacing on atrial flutter cycle length. Evidence of macroreentry with an excitable gap. Am J Cardiol 1981;48:623.
19. Morady F, Scheinman MM, Winston SA, DiCarol LA Jr, Davis JC. Dissociation of atrial electrograms by right and left atrial pacing in patients with atrial ventricular reciprocating tachycardia. J Am Coll Cardiol 1984;4:1283.
20. Saoudi NC, Castellanos SA, Zaman L, Portillo B, Schwartz A, Myerburg RJ. Attempted entrainment of circus movement tachycardias by ventricular stimulation. PACE 1986; 9:78.
21. Beckman K, Lin HT, Krafchek J, Wyndham CRC. Classic and concealed entrainment of typical and atypical atrial flutter. PACE 1986;9:826.
22. Chen PS, Lowe JE, German LD, Vidaillet HJ Jr, Greer GS, Smith WM, Ideker RE. Mapping ventricular fusion beats during entrainment. Circulation 1986;74:II-484.
23. El-Sherif N, Gough WB, Restivo M. The mechanism for "entrainment" in termination of reentrant ventricular tachycardia by overdrive pacing (abstr). J Am Coll Cardiol 1986;7:40A.
24. Dillion S, Wit AL. Mechanisms for effects of overdrive on reentrant ventricular tachycardia. Circulation 1986;74:II-118.
25. Frame LH, Page RL, Hoffman BF. Atrial reentry around an anatomic barrier with a partially refractory excitable gap: A canine model of atrial flutter. Circ Res 1986;58:495.
26. Boyden PA, Frame LH, Hoffman BH. Activation patterns during transient entrainment of reentrant excitation in isolated canine atrium (abstr). Circulation 1986;74: II-350.
27. Cranefield PF. The Conduction of the Cardiac Impulse. The Slow Response and Cardiac Arrhythmias. Mt. Kisco, New York, Futura Publishing Co., 1975.
28. Mayer AG. Rhythmical pulsation in Scyphomedusae: II. In Papers from the Tortugas Laboratory of the Carnegie Institution of Washington. 1908;1:113.
29. Mines GR. On circulating excitations in heart muscles and their possible relation to tachycardia and fibrillation. Trans Roy Soc Can, Ser 3, sec 4, 1914;8:43.
30. Wit AL, Hoffman BF, Cranefield PF. Slow conduction and reentry in the ventricular conducting system. I. Return extrasystole in canine Purkinje fibers. Circ Res 1972;30:1.
31. Wit AL, Cranefield PF, Hoffman BF. Slow conduction and reentry in the ventricular conducting system. II. Single and sustained circus movement in networks of canine and bovine Purkinje fibers. Circ Res 1972;30:11.
32. Wellens HJJ. Value and limitations of programmed electrical stimulation of the heart in the study and treatment of tachycardias. Circulation 1978;57:845.
33. Rosen MR, Reder RF. Does triggered activity have a role in the genesis of cardiac arrhythmias? Ann Intern Med 1981;94:794.
34. Brugada P, Wellens HJJ. The role of triggered activity in clinical ventricular arrhythmias. PACE 1984;7:260.
35. Brugada P, Wellens HJJ. Early afterdepolarizations: Role in conduction block, "prolonged repolarization-dependent reexcitation," and tachyarrhythmias on the human heart. PACE 1985;8:889.
36. Wit AL, Rosen MR. Afterdepolarizations and triggered activity. In The Heart and Cardiovascular System. Scientific Foundations. Fozzard HA, Haber E, Jennings RB, Katz AM, Morgan HE, eds. New York, Raven Press, 1986;1449.
37. Lange G. Action of driving stimuli from intrinsic and extrinsic sources on *in situ* cardiac pacemaker tissues. Circ Res 1965;17:449.
38. Waldo AL, Henthorn RW, Epstein AE, Plumb VJ. Significance of transient entrainment in pacing treatment of tachyarrhythmias. Archives des Maladies du Coeur et Vaisseaux 1985;78:23.
39. Waldo AL, Henthorn RW, Plumb VJ. Relevance of telemetry of electrograms and transient entrainment for antitachycardia devices. PACE 1984;7:588–600.

40. Josephson ME, Seides SF. Clinical Cardiac Electrophysiology. Techniques and Interpretation. Philadelphia, Lea & Febiger, 1979;264.
41. Brugada P, Wellens HJJ. Entrainment as an electrophysiologic phenomenon. J Am Coll Cardiol 1984;3:451.
42. Olshansky B, Okumura K, Moreira D, Henthorn RW, Epstein AE, Plumb VJ, Waldo AL. Entrainment of double potentials in human atrial flutter (abstr). PACE 1986;9:306.
43. Olshansky B, Henthorn RW, Waldo AL. Entrainment of double potentials in human ventricular tachycardia (abstr). Circulation (Submitted, 1987)

10

Localization of the Area of Slow Conduction During Ventricular Tachycardia

R. Frank, J.L. Tonet
S. Kounde, G. Farenq
G. Fontaine

Introduction

Catheter endocardial mapping was first used to understand the mechanism of tachycardias, atrial flutter,[1] or Wolff-Parkinson-White syndrome.[2] With the development of surgery for arrhythmias, endocardial mapping has become a preoperative study directed to localize the area of interest during surgery, in patients with WPW syndrome or with ventricular tachycardia (VT). This last application has been particularly developed and studied by Josephson.[3] Endocardial mapping is now of primary importance during catheter ablative procedures because of the need to direct the therapeutic agents to the exact site of origin of the arrhythmia.

The techniques used during catheter endocardial mapping for fulguration of ventricular tachycardia have derived from two previously existing techniques: surgical treatment of ventricular tachycardia and His bundle fulguration. Since 1973, surgical treatment of ventricular tachycardia has demonstrated that sometimes a very limited incision at a site of origin can prevent tachycardia recurrence.[4] This site can be localized during perioperative mapping as the site where the earliest potential is recorded during tachycardia and occurring before the onset of the QRS complex on the surface ECG.[5] Fulguration of the bundle of His also has proved that an electric shock will destroy the tissues from which a recorded potential originates,[6] preventing local conduction. It has been assumed, therefore, that fulguration could prevent the reinitiation of VT when delivered at its site of origin, identified by the earliest endocardial potential during tachycardia.[7] The aim of catheter endocardial mapping during fulguration is to get as close as possible to the endocardial zone earliest activated during tachycardia.

As few simultaneous points can be recorded with catheter techniques, pacing can become an important adjunct to demonstrate that early potential originates close to the site of origin of the arrhythmia.[8,9] By pacing the ventricles from different areas, many different QRS morphologies can be reproduced. When pacing is performed in the area where tachycardia originates or inside a critical tachycardia pathway, morphologies of the QRS similar to the spontaneous tachycardia can be obtained. We call "exact pace mapping" the exact reproduction of VT morphology on the 12 surface ECG leads. The purpose of this presentation is to discuss the phenomena observed during exact pace mapping and its value for the localization of the site of origin of VT.

Methods

Bipolar or multipolar catheters with 1 cm interelectrode distance are inserted transcutaneously in the subclavian and the femoral veins and placed at the right atrium, coronary sinus, right ventricular apex, His bundle, and right ventricular outflow tract. These catheters serve as reference or as pacing electrodes. Catheters previously selected to withstand the fulguration shock[8] are placed at different areas of the ventricles to record bipolar endocardial potentials. A long sheath (Cordis femoral ventricular catheter/sheath set) is inserted via the femoral artery, inside the left ventricle, to allow easier catheter positioning. Filters are set between 10 and 300 Hz. Signals are amplified 1000 to 10,000 times. One-millivolt calibration marks and time marks are automatically and simultaneously generated on the tracing. All data are recorded on analogic tape (EMI tape recorder). The position of the catheters is monitored by bidimensional fluoroscopy and stored on video tape. Hemodynamic monitoring is performed using radial arterial pressure, pulmonary wedge pressure through a Swan-Ganz catheter, and serial cardiac output by thermodilution.

To minimize the time during which the patient remains in ventricular tachycardia and the risk of hemodynamic compromise, the study is always started by pace mapping. This is done by pacing the ventricle at the tachycardia rate at different endocardial sites. Twelve-lead ECGs are recorded and compared to the spontaneous VT morphology. When a good matching is obtained, VT is triggered by programmed pacing, and endocardial potentials are recorded and analyzed. Time measurements are made on the rapid portion of the signal, corresponding to the moment when the activation wave passes under the recording electrode, as suggested by previous simulation studies.[10] The catheter is moved slightly in the same region, and when the earliest occurring potential has been determined, pacing is resumed on that site to try to reproduce the exact morphology of VT.

Mapping may take between 30 minutes and several hours, depending upon the ease with which the leads can be manipulated. VT has to be hemodynamically tolerated during long periods of time, and for this purpose, the patients are usually left under chronic amiodarone therapy (400 mg a day) to have a slower tachycardia.

All Class I antiarrhythmic drugs having negative inotropic effects are discontinued for five half-lives before fulguration. Hemodynamic monitoring is performed continuously during the procedure and VT is terminated if hemodynamic function deteriorates.

Case Report

Patient No. 1 (Figs. 1, 2, 3)

A patient with right and left ventricular dilated cardiomyopathy had a ventricular tachycardia with left axis deviation and left bundle branch block morphology. VT cycle was irregular, with a cycle length between 360 and 430 ms. An early potential preceding the QRS by 100 ms was recorded in the inferior right ventricular wall, under the tricuspid valve. The local potential at this area during sinus rhythm was multiphasic with a duration of 255 ms (Fig. 1). Pacing at that site with a cycle length of 500 ms reproduced VT morphology exactly. A delay of 100 ms between the pacing artifact and the ventricular response was observed (Fig. 2). During VT, an extrastimulus given 260 ms after the previous QRS (that is, 360 ms

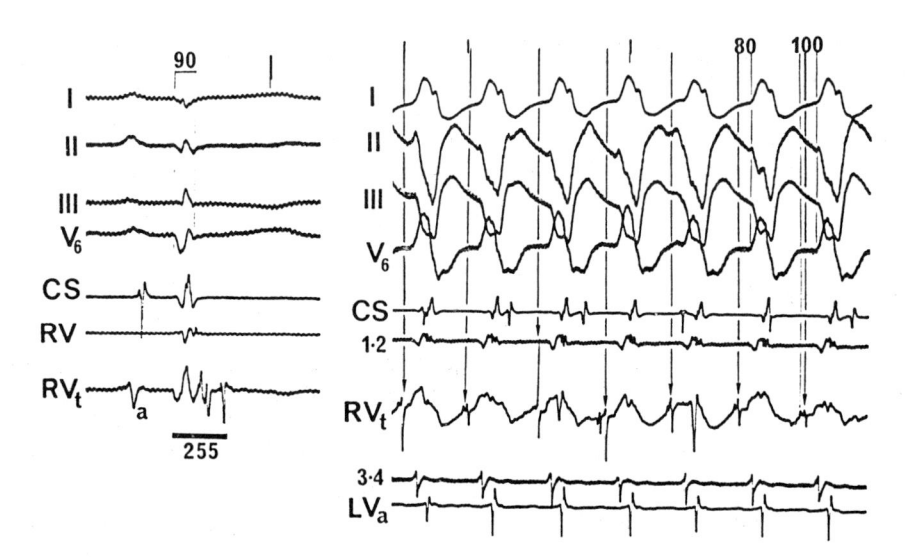

Figure 1: Patient no. 1. Endocardial potentials in sinus rhythm (on the left) and during VT (on the right). See text. CS = Coronary sinus; 1-2, 3-4 = quadripolar apical right ventricular lead; LVa = left ventricular apex; RVt = right ventricular diaphragmatic site under the tricuspid valve, where an atrial (a) potential is also recorded.

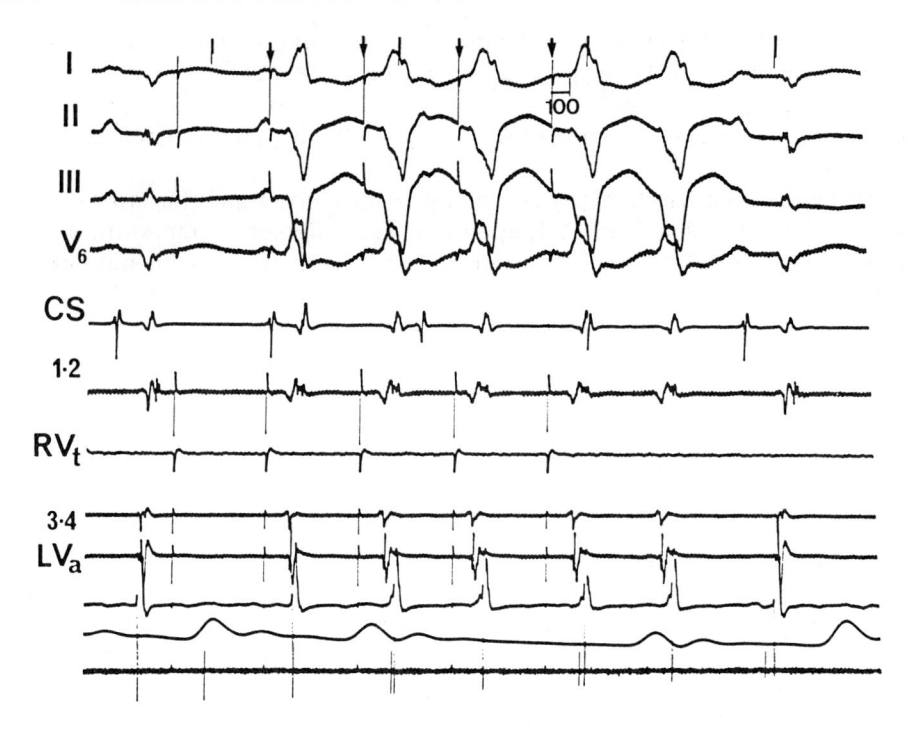

Figure 2: Patient no. 1 (see text). Exact pace mapping in sinus rhythm triggering one spontaneous VT cycle.

after the local endocardial potential) was followed 100 ms later by a QRS with a morphology similar to the spontaneous VT. VT then resumed with a slightly longer cycle length of 406 ms. As can be observed in Figure 3 after a cycle length of 405 ms, the following cycles become regular with a cycle length of 400 ms. A burst of stimuli changed the VT cycle length without changing its morphology. A single fulguration shock at that site was effective on that patient.

Patient No. 2

A patient with the syndrome of right ventricular dysplasia presented with a VT with left axis and right bundle branch pattern, with a stable cycle length of 450 ms.

The earliest potential recorded by endocardial mapping was localized in the mid-right septal area. It preceded the onset of the QRS complex on the surface ECG by 50 ms. Its morphology was unusual. A discrete potential with a sharp deflection resembling a His bundle potential, with an amplitude of 0.4 mV preceded a wider complex, synchronous with the QRS on the surface ECG. Pacing that site at the tachycardia rate reproduced exactly the morphology of the tachycardia on the 12 leads of the ECG. A delay of 50 ms, similar to the prematurity of the endocardial complex, was observed between stimulus and onset of the

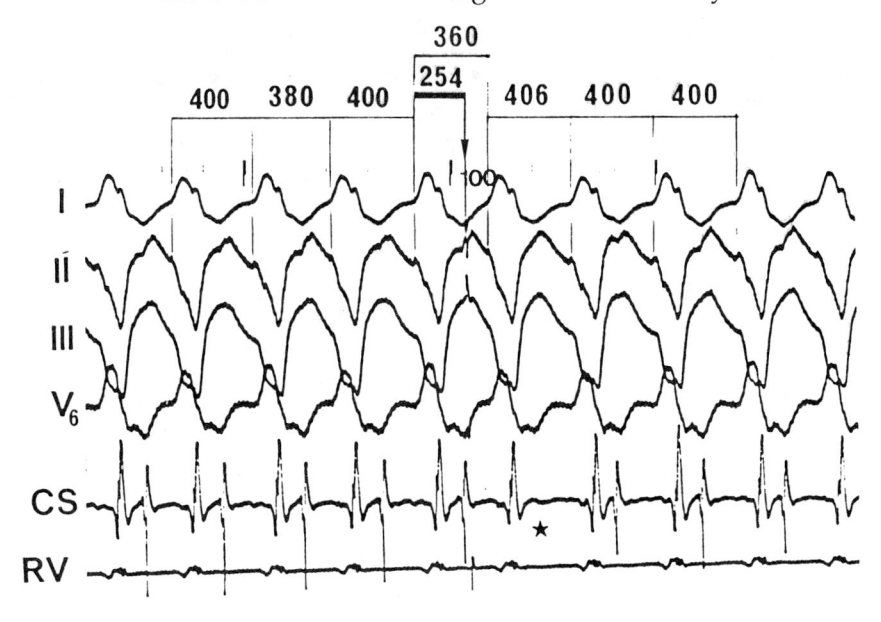

Figure 3: Patient no. 1. Entrainment of VT by one extrastimulus conducted with a delay of 100 ms.

QRS complex on the surface ECG (Fig. 4). When the tachycardia was interrupted, a small, sharp late potential resembling the early one during VT closely followed the endocardial potential (Fig. 5) during sinus rhythm.

Ventricular extrastimuli with increasing prematurity were given at that site during ventricular tachycardia (Fig. 6). When given after 270 ms after the discrete potential, a paced beat was observed 320 ms after the previous ventricular beat. This beat was followed 500 ms later by a new tachycardia beat, the next beat occurring after 440 ms and the tachycardia regaining its original 450 ms cycle length.

When the extrastimulus coupling interval was decreased by 10 ms (260 ms), no ventricular response followed the stimulus falling into the refractory period of the preceding beat. However, a marked prolongation of the ventricular tachycardia cycle length to 550 ms occurred. The two next cycles had a duration of 430 and 460 ms, and the tachycardia cycle again regained a stable cycle length of 450 ms.

When the coupling interval was again decreased by 10 ms (250 ms) no capture was observed and no change occurred in the tachycardia cycles, the ventricle then being truly refractory. That phenomenon could be repeated on that pacing site, without ever interrupting the tachycardia. It was not observed at other right ventricular pacing sites. A single shock on that site was effective to prevent the VT.

Patient No. 3

A patient with an inferolateral left ventricular aneurysm due to an old myocardial infarction had two different morphologies of VT, one with right axis,

196 • CARDIAC ARRHYTHMIAS

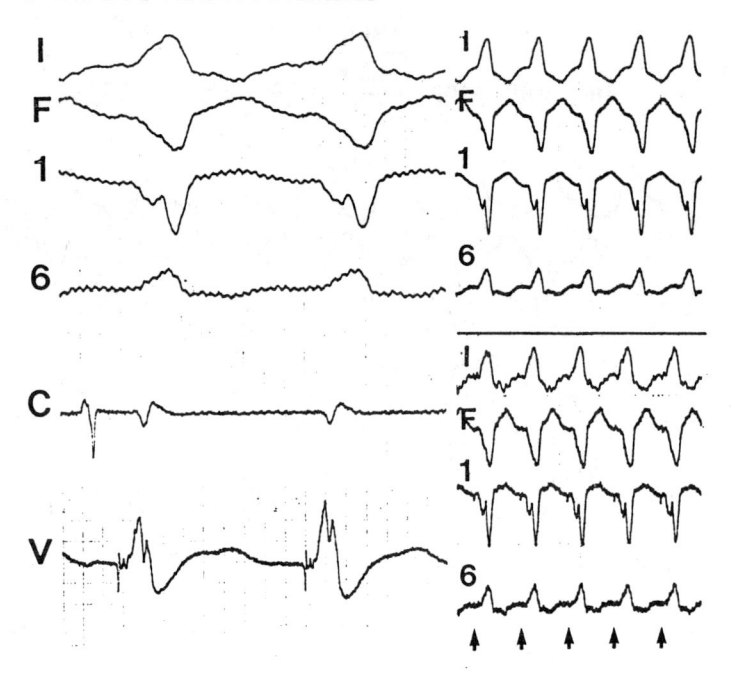

Figure 4: Patient no. 2. Left panel: endocardial right ventricular potential during VT. Right panel: exact pace mapping; upper tracing: spontaneous VT; lower tracing: pace mapping.

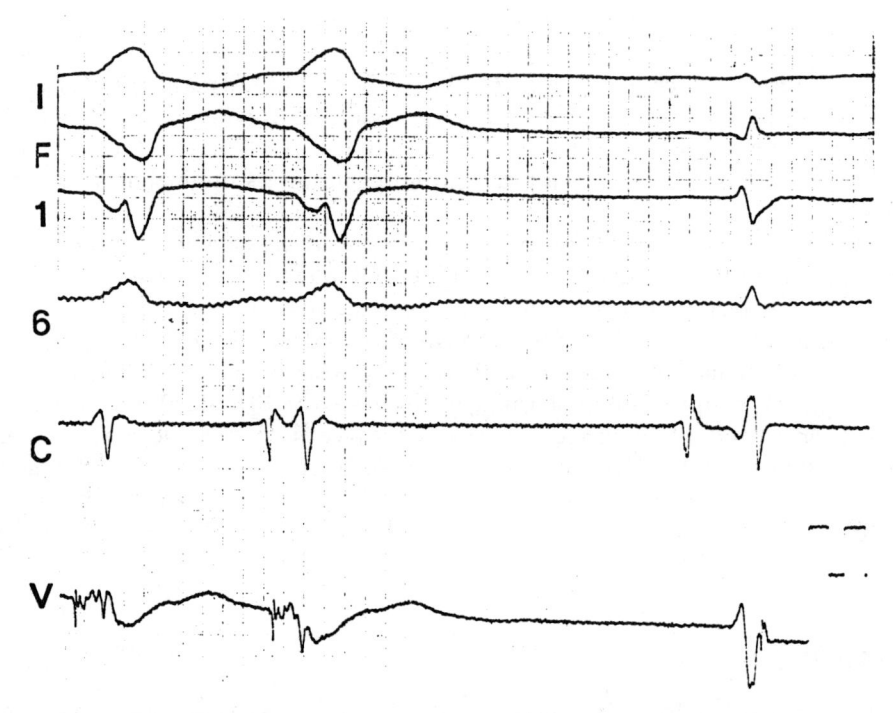

Figure 5: Patient no. 2. endocardial potential during tachycardia and in sinus rhythm (see text).

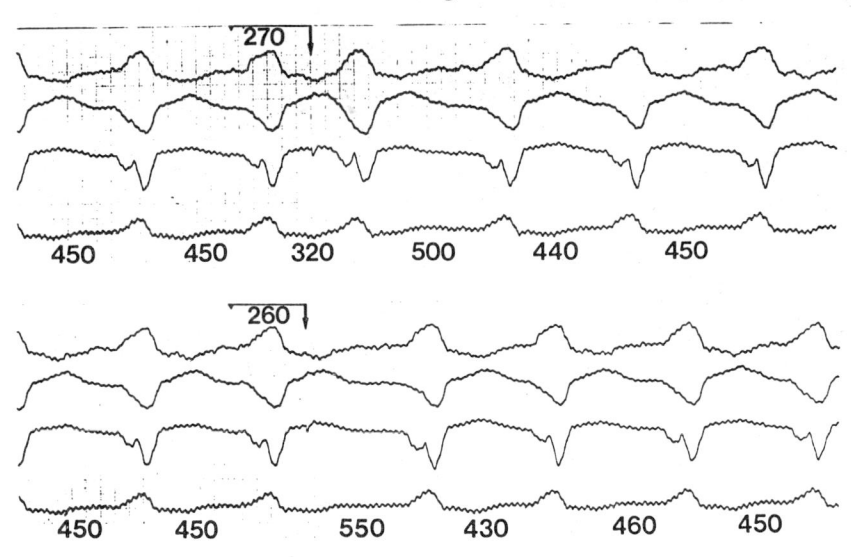

Figure 6: Patient no. 2. scanning of the earliest site during ventricular tachycardia (see text).

and one with left axis deviation, both with a right bundle branch block pattern in lead V$_1$.

Pacing from the lower part of the left ventricle could produce different QRS morphologies depending upon the duration of pacing and the pacing cycle length (Fig. 7). The delay between the pacing artifact and the onset of the surface QRS was different for each morphology. When pacing was interrupted, a tachycardia with left axis deviation having a slightly different pattern was induced. The endocardial potential during tachycardia on that site preceded the surface QRS by 50 ms. The local potential during sinus rhythm was broad with a duration of 100 ms.

A second VT was induced. This VT had a long cycle length of 580 ms. Multiphasic potentials were recorded in the left ventricular inferior wall occurring, however, 180 ms after the onset of the QRS of the returning VT complex when the tachycardia cycle was interrupted by a spontaneous extrasystole (Fig. 8).

Pacing from that site (Fig. 9) required a current strength of 20 mA. During pacing with a cycle length of 480 ms, it can be observed that the fourth stimulus captured the ventricular tachycardia with a 440 ms delay between the pacing artifact and the capture of the QRS (black star), the ulterior ventricular cycles shortening to the same value, demonstrating the capture of the tachycardia by pacing, with an exact pace mapping (Fig. 10). When pacing was interrupted, the immediate short cycle following pacing termination in fact was the last paced beat and the tachycardia resumed its original 580 ms cycle length. This observation could be done while pacing from three other different sites in the left ventricle (Fig. 11).

At each site, late multiphasic potentials were recorded during sinus rhythm.

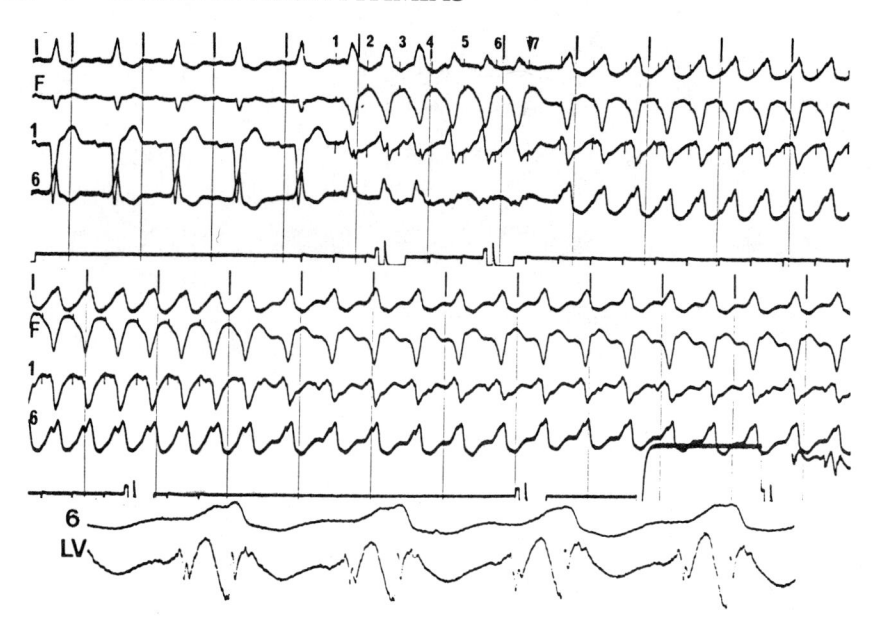

Figure 7: Patient no. 3: (see text). Changing morphologies of the paced beat. Upper ECG: Onset of overdrive pacing. Lower ECG: ECG interruption of overdrive pacing and induction of a ventricular tachycardia with left axis. Bottom traces: lead V_6 and left ventricular (LV) recording from the previously paced site (100 mm/s).

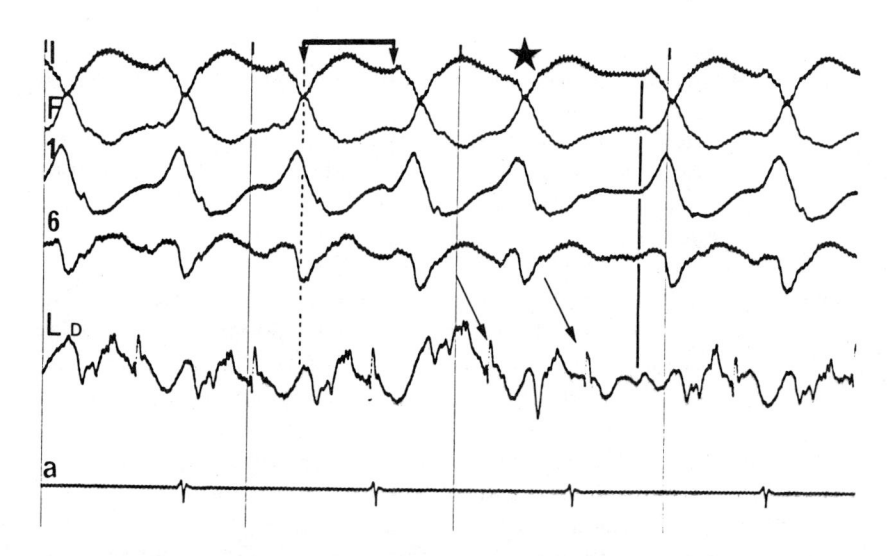

Figure 8: Patient no. 3: ECG and endocardial potential during VT with right axis (no. 2) with a spontaneous extrasystole marked by a star (left ventricular site D, see Fig. 12). The upper black line is the report of the long delay when pacing at that site between the pacing artifact and the onset of the QRS.

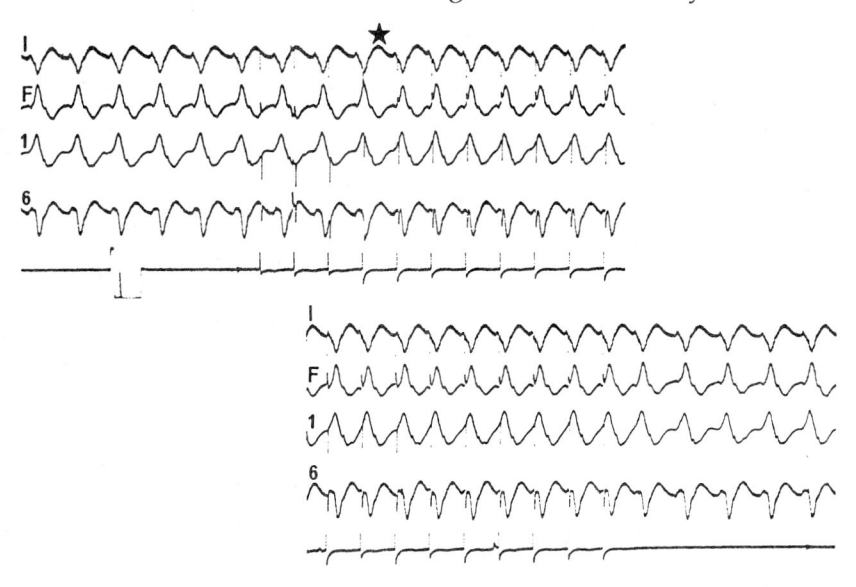

Slow Conduction During Ventricular Tachycardia • 199

Figure 9: Patient no. 3. Capture of VT no. 2 by overdrive pacing with exact pace mapping (see text) (left ventricular site D).

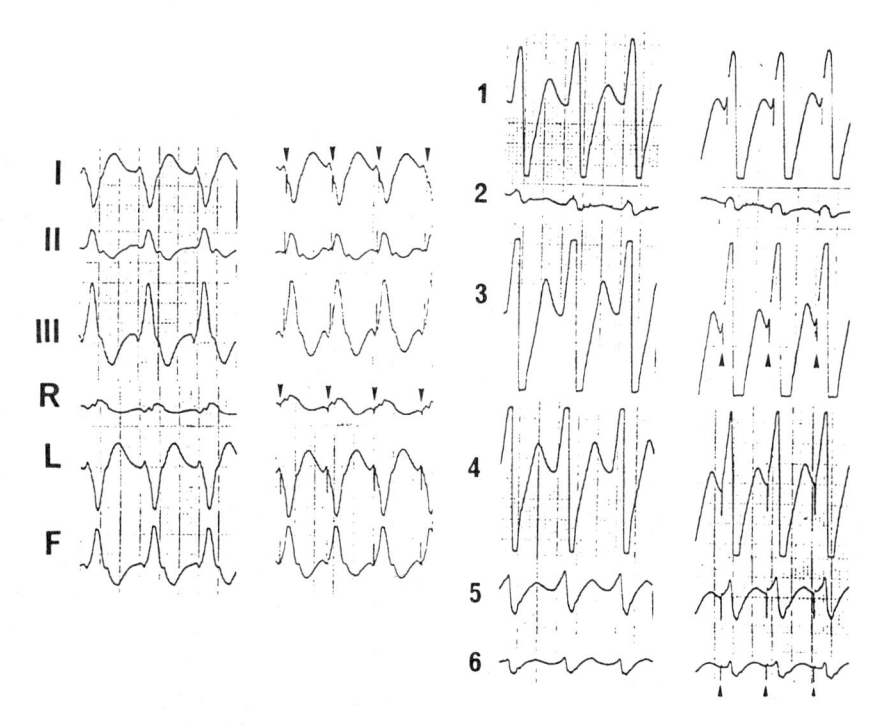

Figure 10: Exact pace mapping at site D (see Fig. 12).

200 • CARDIAC ARRHYTHMIAS

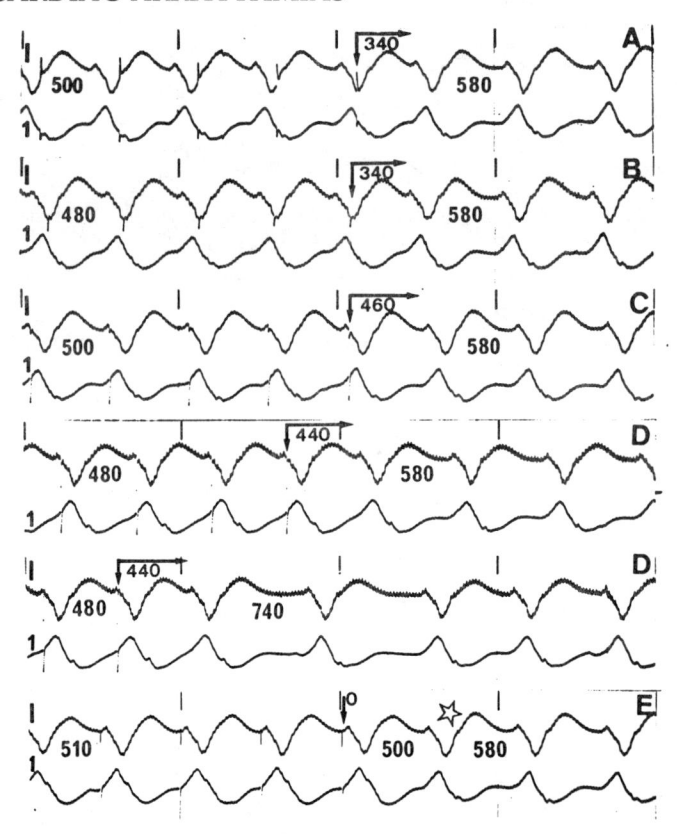

Figure 11: Patient no. 3. VT no. 2 with a 580 ms cycle length. Entrainment at five different ventricular sites (see Fig. 12) by overdrive at a 480, 500, and 510 ms cycle lengths. Sites A to D given an exact pace mapping after a long delay (340 to 460 ms). There is no delay at site E and the overdrive pacing gives only a fusion beat (morphology of lead V_1). The delay has slight variations between 340 to 360 ms at site A. The return VT cycle at site D is exact (580 ms) or prolonged to 740 ms.

During VT, local activation was late in relation to the onset of the QRS complex on the surface ECG (Fig. 12).

Underdrive pacing was then performed from the same sites during stable tachycardia with a constant cycle length of 580 ms. The paced impulse was either ineffective, or captured the VT after a long delay of 420 ms. This happened when the impulse occurred 100 ms after the onset of the QRS on the surface ECG. When the spike was synchronous with the onset of the QRS, the next VT cycle was markedly prolonged to 700 ms in spite of the apparent absence of ventricular capture (Fig. 13). Fulguration had to be applied at each of these sites in this patient to prevent ulterior VT recurrence.

Discussion

Reentry is often described as a circular ring of activation. For reentry to initiate and perpetuate unidirectional block, a slow conducting zone and a good

Slow Conduction During Ventricular Tachycardia • 201

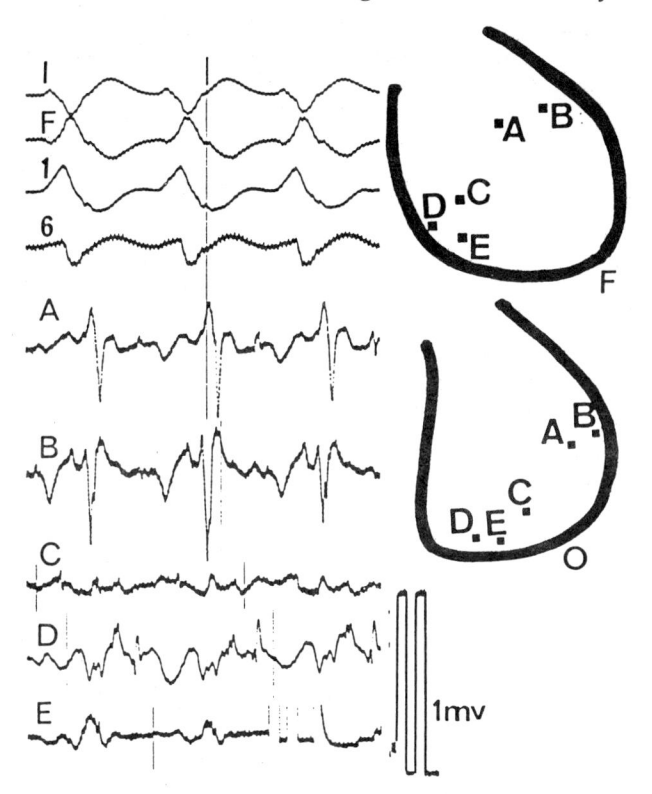

Figure 12: Patient 3. VT no. 2. Low amplitude endocardial potentials in sites A to E. Note the absence of continuous activity at site E. On the right, frontal and oblique radiologic projection of sites A to E.

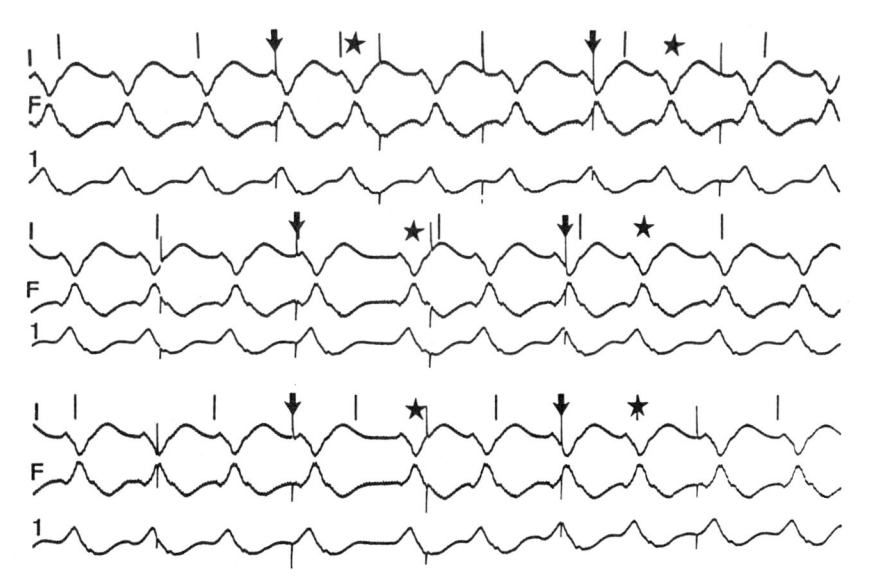

Figure 13: Underdrive pacing in VT no. 2 at site A in patient no. 3 (see text). The arrow shows an impulse followed by change in VT cycle length, marked by a star.

balance between conduction velocity and refractioness is required for the excitatory front to always find excitable tissue ahead. Conduction block at any point of the circuit will interrupt the arrhythmia.

During ventricular tachycardia caused by chronic myocardial infarction, or right ventricular dysplasia, reentry cannot be described in the same way as in the Wolff-Parkinson-White syndrome, since it does not involve specific bundles, but diseased tissue with long refractory periods and slow conduction velocities. Mehra and El-Sherif[11–13] have shown a figure-8 pattern of activation by experimentally mapping ventricular tachycardia occurring some days after experimental infarction in the dog. A common reentrant wavefront with a slow conduction velocity is surrounded at each side by two areas of functional and/or organic block. The activation front divides itself into two fronts moving clockwise and anticlockwise around the two zones of block. Interruption of the tachycardia can be obtained only by blocking conduction on the common reentrant pathway. In their experiments, conduction velocities and refractory periods are particularly prolonged in the common pathway.[14] Interruption of the reentry circuit by cryothermal techniques (allowing very localized modification of the reentry circuit) could only be achieved at the distal part of the common reentrant pathway, proximal to the site of the earliest reactivation of the myocardium.

Localization of that "slow" common pathway is mandatory when ablative techniques are considered for the radical treatment of ventricular tachycardia. A rough determination of the origin of VT by the earliest potential is enough to allow an effective surgical therapy, as multiple recordings are available, and as a large zone of myocardium is removed. By contrast, when fulguration is considered, because of its more limited effect, a more selective site of block is needed.

The earliest recorded endocardial potential can correspond to a zone localized at the exit of the common pathway. This is not always the case, however, either because of lack of catheter mapping, or because of a subepicardial or intraseptal location of the reentry circuit. Pacing can be used to validate the significance of that potential. An exact pace mapping demonstrates that the paced site has the same exit as the VT, and has a possible relation with the common pathway.[9] The delay between the electrical impulse and the ventricular response indicates that pacing is indeed done in an area of slow conduction.[15,16] Modification of the VT cycle length by pacing confirms entrance of the paced impulse in the reentry circuit.

Pace Mapping Morphology

Josephson has shown[9] that pacing at the site of origin of ventricular tachycardia produces an electrogram and an activation sequence similar to those produced by ventricular tachycardia, as in our patients nos. 1 and 2. However, pacing in close proximity to that site can produce either a similar or a grossly different electrocardiographic pattern than during ventricular tachycardia. This is due to conduction disturbances in the pathological zone, with different exit blocks. This is illustrated by the findings in our patient no. 3 (Fig. 7), where ventricular pacing with a perfectly stable endocardial lead could produce three different morphologies. The induced VT had a fourth morphology, and the endocardial potential on that site was recorded 50 ms before the QRS. This suggests that the lead was located at the distal part of the common pathway in a pathological area where the activation front may have had different exits, caused by local conduction disturbances and changes in refractoriness induced by pacing or by the tachycardia activation front.[14]

The Paced Beat Delay

Intraventicular delayed potentials are caused by slow activation of the pathological myocardium. This has been directly demonstrated by mapping[15] and indirectly[16] by the fact that pacing and recording from the same site resulted in a delay between the pacing artifact and the ventricular response on the surface ECG. That delay will increase with the pacing rate until block occurs.[16] If the paced QRS is identical to the VT complex, it may be deduced that the output from that slow conduction zone is at the same site of origin of ventricular activation during VT. This region has to be connected to the slow part of the reentry pathway. Another element in favor of this interpretation is a similar value of the delay between the pacing impulse and the ventricular response, and the prematurity of the endocardial early potential at that area. This is clearly demonstrated in patient no. 1, in whom pacing at the tachycardia rate exactly reproduced the QRS configuration in tachycardia, with a delay of 100 ms, corresponding to the prematurity of the local potential. The same observation could be done in patient no. 2.

Patient no. 3 is a more complex case (Fig. 7). Pacing at a cycle length of 400 ms with a stable catheter position on the posterolateral zone of the ventricle induced three successive morphologies. After three cycles of pacing, the delay between the pacing artifact and the QRS prolonged, and the morphology of the paced QRS markedly changed. After three new cycles, the seventh spike appeared to be nonconducted and was followed 500 ms later by a complex with a new morphology. Its onset clearly preceded the following impulse. The next one was followed after 50 ms by a QRS. When pacing was interrupted, the last driven beat was followed by a beat of the same morphology, after a time equal to the driven cycle. Another VT was then induced, with a longer cycle length and a different morphology in lead V_1. The interpretation of the tracing could be that VT was induced after the seventh spike, and that pacing entrained the tachycardia, which resumed later. However, the last entrained beat still had the same paced morphology which is against the first criteria of entrainment[17] as will be discussed later.

Another interpretation of that tracing should be given. The missed seventh impulse is in fact conducted with a very long delay and induced the next QRS. This is supported by its morphology similar to the next paced beat. Also when pacing was interrupted, the next beat had the same morphology as the paced beat, was exactly separated by the same interval from the preceeding QRS than the previous ones and could represent the response to the last stimulus. Such an important intraventricular delay of 500 ms seems very unusual. However, an extremely long delay was found again in the same patient when pacing during another VT with right axis deviation originating higher in the posterolateral left ventricular wall. "Exact pace mapping" was obtained after the first capture of the tachycardia, with shortening of the RR interval to the pacing cycle. The first delay was 400 ms, and then slowly increased. The delay had a value of 420 ms with the last pacing impulse which seemed to occur before the previous ventricular complex (Fig. 9).

This observation could be repeated from four different sites of the left ventricle during the same VT. Such a long delay may be interpreted as pacing from a pathologic zone, with the same exit point to the rest of myocardium as the VT. As the local endocardial potentials were late and fragmented at each site instead of being early as in the two preceeding cases (Fig. 12), one must then conclude that pacing is not done near the exit of the slow conduction zone, but near its entrance. These sites are localized in the aneurysm as suggested by the low amplitude of these potentials and the high pacing threshold. The exit zone should be nearer the highest site (A and B) as the delay is shorter (320 and 340 ms) than in the lowest sites (440 and 460 ms). Whatever the mechanisms of these blocks, the paced impulse is only able to follow the pathway of the VT. The fact that impulses from four different parts of the left ventricle could give the same configuration suggests that the entrance to the area of slow conduction was widely opened in contrast with its exit which must be a limited area as the paced QRS always had the same morphology. This VT must involve a macroreentry circuit within the ventricular aneurysm. Such a wide circuit, combined with the effect of amiodarone, explains the long VT cycle length.

Effect of Pacing on the Tachycardia Cycle

Entrainment

It has been observed for many years that pacing can interrupt ventricular tachycardia.[18] It has been suggested that this phenomenon supports a reentrant mechanism. However, experimental studies have demonstrated that some automatic tachycardias can also be interrupted by pacing. More recently, the phenomenon of entrainment during overdrive pacing has been described and presented as evidence for a reentrant mechanism of the arrhythmia.[17] It has also been demonstrated that to observe that phenomenon, the site of pacing should be proximal to the area of slow conduction.[19-21] During entrainment, it is assumed that the paced activation front enters the common slow conduction pathway of the reentry circuit defined by its arcs of block, in the same direction as the spontaneous front. Meanwhile, the same paced front depolarizes the rest of the ventricles. In other words, the paced impulse has a *double conduction*, one through the rest of the myocardium and one through the slow conduction zone. This zone cannot be invaded in any other way by the paced activation because of the arcs of block, or from its exit point because the reentry front from the *previous cycle* is running in that area. Conversely, this reentrant front at the exit of the common pathway can only activate a limited ventricular area, as it is blocked by the *next paced front*. Both activation fronts collide resulting in a fusion beat.

Slow Conduction During Ventricular Tachycardia • 205

When pacing is interrupted (Fig. 14), the last paced activation depolarizes the ventricles and also invades the common slow conduction pathway. However, as this slow conduction front is not blocked near its exit by a new paced activation, it will capture the ventricles and reproduce a VT beat. That beat, initiated by the paced impulse, will occur "early" after the last paced QRS, in comparison with the following VT cycle length. In fact, it exhibits a *very long conduction delay between the pacing site and the exit of the common slow pathway*.

These phenomena are observed in patient no. 3 in whom pacing in a normal zone induced a ventricular potential without delay. After interruption of overdrive pacing, the first VT beat is entrained, occurring after a delay of 500 ms (shorter than the spontaneous 580 ms VT cycle) (Fig. 11E).

The situation is different when pacing is performed from the common slow conduction zone. The paced impulse has only a *single* conduction, as it is retrogradely blocked by the reentrant front. It can only anticipate the circular movement, which resumes with its normal 580 ms cycle when pacing is interrupted (Fig. 15). This could be called "exact entrainment."

The effect of a single premature stimulus during tachycardia may be interpreted in the same way as during overdrive pacing. When pacing is performed outside the common reentrant pathway, entrainment is demonstrated by an advanced returning VT cycle with a less than compensatory pause. Long coupling intervals of the premature stimuli do not modify the tachycardia.[22] A single extrastimulus on the common pathway either will be without effect, or will reset the tachycardia. The ventricular cycle following the paced beat equals the spontaneous ventricular cycle length, as after exact entrainment.

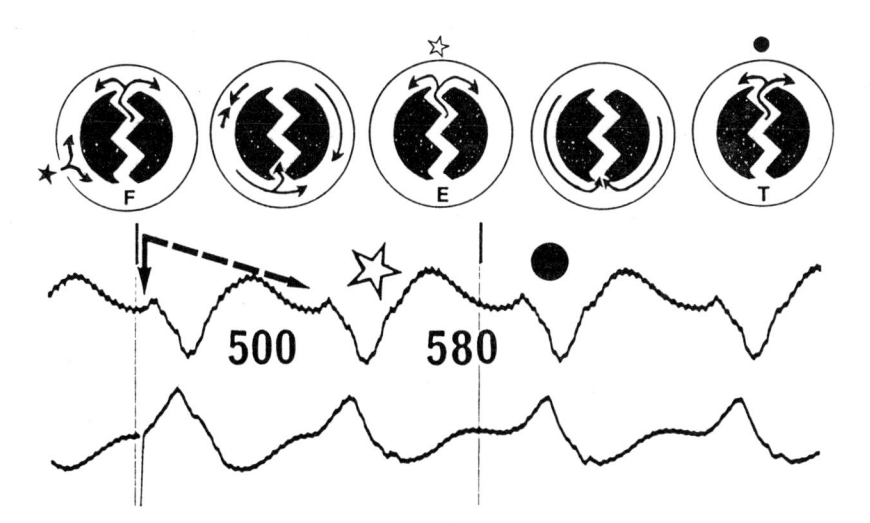

Figure 14: See text. The lower panel shows the last paced beat and the entrainment during VT (site E from Fig. 11). The upper panel is a diagrammatic representation of the reentry circuit during the same event. The white star shows the entrained and not fused beat. The black circle shows the next VT complex.

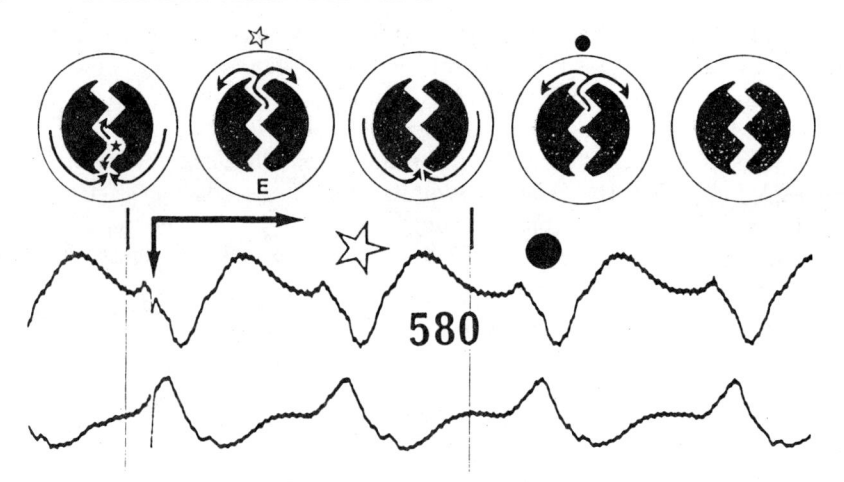

Figure 15: See text. The lower panel shows the last beat of exact pace mapping during overdrive pacing (site C from Fig. 11). The upper panel is a diagrammatic representation of the reentry circuit during the same event. The white star shows the entrained QRS. The black circle shows the next ventricular beat.

Modification of VT Cycle Length

Sometimes the following return cycles are longer than the previous spontaneous VT which then recovers to its original value. This is observed after overdrive pacing in patients nos. 1 and 3 (Fig. 11D) and after a single extrastimulus in patients nos. 1 and 2. This can be interpreted as the induction of conduction delay or change in the slow conduction pathway configuration[12] by the paced activation which keeps the same exit point, as VT morphology is unchanged.

Another effect or a single stimulus can be observed in patient no. 2. During a regular tachycardia, premature stimuli coinciding with the end of the refractory period were not followed by a ventricular response, but by prolongation of the tachycardia cycle. Stimuli given 10 ms later captured the ventricles. This could be called sub-threshold pacing.[23] A similar phenomenon was observed in patient no. 3 (Fig. 13).

Two explanations may be proposed. Electrotonic interaction may impair the transmission of the activation front[24] in a zone of depressed conductivity. The experimental mapping studies[21] favor concealed conduction in the slow pathway, between the arcs of blocks with a still refractory distal pathway for such an early impulse with retrograde conduction block. This situation will again either change the proximal pathway configuration or depress its conduction velocity, and induce a prolongation of the VT cycle, as after overdrive pacing, or after a single extrastimulus in the same zone.

VT interruption by a nonpropagated impulse was observed only once, in both patients 2 and 3, but because the phenomenon was not reproduced, a coincidence could not be excluded.

Conclusion

Pacing in the area of slow conduction of a reentry circuit results in long delays between the stimulus and the surface QRS. Pacing the same site during sinus rhythm can result in multiple ventricular morphologies. However, pacing from different sites in a ventricular aneurysm can give the same "exact pace mapping."

The common slow pathway is the far side of the reentrant circuit when compared to the fast activation which gives rise to the surface QRS. An exact pace mapping during VT at an area with late potentials during VT suggests that the electrode is localized near its entrance as in patient no. 3. When associated with early potentials, it implies a localization near its exit as in patients 1 and 2. Overdrive pacing or a single extrastimulus on that common pathway will give an exact capture of the ventricular tachycardia which immediately resumes its spontaneous cycle. It may also modify the tachycardia cycle length for several beats without any change in QRS configuration. Prolongation of the VT cycle due to a nonpropagated impulse combined with the preceding observations, is highly suggestive for pacing from the area of slow conduction of a reentry circuit.

These data have practical consequences. Using these data, a single shock was effective in patients 1 and 2 to control VT. We believe that the damage produced by the shock was localized to the exit point of the common slow pathway. Fulguration was also effective in patient no. 3 on sites where local potentials were late during VT, but identified as a wide entrance zone to the common pathway.

Acknowledgment: This research was supported by the Centre de Recherche sur les Maladies Cardiovasculaires de l'Association Claude Bernard.

References

1. Peuch P, Latour H, Grolleau R. Le flutter et ses limites. Arch Mal Coeur 1970;61:116.
2. Wallace AG, Boineau JP, Davidson RM, Sealy WC. Wolff-Parkinson-White syndrome: A new look. Am J Cardiol 1971;28:509.
3. Josephson ME, Horowitz LN, Farshidi A, Spear JF, Kastor JA, Moore EN. Recurrent sustained ventricular tachycardia. II. Endocardial mapping. Circulation 1978;57:440.
4. Guiraudon G, Fontaine G, Frank R, Leandri R, Barra J, Cabrol C. Surgical treatment of ventricular tachycardia guided by ventricular mapping in 23 patients without coronary artery disease. Ann Thorac Surg 1981;32:439.
5. Josephson ME, Horowitz LN, Spielman SR, Greenspan AM, Vandepol CJ, Harken AH. Comparison of endocardial catheter mapping with intraoperative mapping of ventricular tachycardia. Circulation 1980;61:395.
6. Scheinman MM, Evans-Bell T. Catheter ablation of the atrioventricular junction: A report of the Percutaneous Mapping and Ablation Registry. Circulation 1984; 70:1024–1029.
7. Hartzler GO. Electrode catheter ablation of refractory focal ventricular tachycardia. J Am Coll Cardiol 1983;2:1107–1113.
8. Curry PVL, O'Keefe DB, Pitcher D, Sowton E, Deverall PB, Yates AK. Localization of ventricular tachycardia by a new technique: Pace mapping (abstr). Circulation 1979; 60:11–25.
9. Josephson ME, Waxman HL, Cain ME, Gardner MJ, Buxton AE. Ventricular activation

during ventricular endocardial pacing. II. Role of pacemapping to localize origin of ventricular tachycardia. Am J Cardiol 1982;50:11.

10. Fontaine G, Pierfitte M, Tonet JL, Fillette F, Frank R, Grosgogeat Y. Interpretation of afterpotentials registered from epicardium, endocardium and body surface in patients with chronic ventricular tachycardia. In: Hombach V, Hilger HH, eds. Signal Averaging Technique in Clinical Cardiology. Stuttgart, F.K. Schattauer, 1981;177.

11. Mehra R, Zeiler RH, Gough WB, El-Sherif N. Reentrant ventriclular arrhythmias in the late myocardial infarction period: Electrophysiologic anatomic correlation of reentrant circuits. Circulation 1983;67:11-24.

12. El-Sherif N, Mehra R, Gough WB, Zeiler RH. Reentrant ventricular-arrhythmias in the late myocardial infarction period: Interruption of reentrant circuits by cryothermal techniques. Circulation 1983;68:644-656.

13. El-Sherif N, Gough WB, Zeiler RH, Hariman RJ. Reentrant ventricular arrhythmias in the late myocardial infarction period: Spontaneous versus induced reentry and intramural versus epicardial circuits. J Am Coll Cardiol 1985;6:124-132.

14. Gough WB, Mehra R, Restivo M, Zeiler RH, El-Sherif N. Reentrant ventricular arrhythmias in the late myocardial infarction period in the dog: Correlation of activation and refractory maps. Circ Res 1985;57:432-442.

15. Fontaine G, Guiraudon G, Frank R. Intramyocardial conduction defects in patients prone to ventricular tachycardia: A dynamic study of the post-excitation syndrome. In: Sandoe E, Julian DG, Bell JW, eds. Management of Ventricular Tachycardia: Role of Mexiletine. Amsterdam, Excerpta Medica, 1978;56-66.

16. Frank R, Fontaine G, Vedel J, Mialet G, Sol C, Guiraudon C, Grosgogeat Y. Electrocardiologie de quatre cas de dysplasie ventriculaire droite arythmogene. Arch Mal Coeur 1978;71:963-972.

17. Waldo AL, Plumb VJ, Arciniegas JC, MacLean WAH, Cooper TB, Priest MF, James TN. Transient entrainment and interruption of the atrioventricular bypass pathway type of paroxysmal atrial tachycardia. Circulation 1983;67:73-83.

18. Wellens HJJ, Schuilenburg RM, Durrer D. Electrical stimulation of the heart in patients with ventricular tachycardia. Circulation 1972;46:216.

19. Okumura K, Henthorn RW, Epstein AE, Plumb VJ, Waldo AL. Further observations on transient entrainment: Importance of pacing site and properties of the components of the reentry circuit. Circulation 1985;72:1293-1307.

20. Mann DE, Lawrie GM, Luck JC, Griffin JC, Magro SA, Wyndham CRC. Importance of pacing site in entrainment of ventricular tachycardia. J Am Coll Cardiol 1985; 5:781-787.

21. El-Sherif N, Gough WB, Restivo M. Mechanisms of "entrainment," acceleration or termination of reentrant ventricular tachycardia by programmed electrical stimulation (abstr). PACE 1986;9:281.

22. Inoue H, Inoue K, Matsuo H, Kuwasi K, Shirai T, Murao S. Resetting of tachycardia cycle by single and double ventricular extrastimuli in recurrent sustained ventricular tachycardia. PACE 1984;7:3-9.

23. Prystowsky EN, Zipes DP. Inhibition in the human heart. Circulation 1983; 8:707-713.

24. Antzelevitch C, Moe GK. Electrotonic inhibition of impulse transmission across inexcitable segments of cardiac tissue (abstr). Circulation 1982;66:358.

11

Effects of Simultaneous Vagal and Sympathetic Stimulation on Spontaneous Sinus Cycle Length, Atrial and Ventricular Refractoriness, and Atrioventricular Nodal Conduction

Hiroshi Inoue
Douglas P. Zipes

Introduction

The vagus and sympathetic nerves exhibit dominance in different areas of the heart and on different electrophysiologic properties. The vagus predominates at the sinus node, and produces a greater absolute increase in the sinus cycle length during tonic adrenergic discharge compared with vagal stimulation during minimal adrenergic activity, a phenomenon known as "accentuated antagonism."[1,2] Such vagal modulation of sympathetic effects probably results from interactions at pre- and post-junctional sites.[3-6] Interestingly, phasic vagal stimulation does not produce accentuated antagonism.[7] Stimulation of both autonomic limbs shortens atrial refractoriness, although vagal stimulation has a more pronounced effect.[8] At the atrioventricular (AV) node, vagal and sympathetic effects are opposite and "algebraically additive,"[9] In the ventricles, the vagus prolongs

From: Brugada P, Wellens HJJ. CARDIAC ARRHYTHMIAS: Where To Go From Here? Mount Kisco, NY, Futura Publishing Company, Inc., © 1987.

210 • CARDIAC ARRHYTHMIAS

ventricular refractoriness, but to a degree far less than adrenergic stimulation shortens it.[10-13]

Considering the vagal dominance at the sinus node, sympathetic dominance in the ventricle, and roughly equivalent effects at the AV node, an increase in both vagal and sympathetic tone, such as might occur during an inferior myocardial infarction,[14,15] might result in no change, or even slowing, of the sinus rate, shortening of ventricular refractoriness, and either slowing or speeding of AV nodal conduction. Thus, the spontaneous sinus cycle length or AV conduction time might be a poor "autonomic barometer" of autonomic input to other cardiac sites such as atrial or ventricular myocardium.

The electrocardiographic example shown in Figure 1 illustrates a clinical situation probably characterized by simultaneous discharge of both autonomic limbs. During a 24-hour ECG recording, the patient developed an episode of atypical angina. ST segments recorded in the inferior ECG lead elevated markedly and the QRS complex took on the appearance of a monophasic action potential

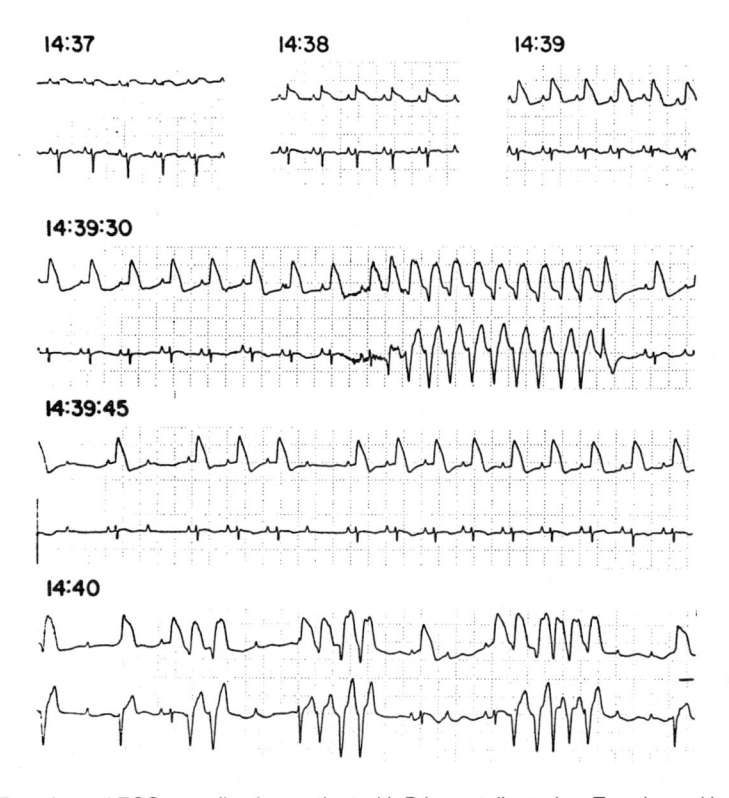

Figure 1: Two channel ECG recording in a patient with Prinzmetal's angina. Top channel is an inferior lead and bottom channel is an anterior lead. Changes in T-wave contour preclude accurate measurement of QT interval duration. ECG recorded by Donald A. Chilson, M.D. (Reproduced with permission from Zipes DP: Specific arrhythmias: Diagnosis and treatment. In Braunwald E. *Heart Disease:* A Textbook of Cardiovascular Medicine. 3rd Edition. W.B. Saunders, Philadelphia, in press.)

(14:38). The sinus cycle length shortened (14:39) and the patient experienced short-lived episodes of nonsustained ventricular tachycardia (14:39:30). Most probably the pain and acute ischemia were accompanied by sympathetic neural discharge which may have played a role in the genesis of the episodes of ventricular tachycardia. Yet, despite the presumptive evidence of increased adrenergic activity, slight lengthening of the sinus nodal cycle length (14:39:30) occurred and Wenckebach second degree AV block resulted (14:39:45). While it is possible that these changes were due to ischemia of the sinus and AV nodes, it is more likely, given the short time interval, that these changes resulted from a vasodepressor reflex response triggered by ischemia from the posteroinferior left ventricular wall.[15] Viewing the sinus slowing and Wenckebach AV block, one would conclude that the clinical situation was characterized by excessive vagal tone and dismiss the possibility of heightened sympathetic tone. However, because of vagal dominance at the sinus node, sympathetic dominance at the ventricular level, and additive effects at the AV node, simultaneous vagal and sympathetic discharge could be responsible for these ECG changes.

The purpose of this study was to test the hypothesis that varying levels of sympathetic and vagal input could yield the same spontaneous sinus cycle length while altering atrial and ventricular effective refractory periods and AV nodal conduction in the canine heart.

Methods

Mongrel dogs of either sex were anesthetized with i.v. alpha chloralose (100 mg/kg), intubated, and ventilated. The chest was opened through a median sternotomy and the heart was suspended in a pericardial cradle, according to our standard procedures.

The cervical vagi were isolated, doubly ligated, and cut in all dogs. Two Teflon-coated wire electrodes were embedded in the cardiac end of each vagal nerve to stimulate efferent vagal nerves. The ansae subclaviae were isolated as they exited from the stellate ganglia, doubly ligated, and cut. Shielded bipolar electrodes were placed on the right and left anterior and posterior ansae subclaviae to stimulate the efferent cardiac sympathetic nerves. The sinus node was not crushed. Hook electrodes made from Teflon-coated wires, insulated except for their tips, were placed in the high and low right atrium, anterior right ventricle, and anterior and posterior left ventricle using a 22-gauge needle. The electrodes served as a cathode for unipolar stimulation. The anode was a 33 mm diameter metal disc placed in the abdominal wall. A quadripolar catheter electrode (USCI, 6F) was advanced from the right carotid artery to the noncoronary cusp of the aorta to record His bundle activation with frequency responses of 30–500 Hz. Bipolar plunge electrodes in the right atrium and left ventricle were used to record atrial and ventricular responses, respectively.

Effective refractory period was determined in a standard fashion[11] by the extrastimulus technique with a 2 ms rectangular unipolar cathodal stimulus at twice diastolic threshold. Surface electrocardiographic lead II, right atrial and His bundle electrograms were recorded at a paper speed of 100 mm/sec. Five consecutive cycle lengths were measured and averaged to obtain the sinus cycle length. After obtaining the spontaneous sinus cycle length, the right atrium was paced at constant pacing cycle lengths of 290–300 ms. The AH interval was measured from the earliest onset of rapid right atrial activity recorded in the His bundle electrogram to the onset of the His potential. The HV interval was measured from the onset of the His bundle deflection to the beginning of ventricular depolarization recorded in the His bundle lead. Five consecutive AH and HV intervals at a constant atrial pacing cycle length were measured and averaged to obtain the AH and HV interval, respectively.

Incremental right atrial pacing was carried out to determine the shortest atrial-paced cycle length at which 1:1 atrioventricular conduction occurred. Pacing cycle length was shortened in steps of 10 ms every 5 sec.

The right and left ansae subclaviae were stimulated with 4 ms rectangular pulses at 3 mA. Frequencies were 1, 2, and 4 Hz. The right and left vagal nerves were stimulated at a current strength set 0.05 mA greater than that required to produce asystole with right vagal stimulation and asystole or complete AV block with left vagal stimulation using 4 ms rectangular pulses at 20 Hz. Pulse width and frequency of vagal stimulation were increased progressively to obtain a constant sinus cycle length or a constant AH interval.

The purpose of the first protocol was to determine the effects of three different levels of simultaneous bilateral ansae subclaviae and vagal stimulation that maintained a constant sinus cycle length. Baseline values were determined first. Five minutes later, bilateral ansae subclaviae were stimulated at 1, 2, or 4 Hz. Two minutes later, the vagi were stimulated bilaterally, adjusting both pulse width and stimulation frequency simultaneously for both right and left vagal nerves to keep sinus cycle length the same as the baseline value. Effective refractory period and AV nodal conduction time were measured 1 minute after the sinus cycle length became stable. Fifteen minutes after terminating all neural stimulation, baseline values were measured again. Then another combination of ansae subclaviae-vagal stimulation was started and refractory periods and AV nodal conduction time were determined as above. The frequency of ansae subclaviae stimulation was selected in a random order, and baseline values were measured both before and after each combination of ansae subclaviae-vagal stimulation.

In the second protocol, we determined the effects of simultaneous unilateral and bilateral ansae subclaviae and vagal stimulation that maintained a constant sinus cycle length. Five minutes after recording the baseline values, stimulation of unilateral ansa subclavia at 2 Hz was started. Two minutes later, the ipsilateral vagus was stimulated, and pulse width and frequency were titrated to keep sinus cycle length the same as the baseline value, as in the first protocol. Fifteen minutes after terminating all neural stimulation, baseline values were measured again. Then the study was repeated stimulating the opposite ansa subclavia at 2 Hz and vagus. The effects of bilateral simultaneous stimulation of ansae subclaviae at 2 Hz and vagi were also determined as in protocol #1.

In the final protocol, we determined the effects of simultaneous bilateral ansae subclaviae and vagal stimulation that maintained AH interval constant at an atrial pacing cycle length of 300 ms. Two minutes after stimulation of bilateral ansae subclaviae at 2 Hz, bilateral vagi were stimulated, and pulse width and frequency were titrated to return the AH interval within ± 4 ms of the baseline value. Then, atrial pacing was terminated. Bilateral vagal and ansae subclaviae stimulation was continued at the same parameters, and spontaneous sinus cycle length and effective refractory periods were measured. The cycle length at which the effective refractory periods were determined was 300 ms.

Results

In the first protocol, while maintaining spontaneous sinus cycle length constant at three different levels of bilateral ansae subclaviae-vagal stimulation, AH interval changed variably from dog to dog. AH interval lengthened by 20 ms or more in three dogs during simultaneous stimulation of the vagi and ansae subclaviae at 1 Hz and at 4 Hz, and in two dogs during stimulation of ansae subclaviae at 2 Hz (Fig. 2). AH interval shortened by 20 ms or more in one, three, and two dogs during stimulation of vagi and ansae subclaviae at 1, 2, and 4 Hz, respectively (Fig. 2). HV interval remained unchanged. The amount of shortening of effective refractory period in the right atrium and ventricle, and anterior and posterior left ventricle increased progressively as the frequency of ansae subclaviae stimulation increased (Fig. 3).

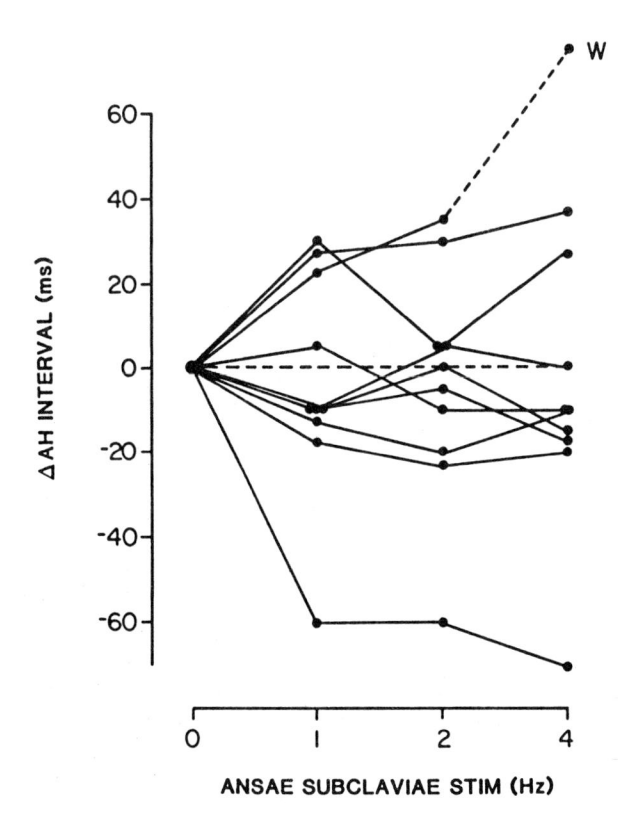

Figure 2: Changes in AH interval in each dog are shown on the ordinate as a function of frequency of ansae subclaviae stimulation shown on the abscissa. Frequency of 0 Hz indicates the baseline state. In one dog, Wenckebach periodicity (W) developed during ansae subclaviae stimulation at 4 Hz with concomitant vagal stimulation. Dotted line shows the baseline level. (Reproduced with permission.[18])

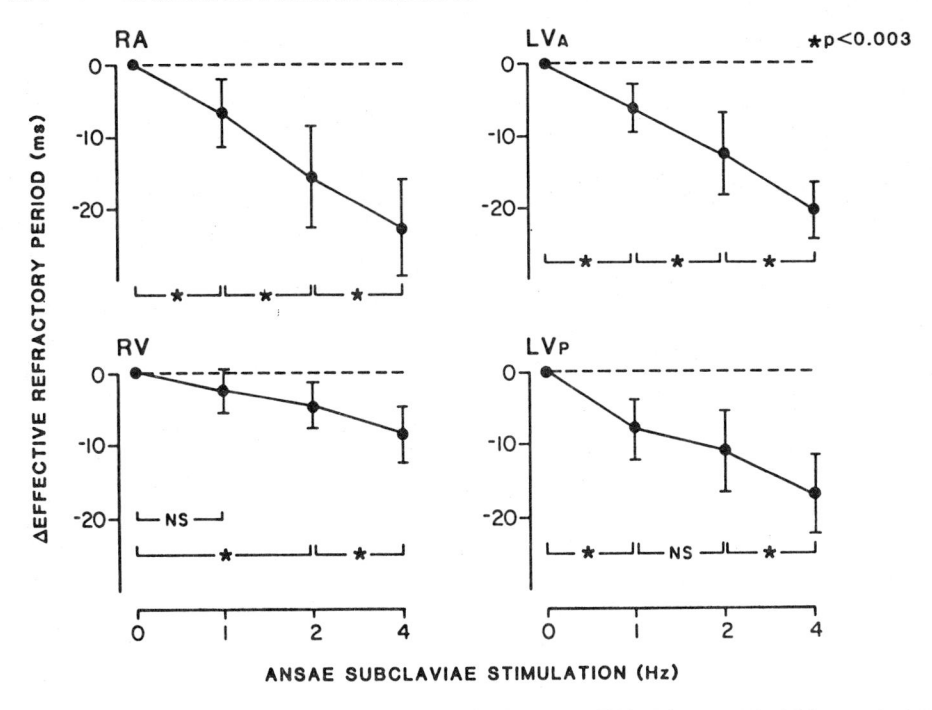

Figure 3: Changes in effective refractory period of right atrium (RA), right ventricle (RV), anterior left ventricle (LVa), and posterior left ventricle (LVp) are shown on the ordinate as a function of frequency of ansae subclaviae stimulation shown on the abscissa. Frequency of 0 Hz indicates the baseline state. Dotted line shows the baseline level. (Reproduced with permission.[18])

In the second protocol, the AH interval lengthened by 15 ms or more in two dogs during stimulation of right ansa subclavia and vagus and during stimulation of bilateral ansae subclaviae and vagi (Fig. 4). During stimulation of left ansa subclavia and vagus, the AH interval shortened in all dogs by 5 to 25 ms. Bilateral ansae subclaviae-vagal stimulation shortened AH interval by 20 ms or more in two dogs. HV interval remained unchanged in all dogs.

Effective refractory period of the right atrium was shortened significantly by stimulation of right ansa subclavia and vagus and by bilateral stimulation, but not by stimulation of the left ansa subclavia and vagus (Fig. 5). The right ventricular refractory period was not shortened by stimulation of unilateral ansa subclavia combined with ipsilateral vagal stimulation, but was shortened significantly by stimulation of bilateral ansae subclaviae and vagi. The refractory period of the anterior left ventricle shortened significantly during each combination of stimulation, and shortened more during bilateral stimulation than during left ansa subclavia-vagal stimulation ($p<0.005$). The refractory period of the posterior left ventricle shortened significantly during stimulation of left and bilateral ansae subclaviae and vagi, but not during right ansa subclavia-vagal stimulation.

In the final protocol, the AH interval at an atrial pacing cycle length of 300 ms was kept constant during bilateral ansae subclaviae-vagal stimulation (Fig. 6). After cessation of atrial pacing, sinus cycle length lengthened in four dogs by 15,

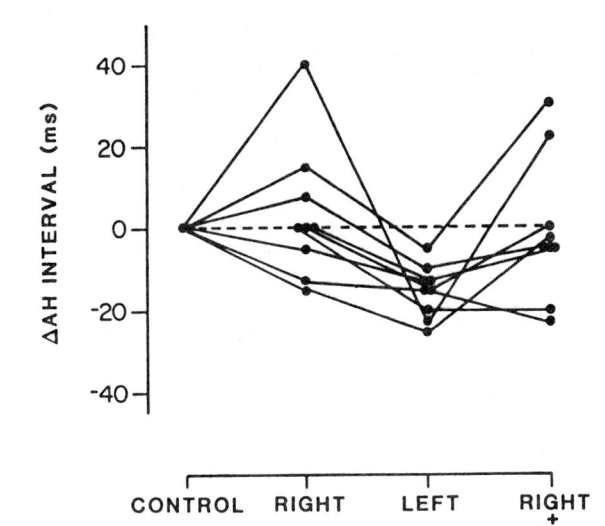

Figure 4: Changes in AH interval in each dog are shown on the ordinate. On the abscissa, site of ansae subclaviae and vagal stimulation is shown. Dotted line shows the baseline level. (Reproduced with permission.[18])

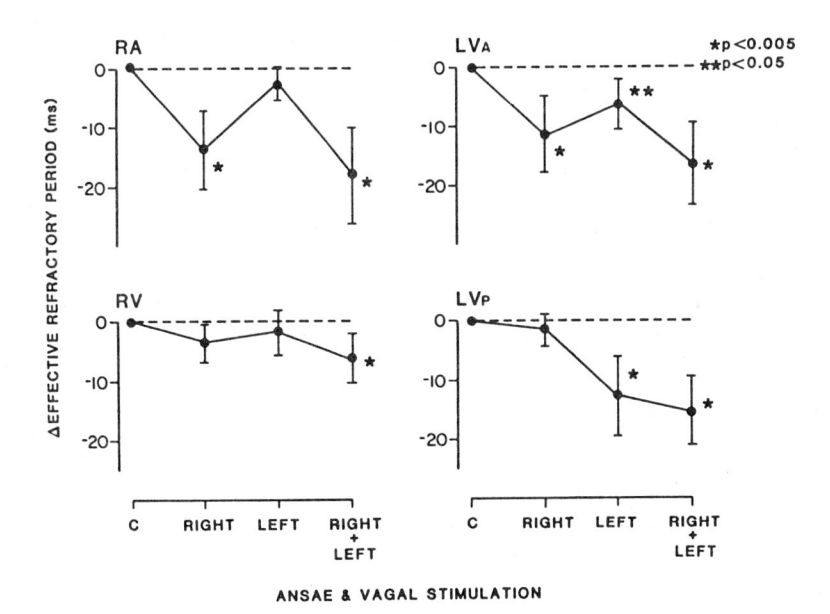

Figure 5: Changes in effective refractory period of right atrium (RA), right ventricle (RV), anterior left ventricle (LVa), and posterior left ventricle (LVp) are shown on the ordinate. On the abscissa, site of ansae subclaviae and vagal stimulation is shown. Dotted line shows the baseline level. P values compared with control value are shown. (Reproduced with permission.[18])

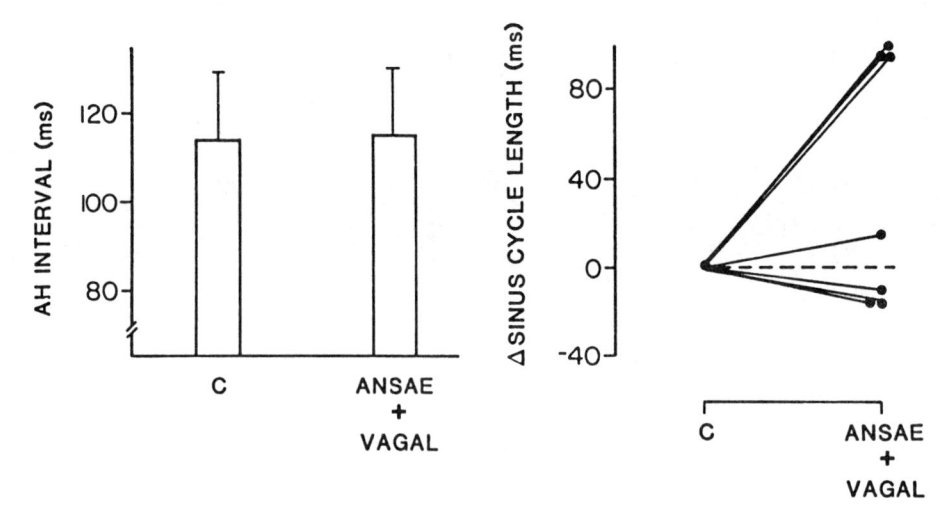

Figure 6: Changes in sinus cycle length induced by bilateral ansae subclaviae (2 Hz) and vagal stimulation (right panel) that resulted in a constant AH interval (left panel).

90, 90, and 95 ms and shortened in three dogs by 10, 15, and 15 ms. Refractory period at each atrial and ventricular test site shortened significantly during simultaneous ansae subclaviae-vagal stimulation (not shown).

Discussion

The major finding of the present study is that, while the spontaneous sinus cycle length was kept constant by titrating levels of vagal stimulation against various combinations and strengths of sympathetic stimulation, effective refractory periods of the right atrium, right ventricle, and left ventricle shortened progressively as the frequency of ansae subclaviae stimulation increased. AV nodal conduction either remained the same, shortened, or delayed, depending on the neural combinations used. When vagal stimulation was titrated against the effects of ansae subclaviae stimulation to maintain AV nodal conduction time constant, atrial and ventricular refractoriness still shortened, while the spontaneous sinus cycle length lengthened in four dogs and shortened in three.

One reason for our study was to investigate the use of the spontaneous sinus nodal cycle length as a kind of "autonomic barometer" for the rest of the heart. Our data provide experimental support for the conclusion that the sinus cycle length or duration of AV nodal conduction may not be an accurate indicator of autonomic "tone" to other cardiac structures, most likely when discharge of both autonomic limbs occurs simultaneously (Fig. 1).

In a previous study, Browne et al.[16] showed that QT interval in humans was significantly longer during sleep than the awake state at the same heart rate. A supporting observation was made by Bexton et al.[17] Browne et al.[16] speculated that the same sinus rate at different times did not necessarily mean the same degree of autonomic input to the ventricle, hence, the change in QT interval. The present data support their speculation. Thus, the same spontaneous sinus rate does not necessarily mean that the autonomic input to the rest of the heart is the same. Situations that may be characterized by increased discharge from both autonomic limbs, e.g., acute inferior myocardial infarction with a vasodepressor reflex response (Fig. 1),[14,15] may show electrocardiographic evidence of vagal effects at the sinus, and possibly AV nodes, which may mask intense adrenergic effects in the ventricle.

Changing our stimulation parameters, e.g., increasing the strength of vagal stimulation, just as easily could have resulted in sinus slowing, possibly prolongation of AV nodal conduction time, but still shortening of atrial and ventricular refractoriness, as long as concomitant ansae subclaviae stimulation resulted. Were these sinus and AV nodal changes to happen clinically, almost certainly it would have been concluded that the patient was experiencing a "vagotonic state" without considering the possibility of simultaneous sympathetic discharge and its effects on atrial and ventricular refractoriness or other properties.

Applied to clinical situations, the results of this study indicate the potential pitfalls of drawing conclusions on the state of autonomic cardiac "tone" based on heart rate or AV nodal conduction time and underscore the complexity of accurately determining the role played by each limb of the autonomic nervous system in the genesis of clinical arrhythmias.

Acknowledgment: Supported in part by the Herman C. Krannert Fund; by Grants HL-06308 and HL-07182 from the National Heart, Lung and Blood Institute of the National Institutes of Health, Bethesda, Maryland; by the American Heart Association, Indiana Affiliate.

References

1. Levy MN, Zieske H. Autonomic control of cardiac pacemaker activity and atrioventricular transmission. J Appl Physiol 1969;27:465–470.
2. Levy MN. Sympathetic-parasympathetic interactions in the heart. Circ Res 1971;29:437–445.
3. Loeffelholz K, Muscholl E. A muscarinic inhibition of the noradrenaline release evoked by postganglionic sympathetic nerve stimulation. Naunyn-Schmiedebergs Arch Pharmacol 1969;265:1–15.
4. Levy MN, Blattberg B. Effect of vagal stimulation on the overflow of norepinephrine into the coronary sinus during cardiac sympathetic nerve stimulation in the dog. Circ Res 1976;38:81–85.
5. Watanabe AM, McConnaughey MM, Strawbridge RA, Fleming JW, Jones LR, Besch HR Jr. Muscarinic cholinergic receptor modulation of beta-adrenergic receptor affinity for catecholamines. J Biol Chem 1978;253:4833–4836.
6. Takahashi N, Zipes DP. Vagal modulation of adrenergic effects on canine sinus and atrioventricular nodes. Am J Physiol 1983;244:H775–H781.
7. Salata JJ, Gill RM, Gilmour RF Jr, Zipes DP. Effects of sympathetic tone on vagally-induced phasic changes in heart rate and AV nodal conduction in the anesthetized dog. Circ Res 1986;58:584–594.
8. Zipes DP, Mihalick MJ, Robbins GT. Effects of selective vagal and stellate ganglion stimulation on atrial refractoriness. Cardiovasc Res 1974;8:647–655.
9. Wallick DW, Martin PJ, Masuda Y, Levy MN. Effects of autonomic activity and changes in heart rate on atrioventricular conduction. Am J Physiol 1982;243:H523–H527.

10. Kolman BS, Verrier RL, Lown B. Effect of vagus nerve stimulation upon excitability of the canine ventricle. Role of sympathetic-parasympathetic interactions. Am J Cardiol 1976;37:1041–1045.
11. Martins JB, Zipes DP. Effects of sympathetic and vagal nerves on recovery properties of the endocardium and epicardium of the canine left ventricle. Circ Res 1980;46:100–110.
12. Nattel S, Euler DE, Spear JF, Moore EN. Autonomic control of ventricular refractoriness. Am J Physiol 1981;241:H878–H882.
13. Takahashi N, Barber MJ, Zipes DP. Efferent vagal innervation of canine ventricle. Am J Physiol 1985;248:H89–H97.
14. Webb SA, Adgey AAJ, Pantridge JF. Autonomic disturbance at onset of acute myocardial infarction. Br Med J 1972;3:89–92.
15. Thames MD, Klopfenstein HS, Abboud FM, Mark AL, Walker JL. Preferential distribution of inhibitory cardiac receptors with vagal afferents to the inferoposterior wall of the left ventricle activated during coronary occlusion in the dog. Circ Res 1978;43:512–519.
16. Browne KF, Prystowsky E, Heger JJ, Chilson DA, Zipes DP. Prolongation of the Q-T interval in man during sleep. Am J Cardiol 1983;52:55–59.
17. Bexton RS, Vallin HO, Camm AJ. Diurnal variation of the QT interval influence of the autonomic nervous system. Br Heart J 1986;55:253–258.
18. Inoue H, Zipes DP. Changes in atrial and ventricular refractoriness and in ventricular nodal conduction produced by combinations of vagal and sympathetic stimulation that result in a constant spontaneous sinus cycle length. Circ Res (in press).

12

Modification of Electrophysiologic Matrix by Antiarrhythmic Drugs

Brian F. Hoffman

Introduction

When a drug acts on the heart, it may change the electrophysiological properties of cardiac cells so that the likelihood, severity, or persistence of certain arrhythmias is altered.[1,2] The actions may be such as to decrease the likelihood of occurrence or persistence of the arrhythmia responsible for drug administration. However, the same drug may simultaneously increase the likelihood, nature, and severity of other arrhythmias that had or had not been observed prior to drug administration. The question of interest is if we can predict, from an understanding of the actions of a drug and the electrophysiologic state of the heart, whether or not the drug will have both antiarrhythmic and arrhythmogenic effects.

A number of factors must be considered in evaluating this question. The first is the meaning we chose to assign to drug actions. It is possible to describe the actions of a drug in terms of induced alterations in excitability, conduction, and refractoriness, the traditional measures of cardiac electrical activity. This provides only a very general and qualitative indication of the outcomes of drug administration. It also is possible to describe effects on specific arrhythmogenic mechanisms such as automaticity or the occurrence of afterdepolarizations, the presence or absence of unidirectional conduction block, and the presence or absence of abnormal forms of the propagating impulse such as the slow response.[3] To help the clinician, this information must be coupled with satisfactory evidence that the particular arrhythmogenic factor is in fact operative in a given patient. It also is possible to quantify drug effects on the passive electrical properties of the cardiac

From: Brugada P, Wellens HJJ. CARDIAC ARRHYTHMIAS: Where To Go From Here? Mount Kisco, NY, Futura Publishing Company, Inc., © 1987.

fibers and syncytium and efforts have been made to relate actions on passive properties to antiarrhythmic action.[4] A more useful understanding of drug actions—one that sometimes permits reasonably accurate predictions—is provided by studies using voltage clamps to quantify drug actions in terms of induced alterations in sarcolemmal ionic currents, i.e., their voltage dependence, their magnitude, and the kinetics of the processes that regulate them.[5,6] Application of the patch clamp technique adds to the information available as it permits a description of changes in ionic currents through single sarcolemmal channels and identifies mechanisms for these changes in terms of alterations in opening probability, open and closed times, or single channel conductance.[7] Measurement of single channel currents also provides information on channel state and the effects of drugs thereon. The technique of intracellular perfusion during voltage clamp and patch clamp experiments has begun to provide information on the metabolic control of channel function.[8,9]

Unfortunately there have not yet been any satisfactory systematic tests of the accuracy and general applicability of predictions based either on one or the other of these approaches or on sets including data from several of the methods mentioned. For arrhythmias of the human heart, an attempt to predict antiarrhythmic efficacy from a drug classification based on the presence or absence of prominent blockade of fast channels and net change in duration of action potentials and refractoriness have not been associated with impressive success.[10] A few studies on arrhythmias induced in the hearts of experimental animals have suggested a correlation between demonstrated actions on specific arrhythmogenic mechanisms and in vivo antiarrhythmic efficacy. For example, lidocaine suppresses normal automaticity of canine Purkinje fibers but has little effect on abnormal automaticity arising in partially depolarized fibers. In contrast, ethmozine has little or no effect on the slope of phase 4 depolarization in normal canine Purkinje fibers but is reasonably effective in suppressing abnormal automaticity.[11] These differences have been shown to correlate well with the ability of each drug to influence ventricular arrhythmias in the canine heart thought to be caused by either normal or abnormal automaticity.[12] However, in general, the success rate of predictions has not been impressive.

A major factor that must be considered in an attempt to predict the effects of a drug on an arrhythmia is the mechanism assumed for the arrhythmia. Clearly drug actions that tend to make afterdepolarizations unlikely may not have much effect on an arrhythmia such as atrial fibrillation that does not depend on afterdepolarizations for its continuation. Conversely, a parasystolic rhythm might result from automatic impulse generation in a protected focus, and a drug that had little effect on automaticity but acted mainly to block fast channels and reduce the stimulating efficacy of the propagating action potential might prevent impulses generated by the parasystolic focus from exciting the heart.

A good general example of this sort of problem is provided by triggered rhythms resulting from delayed afterdepolarizations. The afterdepolarization is caused by a transient inward current and this current is induced when there is an increase in intracellular calcium. The sequence most often assumed is that calcium overload of the sarcoplasmic reticulum (SR) causes an oscillatory release and re-uptake of calcium by the SR. The resulting oscillatory change in free calcium concentration in the cytoplasm causes an oscillatory inward or depolarizing current and gives rise to one or more afterdepolarizations. These, if they are large enough to reduce membrane potential to the threshold firing level, initiate "triggered" premature impulses or a sustained triggered rhythm during which each action potential triggers the next action potential.[13]

There have been many studies in isolated cardiac tissues on the effects of different classes of antiarrhythmic drugs on delayed afterdepolarizations and triggered impulses and, in general, they have failed to reveal any clear and important specificity of antiarrhythmic drug action.[14] Since calcium overload apparently is a necessary condition for afterdepolarizations, or at least when they are caused by digitalis excess, one might assume that a calcium channel blocking drug should diminish or abolish the afterdepolarization and prevent the triggered arrhythmia. This often happens.[15] At the same time, regulation of intracellular calcium concentration depends on exchange of extracellular sodium for intracellular calcium and this exchange is decreased when intracellular sodium concentration rises. One thus might anticipate that partial block of sodium channels by a local anesthetic antiarrhythmic drug would reduce sodium influx during each action potential, reduce intracellular sodium concentration, and decrease the amplitude of delayed afterdepolarizations. Experiments have shown that this does happen.[16] Also, local anesthetics can prevent delayed afterdepolarizations from initiating action potentials by shifting the threshold potential to a more positive voltage. Finally, inward calcium current is enhanced by activation of β-adrenergic receptors and β-blockade can decrease the amplitude of delayed afterdepolarizations under certain conditions.

This summary might suggest that a great variety of antiarrhythmic drugs would or could terminate a triggered rhythm caused by delayed afterdepolarizations; the data certainly indicate that for this cause of arrhythmia the efficacy of a particular type of drug tells little or nothing about the arrhythmogenic mechanism. Unfortunately, the converse has received little attention. An increase in action potential duration augments delayed afterdepolarizations[17] and it would be interesting to know if antiarrhythmic drugs with this as their predominant effect are more likely than drugs from other classes to cause triggered rhythms.

Two other problems contribute to the difficulty of the analysis. The actions of the drug may not be uniform among different cardiac tissues. Thus, extrapolation of results obtained by studies on a particular tissue to other parts of the heart may not be permissible. Also, alterations in electrophysiological properties or structure caused by disease may significantly change response to drugs and, if these are unknown, it may not be possible to study a suitable experimental analogue.

Finally, it is clear that drug actions unrelated to direct effects on cardiac electrophysiological properties may modify antiarrhythmic efficacy;[18] for example, a reflex increase in heart rate will tend to suppress ectopic impulses caused by an automatic focus, favor the appearance of impulses trigged by delayed afterdepolarizations, and decrease the likelihood of arrhythmias due to early afterdepolarizations.

Most of these uncertainties encountered in trying to relate drug-induced changes in electrophysiological properties to antiarrhythmic or arrhythmogenic actions are well known. Few experiments, however, have been directed towards the possibly crucial role of interactions between local differences in the electrical properties of the myocardium and the actions of antiarrhythmic drugs.

Local Differences in Electrophysiologic State

Local differences in the electrophysiologic state of the myocardium can result from several different types of mechanisms. There may be underlying functional abnormalities of the myocardial cells that alter their ability to generate and conduct action potentials or that induce them to generate action potentials as a result of automaticity or triggering. There may be local differences in passive membrane properties that modify local conduction or the time of local repolarization. There may be local abnormalities of structure that modify the electrical coupling between different segments of the myocardium, and there obviously can be local abnormalities of perfusion that influence extracellular ion concentrations. Each of these general classes of abnormalities most likely can, under the proper conditions, lead to the appearance of arrhythmias of different sorts. Only a few examples will be considered here to indicate some of the different ways in which arrhythmias can come about.

Local Slowing of Conduction and Asynchronous Repolarization

It seems reasonable to draw two examples of the arrhythmogenic role of local inhomogeneity of the myocardium from studies on experimental myocardial infarction. There is general acceptance of the concept that after infarction, some arrhythmias result from reentrant excitation. Recent studies on the infarcted canine heart have clearly demonstrated reentry during both sustained and non-sustained ventricular tachycardia.[19,20] More important, when the site of reentry was localized to surviving subepicardial muscle, it has been shown that the necessary conduction block resulted not from the presence of a permanently inexcitable zone but rather from an activity-dependent change in the properties of a group of fibers that greatly slows conduction in them.[21]

Several different sequences of events might bring about the changes in function needed to cause local block and circus movement in this model. First, as has been known for some time, in tissues surviving after infarction, there typically is a decrease in resting potential and a consequent slowing of the recovery of responsiveness after each action potential.[22] The recovery of responsiveness is slowed because the removal of inactivation of sodium channels depends on the transmembrane potential and is greatly slowed at potentials significantly positive to the resting potential.[23]

If the recovery of responsiveness is delayed in an abnormal segment of the myocardium, that segment may conduct impulses normally if the cycle length is sufficiently long but generate slowly conducting impulses or impulses that block when the cycle length is shortened. The ability to induce reentry by premature or rapidly repeated impulses thus might be explicable.

However, the abnormal zone should not be considered the site of a static abnormality; a number of dynamic processes will alter impulse generation and conduction in it. It has been known for some time that changes in conduction will influence action potential duration. As shown by studies on bundles of Purkinje fibers, a local slowing of conduction can result in quite marked delay of repolarization.[13,24] This effect is particularly marked if a slow response replaces the fast response and, as a result, the speed of propagation is markedly reduced. In contrast, if there is local failure of conduction proximal to the site of block action potential duration is greatly abbreviated.[24-25] These changes in action potential duration result from the electrotonic interaction between different parts of the syncytium. With slowing of propagation, the persistent depolarization in downstream segments delays repolarization of proximal segments, whereas with block the polarized, unexcited segments speed repolarization of proximal areas.

If an impulse propagated from normal myocardium up to a zone in which recovery of responsiveness was delayed, along part of the border between normal and abnormal fibers conduction might slow and along another part of the border it might fail. As a consequence, in the first area the action potential would prolong and in the other area it would shorten. The result, an area of slow conduction bounded by areas of prolonged and abbreviated refractoriness, seems well suited to permit reentrant excitation. Obviously, the changes described might develop gradually over several beats or abruptly as a consequence of a single premature beat. Parenthetically, it is not necessary to assume that an increase in rate or a premature impulse is needed to initiate the sequence of events just described. A sufficient cause might be a local change in adequacy of perfusion due to local vascular obstruction, flow redistribution, or an increase in metabolic requirement not accompanied by a proportionate increase in local perfusion.

Many antiarrhythmic drugs will modify the electrophysiological state of abnormal segments of the myocardium in a manner that differs from the changes brought about in normal myocardium. For most, if not all, of the local anesthetic type antiarrhythmic drugs, i.e., those that block fast (sodium) channels in a dose-dependent manner, the intensity of block is a function of the magnitude of the resting potential, the duration of the action potential, and the rate of repetition of propagated impulses. This relationship exists because for most of these drugs, binding to the inactivated sodium channel is stronger than binding to the resting or open channel.[6,26] When a cell develops an action potential, the sodium channels first open and then inactivate. Some channels may be blocked by drug when they open but in general the major fraction of block occurs after the channels have inactivated. The channels remain inactivated until the cell repolarizes and thus, since equilibrium block generally is attained rather slowly, the longer the action potential the greater the fraction of blocked channels. On repolarization the unblocked channels recover from inactivation at the normal rate but the drug-blocked channels do not. Dissociation of drug from blocked channels is slow. Also, local anesthetic antiarrhythmic drugs shift the relationship between membrane potential and recovery from inactivation to more negative potentials[27] and so, if resting potential is reduced, recovery from block may be incomplete even with quite long diastolic intervals. These characteristics of drug-channel interaction are such that for a given plasma drug concentration, the block of fast channels will be greater in areas that are partially depolarized. Also, since after repolarization the dissociation of drug from channel may be relatively slow, if the cycle length is decreased, the intensity of block will increase. This usually is referred to as use-dependence. If the time constant for dissociation of drug from channel is short, as with lidocaine, a use-dependent increment in block will appear only at very rapid rates,[26] but if the time-constant is longer, as it is for most antiarrhythmic drugs, some use-dependent block will be present at normal rates and an increase will occur with a modest decrease in cycle length. The relationship obviously is a complex one. The development of block depends not just on the drug concentration but also on the duration of the action potential, the time constant for dissociation of drug from channel, the cycle length, and the resting potential. A decrease in cycle length will decrease potential duration but in depressed tissues also may reduce the resting potential. Although use-dependence most often is considered in relation to local anesthetic antiarrhythmic drugs of class I, amiodarone also shows clear use-dependent block of fast channels[28] and some calcium channel blocking drugs also demonstrate marked use-dependence.[29]

In summary, the presence of an antiarrhythmic drug is likely to modify or exaggerate local differences in electrophysiological properties that had been present in the drug-free state and thus either decrease or increase the likelihood of arrhythmia.

Local Abnormalities of Perfusion

The electrical activity of cardiac cells is strongly dependent on the integrity of their metabolic support. During each action potential, sodium enters the cell during depolarization and potassium leaves during repolarization. After each action potential there thus has been an increase in intracellular sodium concentration and an increase in extracellular potassium concentration. Normally the sodium is pumped out of the cell and the potassium pumped in by an energy-dependent mechanism, the sodium-potassium pump.[30] The rate of pumping is controlled mainly by the intracellular sodium concentration.[31] Because three sodium ions are transported out across the membrane for each two potassium ions transported in the opposite direction, the pump generates an outward or hyperpolarizing current.[32]

If the function of the pump is impaired, significant changes in intracellular and extracellular ion concentration can result. As a result of diminished pump function, and also as a direct consequence of reduced perfusion, the average concentration of potassium outside the cells will increase and the intracellular concentration will decrease. This will lead to a decrease in resting potential and a local decrease in action potential duration. If the loss of resting potential is large enough, there will be voltage-dependent inactivation of sodium channels, slowing of conduction, and slowing of the recovery of responsiveness after repolarization. The increase in intracellular sodium also will attenuate the action potential upstroke and impair conduction. These changes more or less mimic those described above for an abnormal segment of the myocardium.

If the local depolarization due to impaired active transport of Na and K is sufficient, even depressed fast responses may fail to develop and local conduction will block. Under these conditions, the fast response sometimes is replaced by a slow response.[13] Usually, when extracellular potassium is elevated, the action of catecholamines is needed to permit the generation of a propagating slow response. However, the extracellular K accumulation may cause depolarization of sympathetic efferent terminals and release of norepinephrine from them. If, as well may be the case, local ischemic damage has interrupted efferent sympathetic fibers in some areas but not in others, a slow response might develop only in some fibers. The conjunction of a propagating slow response and adjacent areas of block seems sufficient to initiate reentrant excitation. Obviously, if slow responses have replaced fast responses, drugs acting mainly on sodium channels will lose their effectiveness.

Impaired pump function, due to local ischemia, might well initiate arrhythmias by another mechanism. During each action potential there is a net influx of calcium into the cell and this calcium is for the most part removed by sodium-for-calcium exchange.[33] The exchanger transfers three sodium ions into the cell for each calcium ion moved from the cell into the extracellular phase. The driving force for this transport is a result of the concentration gradients for sodium and calcium across the membrane and the transmembrane potential. If, because of depression of the sodium-potassium pump, intracellular sodium concentration increases, then sodium-for-calcium exchange will decrease and intracellular calcium concentration will rise. Indeed, this is the mechanism by which digitalis exerts its positive inotropic effect. The possible consequences of the increase in intracellular calcium are numerous but one deserves attention here. As mentioned above, abnormal increase in intracellular calcium content seems to be the most frequent cause of delayed afterdepolarizations.[34] It thus seems possible that one consequence of a local inadequacy of perfusion may be the local appearance of delayed afterdepolarizations and triggered rhythms. Even if, because of an elevated extracellular potassium concentration, the afterdepolarizations fail to reach the threshold potential and trigger action potentials, they still can have important effects on impulse conduction.[35] This occurs because the afterdepolarization shifts the resting potential in a positive direction and this depolarization causes some inactivation of fast channels and attenuation or block of the fast response. Obviously the effect will be more likely in partially depolarized fibers.

Local Differences in Repolarization

Two clear examples of large, localized differences in action potential duration have been provided by studies on infarction of the canine heart. Ligation of the left anterior descending coronary artery sometimes causes an infarct that appears to be transmural. However, the subendocardial Purkinje fibers subtended by the infarct survive.[36] With time the duration of action potentials generated by these fibers increases markedly until a premature impulse in normal fibers is blocked in the area of delayed repolarization. In vitro this has been shown to result in what appears to be a sustained reentrant rhythm. In the same canine model of infarction, a zone of subepicardial muscle often survives.[19] With time, fibers in this zone regain almost normal resting potentials and generate action potentials of reasonable amplitude. However, the duration of the action potentials is markedly decreased.[37] This change may persist for weeks after the onset of ischemia. In summary, in fibers that survive infarction, there may be long-lasting and marked abnormalities of action potential duration.

Local changes in propagation, either slowing or block, can cause local changes in action potential duration as described in a prior section. In addition, it is possible to think of other mechanisms that could alter action potential duration in a localized area. A local increase in extracellular potassium concentration, mentioned above, will abbreviate the plateau whereas a decrease in outward current generated by the sodium-potassium pump will prolong it. In most cases several mechanisms operate simultaneously and thus the net change in action potential duration must be determined directly. If transport of ions by the sodium-potassium pump were reduced, there would be an immediate decrease in resting potential and an increase in action potential duration due to loss of pump current. The decrease in pump rate would be accompanied by a transient increase in extracellular potassium concentration. As extracellular potassium concentration rose, there would be a further decrease in resting potential and a decrease in action potential duration. The increase in extracellular potassium would decrease membrane resistance and, as a result, whatever its magnitude the pump current would cause a reduced change in membrane potential. An increase in intracellular calcium concentration and intracellular acidification would tend to decrease the conductance of the gap junctions and partially uncouple cells.[38] This would not only modify conduction but attenuate electrotonic interactions among cells during repolarization. It is possible, therefore, to enumerate a number of mechanisms that might operate to cause transient local abnormalities of repolarization but it is not possible to make any general predictions about the actual direction or magnitude of the change.

The role of antiarrhythmic drugs as a cause of local differences in repolarization should not be ignored. We have presented data elsewhere indicating that quinidine can cause a delay in repolarization and early afterdepolarizations[39] and that these may be a cause of torsades-like arrhythmias. The same reasoning applies to any antiarrhythmic drug that blocks both fast channels and the delayed rectifier channel that carries repolarizing potassium current as long as the kinetics of use-dependent block of fast channels are appropriate. Quinidine blocks fast channels and the intensity of block increases as the cycle length decreases. Quinidine also blocks the repolarizing current carried by the delayed rectifier channel and thus slows repolarization. However, the effect on repolarization is less than might be expected because the blockade of fast channels by quinidine reduces window current, i.e., inward depolarizing current carried by fast channels during the plateau. The result is a somewhat prolonged action potential. With a decrease in rate, the block of fast channels diminishes, the magnitude of window current increases, and the delay of repolarization may be greatly enhanced. In this setting, an early afterdepolarization often appears and gives rise to a sustained rhythm due to what we have called abnormal automaticity.[40] The likelihood of this sequence of events is enhanced when the extracellular potassium concentration is low. It seems likely that is so because of the strong effect of extracellular potassium on current carried by the inward rectifier i_{K1}. The lower the extracellular potassium concentration the smaller the outward (repolarizing) current carried by this channel and the greater the delay in repolarization. In our experiments, an increase in cycle length was needed to induce the early afterdepolarizations and arrhythmia. However, this need not be the only suitable mechanism. Several sequences of events can be postulated to cause early afterdepolarizations in the presence of drugs that block the delayed rectifier. It must be emphasized that repolarizing current in this channel increases as membrane potential is made more positive. Thus a negative shift in plateau voltage might elicit less delayed rectifier current and either delay or prevent repolarization. Such a shift in plateau voltage also would tend to augment window current and this inward current would prolong the plateau. Such a change in voltage-time course of the plateau is often a consequence of ischemia. We do not know if block of the delayed rectifier by antiarrhythmic drugs is use-dependent or voltage-dependent but this may well be the case.

It also is possible to assume that the effect of an antiarrhythmic drug is not sufficient to elicit delayed afterdepolarizations in an abnormal segment of the myocardium because perfusion of that segment is somewhat inadequate and extracellular potassium concentration is somewhat elevated. In this case an *improvement* of local perfusion and the resulting *reduction* in extracellular potassium towards normal might be sufficient to elicit early afterdepolarizations and arrhythmia.

Structural Abnormalities

Ischemic damage to the myocardium causes changes in structure and these may contribute to an increased likelihood of arrhythmias. In infarcts caused by ligation of the left anterior descending coronary artery in dogs, typically there is an increase in the anisotropy of surviving subepicardial muscle due at least in part to separation of surviving muscle bundles by collagen.[21] Conduction velocity is much slower at right angles to the long axis of the fibers then parallel to the long axis and block of conduction is more often associated with propagation perpendicular to the fiber axis. There seems little doubt that this localized increase in the degree of anisotropy is associated with an increased likelihood of reentrant rhythms.

Arrhythmogenic Potentials of Antiarrhythmic Drugs

The potential for an antiarrhythmic drug to induce arrhythmias or to increase the incidence or severity of existing arrhythmias often will be a function of the electrophysiologic condition of the myocardium and always will be a function of the drug concentration. A local anesthetic antiarrhythmic drug that has a much higher affinity for inactivated fast channels than for resting channels will cause greater depression of conduction in a partially depolarized area than in the normal myocardium. Also, typically any delay in the recovery of responsiveness after an action potential will be greater in the partially depolarized area. Whether or not these regional differences in intensity of effect will be arrhythmogenic depends on the starting conditions. At one extreme both normal and premature impulses can be assumed to conduct throughout both the normal and depressed myocardium in the drug-free state although with some slowing of conduction in the depressed area. After administration of drug, the more intense effect on the depressed area might result in markedly slow conduction in some areas and conduction block in others. This effect might predispose to a reentrant rhythm. At the other extreme, one can assume that in the drug-free state, slow conduction and areas of block already are present in the depressed area. Now a drug concentration that does not greatly influence conduction in normal myocardium may completely suppress conduction in the abnormal area and thus prevent reentry from occurring there.

Another possibility seems equally likely. In the presence of a fixed concentration of antiarrhythmic drug, there may be unidirectional block along one border of a depressed area and slow conduction through the depressed area. However, conduction is not quite slow enough and consequently the impulse spreading through the depressed area encounters refractoriness of normal surrounding myocardium, and thus blocks. If the block of fast channels of the drug shows use dependence, an increase in heart rate can further slow conduction in the abnormal segment. Because of the slower conduction, the impulse may reach the border of the depressed segment with a delay sufficient to permit reexcitation of the normal myocardium and generation of reentrant excitation. For this to happen, the effect on conduction would have to be great enough to compensate for any drug-induced prolongation of refractoriness in the normal myocardium.

Conclusions

It seems clear that under many conditions, there may be localized differences in the electrophysiological state of the myocardium and that these differences may be activity-dependent and perfusion-dependent. Moreover, the differences in electrophysiological state are such that they can be the cause of arrhythmias. When antiarrhythmic drugs act on the heart, local differences in electrophysiological state can and will modify the drug actions and this also can lead to the development of arrhythmias. The problems presented by these considerations are difficult since, for the in situ heart, it is often not possible to detect and quantify local differences in electrophysiologic state.

References

1. Hoffman BF. Modification of the electrophysiologic matrix by antiarrhythmic drugs. J Am Coll Cardiol 1985;5:28B–30B.
2. Hoffman BF, Dangman KH. The role of antiarrhythmic drugs in sudden cardiac death. J Am Coll Cardiol 1986;8:104A–109A.
3. Bigger JT Jr, Hoffman BF. Antiarrhythmic drugs. In Gilman A, ed. The Pharmacological Basis of Therapeutics. New York, MacMillan Company, 1985;748–783.

4. Arnsdorf MF, Wasserstrom JA. Mechanisms of action of antiarrhythmic drugs: A matrical approach. In Fozzard HA, ed. The Heart and Cardiovascular System: Scientific Foundations. New York, Raven Press, 1986;1259–1316.
5. Bean BP, Cohen CJ, Tsien RW. Lidocaine block of cardiac sodium channels. J Gen Physiol 1983;81:613–642.
6. Colatsky TJ. Mechanisms of action of lidocaine and quinidine on action potential duration in rabbit cardiac Purkinje fibers: an effect on steady state sodium currents? Circ Res 1982;50:17–27.
7. Hess PJ, Lansman B, Tsien RW. Different modes of Ca channel gating behaviour favoured by dihydropyridine agonists and antagonists. Nature 1984;309:453–456.
8. Kameyama M, Hofmann F, Trautwein W. On the mechanism of beta-adrenergic regulation of the Ca channel in the guinea pig heart. Pflugers Arch 1985;405:285–293.
9. Noma A, Shibasaki T. Membrane current through adenosine-triphosphate-regulated potassium channels in guinea-pig ventricular cells. J Physiol 1985;363:463–480.
10. Zipes DP, Prystowsky EN, Heger JJ. Electrophysiologic testing of antiarrhythmic agents. Am Heart J 1982;103:610–614.
11. Dangman KH, Hoffman BF. Antiarrhythmic effects of ethmozin in cardiac Purkinje fibers: suppression of automaticity and abolition of triggering. J Pharmacol Exp Ther 1983;227:578–586.
12. Ilvento JP, Provet J, Danilo P Jr, Rosen MR. Fast and slow idioventricular rhythms in the canine heart: A study of their mechanism using antiarrthymic drugs and electrophysiologic testing. Am J Cardiol 1982;49:1909–1916.
13. Cranefield PF. The Conduction of the Cardiac Impulse. Mt Kisco, NY, Futura Publishing Co., 1975.
14. Rosen MR, Danilo P. Effects of tetrodotoxin, lidocaine, verapamil and AHR-2666 on ouabain-induced delayed afterdepolarizations in canine Purkinje fibers. Circ Res 1980; 46:117–124.
15. Gough WB, Zeiler RH, El-Sherif N. Effects of diltiazem on triggered activity in canine 1-day-old infarction. Cardiovasc Res 1984;18:339–343.
16. Sheu SS, Lederer WJ. Lidocaine's negative inotropic and antiarrhythmic actions: Dependence on shortening of action potential duration and reduction of intracellular sodium activity. Circ Res 1985;57:578–590.
17. Henning B, Wit AL. The time course of action potential repolarization effects delayed afterdepolarization amplitude in atrial fibers of the canine coronary sinus. Circ Res 1984;55:110–115.
18. Hoffman BF. Mechanisms of antiarrhythmic action. In Zipes DP, Jalife J, eds. Cardiac Electrophysiology and Arrhythmias. New York, Grune & Stratton, Inc., 1985;193–205.
19. El-Sherif N, Rahul Gough WB, Zeiler RH. Ventricular activation patterns of spontaneous and induced ventricular rhythms in canine one-day-old myocardial infarction: evidence for focal and reentrant mechanisms. Circ Res 1982;51:152–166.
20. Wit AL, Allessie MA, Bonke FIM, Vammers W, Smeets J, Fenoglio JJ Jr. Electrophysiologic mapping to determine the mechanism of experimental ventricular tachycardia initiated by premature impulses: Experimental approach and initial results demonstrating reentrant excitation. Am J Cardiol 1982;49:166–185.
21. Gardner PI, Ursell PC, Pham TD, Fenoglio JJ Jr, Wit AL. Experimental chronic ventricular tachycardia: Anatomic and electrophysiologic substrates. In Josephson ME, ed. Tachycardias: Mechanisms, Diagnosis and Treatment. Philadelphia, Lea & Febiger, 1984;29–60.
22. Lazzara R, El-Sherif N, Scherlag BJ. Disorders of cellular electrophysiology produced by ischemia of the canine His bundle. Circ Res 1975;36:444–454.
23. Carmeliet E, Vereecke J. Electrogenesis of the action potential and automaticity. In Handbook of Physiology: The Cardiovascular System I. American Physiological Society, 1979;269–334.
24. Cranefield PF, Klein HO, Hoffman BF. Conduction of the cardiac impulse. I. Delay, block, and one-way block in depressed Purkinje fibers. Circ Res 1971;28:199–219.
25. Mendez C, Mueller WJ, Meredith J, Moe GK. Interaction of transmembrane potentials

in canine Purkinje fibers and of Purkinje fiber-muscle junction. Circ Res 1969;24: 361–372.
26. Hondeghem LM, Katzung BG. Antiarrhythmic agents: the modulated receptor mechanism of action of sodium and calcium channel-blocking drugs. Ann Rev Pharmacol Toxicol 1984;24:387–423.
27. Weidmann SL. Effects of calcium ions and local anesthetics on electrical properties of Purkinje fibers. J Physiol (Lond) 1955;129:568–582.
28. Mason JW, Hondeghem LM, Katzung BG. Block of inactivated sodium channels and of depolarization-induced automaticity in guinea pig papillary muscle by amiodarone. Circ Res 1984;55:277–285.
29. Sanguinetti MC, Kass RS. Voltage-dependent block of calcium channel current in the calf cardiac Purkinje fiber by dihydropyridine calcium channel antagonists. Circ Res 1984;55:336–348.
30. Gadsby DC. The Na/K pump of cardiac cells. Ann Rev Biophys Bioeng 1984;13:373–398.
31. Eisner DA and Lederer J. Characterization of the electrogenic sodium pump in cardiac Purkinje fibres. J Physiol (Lond) 1980;303:441–474.
32. Gadsby DC, Cranefield PF. Electrogenic sodium extrusion in cardiac Purkinje fibers. J Gen Physiol 1979;73:819–837.
33. Mullins LJ. The generation of electric currents in cardiac fibers by Na/Ca exchange. Am J Physiol 1979;236:C103–C110.
34. Lederer WJ, Tsien RW. Transient inward current underlying arrhythmogenic effects of cardiotonic steroids in Purkinje fibers. J Physiol (Lond) 1976;263:73–100.
35. Rosen MR, Wit AL, Hoffman BF. Electrophysiology and pharmacology of cardiac arrhythmias. IV. Cardiac antiarrhythmic and toxic effects of digitalis. Am Heart J 1975;89:391–399.
36. Friedman PL, Stewart JR, Fenoglio JJ Jr, Wit AL. Survival of subendocardial Purkinje fibers after extensive myocardial infarction in dogs. In vitro and in vivo correlations. Circ Res 1973;33:597–611.
37. Ursell PC, Gardner PI, Albala A, Fenoglio JJ Jr, Wit AL. Structural and electrophysiological changes in the epicardial border zone of canine myocardial infarcts during infarct healing. Circ Res 1985;56:436–451.
38. Spray DC, White RL, Mazet F, Bennett MVL. Regulation of gap junctional conductance. Am J Physiol 1985;17:H753–H764.
39. Roden DM, Hoffman BF. Action potential prolongation and induction of abnormal automaticity by low quinidine concentrations in cardiac Purkinje fibers. Circ Res 1985;56:857–867.
40. Dangman KH, Hoffman BF. Studies on overdrive stimulation of canine cardiac Purkinje fibers: Maximal diastolic potential as a determinant of the response. J Am Coll Cardiol 1983;2:1183–1190.

III

SUPRAVENTRICULAR ARRHYTHMIAS

13

Role of Electrophysiologic Studies in Supraventricular Tachycardia

Masood Akhtar
Mohammad Shenasa
Patrick J. Tchou
Mohammad Jazayeri

Introduction

Supraventricular tachycardia (SVT) has fascinated clinicians and electrophysiologists for some time.[1-13] The introduction of invasive electrophysiologic studies (EPS) and programmed electrical stimulation have immensely improved our understanding of the underlying mechanisms and helped map out the reentrant circuits.[2-13] In addition, the knowledge obtained in the clinical laboratory has helped in formulating a rational basis for pharmacologic and nonpharmacologic therapy of SVT.[14-19] Since electrophysiologic studies have represented the most definitive method for the diagnosis of specific arrhythmias, the laboratory knowledge has been subsequently translated onto surface ECG to improve diagnostic accuracy in dealing with the variety of SVTs that are encountered in clinical practice.[10-13,20] For accurate detection of various types of SVT, several new criteria have been proposed and many of the earlier ones have been revised, modified, or accepted with some degree of confidence. At the present time, an EPS constitutes an important part of the clinical evaluation in problem cases with SVT from both diagnostic and therapeutic perspectives. It goes without saying that without the availability of EPS and PES, our ability to make a correct diagnosis and select appropriate therapy would have been limited.

From: Brugada P, Wellens HJJ. CARDIAC ARRHYTHMIAS: Where To Go From Here? Mount Kisco, NY, Futura Publishing Company, Inc., © 1987.

Nonetheless, with the current body of knowledge, albeit materialized by invasive EP testing, is it still necessary to perform such studies for either diagnostic and/or therapeutic purposes? To address some of these issues, we looked at the SVT cases referred to our services during the last 2 years. The purpose of this analysis was to see how often an accurate diagnosis of SVT was initially made from available electrocardiographic and clinical data to the primary physician. Subsequently all clinical and ECG data were evaluated and a diagnosis of specific type of SVT was made by the authors. To be included in this series, the main requirement was availability of a 12-lead electrocardiogram (ECG) during the tachycardia ECG diagnosis initially made by the primary physician. Final diagnosis of specific arrhythmia utilizing the EPS was available in all patients included in the series.

Since SVT presented either a narrow or a wide QRS tachycardia, our findings are separately outlined under the two subgroups.

SVT Presenting as a Narrow QRS Tachycardia

There was a total of 30 cases and the majority of these had either atrioventricular nodal (AVN) reentry (13 patients) or orthodromic tachycardia (12 patients) when documented by EPS. Some relevant clinical and electrocardiographic data are depicted in Table I. In the vast majority of these cases, the impression of PAT or SVT was used by the primary physician. A specific and accurate diagnosis of orthodromic tachycardia (OT) was mentioned in 3/12 and atrial flutter in 1/3 patients. For OT, however, it was not clear from the notes if the diagnosis was based on the known association between OT and the Wolff-Parkinson-White syndrome or whether it was made from 12-lead ECG alone.

Our own analysis of the 12-lead ECG revealed the following findings. The tachycardia cycle length (CL) was shorter during OT, but there was a significant overlap between OT, AVN reentry, and atrial tachycardias such that the use of CL alone made it difficult for us to make correct diagnoses in individual cases. The P

Table I
Narrow QRS Tachycardial (Total Number of Patients: 30)

	Common AVN Reentry	Orthodromic Tachycardia	Long RP Tachycardia	Atrial
Number of Pts.	13	12	2	3
Age-Yrs.	56 ± 19	35 ± 15	56 ± 24	61.5 ± 6
(Range)	(19–80)	(19–56)	(22–78)	(56–70)
Sex M/F	4/9	5/7	1/1	2/1
CL msec (Mean ± SD)	357.5 ± 56.8	321.25 ± 60	510 ± 10	373.3 ± 37.7
(Range)	(230–450)	(220–420)	(500–520)	(320–400)
P Polarity	—	—	2	2
Typical P Location	13	5	2	2
QRS Alternation	1	4	0	0

The diagnostic categories listed in the table represent the final diagnosis made at EPS. CL=cycle length.

wave polarity could be discerned with confidence in only the four cases where the P wave was identified outside the ST-T segment. The typical P wave location was suggested by a lack of identifiable P wave in all 11/13 cases of AVN reentry, whereas in 2/13 patients the P wave was identified at the end of the QRS complex.[10-13,20] In only 5/12 cases with OT, a P wave was clearly identified in the ST-T segment.[10-13,20] In the remaining 7/12 cases, although the atrial activation did follow the QRS, it could not be appreciated on the surface ECG and incorrect diagnosis of AVN reentry was suggested. As pointed out above and depicted in the table, the P wave location (and polarity) was clearly identified in the two patients with long RP tachycardia.[21-23] EPS revealed uncommon AVN reentry as the mechanism in one, and accessory pathway with long VA conduction time in the other. In 1/3 cases with atrial tachycardia, the P wave location was not clearly detectable, whereas in the remaining two patients with intra-atrial reentry, a combination of clearly identifiable P waves and their polarity permitted a correct diagnosis of atrial origin for the arrhythmias.

A QRS alternans was seen in 4/12 cases with OT and 1/13 patients with AVN reentry and in none of the cases in other categories.[20] Interestingly, all cases with QRS alternans had CL of the tachycardia which were among the shortest in this series.

In none of the cases in this series was a transition from a bundle branch block (BBB) to narrow QRS (or vice versa) recorded during spontaneous SVT, making this criterion of little practical value to distinguish narrow QRS OT from other varieties.

SVT Presenting as a Wide QRS Tachycardia

Among the 21 patients in whom a final diagnosis of wide QRS SVT was made, there were 10 who had BBB or aberrant conduction during SVT and the remaining 11 had conduction over an accessory pathway. Clinical presentation in these two groups is separately outlined below.

SVT with Aberrant Conduction (10 Patients)

A diagnosis of VT was made in 4/10 patients by the primary physician whereas the remaining cases carried a diagnosis of wide QRS tachycardia without any further specification. The 12-lead ECG analysis suggested SVT with aberrant conduction in 8/10, two of whom had preexisting BBB, making this diagnosis easier.[24] In the remaining two cases, the diagnosis of VT was made due to negative concordance across the precordium. On the basis of P wave location or other criteria for SVT (used in narrow QRS SVT), a precise diagnosis of the underlying rhythm was suggested in only 2/10, one with OT and one with atrial tachycardia. The underlying EP mechanism was OT in 6/10 whereas two had AVN reentry and the remaining two had atrial tachycardia.

Based on prior history of preexcitation during sinus rhythm, a correct diagnosis of OT (by simple association) could have been made in 5/6 cases.

SVT with Conduction over AP (11 Patients)

Nine of the 11 cases had atrial flutter-fibrillation as the underlying rhythm abnormality, one had antidromic tachycardia, and the remaining one had antegrade conduction over a nodoventricular Mahaim. The primary physician made the diagnosis of VT in 3/11, SVT in 5/11, and labeled the tachycardia as wide QRS in the remaining three. The diagnosis of SVT in these five cases does not necessarily reflect identification of the exact underlying arrhythmia problem since 4/5 received IV verapamil with deleterious consequences. The electrocardiograms in all cases were quite typical and our assessment was that an accurate diagnosis of the underlying arrhythmia could be made in 9/11 cases from the 12-lead ECG alone.

Since wide QRS SVT is often diagnosed as VT and vice versa, we analyzed some of the clinical data in 85 cases with VT even though this chapter deals primarily with evaluation of SVT. A comparison of these data is presented in Table II. A correct diagnosis of VT was made by the primary physicians in 25/85 (29%) of the cases. In 38/85 cases (45%), a diagnosis of SVT was applied whereas the remaining 22/85 (26%) were labeled as having wide QRS tachycardia.

Evaluation of some of the clinical parameters revealed that patients presenting with wide QRS tachycardia associated with anterograde conduction over the AP were clearly younger. Except for one patient, all were younger than 40 years of age. On the other hand, there was significant overlap of ages between patients with aberrant conduction and those who had VT even though the average patient with VT was significantly older.

A strong association was apparent between the history of prior MI and the occurrence of wide QRS tachycardia of ventricular origin. In fact, in 73% of cases, the diagnosis of VT could be made on the basis of previous history of MI alone. None of the patients with preexcitation during SVT had prior documented myocardial infarction (MI). Two of the cases with aberrant conduction had a prior documented MI. Furthermore, only 4/85 patients with VT had no detectable structural heart disease (SHD) whereas none of the cases with wide QRS tachycardia due to anterograde preexcitation had SHD, and 3/10 patients with aberrant conduction had demonstrable SHD.

Table II
Wide QRS Tachycardia (Total Number of Patients: 106)

	Aberrant Conduction	Conduction over AP	VT
Number of Pts.	10	11	85
Age (Yrs.)	51.7 ± 23	30.2 ± 14.5	60.8 ± 12.8
	(8–81)	(20–73)	(22–81)
M/F	4/6	8/3	68/17
SHD	3/10 (30%)	0 (0%)	81 (95%)
H/O MI	2 (20%)	0 (0%)	62 (73%)

AP = accessory pathway; SHD = structural heart disease; VT = ventricular tachycardia.

Application of Surface ECG Criteria for the Diagnosis of Wide QRS Tachycardia

We utilized the often used, existing criteria for distinction between the SVT and VT and the results are outlined below.[25-28]

QRS Complex Duration (Table III)

The mean QRS duration in the three groups with wide QRS tachycardia are depicted in Table III and it can be appreciated that mean QRS duration was longest in VT and shortest in aberrant conduction. Using a cut-off of 140 ms, only 6/85 (7%) with VT had a QRS complex measuring < 140 ms. All except one patient (with Mahaim) had a QRS duration >140 ms among the cases with anterograde preexcitation during the tachycardia. During aberrant conduction, three of the five cases with left (L)BBB had a QRS complex exceeding >140 ms (160 ms in each case). On the basis of QRS duration alone, a clear distinction between preexcited tachycardia, aberrantly conducted QRS complexes with a LBBB morphology, and complexes of ventricular origin could not be made in this series of cases. Excluding preexcitation, QRS complexes showing a right (R)BBB morphology and a duration of >140 ms were primarily seen in patients with VT. It is of interest to note that in four cases of VT, the QRS duration was ≤ 120 ms.

QRS Complex Morphology (Table III)

As can be seen from the table, the mere classification of QRS complex into a RBBB or LBBB pattern was not useful in distinguishing the various mechanisms for wide QRS complexes. A typical triphasic complex of RBBB aberrancy was seen in all five cases with RBBB. This appearance of QRS complex was seen in 3/47 (6%)

Table III
Wide QRS Tachycardia (Total Number of Patients: 106)

	Aberrant Conduction	Conduction over AP	VT
ECG Parameters			
QRS duration (ms)	139.5 ± 14.6 (120–160)	160.9 ± 23.9 (120–200)	168.9 ± 28 (90–300)
CL (ms) (R-R)	349 ± 66.5 (240–450)	300 ± 67.9 (200–400)	360.8 ± 54 (240–560)
LBBB Pattern	5 (50%)	3 (27%)	38 (45%)
RBBB Pattern	5 (50%)	8 (73%)	47 (55%)
QRS Concordance			
Positive	0 (0%)	0 (0%)	8 (9%)
Negative	2 (20%)	0 (0%)	8 (9%)

LBBB = left bundle branch block; RBBB = right bundle branch block.

cases with VT. In 4/5 cases with LBBB type of aberrancy, accurate diagnosis was suggested by the surface ECG. A QRS morphology showing a typical LBBB pattern was seen in 2/38 (5%) of patients with VT. On the other hand, monophasic or biphasic complexes were seen primarily during preexcitation or VT. The latter two were indistinguishable on the basis of QRS morphology alone. A positive QRS concordance in leads V_1-V_6 was seen only in VT in eight cases (9%), whereas a negative concordance was observed in 8/85 (9%) patients with VT, and 2/10 (20%) cases with aberrant conduction. Interestingly, neither a positive nor a negative QRS concordance was seen in any of the preexcited complexes.

The presence of preexisting BBB was extremely helpful in arriving at an accurate diagnosis.[24] In all 14 patients with VT and preexisting BBB, the QRS morphology was different during the tachycardia as compared to sinus beats, whereas in two patients with preexisting LBBB, the QRS morphology did not change during SVT.

Cyle Length of the R-R Interval (Table III)

There was a significant difference in the mean cycle length of RR intervals in patients with preexcited complexes versus those with VT or aberrant induction. However, an appreciable amount of overlap existed in the various categories which made a clear distinction difficult in individual cases. It should be mentioned here that as expected, the RR intervals were appreciably irregular (albeit the changes were often subtle) in patients with atrial fibrillation and conduction over the AP.

QRS Complex Axis (Table IV)

Although a QRS axis in the normal range was seen in almost 40% of the cases with aberrant conduction and in less than 20% of the patients with VT or preexcited complexes, this parameter was clearly not very useful for determination of tachycardia origin in any of the three categories. Right, left, and extreme westward axis was equally frequent in VT. The distribution of axis among the patients with preexcited complexes was essentially a function of the AP location and therefore was often oriented superiorly (posteroseptal) or inferiorly directed (left free wall), i.e., the two most common AP locations. In all patients with aberrant

Table IV
Wide QRS Tachycardia (Total Number of Patients: 106)

	Aberrant Conduction	Conduction over AP	VT
QRS Axis			
−30 to +90	4 (40%)	2 (18.1%)	14 (16.4%)
<−30 to −90	4 (40%)	4 (36.4%)	26 (30.6%)
<−90 to ± 180	0 (0%)	1 (9.1%)	22 (25.9%)
>+90 to + 150	2 (20%)	4 (36.4%)	23 (27.1%)

conduction, the axis seen during sinus rhythm did not significantly change with the wide QRS tachycardia.

AV Dissociation

Dissociation between atrial and ventricular activity that could be discerned on the surface ECG was noted in 18/85 (21%) cases. In the remainder, either there was a 1-1 P-QRS relationship or the P wave simply could not be clearly identified. Although in all patients with AVN reentry or OT, a 1-1 P-QRS relationship existed; the P wave on the surface ECG was seen only in a minority.

Discussion

The analysis just presented suggests that an initial misdiagnosis concerning the origin of wide QRS complex tachycardia or a specific type of a narrow QRS tachycardia is frequent despite availability of various surface ECG criteria. In patients with VT, the diagnosis of SVT was made more often than VT and conversely VT was commonly diagnosed in patients with SVT with either aberrant conduction or anterograde preexcitation.

On the surface ECG, the QRS duration, positive QRS concordance, and a monophasic or biphasic QRS morphology were the most useful criteria for distinction between VT and aberrant conduction as has been pointed out previously by Wellens et al.[26] However, in all categories, exceptions were seen in at least 5% of the cases. The most accurate criteria for the diagnosis of VT were identifiable presence of AV dissociation and different QRS appearance during tachycardia in patients with preexisting BBB (no exceptions seen).[24] However, the inability to see the P wave clearly during wide QRS tachycardia and relatively infrequent occurrence of preexisting BBB, i.e., 14/85 (16%), made these findings of limited practical use. Considering that demonstration of AV dissociation is almost diagnostic of VT, other methods of atrial activity detection such as esophageal electrogram, etc. should prove useful. Various other criteria including axis orientation were not found useful for reliable distinction between the three categories of wide QRS tachycardia presented here.

The absence of SHD and/or a positive history of preexcitation made the diagnosis of SVT more likely. On the other hand, a history of prior MI markedly increased the probability of VT.

Despite these clinical and surface ECG criteria, an accurate diagnosis of a specific mechanism of wide QRS arrhythmias could not be made in all cases. When one combines the various surface ECG criteria, a correct diagnosis of VT or SVT could be made in more than 90% of the cases. This degree of accuracy, however, may not be sufficient to distinguish relatively benign SVT (aberrant conduction) from potentially life-threatening arrhythmias seen in preexcitation syndromes and VT. It would seem, therefore, that in difficult cases, an accurate diagnosis would require EPS. In addition, the EPS would also seem useful for prognostication which cannot be done unless a reliable diagnosis can be made.

In patients presenting with narrow QRS complex tachycardia, an initial diagnosis of SVT is the rule and the possibility of VT is seldom entertained. This represents an accurate diagnosis in better than 98% of the cases. However, the surface ECG criteria which utilizes P wave analysis to distinguish various subsets of SVT have limited practical value since P waves cannot be accurately placed in many of these cases. In this study, we also did not find the presence of QRS alternans very useful in distinguishing rapid AVN reentry from OT. It seemed as if the QRS alternans was a function of short CL rather than AVN versus AV reentry.

If a precise diagnosis of specific reentry circuit is important for whatever reason, invasive EPS will remain the most definitive approach.

EPS for Therapeutic Considerations

An incorrect diagnosis in patients with wide QRS tachycardia is of more than an academic interest. Inappropriate therapy is a consequence of such diagnosis and often leads to inappropriate (and often hazardous) therapy both in the acute termination and subsequent prevention of the tachycardia. If the correct diagnosis of a specific mechanism of wide or narrow QRS complex tachycardia is made, one can rationally avoid drugs traditionally ineffective in the specific type of SVT. For some of the reasons listed below, EPS may provide the best option for assessment of efficacy or failure in certain categories of patients.

1. In patients with severe symptoms during SVT, such as presyncope, syncope, angina, congestive heart failure, etc., a trial with empiric therapy may not be advisable. Following the serial drug testing approach initially used by Wu et al., effectiveness, or lack thereof, of pharmacologic therapy can be demonstrated safely and in a relatively short period of time.[14] Drugs that prevent induction of SVT in the laboratory are often effective in the prevention of clinical recurrences.[14-16] Our own experience has been that pharmacologic agents that produce retrograde block are far more effective in prevention of clinical tachycardia compared to those that only influence antegrade conduction along the AV node. This seems true for both OT, as well as for AVN reentry tachycardia.[29,30] A slowing of ventricular response via the accessory pathway during induced atrial fibrillation following an oral agent has also been consistently rewarding in our experience even when a pharmacologic agent does not seem to produce any significant prolongation in the effective refractory period of the Kent bundle.[31] A reversal of drug effects can often be demonstrated with isoproterenol in the laboratory[32] and frequently translates into clinical recurrences that can be treated with the addition of beta-blockers.[33] An isoproterenol infusion test is currently a part of the routine assessment of drug therapy evaluation of SVT in our laboratory. Drugs capable of preventing tachycardia induction despite isoproterenol infusion have been quite reliable in preventing clinical recurrences in our experience.

2. For patients with drug-resistant SVT or those considered better suited for nonpharmacologic therapy, such as ablation or surgery, EPS constitute the essential initial step.

Patients with narrow QRS SVT not included in the above two categories can often be managed safely with empiric drug therapy. In many cases the knowledge of the exact underlying mechanism is not essential for successful therapy. Furthermore, class 1A and 1C drugs depress retrograde conduction in both the AV node as well as in the AP and are quite effective in controlling the reentry process. In addition, these agents also are capable of preventing the triggering mechanism which compliments their depressant effect on reentrant circuits.[34]

On the other hand, without availability of a definitive diagnosis, a considerable degree of uncertainty exists concerning the exact origin in patients presenting as a wide QRS complex tachycardia. Therefore, invasive electrophysiological studies are still the best technique for diagnosis, prognostication, as well as selection of pharmacologic and nonpharmacologic therapeutic modalities in patients with wide QRS SVT.

References

1. Mendez C, Moe GK. Demonstration of a dual A-V nodal conduction system in the isolated rabbit heart. Circ Res 1966;19:378.
2. Durrer D, Schoo L, Schuilenburg RM, Wellens HJJ. The role of premature beats in the initiation and termination of supraventricular tachycardia in the Wolff-Parkinson-White syndrome. Circulation 1967;36:644.
3. Goldreyer BN, Damato AN. The essential role of atrioventricular conduction delay in the initiation of paroxysmal supraventricular tachycardia. Circulation 1971;43:679.
4. Denes P, Dhingra RC, Chuquimia R, et al: Demonstration of dual A-V nodal pathways in patients with paroxysmal supraventricular tachycardia. Circulation 1973;43:549.
5. Wellens HJJ. Unusual examples of supraventricular re-entrant tachycardia. Circulation 1975;51:997–1002.
6. Gallagher JJ, Gilbert M, Svenson RH, et al. Wolff-Parkinson-White syndrome: the problem, evaluation and surgical considerations. Circulation 1975;51:767–785.
7. Goldreyer BN, Gallagher JJ, Damato AN. The electrophysiologic demonstration of atrial ectopic tachycardia in man. Am Heart J 1973;85:205.
8. Josephson ME, Kastor JA. Paroxysmal supraventricular tachycardia. Is the atrium a necessary link? Circulation 1976;54:430.
9. WU D, Denes P, Amat-y-Leon F, et al. An unusual variety of atrioventricular nodal re-entry due to retrograde dual atrioventricular nodal pathways. Circulation 1977;56:50–59.
10. Akhtar M, Damato AN. Determination of site of re-entry from antegrade and retrograde conduction ratios in paroxysmal atrioventricular junctional re-entrant tachycardia (abstr). Clin Res 1976;24:204A.
11. Akhtar M, Damato AN, Ruskin JN, Batsford WP, Reddy CP, Ticzon AR, Dhatt M, Gomes JAC, Calon AH. Antegrade and retrograde conduction characteristics in three patterns of paroxysmal atrioventricular junctional reentrant tachycardia. Am Heart J 1978;95:22–42.
12. Wu D, et al. Clinical electrocardiographic and electrophysiologic observations in patients with paroxysmal supraventricular tachycardia. Am J Cardiol 1978;41:1045–1051.
13. Josephson ME. Paroxysmal supraventricular tachycardia. An electrophysiologic approach. Am J Cardiol 1978;41:1123–1126.
14. Wu D, et al. Chronic electrophysiological study in patients with recurrent paroxysmal tachycardia: A new method for developing successful oral antiarrhythmic therapy. In Kulbertus HE, ed. Reentrant Arrhythmias. Baltimore, University Park Press, 1976.
15. Bauernfeind RA, Wyndham CR, Dhingra RC, et al. Serial electrophysiologic testing of

multiple drugs in patients with atrioventricular nodal reentrant paroxysmal tachycardia. Circulation 1980;62:1341–1349.
16. Akhtar M. Supraventricular tachycardias. Electrophysiologic mechanisms, diagnosis and pharmacologic therapy. In Josephson ME, Wellens HJJ, eds. Tachycardias: Mechanisms, Diagnosis, Treatment. Philadelphia, Lea and Febiger, 1984:137–169.
17. Gallagher JJ, Sealy WC, Cox JL, German LD, Kasell JH, Bardy GH, Packer DL. Results of surgery for preexcitation caused by accessory atrioventricular pathways in 267 consecutive cases. In Josephson ME, Wellens HJJ, eds. Tachycardias: Mechanisms, Diagnosis, Treatment. Philadelphia, Lea and Febiger, 1984;259–269.
18. Scheinman MM, Morady F, Hess DS, Gonzalez R. Catheter-induced ablation of the atrioventricular junction to control refractory supraventricular arrhythmias. JAMA 1982;242:851.
19. Gallagher JJ, Cox JL, German LD, Kasell JH. Nonpharmacologic treatment of supraventricular tachycardia. In Josephson ME, Wellens HJJ, eds. Tachycardias: Mechanisms, Diagnosis, Treatment. Philadelphia, Lea and Febiger, 1984;271–285.
20. Bar FW, Brugada P, Dassen WRM, Wellens HJJ. Differential diagnosis of tachycardia with narrow QRS complex (shorter than 0.12 second). Am J Cardiol 1984;54:555–560.
21. Coumel P, Attuel P, Leclerq JF. Permanent form of junctional reciprocating tachycardia: mechanism, clinical and therapeutic implications. In Narula OS, ed. Cardiac Arrhythmias: Electrophysiology, Diagnosis and Management. Baltimore, Williams & Wilkins, 1979:347.
22. Farre J, Ross D, Wiener I, Bar FW, Vanagt EJ, Wellens HJJ. Reciprocal tachycardias using accessory pathways with long conduction times. Am J Cardiol 1979;44:1099–1109.
23. Gallagher JJ, Sealy WC. The permanent form of junctions reciprocating tachycardia. Further elucidation of the underlying mechanism. Eur J Cardiol 1978;8:413.
24. Dongas J, Lehmann MH, Mahmud R, Denker S, Soni J, Akhtar M. Value of pre-existing bundle branch block in the electrocardiographic differentiation of supraventricular from ventricular origin of wide QRS tachycardia. Am J Cardiol 1985;55:717–721.
25. Marriott HJL, Sandler IA. Criteria, old and new, for differentiating between ectopic ventricular beats and aberrant ventricular conduction in the presence of atrial fibrillation. Prog Cardiovasc Dis 1966;9:18.
26. Wellens HJJ, Bar FWHM, Lie KI. The value of the electrocardiogram in the differential diagnosis of a tachycardia with a widened QRS complex. Am J Med 1978;64:27–33.
27. Akhtar M. Electrophysiologic bases for wide QRS complex tachycardia. PACE 1983;6:81–98.
28. Benditt DG, Pritchett ELC, Gallagher JJ. Spectrum of regular tachycardias with wide QRS complexes in patients with accessory atrioventricular pathways. Am J Cardiol 1978;42:828–838.
29. Prystowsky EN, Klein GJ, Rinkenberger RL, Heger JJ, Naccarelli GV, Zipes DP. Clinical efficacy and electrophysiologic effects of encainide in patients with Wolff-Parkinson-White syndrome. Circulation 1984;69:278–287.
30. Naccarelli GV, Dougherty AH, Berns E, Rinkenberger RL. Assessment of antiarrhythmic drug efficacy in the treatment of supraventricular arrhythmias. Am J Cardiol 1986;58:31C–36C.
31. Wellens HJJ, et al. Effect of drugs in the Wolff-Parkinson-White syndrome: Importance of initial length of effective refractory period of the accessory pathway. Am J Cardiol 1980;46:665–669.
32. Wellens HJJ, et al. Effect of isoproterenol on the anterograde refractory period of the accessory pathway in patients with the Wolff-Parkinson-White syndrome. Am J Cardiol 1982;50:180–184.
33. Dongas J, Tchou P, Mahmud R, Lehmann MH, Denker S, Akhtar M. Catecholamine-mediated reversal of procainamide induced retrograde block in paroxysmal supraventricular tachycardias: possible cause of treatment failures (abstr). Circulation 1985;72(Pt.II):III-126.
34. Wellens HJJ, Brugada P. Electrophysiology in assessing supraventricular arrhythmias: value of programmed stimulation in predicting and understanding efficacy of encainide. Am J Cardiol 1986;58:37C–40C.

14

Atrial Unipolar Waveform Analysis During Retrograde Conduction Over Left-Sided Accessory Atrioventricular Pathways

Jerónimo Farré, Angel Grande
Jorge Martinell, Julián Fraile
José A Ramirez, Gregorio Rábago

Introduction

The understanding of the mechanisms and clinical consequences of tachycardia in man and the design of a successful therapeutic strategy requires the identification of the anatomic and/or physiologic arrhythmogenic substrate, the natural triggers of the arrhythmia, and the possible modulating bystanders. Supraventricular tachycardia, in its various forms, is not only a very frequent type of arrhythmia, but also an investigational model to study electrophysiologic concepts that can subsequently be extended to the field of ventricular tachyarrhythmias. AV junctional tachycardias utilizing extranodal accessory pathways (AP) offer us an unparalleled substrate to explore mechanisms, triggers, and modulating factors with the aid of direct cardiac stimulation and recording techniques. As repeatedly stated throughout this book, programmed electrical stimulation of the heart was first used in the human cardiac laboratory to study patients with AP.[1] Similar principles were subsequently applied to explore the mecha-

From: Brugada P, Wellens HJJ. CARDIAC ARRHYTHMIAS: Where To Go From Here? Mount Kisco, NY, Futura Publishing Company, Inc., © 1987.

nisms underlying ventricular tachycardia in man.[2] The yield of stimulation studies during the last 20 years can probably be evaluated best by balancing their contribution to the understanding of the arrhythmias related to the existence of bypass tracts. Stimulation studies cannot be viewed apart from intracardiac electrocardiography. Recording techniques, despite the impressive, almost sparkling, appearance of multichannel analogic displays of intracardiac electrograms that usually illustrate electrophysiologic papers and monographs, have received relatively little attention. The history of medicine shows examples of instances in which methods are used without a sufficient understanding of their underlying principles. One such situation is that of the recording techniques utilized to perform electrophysiologic studies. In this paper, we will review some methodologic concepts regarding the use of intracardiac recordings and offer our preliminary views on how the analysis of intracardiac waveforms can help to open new avenues in clinical electrophysiology.

Can We Expect to Grasp New Information From Invasive Electrophysiologic Tests?

A major question asked by the organizers of this meeting is where to go in the future in the field of invasive electrophysiologic testing. We certainly need some fresh ideas to maintain the pace of progress in clinical electrophysiology. The innovative ideas have to come from new methodologic refinements and/or conceptual views. The way in which they will arrive is impossible to predict. During the initial days of clinical electrophysiology, programmed electrical stimulation was introduced in the human cardiac laboratory imitating the methods utilized by the basic electrophysiologists and to answer questions posed by clinical arrhythmias. Inspiration from work at the cellular and animal electrophysiology level is still not only a valid approach, but a "must" to enhance our understanding of tachycardia, its site of origin, substrate, triggers, modulating influences, and the beneficial and deleterious effects of antiarrhythmic drugs.

In 1970, only 3 years after the introduction of programmed electrical stimulation as a new clinical method of investigation, Durrer and co-workers in their classic paper, "Pre-excitation Revisited,"[3] made the first appraisal of the state of the art of invasive electrophysiologic tests in the study of the AV junction. Concepts discussed in that article, such as supernormal conduction in the AP, spatial relation of the bypass tracts to the specific conduction system, and mode of transition from the anomalous bundle to the receiving structure, remain today relatively unexplored.[3] The topic of how the AP is proximally connected to the atrial myocardium and the way in which the excitation wave propagates during VA conduction over the bypass tract is the major issue of this chapter.

Anisotropic Conduction at the Sites of Insertion of Accessory Pathways

Propagation of the cardiac impulse within the myocardium rather than being uniform seems frequently to follow an uneven pattern that depends on various factors such as: (1) the orientation of the muscular fibers relative to the site of impulse formation, (2) the size of the individual myocardial bundles, (3) the quantity of the conjunctive tissue encircling those bundles, (4) the pattern of branching, and (5) the number and disposition of junctions with adjacent muscular fascicles. The myocardium, being a tridimensional structure, offers a number of possibilities. Spach et al. have shown that the conduction velocity within a myocardial bundle is faster in the longitudinal than in the transverse direction, a phenomenon that has been called "uniform anisotropic propagation."[4] In addition, packing of myocardial fibers into bundles may lead to a "nonuniform anisotropic conduction" in which propagation perpendicular to the longitudinal axis of these bundles is discontinuous so that adjacent fascicles are activated irregularly resulting in fragmentation of the extracellularly recorded unipolar electrograms.[5] The junctions between myocardial bundles represent an additional level of structural complexity that results in a reduction of the conduction velocity, changes in the configuration of the unipolar extracellular excitation wavefront, and a modification in the safety factor of propagation of the cardiac impulse.[5]

The proximal and distal insertion of an AP provide relatively simple models to study anisotropic conduction. The very strategic situation of the coronary sinus (CS) and the recording of unipolar "unfiltered" atrial electrograms along this structure during orthodromic circus movement tachycardia (CMT) and/or ventricular pacing could enable us to study whether signals consistent with the existence of an anisotropic propagation of the cardiac impulse during retrograde conduction over an AP can be identified at the vicinity of the atrial insertion of the bypass tract.

Cardiac Electrogram Waveform

The recording of unipolar and bipolar electrograms has been utilized to date to perform activation maps at the atrial and ventricular level.[6,7] Several investigators have studied the waveforms of the recorded bipolar electrograms both in the normal and infarcted ventricular myocardium.[8-12] The shape of the waveform recorded with bipolar electrodes depends on several variables such as the interelectrode distance, the orientation of both electrodes relative to the spread of the electric field generated during the activation process of the underlying myocardium, and the characteristics of the electronic filters of the amplifiers used to handle the generated biopotentials.[13] The morphologic characteristics of the unipolar waveforms depend on the location of the exploring (positive) electrode relative to the myocardial tissue, the direction of the propagating electric wavefront, and the filter settings of the amplifier. In unipolar recordings, the indifferent electrode is placed far away from the exploring electrode to prevent changes in the position of the former electrode from resulting in significant modifications in the shape of the recorded electrogram.

The use of frequency cutoffs below 0.1 Hz for the high-pass filter and above 400–1000 Hz for the low-pass setting gives us signals in which slow and fast components are not "artifactually" lost or enhanced. In addition, these undifferentiated recordings allow us to measure the amplitude (voltage) of the signal, something that cannot be done with "filtered" bipolar (or unipolar) electrograms. Bipolar recordings, as performed in most laboratories, are more suitable for measuring activation times than for waveform interpretation. To analyze the configuration and voltage of endocardial or epicardial electrograms, unipolar DC recordings or AC recordings using ample bandwidth filters, are more appropriate.

The Role of the Electronic Filters Utilized in Bioelectric Amplifiers

Amplifiers used in clinical electrophysiology may be AC- or DC-coupled. Most of the time, near DC amplifiers are used instead of true DC amplifiers. In true DC amplifiers, the low frequency response is 0 Hz whereas the near-DC version of an AC amplifier has frequency responses from 0.05 Hz to 0.1 Hz. Surface ECG and so-called "unfiltered" recordings utilize near-DC amplifiers with a high-pass filter (low frequency response) between 0.05 and 0.1 Hz. As shown in panels A, B, and C of Figure 1, DC or almost-DC recordings do not modify the shape of the input signal. Bipolar intracardiac recordings are usually obtained using a high-pass filtering setting of 30, 50, 80, or 100 Hz. These high-pass filters (lower frequency limit) function as an analogic differentiator producing an output whose voltage is proportional to the rate of change in voltage of the input signal. In panels D, E, and F, an input signal having a constant amplitude (voltage) but different rates of rise is fed into an AC amplifier having a lower frequency limit of 80 Hz. As shown, the resulting output signal has a voltage that is a function of the rate of rise of the input voltage and not of the magnitude of that voltage. Using this type of setting for the high-pass filter makes it inappropriate to speak about voltages of the recorded signals. In panels G and H, this point is illustrated with real electrograms. In panel G, a unipolar "unfiltered" signal recorded from within the CS during right atrial pacing has been fed into a DC amplifier, the output signal being identical in configuration to the input voltage. When the same signal is introduced in an AC amplifier (panel H), the input information is differentiated; the resulting sharp atrial deflection is a derivative of the input atrial potential; its peak corresponds to the maximal change in rate of the intrinsic deflection of the unipolar potential; its amplitude is proportional to the frequency characteristics of the input signal, not to the input amplitude. As shown in panel H, the input ventricular electrogram consists of two negative deflections; the first is large and slow and the second is of a very low amplitude but its intrinsic deflection is almost as fast as that of the preceding wave. The differentiated ventricular output consists of two waves of a similar amplitude since the rate of change of the input deflections was analogous.

AC amplifiers also have a low-pass filter (high frequency cutoff) that creates a "time-rise" in the input signals. The waves depicted in the upper tracing of panels A, B, and C of Figure 1 have been created by modifying the upper frequency limit of the generated "square" wave, from 400 Hz (panel A) to 30 Hz (panel B) and 5 Hz (panel C). Very fast deflections will be lost if the high frequency cutoff is set too low. In clinical electrophysiology, the upper frequency limit is usually set between 400 and 1200 Hz but cutoffs above 120 Hz are acceptable for most purposes.

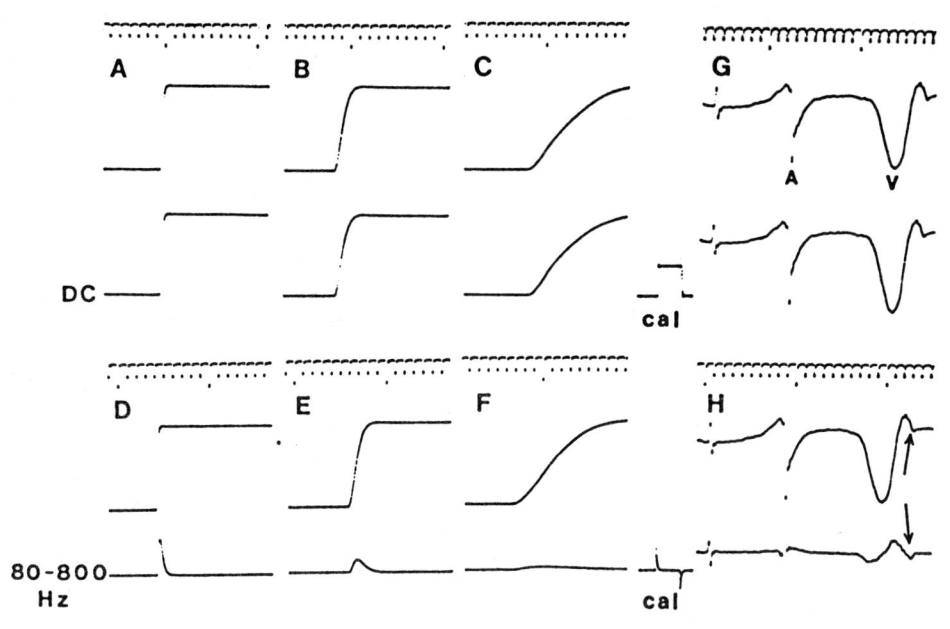

Figure 1: Role of the high-pass (lower frequency cutoff) filter setting in the recording of biopotentials. The rate of rise of the signal shown in the upper tracing of panels A, B, and C progressively diminishes but its amplitude is maintained constant. This signal is fed into the input of a DC amplifier (lower tracing); the output signal is identical in configuration and amplitude to the input signal. The calibration signal is a square wave and the same for panels A–G. In panel G, an actual AV recording in the CS is fed into the same DC amplifier and the resulting deflection maintains the same characteristics as the incoming potentials. In panels D–H, the same input signals are fed into the input of an AC amplifier whose low frequency limit has been set at 80 Hz (-3dB). The calibration signal was also the same for the four panels. In spite of a constant input voltage in panels D–F, the recorded output was very different since the latter was an expression of the slope of the original signal (see text). These three panels illustrate that measuring the voltage of signals recorded with conventional filtering settings (low frequency limit between 30 and 100 Hz) is incorrect since the actual dimensions of the measurement is Volt/sec. In panel H, the intrinsic deflection of the atrial electrogram results in a sharp spike whereas the largest deflection of the ventriculogram (which originally was of a similar or larger amplitude) because of its slow characteristics is transformed into a much smaller wave in the AC recording. Moreover, the second deflection of the input ventriculogram, which in the above top tracing is of a very small voltage, in the differentiated output has a similar amplitude to the first ventricular wave reflecting that the slope of both incoming signals was the same.

The Waveform of the Unipolar Electrogram

The shape of the unfiltered unipolar myocardial electrogram depends on various factors such as: (1) the distance between the recording point and the site of impulse formation, (2) the distance between the exploring electrode and the surface of the excitable myocardium, (3) the orientation of the underlying myocardial bundles relative to the direction of the propagating excitation wavefront, (4) the size of the probing electrode, (5) the anatomic characteristics of the investigated myocardium (diameter of bundles of fibers, presence of conjunctive tissue and/or Purkinje fibers), and (6) the functional status of the explored area secondary to various influences (hypoxia, electrolyte changes, catecholamine

248 • CARDIAC ARRHYTHMIAS

level, etc.). Spach et al. have shown that the extracellularly recorded unipolar potential at a certain point is influenced by the electric currents up and down the myocardial fiber, by those immediately beneath the electrode, and by those generated by fibers in the vicinity of the recording site.[13,14] The distance between the recording electrode and the activating myocardium influences both the shape and amplitude of the unipolar electrogram. As the exploring electrode is moved away from the myocardial surface, the amplitude of the recorded unipolar potential decreases and the time between the positive and negative peaks of the biphasic waveform increases.[14] Not infrequently the extracellular unipolar electrogram has a polyphasic waveform which, according to Spach et al., is due to the superimposition of currents from different electrically isolated strands of muscle that are activated asynchronously and that are situated at varying distances from the recording electrode.[14] The time of the maximum negative slope of the unipolar extracellular potential (intrinsic deflection) has been shown to be coincidental with the value of $t(V_{max})$ of the cell (or group of fibers) immediately underneath the recording site.[15]

Spach et al. have also established that in the uniform anisotropic cardiac muscle, conduction along the longitudinal axis of the fibers produces a characteristic biphasic smooth unipolar waveform.[16] In the transverse direction, the unipolar extracellular recording is of a smaller amplitude and its positive-negative deflection is preceded by a negative, relatively slow deviation of the base line. Figure 2 displays the configuration of the "normal" atrial electrograms recorded

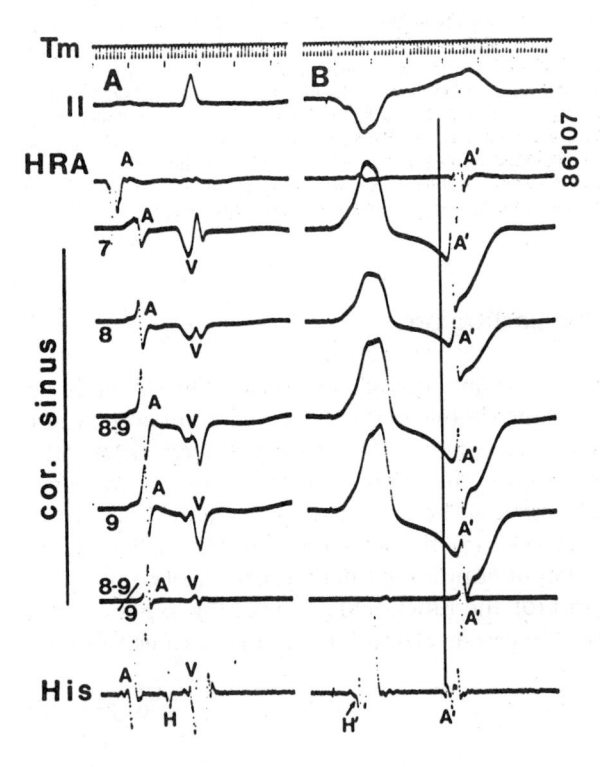

Figure 2: Recordings obtained during sinus rhythm (panel A) and pacing from the right ventricular apex (panel B). Tracings are organized in a similar manner throughout the chapter. From top to bottom: time marks (10 and 100 ms) and recordings from the high right atrium (filtered bipolar), CS (unfiltered unipolar and filtered bipolar), and His (filtered bipolar). The numbers in the CS leads indicate the sites at which the exploring electrodes were located (7=posterior free wall; 8=posterolateral; 9=lateral; 8-9=intermediate position between points 8 and 9). In this patient, retrograde conduction was over a slow AV nodal pathway. The unfiltered CS unipolar retrograde atrial electrograms (A') show a normal smooth biphasic deflection.

with a quadripolar catheter from within the CS during VA conduction over the normal His-AV nodal pathway. These electrograms are consistent with longitudinal propagation over a uniform anisotropic myocardium.

The same investigators have also shown that in the nonuniform anisotropic cardiac muscle, the waveform of the unipolar electrograms recorded parallel to the longitudinal axis of the preparation consists of a large positive-negative deflection with additional small fast spikes superimposed on the negative component of the electrogram.[16] When propagation occurs in the transverse direction, the waveform is of a lower amplitude and shows a fragmented pattern due to the superimposition of small fast deflections.[5,16]

Other waveforms observed when obtaining unipolar recordings deserve a further comment. Spach et al. have demonstrated that positive uniphasic unipolar extracellular electrograms are characteristic of terminating propagation or collision.[4] The latter waveforms represent zero velocity or, in other words, no propagation away from the recording site. In addition, work from the same laboratory has established that the unipolar waveform is negative within a very small area (100–200 μm along the fast axis) in the immediate vicinity of the site of onset of excitation.[17]

According to the above experimental observations, unipolar electrograms recorded close to the atrial junction of an AP during retrograde conduction might reflect several features depending on a number of individual circumstances (Fig. 3) such as:

1. the spatial relation between the recording electrode and the insertion of the AP,
2. the orientation of the fibers of the AP relative to that of the atrial myocardium at the site of junction,
3. the orientation of the atrial fibers relative to the location of the exploring unipolar electrodes in the CS,
4. the gross anatomic characteristics of the AP (epicardial versus endocardial course and width and/or branching pattern of the atrial end).

The Technique of Recording Unipolar Atrial Electrograms

We have analyzed the waveforms of the unipolar atrial electrograms recorded within the CS in 23 consecutive patients with left-sided retrogradely conducting atrioventricular AP and without associated organic heart disease. All patients had CMT of the common (orthodromic) type and 15 patients also had atrial fibrillation, either as a spontaneously occurring clinical arrhythmia (six patients) or developing during the electrophysiologic study. The age of the patients was 32 ± 14 years and there were 13 males. In all patients the CS was mapped by means of a quadripolar catheter-electrode that was moved within the great cardiac vein to identify the area of earliest atrial excitation (bracketing) during retrograde conduction. In two female patients aged 11 and 13 years, the CS was mapped with a 5F bipolar catheter-electrode. Unipolar CS atrial electrograms were obtained from each electrode of the mapping catheter against a Wilson terminal during orthodromic CMT and/or ventricular pacing. These electrograms

250 • CARDIAC ARRHYTHMIAS

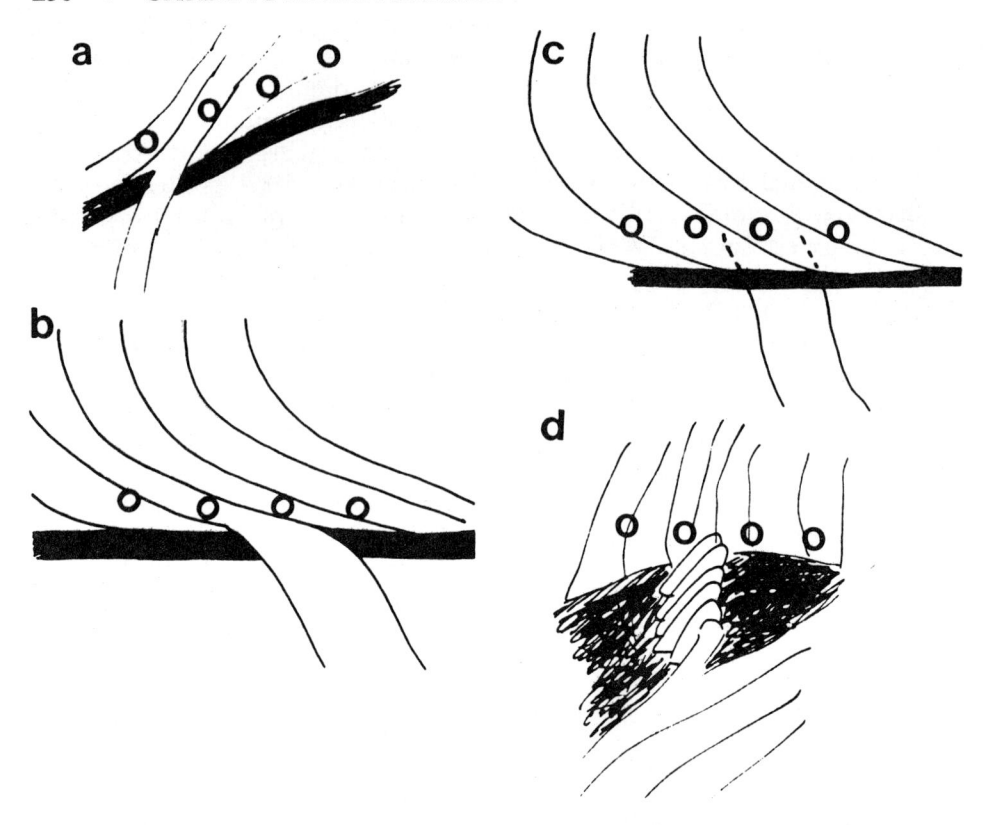

Figure 3: Schematic representation of different theoretical relations between the atrial myocardium and the upper insertion of an AP. Panels "a," "b," and "d" represent epicardially located bypass tracts; panel "c" exemplifies an AP with en endocardial course. Panel "d" depicts a hypothetical AP whose fibers are almost perpendicular to its longitudinal axis. The open circles represent the exploring electrodes of a quadripolar catheter. See text for further discussion.

were amplified and filtered between 0.1 and 1000 Hz to be directly recorded on paper at a speed of 250 mm/sec by means of a Mingograf ink-jet recorder whose galvanometers have a flat frequency response up to 1200 Hz. Although this analogic information was also stored on magnetic tape (recording speed 0.937 or 1.875 inches/sec), only the real time direct recordings obtained during the electrophysiologic study were used in this investigation. Most of the illustrations in this paper are made from these directly obtained recordings. When, for the sake of clarity, tracings have been played back from the tape, that statement is made in the corresponding legend of the figure.

Atrial Unipolar Waveforms During VA Conduction Over an Accessory Pathway

From the foregoing discussion, a number of atrial unipolar waveforms can be anticipated during VA conduction over an AP. We have examined separately the

Retrograde Atrial Unipolar Waveforms at the Bracketing Site

Close to the atrial insertion of the bypass tract, we have been able to register two major types of unipolar waveforms in the 20 patients in whom a clear bracketing could be demonstrated during CS mapping:
1. monophasic ("QS"-like) negative deflections lasting for 41 ± 11 ms in 10 patients (50%),
2. biphasic ("rS" or "RS"-like) positive-negative deflections lasting for 34 ± 8 ms in the remaining 10 patients.

Monophasic and biphasic deflections at the site of the shortest VA conduction time during CMT could consist of smooth or almost smooth waveforms (Fig. 4) or exhibit fragmentation, polyphasic forms, or a multimodal configuration (Fig. 5). QS-like deflections at the site of bracketing during CMT were smooth in three

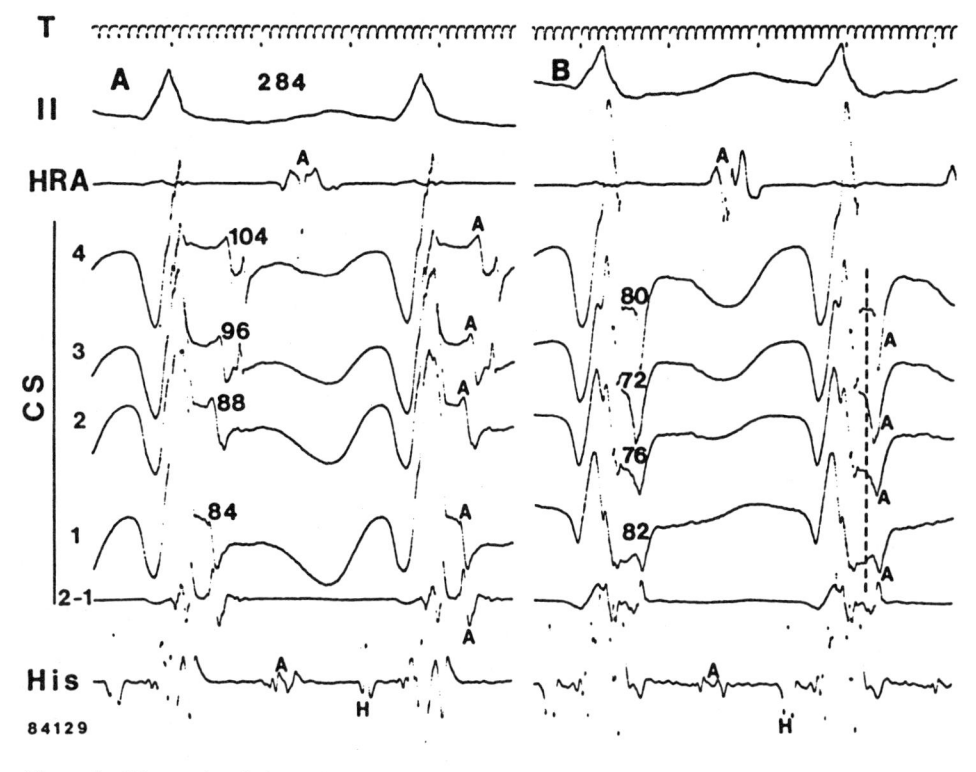

Figure 4: CS mapping during orthodromic CMT. The CS catheter is moved from a more proximal (panel A) to a more distal location (panel B). The atrial unipolar waveform at the site of bracketing is a QS-like almost smooth deflection. Note that in the proximal direction (panel A), the unipolar atrial electrogram is polyphasic. The filtered bipolar CS lead between electrodes #1 and #2 shows a fast deflection at the end of the local ventriculogram (panel B). This spike can be taken as the AP potential; as explained in the text, an alternative explanation is that such a spike represents local ventricular activation. As the CS catheter is progressed laterally it gets closer to the ventricular aspect of the AV groove (see text).

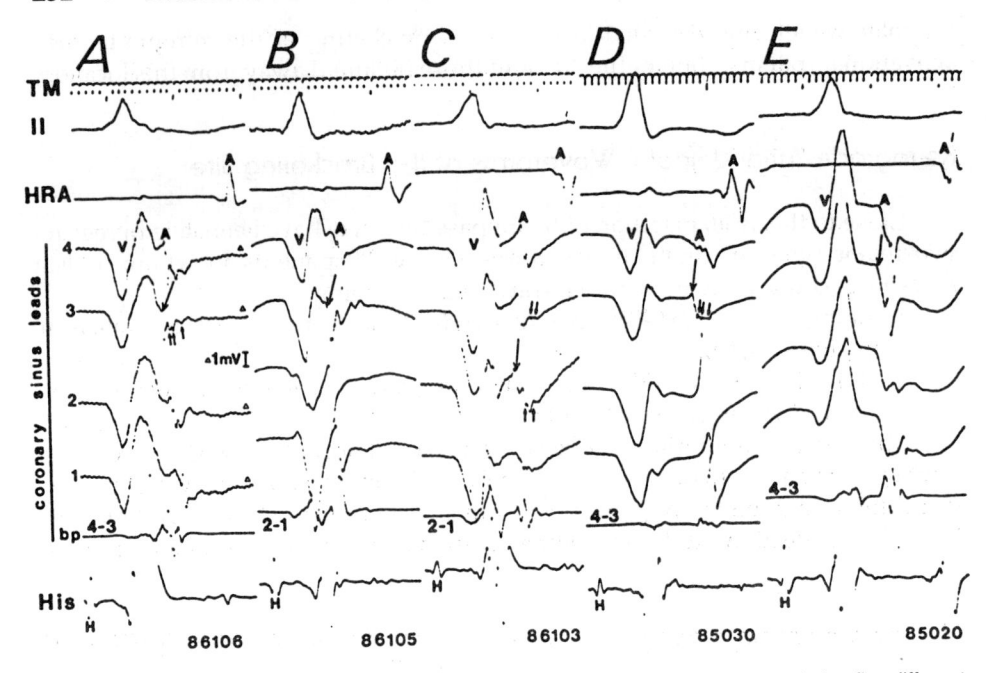

Figure 5: Recordings at the site of bracketing of the retrograde atrial excitation front during five different CMT (long arrow) showing fragmented, polyphasic, or bimodal unipolar atrial waveforms. Small arrows indicate the presence of fragmented or superimposed deflections. The numbers of the CS leads simply indicate the order of the individual electrodes (4 is the most proximal and 1 the most distal) and not definite anatomic positions.

patients (15%) (Fig. 4) and fragmented or polymodal in seven instances (35%) (Figs. 5A, 5E, and 6). Biphasic rS-like deflections at the site of bracketing were smooth in two patients and fragmented or multimodal in the remaining eight cases (Figs. 5B, 5C, 5D, 7, and 8). Therefore, smooth atrial waveforms at the site of bracketing (QS or rS-like) were present in only five patients.

Unipolar Waveforms During the Spread of Retrograde Atrial Activation Over the Accessory Pathway

The spread of the retrograde atrial activation front resulted in several different unipolar waveforms. Two of the three patients in whom the site of bracketing could not be reached had a left anterolateral AP. In both of them the most laterally obtained unipolar atrial electrogram was a monophasic negative waveform ("QS"-like pattern) thus suggesting it as the site of insertion of the AP or an area very close to it. From that site towards the posterior AV groove, the activation front resulted in biphasic smooth waveforms in one patient and in a biphasic wave with notches in the negative deflection in the other. The remaining patient with a posteroseptal AP showed biphasic smooth waveforms all over the CS.

In three patients in whom the earliest retrograde unipolar atrial electrogram

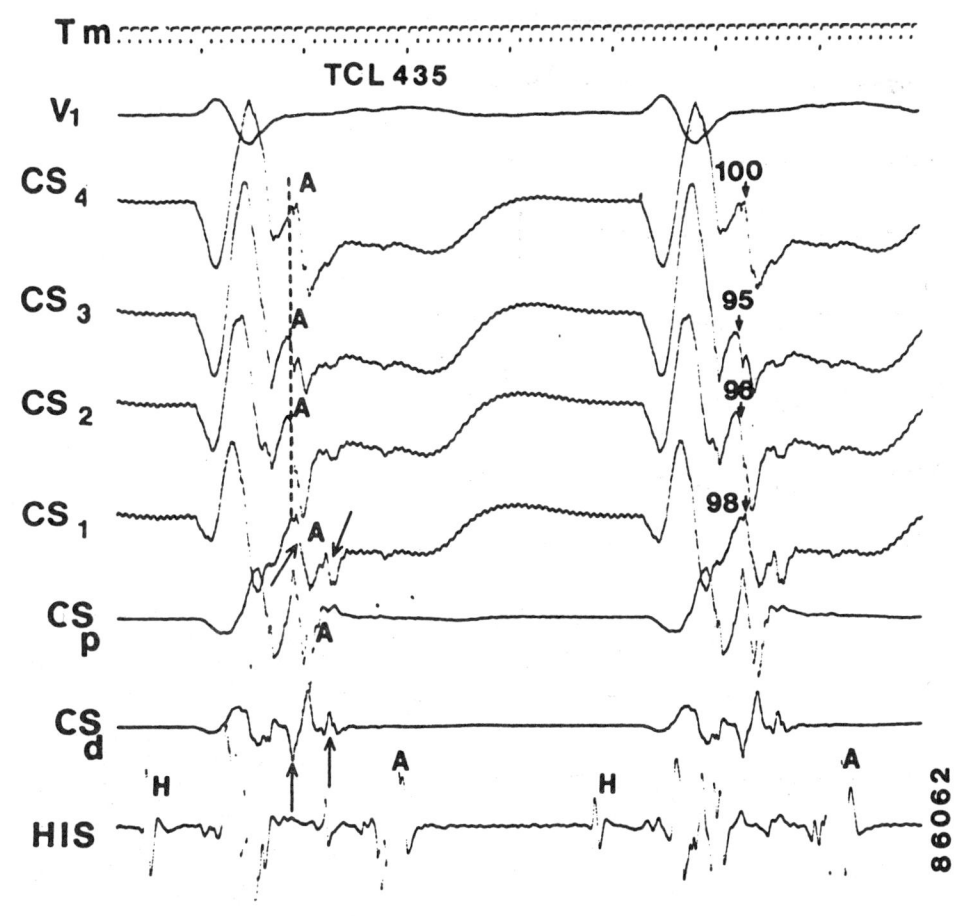

Figure 6: Bimodal QS-like unipolar atrial waveform at the site of bracketing of the retrograde atrial excitation during CMT. In CS_1, the atrial electrogram is a polyphasic rS-like deflection. In the filtered bipolar distal CS lead, a pseudo AP potential is recorded; the first peak corresponds to the intrinsic deflection of CS_2 and the second to that of the late deflection of CS_1 (see text).

had a monophasic negative configuration, the spread of activation, particularly in the direction towards the ostium of the CS, resulted in multiphasic waveforms (Fig. 4). The propagation of the retrograde atrial activation in the two patients with a biphasic smooth unipolar wavefront at the site of bracketing resulted in similar positive-negative "rS"-like deflections in the direction towards the lateral aspect of the ostium of the CS. In one of them, however, multiphasic rS-like deflections were recorded at the vicinity of the bracketing site towards the ostium of the CS.

In five of the 15 patients with multiphasic or multimodal "rS" or "QS"-like waveforms at the site of insertion of the AP, propagation of the retrograde activation front produced smooth "RS" deflections either to the right or to the left of the bracketing electrode (Figs. 5D and 8). It is interesting to note that in four patients and within 0.5–1.0 cm of the atrial insertion of the AP, "QS"-like

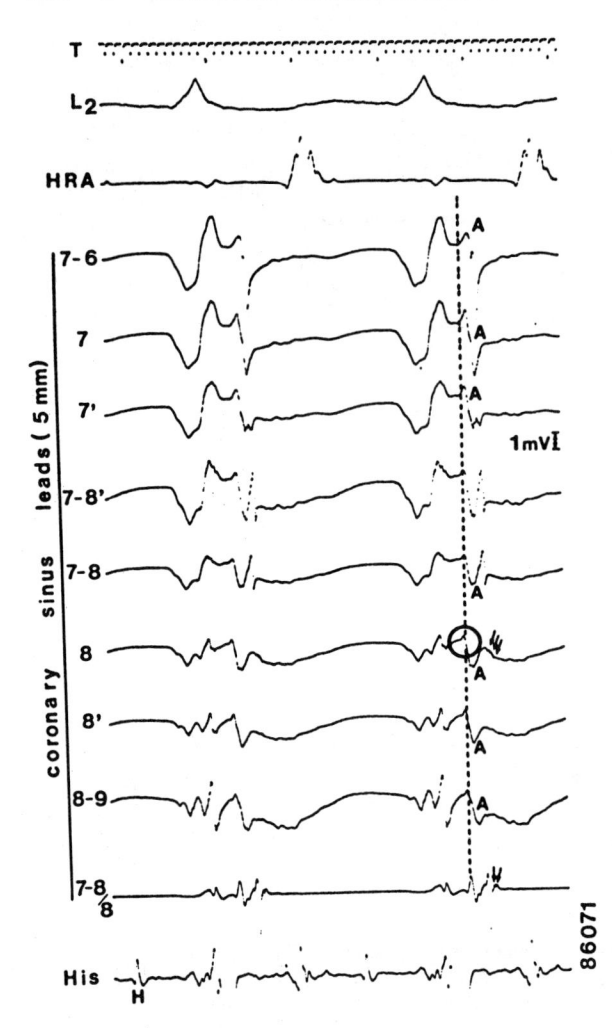

Figure 7: The numbers in the CS leads correspond to the anatomic positions defined in the legend of Figure 1. At the site of bracketing (CS_8) the atrial electrogram is biphasic (rS-like); a low amplitude fragmentation (arrows) is recorded at the offset of this atrial electrogram. In the position estimated between points 7 and 8, the unipolar electrogram is triphasic with two relatively fast deflections. The bipolar lead (7–8/8) shows a pseudo AP potential that can be easily differentiated from a true electrogram of the bypass with the aid of the unfiltered unipolar recordings.

fragmented deflections were recorded; the waveform at the site of shortest VA time during CMT was "QS"-like in two of these four patients (Fig. 9) and "rS"-like in the other two cases (Fig. 10).

Relation Between Fragmentation and Atrial Fibrillation

Since fragmentation of the recorded atrial unipolar electrogram during CMT either at the site of bracketing or at its vicinity was present in all but three patients, no relation could be established between this finding and the documentation of clinical- or laboratory-induced atrial fibrillation.

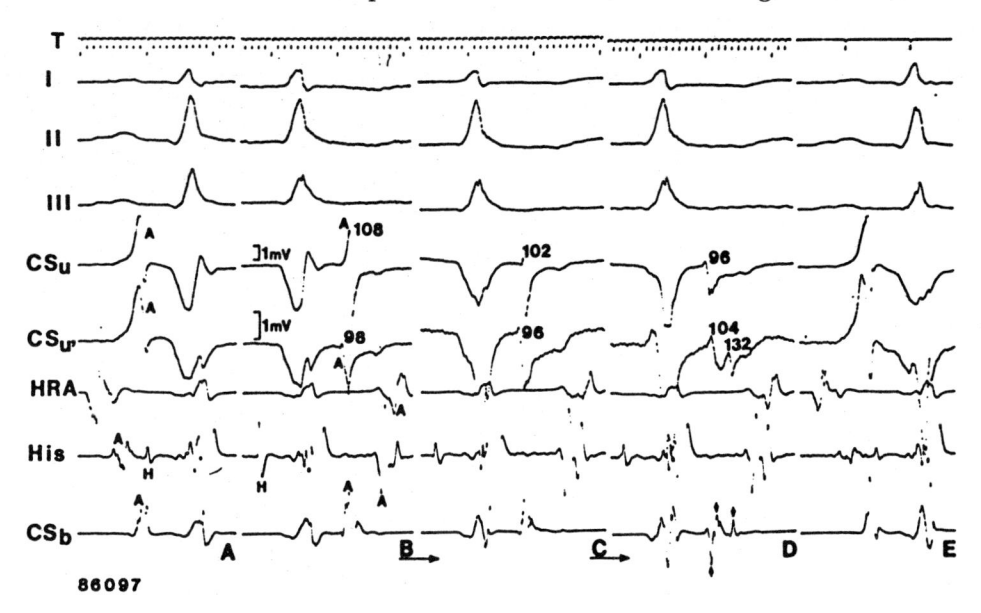

Figure 8: From top to bottom: time marks (10 and 100 ms), leads I, II, and III, unfiltered unipolar recordings from the electrodes of a bipolar catheter, bipolar filtered high right atrial lead, His bundle lead, and bipolar filtered CS lead. These tracings were taken in a 13-year-old patient in whom a 5F bipolar catheter was introduced in the CS. Panels A and E are recordings during sinus rhythm and panels B to D during CMT. In this patient, instead of searching for bracketing, the CS catheter was progressed looking for the site having the shortest VA conduction time. The latter value was found to be 96 ms. The filtered bipolar lead in panel D shows a pseudo AP potential that, as in previous figures, is due to the multiphasic nature of one of the contributing unipolar waveforms. The AP was laterally located and the unipolar CS atrial electrograms during sinus rhythm are mainly positive suggesting collision (see text).

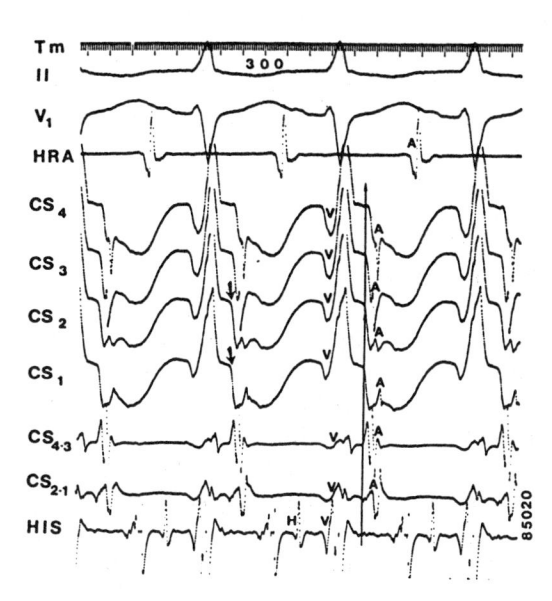

Figure 9: Tracing obtained from the tape on paper at an effective running speed of 200 mm/sec. Time marks (5 and 50 ms), leads II and V1, filtered bipolar HRA, unfiltered unipolar CS from electrode 4 (proximal) to 1 (distal), filtered bipolar CS leads (proximal and distal pairs), and His bundle lead. QS-like waveforms were recorded at sites 2 and 1 (arrows).

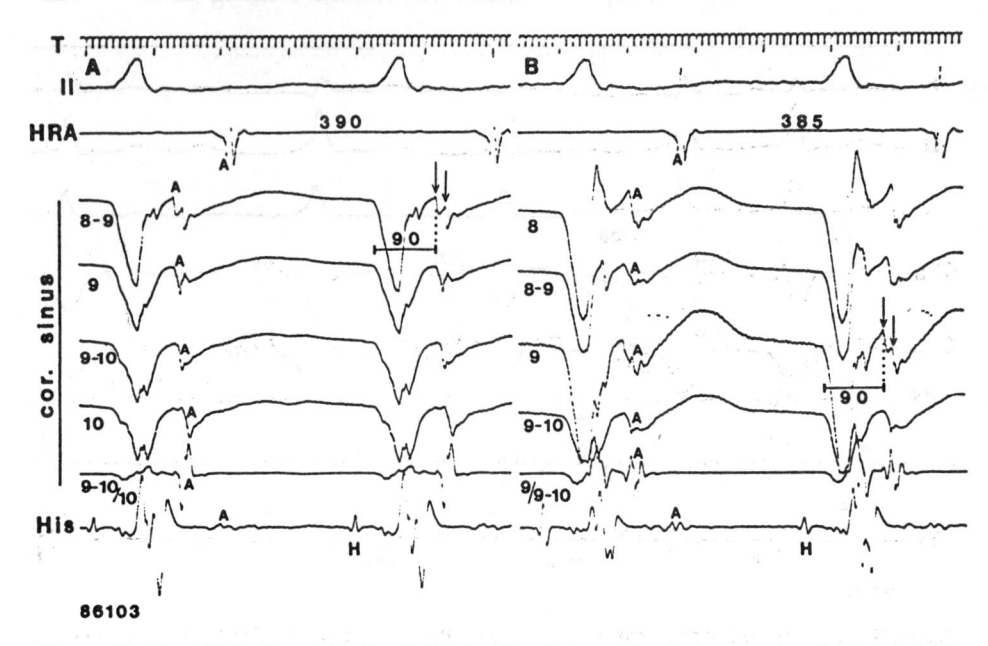

Figure 10: The distribution of leads, similar to other figures. Numbers are approximate anatomic locations within the CS (see legend of Figure 2; point 10 is anterolateral). In panel B, the CS catheter has been withdrawn slightly to reach the site of bracketing (shortest VA time, 90 ms). Although the atrial unipolar electrogram at the bracketing point shows a polymodal rS-like configuration, the waveform at its lateral vicinity is a QS-like complex (see text).

Relation Between the Width of the Unipolar Atrial Electrogram and the Retrograde AP Conduction Time and Refractory Period

The width of the unipolar atrial electrogram at the site of bracketing was 36 ± 11 ms (from 20 to 58 ms). In addition, the shortest VA conduction time was 87 ± 22 ms (60 to 156 ms) and the retrograde refractory period of the AP was 267 ± 53 ms (200 to 410 ms). Neither univariate nor multivariate regression analysis demonstrated any relation among these three variables.

Meaning of the Shape of the Major Deflection of the Unipolar Electrogram

Postmortem histologic studies in patients with the WPW syndrome as well as the anatomic experience derived from surgical interventions in patients with AP have led to the conclusion that bypass tracts can cross the AV groove at any level from the endocardium to the epicardium.[18,19] In addition, it can be postulated that the spatial relation between the CS (our recording site) and the uppermost portion of the AP can also be variable (Fig. 3C). Gallagher et al. have reported on the value of the morphology of the unipolar ventricular electrogram recorded during intraoperative epicardial ventricular mapping to differentiate epicardial and endocardial AP.[6] A similar remark as to the waveform of the unipolar atrial electrogram during VA conduction over the AP has not been made in mapping studies performed at the electrophysiology laboratory or the operating room. Our observation of two major unipolar atrial waveforms at the site of bracketing during retrograde conduction over the AP, "QS" and "rS"-like deflections, is consistent with an epicardial and endocardial location of the AP, respectively. Recording close to the atrial insertion of the bypass tract during retrograde conduction over the AP should generate a monophasic "QS"-like unipolar waveform if the anomalous bundle is epicardially located.

The observation of an "rS"-like morphology allows other interpretations apart from an endocardial situation. According to the experimental work of Spach et al., an epicardially located AP could also result in "rS"-like waveforms should the position of the closest exploring CS electrode be relatively distant from the actual insertion of the bypass tract.[17] If this is true, more than 50% of the left-sided AP could have an epicardial course, a figure that is in accord with the impression expressed by Becker et al. based on their pathologic observations in four patients with left-sided AP.[19] In the latter study it was found that the AP in each of the four patients skirted the annulus on its epicardial aspect.[19]

The fact that in certain patients "QS"-like unipolar atrial waveforms were recorded not only at the site of bracketing but also in its vicinity is compatible with a wide and/or branching atrial insertion of an epicardially located AP. This is the most likely interpretation in the light of the experiments of Spach et al. where "QS" monophasic waveforms could be recorded in a very small area around the site of onset of excitation.[17] Durrer et al. and Davies, Anderson, and Becker had previously suggested that the AP frequently arborizes close to its ventricular insertion.[20,21] However, the latter group of cardiac anatomists support the view that the atrial attachment of the AP is a single trunk 1 to 2 mm wide.[21] Our observations are not in accord with the latter opinion; we expect that wider or branching atrial junctions of the bypass tract will be anatomically demonstrated.

More difficult to explain is the observation of "QS"-shaped unipolar electrograms close to the site of insertion in patients in whom the atrial waveform at the site of bracketing is of the "rS" type; the latter observation is consistent with an AP having a rather wide and/or branching atrial insertion extending from the epicardium towards the endocardium. It is also possible in these patients that the real site of bracketing has been lost and that if an exploring electrode could have been positioned at that point, a negative "QS"-like waveform would have been obtained.

Relation Between Atrial Unipolar Waveform and Route of the Activation Front

Fragmentation of the unipolar atrial "unfiltered" waveform during VA conduction over the AP can be the reuslt of the asynchronous excitation of underlying muscular fascicles reflecting a nonuniform anisotropic propagation of the activation front.[4,5,13,14,16,17] That the presence of these multimodal "fragmented" waveforms was related to the direction of the retrograde atrial activation front could be demonstrated in two patients in this series. As shown in Figure 11, the introduction of single ventricular premature stimuli during ventricular pacing enabled us in one patient with two AP, one posteroseptal and the other left lateral, to observe that the atrial unipolar electrogram was fragmented only when VA conduction was over the posteroseptal AP. When VA conduction proceeded via either the left lateral AP or over the normal His-AV nodal axis, the atrial unipolar waveform was a smooth "RS"-like deflection in the same leads that depicted fragmented electrograms. The other ptaient had a left lateral AP and during CMT the unipolar atrial waveform at the site of bracketing as well as in its vicinity was multimodal or polyphasic (Fig.6). After the surgical division of this AP retrograde conduction via the normal His-AV nodal pathway was present and as shown in Figure 12, the waveform of the unipolar atrial electrograms recorded all over the CS, and particularly at the site where the AP was located preoperatively, consisted of a smooth biphasic deflection.

Comparison of the atrial waveforms recorded during sinus rhythm and CMT can be misleading since, theoretically speaking, fragmentation (multimodal, polyphasic or truly fragmented electrograms) could be due to fusion of two excitation fronts. In practice, when the latter occurs, the unipolar electrogram at that site should be predominantly positive as expected from a situation in which collision exists.[17] An example of the latter phenomenon is presented in Figure 13 where recordings during sinus rhythm (left panel) and CMT (right panel) are displayed. The most proximal and most distal electrodes (CS_4 and CS_1, respectively) are activated, during sinus rhythm, earlier than electrodes #3 and #2. This situation, which is frequently observed when the CS catheter is located laterally in the AV groove, results in the recording of a predominantly positive deflection (CS#3), and if fragmentation occurs, the possibility of fusion cannot be excluded (arrow). During CMT, fusion cannot be alleged since atrial activation is via the AP exclusively. Despite the theoretical considerations on the interpretation of fragmented and/or polyphasic unipolar waveforms during sinus rhythm, most of the time, the latter electrograms are smooth where wider, lower in the amplitude and fragmented or multiphasic deflections are recorded during CMT. This is true even at sites where the pattern of collision during sinus rhythm is present (Fig. 14).

Implications of Anisotropic Propagation of the Cardiac Impulse During CMT

In this study, we have found that during retrograde conduction over an AP, the atrial waveform close to the insertion of the bypass tract is frequently fragmented, multiphasic, or multimodal. The absence of smooth monophasic or biphasic waveforms suggests that the bundles of atrial fibers underlying the exploring electrode are activated asynchronously. In addition, in two of our patients we could demonstrate that the presence of these "superimposed" waveforms depends on the course of the excitation front. These observations are consistent with a nonuniform anisotropic propagation of the cardiac impulse. Further signs of anisotropy could have been identified if unipolar recordings had been obtained at different left and right atrial sites. This point is illustrated by the

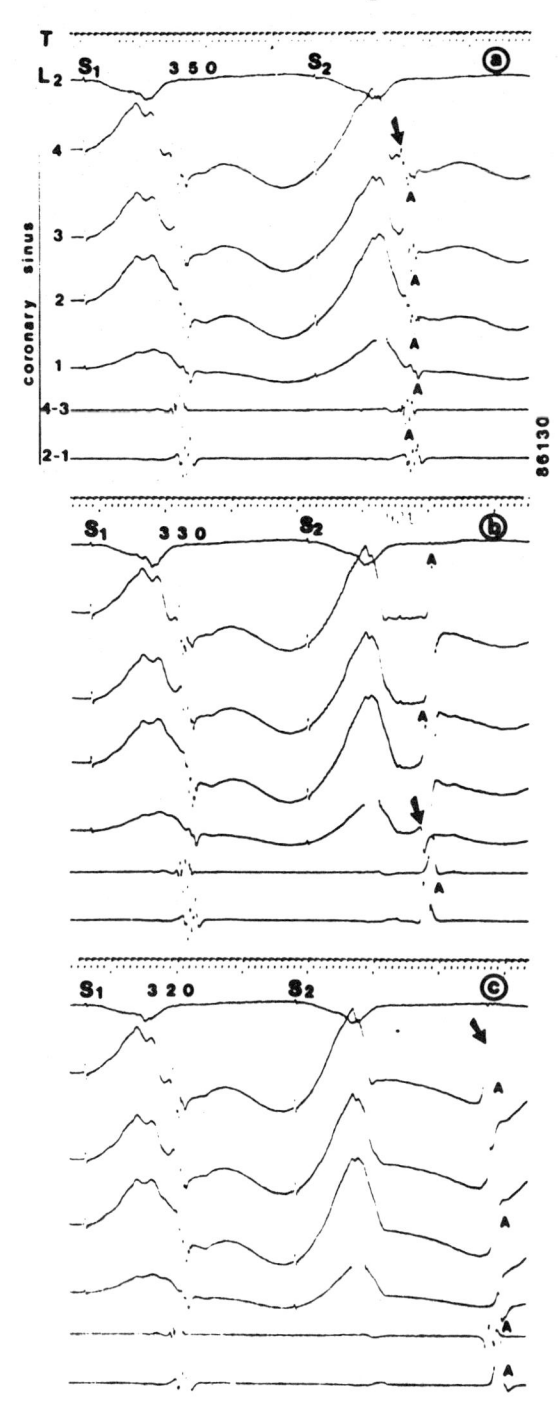

Figure 11: Panels "a", "b," and "c" show from top to bottom, time marks (10 and 100 ms), lead II, four unipolar CS leads, and two bipolar CS leads. The patient is being paced from the right ventricular apex, and the extrastimulus plus the last beat of the driving train are shown in the three panels. In panel "a," VA conduction after S_1 and S_2 is via a posteroseptal AP and the waveform of the CS unipolar atrial electrograms is fragmented (or multiphasic). At a premature beat interval of 330 ms (panel "b"), the posteroseptal AP blocks and VA conduction after S_2 is via an additional, laterally placed, bypass tract. The earliest retrograde atrial activity is now recorded in the most distal electrode of the C_S (CS_1) (arrow). By reducing the extrastimulus coupling interval in 10 ms (panel "c," S_1S_2 320 ms) that second AP also blocks and now VA conduction is via a slow AV nodal pathway; note that the earliest atrial electrogram is again the most proximal one (CS_4). During VA conduction over the lateral extranodal AP or the slow AV nodal pathway, the atrial unipolar electrogram consists of biphasic smooth waveforms that are of a larger amplitude than the multiphasic atrial deflections recorded at the same sites when VA conduction is over the posteroseptal AP. These findings demonstrate that the direction in which the activation front propagates plays an important role in the configuration of the recorded unipolar atrial electrograms.

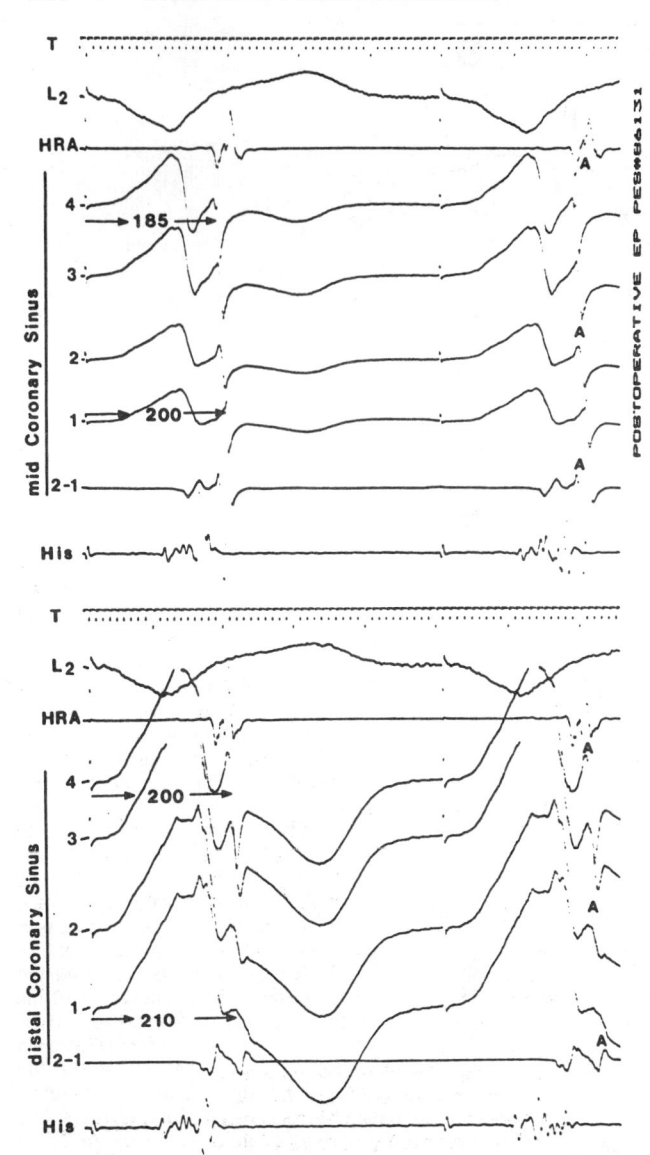

Figure 12: Same patient as in Figure 6. After the surgical section of the lateral AP, the patient underwent a new electrophysiologic study in which VA conduction over the AP was absent while retrograde conduction via the normal His-AV nodal pathway was maintained. The CS was extensively mapped during ventricular pacing and the recorded unipolar atrial waveforms were smooth and biphasic and lacking the polyphasic and fragmented configuration that was demonstrated in the preoperative study when conduction over the AP was present.

fact that the most widely fragmented or markedly polyphasic waveform was not always the one recorded at the site of bracketing. Figures 4, 7, and 8 show that multiphasic atrial waveforms were registered at some distance from the site at which the shortest VA time during CMT was measured. This finding mostly likely reflects that the exploring electrode is recording the asynchronous activation of two adjacent atrial bundles, one of them excited by a longitudinally propagating wavefront that spreads transversely to reach the second bundle (Fig. 3a, first electrode).

In this series, no relation could be established between the identification of

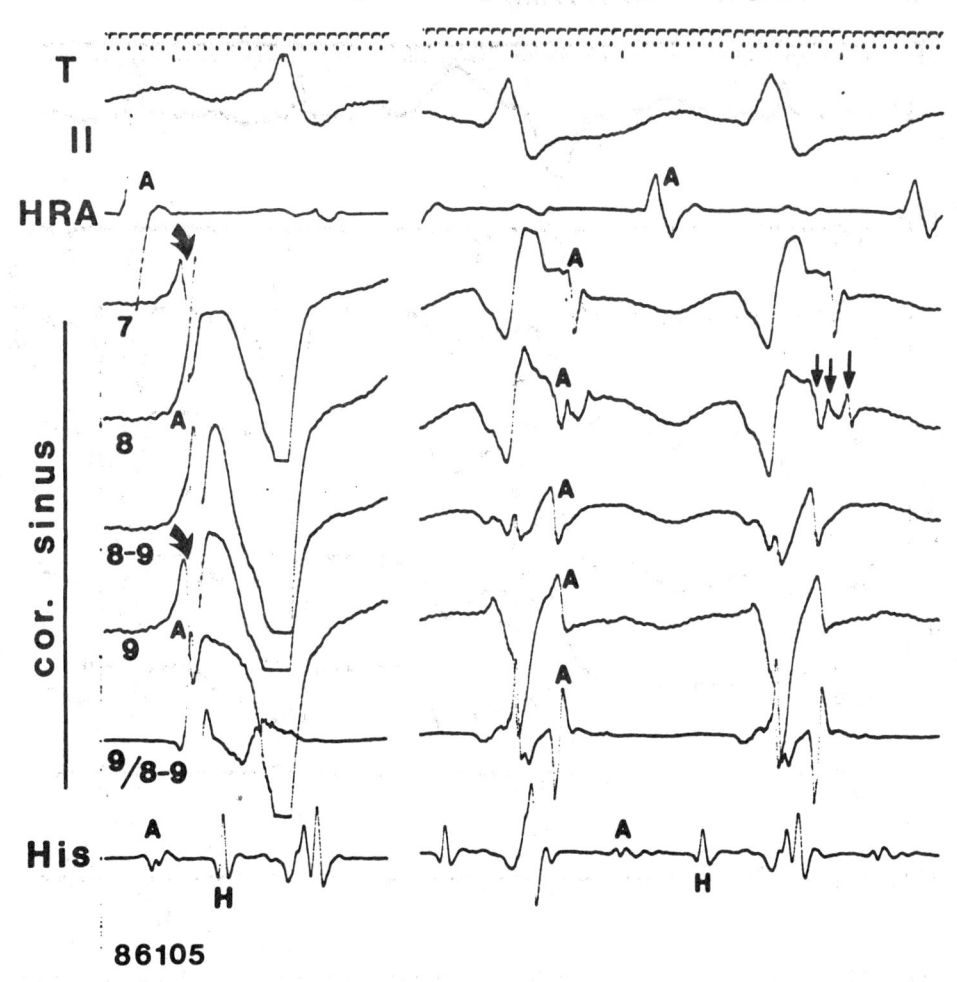

Figure 13: Recordings during sinus rhythm (left) and CMT. During sinus rhythm the filtered bipolar lead shows a very small deflection (arrow) between the atrial and ventricular electrograms. This spike represents a low amplitude deflection in one of the unipolar leads (CS_3, second arrow). The latter spike cannot be caused by the AP since it is registered after the onset of the delta wave. During CMT (right panel), the site of bracketing is identified under electrode #3 (thick arrow). In the filtered bipolar lead, a spike that could be caused by the AP electrogram is recorded between the atrial and ventricular deflections. In the four unipolar leads, a fast deflection is recorded at the offset of the ventriculogram thus suggesting the local ventricular activation rather than the potential of the AP.

fragmented or multimodal unipolar waveforms and the presence of clinical- and/or laboratory-induced atrial fibrillation. This, by no means, excludes that the relatively high incidence of atrial fibrillation in patients with AP is unrelated to nonuniform anisotropic conduction particularly if we take into account that fragmentation of the unipolar atrial electrograms in the neighborhood of the AP insertion was present in all but three patients in our series. According to Spach et al., the safety factor of propagation of the cardiac impulse is lowest in the direction parallel to the longitudinal axis of the myocardial fibers.[5] Under certain condi-

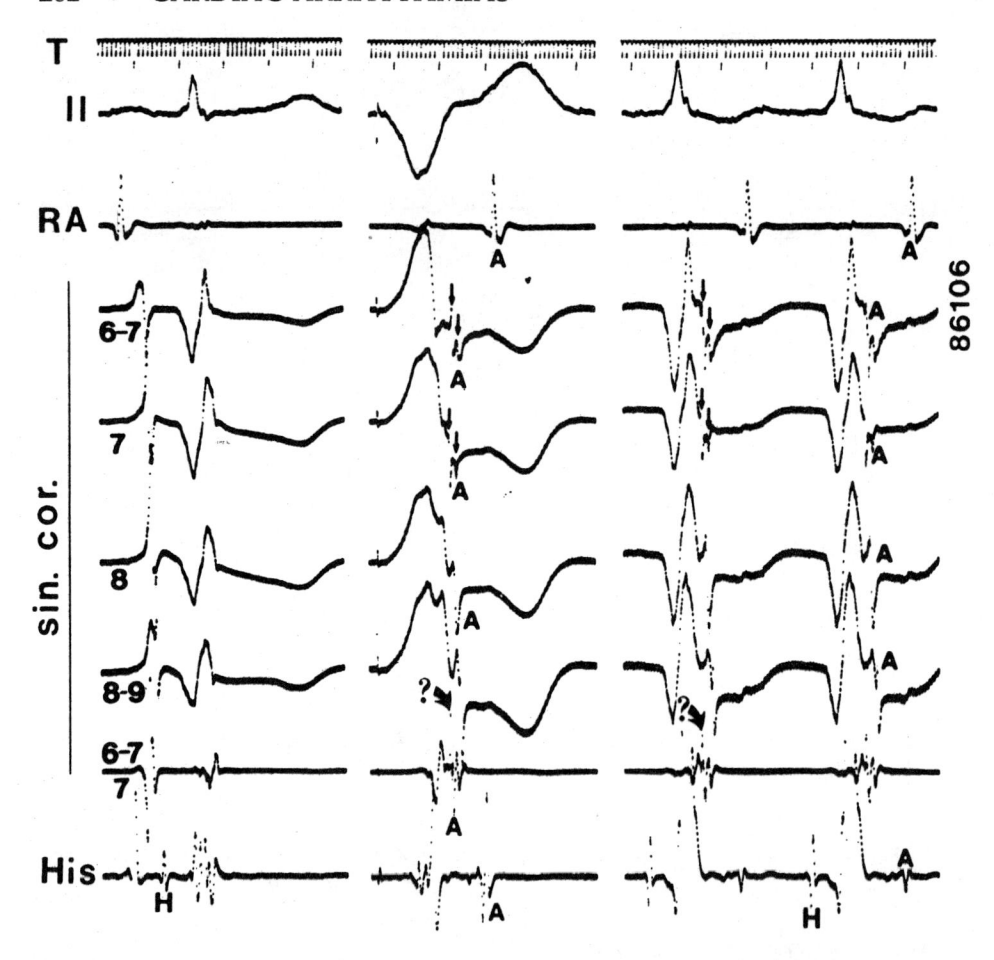

Figure 14: Normal (smooth biphasic) unipolar atrial electrograms are recorded during sinus rhythm at sites where during CMT the unipolar waveforms are multiphasic and of a lower amplitude (see text).

tions (such as during the sudden increase in rate at the start of CMT), propagation in the longitudinal direction could fail within a bundle of atrial myocardium and reexcitation of the latter area could occur through activation fronts propagating at a slower velocity in the transverse direction so that the condition for multiple functional reentry loops has been generated. Allessie et al. in their very detailed studies on the spread of the excitation waves in the dog's atrial flutter have postulated that small areas of conduction block may be sufficient to permit reentry.[22] They also conclude that the same mechanism can produce atrial flutter and atrial fibrillation depending on whether one or more circuits are established. Although these investigators do not mention the role of anisotropic conduction in the genesis and/or perpetuation of atrial tachyarrhythmias in the dog's heart, it seems to us that the existence of a route of safer and slower conduction facilitates the production of reexcitation if conduction block develops at a given atrial site.

Also of interest is the lack of a relation between the width of the unipolar atrial electrogram at the site of bracketing and the shortest VA time and retrograde refractory period of the AP. Theoretically speaking, such a relation could exist in several ways; for instance, if activation transverse to the direction of the fibers results in a slower conduction and a better safety factor of propagation, longer VA conduction times would be expected in patients with a short refractory period of the AP. In addition, if the width of the unipolar electrogram is an index of the degree of anisotropy, positive relations could be expected with the AP retrograde refractory period and conduction times. The lack of evident relationships most likely reflects the very complex nature of the issue. The unipolar atrial electrogram close to the proximal end of the AP does not reflect the conduction characteristics within the bypass tract itself or at its junction with the ventricular myocardium.

The Recording of the Potential of Accessory Pathways

Takashi Iwa first reported on the recording of a fast potential considered to represent the excitation of a right-sided AP in a patient with Ebstein's anomaly of the tricuspid valve and the WPW syndrome.[23] Gallagher et al. illustrated an example of what they had interpreted as the electrogram of a superficial posterior right ventricular free-wall AP.[24] Most of the examples reported thus far in which a sharp bipolarly recorded spike was found between the atrial and ventricular major deflections and considered to represent the AP electrogram also belong to patients with right-sided bypass tracts.[25-27] Durrer et al. were unable to register AP electrograms during careful epicardial mapping close to the ventricular insertion of the bypass tract except for one instance in which an intramural electrode, introduced into the ventricular wall of an early activated area, revealed a low voltage deflection that could not be recorded from a terminal located 2 mm deeper in the wall.[20]

The analysis of our unipolar recordings enabled us to demonstrate in ten of our patients (50%) that fast deflections registered by means of filtered bipolar leads between the "major" ventricular and atrial electrograms are the result of combining two waves that are atrial in origin (Figs. 6–8, 15, 16).

When fast deflections are recorded at the vicinity of the offset of the ventricular complex, more doubts can arise as to their origin. They could reflect the activation of the AP or of the underlying ventricular myocardium. In this regard, it is important to remember that the CS is near the atrium in its posterior region and runs closer to the left ventricle as it turns towards the anterior and septal areas. It is therefore not surprising that in the posteroseptal and posterior regions of the CS, the unipolar recordings would be devoid of fast deflections. As previously mentioned, Spach et al. have shown that the rate of the intrinsic deflection decreases as the exploring electrode is moved away from the myocardial surface.[14] Fast deflections within the terminal half of the CS lead ventriculogram were recorded at the vicinity of the site of bracketing in 13 patients, 10 with an anterolateral or left-lateral AP (Figs. 4, 10, and 17), two patients with a left posterior free-wall bypass (Figs. 12 and 15), and the remaining case with a posteroseptal anomalous tract. This estimation is conservative since, as previously mentioned, the site of bracketing could not be reached in two patients

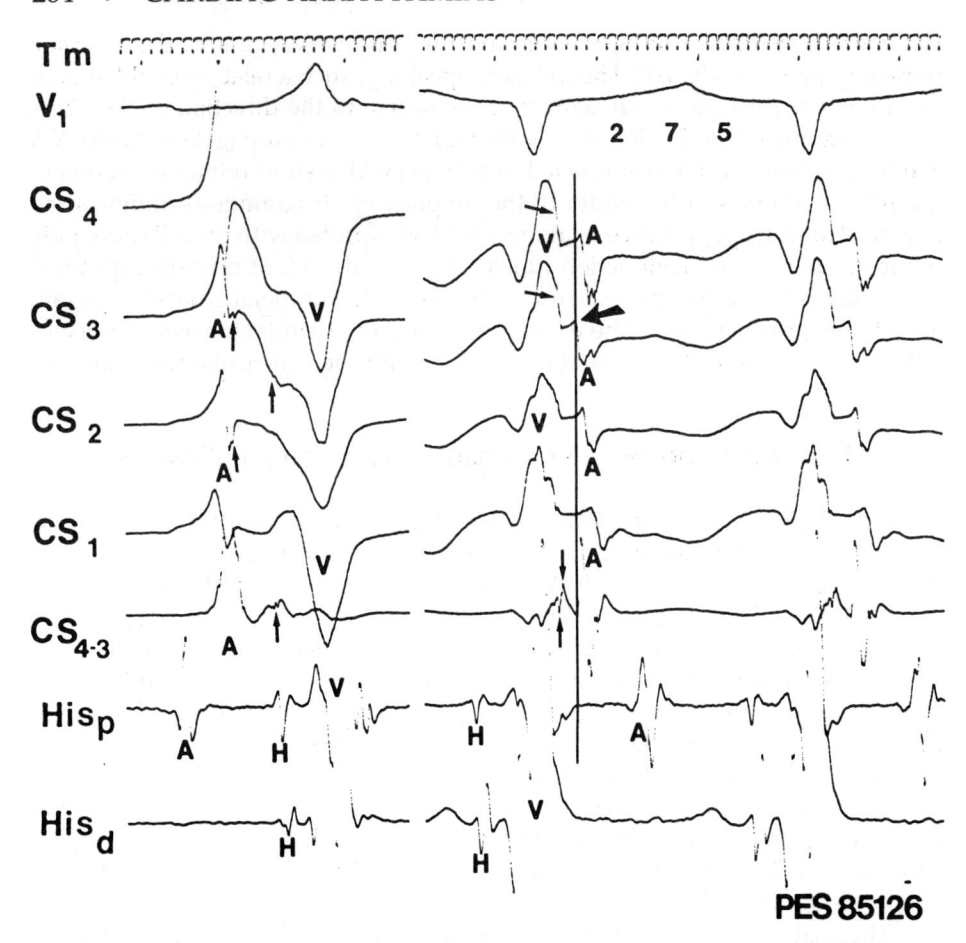

Figure 15: Recordings obtained at a paper speed of 100 mm/sec. The three panels show sinus rhythm (left), right ventricular pacing (middle), and CMT (right). In the filtered bipolar CS lead (between electrodes at sites 6–7 and 7), a tall and sharp spike is recorded between the major atrial and ventricular electrograms (arrow). This spike corresponds to the initial fast intrinsic deflection of the unipolar waveform at the site of bracketing.

with lateral AP. In one of them, the most laterally placed unipolar electrode showed a fast deflection in the ventriculogram during CMT. This distribution is statistically significant (P= 0.04).

Bipolarly recorded similar spikes can originate from fast deflections in the corresponding unipolar ventriculograms at some distance from the site of bracketing. The latter situation was found in two of the six patients with posteroseptal AP and in three of the four subjects with posterior free-wall AP. The incidence in the group of posteroseptal AP could have been higher if mapping of the lateral and anterolateral regions of the CS would have been performed systematically. Figure 16 shows (upper panel) a fast spike (thick arrow) in the bipolar proximal CS lead which coincides with a fast deflection at the end of the ventriculogram recorded in

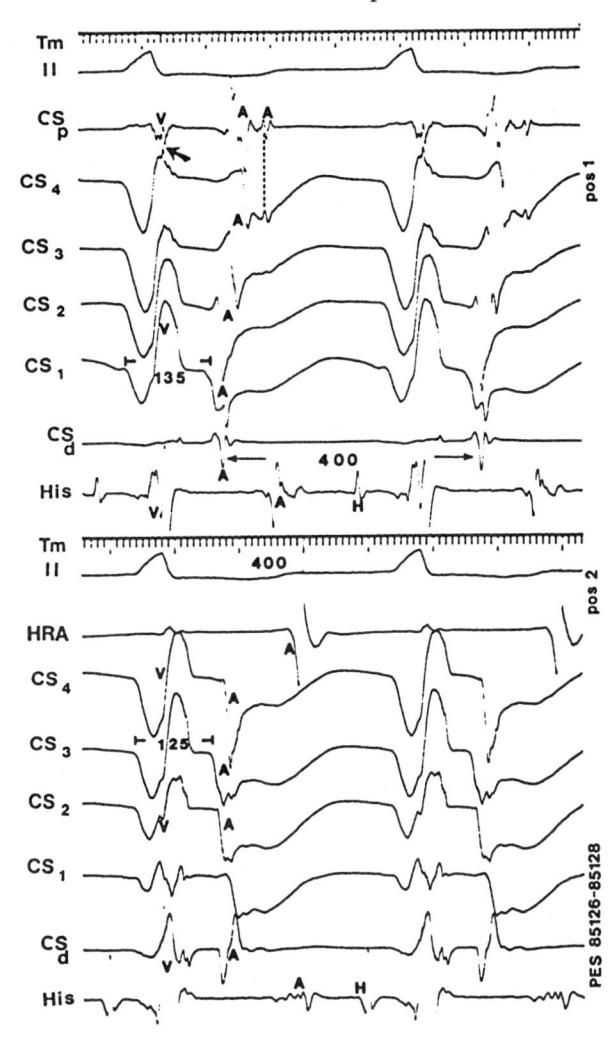

Figure 16: Shown in the upper panel are simultaneously recorded time marks, lead II, CS proximal (filtered and bipolar), the individual unfiltered unipolar leads, the distal CS (filtered bipolar), and the His. In the lower panel, the proximal bipolar CS has been replaced by the HRA. Both panels represent different positions of the mapping catheter during CMT. The interesting finding is that the pseudo AP potential recorded in the proximal CS bipolar lead reflects the presence of a fast deflection late in the unipolar ventriculogram under electrode 4 (upper panel), a site well apart from the point of bracketing (electrode 3, lower panel) (see text).

the unipolar CS lead #4, a point far away from the site of bracketing (lower panel, position #2). Figure 13 exemplifies a different situation; in the proximal bipolar lead (CS 4–3), a fast spike is registered between the major ventricular and atrial electrograms during VA conduction over the AP that corresponds to fast deflections in the unipolar ventriculograms (small arrows). These fast signals are present in the four unipolar leads displayed in this illustration thus suggesting to represent local activation of the ventricular myocardium rather than the AP electrogram. In the same patient, during sinus rhythm, the bipolar CS lead shows a tiny spike between the atria and the ventricles. It is very unlikely that the latter deflection represents an AP electrogram since it occurs in the unipolar lead well after the onset of the delta wave (Fig. 13).

266 • CARDIAC ARRHYTHMIAS

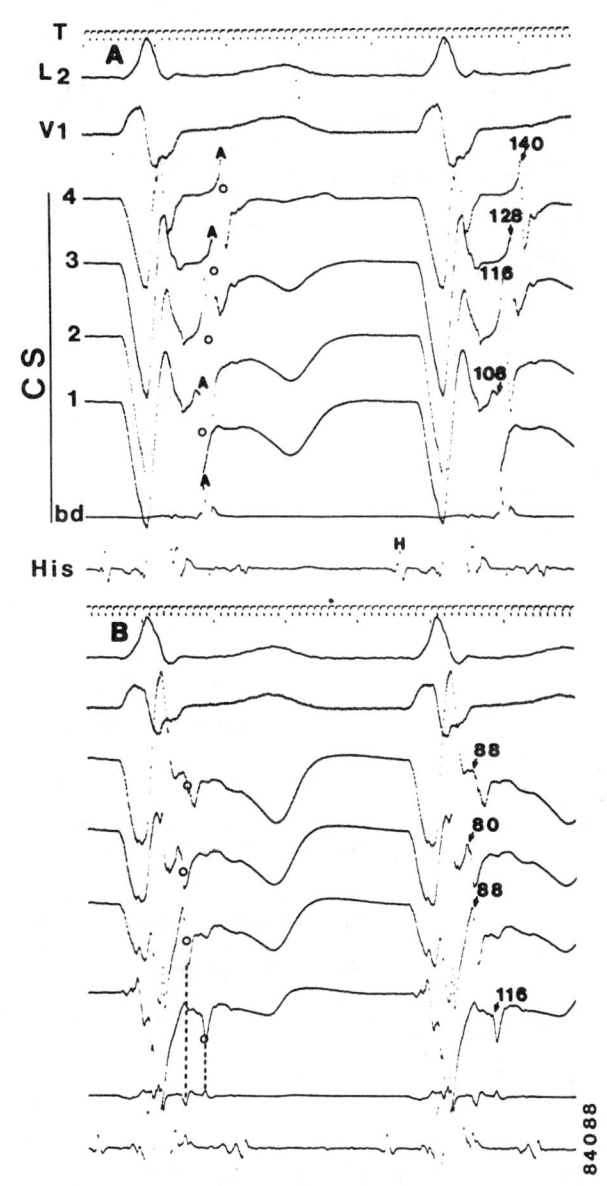

Figure 17: Panels A and B depict leads II, V1, four unipolar CS leads, a filtered bipolar CS recording from the distal pair of electrodes (bd) and the His lead. The site of bracketing during CMT is shown in panel B. The filtered bipolar CS lead of this panel shows a split atrial electrogram (the differentiation with an AP potential is easily made with the aid of the unipolar recordings). The circles mark the fastest portion of the intrinsic deflection. Fast deflection are also recorded at the offset of the unipolar ventriculogram in the lead where bracketing is observed (see text).

Conclusions and Reflections

We would like to end this presentation with conclusions and speculative reflections. For a publication aimed at meditating on "Where to go in the Future," conclusions are required that lead to new questions and ideas which should be tested in the coming years.

Conclusions

The recording of unfiltered unipolar atrial electrograms from the CS during CMT and/or ventricular pacing in patients with left-sided AP frequently displays fragmented, multimodal, or multiphasic waveforms either at the site of insertion of the AP or in its vicinity. That the latter waveforms are due to a nonuniform anisotropic propagation of the cardiac impulse and not to intrinsic characteristics of the atrial fibers underlying the exploring electrode is demonstrated by the recording of smooth deflections when the site of impulse formation is changed. In addition, "QS"-like waveforms, suggesting an epicardial location of the atrial insertion of the AP, are recorded in at least 50% of the instances. When the site of bracketing is not reached due to the inability to progress the catheter within the CS, the finding of a "QS"-like deflection in the most distal electrode may be taken as evidence favoring a very close situation of the atrial insertion of the AP. The recording of these unfiltered unipolar waveforms enables us to define with precision that certain fast deflections that are registered in conventionally filtered bipolar leads represent atrial activity and not the electrogram of the bypass tract. Our observations also support that sharp spikes frequently registered at the end of the QRS complex in filtered bipolar leads most likely represent the local activation of ventricular fibers in the neighborhood of the recording electrodes. The latter interpretation is supported by two facts: (1) such deflections are sometimes recorded at some distance from the site of bracketing of the retrograde atrial activity during CMT, and (2) their presence at the site of bracketing increases as the AP is more laterally located perhaps secondarily to a closer anatomic relation of the lateral and anterior CS to the left ventricular epicardium.

Recording the unfiltered unipolar electrogram is the only possible method to analyze the electrophysiologic implications of the waveform of myocardial excitation and to measure the actual voltage of the potentials generated by the underlying fibers. Filtered bipolar electrograms as utilized in ventricular mapping studies do not reflect voltage but the difference in the rate of change of the voltage registered by each electrode.

Speculations

The anisotropic propagation of the atrial excitatory wavefront during CMT might favor the development of atrial tachyarrhythmias such as flutter or fibrillation. That this is not the only cause for the relatively frequent occurrence of atrial fibrillation in patients with AP is exemplified though by the development of the latter arrhythmias even in patients in whom the bypass tract only conducts in the anterograde direction. Despite the lack of statistical relation between the presence of signs consistent with anisotropic conduction and the retrograde conduction time and refractory period of the AP, anisotropic propagation of the cardiac impulse at the ventricular junction, within the AP itself and at the atrial insertion of the anomalous tract, may play a very important role in many of the still-intriguing features of the electrophysiologic and electropharmacologic behavior of bypass fibers.

Near-DC unipolar ventricular mapping may enhance our abilities to localize the site of origin of ventricular tachycardia by discarding as such those areas in which, despite showing "presystolic" activity, the unipolar waveform is not of a "QS"-like configuration. The validation of that concept is currently under way at our laboratory.

Acknowledgment: JF wishes to dedicate this chapter to Dr. Hein Wellens, teacher, coach, researcher, clinician, and loyal friend. His contributions to the development of clinical electrophysiology and his efforts to enhance the diagnostic value of the 12-lead ECG are quite evident and do not need to be stressed here. But it is for his capacity to listen critically, his determination to reach his goals, and his generosity that I admire the man behind the scientist, educator, and physician. To him I am materially and immaterially indebted and I hope that he will accept the challenge of evaluating over 10 years what the impact has been of this book and the 1987 Maastricht meeting on the course of clinical electrophysiology.

References

1. Durrer D, Schoo L, Schuilenburg RM, Wellens HJJ. The role of premature beats in the initiation and termination of supraventricular tachycardia in the Wolff-Parkinson-White syndrome. Circulation 1967;36:644–662.
2. Wellens HJJ, Schuilenburg RM, Durrer D. Electrical stimulation of the heart in patients with ventricular tachycardia. Circulation 1972;46:216–226.
3. Durrer D, Schuilenburg RM, Wellens HJJ. Pre-excitation revisited. Am J Cardiol 1970;25:690–697.
4. Spach MS, Miller WT, Geselowitz DB, Barr RC, Kootsey JM, Johnson EA. The discontinuous nature of propagation in normal canine cardiac muscle: Evidence for recurrent discontinuities of intracellular resistance that affect the membrane currents. Circ Res 1981;48:39–54.
5. Spach MS, Miller WT, Dolber PC, Kootsey JM, Sommer JR, Mosher CE. The functional role of structural complexities in the propagation of depolarization in the atrium of the dog: Cardiac conduction disturbances due to discontinuities of effective axial resistivity. Circ Res 1982;50:175–191.
6. Gallagher JJ, Kasell J, Sealy WC, Pritchett ELC, Wallace AG. Epicardial mapping in the Wolff-Parkinson-White syndrome. Circulation 1978;57:854–866.
7. Gallagher JJ, Kasell JH, Cox JL, Smith WM, Ideker RE, Smith WM. Techniques of intraoperative electrophysiologic mapping. Am J Cardiol 1982;49:221–240.
8. Cassidy DM, Vassallo JA, Buxton AE, Doherty JU, Marchlinski FE, Josephson ME. The value of catheter mapping during sinus rhythm to localize site of origin of ventricular tachycardia. Circulation 1984;69:1103–1110.
9. Cassidy DM, Vassallo JA, Marchlinski FE, Buxton AE, Untereker WJ, Josephson ME. Endocardial mapping in humans in sinus rhythm with normal left ventricles: Activation patterns and characteristics of electrograms. Circulation 1984;70:37–42.
10. Kienzle MG, Miller J, Falcone RA, Harken A, Josephson ME. Intraoperative endocardial mapping during sinus rhythm: Relationship to site of origin of ventricular tachycardia. Circulation 1984;70:957–965.
11. Josephson ME, Wit AL. Fractionated electrical activity and continuous electrical activity: fact or artifact? Circulation 1984;70:529–532.
12. Gardner PI, Ursell PC, Fenoglio JJ, Wit AL. Electrophysiologic and anatomic basis for fractionated electrograms recorded from healed myocardial infarcts. Circulation 1985;72:569–611.
13. Spach MS, Barr RC, Serwer GA, Kootsey JM, Johnson EA. Extracellular potentials related to intracellular action potentials in the dog Purkinje system. Circ Res 1972;30:505–519.
14. Spach MS, Barr RC, Johnson EA, Kootsey JM. Cardiac extracellular potentials. Analysis of complex wave forms about the Purkinje networks in dogs. Circ Res 1973;33:465–473.

15. Roberge FA, Vinet A, Victorri B. Reconstruction of propagated electrical activity with a two-dimensional model of anisotropic heart muscle. Circ Res 1986;58:461–475.
16. Spach MS, Dolber PC. The relation between discontinuous propagation in anisotropic cardiac muscle and the "vulnerable period" of reentry. In Zipes DP, Jalife J, eds. Cardiac Electrophysiology and Arrhythmias. Orlando, Grune & Stratton, 1985;241–252.
17. Spach MS, Miller WT, Miller-Jones E, Warren RB, Barr RC. Extracellular potentials related to intracellular action potentials during impulse conduction in anisotropic canine cardiac muscle. Circ Res 1979;45:188–204.
18. Gallagher JJ, Sealy WC, Cox JL, German LD, Kasell JH, Bardy GH, Packer DL. Results of surgery for preexcitation caused by accessory atrioventricular pathways in 267 consecutive cases. In: Josephson ME, Wellens HJJ, eds. Tachycardias: Mechanisms, Diagnosis and Treatment. Philadelphia, Lea & Febiger, 1984;259–269.
19. Becker AE, Anderson RH, Durrer D, Wellens HJJ. The anatomical substrates of Wolff-Parkinson-White syndrome: A clinicopathologic correlation in seven patients. Circulation 1978;57:870–879.
20. Durrer D, Janse MJ, Van Dam RT, Van Capelle FJL, Moulijn A, Meyne NG. Electrophysiologic observations during cardiac surgery of patients with the Wolff-Parkinson-White syndrome. In: Bircks W, Loogen F, Schulte HD, Seipel L (eds). Medical and Surgical Management of Tachyarrhythmias. Berlin, Springer-Verlag, 1980;107–113.
21. Davies MJ, Anderson RH, Becker AE. The Conduction System of the Heart. London, Butterworths, 1983;181–202.
22. Allessie MA, Lammers WJEP, Bonke FIM, Hollen J. Intra-atrial reentry as a mechanism for atrial flutter induced by acetylcholine and rapid pacing in the dog. Circulation 1984;70:123–135.
23. Iwa T: Surgical management of Wolff-Parkinson-White syndrome. In: Narula OS, ed. His Bundle Electrocardiography and Clinical Electrophysiology. Philadelphia, FA Davis, 1975;387–405.
24. Gallagher JJ, Sealy WC, Kasell JH. Intraoperative localization and division of accessory pathways associated with the Wolff-Parkinson-White syndrome. In: Bircks W, Loogen F, Schulte HD, Seipel L, eds. Medical and Surgical Management of Tachyarrhythmias. Berlin, Springer-Verlag, 1980;114–137.
25. Prystowsky EN, Browne KF, Zipes DP. Intracardiac recording by catheter electrode of accessory pathway depolarization. JAAC 1983;2:468–470.
26. Jackman WM, Friday KJ, Scherlag BJ, Dehning MM, Schechter E, Reynolds DW, Olson EG, Berbari EJ, Harrison LA, Lazzara R. Direct endocardial recording from an accessory atrioventricular pathway: Localization of the site of block, effect of antiarrhythmic drugs and attempt at nonsurgical ablation. Circulation 1983;68:906–916.
27. O'Callagham WG, Colavita PG, Kay N, Ellenbogen KA, Gilbert MR, German LD. Characterization of retrograde conduction by direct endocardial recording from an accessory atrioventricular pathway. JAAC 1986;7:167–171.

15

Is Understanding the Mechanism of a Supraventricular Arrhythmia Necessary for Correct Treatment?

Jean Francois Leclercq
Antoine Leenhardt
Robert Slama

Introduction

Over the past 20 years, our knowledge of supraventricular arrhythmias has been constantly growing since the introduction of programmed stimulation and Holter monitoring. However, it remains questionable if this increase in knowledge has any consequences for the management of these arrhythmias in clinical practice. Many physicians or cardiologists think that a supraventricular tachycardia can always be stopped by electrical countershocks and prevented by amiodarone, and necessitates no sophisticated investigations. Stopping a supraventricular arrhythmia is indeed usually easy, by vagal maneuvers for reciprocating tachycardia, or countershock for the atrial arrhythmias. It is also true that the percentage of success obtained with empirical medical treatment using effective drugs, such as amiodarone or class I-C drugs, is very high for a number of supraventricular arrhythmias, and even higher for curative than for preventive treatment.[7,11,14,25] Therefore, empirical therapy can then be accepted in some clinical situations. By contrast, curative treatment by surgical or percutaneous ablation in the Wolff-Parkinson-White syndrome requires the recognition and the precise localization of the involved accessory pathway.

From: Brugada P, Wellens HJJ. CARDIAC ARRHYTHMIAS: Where To Go From Here? Mount Kisco, NY, Futura Publishing Company, Inc., © 1987.

272 • CARDIAC ARRHYTHMIAS

Thus, there are some situations in which a precise knowledge of the mechanism of arrhythmia is useful, and others in which it remains of little interest. This chapter reviews the different clinical situations and their possible implications for treatment.

The first step of a precise diagnosis of a tachyarrhythmia is usually the differential diagnosis between a ventricular and a supraventricular tachycardia. This is usually very simple, but some well-known difficulties can necessitate the use of vagal maneuvers or the recording of the atrial activity. The ventricular tachycardias with almost narrow QRS complex or the supraventricular tachycardias with wide QRS because of preexistent or rate-dependent bundle branch block are usually easily recognized using these simple maneuvers. An electrophysiological study is unnecessary for correct diagnosis in the great majority of patients. However, in some rare situations, the diagnosis appears electrocardiographically obvious, until a complete electrophysiological study demonstrates another mechanism of arrhythmia. Figure 1 shows an example of such a situation. This young patient had frequent runs of a wide monomorphic QRS complex, but a normal resting ECG, and no structural heart disease. The obvious diagnosis seems to be runs of benign idiopathic ventricular tachycardia. Surprisingly, the electrophysiological study (EPS) demonstrates a mechanism of an antidromic reciprocating tachycardia initiated by an extrasystole originating near the ventricular part of the accessory pathway.[18] This rare etiology cannot be diagnosed without EPS in the

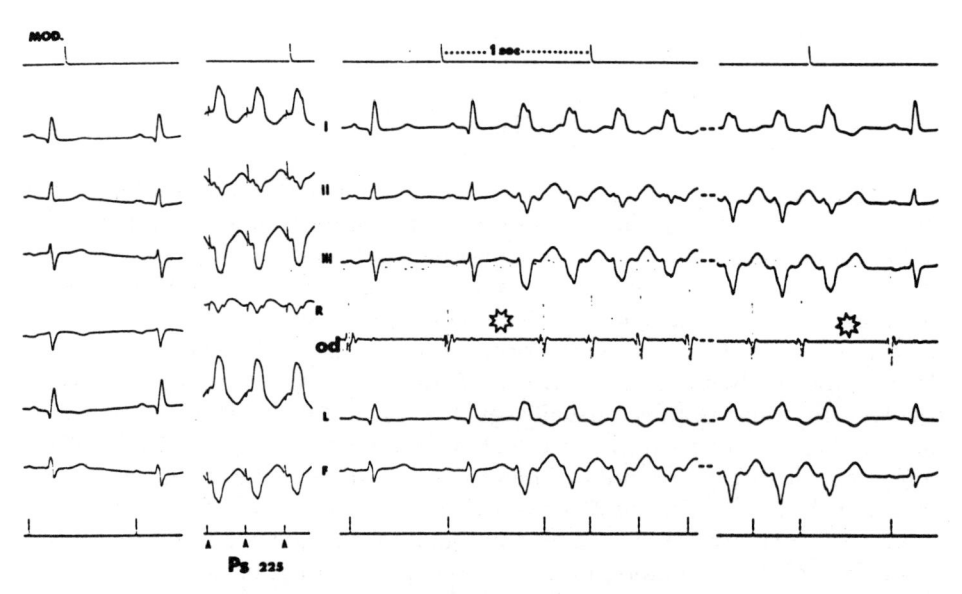

Figure 1: Spontaneous self-terminating monomorphic tachycardia with wide QRS complexes (right). Despite the absence of visible preexcitation during sinus rhythm (left), the mechanism is an antidromic reciprocating tachycardia. Note the similarity in QRS during tachycardia and during fast right atrial pacing (middle). The spontaneous runs of tachycardia were initiated without atrial activity and terminated when retrograde conduction was blocked in the AV node (stars). Thus, the mechanism of the arrhythmia is: an antidromic reciprocating tachycardia initiated by an extrasystole originating within the Kent bundle or its ventricular end, and not runs of ventricular tachycardia.

absence of visible antegrade preexcitation during sinus rhythm in this unapparent Wolff-Parkinson-White syndrome.

Junctional Arrhythmias

When interruption of an accessory pathway is required, either by surgery or by electrical ablation, it seems important to know, as accurately as possible, the number and the localization of the accessory pathways (AP) that have to be divided. If the clinical problem is a high ventricular rate during atrial arrhythmia, the only problem is the accurate localization of the accessory pathways. In the example presented in Figures 2 and 3, we were not able to differentiate two separate left-sided AP during the preoperative EP study. However, the spontaneous tracing during atrial fibrillation (Fig. 2) is probably sufficient to suspect that a septal posterior AP was associated with the obvious left lateral AP, because of the polymorphism of the QRS complexes. This diagnosis was not made preoperatively, and after the dissection of the left free wall AV sulcus, it was found that it was still possible to induce and stop a reciprocating tachycardia using a retrograde posterior septal AP (Fig. 3). We decided to perform immediately the surgical cure of this second AP, but unfortunately the patient died from acute myocardial ischemia at the sixth hour postoperatively, probably due to the extensive dissection (2/3 of the left AV groove) requiring two cardiopulmonary bypasses in

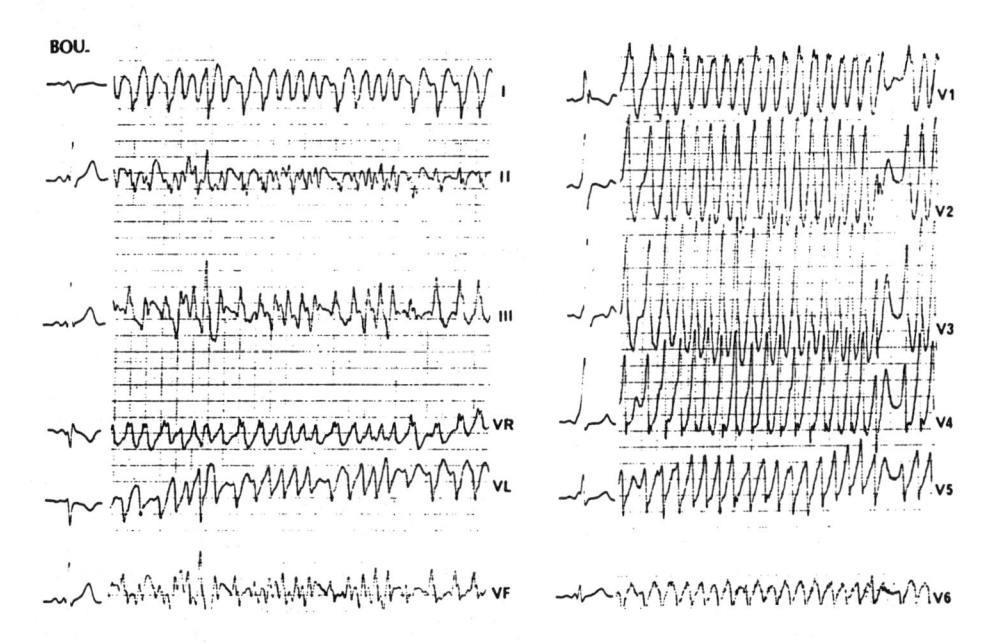

Figure 2: Comparison of QRS morphology during atrial fibrillation and sinus rhythm in a case of left atrioventricular preexcitation. Sinus rhythm revealed a left lateral AP. However, during atrial fibrillation, while all complexes have a QS pattern in leads I and L, some have a QR pattern and some a R pattern in leads III and F. This finding should suggest that a left posteroseptal AP is associated with the left lateral one.

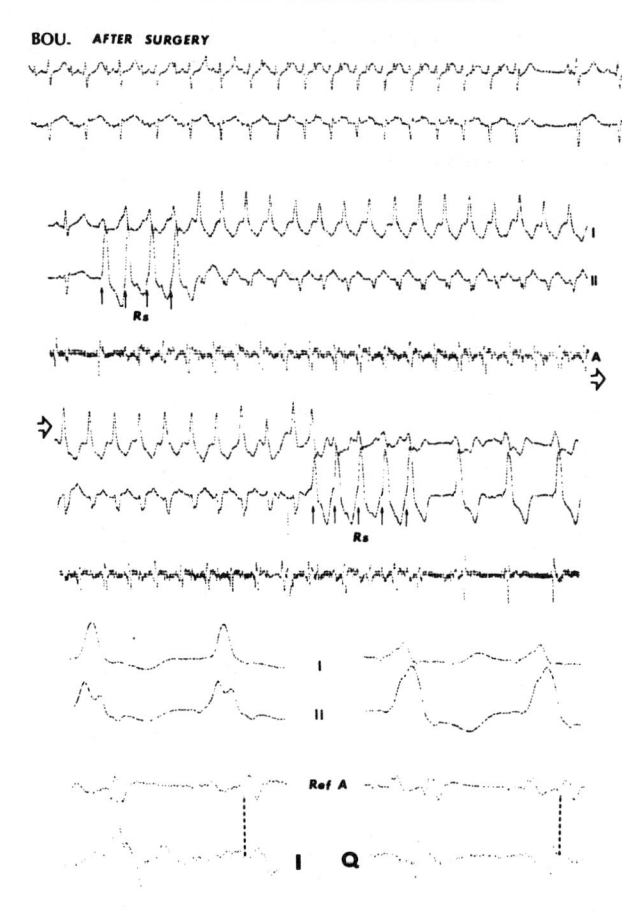

Figure 3: Same patient as in Figure 2. Intraoperative EP testing after surgical cure of the left lateral AP: no antegrade preexcitation was evidenced by atrial pacing (top), but reciprocating tachycardia could be triggered and stopped by ventricular extrastimulation (middle). Mapping of the atrial site of the AV groove during reciprocating tachycardia (bottom) showed that the left side of the crux (Q point) preceded the anterior part of the septum (I point), proving that the retrograde pathway is a left posteroseptal AP and not the His bundle.

succession. It was our only death during surgery for WPW syndrome in 44 cases during the last 3 years. This example clearly shows how important it is to delineate as precisely as possible the number and location of the AP before surgical treatment.

The same holds true when the technique of catheter ablation is considered. These techniques are still experimental and their safety is not well demonstrated. It is then important to know exactly the type of arrhythmia to be treated before an attempt to fulgurate of an AP. The example shown in Figures 4 and 5 concerns a 26-year-old patient with Ebstein's disease and reciprocating tachycardias using a right posterior septal AP. However, this patient had two types of tachycardias, one with narrow QRS complexes, and one with wide QRS complexes resembling those with major preexcitation, but with some slight differences in morphology. Extensive EP study shows the coexistence of two AP, one Kent bundle, and one of the nodoventricular Mahaim's type. In this case, a surgical attempt appeared difficult and hazardous because of the Ebstein's disease. During this EP, we performed a mapping of the AV region and two shocks of 250 joules were delivered at the earliest recorded site of depolarization of the right atrium during tachycardia. Comparison of EP studies before and after ablation (Fig. 4) shows a

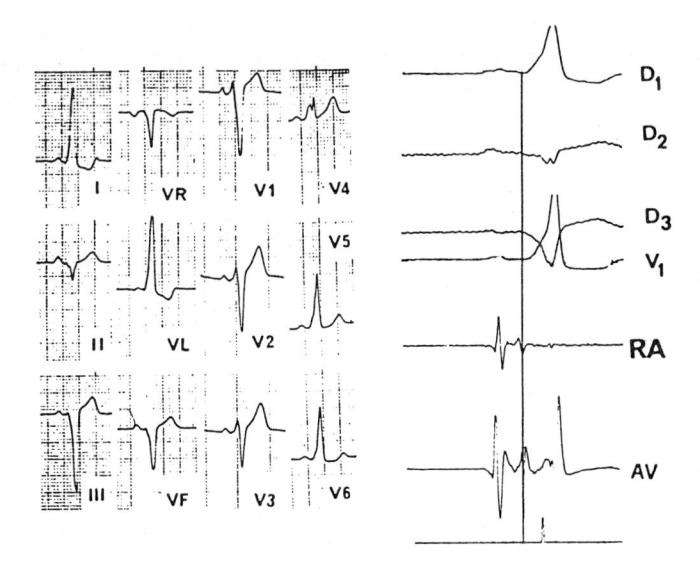

Therapeutic Consequences of SVT Mechanisms • 275

FULGURATION

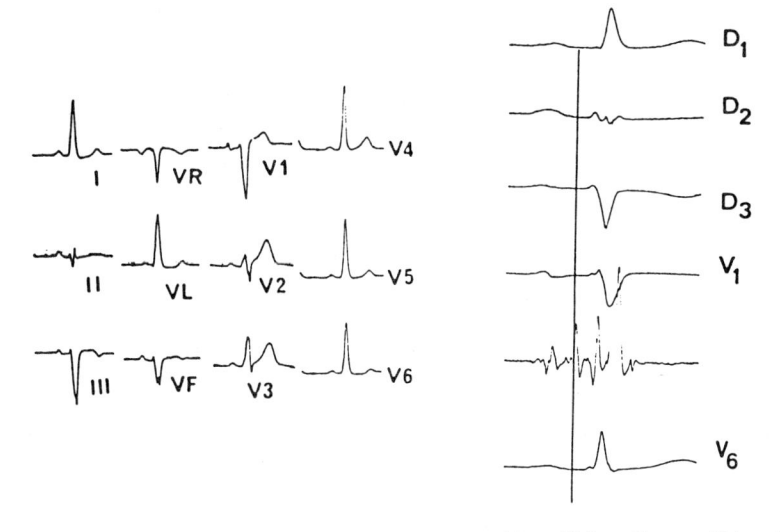

Figure 4: Results of fulguration procedure of AP in a case with multiple pathways. This patient with Ebstein's disease had two AP: a right posteroseptal Kent bundle, and nodoventricular Mahaim fibers. Before fulguration, the ECG showed a short PR interval and a delta wave which is clearly negative in lead II and positive in leads V4, V5, and V6. The His bundle is recorded simultaneous with the onset of the delta wave. After mapping during orthodromic reciprocating tachycardia, shocks were delivered in the intermediate chamber at the earliest site of depolarization. After fulguration (bottom), the PR interval increased and the delta wave was less obvious. The His bundle electrogram now precedes the R wave (HV = 35ms).

less marked preexcitation during sinus rhythm with an increase in the PR and HV intervals, but minor changes in QRS complexes morphology. Atrial pacing (Fig. 5) is able to increase the wideness of QRS complexes through the nodoventricular AP, but ventricular pacing shows an absence of retrograde VA conduction, and the patient remained free of any tachycardia during a follow-up period of 6 months.

These two examples clearly demonstrate the necessity of recognizing as precisely as possible the exact structures and mechanisms of a supraventricular arrhythmia, when an etiologically curative treatment is proposed.[10,27,28] The presence of multiple AP in about 5 to 10% of the series in the literature[8,9,15,22,23] justifies the practice of complete EP studies before and during surgical or electrical ablation procedures.

When the physician chooses to use a palliative treatment, namely antiarrhythmic drugs, precise knowledge of the mechanisms of the arrhythmia often seems less necessary. This is evidenced by the example initially presented in Figure 1. The mechanism of the arrhythmia is particularly complex, and the EP study revealed a completely unexpected etiology. However, efficient therapy could be predicted by the simple examination of the Holter recording, showing a particular behavior of the arrhythmia: attacks of tachycardia were present only during the day. Thus, beta-blockers proved to be completely effective in this case, as shown in Figure 6. This accurate prediction is completely independent of the site of origin or mechanism of the arrhythmia and comes only from the observation of the behavior of the arrhythmia.

This latter example is of course schematic, and Holter monitoring is in fact useful only in a limited number of reciprocating tachycardias, because the sponta-

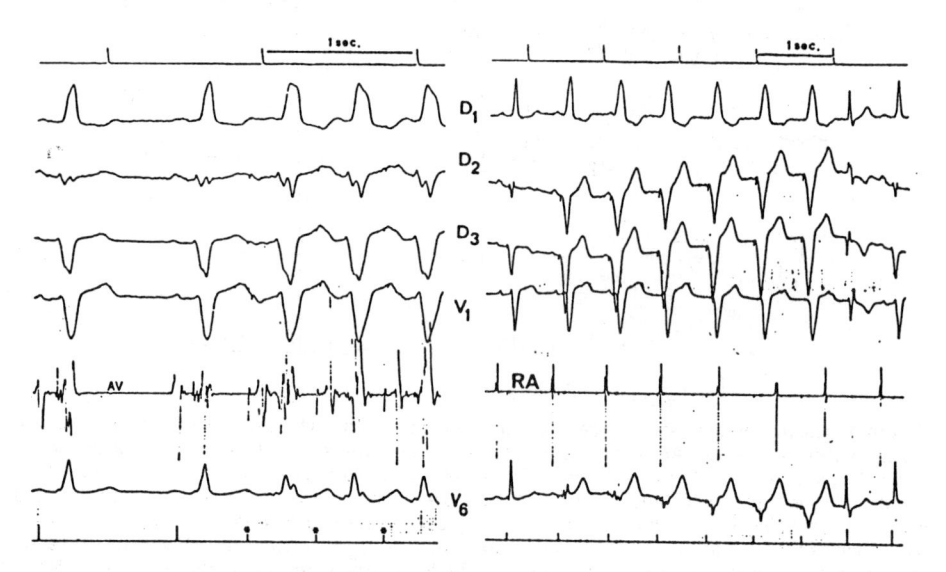

Figure 5: Same patient as Figure 4. After ablation, atrial pacing still evidenced an increase of the preexcitation pattern, due to the persistence of nodoventricular Mahaim fibers (left), but ventricular pacing (right) showed absence of retrograde VA conduction and the patient remains free of reciprocating tachycardia.

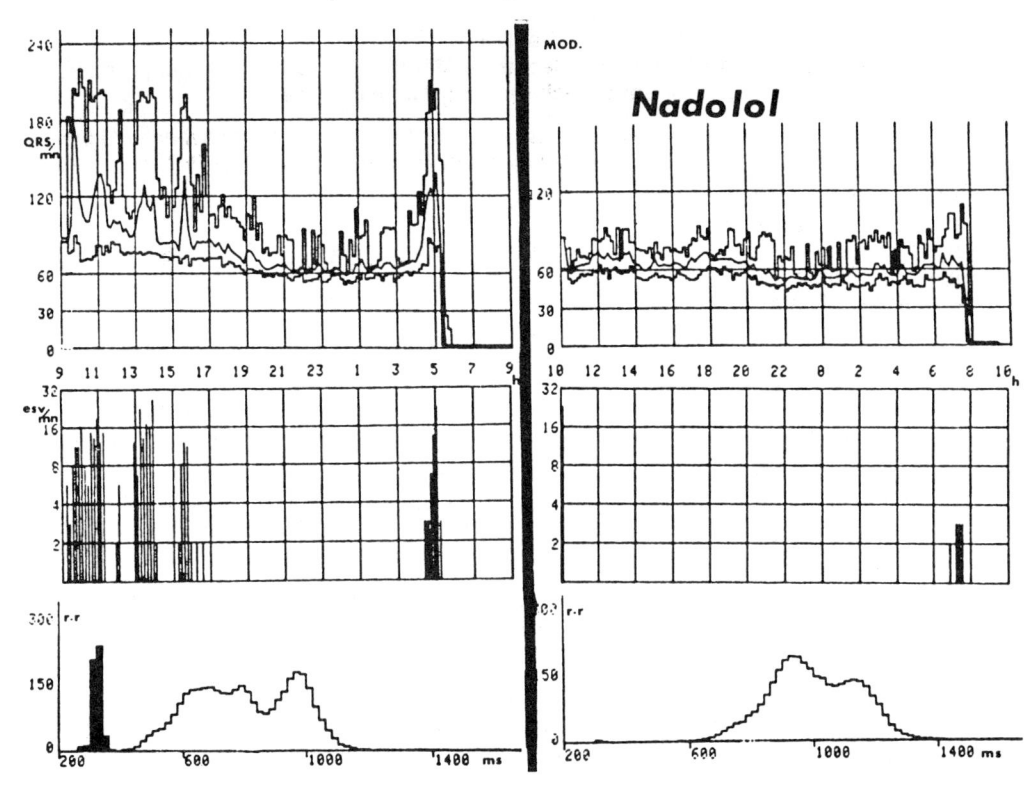

Figure 6: Same case as in Figure 1. Holter recording before treatment (left) showed that all runs of antidromic tachycardia occurred during daytime (5 am to 5 pm). Under beta-blocking therapy (right), almost all attacks disappeared, except for some upon waking.

neous attacks are paroxysmal and rarely recorded. Nevertheless, if we were able to record the spontaneous initiation of the attack, some therapeutic implications could ensue.[6] Table I shows the respective frequency of the five different modes of spontaneous onset of reciprocating tachycardias in our experience.[19] In case of initiation by His escape beats,[1] usually because of a sinoatrial block, a pacemaker can be useful. The onset by sinus tachycardia (due to a phase III block in the concealed antegrade conduction in the AP) invites the use of beta-blockers or amiodarone. When the tachycardia follows a run of ventricular premature beats, class I antiarrhythmic drugs are probably useful, since they are more effective on the repetitive phenomena than on isolated extrasystoles.[24] However, the vast majority of reciprocating tachycardias are initiated by isolated atrial premature beats, the most difficult arrhythmia to treat in clinical practice. Thus, recording of the spontaneous onset of the reciprocating tachycardia remains often without clinical implications for therapy.

Knowing the location of the reentrant circuit may provide some guidelines for the choice of medical treatment. This is why some groups systematically perform an EP study in reciprocating tachycardias necessitating chronic antiar-

Table I
Initiating Events and Sustaining Reentrant Mechanism in 46 Recordings of Spontaneous Reciprocating Tachycardias

	Reentry using an AP (35 pts) Modes of initiation = 36	AV nodal reentry (9 pts) Modes of initiation = 10
Atrial premature beats	6	26
Ventricular premature beats	4	2
Sinus tachycardia	—	5
Sinus bradycardia	—	1
Hisian escape beats	—	4

rhythmic therapy. If we compare the long-term results of chronic antiarrhythmic therapy in relation to the reentry pathway,[21] we can make two relevant considerations (Table II): (1) reciprocating tachycardias using an AP are less sensitive to antiarrhythmic therapy than AV nodal reentrant tachycardias (AVNRT), and (2) verapamil and digoxin, drugs acting only on the AV node, are statistically more effective in AVNRT than in tachycardias using an AP.[12,13,17,29] Also, some reports in the literature demonstrate a relationship between the effects of acute drug testing during EP study and the efficacy during long-term oral treatment.[16,25]

A perfect knowledge of the mechanism of a reciprocating tachycardia, i.e. the site of reentry and the mechanism of spontaneous initiation, is probably useful in some cases, but it is not always necessary in order to obtain a satisfactory result. The simple observation that the arrhythmia occurred always during exercise or stress may provide sufficient arguments in favor of the usefulness of beta-blocking agents (alone or combined with other antiarrhythmic drugs), without knowing precisely the type of tachycardia, or the mechanism of initiation and maintenance.

Atrial Arrhythmias

The difference between atrial and junctional arrhythmias is not always easy, and some arrhythmias are direct consequences of junctional tachycardias. This is particularly true in the WPW syndrome, but it can also occur in other situations. It then becomes important to recognize that the reciprocating tachycardia induces the atrial arrhythmia, since junctional arrhythmia may require specific treatment. This transformation of reciprocating tachycardias into atrial arrhythmia[26] is a function of the rate of the tachycardia and explains why it is more frequent in tachycardias using an AP than in intranodal tachycardias which usually have a lower cardiac atrial arrhythmic rate during ventricular pacing at increasing rates (Fig. 7). As shown, this includes a high atrial rate because of retrograde conduction over the AP, and atrial fibrillation ensues. The same applies to some cases in which a ventricular tachycardia is able to trigger an atrial arrhythmia if 1/1 retrograde VA conduction is possible. It explains some cases of bitachycardias.

The presence or absence of synchronization of the atria during an atrial arrhythmia is important to note if we want to attempt to restore sinus rhythm by

Table II
Effects of Preventive Antiarrhythmic Treatment in Relation to the Reentrant Circuit in Patients with Paroxysmal Tachycardia Based on AV Nodal Reentry or Using an Accessory Pathway (AP)

Drugs	AV Nodal Reentry			Reentry Using an AP		
	+	±	−	+	±	−
Class IA	3	2	8	4	15	31
Beta-blockers	1	4	3	3	5	33
Amiodarone	4	1	1	27	10	10
Verapamil, Digitalis	9	0	2	1	3	18

Results are considered as + when the reduction of attacks is > 90%, and as ± if it is reduced by 50–90%.

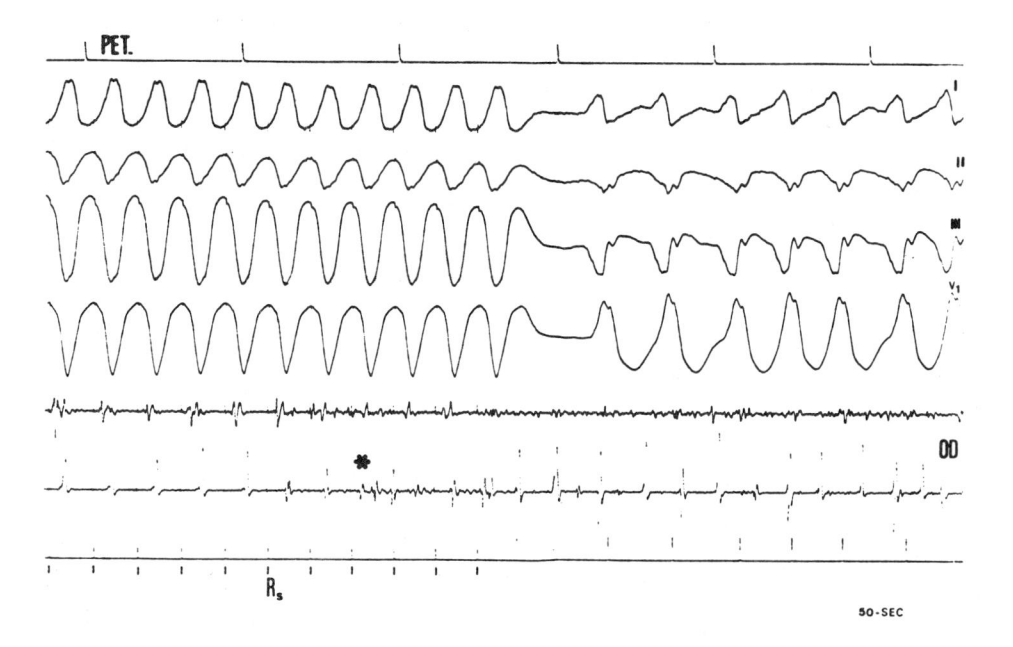

Figure 7: Triggering of atrial fibrillation by fast retrograde VA conduction through an AP during ventricular pacing at increasing rates. This mode of onset is frequently found in patients with rapid atrioventricular reciprocating tachycardias.

atrial stimulation (endocavitary or transesophageal pacing). Atrial flutter, intra-atrial reentry, and more generally speaking, all regular atrial tachycardia can be restored into sinus rhythm or transformed in atrial fibrillation by fast atrial pacing and do not systematically require electrical countershock, in contrast to atrial fibrillation. But this is in relation more to the electrocardiographic pattern than the mechanism of arrhythmia itself.

Preventing the relapses of paroxysmal atrial fibrillation or atrial tachycardia is often difficult. It is probably one of the most difficult arrhythmias to prevent by

280 • CARDIAC ARRHYTHMIAS

the presently available antiarrhythmic therapy. This is why knowledge of the mechanism of the arrhythmia, or more simply, the observation of the behavior of the arrhythmia in relation to the function of the autonomic nervous system, is important to guide the therapy.

In patients without apparent heart disease, paroxysmal atrial fibrillation is often what we call a "vagally induced atrial arrhythmia."[2,3] This syndrome can be recognized clinically, simply by an accurate case history. Most of these patients, usually middle-aged men, spontaneously say that the onset of their arrhythmia occurs at rest, never during physical activity, and especially in the evening or during the night. They fall asleep in sinus rhythm, and awake in atrial fibrillation or flutter. In addition, the occurrence of this frequent arrhythmia (many episodes every week, sometimes with a follow-up of many years) is favored by stress, alcohol intake or exercise, but occurs after it. In most of the cases, minor digestive disorders are the most common way to trigger the arrhythmia in the vagotonic state. Holter recordings provide important data, confirming this mechanism, namely the occurrence at evening or night, and after a slight decrease in sinus rate, but usually the arrhythmia occurs at a "normal" sinus frequency, i.e. between 50 and 60 beats/min. A short sequence of bigeminism is usual, the post-extrasystolic pause favoring the genesis of the arrhythmia. Atrial fibrillation can often easily be reproduced by vagal maneuvers, or adenosine triphosphate infusion, if they are used in the afternoon or evening, i.e., if the vagotonic drive is sufficient. Figure 8 shows an example of this setting.

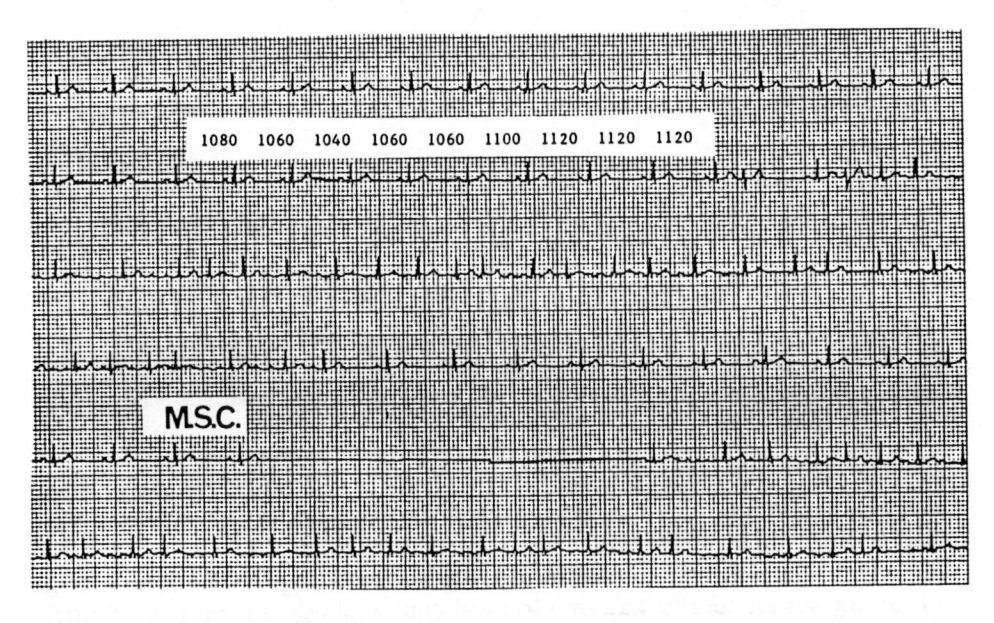

Figure 8: Vagally induced atrial tachyarrhythmia. The first attack of arrhythmia (2nd line) is preceded by a progressive increase in sinus cycle length reflecting an increase in vagal tone. After spontaneous recurrence of sinus rhythm, atrial fibrillation can be provoked by a vagal maneuver, i.e., carotid sinus compression (M.S.C.). After a prolonged sinus pause (5th line), atrial fibrillation starts again.

Therapeutic consequences of this diagnosis of vagally induced arrhythmia are that digitalis, verapamil, beta-blockers, and propafenone are always ineffective, or deleterious, favoring the onset of the arrhythmia. Class IA drugs, namely disopyramide (because of its vagolytic side effect) have little efficacy at the initial stage of the disease. Amiodarone and flecainide are the only drugs that are really useful, able to control the arrhythmia, separately or frequently in combination. Permanent AAI pacing at 80 or 90 beats/min is also useful in refractory cases,[4] providing probably a better synchronization of the refractory periods of the atria.

The reverse situation, i.e., catecholamine-sensitive atrial arrhythmias, are less commonly encountered in clinical practice.[5] They are more frequently organized atrial tachycardias than true atrial fibrillation, and occur more often in young women. The clinical history is usually clear: palpitations occur during stress, exercise, never at rest, and can be provoked by caffeine intake.

Some of these arrhythmias are found in relationship with minor hyperthyroidism, but in the majority of cases, no hormonal dysfunction can be evidenced. Infusion of catecholamines or stress provocation are able to reproduce the arrhythmia, more easily than a routine exercise test. Holter recordings show that the arrhythmia occurs in the daytime, usually the morning, and is preceded by a sinus rate increase, as in the example given in Figure 9.

The usefulness of beta-blocking agents in these cases appears obvious, since this arrhythmia is clearly favored by an increase in the sympathetic drive. However, beta-blockers having an intrinsic sympathomimetic activity are unable to induce a sufficient degree of sinus bradycardia,[20] and are ineffective in this setting, as shown in the example in Figure 9. Only beta-blocking drugs without any intrinsic sympathetic activity can be used to obtain a significant sinus bradycardia, and do control the arrhythmia. Moreover, beta-blockers alone become ineffective after several weeks or months, probably because of the modifications of sympathetic receptors, and these patients require additional Class I antiarrhythmic therapy, or drugs having nonselective beta-inhibition properties, such as amiodarone or propafenone.[5]

Thus, this distinction between vagally induced and adrenergic-induced paroxysmal atrial arrhythmias has clear therapeutic implications. Nevertheless, it should be noted that amiodarone is effective in both situations, and that some atrial arrhythmias have no clear relationship with the autonomic nervous system. This distinction is of course sometimes schematic, and empiric therapy using amiodarone is effective in the vast majority of cases.

Finally, some therapies can be effective, whatever the mechanism of the arrhythmia, and whatever the type of supraventricular arrhythmia. Electrical His bundle ablation or fulguration is certainly the best example of this possibility. However, it is shocking to think that cardiologists specializing in arrhythmias would destroy this normal structure, necessitating a pacemaker implantation, in order to control the consequences of disease of another structure. This effective therapy is therefore usually reserved for patients really refractory to any antiarrhythmic drug combination. They should not be candidates for direct surgery, and pacemaker implantation should be possible. These important limitations explain why its use remains yet limited to less than 1% of patients.

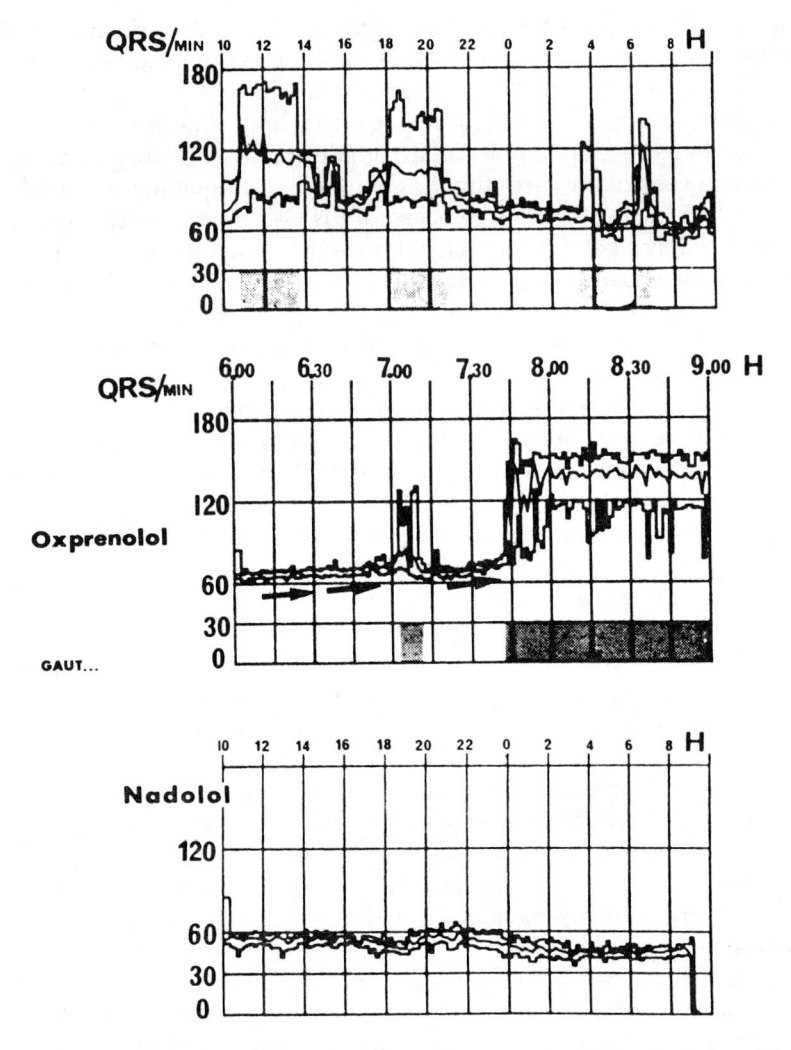

Figure 9: Adrenergic-induced atrial tachyarrhythmia. Twenty-four hour Holter recording without treatment (top) shows a daytime predominance of the atrial tachycardia (shadow zones). Under oxprenolol therapy, a beta-blocker with intrinsic sympathetic activity (middle), the sinus rate increase upon waking-up again triggers the atrial tachycardia. With nadolol treatment (without intrinsic adrenergic properties), a more pronounced sinus bradycardia is obtained, and no atrial arrhythmias recur (bottom).

References

1. Coumel P, Attuel P, Slama R, Curry P, Krikler D. "Incessant" tachycardias in Wolff-Parkinson-White syndrome. II. Role of atypical cycle length dependency and nodal-His escape beats in initiating reciprocating tachycardias. Br Heart J 1976;38:897–905.
2. Coumel P, Attuel P, Lavallee JP, Flammang D, Leclercq JF, Slama R. Syndrome d'arythmie auriculaire d'origine vagale. Arch Mal Coeur 1978;71:645–656.
3. Coumel P, Leclercq JF, Attuel P, Lavallee JP, Flammang D. Autonomic influences in the genesis of tachycardias: atrial flutter and fibrillation of vagal origin. In Narula, OS,

ed. Cardiac Arrhythmias: Electrophysiology, diagnosis and management. Baltimore, Williams & Wilkins, 1979;347–359.
4. Coumel P, Friocourt P, Mugica J, Attuel P, Leclercq JF. Long-term prevention of vagal atrial arrhythmias by atrial pacing at 90/minute. Experience with 6 cases. PACE 1983;6:552–560.
5. Coumel P, Attuel P, Leclercq JF, Friocourt P. Arythmies auriculaires d'origine vagale ou catécholergique. Effets comparés du traitement béta-bloqueur et phénomènes d'échappement. Arch Mal Coeur 1982;75:373–388.
6. Dunnigan A, Benditt DG, Benson DW. Modes of onset ("Initiating events") for paroxysmal atrial tachycardia in infants and children. Am J Cardiol 1986;57:1280.
7. Escoubet B, Coumel P, Poirier JM, Maisonblanche P, Jaillon P, Leclercq JF, Menasche P, Cheymol G, Piwnica A, Lagier G, Slama R. Suppression of arrhythmias within hours after a single oral dose of amiodarone and relation to plasma and myocardial concentrations. Am J Cardiol 1985;55:696–702.
8. Gallagher JJ, Sealy WC, Cox JL, German LD, Kasell JH, Bardy GH, Packer DL. Results of surgery for prexcitation caused by accessory atrioventricular pathways in 267 consecutive cases. In Josephson ME, Wellens HJJ, eds. Tachycardias, Mechanisms, Diagnosis, Treatment. Philadelphia, Lea & Febiger, 1984.
9. Gallagher JJ, Sealy WC, Kasell J, Wallace AG. Multiple accessory pathways in patients with the pre-excitation syndrome. Circulation 1976;54:571–591.
10. Gallagher JJ, Selle JG, Sealy WC, Fedor JM, Svenson RH, Zimmern SH. Intermediate septal accessory pathways: a subset of preexcitation at risk for complete heart block/failure during WPW surgery (abstr). Circulation 1986;74:II–387.
11. Gilbert EM, Anderson JL, Anastasiou-Nana MI, Heath BM. Flecainide for prophylaxis of paroxysmal atrial fibrillation or tachycardia, double-blind, placebo-controlled, crossover study (abstr). Circulation 1986;74:II–102.
12. Haissaguerre M, Leclercq JF, Chouty F, Cauchemez B, Maisonblanche P, Coumel P, Slama R. La conduction ventriculo-auriculaire dans l'étude des rythmes réciproques intranodaux: intérêt pratique. L'Info Cardiol 1984;6:289–293.
13. Hamer A, Peter J, Mandel WJ. Atrio-ventricular node reentry: intravenous verapamil as a method of defining multiple electrophysiologic types. Am Heart J 1983;105:629.
14. Hellestrand KJ, Nathan AW, Bexton RS, Camm AJ. Electrophysiologic effects of flecainide acetate on sinus node function, anomalous atrioventricular connections, and pacemaker thresholds. Am J Cardiol 1984;53:30B–38B.
15. Iwa T, Mitsui T, Misaki T, Mukai K, Magara T, Kamata E. Radical surgical cure of Wolff-Parkinson-White syndrome: the Kanazawa experience. J Thorac Cardiovasc Surg 1986;91:225–233.
16. Klein GJ, Gulamhusein S, Prystowsky EN, Carruthers SG, Donner AP, Ko PT. Comparison of the electrophysiologic effects of intravenous and oral verapamil in patients with paroxysmal supraventricular tachycardia. Am J Cardiol 1982;49:117.
17. Krikler D, Rowland E. Management of supraventricular tachycardia with drugs and artificial pacing. In Narula OS, ed. Cardiac Arrhythmias: Electrophysiology, Diagnosis and Management. Baltimore, Williams & Wilkins, 1979.
18. Leclercq JF, Cauchemez B, Attuel P, Childers R, Coumel P, Slama R. Rythme réciproque antidromique sur W.P.W. déclenché par une extrasystole ventriculaire provenant du lieu d'émergence de la voie de préexcitation. Arch Mal Coeur 1983;76:95–103.
19. Leclercq JF, Slama R. Clinical relevance of supraventricular arrhythmias detected by Holter electrocardiography. In Roelandt J, Hugenholtz PG, eds. Long-term Ambulatory Electrocardiography. The Hague, Martines Nijhoff publ., 1982;40–50.
20. Leclercq JF, Rosengarten MD, Kural S, Attuel P, Coumel P. Effects of betablocker's sympathetic activity on SA and AV nodes in man. Europ J Cardiol 1981;12:367–375.
21. Leclercq JF, Coumel P. The role of the A-V node in supraventricular tachycardias. In Rosenbaum MB, Elizari MV, eds. Frontiers of Cardiac Electrophysiology. The Hague, Martines Nijhoff, 1983;376–396.
22. Leclercq JF, Menasche P, Guiraudon G, Coumel P. Results of surgery in W.P.W. syndrome. New Trends Arrhyth 1986;79:113.

23. Morady F, Scheinmann MM, DiCarlo LA, Winston SA, Davis JC, Baerman JM, Krol RB, Crevey BJ. Coexistent posteroseptal and right-sided atrioventricular bypass tracts. J Am Coll Cardiol 1985;5:640.
24. Myerburg RJ, Kessler KM, Pefkaros KC, Cooper D, Kiem I, Castellanos A. Effects of antiarrhythmic agents on premature ventricular contractions and on potentially lethal arrhythmias. In Harrison, DC, ed. Cardiac Arrhythmias: A Decade of Progress. Boston, GK Hall, 1981;571.
25. Prystowsky EN, Klein GJ, Rinkenberger RL, Heger JJ, Naccarelli GV, Zipes DP. Clinical efficacy and electrophysiologic effects of encainide in patients with Wolff-Parkinson-White syndrome. Circulation 1984;69:278.
26. Roark SF, McCarthy EA, Lee KL, Pritchett ELC. Observations on the occurence of atrial fibrillation in paroxysmal supraventricular tachycardia. Am J Cardiol 1986;57:571.
27. Ross DL, Johnson DC, Denniss AR, Cooper MJ, Richards DA, Uther JB. Curative surgery for atrioventricular junctional ("AV nodal") reentrant tachycardia. J Am Coll Cardiol 1985;6:1383.
28. Warin JF, Haissaguerre M, Belhassen B, Lemetayer P, Blanchot P. Electrical catheter ablation of accessory pathways: beneficial effects using a direct approach in 10 patients (abstr). Circulation 1986;74:II-387.
29. Wellens HJJ, Duren DR, Liem KL, Lie KI. Effect of digitalis in patients with paroxysmal atrioventricular nodal tachycardia. Circulation 1975;52:779.

16

Antitachycardia Pacing: Is There a Universal Pacing Mode to Terminate Supraventricular Tachycardia?

Karel den Dulk, Paolo Della Bella
Willem Dassen, Thierry Dugernier
Pedro Brugada, Hein J.J. Wellens

Introduction

Symptomatic paroxysmal reentrant ventricular tachycardia and supraventricular tachycardia (SVT) can be treated by drugs, a pacemaker, surgery, fulguration techniques, or a combination of these. The usefulness of antitachycardia pacemakers in the management of reentrant tachycardias has been well demonstrated.[1-4] Antitachycardia pacing may be the therapy of choice in patients who do not respond to or cannot tolerate drug therapy, patients who do not take their medication, patients who are not suited for or refuse surgery, or for whom elective surgery is not readily available, and patients who cannot tolerate prolonged episodes of tachycardia because of the development of cardiac failure, angina pectoris, or dizziness. Many patients may prefer treatment with small reliable pacemakers above the chronic intake of antiarrhythmic drugs with possible side effects and accumulating expense. In addition, fully automatic pacemakers usually terminate tachycardia so rapidly that the tachycardia is not noticed or only experienced as a premature beat by the patient.

286 • CARDIAC ARRHYTHMIAS

In this chapter we describe our further experience with a pacing mode using adaptive coupling intervals and an automatically increasing number of stimuli.[5] The benefit of such a mode is the rapid termination of reentrant tachycardias irrespective of rate, site of origin, and body position. This could also be of importance in patients in whom a reentrant tachycardia other than the tachycardia for which the device was implanted occurs. We therefore also reviewed our antitachycardia pacing experience in respect to the occurrence of reentrant tachycardias other than the tachycardia for which the pacemaker was implanted. Finally, we will report on our overall, long-term antitachycardia pacing experience in 31 patients with supraventricular tachycardia.

Methods

Adaptive Mode Using an Automatically Increasing Number of Stimuli

Pacing Mode

This pacing mode was tested with the Medtronic Interactive Tachy System.[3,4] This system consists of three parts: (1) model sp0500 implantable pacemaker; (2) model sp0501 pacemaker activator, and (3) model sp0503 prescription formulator (sophisticated, portable stimulator). The prescription formulator can be directly connected to a temporary endocavitary lead or it can be coupled to an implanted model sp0500 pulse generator through the bidirectional radiofrequency link. Tachycardia is recognized if the intervals between sensed depolarizations are shorter than the tachycardia trigger interval (selectable from 190 to 966 ms) for a programmable number of consecutive intervals (selectable from 1 to 99). On recognition of tachycardia, a treatment that may consist of one to 99 stimuli will be delivered. The first stimulus, S_1, is synchronized to the last sensed event R. The RS_1 interval and S_1S_2 interval can be individually selected, as can the remaining (S_2Sn) intervals. For the mode to be tested, these three interval values are selected as a percentage of the last sensed tachycardia interval. Interval values between 3% and 97% can be chosen. The last stimulus of the treatment activates a delay, selectable from 0 to 9 seconds, after which the tachycardia recognition system is again activated. If the tachycardia persists, the number of stimuli can be automatically increased for each treatment from one to the selected "maximum number of pulses in treatment" (one to 99). Figure 1 illustrates termination of two episodes of tachycardia with different rates in the same patient.

In this study, the adaptive mode using an automatically increasing number of stimuli was evaluated with short and long coupling intervals ($RS_1 = 75\%$, $S_1S_2 = 69\%$, $S_2Sn = 66\%$ and $RS_1 = 91\%$, $S_1S_2 = 81\%$, $S_2Sn = 75\%$). The following settings were chosen: number of consecutive intervals to trigger = 4, delay after treatment = 0, maximum number of pulses in treatment = 10. In patients where the number of consecutive intervals to trigger was > 4, this was corrected to equal 4 to calculate the mean time required to terminate tachycardia.

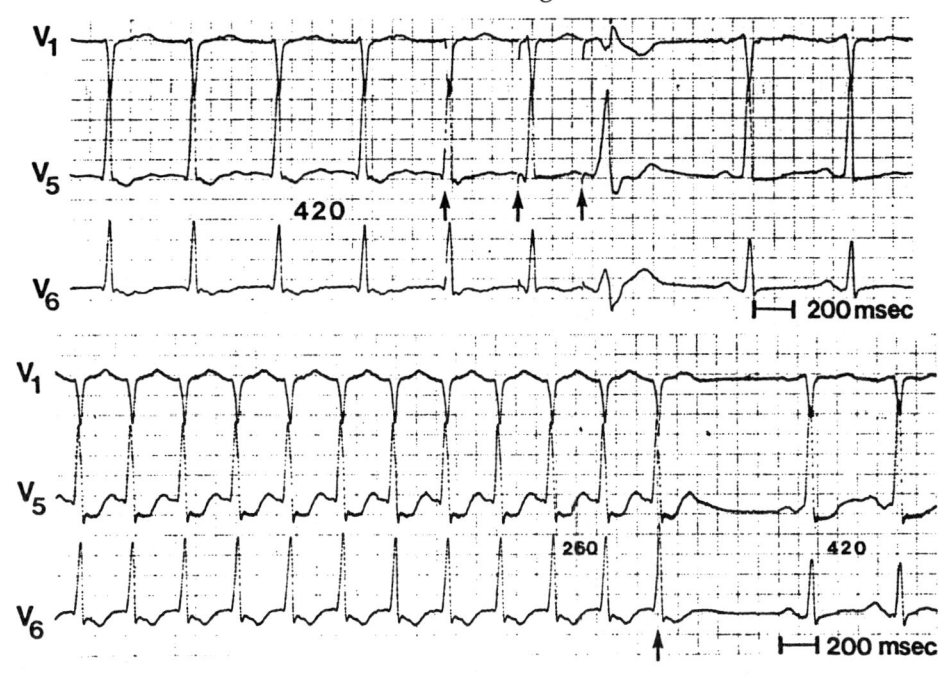

Figure 1: Two three-channel electrocardiographic recordings of termination of two episodes of circus movement tachycardia with different rates in a patient with WPW syndrome and dual AV nodal pathways. The adaptive mode (RS_1 = 91%, S_1S_2 = 81%, S_2Sn = 75%) with an increasing number of stimuli was used to terminate tachycardia. Top Strip: Three stimuli from the coronary sinus were required to terminate tachycardia using the slowly conducting AV nodal pathway for AV conduction. The third stimulus is anterogradely conducted over the left-sided accessory pathway. We cannot therefore exclude that tachycardia was terminated by the second stimulus. Bottom Strip: One stimulus from the coronary sinus was required to terminate tachycardia using the fast conducting AV nodal pathway for AV conduction.

Patients

The pacing mode was tried prospectively with short (RS_1 = 75%, S_1S_2 = 69%, S_2Sn = 66%) and long (RS_1 = 91%, S_1S_2 = 81%, S_2Sn = 75%) coupling intervals in two groups of patients. Group I consisted of 19 patients who underwent electrophysiologic study for supraventricular tachycardia in our laboratory according to methods described previously.[6] In this group of patients, termination was attempted from high right atrium, coronary sinus, and right ventricle. Each mode (RS_1 = 75%, S_1S_2 = 69%, S_2Sn = 66%, and RS_1 = 91%, S_1S_2 = 81%, S_2Sn = 75%) was tried once from a single stimulation site. Group II consisted of 11 patients who came to the outpatient clinic for check-up of their Medtronic Interactive Tachy pacemaker every 3–4 months. The adaptive mode using an automatically increasing number of stimuli had not been tried in the electrophysiology laboratory prior to implantation of the pacemaker. Tachycardia was initiated noninvasively by means of the Medtronic Prescription Formulator (model sp0503) using a radiofrequency link with the implanted pacemaker. Each antitachycardia pacing mode was tried once at each follow-up visit, so that in this group of patients, the two modes were tried several times on different occasions from the same stimulation site.

Antitachycardia Pacemaker Experience

Patients

Thirty-one patients had pacemakers implanted for termination of their paroxysmal-reentrant SVT. Eighteen had a Medtronic model sp0500 (patient-activated), five had a Cordis model 284 (automatic and/or patient-activated), five had an Intermedics model 262-12 (automatic and/or patient-activated) of which one electively replaced a Medtronic model sp0500 during breast surgery, two had a Medtronic model 7008 (automatic), and one a Medtronic model 7000. Fifteen of the patients were women, 16 were men. They were 22 to 70 years old (mean 52). Long-term oral drug trials had failed to control their tachycardias. A DDD pacemaker was implanted in three patients, in two for bradycardia support, prevention, and termination of tachycardia, in one for prevention and termination. In each patient, an electrophysiological study was performed to determine the mechanism of tachycardia and the pacing site from which the tachycardia could be safely terminated. The pacing catheter was placed as close to the circuit as possible, using the pacing site that was most successful during the electrophysiological study. Atrial stimulation was avoided wherever possible if atrial fibrillation or flutter was easily induced. Fifteen patients were paced from the right atrium, five from the coronary sinus, eight from the right ventricle, and three had a DDD pacemaker implanted for prevention as well as termination of tachycardia.

System Description

Devices used have been described extensively elsewhere.[3,4,8–10]

Work-Up

A symptom-limited maximal exercise test and a 24-hour Holter recording during daily activity before pacemaker implantation were used to evaluate if tachycardia recognition by rate would be able to distinguish sinus tachycardia from the reentrant tachycardia. After implantation, tachycardias were repeatedly initiated and terminated in supine and upright positions as well as after exercise to ensure safe and reproducible termination with the least number of stimuli with maximal coupling intervals.

Follow-Up

During outpatient clinic visits, the number of episodes of tachycardia, success rate of the system, complications, and problems that had occurred in the interim were recorded. During each visit, tachycardias were initiated several times and adequate termination by the pacemaker was checked. If pacing treatment was inadequate, the mode was tailored and retested to ensure prompt and safe termination of tachycardia.

Results

Adaptive Mode Using an Automatically Increasing Number of Stimuli

An antitachycardia pacing mode using an automatically increasing number of stimuli with adaptive coupling intervals was tested in 31 patients. One hundred and fifteen tachycardias were initiated (36 in the outpatient clinic and 79 in the electrophysiology laboratory). Tables I and II summarize the results.

Group I

In patients with AV nodal tachycardia, tachycardia cycle length ranged from 255 to 420 (mean 340) ms. In patients with WPW syndrome, tachycardia cycle length ranged from 240 to 460 (mean 315) ms. In the patients with a concealed accessory pathway, it ranged from 260 to 330 (mean 305) ms. During 79 episodes of tachycardia, termination was attempted with an increasing number of stimuli and adaptive coupling intervals.

As shown in Table II, 43 terminations were attempted with coupling intervals 75% (RS_1), 69% (S_1S_2), 66% (S_2Sn). One episode of AV nodal tachycardia was not terminated from the right ventricle in a patient with complete right bundle branch block. The arrhythmia could, however, be terminated with longer coupling intervals of 91%, 81%, and 75%. The mean time required and mean number of

Table I
Number of Patients, Tachycardia Mechanism, and Incidence of Successful Termination in the Electrophysiology Laboratory (Group I)

	mode RS_1 = 75%, S_1S_2 = 69%, S_2Sn = 66%		
	AVN	CAP	WPW
RA	7/7	3/3	7/7
CS	—	3/3	5/5
RV	6/7*	5/5	6/6
No pat	7	5	7
	mode RS_1 = 91%, S_1S_2 = 81%, S_2Sn = 75%		
	AVN	CAP	WPW
RA	5/5	2/2	7/7
CS	—	3/3	5/5
RV	5/5	4/4	4/5**
No pat	6	4	7

AVN = AV nodal tachycardia; CAP = concealed accessory pathway; WPW = Wolff-Parkinson-White syndrome; RA = right atrium; CS = coronary sinus; RV = right ventricle; pat = patients; * = tachycardia could not be terminated in one patient; ** = atrial fibrillation was induced in one patient.

Table II
Number of Patients, Tachycardia Mechanism, and Incidence of Successful Termination in the Out-Patient Clinic (Group II)

	mode RS_1 = 75%, S_1S_2 = 69%, S_2Sn = 66%		
	AVN	CAP	WPW
RA	6/6	—	—
CS	3/3	3/3	3/3
RV	—	2/2	2/2
No pat	5	3	2
	mode RS_1 = 91%, S_1S_2 = 81%, S_2Sn = 75%		
	AVN	CAP	WPW
RA	4/4	—	1/1
CS	2/2	4/4	2/2
RV	—	2/2	2/2
No pat	5	3	3

AVN = AV nodal tachycardia; CAP = concealed accessory pathway; WPW = Wolff-Parkinson-White syndrome; RA = right atrium; CS = coronary sinus; RV = right ventricle; pat = patients.

premature beats to terminate tachycardia were 7203 ms, 3.5 beats from the right atrium; 2685 ms, 1.6 beats from the coronary sinus; and 5880 ms, 3.2 beats from the right ventricle.

Thirty-six terminations were attempted using coupling intervals 91% (RS_1), 81% (S_1S_2), 75% (S_2Sn). In one patient, who was studied because of repeated episodes of collapse due to atrial fibrillation in the presence of a WPW syndrome, atrial fibrillation was induced during circus movement tachycardia by two stimuli from the right ventricle (which induced two repetitive ventricular responses). The mean time required and mean number of premature beats to terminate tachycardia were 10110 ms, 4.6 beats from the right atrium; 6478 ms 3.4 beats from the coronary sinus; and 6506 ms, 3.4 beats from the right ventricle.

Comparison of the two test modes suggests that the mode with shorter coupling intervals requires less time and less stimuli to terminate tachycardia.

Group II

Tachycardia cycle length ranged from 280 to 400 (mean 340) ms in patients with AV nodal tachycardia, from 320 to 440 (mean 395) ms in patients with WPW syndrome, and from 270 to 400 (mean 345) ms in patients with a concealed accessory pathway. In this group of 11 patients, all episodes of tachycardia (36 episodes) were terminated promptly. The mean time required and mean number of premature beats to terminate tachycardia was 5150 ms, 2.5 premature beats for the 75%, 69%, 66% coupling intervals and 6510 ms, 2.8 premature beats for coupling intervals 91%, 81%, and 75%.

Success of Termination

Of the 115 attempted terminations of tachycardia, two were not successful. In one patient with AV nodal tachycardia with complete right bundle branch block, coupling intervals of 75%, 69%, and 66% were too short to reach the circuit to terminate tachycardia from the right ventricle. Tachycardia was terminated, however, with coupling intervals 91%, 81%, and 75%. In one patient with WPW and several clinical episodes of atrial fibrillation, two stimuli ($RS_1 = 91\%$, $S_1S_2 = 81\%$) delivered in the right ventricle (gave rise to two repetitive ventricular responses) induced atrial fibrillation. All other episodes were terminated promptly with the test mode without having prior knowledge about the required coupling intervals or number of stimuli.

Antitachycardia Pacing Experience

Table III is a summary of the data from our 31 patients who underwent pacemaker implantation for SVT. Two patients died during follow-up. One died from congestive failure in the presence of dextrocardia, monoatrium, monoventricle, and transposition of the great arteries. The other patient died in a terminal stage of metastasized carcinoid syndrome. A third patient, who initially preferred pacemaker therapy, recently underwent sectioning of a concealed accessory pathway after having required two lead replacements because of lead insulation problems within 5 years.

Tachycardias at Home

During a total follow-up period of 955 months, an estimated 10,016 episodes of tachycardia occurred spontaneously; 9921 were terminated promptly by the pacemaker. Fifty-one were prolonged and required several attempts to terminate; 36 episodes were sustained and lasted longer than 30 minutes. Episodes lasting longer than 30 minutes occurred in five patients. In one patient, three episodes occurred because of intermittent capture (for which the pulse width was reprogrammed). In three patients, 32 episodes occurred during emotional stress and tachycardia was terminated 30–45 minutes after taking an antiarrhythmic agent. One patient did not have a spare battery for the pacemaker activator. Eight of the remaining episodes of tachycardia required admission to hospital for termination of tachycardia; one patient was admitted twice with atrial fibrillation, one because the tachycardia trigger interval was too short after prescribing a beta-blocker for hypertension, one because of a lead dislocation, one because of improper use of the pacemaker activator, one was admitted with atrial flutter (adaptive mode with increasing stimuli could subsequently be used to terminate circus movement tachycardia as well as atrial flutter), one because of inadequate intake of antiarrhythmic medication, and one because of a defective pacemaker activator.

Table III
Type of Tachycardia, Age, Sex, Presence or Absence of Associated Cardiac Disease and Antiarrhythmic Therapy, Pacing Site, Number of Hospital Admissions in the 3 Months Prior to Pacemaker Implantation and During Follow-Up After Implantation in 31 Patients with Supraventricular Tachycardia

Case	Age, Sex	Associated Cardiac Disease	Pacing Site	Antiarr. Therapy	Hospital Admission Before impl. (3 mo)	after impl	Follow-up (months)
AV Nodal Tachycardia							
1	61m	...	ra	+	2	0	24
2	55f	...	ra	+	3	0	22
3	62f	...	rv	+	0	0	18
4	50m	Carcin Syn	rv	−	3	0	16
5	70f	...	ra	−	2	1	44
6	60m	...	ra	+	2	2	10
7	42f	...	ra	−	9	0	36
8	37f	...	ra	−	2	1	30
9	56f	par. af	cs	+	6	1	55
10	67f	...	ra	−	1	0	5
11	61f	...	cs	−	2	0	24
12	60f	...	ra	−	2	0	30
Concealed Accessory Pathway							
13	61f	...	ra	−	1	0	15
14	37m	...	rv	+	5	0	67
15	52m	...	ra	+	0	0	27
16	22m	Complex cong defect	ra	+	4	1	43
17	46m	...	cs	+	5	1	69
18	51m	...	rv	−	3	0	24
26	53m	mi	cs	+	2	0	66
27	35m	...	ra	−	2	0	12
28	59f	...	rv	+	1	0	30
Atrial Tachycardia							
29	49f	...	ra	−	1	0	9
30	66f	...	ra	−	0	0	8
Atrial Flutter							
31	43m	SSS + AV cond dist	a + v	+	1	0	30

Antiarr = antiarrhythmic; impl. = implantation; mo = months; m = male; f = female; Carcin Syn = carcinoid syndrome; par. af = paroxysmal atrial fibrillation; ra = right atrium; cs = coronary sinus; rv = right ventricle; a + v = atrium and ventricle; cong = congenital; mit. insuff = mitral insufficiency; SSS = sick sinus syndrome; DC = dilated cardiomyopathy; cond dist = cnduction disturbance; + = yes; − = no.

Patient Opinion

For 30 patients, pacemaker implantation has been a very satisfactory mode of therapy. It has changed their lifestyle completely, avoiding repetitive hospital admissions and the inconvenience of many prolonged episodes of tachycardia. In fact, most of the patients with an automatic pacemaker (as documented by Holter recordings) either do not feel tachycardia at all or only have a premature beat sensation when tachycardia is terminated rapidly. Two patients were temporarily dissatisfied because of prolonged episodes of tachycardia. One of these two patients has now undergone sectioning of a concealed accessory pathway after requiring a second lead replacement within 5 years. In one patient, the clinical result has been less than satisfactory. After implantation of a pacemaker for AV nodal tachycardia he had to be admitted twice with atrial fibrillation.

Additional Tachycardias

Tachycardias other than the tachycardia for which the pacemaker was implanted or tachycardias in which the reentry circuit changed occurred in nine patients. In four patients, another tachycardia occurred; in two, the additional tachycardia was an atrial tachycardia, in one it was an atrial flutter, and one patient had atrial tachycardia, AV nodal tachycardia, and tachycardias with marked rate changes because of reentrant circuits using an accessory pathway and dual AV nodal pathways. Rate of tachycardia changed markedly with change in the reentrant circuit in the remaining five patients due to bundle branch block in two, WPW syndrome and dual AV nodal pathways in one, and 2:1 subnodal block during AV nodal tachycardia in two (Fig. 2).

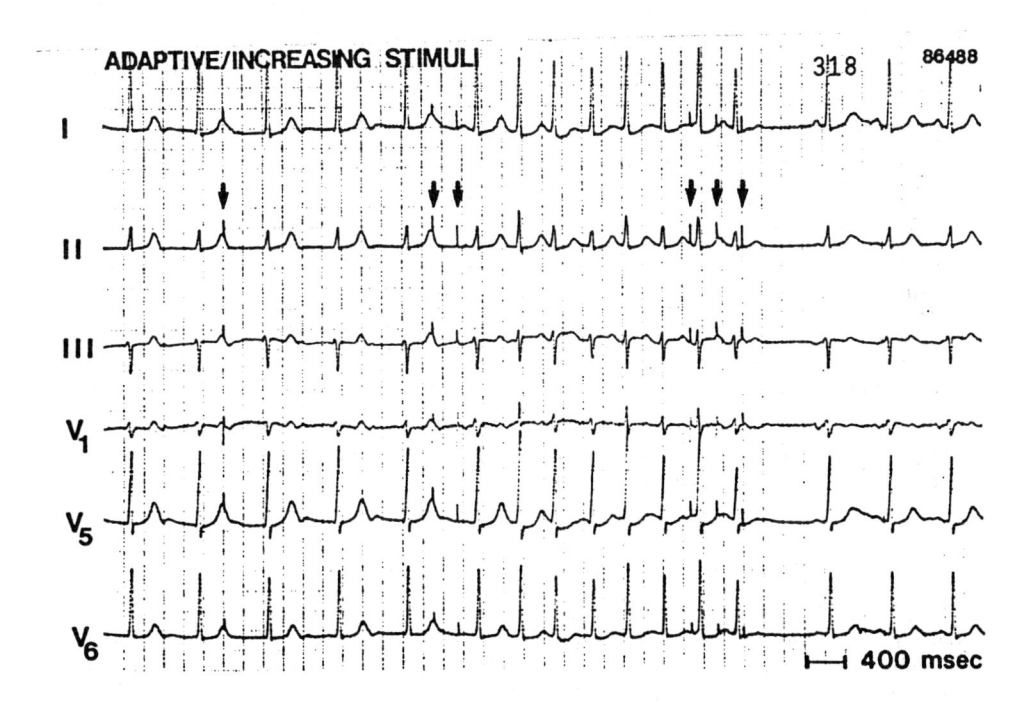

Figure 2: Six-channel electrocardiographic recording illustrating termination of an AV nodal tachycardia with 2:1 subnodal block (left part of the figure) with the universal antitachycardia pacing mode. After delivering two APBs, 1:1 conduction is restored and tachycardia is subsequently terminated with three APBs.

Discussion

Antitachycardia pacing has previously been found to be very effective over the short term.[3,4] In addition, as shown in this report, the long-term results appear to be as good. The pacemakers are safe, reliable, and effective in terminating paroxysmal reentrant tachycardias. This mode of therapy has improved the quality of life significantly in these patients by rapidly terminating previously prolonged episodes of tachycardia and by avoiding repetitive hospital admissions. Most patients with automatic devices either don't feel the short episodes of pacemaker-terminated tachycardia or recognize the episode as a premature beat.

After implantation of an antitachycardia pacemaker, the mode selected needs to be tested and tailored under various circumstances because number and timing of required stimuli may change with changes in posture, autonomic tone, tachycardia rate, refractory period, drug level, or for other reasons. This testing and tailoring takes a long time. An adaptive pacing mode with increasing number of stimuli adapts to these changes by adjusting the coupling intervals to the tachycardia rate and by delivering the required number of stimuli to terminate tachycardia.

As discussed, additional supraventricular tachycardias occur commonly (9 of 31 patients). The benefit of an adaptive antitachycardia pacing mode using an increasing number of stimuli lies not only in the time saved during testing and tailoring but also in the ability to cope with additional reentrant tachycardias easily, because, as shown, this mode of pacing rapidly terminates reentrant supraventricular tachycardias without having prior knowledge about required coupling intervals or number of stimuli. Our results support an approach that during the invasive electrophysiological study the mechanism of tachycardia, safety, and applicability of antitachycardia pacing be studied and not the reproducibility of termination under various circumstances. This can be studied after pacemaker implantation. In the electrophysiology laboratory, the test mode with short coupling intervals terminated tachycardia quicker and required less stimuli to terminate. In the out-patient clinic group, this difference was not seen and could be due to patient selection as well as the fact that the best stimulation site was selected for chronic antitachycardia pacing.

We conclude that a pacing mode using adaptive coupling intervals with an automatically increasing number of stimuli represents a universal antitachycardia pacing mode for rapid termination of reentrant supraventricular tachycardias irrespective of rate or site of origin.

References

1. Barold SS, Falkoff MD, Ong LS, Heinle RA. New pacing techniques for the treatment of tachycardias. The golden age of cardiac pacing. In Barold SS, Mugica JM, eds. The Third Decade of Cardiac Pacing. New York, Futura Publishing Co, 1982;309–332.
2. Fisher JD, Kim SG, Furman S, Matos JA. Role of implantable pacemakers in control of recurrent ventricular tachycardia. Am J Cardiol 1982;49:194–206.
3. den Dulk K, Bertholet M, Brugada P, Bar FW, Richards D, Demoulin JC, Waleffe A, Bakels N, Lindemans FW, Bourgeois I, Kulbertus HE, Wellens HJJ. A versatile pacemaker system for termination of tachycardias. Am J Cardiol 1983;52:731–738.

4. den Dulk K, Bertholet M, Brugada P, Bar FW, Demoulin JC, Waleffe A, Bakels N, Lindemans FW, Bourgeois I, Kulbertus HE, Wellens HJJ. Clinical experience with implantable devices for control of tachyarrhythmias. PACE 1984;7:548–556.
5. den Dulk K, Kersschot IE, Brugada P, Wellens HJJ. Is there a universal antitachycardia pacing mode? Am J Cardiol 1986;57:950–955.
6. Ross DL, Farre J, Baer FWHM, Vanagt E, Dassen WRM, Wiener I, Wellens HJJ: Comprehensive clinical electrophysiological studies in the investigation of documented or suspected tachycardias. Time, staff, problems and costs. Circulation 1980;61:1010–1016.
7. den Dulk K, Brugada P, Waldecker B, Begemann M, van der Schatte O, Wellens HJJ: Automatic pacemaker termination of two different types of supraventricular tachycardia. J Am Coll Cardiol 1985;6:201–5.
8. Nathan AW, Creamer JE, Davies DW, Camm AJ. Clinical experience with a software based tachycardia reversion pacemaker. PACE 1986;9:1312–1315.
9. Zipes DP, Prystowsky EN, Miles WM, Heger JJ. Initial experience with Symbios model 7008 pacemaker. PACE 1984;7:1301–1305.
10. den Dulk K, Lindemans FW, Wellens HJJ. Noninvasive evaluation of pacemaker circus movement tachycardias. Am J Cardiol 1984;53:537–543.

IV

Ventricular Tachycardia and Sudden Death

17

Signal Averaging of the ECG in the Management of Patients with Ventricular Tachycardia: Prediction of Antiarrhythmic Drug Efficacy

Michael B. Simson
Elizabeth Kindwall
Alfred E. Buxton
Mark E. Josephson

Introduction

In the last decade, investigators have recorded distinctive, high frequency potentials on the body surface of patients with ventricular tachycardia (VT) after myocardial infarction.[1-7] These waveforms, frequently termed "late potentials," are continuous with the QRS complex and generally require a signal averaged electrocardiogram (ECG) to detect because the amplitude is less than 20 microvolts. Late potentials are rarely recorded from normal patients and appear to correlate with delayed and disorganized activation in small areas of the myocardium.[8]

Successful surgical control of VT often normalizes the signal averaged ECG and eliminates the late potential.[9,10] The effects of antiarrhythmic drug therapy on the signal-averaged ECG is less clear and it has been reported that effective drug therapy is associated with a decrease in high frequency components in the terminal QRS and early ST segment.[11] This study was undertaken to evaluate the effects of antiarrhythmic drugs on the signal-averaged ECG in patients with VT

From: Brugada P, Wellens HJJ. CARDIAC ARRHYTHMIAS: Where To Go From Here? Mount Kisco, NY, Futura Publishing Company, Inc., © 1987.

and to test whether drug-induced changes in the signal-averaged ECG could predict successful control of the arrhythmia.

Methods

The patient population consisted of 49 patients with a history of spontaneous, recurrent sustained VT. All patients had suffered a myocardial infarction more than 1 month prior to study. The VT occurred at least 1 week after myocardial infarction. The infarcts were inferior in 26, anterior in 22, and non-Q wave in one patient. All patients were in sinus rhythm and none had bundle branch block. There were 38 men and 11 women with a mean age of 57 years (range 37–69 years of age).

Each patient underwent electrophysiologic testing using previously described techniques while on no antiarrhythmic medications (control study).[12] Sustained (>30 sec) VT of uniform morphology was inducible by one to three premature ventricular depolarizations in each patient. Electrophysiologic testing and a signal-averaged ECG were repeated after oral administration of antiarrhythmic drugs. Six agents were used, alone and in combination (amiodarone, procainamide, quinidine, phenytoin, mexiletine, and disopyramide). A total of 70 trials were performed and each drug was used in four to 22 trials. Serum concentrations were available and were within the "therapeutic range" at the time of the repeat electrophysiologic evaluation and signal-averaged ECG, (Table I). Patients on amiodarone were tested after receiving a loading dose 1400 mg daily for 1 week, and after at least 1 week of therapy at 400–800 mg daily.

For all drugs except amiodarone, successful therapy was defined as no inducible VT and no recurrence of VT for at least 1 year. If a patient had inducible VT, then the trial was judged a failure and another antiarrhythmic agent was tried. For patients on amiodarone, successful therapy was defined as no VT recurrence during a 1 year follow-up. There were 21 successful and 49 unsuccessful trials.

A signal-averaged ECG was recorded within 1 day of each electrophysiologic stimulation test. Signal averaging is a computer-based process which reduces extraneous noise, primarily from skeletal muscle, which contaminates the ECG. The technique averages together multiple samples of a repetitive waveform, such as the QRS complex. Nonrepeating, random noise tends to cancel and is reduced.[13]

Table I
Antiarrhythmic Drugs Used (Alone and in Combination)

Drug	Number of Trials	Serum Level ($\mu g/ml$)
Amiodarone	22	
Procainamide	19	11.1 ± 4.6
Quinidine	17	3.8 ± 1.5
Phenytoin	11	11.5 ± 6.5
Mexiletine	6	
Disopyramide	4	3.7 ± 1.8

Bipolar X, Y, Z leads were averaged during sinus rhythm. The X lead was between the right and left midaxillary lines at the 4th intercostal space. The Y leads were placed at the superior aspect of the manubrium and the proximal left leg. The anterior Z lead was at the V_2 position and the other electrode was at an identical position on the posterior chest. The three leads were amplified and then converted into digital format with a resolution of 1 or 2.5 µV. The band width was 0.05 to 250 Hz.

The ECG waveforms were signal averaged after being matched against a template of previous beats in order to reject ectopic or grossly noisy beats.[5] Approximately 140 beats were averaged. The reference time for the averaging process was derived from one lead, usually the Z lead, at a time when the slope of the QRS complex was rapid. The variation in the reference time or "trigger jitter" was measured at 0.5 ms (standard deviation), thereby ensuring a high frequency response of greater than 200 Hz.[5,13]

Each averaged lead processed with a high pass filter in order to eliminate the low frequencies contained in the QRS complex and the ST segment. A specially designed, bidirectional filter was used in order to eliminate filter ringing or artifacts which would impair the detection of low level signals that occur at the end of the QRS complex.[5] The filter was based on a 4 pole Butterworth design which has a maximally flat response above 25 Hz and sharp attenuation characteristics below 25 Hz, −24 dB/octave. The filtered leads were then combined into a vector magnitude, $\sqrt{(X^2 + Y^2 + Z^2)}$, a measure which sums the high frequency voltage contained in each lead and which is referred to as the "filtered QRS complex" in this chapter (Fig. 1).

Six measurements were made on the filtered QRS complex. First, the total duration was determined; the end-points of the filtered QRS complex were identified by a computer algorithm. Second, the time that the terminal portion of the filtered QRS complex remained under 40 µV was determined. The voltage in the first 80 ms of the filtered QRS complex and in the last 40 ms was calculated using the root mean square method. A vector magnitude was also formed from the unfiltered leads. The voltage in the first 80 and the last 40 ms was measured so that the amount of high frequency (>25Hz) components could be expressed as a fraction of the total voltage at the same portion of the QRS complex.

A late potential was defined as a low amplitude signal (<25 µV) in the last 40 ms of the filtered QRS complex. An abnormal signal-averaged ECG was defined as a filtered QRS complex longer than 110 ms or the presence of a late potential. All data is presented as the mean ± standard deviation and comparisons were made by the paired and unpaired Student's *t*-test.

Results

In the control recordings, 42 patients (86%) had an abnormal signal-averaged ECG. The filtered QRS duration was prolonged (136 ± 27 ms) and the voltage in the last 40 ms of the filtered QRS complex was low (18 ± 16 µV). The filtered voltage remained <40 µV in the terminal QRS for 55 ± 30 ms (normal is <39 ms).

Figure 2 illustrates the effect of amiodarone and procainamide on the filtered

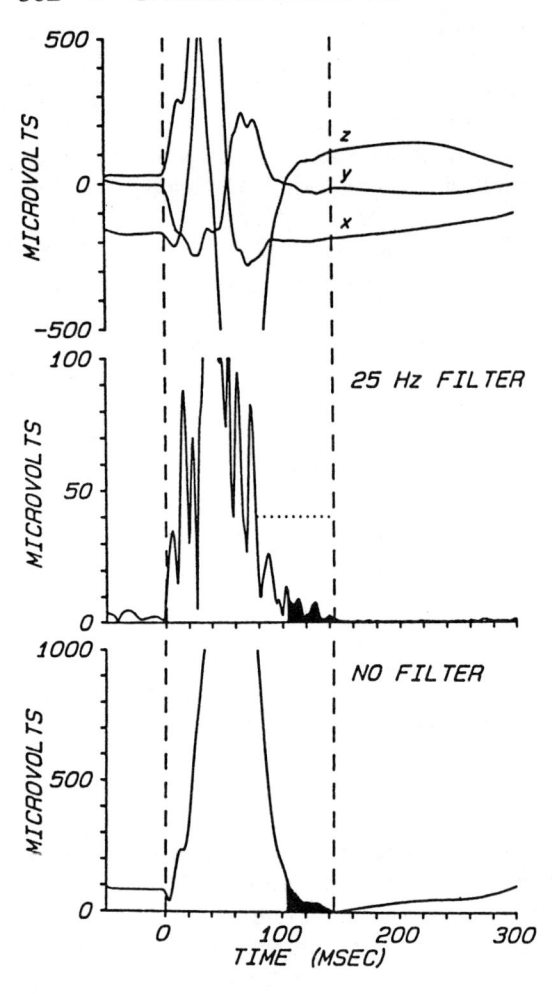

Figure 1: An example of the signal processing. On the top are signal averaged X, Y, and Z leads. The middle panel shows the filtered QRS complex, a vector magnitude of the filtered leads. The end-points of the filtered QRS are shown by the dashed lines. The duration that the filtered QRS complex remains below 40 μV is indicated by the dotted line. The bottom panel shows the vector magnitude of the unfiltered leads. The amplitude is much larger than the filtered QRS complex (middle) because large amplitude, low frequency components are included. The shaded areas show the last 40 ms of both vector magnitudes.

QRS complex. Off medication, the patient had a long filtered QRS complex (117 ms) and low voltage in the terminal portions of the filtered QRS complex (12 μV in the last 40 ms). The drug therapy prolonged the filtered QRS duration and the low amplitude signal at the terminal portion of the filtered QRS complex. The arrhythmia was not controlled by the antiarrhythmic agents in this patient.

The changes that occurred in the measured parameters with all the drug trials are presented in Figures 3–6. In general, the changes were small but statistically significant by paired analysis. With drug therapy, the mean filtered QRS duration increased by 10.1 ± 16.7 ms ($P < 0.001$), a change of 7.4%. The duration that the amplitude remained under 40 μV in the terminal portion of the filtered QRS complex increased by 3.5 ± 13.4 ms ($P = 0.02$), a change of 6.5%. Hence, both the low amplitude, terminal portion of the filtered QRS complex, and the overall filtered QRS duration prolonged by a similar degree with drug therapy.

The voltage in the first 80 ms of the filtered QRS complex, the initial high amplitude portion, decreased by 7.8% or 9.8 ± 31.9 μV ($P = 0.006$) (Fig. 4). The voltage in the last 40 ms of the filtered QRS complex decreased by 9.6% or

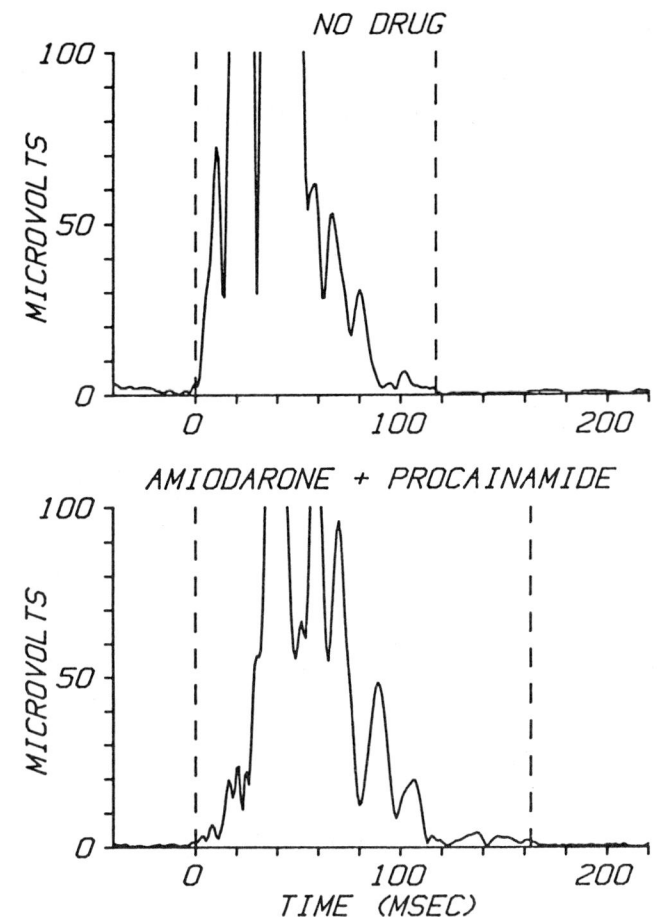

Figure 2: The effects of amiodarone and procainamide on the filtered QRS complex. With therapy, the filtered QRS complex prolongs from 117 to 164 ms and the voltage late in the filtered QRS complex decreases from 12 to 3 μV. The terminal portion of the filtered QRS complex remains below 40 μV for 44 ms in the control recording and 70 ms after antiarrhythmic agents were administered.

1.7 ± 8.6 μV (P = 0.05). When the filtered QRS voltage was normalized for the total voltage in the same segment, there was a 20.4% decrease with therapy in the first 80 ms of the QRS (Fig. 5). The high frequency (>25 Hz) components represented 0.14 ± 0.07 of the total voltage before therapy and those components decreased 0.11 ± 0.05 with drug administration (P =0.001). The relative amplitude of the filtered QRS voltage in the last 40 ms decreased by 11.6% with drug therapy (0.10 ± 0.06 vs 0.09 ± 0.06, P =0.003). The antiarrhythmic agents decreased the high frequency components in the initial and terminal portions of the QRS both relatively and absolutely.

In 21 trials, the VT was successfully controlled by the antiarrhythmic agents. The agents failed to control the arrhythmia in 49 trials, most frequently because VT remained inducible. The signal-averaged ECG did not predict the outcome of the drug trial. Similar changes were found in each measured parameter regardless of whether the trial succeeded or failed. The QRS duration during therapy increased by 8.9 ± 17.8 ms in the successful and 10.6 ± 16.4 ms in the unsuccessful trials (P = 0.35) (Fig. 6). When the duration of signal less than 40 μV in the terminal portion of the filtered QRS complex was considered, there was a 5.3 ± 17.3

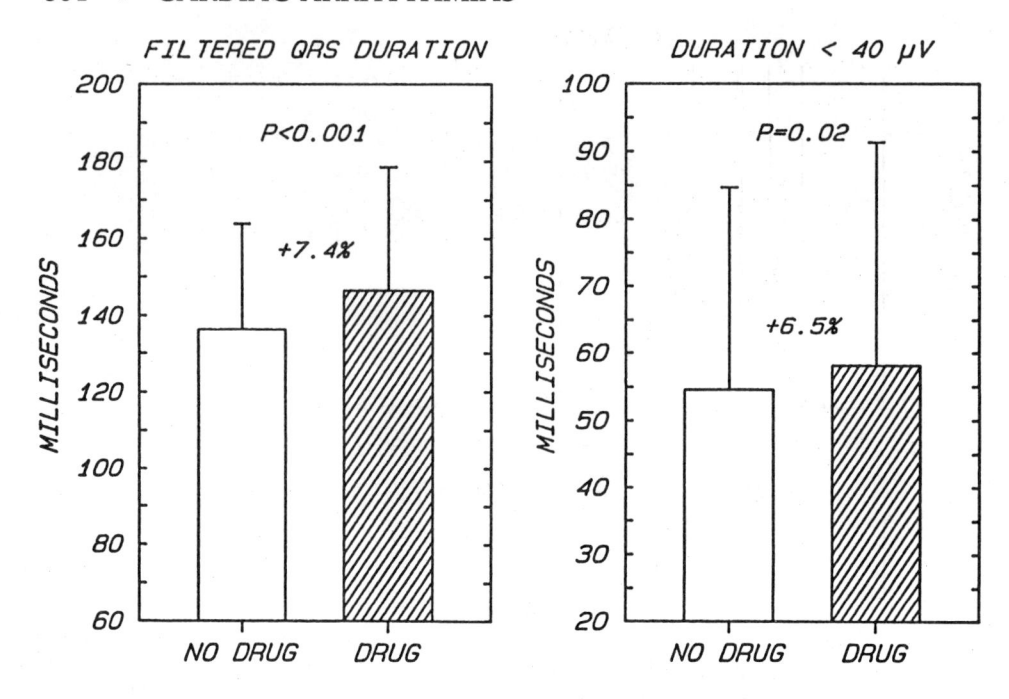

Figure 3: The filtered QRS duration and the duration that the amplitude remains less than 40 μV for the control recordings and those during drug administration (shaded bars). The percent change in the mean is indicated. The bar indicates the mean and standard deviation.

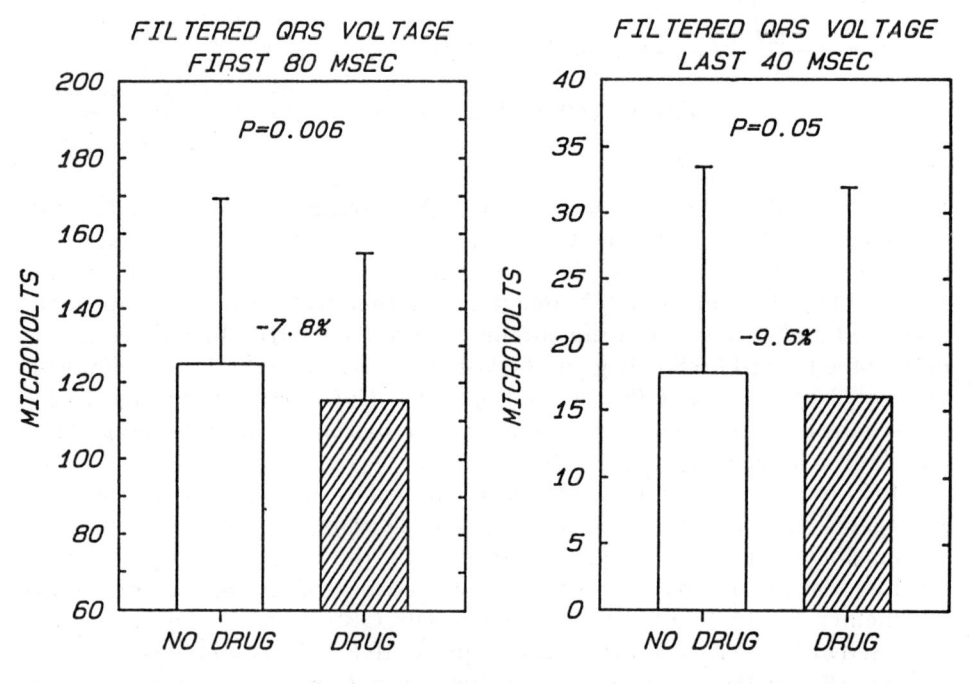

Figure 4: The filtered QRS voltage for the first 80 ms and the last 40 ms of the filtered QRS complex.

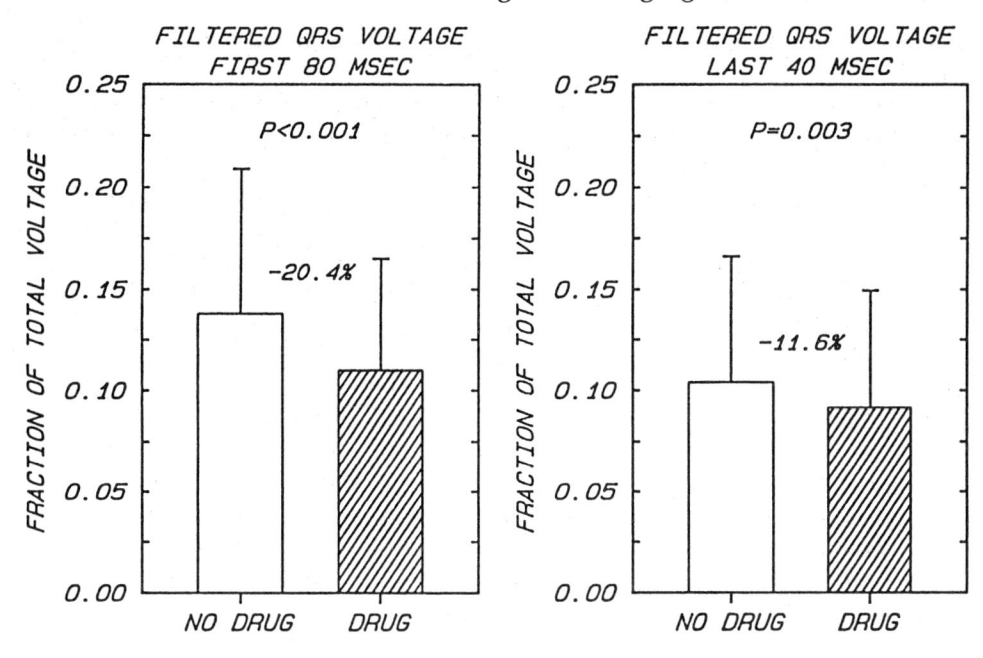

Figure 5: The filtered QRS voltage for the first 80 ms and the last 40 ms as expressed as a fraction of the total voltage in the same segments.

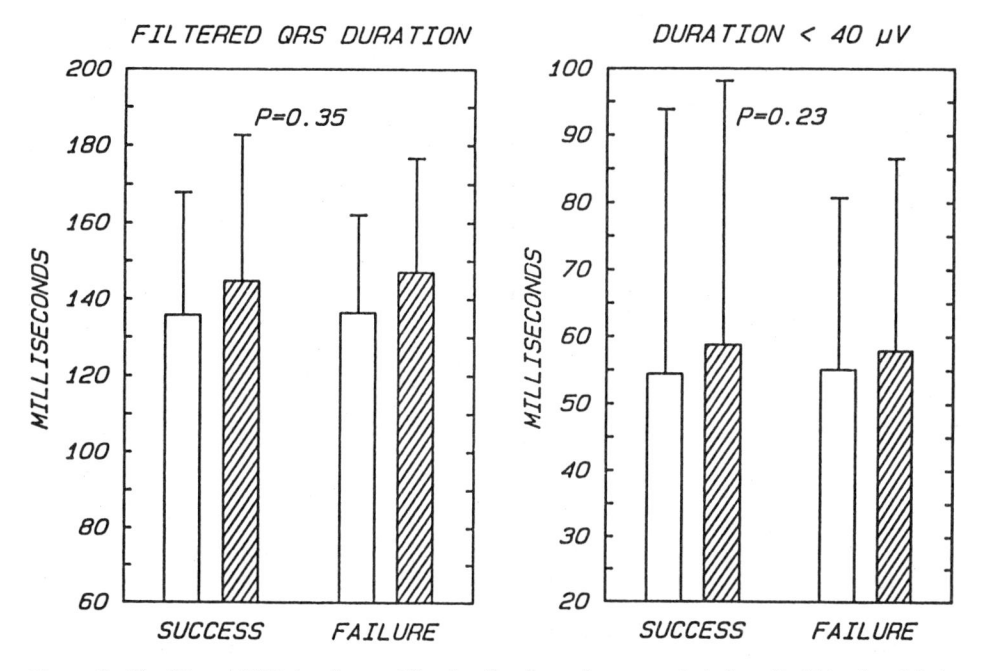

Figure 6: The filtered QRS duration and the duration the voltage remain below 40 μV for the trials in which the antiarrhythmic agents succeeded and failed to control VT. The clear bar is the control recording and the shaded bar is the measurement after drug is administered. The P-value refers to a comparison of the changes induced by the drugs in the successful and unsuccessful drug trials.

ms increase in the successful trials and a 2.8 ± 11.4 ms increase in the trials that failed (P = 0.23).

The filtered QRS voltage in the first 80 ms decreased in both the successful and unsuccessful trials by similar amounts (12.4 ± 38.1 µV vs 8.6 ±29.2 µV, P = 0.33) (Fig. 7). The filtered QRS voltage late in the QRS complex decreased in both the successful and unsuccessful trials; no significant difference could be detected between the changes (−2.4 ± 11.5 vs 1.4 ± 7.1 µV, P = 0.33). When the high frequency voltage of the filtered QRS was expressed as a fraction of total QRS voltage, there was a similar decrease in the initial portion of the QRS (Fig. 8). In both cases the fraction of high frequency energy decreased by a mean of 0.03 (P = 0.48). In the last 40 ms of the filtered QRS complex, there was a larger decrease in the successful drug trials (0.02 ± 0.03) than in the unsuccessful trials (0.008 ± 0.03). This trend, however, did not reach significance (P = 0.073).

In summary, a comparison of the changes in the six parameters measured on the signal-averaged ECG revealed no significant differences between the 21 successful trials and the 49 trials that failed to control VT. When two subgroups were analyzed, a similar lack of predictive value was detected. Amiodarone successfully controlled the arrhythmia in 14 trials and it failed in eight. Amiodarone altered the parameters in similar directions to those detected for all drugs (Figs. 6–8) and a comparison of the changes in the six parameters revealed insignificant differences (P= 0.14–0.48). When procainamide, quinidine, and disopyramide were examined as a group, they were successful in six trials and failed in 35 trials.

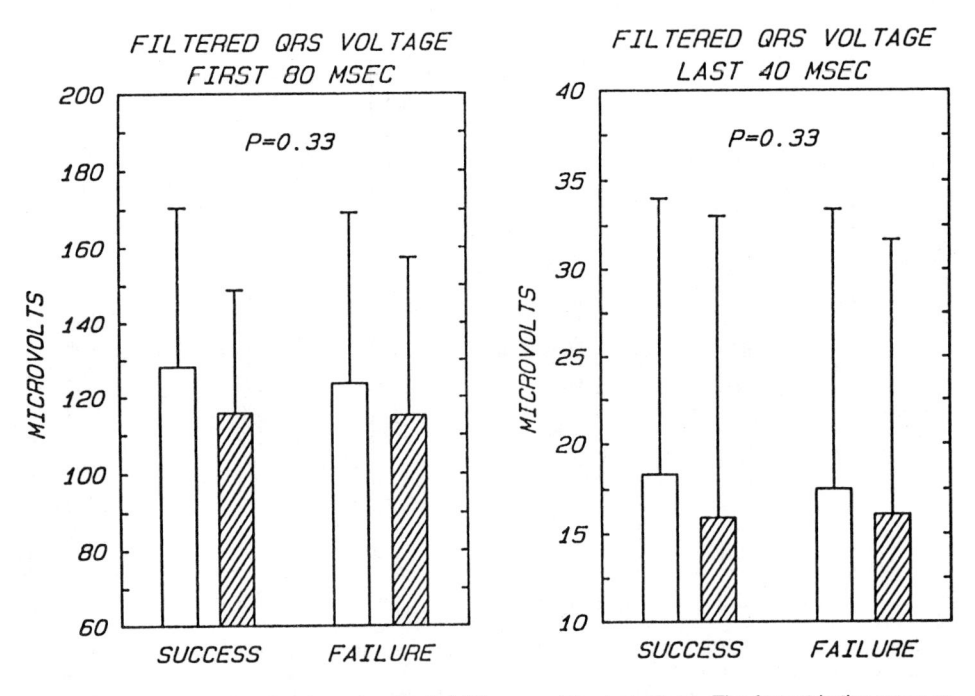

Figure 7: The filtered QRS voltage for the first 80 ms and the last 40 ms. The format is the same as Figure 6.

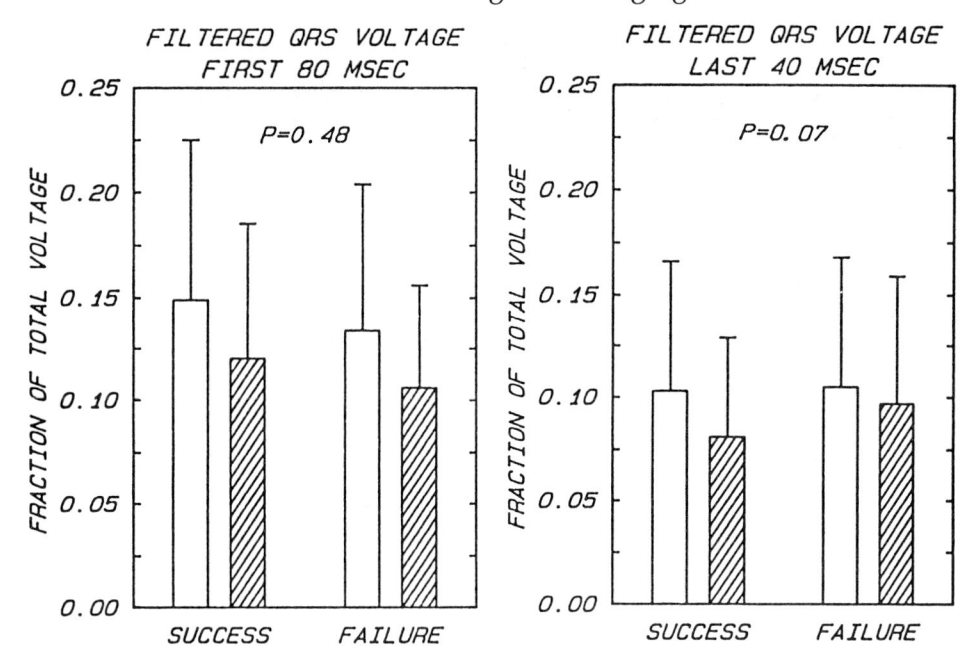

Figure 8: The filtered QRS voltage for the first 80 ms and the last 40 ms as expressed is a fraction of the total voltage in the same segment. The format is the same as Figure 6.

A comparison of changes in the six measured parameters revealed no meaningful differences between the successful and unsuccessful trials (P= 0.20–0.36).

Discussion

The purposes of this study were to evaluate the effects of antiarrhythmic agents on signal-averaged ECG and to determine whether drug-induced changes in the signal-averaged ECG predicted successful control of VT. Antiarrhythmic drug therapy, in general, prolongs the filtered QRS duration and decreases the filtered QRS voltages in the initial and terminal portions of the QRS complex. No pattern of change in the filtered QRS complex was identified, however, which would identify those patients for whom the VT could be controlled by antiarrhythmic agents.

Computerized signal averaging has been applied to the ECG in the last decade in order to reduce random noise, which arises primarily from skeletal muscle activity, and to allow the reliable detection of microvolt level waveforms on the body surface. In most studies, the noise level, after averaging, is approximately 1 μV or less, or 10–20 times lower than the noise level of a conventional ECG. A high pass filter is commonly applied to the signal-averaged ECG in order to reject the low frequency, large amplitude signal in the ECG associated with the plateau and repolarization phases of the action potential. The filter enhances relatively the high frequencies corresponding to the movement of wavefronts of activation.[14] The filter used in this study was designed to eliminate artifacts or ringing at the end of the QRS complex so that valid measurements of high frequencies in the terminal portion of the QRS could be made.[5] The Fourier transform has also been applied to signal-averaged ECGs in order to extract diagnostic high frequency content.[7]

Many groups have recorded abnormal signal-averaged ECGs from patients with VT.[1-7] The most commonly reported findings are an increase in the total duration of the filtered QRS complex and a low amplitude, high frequency waveform (late potential) in the terminal QRS complex. Seventy-three to 92% of patients with sustained and inducible VT after MI have abnormal signal-averaged ECGs. Only 0–6% of normal volunteers, and 7–15% of patients without VT after MI and Lown class 0-1 ectopy have abnormal signal-averaged ECGs.[5-7,15,16] Late potentials have also been recorded from patients with VT and arrhythmogenic right ventricular dysplasia or nonischemic cardiomyopathy.[15,17,18]

Late potentials appear to be a manifestation on the body surface of delayed activation in small areas of the myocardium. They have been recorded from dogs with experimental infarcts and the late potential correlated in time with fragmented and delayed electrograms recorded directly from the epicardium.[19,20] In patients with VT after myocardial infarction, the late potential has been shown to correspond to delayed and fragmented electrograms recorded from endocardial and epicardial sites within the zone of infarction.[3,4,17,21] In order to be recorded on the body surface as a late potential, the delayed activity must outlast the activation of most or all of the normal myocardium. When the fragmented electrograms were of brief duration, then late potentials could not be recorded on the body surface because they were masked by activation of normal myocardium.[21] After successful surgical control of VT in man, the late potential is commonly abolished or reduced in duration, and the signal-averaged ECG is often normalized.[2-4,9-10] In our experience, 90% of patients who lose the late potential after surgery will have the arrhythmia controlled.[10]

In this study, we found that late potentials were not abolished by antiarrhythmic agents and that successful pharmacologic control of the arrhythmia could be achieved despite persistence of late potentials. Our study provides indirect evidence that the antiarrhythmic drug study did not eliminate the delayed and disorganized ventricular activation which appears to be responsible for the late potential. The agents we investigated prolonged the total filtered QRS duration and the duration of low level signals in the terminal portion of the QRS complex by a similar degree (Fig. 3); this evidence suggests that the slowing of conduction by the antiarrhythmic agents occurred throughout the QRS complex.

VT after myocardial infarction is most likely due to a reentrant mechanism since the arrhythmia can be induced reliably with premature stimulation and it is associated with evidence of slow conduction.[12,22-27] Initiation of reentry requires unidirectional block, slow conduction, and a circuitous pathway. The persistence of the late potential with successful drug therapy argues that slow conduction in damaged tissue remains during sinus rhythm. There are several possible mechanisms by which the antiarrhythmic agents could disrupt a reentrant rhythm without affecting slow conduction during sinus rhythm. First, the drugs could prolong the refractory period of normal myocardium and thereby isolate the slowly conducting tissue and prevent reexcitation of normal myocardium. Second, a prolongation of conduction time in infarcted tissue has been noted in response to premature beats;[24] if the antiarrhythmic agents prevented early ectopic beats from occurring, then a sufficient degree of conduction delay may not be achieved to allow a reentrant arrhythmia to be established. Third, the agents could promote block within a slowly conducting tissue with premature stimulation or only during rapid rates of stimulation because of use-dependent properties. Studies during sinus rhythm may not reveal evidence of block. Finally, the agents could cause excessive degrees of conduction slowing with premature beats which can destabilize a reentrant circuit.[28] These possibilities and others require further investigation. The use of the signal averaging technique offers a noninvasive method of indirectly studying slow conduction and may provide insight into the mechanisms of action of antiarrhythmic agents. The signal-averaged ECG during sinus rhythm, however, does not appear to predict effective pharmacologic control of VT after myocardial infarction.

Acknowledgments: This research was supported in part by Grant HL27925 from the National Heart, Lung and Blood Institute. Dr. Simson is the Samuel Bellet Associate Professor of Medicine at the Hospital of the University of Pennsylvania. Dr. Josephson is the Robinette Professor of Medicine, University of Pennsylvania.

References

1. Fontaine, G, Guiraudon, G, Frank R, Vedel J, Grosgogeat Y, Cabrol C, Facquet J. Stimulation studies and epicardial mapping in ventricular tachycardia. Study of mechanisms and selection for surgery. In Kulbertus HE, ed. Reentrant Arrhythmias. Lancaster, MTP Press, 1977;334–350.
2. Uther JB, Dennett CJ, Tan A. The detection of delayed activation signals of low amplitude in the vectorcardiogram of patients with recurrent ventricular tachycardia by signal averaging. In Sandor E, Julian DJ, Bell JW, eds. Management of Ventricular Tachycardia—Role of Mexiletine. Amsterdam-Oxford, Excerpta Media, 1978;80.
3. Rozanski JJ, Mortara D, Myerburg RJ, Castellanos A. Body surface detection of delayed depolarization in patients with recurrent ventricular tachycardia and left ventricular aneurysm. Circulation 1981;63:1172–1178.
4. Breithardt G, Becker R, Seipel L, Abendroth R, Ostermeyer J. Noninvasive detection of late potentials in man - a new marker for ventricular tachycardia. Europ Heart J 1981;2:1–11.
5. Simson MB. Use of signals in the terminal QRS complex to identify patients with ventricular tachycardia after myocardial infarction. Circulation 1981;64:235–242.
6. Denes P, Santarelli P, Hauser RG, Uretz EF. Quantitative analysis of the high-frequency components of the terminal portion of the body surface QRS in normal subjects and in patients with ventricular tachycardia. Circulation 1983;67:1129–1138.
7. Cain ME, Ambos D, Witkowski FX, Sobel BE. Fast-Fourier transform analysis of signal-averaged electrocardiograms for the identification of patients prone to sustained ventricular tachycardia. Circulation 1984;69:711–720.
8. Simson MB, Untereker WJ, Spielman SR, Horowitz LN, Marcus NH, Falcone RA, Harken AH, Josephson ME. The relationship between late potentials on the body surface and directly recorded fragmented electrograms in patients with ventricular tachycardia. Am J Cardiol 1983;51:105–112.
9. Breithardt G, Seipel L, Ostermeyer J, Karbenn U, Abendroth R-R, Borggrefe M, Yeh HL, Bircks W. Effects of antiarrhythmic surgery on late ventricular potentials recorded

by precordial signal averaging in patients with ventricular tachycardia. Am Heart J 1982;104:996–1003.
10. Marcus NH, Falcone RA, Harken AH, Josephson ME, Simson MB. Body surface late potentials: Effects of endocardial resection in patients with ventricular tachycardia. Circulation 1984;70:632–637.
11. Cain ME, Ambos HD, Fischer AE, Markham J, Schectman KB. Noninvasive prediction of antiarrhythmic drug efficacy in patients with sustained ventricular tachycardia from frequency analysis of signal-averaged ECGs (abstr). Circulation 1984;70:II–252.
12. Buxton AE, Waxman HL, Marchlinski FE, Untereker WJ, Waspe LE, Josephson ME. Role of triple extrastimuli during electrophysiologic study of patients with documented sustained ventricular tachyarrhythmias. Circulation 1984;69:532–540.
13. Ros HH, Koeleman ASM, Akker TJV. The technique of signal averaging and its practical application in the separation of atrial and His Purkinje activity. In Hombach V, Hilger HH, eds. Signal Averaging Technique in Clinical Cardiology. Stuggart, New York, F.K. Schattauer Verlag, 1981;3.
14. Plonsey R: Bioelectric Phenomena. New York, McGraw Hill, 1969;281–299.
15. Breithardt G, Borggrefe M. Karbenn U, et al. Prevalence of late potentials in patients with and without ventricular tachycardia: Correlation and angiographic findings. Am J Cardiol 1982;49:1932–1937.
16. Coto H, Maldonado C, Palakurthy P, Flowers NC. Late potentials in normal subjects and in patients with ventricular tachycardia unrelated to myocardial infarction. Am J Cardiol 1985;55:384–390.
17. Fontaine G, Guiraudon G, Frank R, et al: Stimulation studies and epicardial mapping in ventricular tachycardia: Study of mechanisms and selection for surgery. In Kulbertus H, ed. Reentrant Arrhythmias. Lancaster, MTP Press, 1977;334.
18. Poll DS, Marchlinski FE, Falcone RA, Simson MB. Abnormal signal averaged ECG in nonischemic congestive cardiomyopathy: Relationship to sustained ventricular tachyarrhythmias. Circulation 1985;72:1308–1313.
19. Berbari EJ, Scherlag BJ, Hope RR, et al. Recording from the body surface of arrhythmogenic ventricular activity during the ST segment. Am J Cardiol 1978;41:697.
20. Simson MB, Euler D, Michelson EL, et al. Detection of delayed ventricular activation on the body surface in dogs. Am Physiol 241 (Heart Circ Physiol 1981;10:H363–H369.
21. Simson MB, Untereker WJ, Spielman SR, et al. The relationship between late potentials on the body surface and directly recorded fragmented electrograms in patients with ventricular tachycardia. Am J Cardiol 1983;51:105–112.
22. Boineu JP, Cox JL. Slow ventricular activation in acute myocardial infarction: A source of reentrant premature ventricular contraction. Circulation 1973;48:702–713.
23. Waldo AL, Kaiser G. A study of ventricular arrhythmias associated with acute myocardial infarction in the canine heart. Circulation 1973;3:1222.
24. El-Sherif N, Scherlag BJ, Lazzara R, et al. Reentrant ventricular arrhythmias in the late myocardial infarction period. II. Patterns of initiation and termination of reentry. Circulation 1977;55:702.
25. Josephson ME, Horowitz LN, Farshidi A. Continuous local electrical activity: A mechanism of recurrent ventricular tachycardia. Circulation 1978;57:659.
26. Klein H, Karp RB, Kouchoukos NT, Zorn GL, James TN, Waldo AL. Intraoperative electrophysiologic mapping of the ventricles during sinus rhythm in patients with previous myocardial infarction: Identification of the electrophysiologic substrate of ventricular arrhythmias. Circulation 1982;66:847–853.
27. Wiener I, Mindich B, Pitchon R. Determinants of ventricular tachycardia in patients with ventricular aneurysms: Results of intraoperative epicardial and endocardial mapping. Circulation 1982;65:856–861.
28. Simson MB, Spear JF, Moore NE. Stability of an experimental A-V reentrant tachycardia in dogs. Am J Physiol 1981;240:H947–H952.

18

Fast Fourier Transform Analysis of the Signal-Averaged Electrocardiogram in the Management of Patients with or Prone to Ventricular Tachycardia or Fibrillation

Michael E. Cain
H. Dieter Ambos
Bruce D. Lindsay

Introduction

Each year, more than 400,000 Americans die suddenly from malignant ventricular arrhythmia. Most have multivessel coronary artery disease and ventricular dysfunction.[1] Although basic and clinical research has helped to delineate the electrophysiologic derangements underlying sustained ventricular tachycardia (VT) and ventricular fibrillation (VF), accurate noninvasive detection of the patient at risk after myocardial infarction is not yet possible. Prediction has been attempted with clinical and electrocardiographic criteria including frequent and

From: Brugada P, Wellens HJJ. CARDIAC ARRHYTHMIAS: Where To Go From Here? Mount Kisco, NY, Futura Publishing Company, Inc., © 1987.

complex ventricular ectopy detected in the course of ambulatory monitoring and exercise testing.[1-11] Although certain patterns of ventricular ectopy predict higher cardiac mortality in large groups, none specifically predicts risk for developing sustained VT or VF when applied to individuals.

Results of clinical[12-17] and laboratory[18-24] studies implicate reentrant mechanisms, at least in part, for the genesis of ventricular arrhythmias complicating ischemic heart disease. Derangements of ventricular conduction during sinus rhythm have been observed consistently in regions bordering the infarct and overlying epicardial regions and appear temporally related to the development of sustained ventricular arrhythmias.[19-29] Unfortunately, surface electrocardiographic signals obtained conventionally during sinus rhythm do not distinguish patients with and without sustained VT or VF despite the occult derangements in ventricular activation presumably present.

Recently, several groups have used advanced signal-processing techniques to extract this concealed yet clinically relevant information from the surface electrocardiogram (ECG).[30-40] We have developed, tested, and implemented a signal-processing system using fast Fourier transform (FFT) analysis in order to determine whether frequency analysis facilitates objective, noninvasive identification of a substrate conducive to the development of reentrant ventricular arrhythmias and to determine whether results of frequency analysis can be used to prospectively stratify patients with structural heart disease at high and low risk for developing sustained ventricular arrhythmias.[36-40] This selected review describes the evolution of this approach and summarizes the results of clinical studies.

Methods

Rationale for Using Frequency Analysis

FFT analysis is a powerful analytic method for signal processing in the frequency domain that allows some of the inherent limitations of high gain amplification and signal filtering required for analysis in the time domain to be avoided.[41,42] Moreover, frequency analysis facilitates identification and characterization of frequencies independent of signal amplitude and provides flexibility for analyzing different electrocardiographic segments. Any periodic signal, such as the QRS complex, may be represented by the mathematical summation of a series of sine waves of differing frequencies and amplitudes. The sinusoidal component with the lowest frequency is called the fundamental and has a repetition rate equal to the repetition rate of the periodic signal under evaluation (Fig. 1). All higher sinusoidal components, or harmonics, have frequencies that are integer multiples of the fundamental frequency. FFT analysis is a computer-based mathematical algorithm whereby the amplitudes of the various harmonics that comprise a complex periodic waveform are determined. The Fourier transform is unique since for each time-domain signal there is one and only one frequency-domain presentation.

To test the hypothesis that FFT analysis would facilitate identification of low

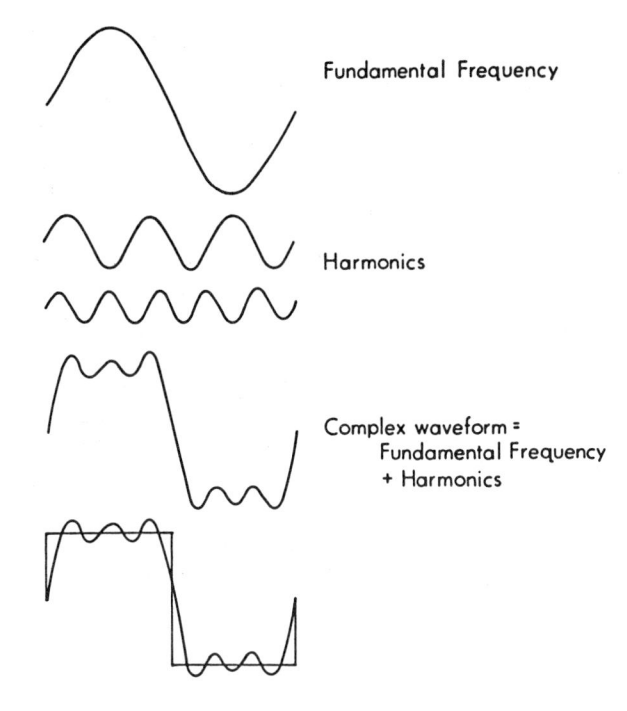

Figure 1: Schematic diagram depicting a series of sine waves representing the fundamental frequency and the 3rd and 5th harmonics of the fundamental frequency. Any periodic complex waveform in the time-domain, such as a square wave, can be represented by a fundamental frequency and various harmonics of the fundamental frequency. Conversely, if the fundamental frequency and its harmonics are known, the time-domain signal can be reconstructed. For each time-domain presentation, there is one and only one frequency-domain presentation.

amplitude potentials in the ECG, we first implemented a computer-based mathematical model and then subjected it to rigorous testing before constructing the signal-processing unit for patient use.[36] To simulate a small oscillatory waveform superimposed on the trailing edge of a QRS complex, two complete cycles of a 40 Hz sine wave of variable voltage and onset were superimposed on a ramp function with a negative voltage vs time slope starting at a fixed voltage of 1 mV and reaching 0 mV at 50 ms. After multiplication by a window function, classic Fourier series analysis was performed on both functions. A comparison of results of time- and frequency-domain analyses is shown (Fig. 2). The spectral analyses of the ramp function, 40 Hz sine burst, and the sum of the ramp and sine burst functions are shown along with both the original time-domain waveforms and the time-domain reconstruction from the Fourier series. As shown in Figure 2C, the amplitude (0 to peak) of the sine burst was 0.1 mV and the peak amplitude of the ramp function was 1 mV. The time-domain perturbation that reflected the 40 Hz sine burst contribution was minimal but clearly detectable in the frequency domain. Moreover, the sine burst component was easily detected at levels as low as 10 μV in the frequency domain as a bump in the spectra near 40 Hz. However, it was not evident at these low levels in the time domain without prefiltering regardless of gain. A limitation of filtering is that the selection of the high and low pass filters requires a priori knowledge of the frequency content of the signal of interest. Furthermore, filtering may exclude signals of potential interest. Frequency analysis avoids some of the inherent limitations of filtering used commonly for time-domain analysis.

Results of clinical studies using catheter mapping techniques during sinus rhythm have shown that patients with prior myocardial infarction who subse-

314 • CARDIAC ARRHYTHMIAS

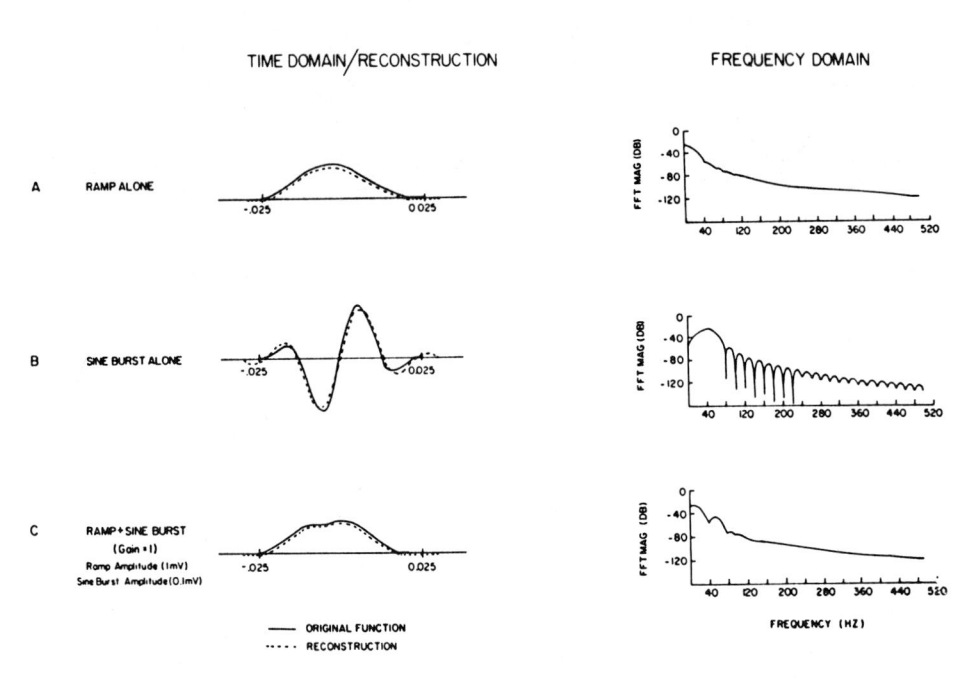

Figure 2: Comparison of results of time- and frequency-domain analyses. Right, the spectral analysis of the ramp function (A), 40 Hz sine burst function (B), and the sum of the ramp and sine burst functions (C) are shown. Left: the original time-domain waveforms (solid lines) of these functions are shown along with the time-domain reconstruction (broken lines) from the Fourier series. C: the amplitude (0 to peak) of the sine burst is 0.1 mV, and the peak amplitude of the ramp function is 1 mV. The time-domain perturbation that reflects the sine burst contribution is minimal without pre-filtering. However, the contribution from the 40 Hz sine wave is easily detectable in the frequency domain. (Reproduced by permission of the American Heart Association, Inc., from Cain ME, Ambos HD, Witkowski FX, et al.[36])

quently develop sustained VT have a greater number of ventricular sites demonstrating abnormal fragmented electrograms (Fig. 3) when compared with the results from patients with prior infarction without sustained VT.[43] Because the surface ECG reflects total activation of the heart, we hypothesized that the frequency content of signal-averaged ECGs from patients with sustained VT would differ quantitatively from that from patients without sustained VT. We have stressed previously that when using FFT methods, several major sources of artifactual frequency shifts must be excluded before reliable differences in the spectral content in signals from patients with and without sustained VT can be accepted.[36–38,40]

Hardware

Standard Frank X, Y, and Z leads are recorded simultaneously using a Hewlett-Packard HP 1507A vectorcardiograph modified to give a specific frequency response of 0.05 to 470 Hz with a rolloff of 18 dB per octave. The electrocardiographic signals are amplified approximately 1000-fold to optimize

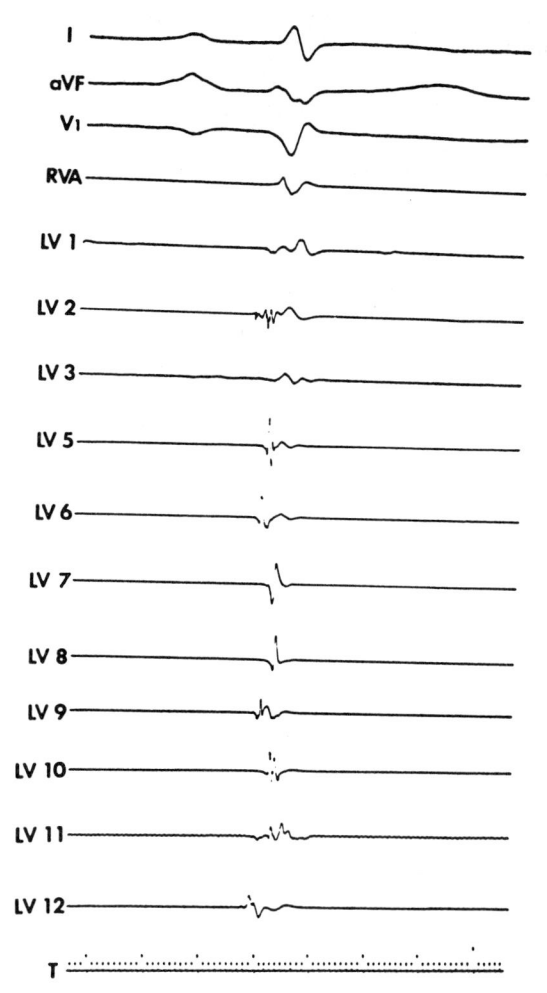

Figure 3: Results of catheter endocardial ventricular mapping during sinus rhythm from a patient with a history of prior myocardial infarction and subsequent sustained ventricular tachycardia (VT). The figure is organized from top to bottom with surface electrocardiographic leads I, aVF, V_1 and intracardiac electrograms from the right ventricular apex (RVA) and 11 preselected left ventricular (LV) sites. Electrograms from septal and anterior LV sites (1, 2, 3, and 11) are fragmented, prolonged, and have lower amplitudes when compared to more normal electrograms recorded from posterior-lateral sites (5,6,7,8). These derangements in ventricular activation are found more commonly in patients with compared to those without sustained VT and alter the frequency content of the surface ECG.

the maximum ± 2.5 V input range of the A/D converter. Each lead is digitized at 1 KHz using a 12 bit A/D converter providing a 72 dB range. The digitized data are processed utilizing a DEC VT103 LSI 11/23 microcomputer system running with the RT 11 operating system. During signal averaging, the amplified X, Y, and Z leads are displayed simultaneously for continuous real time visual monitoring.

Signal Averaging

The X, Y, and Z leads are recorded during sinus rhythm and 3 seconds of data are digitized. The lead having the largest R-wave in relation to the P- and T-waves is selected. The polarity of the signal can be negative or positive. The R-R interval and fiducial point are identified. The R-R interval, fiducial point, and 20 points on either side of the fiducial point of the lead selected initially as well as the peak-to-peak amplitudes of all three leads are stored as a template in the microprocessor memory. During averaging, 3 seconds of X, Y, and Z lead data are stored in a circular memory buffer consisting of three individual 1K word buffers per lead. Usually, the data contained in the center buffer are compared with the template beat generated previously. The R-R interval is checked forward and backward with the beat in the first and last buffers, respectively. If the R-R interval is not within 20% of the template value, the beat is rejected. Otherwise, the peak-to-peak amplitudes of the X, Y, and Z leads are compared with the stored template values. The amplitudes must be within 5% of the template values for the beat to be considered further for averaging. If the R-R interval and amplitudes are acceptable, a 40-point cross-correlation of the R-wave is performed about the fiducial point. If the correlation coefficient is <98%, the beat is rejected. The beat immediately following a rejected beat is rejected also. Signal averaging is performed in real time and uses double precision arithmetic. Routinely, 100 sinus beats are averaged. The analog system has an input noise level of 15 to 18 μV peak-to-peak. A 100 beat average reduces inherent noise to 1.8 μV, approximately equal to the 1.2 μV quantization error of the A/D converter. After averaging is complete, the double precision values are changed to single precision values and stored on floppy disc.

Fast Fourier Transform Analysis

We have performed FFT analysis on the entire QRS complex, the terminal 40 ms of the QRS complex, the ST segment, and the T-wave of each signal-averaged X, Y, and Z lead. For each region of interest, a 512 point FFT is calculated after multiplication by a four-term Blackman-Harris window to reduce spectral leakage.[44] After multiplication by the window function, the selected sample values are placed at the beginning of the 512 point array and the remaining values set to zero. Since data are obtained at 1 ms intervals, samples up to 512 ms in length can be analyzed.

Data Analysis

For each electrocardiographic region of interest, frequency plots have been generated from the X, Y, and Z leads. Initially, spectral plots were compared only qualitatively to confirm our hypothesis that results of FFT analysis differentiate patients with from those without sustained VT.[36]

To quantify and characterize the differences in frequency content between patients with and without sustained VT, the energy spectrum was computed by squaring the magnitudes of the FFT data.[38] This computation is generally used in mathematical analysis of waveforms to expose frequencies with high amplitude components and differentiate their contributions to the signal-averaged raw data from the contributions of frequencies with lower amplitude components.[42] Moreover, to enhance frequency resolution, FFT analysis was performed on the terminal QRS and ST segment as a single unit. The windowed signal was scaled before computation of the FFT to reduce variations in magnitude of the transformed data and the maximum magnitude identified and scaled to unity. Data were plotted on a scale defined by the maximum of the data curve. To visualize smaller peaks that might be obscured by the dominant amplitudes of low frequency components, a second plot was generated by dividing the initial scale by 500. Data were analyzed for peaks between 20 to 50 Hz after analysis over the entire bandwidth (0.05 to 470 Hz) demonstrated that frequencies above 70 Hz did not contribute substantially in distinguishing patients with and without sustained ventricular tachycardia. The relative contributions of frequencies between 20 and 50 Hz to the terminal QRS and ST segments have been expressed as magnitude and area ratios as described previously.[38,39]

Effects of ST Segment Length

Studies published to date have been performed in patients during sinus rhythm having comparable signal durations.[36-39] Frequency resolution, however, is proportional to the duration of the signal analyzed. Before the clinical application of this noninvasive approach can be expanded, methods of data analysis must be relatively insensitive to physiologic and pathologic variations in ST segment length. To determine the effect of the ST segment length on the FFT in order to develop a method of analysis that would enable the reliable comparison of FFT results in patients over a broad range of physiologic and pathologic ST segment lengths, changes in the energy distribution between 0 to 50 Hz were computed at 10 Hz intervals from the energy spectrum and FFT magnitude during progressive shortening of the ST segment.[40] The area under the curve for each 10 Hz interval was calculated and normalized by dividing the area of each interval by the value of the maximum magnitude. In addition, the data were examined for peaks between 20 and 50 Hz as described previously.[38] The relative contribution of peak magnitudes in this range to the frequency content of the entire interval of interest was computed by dividing the peak magnitudes by the maximum magnitude.

Results

Qualitative Differences in Frequency Content

Prior to performing studies in patients, our signal-processing system was validated by analyzing test signals of known amplitudes and frequency.[36,37] Results of initial clinical studies demonstrated significant ($p < 0.0001$) qualitative differences in the frequency content of the terminal 40 ms of the QRS complex and of the ST segment of sinus beats from patients with histories of prior myocardial infarction and subsequent sustained VT when compared with results from patients with prior infarction without sustained VT and with those from normal subjects.[36] Representative plots of results of FFT analysis of the terminal QRS complex from patients with and without sustained VT are shown in Figure 4. Each panel depicts power vs frequency plots of the terminal 40 ms of signal-averaged X, Y, and Z electrocardiographic leads. From each frequency plot, the computer defined the decibel drop at 40 Hz and the area under the curve from the fundamental frequency to the frequency at which the amplitude of the spectrum was 60 dB lower than peak. The 40 Hz intercept was chosen because most of the energy of a normal QRS is less than 35 Hz. The 60 dB area chosen was well within the 72 dB range of the 12 bit A/D converter. In each lead, the terminal 40 ms of the QRS complex from the patient who had manifest sustained VT contained relatively more high frequency components than the complex from the patient who had not, which was reflected by a greater value for the 60 dB area and a lesser decibel drop at the 40 Hz intercept. Similar differences in the frequency content of the ST segment were observed between patients with and without sustained VT. Comparisons between the mean value of the 60 dB areas of the terminal 40 ms of the QRS complex, the ST segment, the entire QRS complex, and the T-wave for patients with infarction with sustained VT, patients with infarction without sustained VT, and normal subjects are summarized in Figure 5. There were no significant differences in the 60 dB areas or the 40 Hz intercepts of the total QRS complex or of the T-waves among the three groups.

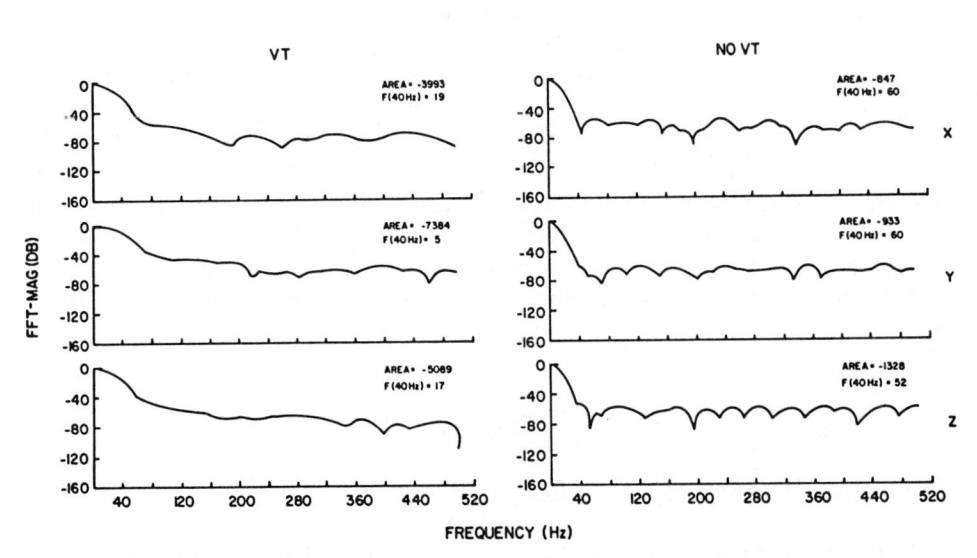

Figure 4: Representative FFT results of the terminal QRS complex from a patient with prior myocardial infarction with sustained ventricular tachycardia (VT) (left) and from a patient with prior myocardial infarction without sustained VT (right). Shown in each panel are power vs frequency plots of the terminal 40 ms of signal-averaged QRS complexes recorded from orthogonal X, Y, and Z leads, values for the 60 dB area, and values for the 40 Hz intercept. In each lead, the terminal QRS complex from the patient with VT contains relatively more high frequency components than the complex from the patient without VT.

60 dB AREA

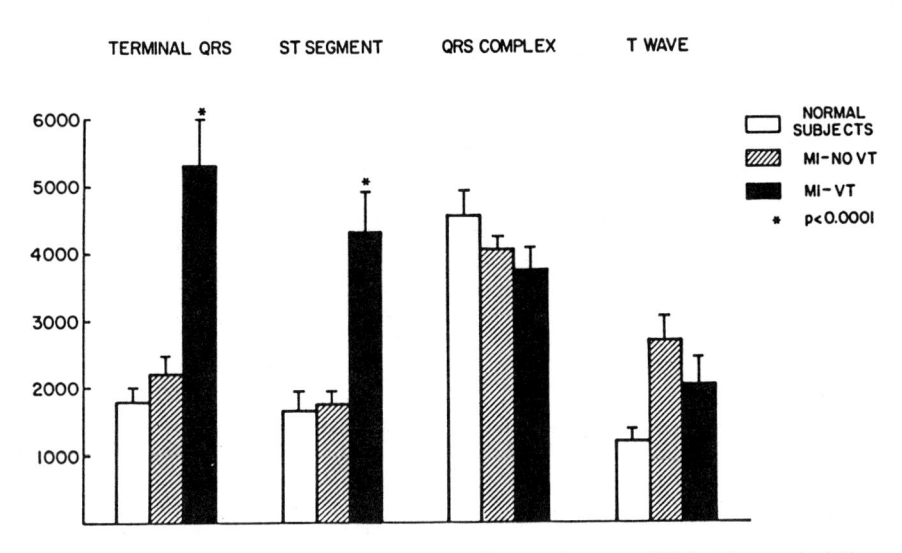

Figure 5: Comparisons of the mean values for the 60 dB areas (mean ± SEM) of the terminal 40 ms of the QRS complex, ST segment, total QRS complex, and T-wave from patients with prior myocardial infarction (MI) having sustained ventricular tachycardia (VT), patients with prior MI without VT, and normal subjects. Values for the 60 dB area of the terminal QRS and the ST segment in patients with sustained VT were significantly higher ($p < 0.0001$) when compared to those from patients with prior MI without VT and from normal subjects.

Quantitative Analysis of Frequency Content

The results of quantitative analysis of the terminal QRS and ST segments from patients with sustained VT have demonstrated a greater proportion of components in the 20 to 50 Hz range compared with the proportion in corresponding electrocardiographic segments of patients without VT.[38] Figure 6 illustrates the results of quantitative FFT analysis from a patient with and from a patient without sustained VT. The data are expressed as a ratio (area ratio) of the area under the spectral plot between 20 to 50 Hz divided by the area under the spectral plot between 0 to 20 Hz and as a magnitude ratio that quantifies the relative magnitudes of frequency peaks identified between 20 to 50 Hz. In each lead the terminal QRS and ST segment from the patient with VT contains a 10- to 100-fold greater proportion of frequencies in the 20 to 50 Hz range compared with corresponding values in the patient without VT. These distinguishing features are independent of QRS duration, left ventricular ejection fraction, or complexity of spontaneous ventricular ectopy. Moreover, these indexes are reproducible over time and among observers (Fig. 7). Overall, results of quantitative analysis have demonstrated that differences in the energy spectra in patients with and without sustained VT do not result primarily from differences in the frequencies of

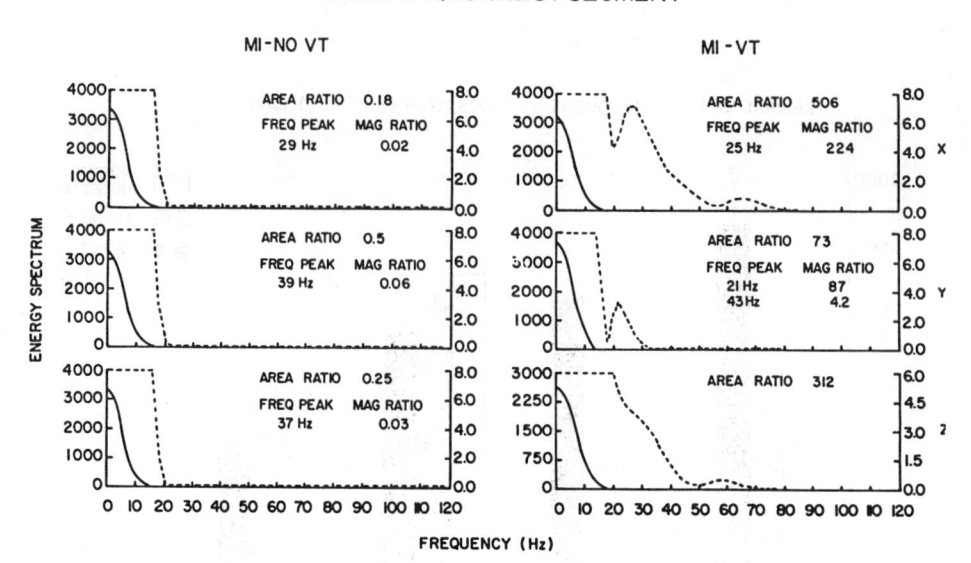

Figure 6: Energy spectra of the terminal QRS and ST segments from a patient with prior myocardial infarction (MI) and sustained ventricular tachycardia (VT) (right) and from a patient with prior MI without sustained VT (left). Shown in each panel are the initial (left scale-solid curve) and magnified (right scale-broken curve) energy vs frequency plots of the terminal QRS and ST segment of signal-averaged X, Y, and Z electrocardiographic leads, values for the area ratio (20–50 Hz/0–20 Hz), peak frequencies and values for the magnitude ratios. In each lead, the combined terminal QRS and ST segment from the patient with sustained VT contains a 10- to 100-fold greater proportion of components in the 20 to 50 Hz range compared with corresponding values form the patient without VT.

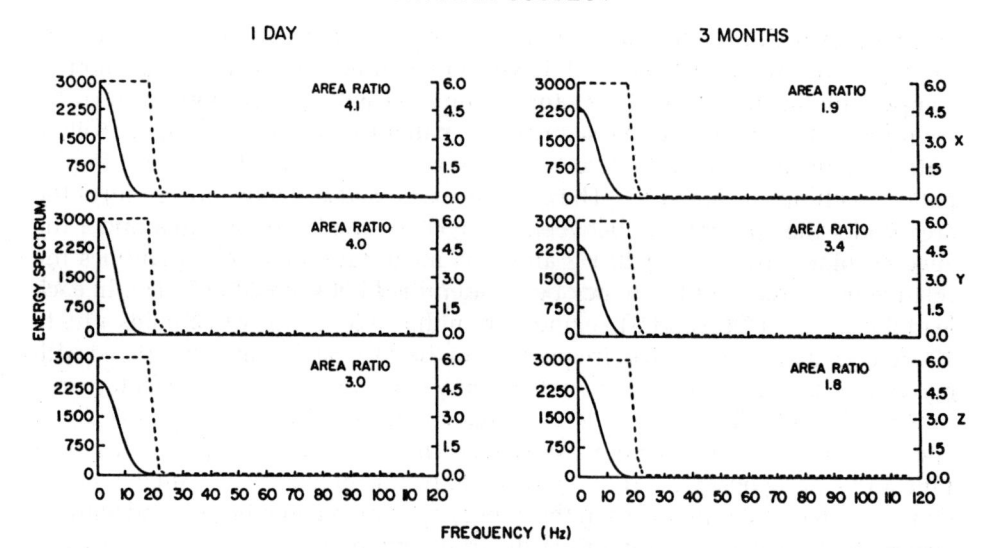

Figure 7: Reproducibility of results of frequency analysis from a normal subject during an interval of 3 months.

Relation to Results of Programmed Ventricular Stimulation

The clinical value of this approach depends ultimately on whether results prospectively detect vulnerability to the development of sustained ventricular arrhythmias. Recently, we tested the hypothesis that FFT results would improve selection of patients for programmed ventricular stimulation.[39] FFTs of signal-averaged ECGs were obtained first from patients with spontaneous sustained VT (group I) and compared with the results of programmed stimulation. A logistic regression with inducibility as the dependent variable was used to define abnormal FFT results. Sustained monomorphic VT was induced in 18 patients; each had an abnormal FFT value. Sustained VT was not induced in two patients; each had normal FFT data. FFT results were then compared prospectively with the results of programmed stimulation in patients (group II) with nonsustained VT or syncope referred for electrophysiologic study. Comparisons between results of FFT analysis and results of programmed stimulation for patients in groups I and II are shown in Figure 8. Five of the 12 patients in group II with abnormal FFT results had sustained monomorphic VT induced; all had organic heart disease. Seven patients had abnormal FFT values, but sustained VT was not induced.

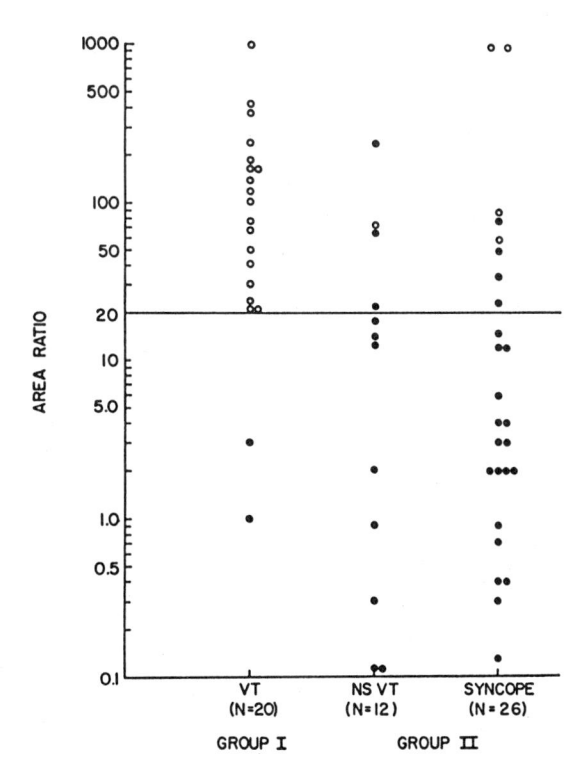

Figure 8: Comparison of values for the area ratio and the results of programmed stimulation in patients having sustained ventricular tachycardia (VT) clinically (group I) and patients (group II) having nonsustained VT (NSVT) or syncope. Open circles represent patients in whom sustained VT was induced. Closed circles represent patients in whom sustained VT was not induced. Area ratio values greater than 20 (horizontal line) were defined as abnormal. (Reproduced by permission of the American Heart Association, Inc., from Lindsay BD, Ambos HD, Schechtman KB, et al.[39])

322 • CARDIAC ARRHYTHMIAS

Asymptomatic nonsustained VT was induced in four of these patients, nonsustained VT with symptoms of lightheadedness was induced in one patient, and no arrhythmias were induced in two patients. None of the patients in group II with normal FFT results had sustained VT induced. Thus, the results of FFT analysis correctly predicted the response to programmed stimulation in 88% of patients studied and in 82% of patients with nonsustained VT or syncope. The sensitivity of the prediction of inducibility was 100%, and specificity was 77%. Results of multivariate analysis demonstrated that results of FFT analysis were independent of other determinants of inducibility, including ejection fraction and prior myocardial infarction. This approach offers promise for improving identification of patients in whom sustained VT will be induced during programmed ventricular stimulation.

Effect of ST Segment Length

Tables I and II demonstrate the effects of shortening ST segment length by 12 ms and 25 ms on values for the area and magnitude ratios computed using the energy spectrum (left columns). As shown, shortening the data segment from 160 to 135 ms increased the value of the area ratio by 247% from 15 to 52. Values for the peak magnitude were less dramatically affected and changed by 42%. We have demonstrated recently that shortening the ST segment increases substantially the proportion of frequency components in the 10 to 20 Hz and 20 to 30 Hz ranges while the proportion of components in the 0 to 10 Hz range decreases.[40] Values for the area under the curve between 30 to 50 Hz changed only modestly. The

Table I
Mean Area Ratio

	Energy Spectrum (squared data)	FFT Magnitude (natural data)
160 points	15	96
148 points	23 (53%)	99 (3%)
135 points	52 (247%)	105 (9%)

$$\text{Area Ratio} = \frac{20-50 \text{ Hz Area}}{0-20 \text{ Hz Area}} \times 10000 \qquad \text{Area Ratio} = \frac{20-50 \text{ Hz Area}}{10-50 \text{ Hz Area}} \times 1000$$

Table II
Peak Magnitudes

	Energy Spectrum (squared data)	FFT Magnitude (natural data)
160 points	.000043	.0041
148 points	.000025 (42%)	.0039 (7%)
135 points	.000025 (42%)	.0038 (10%)

largest relative change occurred between 20 to 30 Hz where area values increased by 200% to 1400%. Since the ST segment is composed predominantly of low frequency components, shortening the ST segment results in a change in the proportions of low and high frequencies. However, when the same data were expressed as a FFT magnitude and not as the energy spectrum, the shifts in the energy distribution from 0 to 50 Hz observed during ST segment shortening are much less marked when compared with the changes observed in the energy spectrum.

Previously, in studies of patients having comparable data segment lengths, we calculated an area ratio, 20–50 Hz/0–20 Hz, from the energy spectrum.[38,39] Importantly, results of studies in several subjects demonstrated that as the ST segment was progressively shortened, the energy distribution from 0 to 10 Hz changed disproportionately to that observed from 10 to 30 Hz. As a result, the 20–50 Hz/0–20 Hz ratio computed from the energy spectrum changes dramatically with changes in ST segment length (Table I). To avoid this inherent variable so that results of FFT analysis from patients having a broad range of physiologic and pathologic ST segment lengths can be compared, a new ratio was calculated from the FFT magnitude whereby the area between 20 to 50 Hz was divided by the area from 10 to 50 Hz. Thus, the numerator and denominator contain data pertinent to the frequency distribution between 20 to 30 Hz, the range of frequencies most affected by changes in the length of the ST segment. Tables I and II also demonstrate the effects of shortening the ST segment on values for the area ratio and magnitude ratio computed using the FFT magnitude and not as the energy spectrum. As demonstrated, values for the new ratio changed by only 9% from 96 to 105 when the ST segment was shortened by 25 ms.

Comparison of the results of analysis of FFT magnitudes between patients with and without sustained VT demonstrate, as expected, that patients with VT have significantly higher area ratio values and peak magnitude indexes when compared to patients without VT and with normal subjects. Representative FFT magnitudes from a patient with and a patient without sustained VT are shown in Figure 9. Values for the area ratio and peak magnitude index are independent of the length of the data segment.

Discussion

Sudden cardiac death remains a major health issue throughout the world. Optimal management requires accurate detection of the patient at risk for developing sustained ventricular arrhythmias as well as the appropriate selection of an effective therapeutic intervention. Judging from the results of our studies, FFT analysis of signal-averaged orthogonal ECGs is an accurate, noninvasive method for distinguishing patients with prior myocardial infarction with and without sustained ventricular arrhythmias. Overall, abnormal FFT results have been identified in 91% of patients with prior myocardial infarction and subsequent sustained VT, 15% of patients with prior myocardial infarction without documented sustained VT, and 4% of normal subjects. In addition, the approach developed is a sensitive method for identifying patients who may have sustained

324 • CARDIAC ARRHYTHMIAS

TERMINAL QRS and ST SEGMENT

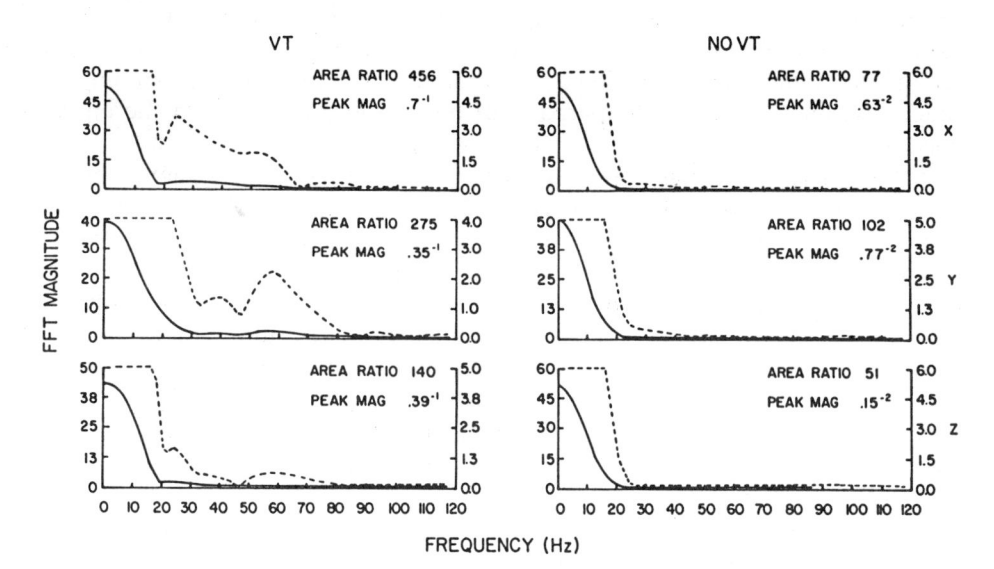

Figure 9: Comparison of fast Fourier transform (FFT) magnitudes from a patient with prior myocardial infarction and subsequent sustained ventricular tachycardia (VT) and from a patient with prior infarction without sustained VT (right). The format of the figure is similar to that used in Figure 6 except the FFT data are expressed as magnitudes (natural data) and not energy spectra (squared data). In each lead, values for the area ratio (20–50 Hz/10–50 Hz) are 2- to 3-fold higher and values for the peak magnitude are 10-fold greater from the patient with VT when compared to values from the patient without VT. Area ratios and peak magnitude ratios calculated from FFT magnitudes provide the best discrimination of patients with and without sustained VT and are applicable to patients having a broad range of physiologic and pathologic ST segment lengths.

VT induced during programmed stimulation. Importantly, FFT results are independent of more conventional determinants of prognosis and inducibility. These findings are indicative that abnormal FFT results reflect an anatomic/electrophysiologic substrate conducive to the development of sustained VT or VF. Results of studies using signal-processing systems in the time domain have demonstrated a correlation between abnormal late potentials detected in the signal-averaged ECG and delayed ventricular activation detected during the course of epicardial mapping.[31,43,45] Studies are in progress in our laboratory utilizing a recently developed computer mapping system[46,47] and morphometric analytic techniques to define the anatomic/electrophysiologic substrate responsible for the genesis of the abnormal frequencies detected by FFT analysis of the terminal QRS and ST segments of signal-averaged ECGs. Although delayed ventricular activation is likely to be responsible in part for the differences in frequency content between patients with and without sustained VT, our finding that results of FFT analysis are independent of QRS width[36,38] indicates that derangements in ventricular conduction in addition to the total duration of ventricular activation contribute to the generation of abnormal frequency components. Heterogeneity in the pattern and phase of ventricular activation caused by the concomitant excitation of normal myocardium and myocardium that has undergone infarction will generate QRS complexes comprised of frequency components that differ from QRS complexes resulting from more homogeneous activation even though the total duration of ventricular activation may be comparable. Accordingly, late potentials may not be the only hallmark of an anatomic/electrophysiologic substrate conducive to the development of sustained ventricular arrhythmias; and such a substrate may be present despite the absence of late potentials. Results of preliminary studies comparing time- and frequency-domain techniques in the same patients help support these assumptions.[48]

Future Directions

Methods of frequency analysis of signal-averaged ECGs have evolved from qualitative to quantitative techniques having broad clinical applicability. As discussed previously, the clinical value of this and other signal-processing techniques depends ultimately on whether results prospectively detect patients who develop sustained VT or VF spontaneously. The largest number of patients at increased risk for developing sustained ventricular arrhythmias are those recovering from myocardial infarction. In this group, the incidence of sudden cardiac death is highest during the first 3 months following infarction. Obviously, accurate noninvasive identification of patients prior to hospital discharge who are destined to develop sustained VT or VF would improve patient management. Studies in patients during the acute and convalescent phases of myocardial infarction are being performed to characterize the serial changes in FFT results that occur during evolving myocardial infarction and to determine if the results of this approach can be relied on to prospectively identify patients who develop sustained VT or VF. Preliminary findings demonstrate that FFT results obtained at the time of hospital discharge presage those observed 3 months after infarction and support the concept that stratification of risk may be possible based on FFT results obtained 10 to 14 days following acute myocardial infarction.[49]

A second potential application of results of interrogation of signal-averaged ECGs is assessment of the salutary effects of antiarrhythmic interventions. Results of studies using time-domain techniques have failed to demonstrate a correlation between the efficacy of antiarrhythmic drugs and changes in late potential characteristics.[50] In contrast, results of preliminary studies using frequency-domain analysis have demonstrated that antiarrhythmic drugs may alter the frequency composition of the terminal QRS and ST segment and that these changes correlate with drug efficacy.[51] Understanding the pathophysiologic derangements responsible for the relative increase in 20 to 50 Hz frequencies identified in the terminal QRS and ST segments from patients with prior infarction and subsequent sustained VT will be paramount to interpreting the effects of medical and surgical antiarrhythmic interventions that alter the electrophysiologic milieu.

Finally, we have implemented studies to determine whether this approach is applicable to patients having bundle branch block during sinus rhythm and to examine the optimal electrocardiographic lead system for performing FFT analysis.

Noninvasive interrogation of the signal-averaged ECG continues to offer promise as a clinically relevant approach that will provide the practicing physician with data pertinent to the management of patients with or prone to sustained ventricular arrhythmias.

Acknowledgment: This research was supported in part by NIH Grant HL 17646, SCOR in Ischemic Heart Disease. We gratefully appreciate the expert technical assistance of Albert Fischer and the expert secretarial assistance of Elaine Zuzack.

References

1. Bigger JT Jr, Fleiss JL, Kleiger R, Miller JP, Rolnitzky LM, and the Multicenter Post-infarction Research Group. The relationships among ventricular arrhythmias, left ventricular dysfunction, and mortality in the 2 years after myocardial infarction. Circulation 1984;69:250–258.
2. Tominaga S, Blackburn H. The coronary drug project research group: prognostic importance of premature beats following myocardial infarction. JAMA 1973;223:1116–1124.
3. Schulze RA Jr, Rouleau J, Rigo P, Bowers S, Strauss HW, Pitt B. Ventricular arrhythmias in the late hospital phase of acute myocardial infarction: relation of left ventricular function detected by gated cardiac blood pool scanning. Circulation 1975;52:1006–1011.
4. Vismara LA, Vera Z, Foerster JM, Amsterdam EA, Mason DT. Identification of sudden death risk factors in acute and chronic coronary artery disease. Am J Cardiol 1977;39:821–828.
5. Anderson KP, DeCamilla J, Moss AJ. Clinical significance of ventricular tachycardia (3 beats or longer) detected during ambulatory monitoring after myocardial infarction. Circulation 1978;57:890–897.
6. Califf RM, Burks JM, Behar VS, Margolis JR, Wagner GS. Relationships among ventricular arrhythmias, coronary artery disease, and angiographic and electrocardiographic indicators of myocardial fibrosis. Ciruclation 1978;57:725–732.
7. Moss AJ, Davis HT, DeCamilla J, Bayer LW. Ventricular ectopic beats and their relation to sudden and nonsudden cardiac death after myocardial infarction. Circulation 1979;60:998–1003.
8. Ruberman W, Weinblatt E, Goldberg JD, Frank CW, Chaudhary BS, Shapiro S. Ventricular premature complexes and sudden death after myocardial infarction. Circulation 1981;64:297–305.
9. Bigger JT Jr, Weld FM, Rolnitzky LM. Prevalence, characteristics and significance of ventricular tachycardia (three or more complexes) detected with ambulatory electrocardiographic recordings in the late hospital phase of acute myocardial infarction. Am J Cardiol 1981;48:815–823.
10. Moss AJ and the Multicenter Postinfarction Research Group. Risk stratification and survival after myocardial infarction. N Engl J Med 1983;309:331–336.
11. Mukharji J, Rude RE, Poole WK, Gustafson N, Thomas LJ Jr, Strauss HW, Jaffe AS, Muller JE, Roberts R, Raabe DS, Croft CH, Passamani E, Braunwald E, Willerson JT, and the MILIS Study Group. Risk factors for sudden death after acute myocardial infarction: two year follow-up. Am J Cardiol 1984;54:31–36.
12. Wellens HHJ, Duren DR, Lie KI. Observations on the mechanisms of ventricular tachycardia in man. Circulation 1976;54:237–244.
13. Josephson ME, Horowitz LN, Farshidi A, Kastor JA. Recurrent sustained ventricular tachycardia. 1. Mechanisms. Circulation 1978;57:431–440.
14. Josephson ME, Horowitz LN, Farshidi A. Continuous local electrical activity: a mechanism of recurrent ventricular tachycardia. Circulation 1978;57:659–665.

15. Josephson ME, Spielman SR, Greenspan AM, Horowitz LN. Mechanisms of ventricular fibrillation in man: Observations based on electrode catheter recordings. Am J Cardiol 1979;44:623–631.
16. MacLean WAH, Plumb VJ, Waldo AL. Transient entrainment and interruption of ventricular tachycardia. PACE 1981;4:358–366.
17. Almendral JM, Stamato NJ, Rosenthal ME, Marchlinski FE, Miller JM, Josephson ME. Resetting response patterns during sustained ventricular tachycardia: relationship to the excitable gap. Circulation 1986;74:722–730.
18. Garan H, Farrow JT, Ruskin JN. Sustained ventricular tachycardia in recent canine infarction. Circulation 1980;62:980–987.
19. El-Sherif N, Scherlag BJ, Lazzara R, Hope RR. Reentrant ventricular arrhythmias in the late myocardial infarction period. 1. Conduction characteristics in the infarction zone. Circulation 1977;55:686–701.
20. El-Sherif N, Hope RR, Scherlag BJ, Lazzara R. Reentrant ventricular arrhythmias in the late myocardial infarction period. 2. Patterns of initiation and termination of reentry. Circulation 1977;55:702–719.
21. Karaguezian HS, Fenoglio JJ, Weiss MB, Wit AL. Protracted ventricular tachycardia induced by premature stimulation of the canine heart after coronary artery occlusion and reperfusion. Circ Res 1979;44:833–846.
22. Klein GJ, Ideker RE, Smith WM, Harrison LA, Kasell J, Wallace AG, Gallagher JJ. Epicardial mapping of the onset of ventricular tachycardia initiated by programmed stimulation in the canine heart with chronic infarction. Circulation 1979;60:1375–1384.
23. Wit AL, Allessie MA, Bonke FIM, Lammers W, Smeets J, Fenoglio JJ. Electrophysiologic mapping to determine the mechanism of experimental ventricular tachycardia initiated by premature impulses: Experimental approach and initial results demonstrating reentrant excitation. Am J Cardiol 1982;49:166–185.
24. Kramer JB, Saffitz JE, Witkowski FX, Corr PB. Intramural reentry as a mechanism of ventricular tachycardia during evolving canine myocardial infarction. Circ Res 1985;56:736–754.
25. El-Sherif N, Smith RA, Evans K. Canine ventricular arrhythmias in the late myocardial infarction period. 8. Epicardial mapping of reentrant circuits. Circ Res 1981;49:255–265.
26. Josephson ME, Horowitz LN, Farshidi A, Spear JF, Kastor JA, Moor EN. Recurrent sustained ventricular tachycardia. 2. Endocardial mapping. Circulation 1978;57:440–447.
27. Horowitz LN, Josephson ME, Harken AH. Epicardial and endocardial activation during sustained ventricular tachycardia in man. Circulation 1980;61:1227–1238.
28. Weiner I, Mindick B, Pitchon R. Determinants of ventricular tachycardia in patients with ventricular aneurysms: results of intraoperative epicardial and endocardial mapping. Circulation 1982;65:856–861.
29. Klein H, Karp RB, Kouchoukos NT, Zorn GL, James TN, Waldo AL. Intraoperative electrophysiologic mapping of the ventricle during sinus rhythm in patients with a previous myocardial infarction. Identification of the electrophysiologic substrate of ventricular arrhythmias. Circulation 1982;66:847–853.
30. Uther JB, Dennet CJ, Tan A. The detection of delayed activation signals of low amplitude in the vectorcardiogram of patients with recurrent ventricular tachycardia by signal averaging. In Sandoe E, Julian DG, Bell JW, eds. Management of Ventricular Tachycardia: Role of Mexiletine. Amsterdam, Excerpta Medica, 1978;80–82.
31. Berbari EJ, Scherlag BJ, Hope RR, Lazzara R. Recording from the body surface of arrhythmogenic ventricular activity during the S-T segment. Am J Cardiol 1978;41:697–702.
32. Rozanski JJ, Mortara D, Myerburg RJ, Castellanos A. Body surface detection of delayed depolarizations in patients with recurrent ventricular tachycardia and left ventricular aneurysm. Circulation 1981;63:1172–1178.
33. Simson MB. Use of signals in the terminal QRS complex to identify patients with ventricular tachycardia after myocardial infarction. Circulation 1981;64:235–242.

34. Breithardt G, Borggrefe M, Karbenn U, Abendroth RR, Yeh HL, Seipel L. Prevalence of late potentials in patients with and without ventricular tachycardia: Correlation with angiographic findings. Am J Cardiol 1982;49:1932–1937.
35. Denes P, Santarelli P, Hauser RG, Uretz EF. Quantitative analysis of the high frequency components of the terminal portion of the body surface QRS in normal subjects and in patients with ventricular tachycardia. Circulation 1983;67:1129–1138.
36. Cain ME, Ambos HD, Witkowski FX, Sobel BE. Fast-Fourier transform analysis of signal-averaged electrocardiogram for identification of patients prone to sustained ventricular tachycardia. Circulation 1984;69:711–720.
37. Ambos HD, Markham J, Cain ME. Use of fast-Fourier transform analysis to detect patients prone to sustained ventricular arrhythmias. Comput Cardiol 1984;181–184.
38. Cain ME, Ambos HD, Markham J, Fischer AE, Sobel BE. Quantification of differences in frequency content of signal-averaged electrocardiograms between patients with and without sustained ventricular tachycardia. Am J Cardiol 1985;55:1500–1505.
39. Lindsay BD, Ambos HD, Schechtman KB, Cain ME. Improved selection of patients for programmed ventricular stimulation by frequency analysis of signal-averaged electrocardiogram. Circulation 1986;73:675–683.
40. Ambos HD, Markham J, Lindsay BD, Cain ME. Spectral analysis of signal-averaged electrocardiograms from patients with and without ventricular tachycardia. Comput Cardiol (in press).
41. Brigham EO. The Fast-Fourier Transform. Englewood Cliffs, Prentice-Hall, 1974; 11–28.
42. Bracewell RN. The Fourier Transform and Its Application, 2nd ed. New York, McGraw-Hill, 1978;46–47.
43. Simson MB, Untereker WJ, Spielman SR, Horowitz LN, Marcus NH, Falcone RA, Harken AH, Josephson ME. Relation between late potentials on the body surface and directly recorded fragmented electrograms in patients with ventricular tachycardia. Am J Cardiol 1983;51:105–112.
44. Harris FJ. On the use of windows for harmonic analysis with the discrete Fourier transform. Proc IEEE 1978;66:51–83.
45. Simson MB, Eule D, Michelson EL, Falcone RA, Spear JF, Moore EN. Detection of delayed ventricular activation on the body surface in dogs. Am J Physiol 1981;241: H363–H369.
46. Witkowski FX, Corr PB. An automated transmural cardiac mapping system. Am J Physiol 1984;247:H661–H668.
47. Kramer JB, Corr PB, Cox JL, Witkowski FX, Cain ME. Simultaneous computer mapping to facilitate intraoperative localization of accessory pathways in patients with Wolff-Parkinson-White syndrome. Am J Cardiol 1985;56:571–576.
48. Cain ME, Lindsay BD, Fischer AE, Ambos MD, Sobel BE. Prospective comparison of frequency- and time-domain analysis of signal-averaged ECGs from patients with ventricular tachycardia (abstr). Circulation 1986;74:II–471.
49. Lindsay BD, Ambos HD, Fischer AE, Cain ME. Predictive value of frequency analysis of signal averaged ECGs at specific intervals after myocardial infarction (abstr). Circulation 1986;72:III–164.
50. Simson MB, Falcone R, Kindwall E. The signal averaged electrocardiogram does not predict antiarrhythmic drug success (abst). Circulation 1985;72:III–7.
51. Cain ME, Ambos HD, Fischer AE, Markham J, Schechtman KB. Non-invasive prediction of antiarrhythmic drug efficacy in patients with sustained ventricular tachycardia from frequency analysis of signal averaged ECGS (abst). Circulation 1984;70:II–253.

19

Identification of Patients at Risk of Sudden Death After Myocardial Infarction: The Continued Australian Experience

David Richards, Amanda Taylor
Paul Fahey, Les Irwig
Chee Choong Koo, David Ross
Mark Cooper, Hosen Kiat
Michael Skinner, John Uther

Introduction

Previous prospective studies in Australia of survivors of acute myocardial infarction have demonstrated that patients with inducible ventricular arrhythmias are subsequently more likely to exhibit spontaneous ventricular tachycardia than patients without inducible ventricular arrhythmias.[1-3] We have also demonstrated that prolonged ventricular activation, measured on the signal averaged electrocardiogram, has a predictive value similar to that of inducible ventricular tachycardia.[3] Other studies have suggested a relationship between high grade ventricular ectopy and or low ejection fraction, with poor prognosis after infarction.[4,5] We have shown that patients without inducible ventricular tachycardia and without evidence of reversible myocardial ischemia at exercise testing are very unlikely to die during the first year after infarction.[6]

From: Brugada P, Wellens HJJ. CARDIAC ARRHYTHMIAS: Where To Go From Here? Mount Kisco, NY, Futura Publishing Company, Inc., © 1987.

The purpose of the present prospective study was to examine in a single cohort of myocardial infarction patients the predictive values of different methods of programmed stimulation, signal averaged electrocardiogram, grade of ventricular ectopy, magnitude of left ventricular ejection fraction, and presence of ST-segment displacement at exercise testing.

Methods

Two hundred consecutive patients aged less than 71 years who fulfilled the following criteria were recruited: admission to Westmead Hospital because of acute myocardial infarction; no spontaneous ventricular tachycardia or ventricular fibrillation beyond 48 hours after infarction; no persistent angina at rest; no cardiac failure, or cardiac failure controlled with digitalis and diuretics; no significant comorbidity and written informed consent.

Programmed Stimulation

Each patient underwent programmed stimulation 6–28 days following infarction. All cardioactive medications (other than digitalis and diuretics) were suspended at least 5 days prior to programmed stimulation. No patient had taken amiodarone. Each patient underwent programmed stimulation utilizing two separate protocols, applied in random order, with a break of 5–10 minutes between the completion of one protocol and the commencement of the other. Protocol 1 comprised right ventricular stimulation, with a drive train of eight ventricular paced beats and a single extrastimulus (from 300 ms in 10 ms decrements to ventricular refractoriness), then paired extrastimuli applied first at the right ventricular apex at twice diastolic current threshold, then repeated at the right ventricular outflow tract at twice diastolic current threshold.[7] The entire protocol was then repeated at 20 milliamps current intensity first at the right ventricular apex and then at the right ventricular outflow tract. End-points for stimulation were completion of the protocol, or induction of ventricular fibrillation, or induction of ventricular tachycardia lasting at least 10 seconds.

Protocol 2 also utilized right ventricular stimulation but differed from the first protocol in that only the right ventricular apex was stimulated and all stimuli were at twice diastolic current threshold. Each extrastimulus (from 300 ms in 10 ms decrements to ventricular refractoriness) was applied three times at each coupling interval before proceeding to the next coupling interval. Up to five extrastimuli were applied. End points for the second protocol were the same as for the first.

Signal Averaging

Ventricular activation time was measured from averaged digitized recordings as the difference between latest offset of ventricular activation in any of the Frank vectorcardiogram leads X, Y, and Z and earliest onset of ventricular activation in any of the same leads, using a method described in detail previously.[8]

Ambulatory Monitoring

Ambulatory electrocardiographic monitoring was performed for 24 hours in each patient. Ventricular ectopy was recorded as the maximum Lown grade:[9] grade 0: zero ventricular ectopics; grade 1: 1–29 ventricular ectopics per hour; grade 2: 30 or more ventricular ectopics per hour; grade 3: multiform ventricular ectopics; grade 4a: paired ventricular ectopics; grade 4b: three or more ventricular ectopics consecutively; and grade 5: R on T ventricular ectopics.

Gated Heart Pool Scanning

Left ventricular ejection fraction was estimated at radionuclide gated heart pool scanning 6–28 days after infarction. Left ventricular aneurysm was defined as paradoxical systolic motion of a part of the left ventricular wall.

Exercise Testing

Exercise testing[10] was performed 1 week and 7 weeks following hospital discharge. ST-segment displacement of at least 2 mm at either test was considered to represent a positive result.

Follow-Up

Patients were followed (median 12 months) utilizing regular telephone contact with patients, families, or medical attendants or a combination of these. No patient was lost to follow-up. Two end-points for follow-up were considered separately: first, electrical events (spontaneous nonfatal ventricular tachycardia or ventricular fibrillation in the absence of fresh myocardial ischemia, witnessed instantaneous death without prodrome and with no postmortem evidence for another cause of death), and second, cardiac death (witnessed instantaneous death, death due to cardiac failure, death following coronary artery bypass surgery, death due to any other cardiac cause).

Statistics

Data were analyzed using the statistical package SPSS X.[11]

Results

Table IA summarizes the clinical characteristics (including the coronary prognostic index of Norris[12]) of patients separated by stimulation Protocol 1 into those with inducible slow ventricular tachycardia (cycle length at least 230 ms) and the remainder. Table IB is constructed similarly with patients separated by pro-

Table I

A — Protocol 1

	Rhythm induced				
	Slow VT (Cycle length at least 230 ms)		All others		p
n	11		189		
Age ± SD years	59 ± 6		56 ± 10		NS
Previous AMI	7	(64%)	41	(22%)	<0.01
Cardiomegaly (CXR)	5	(46%)	22	(12%)	<0.01
CPI ± SD	7 ± 3		4 ± 3		<0.0005
Aneurysm	2	(18%)	6	(3%)	<0.02
LVEF ± SD	0.34 ± 0.13		0.44 ± 0.18		NS
Peak CK (IU/1) ± SD	2194 ± 1016		1756 ± 1260		NS

B — Protocol 2

n	18		182		
Age ± SD years	58 ± 8		56 ± 10		NS
Previous AMI	7	(39%)	41	(23%)	NS
Cardiomegaly (CXR)	7	(39%)	20	(11%)	<0.005
CPI ± SD	6 ± 3		4 ± 3		<0.01
Aneurysm	3	(17%)	5	(3%)	<0.005
LVEF ± SD	0.31 ± 0.16		0.45 ± 0.17		<0.005
Peak CK (IU/1) ± SD	2604 ± 2013		1702 ± 1127		<0.005

A = patients separated according to rhythm inducible at programmed stimulation Protocol 1; B = patients separated according to rhythm inducible at programmed stimulation Protocol 2.
AMI = acute myocardial infarction, CK = creatine phosphokinase, CPI = coronary prognostic index of Norris,[12] CXR = chest X-ray, LVEF = left ventricular ejection fraction, Slow VT = ventricular tachycardia, cycle length at least 230 ms inducible at programmed stimulation.

grammed stimulation Protocol 2. There were no significant differences between patients with inducible slow ventricular tachycardia and the remainder in terms of site of infarction, transmural extent of infarction, presence of pulmonary congestion on chest X-ray, occurrence of ventricular tachycardia or ventricular fibrillation within the first 48 hours after infarction, pericarditis following infarction, development of atrioventricular block of any degree, development of bundle branch block of any type, atrial fibrillation, duration of chest pain prior to admission, or right ventricular ejection fraction measured at gated heart pool scanning.

Inducible Ventricular Tachycardia

Figure 1A depicts the incident-free survival in terms of electrical events for patients with ventricular tachycardia of cycle length at least 230 ms inducible with Protocol 1 compared with the remainder. Figure 1B depicts the incident-free survival in terms of cardiac mortality. Figure 2 depicts the corresponding incident-free survivals for patients separated according to the results of programmed stimulation with Protocol 2.

Table II is a contingency table of raw data (not adjusted for duration of follow-up) summarizing the predictive value of each step of Protocols 1 and 2 in

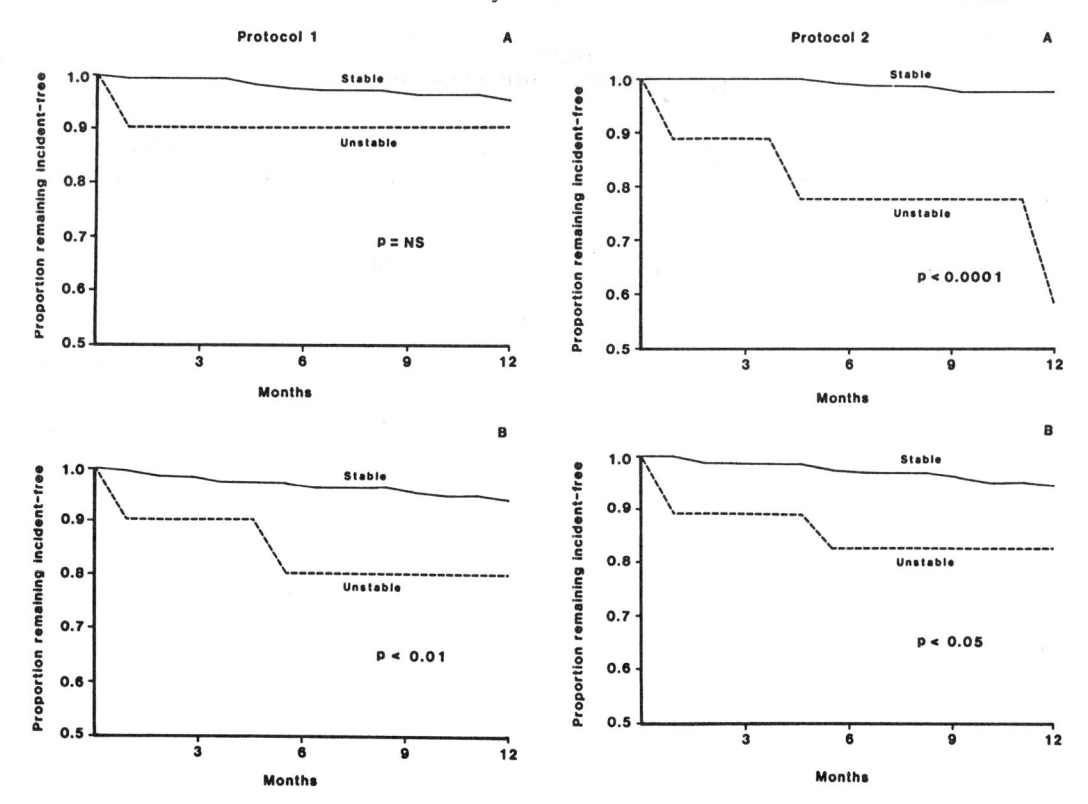

Figure 1: (left) Life table analysis of incident-free survival for patients separated according to the results of programmed stimulation Protocol 1. Broken curves depict patients with inducible ventricular tachycardia with cycle length at least 230 ms (unstable). Solid curves depict the remaining patients (stable). Panel A: analysis in terms of electrical events (spontaneous nonfatal ventricular tachycardia or ventricular fibrillation in the absence of fresh myocardial ischemia, witnessed instantaneous death without prodrome and with no postmortem evidence for another cause of death). Panel B: analysis in terms of cardiac death (witnessed instantaneous death, death due to cardiac failure, death following coronary artery bypass surgery, death due to any other cardiac cause).

Figure 2: (right) Life table analysis of incident-free survival for patients separated according to the results of programmed stimulation Protocol 2. Layout of Figure 2 is otherwise the same as for Figure 1.

terms of identification of patients at risk for sudden death or nonfatal ventricular tachycardia within the first year after infarction (Table IIA) and in terms of identifying patients at risk of cardiac death within 1 year of myocardial infarction (Table IIB). In this table, patients have been separated into three groups accoring to the results of programmed stimulation (slow VT = ventricular tachycardia, cycle length at least 230 ms; fast VT = ventricular tachycardia, cycle length less than 230 ms; VF = ventricular fibrillation; no arrhythmia = no arrhythmia inducible at programmed stimulation).

Table III was derived from Table II. A positive result of programmed stimulation was taken as induction of slow VT (cycle length at least 230 ms) and a negative result as any other response.

Table II

A. Electrical Events During Follow-up

	Inducible Slow VT		Inducible Fast VT or VF		No inducible arrhythmia	
	Yes	No	Yes	No	Yes	No
Protocol 1						
LCA	1	5	2	13	6	173
LCO	1	9	2	25	6	157
HCA	1	10	3	35	5	146
HCO	1	10	3	51	5	130
Protocol 2						
1 extra	1	0	0	2	8	189
2 extras	3	4	0	25	6	162
3 extras	5	10	1	82	3	99
4 extras	5	11	2	128	2	52
5 extras	5	13	3	148	1	30

B. All Cardiac Mortality During Follow-Up

	Inducible Slow VT		Inducible Fast VT or VF		No inducible arrhythmia	
	Yes	No	Yes	No	Yes	No
Protocol 1						
LCA	2	4	1	14	10	169
LCO	2	8	2	25	9	154
HCA	3	8	3	35	7	144
HCO	3	8	4	50	6	129
Protocol 2						
1 extra	1	0	0	2	12	185
2 extras	2	5	1	24	10	158
3 extras	3	12	5	78	5	97
4 extras	4	12	7	123	2	52
5 extras	4	14	9	142	0	31

A = data analyzed in terms of electrical events during follow-up, Yes = witnessed instantaneous death without prodrome and with no postmortem evidence for another cause of death, spontaneous nonfatal ventricular tachycardia or ventricular fibrillation in the absence of fresh myocardial ischemia, No = no electrical events.

B = data arranged in terms of cardiac death during follow-up, Yes = witnessed instantaneous death, death due to cardiac failure, death following coronary artery bypass surgery, death due to any other cardiac cause, No = no cardiac death.

Slow VT = ventricular tachycardia, cycle length at least 230 ms inducible at programmed stimulation, Fast VT = ventricular tachycardia, cycle length less than 230 ms, VF = ventricular fibrillation, No arrhythmia = no arrhythmia, or any arrhythmia other than VT or VF induced at programmed stimulation, LCA = low current (twice diastolic threshold) stimulation at right ventricular apex, LCO = low current stimulation at right ventricular outflow tract, HCA = high current (20 mA) stimulation at right ventricular apex, HCO = high current stimulation at right ventricular outflow tract, extra = extrastimulus, extras = extrastimuli, Event = event during follow-up.

Signal Averaging

Figure 3A depicts the incident-free survival in terms of electrical events for patients with ventricular activation time greater than 120 ms compared with the remainder. Figure 3B depicts the incident-free survival in terms of cardiac mortality.

Table III
Electrical Events

A

	Sensitivity	Specificity	Predictive accuracy	
			Positive	Negative
	%	%	%	%
Protocol 1				
LCA	11	97	17	96
LCO	11	95	10	96
HCA	11	95	10	96
HCO	11	95	10	96
Protocol 2				
1 extra	11	100	100	96
2 extras	33	98	43	97
3 extras	56	95	33	98
4 extras	56	94	31	98
5 extras	56	93	28	98

B — All Cardiac Mortality

	Sensitivity	Specificity	Positive	Negative
Protocol 1				
LCA	15	98	33	94
LCO	15	96	20	94
HCA	23	96	27	95
HCO	23	96	27	95
Protocol 2				
1 extra	8	100	100	94
2 extras	15	97	29	94
3 extras	23	94	20	95
4 extras	31	94	25	95
5 extras	31	93	22	95

A = data arranged in terms of electrical events during follow up, B = data arranged in terms of cardiac deaths. Predictive indices (sensitivity, specificity, positive predictive accuracy and negative predictive accuracy) are based on the results of programmed stimulation: Positive result = inducible VT cycle length at least 230 ms, Negative result = any other response to programmed stimulation. See Table II legend for explanation of abbreviations.

Ambulatory Monitoring

Patients have been separated into those with Lown grade 0–3 and those with Lown grade 4–5 ventricular ectopy. The incident-free survival in terms of electrical events and cardiac mortality are given in Figure 4.

Left Ventricular Ejection Fraction

Figure 5A depicts the incident-free survival in terms of electrical events of patients with left ventricular ejection fraction equal to or greater than 0.40 compared with those whose left ventricular ejection fraction was less than 0.40. Figure 5B depicts the corresponding analysis in terms of cardiac mortality.

The overall incidence of electrical events among patients with inducible slow

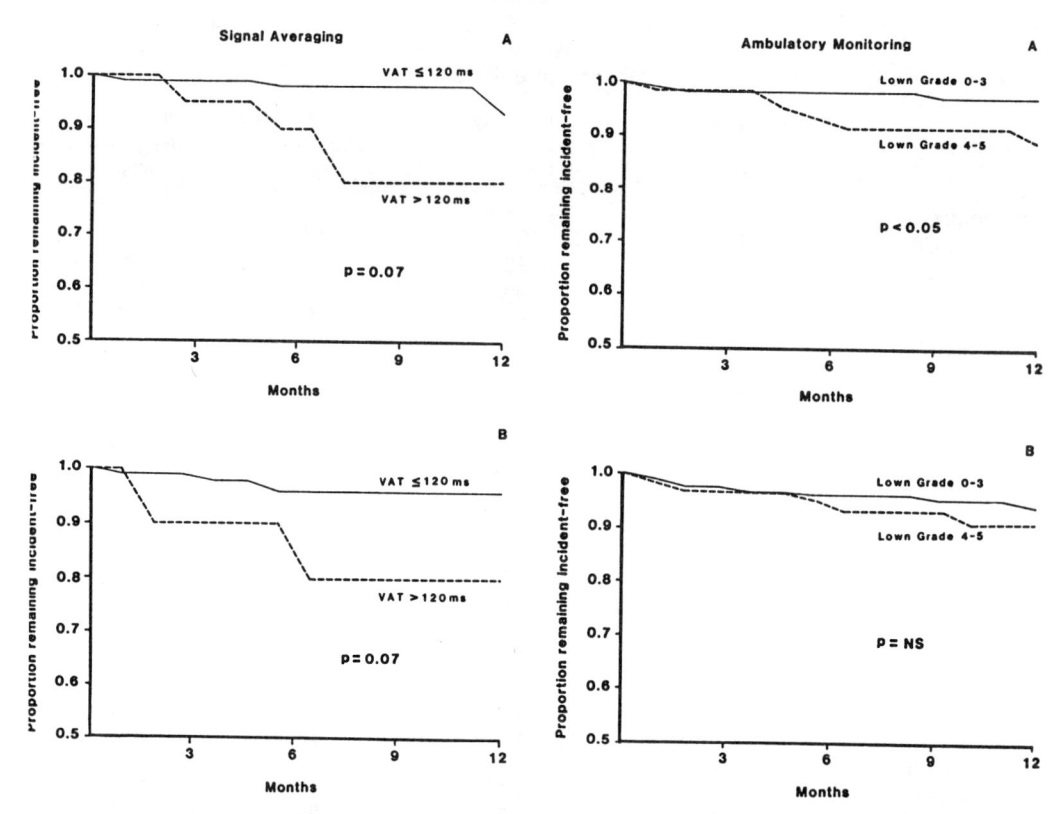

Figure 3: (left) Life table analysis of incident-free survival for patients with ventricular activation time (VAT) greater than 120 ms (broken curves) compared with the remaining patients (solid curves). Panel A: analysis in terms of electrical events. Panel B: analysis in terms of cardiac mortality.

Figure 4: (right) Life table analysis of incident-free survival in terms of grade of ventricular ectopy, Lown 0–3 (solid curves) and Lown 4–5 (broken curves). Panel A: analysis in terms of electrical events. Panel B: analysis in terms of cardiac mortality.

ventricular tachycardia (cycle length at least 230 ms) at Protocol 2 was 28%, not corrected for duration of follow-up. The incidence of electrical events in the subset of patients who had inducible slow ventricular tachycardia and low ejection fraction was 31%, not significantly different from the probability of electrical events among all patients with inducible slow ventricular tachycardia, irrespective of ejection fraction.

Exercise Testing

Figure 6A depicts the incident-free survival in terms of electrical events of patients with two or more mm of ST-segment displacement at exercise testing is compared with that of patients with less than 2 mm of ST-segment displacement or no ST-segment displacement at exercise testing. Figure 6B depicts the corresponding analysis in terms of all cardiac mortality.

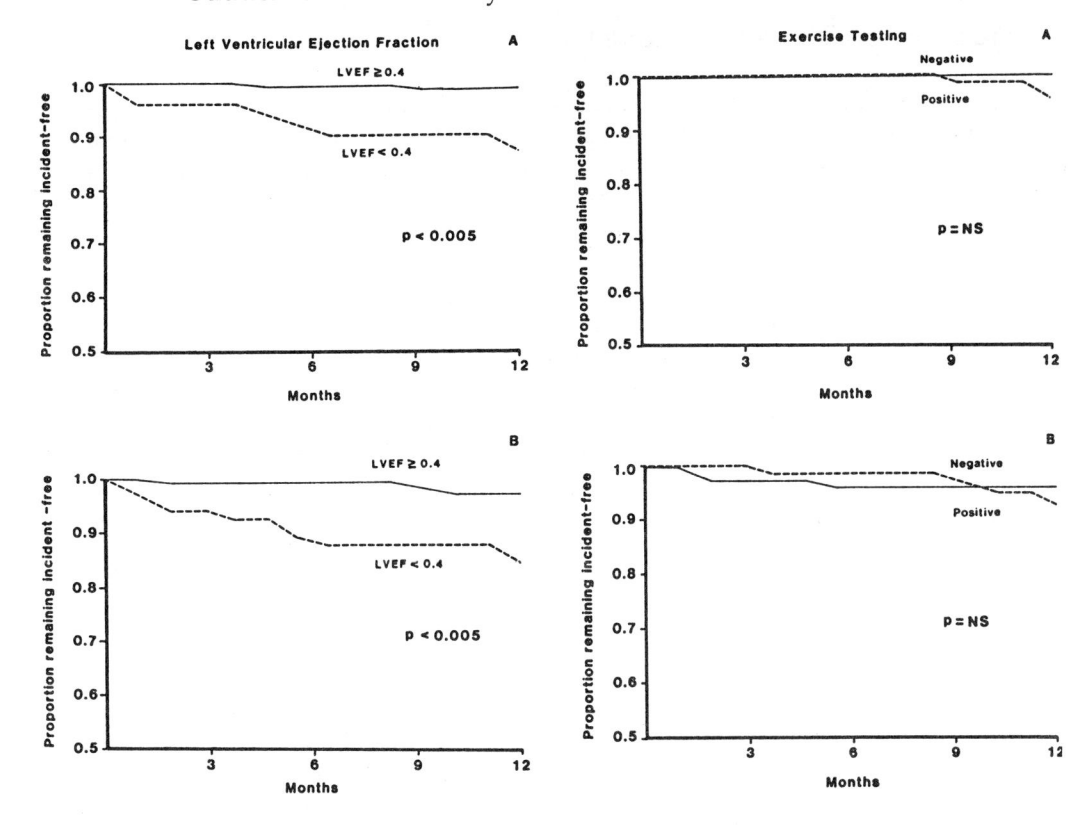

Figure 5: (left) Life table analysis of incident-free survival for patients with left ventricular ejection fraction (LVEF) less than 0.40 (broken curves) compared with the remainder (solid curves). Panel A: analysis in terms of electrical events. Panel B: analysis in terms of cardiac mortality.

Figure 6: (right) Life table analysis of incident-free survival for patients with at least 2 mm ST-segment displacement (positive) at exercise testing (broken curves) compared with the remainder (negative) (solid curves). Panel A: analysis in terms of electrical events. Panel B: analysis in terms of cardiac mortality.

Discussion

This study confirms previous experience that patients with inducible ventricular tachycardia after myocardial infarction are much more likely to exhibit subsequently a spontaneous electrical event than are patients without inducible ventricular tachycardia.[2,3,13] The present study comprises a fresh cohort of patients, none of whom was included in our previous reports.[2,3] We have now studied with programmed stimulation more than 700 patients (three separate cohorts) after myocardial infarction. Our consistent finding that inducible ventricular tachycardia is associated with subsequent spontaneous ventricular tachycardia suggests that our patient samples are unbiased and representative of survivors of uncomplicated myocardial infarction.

Programmed Stimulation After Infarction

The results of the present study suggest that our earlier protocol of programmed stimulation[7] is no longer sufficiently aggressive to obtain an acceptable level of sensitivity to predict sudden death or spontaneous ventricular tachyarrhythmias. This, and the overall lower mortality in the present series compared to our first series,[2] may be because of a change in the nature of our infarct population, or due to variations in therapy which may alter infarct morphology[14] and reduce predisposition to ventricular tachycardia.

Nevertheless, the present study confirms that patients with inducible slow ventricular tachycardia (cycle length at least 230 ms), are at significantly higher risk than patients with any other inducible arrhythmia, or no inducible arrhythmia at all. It would thus appear that it is the type of arrhythmia induced (with three or more ventricular extrastimuli), rather than the exact method of induction of the arrhythmia, which is associated with the increased risk. The indices summarized in Table IIIA suggest that an optimal protocol for programmed stimulation should include at least three extrastimuli, and perhaps no more than three. End-points for study should be ventricular fibrillation, or ventricular tachycardia sustained for at least 10 seconds.

The positive predictive accuracy of programmed stimulation utilizing three extrastimuli remains comparable to that obtained in our original series.[2] The somewhat lower sensitivity than previously found suggests that some patients who have no inducible arrhythmia 1 week following infarction may subsequently undergo structural changes in the infarct which then permit reentry and tachycardia, or that reentrant ventricular tachycardia, precipitated by one or a few spontaneous ventricular premature beats, may not be the mechanism of sudden death in some patients.

Since we have previously shown that changes in inducibility of ventricular tachycardia may occur with time,[3] it is not surprising that some patients may appear to exhibit a "false negative" response to programmed stimulation, just as some other patients exhibit apparently "false positive" responses.

Although the sensitivity of programmed stimulation is lower than our previous series,[2] the specificity and negative predictive accuracy remain very high indeed, and reinforce our contention that patients without inducible ventricular tachycardia are very unlikely to die suddenly or exhibit spontaneous ventricular tachycardia within a year of infarction.

Why have other investigators not confirmed our findings?[15-19] Although the reasons for this may be complex, a few comments seem appropriate. The overall incidence of cardiac events during the year after infarction is today about 10% or less. Even in patients with a history of spontaneous ventricular tachycardia in the context of chronic myocardial infarction, the probability of recurrence (untreated) within a year is only about 35%.[20] Therefore, in order to obtain any useful information from programmed stimulation, one must study relatively large numbers of unselected patients and accept that a positive predictive accuracy on the order of 35% is the maximum to be expected from any single test after infarction. The requirements for adequate methods of programmed stimulation and useful definitions of end-points have been dealt with above.

Other Investigations After Infarction

Measurement of ventricular activation time at signal averaging does not appear as potent a predictor of outcome as does programmed stimulation with three extrastimuli (compare Fig. 3 with Fig. 2). Nevertheless, patients with longer ventricular activation times tend to be more prone to electrical events and cardiac death than do patients with shorter ventricular activation times.

Ventricular ectopy assessed by Lown grading is quite inferior to programmed stimulation with three or more extrastimuli in terms of predicting subsequent electrical events. This is not surprising since ventricular ectopics per se cannot trigger ventricular tachycardia unless an anatomic or functional reentrant circuit is present.

Patients with lower ejection fractions were more likely to sustain electrical events or cardiac death than were patients with higher ejection fractions. However, the probability of electrical events among patients with both low ejection fraction and inducible slow ventricular tachycardia (cycle length at least 230 ms at Protocol 2) was no greater than the probability of an electrical event in the presence of inducible slow ventricular tachycardia (cycle length at least 230 ms at Protocol 2), irrespective of left ventricular ejection fraction. In other words, among these patients, the addition of low ejection fraction did not show an increased risk in those with inducible ventricular tachycardia. The relatively small number of electrical events did not permit any more comprehensive multivariate analysis of the data to be made.

ST-segment displacement at exercise testing did not confirm any significantly increased risk of electrical events or cardiac death in the present series. The absence of an association between reversible myocardial ischemia and spontaneous ventricular tachycardia is in accord with our previous observations.[3] The absence of an association between reversible myocardial ischemia at exercise testing and subsequent cardiac mortality probably reflects our present approach to early revascularization of patients whose ischemia is not readily controlled with medical therapy.

The Real Clinical Value of Programmed Stimulation After Infarction

Approximately 90% of patients after myocardial infarction do not have inducible slow ventricular tachycardia and may be reassured that the risk of spontaneous ventricular tachycardia or sudden death is very low. It is therefore quite inappropriate to prescribe medications to prevent spontaneous ventricular tachycardia in this majority of patients. We see an educational role for programmed stimulation in patients who do have inducible slow ventricular tachycardia. These patients learn to recognize ventricular tachycardia and are counseled that palpitations, presyncope, and syncope should not be ignored after hospital discharge. Extra effort should be undertaken to teach cardiopulmonary resuscitation techniques to the families of patients with inducible ventricular tachycardia in order to increase the probability of survival should ventricular tachycardia occur.

Since conventional "antiarrhythmic" drug therapy in the high-risk group has been demonstrated not to reduce the risk of spontaneous electrical events,[21] we do not prescribe such routine therapy for patients with inducible slow ventricular tachycardia who have not yet exhibited spontaneous ventricular tachycardia. There is obviously a pressing need for well-controlled prospective studies of medical and other interventions (for example, myocardial resection, cryoablation, laser ablation, implantable automatic antitachycardia pacemakers, defibrillators) to prevent spontaneous ventricular tachycardia and sudden death in patients with inducible ventricular tachycardia.

We conclude that the best predictor of sudden death or spontaneous ventricular tachycardia during the first year after infarction is the presence of inducible slow ventricular tachycardia (cycle length at least 230 ms) at programmed stimulation utilizing at least three extrastimuli. Only 58% of such patients are likely to remain incident-free at 1 year. Patients without inducible slow ventricular tachycardia have a 98% probability of remaining incident-free at 1 year.

Acknowledgments: This work was supported by a grant from the National Health and Medical Research Council of Australia. The cooperation of the patients and the expert assistance of our medical and technical colleagues are gratefully acknowledged. We also thank Anita Watts for maintaining patient follow up, and Helen Pinchen, Karen Jones, and Jeanette Walker for their careful preparation of the manuscript.

References

1. Hamer A, Vohra J, Hunt D, Sloman G. Prediction of sudden death by electrophysiologic studies in high risk patients surviving acute myocardial infarction. Am J Cardiol 1982;50:223–229.
2. Richards DA, Cody DV, Denniss AR, Russell PA, Young AA, Uther JB. Ventricular electrical instability: A predictor of death after myocardial infarction. Am J Cardiol 1983;51:75–80.
3. Denniss AR, Richards DA, Cody DV, Russell PA, Young AA, Cooper MJ, Ross DL, Uther JB. Prognostic significance of ventricular tachycardia and fibrillation induced at programmed stimulation and delayed potentials detectable on the signal-averaged electrocardiograms of survivors of acute myocardial infarction. Circulation 1986;74:731–745.
4. Schulze RA, Strauss HW, Pitt B. Sudden death in the year following myocardial infarction. Relation to ventricular premature contractions in the late hospital phase and left ventricular ejection fraction. Am J Med 1977;62:192–199.
5. Bigger JT, Heller CA, Wenger TL, Weld FM. Risk stratification after acute myocardial infarction. Am J Cardiol 1978;42:202–210.
6. Denniss AR, Baaijens H, Cody DV, Richards DA, Russell PA, Young AA, Ross DL, Uther JB. Value of programmed stimulation and exercise testing in predicting one-year mortality after acute myocardial infarction. Am J Cardiol 1985;56:213–220.
7. Richards DA, Cody DV, Denniss AR, Russell PA, Young AA, Uther JB. A new protocol of programmed stimulation for assessment of predisposition to spontaneous ventricular arrhythmias. Eur Heart J 1983;4:376–382.
8. Denniss AR, Richards DA, Farrow RH, Mercer CJ, Scott PJ. Technique for maximising the frequency response of the signal averaged Frank vectorcardiogram. J Biomed Eng 1986;8:207–212.
9. Lown B, Wolf M. Approaches to sudden death from coronary heart disease. Circulation 1971;44:130–142.
10. Sami M, Kraemer H, de Busk RF. The prognostic significance of serial exercise testing after myocardial infarction. Circulation 1979;60:1238–1246.

11. Norusis MJ. SPSS X Advanced Statistics Guide. Chicago, McGraw-Hill Book Company, 1985.
12. Norris RM, Caughey DE, Deeming LW, Mercer CJ, Scott PJ. Coronary prognostic index for predicting survival after recovery from acute myocardial infarction. Lancet 1970;2:485–487.
13. Breithardt G, Borggrefe M, Haerten K. Role of programmed ventricular stimulation and non-invasive recording of ventricular late potentials for the identification of patients at risk of ventricular tachyarrhythmias after acute myocardial infarction. In Zipes D, Jolife J, eds. Cardiac Electrophysiology and Arrhythmias. 1983;553–561.
14. Richards DA, Blake GJ, Spear JF, Moore EN. Electrophysiologic substrate for ventricular tachycardia: correlation of properties in vivo and in vitro. Circulation 1984;69:369–381.
15. Marchlinski FE, Buxton AE, Waxman HL, Josephson ME. Identifying patients at risk of sudden death after myocardial infarction: Value of the response to programmed stimulation, degree of ventricular ectopic activity, and severity of left ventricular dysfunction. Am J Cardiol 1983;52:1190–1196.
16. Santarelli P, Bellocci F, Loperfido F, Mazzari M, Mongiardo R, Montenero A, Manzoli U, Denes P. Ventricular arrhythmia induced by programmed ventricular stimulation after acute myocardial infarction. Am J Cardiol 1985;55:391–394.
17. Waspe LE, Seinfield D, Ferrick A, Fink D, Scanin G, Wanliss M, Kun SG, Mates JA, Fisher JD. Programmed electrical stimulation to predict late sudden death in survivors of complicated myocardial infarction (abstr). J Am Coll Cardiol 1984;3:609.
18. Roy D, Marchand E, Theroux P, Waters DD, Pelletier GB, Bonrassa MG. Reproducibility and significance of ventricular arrhythmias induced after acute myocardial infarction (abstr). Circulation 1984;70:II–18.
19. Gonzales R, Arriagada D, Corbalan R, Chamorro G, Fajuri A, Rodriguez J. Programmed electrical stimulation of the heart does not help to identify patients at high risk post myocardial infarction (abstr). Circulation 1984;70:II–19.
20. Cooper MJ, Hunt LJ, Palmer KJ, Denniss AR, Richards DA, Uther JB, Ross DL. Prediction of proarrhythmic drug effects at electrophysiologic study for ventricular tachycardia (abstr). Circulation 1986;74:II–482.
21. Denniss AR, Ross DL, Cody DV, Richards DA, Russell PA, Young AA, Uther JB. Randomized trial of antiarrhythmic drugs in patients with inducible ventricular tachyarrhythmias after recent myocardial infarction. Circulation 1986;74:II–213.

20

The Canadian Experience on the Identification of Candidates for Sudden Cardiac Death After Myocardial Infarction

Denis Roy, Angel Arenal
Daniel Godin, Etienne Marchand
Dennis Cassidy, Pierre Théroux
David D. Waters

Introduction

In May 1983, a prospective study was undertaken at our institution to evaluate the prognostic significance of programmed ventricular stimulation in survivors of an acute myocardial infarction. We reported[1] that the initiation of a ventricular tachyarrhythmia by electrophysiologic testing was a poor marker of risk for the occurrence of sudden death in the first year after infarction and that prognosis was more related to ejection fraction, exercise-induced ventricular arrhythmias, and presence of a left ventricular aneurysm. This investigation describes the long-term clinical course of our study population.

Methods

Study Population

The study population was selected from 320 patients admitted to the coronary care unit of the Montreal Heart Institute for acute myocardial infarction and who satisfied the following criteria: (1) age 65 years or less, (2) absence of uncontrolled angina or heart failure, and (3) absence of sustained ventricular tachycardia 72 hours or more after the onset of infarction. Of these patients, 150 gave written informed consent to undergo programmed ventricular stimulation before hospital discharge.

Clinical Evaluation

The criteria for acute myocardial infarction included at least two of the following: myocardial ischemic pain lasting more than 30 minutes, serum levels of creatine kinase elevated at least twice above the upper limit of normal with presence of the MB fraction, and Minnesota code electrocardiographic criteria[2] for acute infarction. Patients were observed with continuous visual electrocardiographic monitoring for the first 4 days in the coronary care unit and a 24-hour Holter recording was obtained a mean of 11 ± 9.5 days after myocardial infarction. Counts were made of the total number of ventricular premature complexes during each hour and the arrhythmias were graded according to the system devised by Lown and Wolf.[3] The following tests were also obtained in all patients before hospital discharge: limited exercise test, coronary angiography, and left ventricular radionuclide equilibrium gated scan.

Programmed Ventricular Stimulation

Patients underwent programmed ventricular stimulation while in the postabsorptive state and while receiving no antiarrhythmic medication for at least 72 hours before the study. The tests were performed a mean of 12 ± 2 days (range 8 to 20) after myocardial infarction. A quadripolar electrode catheter was inserted percutaneously and positioned in the right ventricle under fluoroscopic guidance. Stimulation was performed with a programmable stimulator and an isolated constant current source. The stimuli were rectangular pulses 1.5 ms in duration at twice diastolic threshold (0.3 to 1.4 mA). Single and paired ventricular extrastimuli were delivered during two paced ventricular cycle lengths (600 and 400 ms) first at the right ventricular apex and then at the right ventricular outflow tract. The protocol was terminated prematurely if a sustained ventricular tachycardia or ventricular fibrillation occurred.

Definitions

Repetitive responses were defined as one to five ventricular complexes in response to a ventricular stimulus. Ventricular tachycardia was defined as nonsustained if it persisted for six complexes or more but terminated spontaneously within 30 seconds. Ventricular tachycardia was considered sustained if it lasted more than 30 seconds or if it required immediate termination because of hemodynamic collapse. Sustained and nonsustained ventricular tachycardia were considered induced only if they were initiated on two or more occasions and if cardioversion was not required for termination. Ventricular tachycardia degenerating to ventricular fibrillation was characterized as ventricular tachycardia.

Follow-Up

Patients had follow-up contact either by a clinic visit or by phone. Follow-up information was obtained in all patients during the last 4 months of 1986. The end-points of the study were death or the development of documented sustained ventricular tachyarrhythmias. Death was defined as sudden if it occurred within 1 hour of the onset of symptoms.

Statistics

Differences among continuous variables were analyzed by the Student t test. Discrete variables were compared with the chi-square test. For 2×2 tables with cell frequencies of less than 5, analysis was performed with Fisher's exact probability test. All values are expressed as mean ±1 SD. A p value of less than .05 was considered significant.

Results

Response to Programmed Ventricular Stimulation (Table I)

Ventricular fibrillation was initiated in two patients. Sustained ventricular tachycardia was induced in 16 patients. The arrhythmia had a right bundle branch block morphology in 10 patients and a left bundle branch block morphology in six. The mean cycle length of the tachycardia was 246 ms (range 200 to 330) and its mean duration was 40 seconds (range 13 to 180). Nonsustained ventricular tachycardia was initiated in 17 patients. The tachycardia was polymorphic in 13 patients and had a right bundle branch block morphology in four. The mean cycle length of the tachycardia was 214 ms (range 175 to 300) and its mean duration was 16 complexes (range 6 to 43). Two ventricular extrastimuli were required to initiate all sustained and nonsustained ventricular tachycardias. External countershock was required to terminate sustained ventricular tachyarrhythmia in 10 patients.

Table I
Response to Programmed Ventricular Stimulation

Response	n
Group A (n = 35)	
Ventricular fibrillation	2
Sustained ventricular tachycardia	16
Nonsustained ventricular tachycardia	17
Group B (n = 115)	
Repetitive ventricular responses	85
No response	30

Repetitive ventricular responses were induced in 85 patients. Thirty patients had no extra response to programmed ventricular stimulation.

On the basis of programmed stimulation, the patients were divided into two groups. Group A consisted of the 35 patients (23%) with inducible ventricular tachycardia or ventricular fibrillation. Group B comprised the remaining 115 patients (77%), who had either one to five repetitive ventricular responses or no extra response to programmed ventricular stimulation.

Seventeen patients belonging to group A and 56 patients in group B were receiving β-blockers at the time of programmed ventricular stimulation (p = NS). The mean stimulation threshold was 0.71 ± 0.18 mA among patients in group A and 0.62 ± 0.24 mA in group B (p < .05). However, ventricular refractory periods were similar between the two groups (252 ± 20 vs 259 ± 22 ms; p = NS).

Clinical Characteristics (Table II)

The average age of all patients was 52 years; 87% were men and 26% had suffered a previous myocardial infarction. The location of acute infarction was anterior in 45% of the patients and inferior in 47% of patients. Thirty percent of patients had non-Q wave infarction. The mean peak creatine kinase level for all patients was 1989 IU/l. Most patients had no evidence of left ventricular failure at the time of admission. The incidence of inferior infarction was higher in patients in group A (66%) compared with those in group B (41%, p < .01) and anterior infarctions were more frequent in group B (51%) than in group A (26%, p < .01). There was no significant difference in age, sex distribution, incidence of prior myocardial infarction, incidence of non-Q wave infarction, peak creatine kinase levels, or Killip class between the two groups. Thirty-eight (25%) patients had ventricular tachycardia or fibrillation in the first 72 hours after myocardial infarction. Twelve (8%) patients had a sustained ventricular tachyarrhythmia requiring cardioversion and 26 (17%) had nonsustained ventricular tachycardia. The proportion of patients having these acute arrhythmias was not significantly different between group A and group B.

The mean number of ventricular premature complexes per hour recorded during 24 hour Holter monitoring was 4.3 ± 10.9 among patients of group A compared with 2.4 ± 6.5 in patients of group B (p = NS). Only 11 (7%) patients

Table II
Clinical Characteristics

	Group A (n = 35)	Group B (n = 115)	Total (n = 150)	p value
Age (years)	52	52	52	NS
Sex (men)	32 (91%)	99 (86%)	131 (87%)	NS
Prior MI	9 (26%)	30 (26%)	39 (26%)	NS
Location of acute MI				
Anterior	9 (26%)	59 (51%)	68 (45%)	< .01
Inferior	23 (66%)	47 (41%)	70 (47%)	< .01
Undetermined	3 (8%)	9 (8%)	12 (8%)	NS
Non-Q wave MI	8 (23%)	37 (32%)	45 (30%)	NS
Peak creatine kinase (IU/L)	2546 ± 3458	1727 ± 1503	1989 ± 2277	NS
Killip class ⩾ 2	7 (20%)	13 (11%)	20 (13%)	NS

MI = myocardial infarction

in this study had more than 10 ventricular premature complexes per hour. There was also no significant difference in Lown grade classification between patients in group A and group B. Thirteen patients (38%) in group A and 32 patients (28%) in group B had grade 3 or 4 arrhythmias.

Sixty-two (42%) patients developed either angina or ST segment depression during exercise testing. Ventricular premature complexes during or after exercise were observed in 14 patients (9%). Again the incidence of these findings was not significantly different between the two groups.

No significant differences existed between the two groups with respect to the number of coronary vessels with a stenosis of 75% or more (1.5 ± 0.8 vs 1.6 ± 0.8), the mean ejection fraction measured by predischarge radionuclide gated scan (45 ± 12% vs 46 ± 12%), and the number of patients with a left ventricular aneurysm (3 vs. 9 patients).

Follow-Up

In Table III, the results of programmed ventricular stimulation are correlated with clinical outcome during the 31 ± 8 months (range .5 to 42) of follow-up. There were 13 (9%) fatal or near-fatal cardiac events. One group A patient and four patients belonging to group B died suddenly. Four patients belonging to group B suffered nonsudden cardiac deaths. All four deaths were due to cardiogenic shock, two secondary to recurrent myocardial infarction, and two related to coronary bypass surgery. Four patients, one in group A and three in group B, were resuscitated from spontaneous sustained ventricular tachycardia. The arrhythmia occurred 1 week after hospital discharge in the patient in group A and developed in the late hospital course of a recurrent myocardial infarction in two of the three patients in group B. All four patients received specific antiarrhythmic therapy (map-guided subendocardial resection in one, amiodarone in three) and are alive after 30 to 43 months of follow-up. There were no significant differences in the occurrence of sudden death, and/or nonsudden death, and/or spontaneous

Table III
Correlation Between Results of Programmed Ventricular Stimulation and Clinical Outcome (mean follow-up 31 ± 8 months)

	Group A (n = 35)	Group B (n = 115)	Total (n = 150)	p value
Deaths	1	8	9	NS
Sudden	1	4	5	NS
Nonsudden	0	4	4	NS
Spontaneous sustained VT	1	3	4	NS
Recurrent MI	3	14	17	NS
Therapy at end of follow-up				
β-blockers	10	43	53	NS
Coronary bypass surgery or coronary angioplasty	7	19	26	NS
Antiarrhythmic drugs	1	3	4	NS

VT = ventricular tachycardia; MI = myocardial infarction.

sustained ventricular tachycardia between the two groups. There was also no significant difference in the occurrence of these events when the analysis compared only the 18 patients with inducible sustained ventricular tachyarrhythmias with the 132 patients without sustained arrhythmias at electrophysiologic testing. Seventeen patients, 14 belonging to group B and three belonging to group A, experienced recurrent nonfatal myocardial infarction. At the end of the follow-up, 10 group A and 43 group B patients were receiving β-blockers (p = NS). Seven patients in group A and 19 patients in group B underwent coronary bypass surgery or coronary angioplasty for control of angina (p = NS). One patient in group A and three patients in group B were receiving antiarrhythmic drug therapy (p = NS). Of these four patients, one was being treated for paroxysmal atrial fibrillation, and antiarrhythmic therapy was initiated for premature ventricular complexes in three patients.

To determine if other factors could accurately identify high-risk patients, the subjects who died or experienced spontaneous sustained ventricular tachyarrhythmias were compared with those who did not experience these events during the follow-up period with respect to clinical characteristics and results of all available tests. The mean ejection fraction was significantly lower in the 13 patients who suffered cardiac events (sudden death + nonsudden death + sustained ventricular tachyarrhythmias) when compared with the remaining 137 patients ($37 \pm 14\%$ vs $47 \pm 11\%$, $p < .005$). Ventricular arrhythmias occurred during exercise testing in three patients (23%) suffering cardiac events as compared with 11 of the patients (8%) without events ($p < .05$). Three of the 13 patients (23%) with cardiac events had a ventricular aneurysm compared to eight of the 137 patients (6%) without cardiac events ($p < .05$). Similar results were obtained when only patients with primarily arrhythmic events (sudden death + sustained ventricular tachyarrhythmias) were compared with those without these events: the mean ejection fraction was $34 \pm 14\%$ in the nine patients with primarily arrhythmic events as compared with $46 \pm 11\%$ in the remaining 141 patients ($p < .005$) and the incidence of these events was significantly greater in patients with a left ventricular aneurysm than in patients without aneurysm (33% vs. 6%, p < .005).

Reproducibility of Provokable Ventricular Arrhythmias

Of the 35 patients with inducible ventricular tachycardia in the early postinfarction period, 21 agreed to be restudied by programmed ventricular stimulation on an elective basis 4 to 11 months after acute myocardial infarction. Ventricular tachyarrhythmias could be reinitiated in 16 patients (70%): ventricular fibrillation in two, sustained ventricular tachycardia in five, and nonsustained ventricular tachycardia in nine. These patients were followed a mean of 33 ± 7 months (range 14 to 42) and only one patient who had inducible sustained monomorphic ventricular tachycardia died suddenly. The remaining patients have survived follow-up without experiencing an arrhythmic event.

Discussion

The results indicate that the initiation of ventricular tachyarrhythmias in survivors of an acute myocardial infarction was a poor marker of risk for the occurrence of sudden death or spontaneous ventricular tachycardia during the 31 month follow-up period. Despite the reproducible initiation of ventricular tachyarrhythmias, the long-term prognosis was good without antiarrhythmic therapy. Indexes of left ventricular dysfunction were more accurate in distinguishing patients at high and low risk for cardiac events. These findings are in agreement with the initial reports[1,4] of our study.

In the last few years, the ability of programmed ventricular stimulation to reveal propensity for sudden death after infarction has been evaluated in over 1000 patients from nine series.[1,5-12] Five studies[5-7,10,12] have suggested that electrophysiologic testing may be useful while four[1,8,9,11] have not found them to be sensitive predictors of sudden death after infarction. It is difficult to compare or cumulate the results because methods of assessment differed. Study populations, end-points, and definitions of abnormal responses to electrophysiologic testing and stimulation protocols have varied greatly between studies.

Both Hamer et al.[6] and Waspe et al.[10] studied patients with clinical features of a high risk group and found that the response to programmed ventricular stimulation was a sensitive indicator of sudden death after infarction. Most patients in the remaining seven series[1,5,7-9,11,12] were in a low to moderate risk group and the results from four of these studies[1,8,9,11] suggest that electrophysiologic testing was not helpful in identifying patients who suffered arrhythmic events. Thus, differences in study populations may explain some discrepancies in results between studies.

In the present study, only nine patients (6%) died during follow-up. The exclusion of patients with severe heart failure and unstable angina probably accounts for the low mortality. Furthermore, the outcome in our patients may have been influenced by information obtained from exercise testing or coronary angiography and the current attitudes about β-blocking and surgical therapy of survivors of myocardial infarction. Therefore, our data may not be applicable to a high-risk subpopulation of survivors of myocardial infarction. However, no attempt was made to suppress the arrhythmias induced at electrophysiologic testing and only four patients were receiving antiarrhythmic therapy at the end of follow-up. Our results do not encourage antiarrhythmic treatment of ventricular tachyarrhythmias detected at electrophysiologic testing in asymptomatic postinfarction patients.

Several studies[13-15] have suggested that nonsustained ventricular tachycardia and ventricular fibrillation may be nonspecific responses to programmed ventricular stimulation, and Denniss et al.[12] recently reported that inducible sustained ventricular tachycardia was the important variable in prognosis after infarction. In our study, sudden death and near-fatal arrhythmic events occurred in two of the 16 (13%) patients with inducible sustained ventricular tachycardia compared with seven of the remaining 134 (5%) patients (p = NS). None of the 19 patients with either nonsustained ventricular tachycardia or ventricular fibrillation died or developed ventricular tachyarrhythmias during follow-up. The results indicate that although sustained ventricular tachycardia may be a more specific response to programmed ventricular stimulation, the predictive value of this technique for identifying patients prone to sudden death or ventricular tachycardia was only 13%.

The ability to induce ventricular tachycardia did not correlate with the extent of coronary artery disease, the arrhythmias detected either in the coronary care unit or during ambulatory monitoring, and the degree of left ventricular dysfunction. The pathophysiologic significance of susceptibility to tachycardia induction in patients with inferior infarction is unclear.

We conclude that after completion of 2.5 years of follow-up, programmed ventricular stimulation was of limited value in selecting a subset of postinfarction patients at high risk for sudden death. Our data suggest that noninvasive evaluation of left ventricular function provides the greatest prognostic information. Because electrophysiologic testing is associated with some morbidity and potential mortality, we do not recommend it for routine clinical risk stratification of patient recovering from an acute myocardial infarction. However, the prognostic value of this technique in patients with a combination of well-known risk factors needs to be more fully investigated.

Acknowledgment: This research has been supported by the Montreal Heart Institute Research Fund.

References

1. Roy D, Marchand E, Théroux P, Waters DD, Pelletier GB, Bourassa MG. Programmed ventricular stimulation in survivors of an acute myocardial infarction. Circulation 1985;72:487–494.
2. Blackburn H, Keys A, Simonson E, Rautaharju P, Punsar S. The electrocardiogram in population studies: A classification system. Circulation 1960;21:1160–1175.
3. Lown B, Wolf M. Approaches to sudden death from coronary heart disease. Circulation 1971;44:130–142.

4. Roy D, Marchand E, Théroux P, Waters DD, Pelletier GB, Cartier R, Bourassa MG. Long-term reproducibility and significance of provokable ventricular arrhythmias after myocardial infarction. J Am Coll Cardiol 1986;8:32–39.
5. Green HL, Reid PR, Schaeffer AH. The repetitive ventricular response in man: A predictor of sudden death. N Engl J Med 1978;299:729–734.
6. Hamer A, Vohra J, Hunt D, Sloman G. Prediction of sudden death by electrophysiologic studies in high risk patients surviving acute myocardial infarction. Am J Cardiol 1982;50:223–229.
7. Richards DA, Cody DV, Denniss AR, Russell PA, Young AA, Uther JB. Ventricular electrical instability: a predictor of death after myocardial infarction. Am J Cardiol 1983;51:75–80.
8. Marchlinski FE, Buxton AE, Waxman HL, Josephson ME. Identifying patients at risk of sudden death after myocardial infarction: Value of the response to programmed stimulation, degree of ventricular ectopic activity and severity of left ventricular dysfunction. Am J Cardiol 1983;52:1190–1196.
9. Santarelli P, Bellocci F, Loperfido F, Mazzari M, Mongiardo R, Montenero AS, Manzoli U, Denes P. Ventricular arrhythmia induced by programmed ventricular stimulation after acute myocardial infarction. Am J Cardiol 1985;55:391–394.
10. Waspe LE, Seinfeld D, Ferrick A, Kim SG, Matos JA, Fisher JD. Prediction of sudden death and spontaneous ventricular tachycardia in survivors of complicated myocardial infarction: Value of the response to programmed stimulation using a maximum of three ventricular extrastimuli. J Am Coll Cardiol 1985;5:1292–1301.
11. Bhandari AK, Rose JS, Kotlewski A, Rahimtoola SH, Wu D. Frequency and significance of induced sustained ventricular tachycardia or fibrillation two weeks after acute myocardial infarction. Am J Cardiol 1985;56:737–742.
12. Denniss AR, Richards DA, Cody DV, Russell PA, Young AA, Cooper MJ, Ross DL, Uther JB. Prognostic significance of ventricular tachycardia and fibrillation induced at programmed stimulation and delayed potentials detected on the signal-averaged electrocardiograms of survivors of acute myocardial infarction. Circulation 1986;74:731–745.
13. Brugada P, Abdollah H, Heddle B, Wellens HJJ. Results of a ventricular stimulation protocol using a maximum of 4 premature stimuli in patients without documented or suspected ventricular arrhythmias. Am J Cardiol 1983;52:1214–1218.
14. Buxton AE, Waxman HL, Marchlinski FE, Untereker WJ, Waspe LE, Josephson ME. Role of triple extrastimuli during electrophysiologic study of patients with documented sustained ventricular tachyarrhythmias. Circulation 1984;69:532–540.
15. Brugada P, Waldecker B, Kersschot Y, Zehender M, Wellens HJJ. Ventricular arrhythmias initiated by programmed stimulation in four groups of patients with healed myocardial infarction. J Am Coll Cardiol 1986;8:1035–1040.

21

Sudden Death in Hypertrophic Cardiomyopathy: Identification of the "High Risk" Patient

William J. McKenna

Introduction

The natural history of hypertrophic cardiomyopathy is characterized by a slow progression of symptoms and a significant incidence of sudden death.[1,2] The overall annual mortality in adults is approximately 2.5% while in children and adolescents it is even higher, approximately 6%.[3] These figures are from referral centers prior to echocardiography when the diagnosis of hypertrophic cardiomyopathy was based upon clinical, hemodynamic, and angiographic features of the condition. The diagnostic sensitivity has increased with the more widespread availability of M-mode and 2-dimensional echocardiography. In particular, the diagnosis is now more often made in patients who do not have significant symptoms or obvious clinical features of a gradient, who may have otherwise been missed. Natural history studies from nonspecialist referral centers suggest that the proportion of such patients is higher and the annual mortality rate is lower than earlier reports.[4,5] Is hypertrophic cardiomyopathy a common disorder with a benign prognosis? It is probable that the condition is more common and the prognosis better than was previously appreciated. It remains clear, however, that the most important problem in management is the prevention of sudden death; despite an emphasis during the past 5 years on the identification and treatment of the high risk patient, we still have a 4% annual mortality rate from sudden death in children and adolescents.[6]

From: Brugada P, Wellens HJJ. CARDIAC ARRHYTHMIAS: Where To Go From Here? Mount Kisco, NY, Futura Publishing Company, Inc., © 1987.

Patient Studies: Predictions of Sudden Death

Are all patients with hypertrophic cardiomyopathy at risk of sudden death? It has not been practical to assess this important question; however, previous studies have attempted to identify the high risk patient. In a retrospective analysis, we assessed the predictive accuracy of 24 clinical, electrocardiographic, and hemodynamic variables which were recorded at the time of diagnosis in 228 children and adults with hypertrophic cardiomyopathy.[3] During follow-up of 1–23, mean 6 years, 32 patients died suddenly and there were 196 survivors. Discriminant analysis revealed that the combination of young age at diagnosis, syncope, and a family history of hypertrophic cardiomyopathy and sudden death best predicted sudden death with a false negative rate of 30%, a false positive rate of 27%, and a positive predictive accuracy of 24%. It is of interest that readily obtained clinical features were of greater predictive value than electrocardiographic indices of hypertrophy or hemodynamic measurements of filling pressures and left ventricular outflow tract gradients. In a subsequent study in 88 patients, ventricular volumes and their rates of change during the cardiac cycle were derived from digitized cineangiograms recorded at the time of diagnosis and were analyzed to determine the relation of indices of left ventricular function to outcome, particularly sudden death.[7] Ventricular volumes and ejection fraction were similar in survivors and patients who died suddenly. The 11 patients who died suddenly, however, had a lower left ventricular peak ejection rate (5.41 ± 0.69 vs 6.24 ± 1.33 s^{-1}, p = 0.006) and peak filling rate (4.02 ± 0.94 vs 4.88 ± 1.53 s^{-1}; p = 0.02) than the 67 survivors. Stepwise regression analysis revealed that sudden death was best predicted by the combination of increased end-diastolic volume, small end-systolic volume, and low peak filling rate (predictive accuracy 32%, false negative 18%, and false positive 28%). The addition of clinical features and hemodynamic measurements to the analysis improved predictive accuracy to 43% (false negative 18% and false positive 18%). Nevertheless, the predictive power of conventional clinical, hemodynamic, and angiographic features and measurements is relatively poor. The differences in the clinical features (Table I)

Table I
Relation of Age and Clinical Features at Diagnosis to Prognosis

	≤ 14		15–30		31–45		≥ 46	
	D n = 11	A n = 16	D n = 9	A n = 58	D n = 9	A n = 61	D n = 10	A n = 61
No syncope	7 (64)	13 (81)	7 (78)	45 (78)	4 (50)	53 (87)	9 (90)	52 (85)
Syncope	4 (36)	3 (19)	2 (22)	13 (22)	4 (50)	8 (13)*	1 (10)	9 (15)
No chest pain	9 (82)	14 (88)	7 (78)	32 (55)	3 (38)	35 (57)	4 (40)	23 (38)
Exertional chest pain	2 (18)	2 (12)	2 (22)	26 (45)	5 (62)	26 (43)	6 (60)	38 (62)
No dyspnea	7 (64)	11 (69)	4 (44)	25 (43)	1 (12)	25 (41)	2 (20)	21 (34)
Class II	4 (36)	5 (31)	5 (56)	27 (47)	3 (38)	33 (54)	7 (70)	31 (51)
Class III + IV	0	0	0	6 (10)	4 (50)	3 (5)	1 (10)	9 (15)

Adapted from McKenna et al.,[3] Am J Cardiol 1981;47:532–538.
*p = 0.02 for syncope in patients who died vs survivors; D = dead; A = alive.

and hemodynamic and angiographic measurements (Tables II and III) in young and old patients who died suddenly underscores the lack of a homogeneous clinical profile for the high risk patient and also suggests that the mechanism of sudden death may be different in children and in adults.

In both retrospective studies which have been discussed, the variables entered into the discriminant analysis were recorded from evaluations at the time of diagnosis between 1960 and 1978 and did not include echocardiographic data or information from ambulatory electrocardiographic recordings.[3,7] The development of 2-dimensional echocardiography has greatly improved the assessment of the severity and distribution of left ventricular hypertrophy. The role of the echocardiographic assessment of the magnitude and distribution of left and right ventricular hypertrophy in the prediction of sudden death has not been assessed in a discriminant analysis. However, from Maron's work (Fig. 1), it is apparent that septal thickness is similar in patients who die suddenly and in age- and sex-matched control patients who survive and that the absolute septal thickness is unlikely to be useful to predict sudden death in a patient population with hypertrophic cardiomyopathy.[8] Indeed, 16 (26%) of those who died suddenly had a relatively thin ventricular septum (≤ 20 mm) suggesting that other features must be important in determining sudden death.

Table II
Relation of Age and Hemodynamic Features at Diagnosis and Prognosis

	≤ 14		15–30		31–45		≥ 46	
	D n = 11	A n = 14	D n = 8	A n = 57	D n = 7	A n = 61	D n = 9	A n = 61
LVOT gradient								
Yes	5 (45)	9 (64)	6 (75)	32 (56)	5 (71)	38 (62)	7 (78)	42 (69)
No	6 (55)	5 (36)	2 (25)	25 (44)	2 (29)	23 (38)	2 (22)	19 (31)

Adapted from McKenna et al.,[3] Am J Cardiol 1981;47:532–538.
D = dead; A = alive; LVOT = left ventricular outflow tract.

Table III
Comparison of Left Ventricular Volumes and Normalized Peak Ejection and Filling Rates in Young and Older Patients Who Died Suddenly Versus Survivors

	Patients Who Died Suddenly		
	Young (n = 5)	Older (n = 6)	Survivors (n = 67)
EDV (cc)	120 ± 50	171 ± 90	139 ± 42
ESV (cc)	10 ± 7+	42 ± 53	24 ± 12
EF (%)	92 ± 5*	79 ± 17	82 ± 9
PER/EDV (liters/s)	4.83 ± 0.64	4.36 ± 1.16	5.13 ± 1.17
PER/SV (liters/s)	5.28 ± 0.65*	5.52 ± 0.77	6.24 ± 1.33
PFR/SV (liters/s)	4.41 ± 1.07	3.69 ± 0.76**	4.88 ± 1.53
PFR/SV (liters/s)	4.77 ± 0.96	4.73 ± 1.26	5.82 ± 1.70

Adapted from Newman et al.,[7] JACC 1985;5:1064–1074.
*p < 0.05 versus survivors; **p < 0.01.
EDV = end-diastolic volume; ESV = end-systolic volume; EF = ejection fraction; PER = peak ejection rate; PFR = peak filling rate; SV = stroke volume.

356 • CARDIAC ARRHYTHMIAS

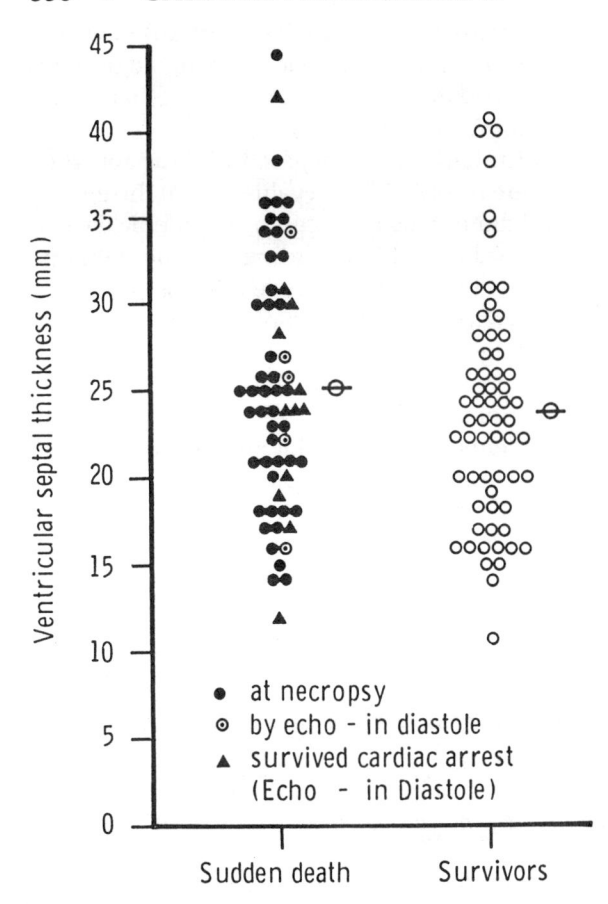

Figure 1: Ventricular septal thickness in 62 patients with hypertrophic cardiomyopathy who died suddenly or had cardiac arrest, compared with a control group of 62 age and sex-matched surviving patients with hypertrophic cardiomyopathy. Mean values are indicated. (Reproduced with permission from Maron et al.,[8] Circulation 1982; 65:1388–1394.)

Arrhythmias as a Determinant of Sudden Death

The importance of arrhythmias as a determinant of sudden death has been emphasized recently.[9–12] Ambulatory electrocardiographic monitoring has revealed that arrhythmias are common (Table IV) and that asymptomatic episodes of nonsustained ventricular tachycardia are detected in approximately 25% of adults with hypertrophic cardiomyopathy.[11,12] These episodes appear benign: they are usually slow (median rate 140 beats/min), follow periods of relative bradycardia (median rate 70 beats/min), and are not associated with ST-segment or QT-interval alteration.[13] Their significance lies in the simultaneous observation from two independent centers that adults with episodes of ventricular tachycardia had an increased annual mortality from sudden death.[12,14] Thirteen of the 170 consecutive unoperated patients from the NIH and the Hammersmith died suddenly during 3 years; nine of these 13 had ventricular tachycardias.[12–14] In both studies, this arrhythmia was significantly more common in those who died suddenly (Fig. 2). This does not indicate a causal relationship but does establish that ventricular tachycardia is a marker of the adult who is at particular risk of sudden death. Indeed, in the adult with hypertrophic cardiomyopathy, non-

Table IV
Arrhythmias Detected During 72-Hour Electrocardiographic Monitoring in 100 Consecutive Patients With Hypertrophic Cardiomyopathy

Arrhythmia	Number
Supraventricular	
Atrial fibrillation	14
Supraventricular tachycardia/paroxysmal atrial fibrillation	
1–3 episodes per day	17
> 3 episodes per day	10
Ventricular	
Ventricular extrasystoles	
> 30 per hour	24
Ventricular tachycardia	
1 episode per day	13
> 1 episode per day	16

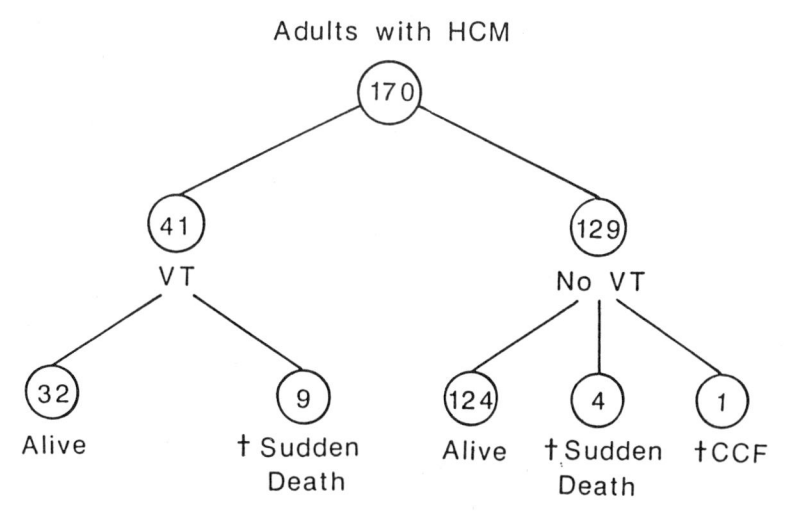

Figure 2: Flow diagram showing clinical outcome in the 170 unoperated patients undergoing 24–72 hour electrocardiographic monitoring. Eighty-four patients are from the series reported by Maron et al;[14] 86 are from McKenna et al.[12] HCM = hypertrophic cardiomyopathy; VT = ventricular tachycardia; CCF = congestive cardiac failure.

sustained episodes of ventricular tachycardia during electrocardiographic monitoring is the best single feature in the prediction of sudden death with a sensitivity of 69% and a specificity of 80% (Table V). The reduced sensitivity, in part, reflects the inclusion of an adolescent who did not have ventricular tachycardia but died suddenly;[14] a recent study reveals that spontaneous arrhythmias are rare in children and adolescents with hypertrophic cardiomyopathy (discussed below) and that other clinical features are of greater predictive value in the young.[6] An 11-year-old girl (patient 1 from Table I, Maron et al.[14]) had recurrent episodes of syncope and presyncope and had clearly shown herself to be at risk of sudden death. In addition, all four of the patients who did not have ventricular tachycar-

Table V
Predictive Accuracy of Ventricular Tachycardia for Sudden Death in Adults with Hypertrophic Cardiomyopathy

Sensitivity	69%
Specificity	80%
Prevalence	7.6%
Positive predictive accuracy	22%
Negative predictive accuracy	97%

The data for the above calculations are presented in Figure 2.

dia but died suddenly (two from NIH and two from Hammersmith) had only 24 hours of electrocardiographic monitoring and thus a sampling error is possible, particularly as ventricular arrhythmias in hypertrophic cardiomyopathy are known to exhibit marked biological variability.[15] We perform 48-hour electrocardiographic monitoring at the time of diagnosis and usually annually thereafter. During the past 6 years, sudden death has occurred in adults who do not have ventricular tachycardia during electrocardiographic monitoring but it is rare (approximate annual mortality rate, 0.6%). The finding of nonsustained ventricular tachycardia during electrocardiographic monitoring identifies adults at high risk with a sensitivity that is probably greater than 69%.

The fact that 32 of the 41 patients with ventricular tachycardia survived is reflected in the low positive predictive accuracy (22%) of ventricular tachycardia for sudden death and it raises the possibility that not all patients with ventricular tachycardia are at increased risk. Though the number of patients in the subset with ventricular tachycardia in each study was small, there did not appear to be features that distinguished patients with ventricular tachycardia who survived from those who died suddenly. In the NIH study, patients with ventricular tachycardia and sudden cardiac catastrophe did not differ from survivors with regard to age or sex distribution, ventricular septal thickness, or occurrence of an abnormal electrocardiogram.[14] In the Hammersmith study, the symptomatic status, the proportion with left ventricular gradients and the incidence of supraventricular and ventricular arrhythmias were similar in the survivors and patients who died suddenly.[12] In another study of the relation of left ventricular function and prognosis in a subset of 14 patients with ventricular tachycardia, digitized angiographic analysis revealed that peak left ventricular ejection rate was significantly reduced in patients with ventricular tachycardia, who died suddenly compared to those who survived (Fig. 3).[7] Impaired left ventricular function may be an important predictor of which patients with ventricular tachycardia are at increased risk and prospective evaluation is warranted.

The Role of Electrophysiological Testing

What is the role of electrophysiological testing in the identification of the high risk patient with hypertrophic cardiomyopathy? Several groups have done electrophysiological studies in adults, many of whom were at "high risk" with previous syncopal episodes or cardiac arrest (Table VI).[16-24]

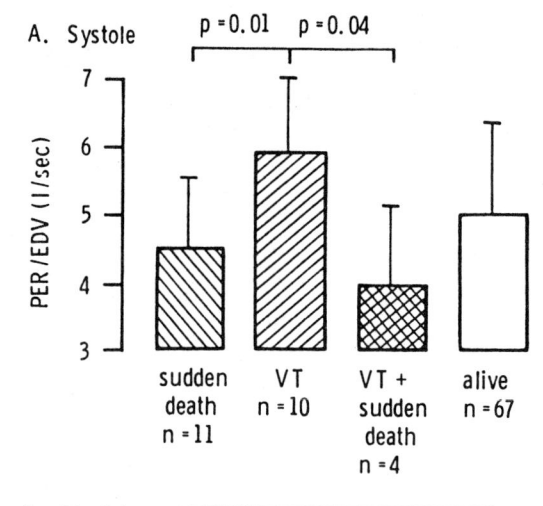

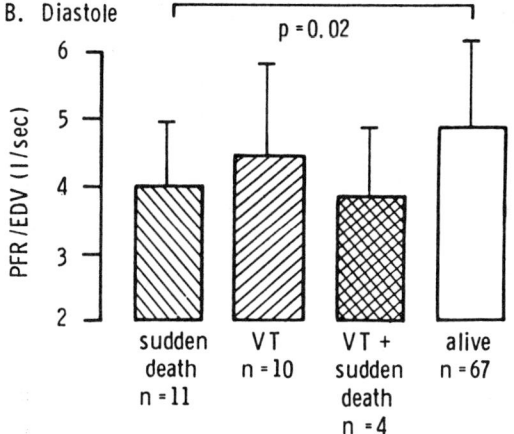

Figure 3: Normalized indexes of ventricular ejection and filling in 10 patients with ventricular tachycardia (VT) who survived and four patients who died suddenly, compared with all 11 patients who died suddenly and with 67 survivors. **A:** Peak ejection rates normalized by end-diastolic volume (PER/EDV) were higher in patients with ventricular tachycardia who survived than in those who died suddenly. **B:** Peak filling rates normalized by end-diastolic volume (PER/EDV) were higher in the survivors than in patients who died suddenly. (Reproduced with permission from Newman et al.,[7] JACC 1985;5:1064–1074.)

Anderson et al. performed right ventricular programmed electrical stimulation in the operating room in 17 symptomatic patients with left ventricular outflow tract gradients who were undergoing myotomy/myectomy and in five control patients who were undergoing coronary artery bypass grafting.[17] In their protocol, which included three premature ventricular stimuli, 14 of the 17 patients had inducible sustained ventricular tachycardia (n = 9) or ventricular fibrillation (n = 5) which was not seen in the five control patients. Their findings indicate that with an aggressive stimulation protocol, inducible life-threatening arrhythmias are more common in patients with hypertrophic cardiomyopathy than in patients without a primary heart muscle disorder.

Watson et al. performed right ventricular programmed electrical stimulation in 17 "high risk" patients with hypertrophic cardiomyopathy who had experienced cardiac arrest (n = 2) or syncope (n = 4), had a malignant family history (n = 2), or had nonsustained ventricular tachycardia during electrocardiographic monitoring (n = 9).[23] Ventricular fibrillation was induced in eight patients (47%) with up to three premature stimuli during programmed ventricular stimulation

Table VI
Programmed Electrophysiological Studies in Patients With Hypertrophic Cardiomyopathy

	Pts	Age (years) mean (range)	History	Holter	PVS 2 ES	PES 3 ES	PAS	FU (months)	Comments
Schiavone[16] 1986	26	51 (18–77)	S : 14	NSVT : 7 SVA : 7	$\frac{26}{VF}$: 1	$\frac{5}{VF}$: 0	$\frac{26}{SVA}$: 17	0	syncope best predicted by hypotension induced during SVA
Anderson[17] 1983	17	46 (15–74)	S : 5 CA : 1	—	$\frac{17}{3}$ - SPVT/VF -	$\frac{14}{11}$	—	0	PVS performed preoperatively under anesthesia
Kowey[18] 1984	7	54 25–75)	CA : 4 (3VF, 1VT) PS : 2 Seizure : 1	NSVT : 3 T de P : 1	$\frac{4}{VT}$: 3	$\frac{1}{VF}$: 1	SVA : 2	6 to 30 (mean 17)	PES useful in identification of cause of symptoms; no events during FU on antiarrhythmic Rx
Ingham[19] 1978	13	51 (25–74)	S, PS or P in all	SVA : 7 NSVT : 3	—	—	dual AV node 7/12 (no inducible SVA)	0	
Geibel[20] 1986	18	—	S : 2 VF : 3 SMVT : 2	—	$\frac{18}{SMVT}$: 2 SPVT : 3		$\frac{12}{SMVT}$: 1 SPVT : 7	0	SMVT induced in 2/2 pts who had D-SMVT
Borgreffe[21] 1986	31	—	S : 21 VT/VF : 5 P : 5	NSVT : 9	$\frac{31}{SMVT}$: 3 SPVT/VF : 5	—	$\frac{31}{Acc P : 2}$ AVNT : 1 AFib : 8 1 : 1 > 200 bpm : 8	0	EPS identified a possible cause of Sx in 52% of pts
Kunze[22] 1986	26	45 (—)	S : 4 VF : 2	—	$\frac{26}{VF}$: 3	$\frac{23}{VF}$: 7	—	32 ± 5	No events during FU (pts with S or VF) Rx with amiodarone
Watson[23] 1986	17	34 (14–63)	S : 4 VT : 9 CA : 2	—	$\frac{17}{VF}$: 5	$\frac{12}{VF}$: 3	VF : 1	0	

Numbers refer to patients unless otherwise stated in the column headings. S = syncope; CA = cardiac arrest; VT = ventricular tachycardia; NSVT = nonsustained ventricular tachycardia; SVA = supraventricular arrhythmia; T de P = torsade de pointes; PVS = programmed ventricular stimulation; PES = programmed electrophysiologic stimulation; PAS = programmed atrial stimulation; SPVT = sustained polymorphic ventricular tachycardia; SMVT = sustained monomorphic ventricular tachycardia; VF = ventricular fibrillation; AV = atrioventricular; Acc P = accessory pathway; AVNT = atrioventricular nodal tachycardia; AFib = atrial fibrillation; FU = follow-up; Rx = treatment; D-SMVT = documented sustained monomorphic ventricular tachycardia; Sx = symptoms.

and in an additional patient during atrial stimulation. Other centers have also shown that programmed electrical stimulation can initiate sustained ventricular tachycardia or fibrillation in a significant proportion of patients (20 of 95, 21% using two premature ventricular stimuli; 16 of 41, 39% using three premature ventricular stimuli or incremental atrial pacing) (Table VI). The high rate of inducible ventricular tachycardia and fibrillation observed by these workers supports the contention that patients with hypertrophic cardiomyopathy may be unusually vulnerable to spontaneous ventricular tachyarrhythmias, particularly in the presence of ischemia or hemodynamic collapse. The prognostic significance of these findings, however, will be uncertain until the clinical outcome has been determined in more patients.

What is the potential for programmed electrical stimulation to improve upon the sensitivity ($\geq 69\%$) of electrocardiographic monitoring for the identification of the high risk adult with hypertrophic cardiomyopathy? As electrocardiographic monitoring identifies most of the adults who are at high risk, electrophysiological studies may be more profitably performed in selected "high risk" patient populations. As discussed above, the predictive accuracy of ventricular tachycardia is low (22%). Programmed stimulation as well as assessment of left and right ventricular function may provide measurements that will improve the predictive accuracy and identify those patients with episodes of nonsustained ventricular tachycardia during electrocardiographic monitoring who are at greatest risk and warrant more vigorous treatment.

Discussion and Summary

Thus far we have reviewed the identification of the adult who is at high risk. Children and adolescents with hypertrophic cardiomyopathy, however, have a much higher annual mortality from sudden death, approximately 6%.[3,25,26] Patients with a family history of multiple sudden deaths are recognized to be at particular risk.[3,27] However, children and adolescents without such a "malignant" family history still have an annual mortality from sudden death of over 4% (Fig. 4).[3,26] Apart from syncopal episodes which are associated with sudden death, other clinical features and electrocardiographic and hemodynamic measurements are similar in those who die suddenly and survive and do not help identify the high risk patient. The majority of children and adolescents who die suddenly do not have any limitation of exercise tolerance nor have they experienced syncope; when syncope does occur, however, this is ominous, and in our retrospective analysis of 37 patients, it was 86% specific for subsequent sudden death.[26] In addition, arrhythmias during electrocardiographic monitoring are uncommon in children and adolescents and do not appear to be of predictive prognostic value.[6] Thus, in the patients with hypertrophic cardiomyopathy who are at greatest risk, many of whom are not only young but also asymptomatic, current clinical and hemodynamic evaluation is of limited value in the identification of most of those who will die suddenly who may not have experienced syncopal episodes or have a "malignant" family history.

Patients with hypertrophic cardiomyopathy are often unable to maintain

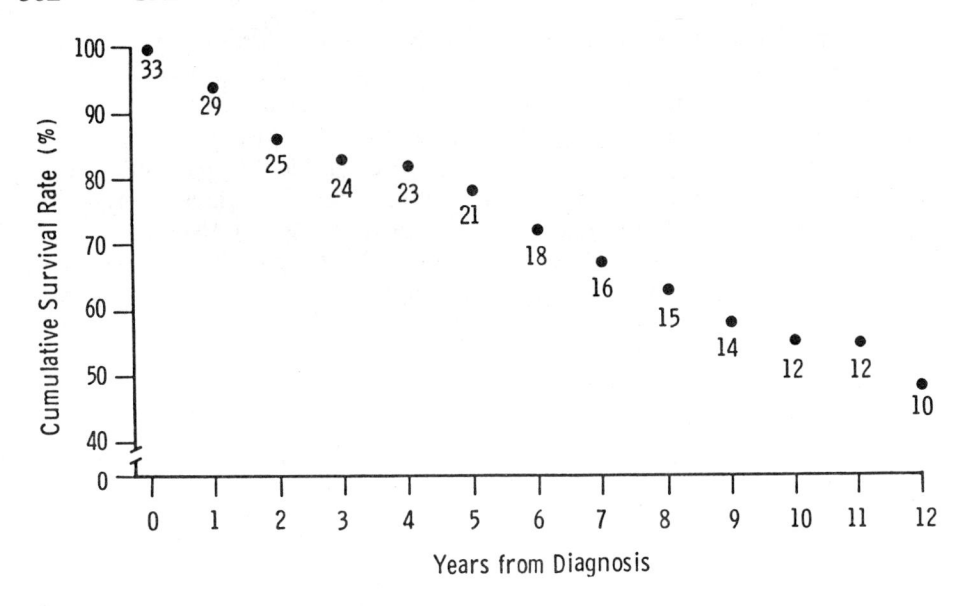

Figure 4: Cumulative survival curve from the year of diagnosis for 33 medically treated patients. The probability of death = the total number of deaths for the year divided by the adjusted number at risk minus the number of deaths due to other causes. (Reproduced with permission from McKenna and Deanfield,[26] Arch Dis Childhood 1984;59:971–975.)

stroke volume and increase cardiac output during exercise, presumably because of the shortened time for filling of a poorly relaxing and noncompliant left ventricle.[28,29] It is well recognized that a physiological tachycardia may be associated with hypotension, ischemia, and symptoms of angina or impaired consciousness (Fig. 5). A recent case report by Stafford et al. is of interest in this regard.[30] A 15-year-old youth, who presented with cardiac arrest and documented ventricular fibrillation, was found to have nonobstructive hypertrophic cardiomyopathy with diffuse left ventricular hypertrophy. Electrophysiological study demonstrated inducible sustained atrial fibrillation with a ventricular response of 180 to 190 beats/min. This rhythm, associated with hypotension and evidence of myocardial ischemia, degenerated into ventricular fibrillation. There was no evidence of an accessory pathway and no ventricular arrhythmias were inducible during programmed ventricular stimulation.[30]

The cause of sudden death in hypertrophic cardiomyopathy is uncertain. The low incidence of spontaneous arrhythmias in the young suggests that in this subgroup of patients, a primary arrhythmia is unlikely. We speculate that in some adults, but particularly in the young, the precipitating event is most often hemodynamic with a decrease in stroke volume and hypotension in relation to emotion or exercise-related tachycardia; a primary supraventricular tachyarrhythmia as the cause of the tachycardia is possible but less likely.[12,14] The outcome, survival versus sudden death, is then determined by the vulnerability of the myocardium to spontaneous life-threatening arrhythmias. In the adult, nonsustained ventricular tachycardia during electrocardiographic monitoring may be a marker of this,

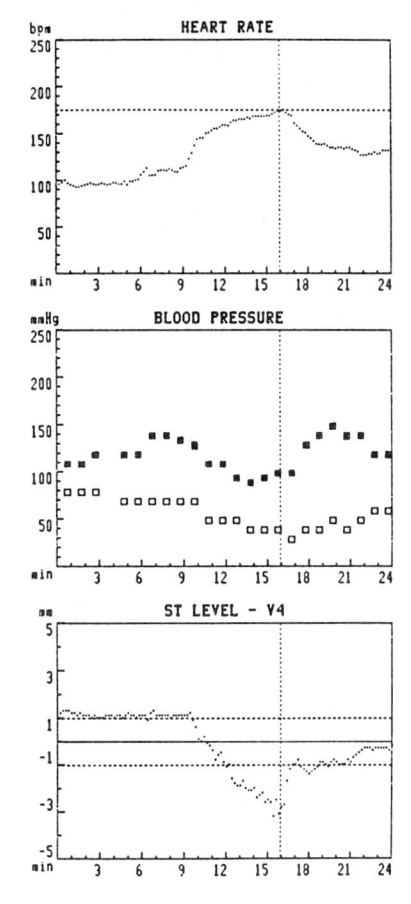

Figure 5: Simultaneous recordings of heart rate, blood pressure, and ST-segment changes during treadmill exercise using a modified Bruce protocol in a 46-year-old man with hypertrophic cardiomyopathy. As heart rate increased, blood pressure fell and ST-segment changes developed in association with mild central chest tightness which resolved quickly. The horizontal dotted line represents the termination of exercise.

while in children and adolescents, to date no such marker has been identified. The extent and severity of myocardial disarray must be an important determinant of the electrical stability of the myocardium. Myocardial disarray is greater in young patients who die suddenly than in adults who die suddenly or from other causes, but the severity and distribution of disarray is not closely related to the severity and distribution of hypertrophy and at present can only be reliably assessed at postmortem examination.[31,32]

In the evaluation of adults and particularly children and adolescents with hypertrophic cardiomyopathy, future studies should evaluate patients in relation to likely mechanisms of sudden death. This should include an assessment of both the propensity for hemodynamic collapse as well as the vulnerability of the myocardium to life-threatening arrhythmias. The optimal method of acquiring this information has not been determined and may differ in patient subgroups, particularly in relation to age and perhaps in relation to the severity of both left ventricular hypertrophy and functional impairment. Noninvasive tests which simulate or record events during normal daily life, such as stress testing, response to physiological maneuvers, and electrocardiographic monitoring, can be broadly applied while invasive investigations, particularly electrophysiological studies, are more appropriate in selected subgroups. It is important that patients with hypertrophic cardiomyopathy are better characterized in relation to likely mechanisms of sudden death as the pharmacological and surgical treatments may significantly improve prognosis if they are applied appropriately.

The role of surgery in the prevention of sudden death remains to be defined. At present it is reserved for symptomatic patients with features of left ventricular outflow tract "obstruction." Whether myotomy/myectomy will prevent hemodynamic collapse and improve prognosis requires evaluation. Though there is no convincing evidence to suggest that symptomatic therapy with beta-blockers or calcium antagonists improves prognosis,[2] the use of low dose amiodarone in patients with nonsustained ventricular tachycardia during electrocardiographic monitoring is associated with improved survival.[33] There have been no deaths in 21 patients who received amiodarone between 1978 and 1980 and who have now been followed for at least 5 years, compared with a 7% annual mortality at 3 years in well-matched control patients. The use of amiodarone in other potentially high risk patients, such as children who may require therapy for many years, is limited by dose/duration-related side effects. The role of amiodarone in these high risk patients is currently under evaulation.

Acknowledgement: With grateful thanks to Dr. Robert Lemery and Ms. Shaughan Dickie for assistance with the preparation of this manuscript.

References

1. Frank S, Braunwald E. Idiopathic hypertrophic subaortic stenosis: Clinical analysis of 126 patients with emphasis on the natural history. Circulation 1968;37:759–788.
2. McKenna WJ, Goodwin JF. The natural history of hypertrophic cardiomyopathy. In Harvey P, ed. Current Problems in Cardiology. Chicago, Year Book Medical Publishers, Vol VI, 1981;5–26.
3. McKenna WJ, Deanfield J, Faruqui A, England D, Oakley CM, Goodwin JF. Prognosis in hypertrophic cardiomyopathy. Am J Cardiol 1981;47:532–538.
4. Shapiro LM, Zezulka A. Hypertrophic cardiomyopathy: a common disease with a good prognosis: Five year experience of a district general hospital. Br Heart J 1983;50:530–533.
5. Wadehra D, Gunnar RM, Scanlon PJ. Prognosis in hypertrophic cardiomyopathy with asymmetric septal hypertrophy. Postgrad Med J 1985;61:1107–1109.
6. McKenna WJ, Deanfield J, Franklin R, Krikler S, Dickie S. Arrhythmia in children and adolescents with hypertrophic cardiomyopathy: incidence and relation to prognosis (abstr). Br Heart J 1985;54:632 (manuscript submitted).
7. Newman H, Sugrue DD, Oakley CM, Goodwin JF, McKenna WJ. Relation of left ventricular function and prognosis in hypertrophic cardiomyopathy: an angiographic study. JACC 1985;5:1064–1074.
8. Maron BJ, Roberts WC, Epstein SE. Sudden death in hypertrophic cardiomyopathy: A profile of 78 patients. Circulation 1982;65:1388–1394.
9. James TN, Marshall TK. De subitaneis mortibus XII. Asymmetrical hypertrophy of the heart. Circulation 1975;51:1149–1166.
10. Goodwin JF, Krikler DM. Arrhythmias as a cause of sudden death in hypertrophic cardiomyopathy. Lancet 1976;2:937–940.
11. Savage DD, Seides SF, Maron BJ, Myers DM, Epstein SE. Prevalence of arrhythmia during 24-hour electrocardiographic monitoring and exercise testing in patients with obstructive and non obstructive hypertrophic cardiomyopathy. Circulation 1979;59:866–875.

12. McKenna WJ, England D, Doi YL, Deanfield JE, Oakley CM, Goodwin JF. Arrhythmia in hypertrophic cardiomyopathy: I. Influence on prognosis. Br Heart J 1981;46:168–172.
13. McKenna WJ, Krikler DM, Goodwin JF. Arrhythmias in dilated and hypertrophic cardiomyopathy. Med Clin N Amr 1984;68:983–1000.
14. Maron BJ, Savage DD, Wolfson JK, Epstein SE. Prognostic significance of 24 hour ambulatory electrocardiographic monitoring in patients with hypertrophic cardiomyopathy: A prospective study. Am J Cardiol 1981;48:252–257.
15. Mulrow JP, Healy MJR, McKenna WJ. Variability of ventricular arrhythmia in hypertrophic cardiomyopathy and implications for treatment. Am J Cardiol 1986;58:615–618.
16. Schiavone WA, Maloney JD, Lever HM, Castle LW, Sterba R, Morant V. Electrophysiologic studies of patients with hypertrophic cardiomyopathy presenting with syncope of undetermined etiology. PACE 1986;9:476–481.
17. Anderson, KP, Stinson EB, Derby GC, Oyer PE, Mason JW. Vulnerability of patients with hypertrophic obstructive cardiomyopathy to ventricular arrhythmia induction in the operating room. Am J Cardiol 1983;51:811–816.
18. Kowey PR, Eisenberg R, Engel TR. Sustained arrhythmias in hypertrophic obstructive cardiomyopathy. N Engl J Med 1984;310:1566–1569.
19. Ingham RE, Mason JW, Rossen RM, Goodman DJ, Harrison DC. Electrophysiologic findings in patients with idiopathic hypertrophic subaortic stenosis. Am J Cardiol 1978;41:811–816.
20. Geibel A, Brugada P, Zehender M, Kersschot I, Wellens HJJ. Results of a standardized ventricular stimulation protocol in patients with hypertrophic cardiomyopathy (abstr). JACC 1986;7:195A.
21. Borggrefe M, Podczeck A, Breithardt G. Electrophysiologic studies in hypertrophic cardiomyopathy (abstr). Circulation 1986;74(Supp II):II–1922.
22. Kunze K-P, Kuck K-H, Geiger M, Bleifeld W. Programmed electrical stimulation in hypertrophic cardiomyopathy - specificity and sensitivity of different stimulation protocols (abstr). JACC 1986;7:195A.
23. Watson RM, Liberati JM, Tucker E, Cannon RO, Rosing DR, Epstein SE, Josephson ME. Inducible ventricular fibrillation in patients with hypertrophic cardiomyopathy (abstr). JACC 1985;5:395.
24. Kuck K-H, Kunze K-P, Dernedde J, Geiger M. Amiodarone in hypertrophic cardiomyopathy - electrophysiologic and long term electrocardiographic study and clinical follow up (abstr). Circulation 1985;72(Supp II):671.
25. Maron BJ, Henry WL, Clark CE, Redwood DR, Roberts WC, Epstein SE. Asymmetric septal hypertrophy in childhood. Circulation 1976;53:9–19.
26. McKenna WJ, Deanfield JE. Hypertrophic cardiomyopathy: an important cause of sudden death. Arch Dis Childhood 1984;59:971–5.
27. Maron BJ, Lipson LC, Roberts WC, Savage DD, Epstein SE. "Malignant" Hypertrophic cardiomyopathy: identification of a subgroup of families with unusually frequent premature death. Am J Cardiol 1978;41:1133–1140.
28. Goodwin JF, Oakley CM. The cardiomyopathies. Br Heart J 1972;34:545–552.
29. Edwards RHT, Kristinsson A, Warrel DA, Goodwin JF. Effects of propranolol on response to exercise in hypertrophic cardiomyopathy. Br Heart J 1970;32:219–225.
30. Stafford WJ, Trohman RG, Bilsker M, Zaman L, Castellanos A, Myerburg RJ. Cardiac arrest in an adolescent with atrial fibrillation and hypertrophic cardiomyopathy. JACC 1986;7:701–704.
31. Maron BJ, Anan TJ, Roberts WC. Quantitative analysis of the distribution of cardiac muscle cell disorganisation in the left ventricular wall of patients with hypertrophic cardiomyopathy. Circulation 1981;63:882–894.
32. Maron BJ, Roberts WC. Quantitative analysis of cardiac muscle cell disorganisation in the ventricular septum of patients with hypertrophic cardiomyopathy. Circulation 1979;59:689–706.
33. McKenna WJ, Oakley CM, Krikler DM, Goodwin JF. Improval survival with amiodarone in patients with hypertrophic cardiomyopathy and ventricular tachycardia. Br Heart J 1985;53:412–416.

22

Programmed Electrical Stimulation in Patients with Hypertrophic Cardiomyopathy: Results in Patients with and without Cardiac Arrest or Syncope

Karl-Heinz Kuck, Klaus-Peter Kunze
Manfred Geiger, Angelika Costard
Michael Schlüter

Introduction

Sudden death is a well-known complication of hypertrophic cardiomyopathy with or without obstruction.[1-3] Nonsustained ventricular tachycardia detected by ambulatory electrocardiography has been associated with subsequent sudden death or cardiac arrest,[4-7] but it is an unspecific finding in the disease. Nonsustained ventricular tachycardia is often slow and asymptomatic and its presence does not provide a causal relationship between ventricular arrhythmias and symptomatic episodes. However, treatment to prevent sudden death is based primarily on findings of ambulatory monitoring. Programmed electrical stimulation has been used in the diagnosis and therapy of patients at risk for syncope or

From: Brugada P, Wellens HJJ. CARDIAC ARRHYTHMIAS: Where To Go From Here? Mount Kisco, NY, Futura Publishing Company, Inc., © 1987.

sudden death and a variety of underlying cardiac disorders.[8-10] The use of this technique in patients with hypertrophic cardiomyopathy has been limited to few reports on selected patients.[11-13] Therefore, we initiated a prospective study in consecutive patients with hypertrophic cardiomyopathy who had either a history of cardiac arrest or syncope, or no history of documented or suspected symptomatic ventricular arrhythmias. All patients underwent programmed electrical stimulation. This report presents the stimulation results of all patients at the time of inclusion into the study.

Methods

The study group consisted of 54 consecutive patients with hypertrophic cardiomyopathy; three patients had a history of cardiac arrest (group A), eight patients had a history of syncope (group B), and 43 patients had no history of either documented or suspected ventricular arrhythmias (group C). In group A, two patients had ventricular fibrillation documented on the electrocardiogram obtained at the time of cardiac arrest. In one patient, cardiac arrest occurred during school sports, in the other patient, it occurred at rest. The remaining patient had documented rapid ventricular tachycardia (rate 300 bpm) at the time of cardiac arrest. In group B, syncopal attacks ranged from one to five episodes per patient. In none of these was the cause of syncope known. An electrocardiographic registration at the time of syncope was not available in any patient. In three patients, syncope was exercise-related; in the other patients, syncopal attacks occurred at rest as well as during exercise. In group C, all patients complained of dyspnea, angina, or occasional episodes of palpitations.

All patients were off any medication for at least seven half-lives before inclusion into the study. M-mode and two-dimensional echocardiographic data were obtained in all but nine patients, in whom the ultrasonic imaging quality was inadequate. The criterion used for the echocardiographic diagnosis of hypertrophic cardiomyopathy was the demonstration of a nondilated hypertrophic left ventricle in the absence of any other cardiac or systemic disease that itself was capable of producing left ventricular hypertrophy.[14,15] The distribution pattern of left ventricular hypertrophy was determined according to Maron.[16]

All patients underwent a standard hemodynamic study including right and left heart catheterization and coronary angiography. Only patients with normal coronary arteries were included in this study. After informed consent had been obtained, a complete electrophysiologic study was performed 1 to 4 days after the hemodynamic investigation. 6-French catheters were passed through both femoral veins and/or through the left brachial or subclavian vein and through the right femoral artery using the Seldinger technique, and were positioned in the heart under fluoroscopic guidance. Quadripolar catheters were placed in the high right atrium, coronary sinus, and right and left ventricles. A bipolar catheter or a hexapolar closely spaced electrode catheter (Mansfield Scientific Inc.) was placed across the tricuspid valve to record the His bundle electrogram. A Siemens 16-channel electrocardiographer was used for continuous display and recording of the endocardial electrograms and of three to six surface electrocardiograms. A stimulator (ERA-HIS, Biotronik GmbH, FRG) was used to deliver rectangular pulses of 1 ms in duration and a constant current of twice diastolic threshold.

Detailed information on the stimulation protocol used in our laboratory has been given previously.[17] Atrial stimulation included right and left atrial stimulation (the latter via coronary sinus) at three different cycle lengths (640, 510, 440 ms) with the single extrastimulus technique. Right atrium and coronary sinus were then paced at increasing rates up to the Wenckebach cycle length. Ventricular pacing was performed first from the right and the from the left ventricle using the extrastimulus technique. A maximum of two extrastimuli was delivered during sinus rhythm and at the same basic cycle lengths as during atrial stimulation. Finally, right ventricular stimulation was performed at increasing rates up to a minimal cycle length of 300 ms.

Definitions

Induced ventricular arrhythmias — Repetitive ventricular response: three to five consecutive ventricular beats. *Nonsustained ventricular tachycardia:* more than five ventricular responses, terminating spontaneously in less than 30 seconds. *Sustained ventricular tachycardia:* duration of more than 30 seconds, unless termination is forced earlier because of hemodynamic deterioration. *Ventricular fibrillation:* ventricular rhythm without identifiable QRS complexes in the surface leads. Ventricular tachycardias with a continuously changing QRS configuration were termed *polymorphic*; those with a uniform QRS complex were termed *monomorphic*. The endpoint of the study was either the initiation of a sustained ventricular tachycardia or ventricular fibrillation or the completion of the stimulation protocol.

Statistical Analysis

Data are expressed as mean ± 1 standard deviation. Comparisons of sets of data were made using Student's *t* test. Differences between distributions were analyzed with the chi-square test. A probability value of $p < 0.05$ was considered statistically significant.

Results

Clinical, electrocardiographic, echocardiographic, and hemodynamic data of patient groups are summarized in Table I. There were no statistically significant differences among patients of groups A, B, and C, except for the echocardiographic ventricular septum/posterior free wall ratio, which was significantly greater in group A than in groups B and C.

Ventricular arrhythmias were induced in two group A patients, in three group B patients, and in 13 group C patients. The type and incidence of induced

Table I
Clinical, Electrocardiographic, Echocardiographic, and Hemodynamic Data of Patients with Hypertrophic Cardiomyopathy

Characteristics			Group A (n = 3)	Group B (n = 8)	Group C (n = 43)
Age			43 ± 20 yrs	45 ± 15 yrs	48 ± 13 yrs
Sex	male		1 pt	5 pts	26 pts
	female		2 pts	3 pts	17 pts
Family history of SD			—	3 pts	12 pts
Electrocardiography					
rythm	sinus		2 pts	8 pts	41 pts
	AFib		1 pt	—	2 pts
QRS morphology	normal		3 pts	2 pts	12 pts
	LVH		—	6 pts	27 pts
	LBBB		—	—	2 pts
	RBBB		—	—	—
	unspecific BBB		—	—	1 pt
	preexitation		—	—	1 pt
QRS width			100 ± 20 ms	95 ± 12 ms	101 ± 18 ms
Echocardiography					
VS thickness			26 ± 2 mm	26 ± 7 mm	24 ± 5 mm
VS/PW			3.1 ± 1.3	2.1 ± 0.8	2.0 ± 0.6
			$\llcorner$——— $p < 0.005$ ———$\lrcorner$ $\llcorner$——— NS ———$\lrcorner$		
			$\llcorner$——————— $p < 0.005$ ———————$\lrcorner$		
Distribution of LVH					
		I	—	1 pt	2 pts
Maron class		II	1 pt	1 pt	11 pts
		III	2 pts	5 pts	21 pts
		IV	—	—	1 pt
Hemodynamics					
LV	no gradient		3 pts	3 pts	17 pts
	gradient	rest	—	73 ± 25 mmHg	82 ± 39 mmHg
		provocable	—	108 ± 49 mmHg	121 ± 60 mmHg
RV	no gradient		—	—	34 pts
	gradient	rest	—	—	16 ± 11 mmHg
Enddiast. pressure	LV		14 ± 2 mmHg	14 ± 8 mmHg	15 ± 9 mmHg
	RV		4 ± 2 mmHg	5 ± 3 mmHg	4 ± 2 mmHg

AFib = atrial fibrillation; BBB = bundle branch block; LBBB = left bundle branch block; LVH = left ventricular hypertrophy; PW = posterior wall; RBBB = right bundle branch block; SD = sudden death; VS = ventricular septum.

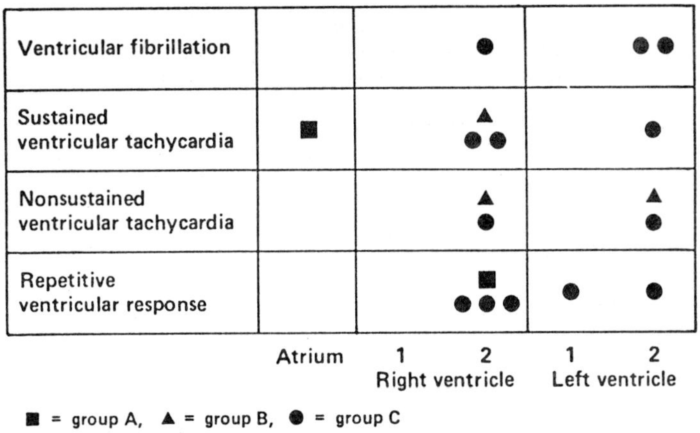

	Atrium	Right ventricle 1	Right ventricle 2	Left ventricle 1	Left ventricle 2
Ventricular fibrillation			●		● ●
Sustained ventricular tachycardia	■		▲ ● ●		●
Nonsustained ventricular tachycardia			▲ ●		▲ ●
Repetitive ventricular response			■ ● ● ●	●	●

■ = group A, ▲ = group B, ● = group C

Figure 1: Incidence of induced ventricular arrhythmias as a function of the stimulation mode in patients with hypertrophic cardiomyopathy. 1,2 = number of extrastimuli.

ventricular arrhythmias did not differ significantly among patients of groups A, B, and C (Fig. 1). The modes of initiation of ventricular tachycardia and fibrillation are shown in Table II. Atrial stimulation induced a ventricular arrhythmia in only one group A patient, who had exercise-induced cardiac arrest. In this patient, right atrial stimulation at a cycle length of 250 ms led to induction of a rapid ventricular tachycardia (cycle length 180 ms), deteriorating into ventricular fibrillation. This patient's Wenckebach cycle length of 250 ms represented the lower limit of all recorded Wenckebach cycle lengths which ranged up to 450 ms. Mean Wenckebach cycle length was 275 ± 35 ms for group A, 333 ± 33 ms for group B, and 320 ± 61 ms for group C. Because of the limited number of patients in group A, no statistical comparison with group B and C Wenckebach cycle lengths was made.

Inducibility of ventricular arrhythmia increased significantly by adding a second extrastimulus during right ventricular pacing and by left ventricular stimulation with two extrastimuli (Fig. 1). The coupling interval of the extrastimulus inducing ventricular arrhythmia was 206 ± 35 ms. This coupling interval was not statistically different from the effective refractory periods during right and left ventricular pacing in patients without induced ventricular arrhythmias (Table III).

Induced sustained ventricular arrhythmias were ventricular tachycardia in five patients and ventricular fibrillation in three patients. Sustained ventricular tachycardia was always rapid, with a mean cycle length of 194 ± 20 ms. Ventricular tachycardia deteriorated always into ventricular fibrillation after 8 ± 3 sec and required DC coutershock for termination.

Patients of groups A, B, and C in whom sustained ventricular arrhythmias were induced did not differ in electrocardiographic, echocardiographic, or hemodynamic data from patients without induced ventricular arrhythmias.

Table II
Mode of Initiation of Ventricular Tachycardia and Fibrillation and Characteristics of Ventricular Tachycardia

	pt.	Stimulation site	Stimulation mode		CL	Ventricular tachycardia morphology	duration
Group A							
sus VT	H. A.	RA	At CL 250 ms during pacing at increasing rates		180	LBBB	VF after 8 s
Group B							
n sus VT	B. G.	RV	BCL 510	S_2S_3 270 / 260	230	polymorphic	6 beats
	M. J.	LV	BCL 510	S_2S_3 230 / 190	250	polymorphic	10 beats
sus VT	S. B.	RV	BCL 510	S_2S_3 240 / 160	180	RBBB	VF after 4 s
Group C							
n sus VT	H. P.	LV	BCL 440	S_2S_3 260 / 230	220	LBBB	9 beats
	J. L.	RV	BCL 510	S_2S_3 290 / 240	350	polymorphic	6 beats
sus VT	H. S.	LV	BCL 640	S_2S_3 260 / 180	180	polymorphic	VF after 8 s
	K. K.	RV	BCL 440	S_2S_3 220 / 190	220	polymorphic	VF after 12 s
	S. H.	RV	BCL 440	S_2S_3 250 / 220	210	polymorphic	VF after 6 s
VF	H. R.	RV	SR	S_1S_2 200 / 250			
	B. H.	LV	SR	S_1S_2 250 / 180			
	H. G.	LV	BCL 510	S_2S_3 250 / 170			

CL = cycle length; LBBB = left bundle branch block; LV = left ventricle; n sus VT = nonsustained ventricular tachycardia; RA = right atrium; RBBB = right bundle branch block; RV = right ventricle; sus VT = sustained ventricular tachycardia; VF = ventricular fibrillation.

Discussion

Several mechanisms may be responsible for sudden death in patients with hypertrophic cardiomyopathy. Sudden increase of the intraventricular pressure gradient in patients with left ventricular outflow obstruction,[18] supraventricular arrhythmias with or without accessory atrioventricular pathways,[13,19,20] bradyarrhythmias,[21] and complete heart block[22] have been reported. A prominent factor possibly related to sudden death is the occurrence of ventricular tachyarrhythmias which, in a high number of patients, are detected during long-term electrocardiographic monitoring.[5-7] Some authors were able to show a close relationship between the occurrence of more than two consecutive premature beats during Holter monitoring and subsequent sudden death.[4,6] However, nonsustained ventricular tachycardia on Holter monitoring is almost always slow and asymptomatic, and therefore the presence of these nonsustained arrhythmias does not establish a causal relationship between arrhythmias and symptomatic episodes. More likely, they seem to be only a marker for subsequent fatal

Table III
Right and Left Ventricular Effective Refractory Periods (ms)

Site	BCL	No. of ES	Group A (n = 3)	Group B (n = 8)	Group C (n = 43)
Right ventricle	640	1	260 ± 15	250 ± 34	264 ± 27
	510	1	247 ± 18	248 ± 39	246 ± 25
	440	1	236 ± 15	225 ± 24	230 ± 22
	640	2	225 ± 40	196 ± 34	210 ± 26
	510	2	210 ± 19	183 ± 31	193 ± 26
	440	2	205 ± 25	178 ± 30	187 ± 25
Left ventricle	640	1	240 ± 13	263 ± 17	263 ± 21
	510	1	230 ± 12	238 ± 31	246 ± 19
	440	1	220 ± 12	234 ± 34	236 ± 25
	640	2	192 ± 14	240 ± 28	209 ± 29
	510	2	195 ± 14	207 ± 66	199 ± 29
	440	2	190 ± 12	210 ± 57	193 ± 28

BCL = basic cycle length; ES = extrastimuli

events. Other variables, in addition to these nonsustained slow ventricular tachycardia, or other arrhythmias may be responsible for the induction of a terminal event.[23]

The inducibility of ventricular tachyarrhythmias by programmed electrical stimulation has been suggested to predict potential sudden death in patients after acute myocardial infarction without previously documented ventricular arrhythmias.[24,25] Few studies on the use of the technique in selected patients with hypertrophic cardiomyopathy have been reported.[11-13] Following reports on the fatal outcome of electrophysiologic studies in patients with hypertrophic cardiomyopthy,[20,26] we were well aware of the potential hazard of this approach, but, because of the limited specificity of ambulatory ECG monitoring and the lack of any other technique to identify patients at risk for sudden cardiac death, we felt that there was the need for such an investigation.

Anderson et al.[11] have reported programmed electrical stimulation of the right ventricle in patients with obstructive hypertrophic cardiomyopathy undergoing myotomy or myectomy, who were studied in the operating room under general anesthesia and under their chronic medication. The stimulation protocol included right ventricular pacing with a maximum of three extrastimuli. Under these conditions, ventricular arrhythmias could be induced in all 17 patients, with ventricular fibrillation in five patients, sustained ventricular tachycardia in nine patients, nonsustained ventricular tachycardia in one patient, and repetitive ventricular response in two patients. In three of the 14 patients with ventricular fibrillation or sustained ventricular tachycardia, the arrhythmias were induced by two extrastimuli, while three extrastimuli had to be applied in the remaining 11 patients. However, the prognostic value of the inducibility of ventricular arrhythmias by three ventricular extrastimuli is not definitely known, and it has been shown that severe ventricular arrhythmias can be induced with more than two extrastimuli, even in normal patients without previously documented ventricular arrhythmias.[27]

The same limitations hold for a recent study in seven symptomatic patients, with cardiac arrest in three patients, syncope in one patient, and presyncope in two patients.[12] Induced arrhythmias were ventricular fibrillation in one patient, ventricular tachycardia in three patients, and supraventricular tachycardia in two patients. Follow-up of these patients was uneventful under a medical therapy guided by electrophysiologic testing. The authors suggested that electrophysiologic investigation may be useful in identifying the cause of symptoms in patients with hypertrophic cardiomyopathy and in selecting prophylactic therapy. However, since no "asymptomatic" patients with hypertrophic cardiomyopathy were included, the specificity of their findings is unknown, particularly with a stimulation protocol which included a maximum of three extrastimuli.

In our investigation, 54 consecutive patients with both obstructive and nonobstructive hypertrophic cardiomyopathy were studied. No patient was under therapy, and the stimulation protocol was limited to two ventricular extrastimuli. The study population included three different groups of patients: (1) patients with a history of cardiac arrest due to ventricular arrhythmias; (2) patients with a history of syncope without documented arrhythmias at the time of syncope; and (3) patients without documented or suspected sustained ventricular arrhythmias. The incidence and type of induced ventricular arrhythmias did not differ among those patients. Interestingly, sustained ventricular arrhythmia always consisted of a rapid ventricular tachycardia or ventricular fibrillation. A slow ventricular tachycardia was never induced.

Induction of a rapid ventricular tachycardia or ventricular fibrillation has been shown to be unspecific in patients with coronary artery disease and myocardial infarction.[27] The fact that these types of arrhythmia were induced in "asymptomatic" and "symptomatic" patients with hypertrophic cardiomyopathy may also indicate the unspecificity of the induction of these arrhythmias by programmed stimulation. In one patient, cardiac arrest caused by exercise-induced ventricular fibrillation was the first documented sign of hypertrophic cardiomyopathy. It is well known that syncope or cardiac arrest may be the first manifestation of the disease.[3] Rapid ventricular tachycardia deteriorating into ventricular fibrillation had been induced in this patient by pacing the right atrium at increasing rates. The inducibility of rapid ventricular tachycardia or ventricular fibrillation by atrial pacing is a very rare finding in patients without an accessory pathway. It has been described in another two patients with hypertrophic cardiomyopathy,[13,28] and possibly this finding is specific for patients with hypertrophic cardiomyopathy.

Repetitive ventricular response or nonsustained ventricular tachycardia was induced in 10 patients. The prognostic value of the inducibility of these types of arrhythmia in normal patients without documented ventricular arrhythmias is low.[29,30] They may be predictive of the spontaneous occurrence of severe ventricular arrhythmias in patients with coronary artery disease.[31] The significance of their occurrence in the setting of hypertrophic cardiomyopathy is uncertain.

The vulnerability of patients with cardiac arrest or of patients with non-documented ventricular tachycardia to the induction of ventricular arrhythmias from the left ventricle is not known. In patients with coronary artery disease, it has been shown that the sensitivity to induce ventricular arrhythmia is higher for a protocol including left ventricular stimulation than for one restricted to right ventricular stimulation.[32] In our study all patients, symptomatic or asymptomatic, underwent left ventricular stimulation when no sustained arrhythmias were induced from the right ventricle. Left ventricular stimulation was included into our protocol intentionally, because hypertrophic cardiomyopathy is primarily a disease of the left ventricle. However, the sensitivity and specificity of left ventricular stimulation in this setting must be assessed in long-term follow-up studies.

Summary

We conclude that programmed electrical stimulation with a maximum of two ventricular extrastimuli in patients with hypertrophic cardiomyopathy cannot distinguish between patients with cardiac arrest or syncope and "asymptomatic" patients. The induction of a rapid ventricular tachycardia by atrial stimulation in the absence of an accessory atrioventricular connection may be a specific finding to identify patients at risk for exercise-induced ventricular fibrillation.

References

1. Frank S, Braunwald E. Idiopathic hypertrophic subaortic stenosis: Clinical analysis of 126 patients with emphasis of the natural history. Circulation 1968;37:759–788.
2. Hardarson T, de la Calzada CS, Curiel R, Goodwin JF. Prognosis and mortality of hypertrophic obstructive cardiomyopathy. Lancet 1973;2:1462–1467.
3. Maron BJ, Roberts WC, Edwards JE, McAllister HA, Foley DD, Epstein SE. Sudden death in patients with hypertrophic cardiomyopathy: Characterization of 26 patients without functional limitation. Am J Cardiol 1978;41:803–810.
4. Maron BJ, Savage DD, Wolfson JK, Epstein SE. The prognostic significance of 24-hour ambulatory electrocardiographic monitoring in patients with hypertrophic cardiomyopathy: A prospective study. Am J Cardiol 1981;48:252–257.
5. McKenna WJ, Chetty S, Oakley CM, Goodwin JF. Arrhythmia in hypertrophic cardiomyopathy: Exercise and 48-hour ambulatory electrocardiographic assessment with and without beta adrenergic blocking therapy. Am J Cardiol 1980;45:1–5.
6. McKenna WJ, England D, Doi YL, Deanfield JE, Oakley C, Goodwin JF. Arrhythmia in hypertrophic cardiomyopathy. I. Influence on prognosis. Br Heart J 1981;46:168–172.
7. McKenna W, England D, Oakley C, Goodwin J. Detection of arrhythmia in hypertrophic cardiomyopathy: prospective study (abstr). Circulation 1980;62(Suppl III):187.
8. DiMarco JP, Garan H, Harthorne JW, Ruskin JN. Intracardiac electrophysiologic techniques in recurrent syncope of unknown cause. Ann Intern Med 1981;95:542–548.
9. Mason JW, Winkle RA. Accuracy of the ventricular tachycardia induction study for predicting long-term efficacy and inefficacy of antiarrhythmic drugs. N Engl J Med 1980;303:1073–1077.
10. Ruskin JN, DiMarco JP, Garan H. Out of hospital cardiac arrest: Electrophysiologic observations and selection of long-term antiarrhythmic therapy. N Engl J Med 1980;303:607–613.
11. Anderson KP, Stinson EB, Derby GC, Oyer PE, Mason JW. Vulnerability of patients with obstructive hypertrophic cardiomyopathy to ventricular arrhythmia induction in the operating room. Am J Cardiol 1983;51:811–816.

12. Kowey PR, Eisenberg R, Engel TR. Sustained arrhythmias in hypertrophic obstructive cardiomyopathy. N Engl J Med 1984;310:1566–1569.
13. Stafford WJ, Trohman RG, Bilsker M, Zaman L, Castellanos A, Myerburg RJ. Cardiac arrest in an adolescent with atrial fibrillation and hypertrophic cardiomyopathy. J Am Coll Cardiol 1986;7:701–704.
14. DeMaria A, Bommer W, Lee G, Mason DT. Value and limitations of 2-dimensional echocardiography in assessment of cardiomyopathy. Am J Cardiol 1980;46:1224–1231.
15. Maron BJ, Epstein SE. Hypertrophic cardiomyopathy: A discussion of nomenclature. Am J Cardiol 1979;43:1242–1244.
16. Maron BJ, Gottdiener JS, Epstein SE. Patterns and significance of distribution of left ventricular hypertrophy in hypertrophic cardiomyopathy. Am J Cardiol 1981;48: 418–428.
17. Kunze KP, Kuck KH, Schlüter M, Kuch B, Bleifeld W. Electrophysiologic and clinical effects of intravenous and oral encainide in accessory atrioventricular pathway. Am J Cardiol 1984;54:323–329.
18. Brock R. Functional obstruction of the left ventricle (acquired aortic stenosis). Guys Hosp Rep 1957;106:221–38.
19. Bonhour JB, Bory M, Bourmayan C, Chiffoleau S, Favereau X, Foussard C, Komajda M, Lassabe G, Morand P, Neiman JL. Tachycardie supraventriculaires au cours des myocardiopathies obstructives. Arch Mal Coeur 1974;74:993–999.
20. Krikler DM, Davies MJ, Fowland E, Goodwin JF, Evans RC, Shaw DB. Sudden death in hypertrophic cardiomyopathy: Associated accessory atrioventricular pathways. Br Heart J 1980;43:245–251.
21. Joseph S, Balcon R, McDonald L. Syncope in hypertrophic obstructive cardiomyopathy due to asystole. Br Heart J 1972;34:974–976.
22. Chmielewski CA, Riley RS, Mahendran A, Most AS. Complete heart block as a cause of syncope in asymmetric septal hypertrophy. Am Heart 1977;J 93:91–93.
23. McKenna WJ, Goodwin JF. The natural history of hypertrophic cardiomyopathy. Curr Prog Cardiol 1981;6:1–25.
24. Hamer A, Vohra J, Hunt D, Sloman G. Prediction of sudden death by electrophysiologic studies in high risk patients surviving acute myocardial infarction. Am J Cardiol 1982;50:223–229.
25. Richards DA, Cody DV, Denniss AR, Russel PA, Young AA, Uther JE. Ventricular electrical instability: A predictor of death after myocardial infarction. Am J Cardiol 1983;51:75–80.
26. Wellens JHH, Bär FW, Vanagt EJ. Death after ajmaline administration (letter). Am J Cardiol 1980;45:905.
27. Kuck KH, Costard A, Schlüter M, Kunze KP. The significance of timing programmed electrical stimulation after acute myocardial infarction. J Am Coll Cardiol 1986; (in press).
28. Wellens HJJ, Bär FWHM, Vanagt EJDM, Brugada P. Medical treatment of ventricular tachycardia: Considerations in the selection of patients for surgical treatment. Am J Cardiol 1982;49:186–193.
29. Brugada P, Abdollah H, Heddle B, Wellens HJJ. Results of a ventricular stimulation protocol using a maximum of 4 premature stimuli in patients without documented or suspected ventricular arrhythmias. Am J Cardiol 1983;52:1214–1218.
30. Akhtar M. The clinical significance of the repetitive ventricular response. Circulation 1981;63:773–775.
31. Breithardt G, Seipel L, Meyer T, Abendroth RR. Prognostic significance of repetitive ventricular response during programmed ventricular stimulation. Am J Cardiol 1982; 49:693–698.
32. Buxton AE, Waxman HL, Marchlinski FE, Unterecker WJ, Waspe LE, Josephson ME. Study of patients with documented sustained ventricular tachyarrhythmias. Circulation 1984; 69:532–540.

23

Late Death After Myocardial Infarction: Mechanisms, Etiologies, and Implications for Prevention of Sudden Death

William G. Stevenson, Gerard C.M. Linssen
Michael G. Havenith, Pedro Brugada
Hein J.J. Wellens

Introduction

Approximately 15% of patients who survive an acute myocardial infarction will die during the following year.[1-5] The majority of these deaths occur suddenly and most are attributed to ventricular fibrillation.[1-5] This arrhythmia appears most frequently to be initiated by either acute ischemia or primary ventricular tachycardia which degenerates to ventricular fibrillation.[6-14] In the latter case, an area of myocardial scar provides the arrhythmogenic substrate, and acute ischemia may not be required for initiation of the arrhythmia. However, the post-myocardial infarction patient is at risk for various complications of atherosclerosis such as stroke and aortic aneurysms which can cause sudden death.

The relative incidence of the various mechanisms of death late after myocardial infarction is difficult to ascertain. Studies of the natural history of myocardial infarction have often been limited by the small number of autopsies.[1-5] Studies of sudden death victims and survivors have included patients with and without prior myocardial infarction.[8-14] To determine the relative frequency of various causes of death late after myocardial infarction, we reviewed clinical and autopsy data from our hospital over a period of 56 months.

From: Brugada P, Wellens HJJ. CARDIAC ARRHYTHMIAS: Where To Go From Here? Mount Kisco, NY, Futura Publishing Company, Inc., © 1987.

Methods

The records of autopsies performed at the Maastricht Academic Hospital from January 1982 to September 1986 were reviewed. This hospital is the only one in the city of Maastricht and the surrounding area encompassing a population of 180,000 people. During the study period, autopsies were performed in 56% of all deaths which occurred in hospital including 69% of deaths which occurred in patients under the care of the cardiology service and 37% of those who died in the emergency room. Autopsies were performed on 27% of people who were dead on arrival to the emergency room.

In 424 patients, the autopsy identified the presence of a myocardial infarction of any age. In 153 (36%) of these patients, death followed a progressive, noncoronary chronic illness or complications of a major surgical procedure (Table I). These patients were excluded from further analysis. Of the remaining 271 autopsies, evidence of an area of old myocardial infarction was identified in 172, which is the subject of this report.

Autopsies included barium angiography of the main epicardial arteries and serial cross-sectioning of these vessels at 4 mm intervals. The maximal luminal narrowing and presence of occlusive thrombi were determined by gross inspection. Cross-sections of the ventricles were stained with nitro blue tetrazolium (NBT).[15] Microscopic examination of sections of the anterior, lateral, and posterior left ventricle, septum and posterior wall of the right ventricle was routinely performed. Examination of the abdominal and thoracic viscera including the main branches of the pulmonary arterial tree was also performed. The brain was examined in only 9% of necropsies, usually if intracranial disease was suspected. Based on the pathologist's review of the NBT stain and gross and histologic examination of the myocardium, the age of each area of infarction was classified as follows:[16]

Acute: less than 24 hrs of age
Recent: 24 hrs to 3 weeks of age
Old: greater than 3 weeks of age.

Table I
Reasons for Exclusion

	N	%
Sepsis	51	20.2
Cancer	26	10.3
Post Surgical	25	9.9
Other Illness*	41	16.3
Inadequate Data	10	4.0
Recent or Acute MI only	99	39.3
Total	252	

*Includes severe lung disease, renal failure, liver failure, pancreatitis, progressive central nervous system diseases.

The locations of left ventricular infarctions were classified as anterior or inferior-posterior.

Following review of the available clinical data and the autopsy results, deaths were classified as follows:

Recurrent MI: Histologic evidence of an acute or recent myocardial infarction was found at autopsy.

Pump Failure: Death was preceded by cardiogenic shock or severe congestive heart failure not due to a dysrhythmia.

Arrhythmia: Death was due to a fatal episode of ventricular tachycardia, ventricular fibrillation, or bradyarrhythmia which was not preceded by severe heart failure or cardiogenic shock and an alternative cause of death such as massive pulmonary embolus, stroke, or cardiac rupture was not identified at autopsy. Witnessed instantaneous deaths and unexpected death during sleep were also classified as arrhythmic deaths.

New MI Unknown Mechanism: For some patients who died after a new infarction, the condition immediately prior to death was not known and it was therefore not possible to distinguish between arrhythmic death and an arrhythmia during severe pump failure. These deaths were classified as due to a new MI–unknown mechanism.

Cardiac Rupture: Spontaneous perforation of the ventricular free wall, septum, or papillary muscle was identified at autopsy.

Noncardiac Death: Stroke, pulmonary embolism occluding approximately 50% or more of the pulmonary circulation, or exsanguination were identified at autopsy.

In-Hospital Death: Fatal cardiac arrest occurred after the patient arrived at the emergency room.

Out-of-Hospital Death: Fatal cardiac arrest occurred prior to arrival in the emergency room. This included patients who were resuscitated out-of-hospital but died later due to direct complications of the initial arrest such as anoxic brain injury.

Statistical analysis was performed using Student's t test, and chi square tests as appropriate. P values less than 0.05 were considered significant. Continuous data are expressed as mean ± 1 standard deviation.

Results

An area of old myocardial infarction was identified at autopsy in 144 in-hospital deaths and 28 out-of-hospital deaths. There was no statistically significant difference between patients who died in hospital as compared to those who died out of hospital in sex, severity of coronary disease, or old infarct location

(Table II). The in-hospital patients were older than those who died out of hospital. Clinical documentation of the date of the first old infarction was available for 83 patients who died in hospital and 12 who died out of hospital. The time from the first infarction to death was not statistically different between the two groups (9.1±7.8 vs. 7.1±6.6 years).

Causes of Death

As shown in Figure 1, recurrent myocardial infarction caused death in 117 (81%) patients who died in hospital and 19 (68%) patients who died out of hospital (p = .18) As shown in Table II, the age of the recurrent infarction was more often recent (1 to 21 days old) in patients who died in hospital (46% vs. 21%, p = .03) as compared to those who died out of hospital. Acute myocardial infarction (less than 24 hours old) without recent infarction was present more often in patients who died out of hospital (39% vs. 19%, p = 0.4). Areas of both recent and acute infarction were present in 16% of in-hospital deaths and 7% of out-of-hospital deaths (p = NS).

The mechanism of death after recurrent infarction was pump failure in 77 (53%) in-hospital deaths and 2 (7%) out-of-hospital deaths (p < .0001). An arrhythmia due to recurrent infarction was the mechanism of death in 26 (18%) in-hospital deaths and 4 (14%) out-of-hospital deaths (p = NS). In 2 (1%) in-hospital deaths and 12 (43%, p < .0001) out-of-hospital deaths with recent or acute infarction, the mechanism of death (pump failure versus arrhythmia) could not be ascertained. Acute infarction was present in 11 of 28 (32%) in-hospital deaths due to arrhythmias or an unknown mechanism. Of the 16 patients who died out of hospital due to an arrhythmia or unknown mechanism, histologic evidence of acute infarction was present in 11 (69%, p = .003). The remainder (31%) had recent but no acute areas of infarction. Ventricular rupture after a recent or acute infarction accounted for 10 (7%) in-hospital and 1 (4%) out of hospital deaths (p = NS).

The relationship of infarct age location and coronary artery disease to the mode of death in the 134 patients who died of a cardiac cause after a new infarction are shown in Table III. The locations of the old infarctions were known for 120 patients (90%). The locations of acute and recent infarcts were known for 125 patients (93%). Recent or acute myocardial necrosis was present in the same general area (anterior or inferior) as an old infarction in 41% of patients. The recent or acute infarction was present in an area clearly separate from that of the old infarction in 31% of patients. Areas of acute or recent infarction were present both in an area remote from the old infarction as well as in the area of the old infarction in 14% of patients. There were no significant differences in infarct age, location, or severity of coronary artery disease between patients who died of pump failure, an arrhythmia, or unknown mechanism. However, patients who died of cardiac rupture tended to have less severe coronary artery disease and more frequently had an area of recent infarction remote from the area of old infarction as compared to patients dying of other causes.

Death was due to an arrhythmia in the absence of a recent or acute infarction

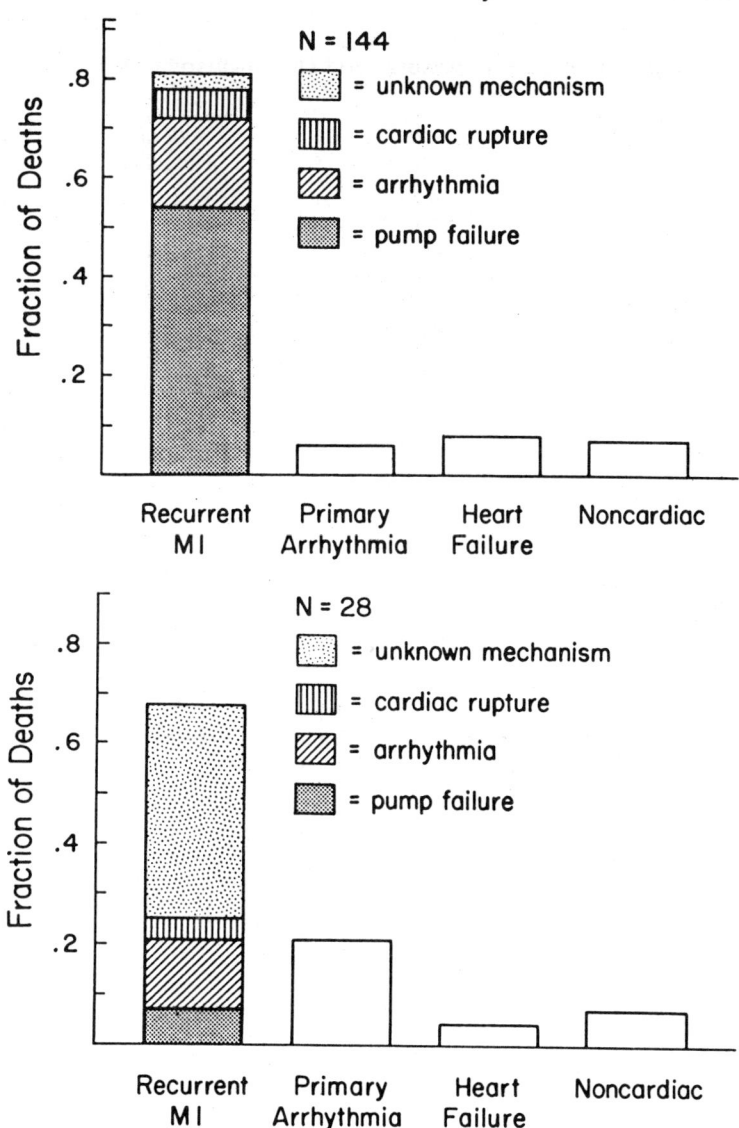

Figure 1: Causes of death in patients with histologic evidence of an old myocardial infarction who died in hospital (top) and out of hospital (bottom). (See text for discussion.)

in 8 (6%) in-hospital and 6 (21%) out-of-hospital deaths (p = .01). However, a fresh coronary thrombus suggesting that death was due to an ischemic arrhythmia was present in 1 of the 8 in-hospital and 1 of the 6 out-of-hospital deaths. Thus, an arrhythmia in the absence of a new ischemic event was a likely cause of death in only 18% of out-of-hospital and 5% of in-hospital deaths.

Progressive heart failure late after infarction without evidence of acute or recent infarction accounted for 12 (8%) in-hospital deaths and 1 (4%) out-of-

Table II
Characteristics of In-Hospital and Out-of-Hospital Deaths

	In Hospital	Out of Hospital	P
N	144	28	
Age (years)	72 ± 10	65 ± 10	.0003
Male	85 (59)	18 (64)	NS
No. CAD	2.7 ± 0.5	2.6 ± 0.6	NS
Old MI Location			
Anterior	56 (39)	5 (18)	.06
Inferior	53 (37)	11 (39)	NS
Both	24 (17)	6 (21)	NS
Unspecified	11 (8)	6 (21)	.06
New MI	117 (81)	19 (68)	NS
Recent MI	66 (46)	6 (21)	.03
Recent + Acute MI	23 (16)	2 (7)	NS
Acute MI	28 (19)	11 (39)	.04

MI = myocardial infarction; No. CAD = number of coronary arteries with > 50% stenoses. Numbers in parentheses are percentages.

Table III
Infarct Location Coronary Artery Disease and Mode of Death in Patients Dying After a New MI

	Total	Pump Failure	Arrhythmia	Unknown Mechanism	Rupture
N	134	79	30	14	11
No CAD					
1	7	3 (42)	2 (29)	1 (14)	1 (14)
2	26	12 (46)	7 (27)	2 (8)	5 (19)+
3	99	64 (65)	20 (20)	11 (11)	4 (4)+
Old MI					
Anterior	43	26 (60)	11 (26)	2 (5)	4 (9)
Inferior	53	31 (58)	12 (23)	6 (11)	4 (8)
Both	24	17 (71)	4 (17)	3 (13)	-0-
New MI					
Anterior	49	30 (61)	12 (24)	3 (6)	4 (8)
Inferior	41	20 (49)	10 (24)	7 (17)	4 (10)
Both	35	24 (69)	7 (20)	1 (93)	3 (9)
Acute	38	24 (63)	7 (18)	6 (16)	1 (3)
Recent	71	39 (55)	19 (27)	5 (7)	8 (11)
Acute + Recent	25	16 (64)	4 (16)	3 (12)	2 (8)
Locations of New versus Old MI					
Same	55	35 (64)	14 (25)	5 (9)	1 (2)°
Separate	41	24 (59)	7 (17)	4 (10)	6 (15)°
Same and Separate	19	13 (68)	5 (26)	-0-	1 (5)

No CAD = number of coronary arteries with > 50% stenosis; MI = myocardial infarction; ° and + = p < .05. Numbers in parentheses are percentages of deaths for that row.

hospital death (p = NS). Noncardiac causes of death were infrequent, occurring in 10 (7%) in-hospital deaths and 1 (4%) out-of-hospital death (p = NS). These consisted of pulmonary emboli (6 patients), exsanguination due to unsuspected gastrointestinal bleeding (1 patient), ruptured abdominal aortic aneurysm (1 patient), spontaneous rupture of an atherosclerotic right coronary artery (1 patient), pulmonary hemorrhage (1 patient), and stroke (1 patient).

Characteristics of patients who died after a new myocardial infarction are compared to those without evidence of a new infarction in Table IV. There were no differences in the severity of the coronary artery stenoses or the location of the old infarct between these two groups.

Previous Arrhythmia History

A nonfatal episode of ventricular fibrillation or sustained ventricular tachycardia during the first 1 to 3 days of an infarction had occurred in 19 patients. Subsequent death was due to pump failure in 18 patients and cardiac rupture in 1 patient.

Four patients had suffered a sustained ventricular arrhythmia late after an acute infarction. Three of these patients had experienced sustained ventricular tachycardia 1 month, 7 months, and 3 years, respectively, prior to death. All were receiving antiarrhythmic medications (bepridil, amiodarone and procainamide, amiodarone and flecainide) at the time of their death. Two of these three died with brady-asystolic cardiac arrests and were found to have acute infarctions at necropsy. The third died of pump failure with mitral valve endocarditis. The fourth

Table IV
Characteristics of Patients Dying With and Without a New MI

	New MI	No New MI	P
N	136	36	
Age (yrs)	71 ± 10	72 ± 10	NS
Male	82 (60)	21 (58)	NS
In Hospital Death	117 (86)	27 (75)	NS
Time From First			
Old MI (yrs)	8.2 ± 7.2	4.1 ± 3.6	NS
Heart Wt (gms)	542 ± 112	563 ± 111	NS
No. CAD			
1	7 (5)	0	NS
2	27 (20)	11 (31)	NS
3	100 (74)	24 (67)	NS
Site of Old MI			
Anterior	45 (33)	16 (44)	NS
Inferior	53 (39)	11 (31)	NS
Both	24 (18)	6 (17)	NS
Unspecified	14 (10)	4 (11)	NS

No. CAD = number of major coronary arteries stenosed > 50%; MI = myocardial infarction; NS = not significant. Numbers in paranthesis are percentages.

patient had been resuscitated from an episode of ventricular fibrillation without acute infarction 4 years prior to death and was treated chronically with procainamide. He died in hospital with refractory congestive heart failure. No histologic evidence of a new infarction was identified at autopsy.

Discussion

Survivors of the acute phase of myocardial infarction comprise an easily identifiable group that is at increased risk for cardiac death.[1-5] Hence a great deal of investigation has been directed toward the identification of high risk postmyocardial infarction subgroups and prophylactic treatment of selected patients. The observation that the majority of late deaths after myocardial infarction occur suddenly has focused a great deal of this effort on the prevention of arrhythmias.[1-5,17-21]

The majority of sudden death victims are found to have ventricular fibrillation at the time of their cardiac arrest.[8,9,11] Two mechanisms appear to predominate as a cause of this arrhythmia: acute ischemia or primary reentrant ventricular tachycardia arising in an area of scar from a previous myocardial infarction. This is supported by several clinical observations. Programmed electrical stimulation can initiate ventricular tachycardia in approximately 60% of patients who have been successfully resuscitated from a cardiac arrest and who do not develop evidence of acute infarction.[12-14] The majority of sudden death survivors who have ventricular tachycardia inducible by programmed stimulation have evidence of an old myocardial infarction.[13] Those with coronary artery disease but without inducible ventricular arrhythmias appear to have a low risk of a recurrent cardiac arrest if subsequent therapy is directed toward preventing episodes of ischemia.[14]

It has been difficult to determine the relative contributions of recurrent ischemia versus primary arrhythmias to sudden death late after a myocardial infarction. Most studies of sudden death have included patients with and without a previous myocardial infarction. Goldstein et al. found that 78% of patients with coronary artery disease who were resuscitated from a cardiac arrest developed ECG or serum enzyme evidence of myocardial infarction or ischemia and classified only 22% of arrests as due to a primary arrhythmic event.[9] An old myocardial infarction was present in 71% of patients who had suffered a primary arrhythmic event compared to 40% of patients whose cardiac arrest was felt to be due to ischemia or infarction. Liberthson et al. found evidence of myocardial infarction or ischemia in 73% of patients resuscitated from a cardiac arrest and 51% had a history of a previous myocardial infarction.[10] Autopsy studies of sudden death victims with coronary artery disease have found histologic evidence of acute myocardial infarction and/or a fresh coronary thrombus in 8–74% of deaths and evidence of old myocardial infarction in 44–82% of deaths.[10,21-30]

All of our patients potentially had the substrate for a primary arrhythmia. That is, they had histologic evidence of a healed myocardial infarction. Therefore we may have anticipated finding a higher incidence of primary arrhythmic deaths than found in previous autopsy studies. Surprisingly, we found evidence of an acute or recent myocardial infarction in over two-thirds of patients who died late after a myocardial infarction, even in the patients who died out of hospital. An arrhythmia in the absence of infarction could account for only 21% of out-of-hospital deaths. This strongly suggests that recurrent infarction is the major cause of sudden death late after myocardial infarction.

Autopsy studies do have several limitations. An infarction less than a few hours old may not produce any detectable histologic changes. We did not perform a detailed microscopic analysis of the coronary arteries to detect atherosclerotic plaque ruptures or microthrombi.[21] However, these factors should lead to an underestimate of the number of acute ischemic cardiac arrhythmias. Examination of the brain and its vasculature were not routinely performed and some deaths due to stroke may have gone undiagnosed. In patients who died after a new infarction, we did not believe that the autopsy data allowed us to reliably distinguish a cardiac arrest precipitated by pump failure from an arrest due to an arrhythmia in the absence of prior hemodynamic deterioration. We required knowledge of the patient's condition immediately prior to death to make this distinction. This information was not available for 43% of the out-of-hospital deaths and 2% of in-hospital deaths which we therefore classified as due to a new infarction but unknown mechanism.

Despite these limitations, recurrent myocardial infarction was found to be the major cause of death in our patients who had survived a previous infarction. Interestingly, the majority of recurrent infarctions occurred in the same general area as an old infarction. Our analysis of infarct locations was not sufficiently detailed to determine if the new infarction was due to reocclusion of a vessel which had recanalized after the previous infarction or if it were due to occlusion of a separate vessel in the same region. However, reocclusion of a vessel whose occlusion and reperfusion or subtotal occlusion had been responsible for a previous infarct has been suggested to be an important cause of reinfarction from studies of non-Q wave infarctions and thrombolytic therapy for acute myocardial infarction.[31-33] The mode of death was to some extent determined by the age of recurrent infarction and the patient's access to medical care. Patients who survived long enough to be hospitalized had a greater incidence of recent (1 day to 3 weeks of age) infarcts than patients who died out of hospital, who were more likely to have acute infarcts (less than 24 hours old). The in-hospital deaths were generally due to pump failure since most serious arrhythmias not precipitated by severe hemodynamic deterioration can be effectively treated in hospital. Noncardiac causes of death were relatively infrequent. However, patients who died after a severe chronic noncoronary illness were excluded from this study.

Our findings are consistent with those of Vedin and co-workers who obtained autopsies in 64 of 70 patients who died during a 2 year follow-up period after an acute myocardial infarction.[34] Death was attributed to recurrent infarction in 54% and a probable primary arrhythmia in 25% of deaths. Noncardiac causes of death were identified in 11% of autopsies. Death occurred within 1 hour of symptoms in 47% of patients. A subsequent study from the same group followed 1306 patients who survived their first myocardial infarction.[35] During a mean follow-up of 6.5 years, autopsies were performed in 160 (85%) patients who died due to complications of coronary artery disease and 43% of these deaths were attributed to reinfarction. The number of deaths due to a primary arrhythmia was not stated.

The predominance of recurrent infarction as the cause of late death after myocardial infarction has important implications for the prevention of sudden death after myocardial infarction. It is consistent with the observations that coronary artery bypass surgery and therapy with beta-adrenergic blocking agents appear to reduce the risk of sudden death, while prophylactic administration of class I antiarrhythmic drugs late after myocardial infarction has not been found to be beneficial.[19,20,36] In a previous study of patients with spontaneous sustained ventricular tachycardia or ventricular fibrillation, we were unable to demonstrate an association between the severity of obstructive coronary artery disease and a history of sudden death or inducible poorly tolerated ventricular tachycardia. The tachycardia rate and underlying ventricular function but not the severity of obstructive coronary artery stenoses were the major determinants of whether inducible ventricular tachycardia produced rapid hemodynamic collapse.[37] We concluded, therefore, that coronary bypass surgery would be unlikely to prevent sudden death in these patients. However, the present study suggests that recurrent ischemia may pose the greatest risk to the post-myocardial infarction patient even if the substrate for a primary ventricular arrhythmia is present as demonstrated by programmed electrical stimulation.[17,18,38,39] This is emphasized by the finding that two of our four patients who had a history of spontaneous sustained ventricular arrhythmias died of recurrent myocardial infarctions and none died of a primary arrhythmia. It is of interest that a preliminary report of a randomized trial by Steinbeck et al. found no difference in the survival of patients with sustained ventricular arrhythmias, comparing those treated empirically with a beta blocker to those who received antiarrhythmic drug therapy guided by electrophysiologic testing.[40]

An antiarrhythmic drug that abolishes ambient ventricular ectopy or ventricular tachycardia inducible by programmed electrical stimulation may not be effective against an ischemic arrhythmia. Some drugs may actually facilitate the occurrence of ischemic ventricular fibrillation, possibly by slowing conduction further in the ischemic border zone.[41,42] Thus, sudden death in a patient receiving an antiarrhythmic drug intended to prevent recurrences of a primary arrhythmia may frequently reflect failure of the drug to prevent an arrhythmia induced by recurrent ischemia rather than failure to prevent a recurrence of the primary arrhythmia. Amiodarone has been found to be very effective in preventing recurrences of sudden death in patients resuscitated from an episode of arrhythmic sudden death despite the fact that it frequently does not prevent inducible ventricular arrhythmias in the electrophysiology laboratory.[43-46] Interestingly, amiodarone appears to be effective against ischemic arrhythmias in some animal models[47,48] and has antianginal activity.[49] It is possible that these effects contribute to its efficacy in the prevention of sudden death.

It is clear that without an autopsy, the cause of death, whether it is sudden or not, cannot be definitely determined. Thus a high autopsy rate is desirable for trials of antiarrhythmic therapy. However, as previously stated, the autopsy is likely to underestimate the number of ischemic events and cannot distinguish death due to cardiogenic shock from that due to an ischemic arrhythmia.

Our findings emphasize the importance of the prevention and treatment of episodes of ischemia in high risk patients. The modification of risk factors for the progression of atherosclerosis has received little emphasis in the management of patients resuscitated from sudden death.[50] Attempts to prevent progression of atherosclerosis, recurrent myocardial infarction, and ischemia deserve continued emphasis and evaluation in patients at high risk for sudden death. These measures are likely to prove of greater benefit to the population at risk for sudden death than antiarrhythmic drug therapy alone.

References

1. Moss AJ, Davis HT, De Camilla J, Bayer LW. Ventricular ectopic beats and their relation to sudden and nonsudden cardiac death after myocardial infarction. Circulation 1979;60:998–1003.
2. Multicenter Postinfarction Research Group. Risk stratification and survival after myocardial infarction. N Engl J Med 1982;309:331–336.
3. Mukharji J, Rude RE, Poole WK, MILIS Study Group. Risk factors for sudden death after acute myocardial infarction: two year follow-up. Am J Cardiol 1984;54:31–36.
4. Goldstein S, Friedman L, Hutchinson R, AMIS Research Group. Timing, mechanism and clinical setting of witnessed deaths in postmyocardial infarction patients. J Am Coll Cardiol 1984;3:1111–1117.
5. Kannel WB, Sorlie P, McNamara PM. Prognosis after initial myocardial infarction: the Framingham study. Am J Cardiol 1979;44:53–59.
6. Nikolic G, Bishop RL, Singh JB. Sudden death during holter monitoring. Circulation 1982;66:218–225.
7. Kempf FC, Josephson ME. Cardiac arrest recorded on ambulatory electrocardiograms. Am J Cardiol 1984;53:1577–1582.
8. Hinkle LE, Thaler HT. Clinical classification of cardiac deaths. Circulation 1982;65:457–464.
9. Goldstein S, Landis JR, Leighton R, Ritter G, Vasu CM, Lantis A, Serokman R. Characteristics of the resuscitated out-of-hospital cardiac arrest victim with coronary heart disease. Circulation 1981;64:977–984.
10. Liberthson RR, Nagel EL, Hirschman JC, Nussenfeld SR, Blackbourne BD, Davis JH. Pathophysiologic observations in prehospital ventricular fibrillation and sudden cardiac death. Circulation 1974;49:790–798.
11. Myerburg RJ, Conde CA, Sung RJ, Mayorga-Cortes A, Mallon SN, Sheps DS, Appel RA, Castellanos A. Clinical, electrophysiologic and hemodynamic profile of patients resuscitated from prehospital cardiac arrest. Am J Med 1980;68:568–576.
12. Ruskin JN, DiMarco JP, Gavan H. Out-of-hospital cardiac arrest: electrophysiologic observations and selection of long-term antiarrhythmic therapy. N Engl J Med 1980;303:607–613.
13. Roy D, Waxman HL, Kienzle MG, Buxton AE, Marchlinski FE, Josephson ME. Clinical characteristics and long-term follow-up in 119 survivors of cardiac arrest: relation to inducibility at electrophysiologic testing. Am J Cardiol 1983;52:969–974.
14. Morady, F, Scheinman MM, Hess DS, Sung RJ, Shen E, Shapiro W. Electrophysiologic testing in the management of survivors of out-of-hospital cardiac arrest. Am J Cardiol 1983;51:85–89.
15. Nachlas MM, Shnitka TK. Macroscopic identification of early myocardial infarcts by alterations in dehydrogenase activity. Am J Pathol 1963;42:379–397.

16. Mallory GK, White PD, Salcedo-Salgar J. The speed of healing of myocardial infarction. Am Heart J 1939;18:647–671.
17. Denniss AR, Richards DA, Cody DV, Russell PA, Young AA, Cooper MJ, Ross DL, Uther JB. Prognostic significance of ventricular tachycardia and fibrillation induced at programmed stimulation and delayed potentials detected on the signal averaged electrocardiograms of survivors of acute myocardial infarction. Circulation 1986;74:731–745.
18. Roy D, Marchand E, Theroux P, Waters DD, Pelletier GB, Bourassa MG. Programmed ventricular stimulation in survivors of an acute myocardial infarction. Circulation 1985;72(3):487–494.
19. May GS, Eberlein KA, Furberg CD, Passamani ER, DeMets DL. Secondary prevention after myocardial infarction: a review of long-term trials. Prog Cardiovasc Dis 1982;24:331–352.
20. Yusuf S, Peto R, Lewis J, Collins R, Sleight P. Beta blockade during and after myocardial infarction: an overview of the randomized trials. Prog Cardiovasc Dis 1985;27:335–371.
21. Davies MJ, Thomas A. Thrombosis and acute coronary-artery lesions in sudden cardiac ischemic death. N Engl J Med 1984;310:1137–1140.
22. Baroldi G, Falzi G, Mariani F. Sudden coronary death. A postmortem study in 208 selected cases compared to 97 "control" subjects. Am Heart J 1979;98:20–31.
23. Penttila A. Sudden and unexpected natural deaths of adult males on analysis of 799 forensic autopsies in 1976. Acta Med Scand 1980;(Suppl)16:249–259.
24. Friedman M, Manwaring JH, Rosenman RH, Donlon G, Ortega P, Grube SM. Instantneous and sudden deaths: clinical and pathological differentiation in coronary artery disease. JAMA 1973;225:1319–1328.
25. Myers A, Dewar HA. Circumstances attending 100 sudden deaths from coronary artery disease with coroner's necropsies. Br Heart J 1975;37:1133–1143.
26. Lovegrove T, Thompson P. The role of acute myocardial infarction in sudden cardiac death: a statistician's nightmare. Am Heart J 1978;96:711–713.
27. Davies MJ. A pathological view of sudden cardiac death. Br Heart J 1981;45:88–96.
28. Schwartz CJ, Walsh WJ. The pathologic basis of sudden death. Prog Cardiovasc Dis 1971;13:465–481.
29. Warnes CA, Roberts WC. Sudden coronary death: relation of amount and distribution of coronary narrowing at necropsy to previous symptoms of myocardial ischemia, left ventricular scarring and heart weight. Am J Cardiol 1984;54:65–73.
30. Roberts WC, Buja LM. The frequency and significance of coronary arterial thrombi and other observations in fatal acute myocardial infarction. Am J Med 1972;52:425–443.
31. Klein LW, Helfant RH. The Q wave and non-Q wave myocardial infarction: differences and similarities. Prog Cardiovas Dis 1986;205–220.
32. Harrison DG, Ferguson DW, Collins SM, Skorton DJ, Ericksen EE, Kroschos JM, Marcus ML, White CW. Rethrombosis after reperfusion with streptokinase: importance of geometry of residual lesions. Circulation 1984;69:991–999.
33. Merx W, Dorr R, Rentrop R, Blanke H, Karsch KR, Mathey DG, Kremer P, Rutsch W, Schmutzler H. Evaluation of the effectiveness of intracoronary streptokinase infusion in acute myocardial infarction: postprocedure management and hospital course in 204 patients. Am Heart J 1981;102:1181–1187.
34. Vedin A, Wilhelmsson C, Elmfeldt D, Save-Soderbergh J, Tibblin G, Wilhelmsen L. Deaths and non-fatal reinfarctions during two years follow-up after myocardial infarction. Acta Med Scand 1975;198:353–364.
35. Ulvenstam G, Aberg A, Bergstrand R, Johansson S, Pennert K, Vedin A, Wedel H, Wilhelmsen L, Wilhelmsson C. Recurrent myocardial infarction. I. Natural history of fatal and non-fatal events. Europ Heart J 1985;6:294–302.
36. Holmes DR, Davis KB, Mack MB, Fisher LD, Gersh BJ, Killip T, Pettinger M. The effect of medical and surgical treatment on subsequent sudden cardiac death in patients with coronary artery disease: a report from the coronary artery surgery study. Circulation 1986;73:1254–1263.

37. Stevenson WG, Brugada P, Waldecker B, Zehender M, Wellens HJJ. Clinical, angiographic, and electrophysiologic findings in patients with sustained ventricular tachycardia after myocardial infarction. Circulation 1985;71:1146–1152.
38. Brugada P, Waldecker B, Kersschot Y, Zehender M, Wellens HJJ. Ventricular arrhythmias initiated by programmed stimulation in four groups of patients with healed myocardial infarction. J Am Coll Cardiol 1986;8:1035–1040.
39. Kuch KH, Costard A, Schluter M, Kunze KP. Significance of timing programmed electrical stimulation after acute myocardial infarction. J Am Coll Cardiol 1986;8:1279–1288.
40. Steinbeck G, Andresen D, Leitner EV, Bach P, Haberl R, Spielberg C. Are antiarrhythmic drugs better than beta-blockers for treatment of sustained ventricular tachyarrhythmias? Circulation 1986;74(Suppl II):100.
41. Temesy-Armos RN, Legenza M, Southworth SR, Hoffman BF. Effects of verapamil and lidocaine in a canine model of sudden coronary death. J Am Coll Cardiol 1985;6:674–681.
42. Elharker V, Gaum WE, Zipes DP. Effect of drugs on conduction delay and incidence of ventricular arrhythmias induced by acute coronary occlusion in dogs. Am J Cardiol 1977;39:544–549.
43. Nademanee K, Singh BN, Cannom DS, Weiss J, Feld G, Stevenson WG. Control of sudden recurrent arrhythmic deaths: role of amiodarone. Am Heart J 1983;106:895–901.
44. Dicarlo LA, Morady F, Sauve MJ, Malone P, Davis JC, Evans-Bell T, Winston SA, Scheinman MM. Cardiac arrest and sudden death in patients treated with amiodarone for sustained venticular tachycardia or ventricular fibrillation risk stratification based on clinical variables. Am J Cardiol 1985;55:372–374.
45. Nademanee K, Hendirckson J, Kannan R, Singh BN. Antiarrhythmic efficacy and electrophysiologic actions of amiodarone in patients with life-threatening ventricular arrhythmias: potent suppression of spontaneously occurring tachyarrhythmias versus inconsistent abolition of induced ventricular tachycardia. Am Heart J 1982;103:950–959.
46. Heger JJ, Prystowsky EN, Jackman WM, Naccarelli GV, Warfel K, Rinkenberger RL, Zipes DP. Clinical efficacy and electrophysiology during long-term therapy for recurrent ventricular tachycardia or ventricular fibrillation. N Engl J Med 1981;305:539–545.
47. Lubbe WF, McFadyen ML, Muller CA, Worthington M, Opie LH. Protective action of amiodarone against ventricular fibrillation in the isolated perfused rat heart. Am J Cardiol 1979;43:533–540.
48. Patterson E, Eller BT, Abrams GD, Vasiliades J, Lucchesi BR. Ventricular fibrillation in a conscious canine model of sudden coronary death: Prevention by short- and long-term amiodarone administration. Circulation 1983;68:857–864.
49. Vastesaeger M, Gillot P, Rasson G. Etude clinque d´une nouvelle medication anti-angoreuse. Acta Cardiol (Brux) 1967;22:483–500.
50. Hallstrom AP, Cobb LA, Ray R. Smoking as a risk factor for recurrence of sudden cardiac arrest. N Engl J Med 1986;314:271–275.

24

Sudden Cardiac Death: A Multifactorial Problem

Hein J.J. Wellens
Pedro Brugada

Introduction

We have learned to live with the fact that in the USA 400,000 people die suddenly each year. In a significant number of them, the sudden demise is the first presentation of cardiovascular disease. Although, as recently discussed by Roberts,[1] many different causes can lead to sudden death; in the majority of victims, coronary artery disease is the culprit. In this chapter we will therefore concentrate on the role of coronary artery disease and its consequences.

What do we know about sudden cardiac death in 1987 and what can possibly be done to prevent this dramatic and unwanted event from occurring?

Can We Recognize High Risk Groups?

While (as shown in Table I) sudden death can be the first manifestation of coronary disease, sudden death victims are frequently known as cardiac patients.[2-4] They should therefore be the group of patients to whom our efforts should be primarily directed especially because in recent years it has become clear that among these patients, risk stratification in predicting those who may die suddenly is possible.

From: Brugada P, Wellens HJJ. CARDIAC ARRHYTHMIAS: Where To Go From Here? Mount Kisco, NY, Futura Publishing Company, Inc., © 1987.

Table I
Background of Patients with Sudden Cardiac Death and Possibility of Identifying High Risk Patients

	Incidence	Recognition
1. Not preceded by symptoms	45%	not possible
2. Short-lasting premonitory symptoms (hours to weeks, specific, aspecific)	20%	partially
3. Longer lasting angina pectoris	15%	possible
4. Myocardial infarction survivor	20%	possible

The Patient with Known Coronary Artery Disease

The literature on sudden death in the patient with coronary artery disease, and emphasized by several contributors to this book, points to the importance of myocardial ischemia, left ventricular function, and ventricular arrhythmias. Figure 1 indicates that these three factors—ischemia, hemodynamic dysfunction, and electrical—instability are closely interrelated. As shown in Figure 1, each of the three main factors is affected by dynamic changes such as changes in degree of ischemia, triggers, blood platelet function, influence of the autonomic nervous system (ANS), etc. The importance of all these different contributing factors may vary, depending upon the stage of coronary artery disease. For example, sudden death in the previously asymptomatic patient is the result of acute myocardial ischemia leading to the lethal cardiac arrhythmia. The mechanism of sudden death can be totally different in the patient with an old myocardial infarction and a large scar. As discussed elsewhere in this book, our knowledge of all the factors contributing to sudden death is far from complete, but in order not to drown in a multifactorial complex situation, a practical approach to the problem requires the analysis of the contributing factors, which are known and can be recognized.

The easiest group to start with are patients who have *suffered from a myocardial infarction in the past*. In these patients, the degree of impairment of left ventricular function has emerged as the most important factor determining prognosis.

The patient with a left ventricular ejection fraction of 20–30% has a 30% 1-year mortality rate as compared to a 5% value in patients with a left ventricular ejection fraction of 50% or more.[5] A critical analysis of the independent value of left ventricular ejection fraction has recently been published.[6] Patients requiring treatment for congestive failure after myocardial infarction have a particular ominous prognosis.[7,8] It is of interest that about half of the patients with symptomatic pump failure after myocardial infarction die suddenly.[7]

Residual ischemia outside the infarcted area is also of prognostic significance. Painful and silent ischemia in rest or during exercise are markers for an increased risk of dying suddenly. Several methods have been advanced to obtain information about the presence or absence of residual ischemia, such as the resting ECG, 24-hour Holter recordings, exercise ECG testing alone or combined with radionuclide techniques, and recently also dobutamine infusion.[9]

Within the residual ischemia group, risk is inversely related to duration of

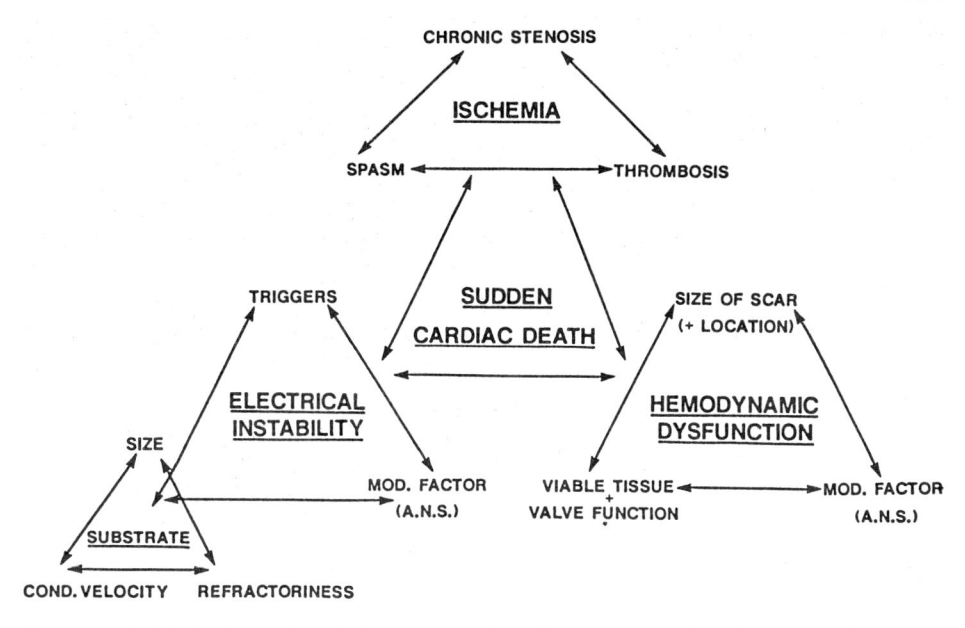

Figure 1: Model showing the factors that play a role in sudden cardiac death in the patient with coronary artery disease. As shown, ischemia, hemodynamic dysfunction, and electrical instability are the three components closely interrelated in producing sudden cardiac death. Several known (and probably other unknown) factors play a role in each of the three main components of the model. Not shown in this figure is the role of time, for example, the age of a myocardial infarction or the duration of ischemia. A.N.S. = autonomic nervous system.

exercise before the onset of complaints or ST segment depression and also inversely related to the rise in blood pressure during exercise.[10,11] The high risk post-MI patient can therefore be recognized by performing an exercise test.

An important area of discussion, as can also be found elsewhere in this book, is the significance of ventricular arrhythmias. There is no question that the occurrence of spontaneous sustained ventricular tachycardia after the acute phase of myocardial infarction worsens prognosis.[12] Discussion centers around the independent prognostic significance of other expressions of ectopic ventricular activity, including frequency of ventricular premature beats, couplets, and nonsustained ventricular tachycardia. While on one hand investigators such as Bigger[13] found prognostic significance of nonsustained ventricular tachycardia independent from left ventricular function, other investigators could not come to the same conclusion.[6,14,15] Studies in which incidence, time of occurrence, and characteristics of ventricular ectopy are carefully related to site and size of infarction and extent of the residual ischemic area are required to give a more definite answer to this question.

The information obtained in patients who have suffered from a myocardial infarction that extent of muscle loss is the prime determinant of the future indicates the extreme importance of reducing infarct size as much as possible when the patient presents *with impending or early myocardial infarction*. Recent data have shown that infarct size can be reduced by early administration of thrombolytic therapy,[16] indicating the importance of the shortest possible time interval between onset of complaints and treatment. Reduction in infarct size is not only of importance for left ventricular function, but also reduces the substrate for malignant ventricular arrhythmias.[17]

The Patient Unknown to Have Coronary Heart Disease

As described, many sudden cardiac death victims have no previous cardiac history,[2,18–20] although somewhat different conclusions were recently reported.[20] In that study it was found that in only a minority of patients resuscitated out of hospital no previous cardiac history was present.[21]

The Asymptomatic Patient

It is possible to recognize groups at higher risk for sudden death in the asymptomatic population. Although risk factors can be identified as smoking, high blood pressure, lipid abnormalities, a familial history of coronary artery disease, and an abnormal rest or exercise electrocardiogram, the predictive value of these abnormalities is too low to justify large scale expensive investigations such as thallium stress testing studies or coronary angiography in the asymptomatic population.

Present Therapeutic Strategies

Depending on the setting and background, different steps have to be taken to reduce sudden death in patients with coronary heart disease.

Sudden Death Outside the Hospital

As indicated in Table II, in the patient dying suddenly outside the hospital, resuscitation has to be started immediately followed by rapid admission to hospital. Resuscitation outside the hospital can be very effective. In areas such as Seattle where a well-organized resuscitation system incorporating citizen-initiated rescue efforts is operative, approximately 1/3 of patients who are resuscitated outside the hospital are discharged alive from hospital.[22] Prehospital resuscitation can therefore lead to a sizable reduction in the number of sudden death victims. This becomes even more important, as discussed by Myerburg et al. elsewhere in this volume, when one realizes that the outlook for the successfully resuscitated patient has improved considerably in recent years. Risk stratification in these patients is possible.[23]

Table II
Steps in Reducing Sudden Cardiac Death

Known CAD Population

Early phase (out of hospital): Resuscitation.
  Required: Personnel and facilities for resuscitation followed by rapid transportation to hospital.
Early phase (in hospital): Aggressive treatment of impending and early MI.
  Required: Awareness by laymen and first line physician of the importance of the shortest possible hospital delay. In hospital knowledge and facilities to recognize high risk subsets.
Late phase (in hospital): Risk stratification
  Required: Information about pumpfunction, residual ischemia, and spontaneous ventricular tachycardia. This should be followed by appropriate therapy (if possible!).
Late phase (out of hospital): Recognition of changes in previously stable condition followed by appropriate action.
  Required: Education of patient and first line physician.

Unknown CAD Population

- Identification of high risk groups (smokers, hypertension, hyperlipemia, familial incidence CAD) followed by counseling.
- General advise on diet (fat, salt, etc.) and exercise.

The Coronary Heart Disease Patient Reaching Hospital

In the patient reaching the hospital with chest pain and developing myocardial infarction, evidence has been presented that infarct size is the most important prognostic predictor in the myocardial infarction survivor.[5] Measures to prevent myocardial infarction or interventions as early as possible after myocardial infarction to reduce infarct size are therefore an important target to reduce sudden death later. Recently much emphasis has been placed on early risk stratification in patients with unstable angina. Questions involving the proper determination of the size of the area at risk,[24] possible profits of thrombolytic therapy, PTCA, or early surgery have only partially been answered. As shown in the study of the Interuniversity Cardiology Institute of the Netherlands (ICIN), 20% of patients admitted with unstable angina develop a myocardial infarction within 48 hours.[24] Regarding the patient admitted to the hospital with an acute myocardial infarction, another study from ICIN demonstrated that thrombolytic therapy is especially useful when electrocardiographic evidence is present of an extensive anterior or inferior wall infarction and the patient is treated within 4 hours after onset of chest pain.[26,27]

If the damage is done, our presently available therapeutic measures for the patient left with limited left ventricular function are disappointing. Approximately 15% of myocardial infarction survivors fall into that category. No randomized studies are available on the effects of inotropic drugs or vasodilators in patients with poor pump function after myocardial infarction, nor are data known on the effect of reconstructive surgery of the left ventricle.

If the combination of poor left ventricular function and residual ischemia is present, revascularization procedures improve prognosis and reduce the incidence of sudden cardiac death.[28,29] It is essential therefore to determine residual ischemia in the myocardial infarction survivor with poor pump function.

Much controversy exists about the value of treating ventricular arrhythmias after myocardial infarction. Secondary prevention trials of antiarrhythmic therapy have thus far been unable to demonstrate a beneficial effect.[30] The problems with these studies include: (1) the absence of stratification according to risk, (2) the absence of individualization of antiarrhythmic drug dose, and (3) the absence of knowledge of the true value of tests used to determine drug efficacy. The study planned by the National Heart, Lung and Blood Institute in which about 4500 survivors of myocardial infarction will be enrolled, will hopefully answer the question of whether effective control of potentially malignant ventricular arrhythmias will improve survival.

In contrast to antiarrhythmic drug therapy, treatment with a beta-blocking agent has been shown to reduce sudden cardiac death.[31] A 25% reduction in sudden death has been demonstrated in the first 2 years after myocardial infarction. The beneficial action seems to be based upon amelioration of ischemia and elimination or blunting of sympathetically mediated modulations in heterogeneity of myocardial repolarization and refractoriness. Presence of cardioselectivity, intrinsic sympathomimetic activity, or membrane depressant action do not seem to play an important role in the protective action of the beta-blocking agent. Since beta-blocking agents after myocardial infarction have been used primarily in patients with reasonable left ventricular function, 100 patients of that type have to be treated for 2 years in order to prevent death in two of them. This suggests that better selection of patients likely to benefit from beta-blocking therapy is necessary. Patients with overt and silent ischemia and/or hypertension seem to be prime candidates for treatment with a beta-blocking drug. An important question is the value of beta-blocking therapy in the patient with mechanical and electrical complications. Furberg et al.[32] suggest beneficial action but more work is needed to define the exact value of beta-blocking therapy in these patients.

While in the whole group of myocardial infarction survivors, antiarrhythmic drug therapy so far has not been shown to be beneficial, as discussed in the chapter on lessons from the parallel study, antiarrhythmic drug therapy does save lives in patients with spontaneously occurring ventricular tachycardia or ventricular fibrillation. As shown in that chapter and also by those reporting on the experience with the implantable defibrillator, subgroups with life-threatening ventricular arrhythmias can be recognized who will profit from that device.

The Coronary Heart Disease Patient after Discharge from Hospital

As pointed out, risk stratification and appropriate therapeutic measures should take place before discharge. In the post-hospital phase, attention should be focused on changes in the stability of the condition. Coronary artery disease is usually a progressive disease and patient and first line physician should be knowledgeable about the necessity of seeking cardiological advice when changes in condition occur. The cardiologist will then perform the necessary investigations to establish its significance and take appropriate action.

The Unknown Coronary Artery Disease Population

In several countries including the USA and the Netherlands, mortality figures for coronary heart disease are decreasing. It is not quite clear which factors are responsible: changes in diet, smoking, or exercise habits, treatment of high blood pressure or the advent of coronary care, bypass surgery, and medication such as beta-blocking and calcium antagonists.

In a large epidemiologic study of employees of the DuPont Company, Pell and Fayerweather reported a fall in incidence of myocardial infarction, sudden death, and total number of cardiac deaths over a 26-year period (1957–1983).[33] The authors conclude that general measures like diet, discontinuation of smoking, etc. contributed more to the decreasing mortality than medication or interventions in the known coronary heart disease patient. For future planning, it seems to be important to be better informed about the role of general versus more specific measures. This could be studied in the following way (Table III). Determine the number of sudden deaths in the population and divide them into those occurring in known cardiac patients (group A) and those in whom sudden death was the first manifestation of cardiac disease (group B). If the same is repeated 10 years later, a decrease in the size of group B will indicate effectiveness of general measures. A decrease in size of group A points to a beneficial effect of specific measures related to individualized information of the cardiac status of the patient.

Epidemiologic studies indicate that in the Western world, 60% of patients suffering from a myocardial infarction fall in 20% of the population, having one or more risk factors including smoking, elevated cholesterol level, or elevated blood pressure. Therefore, 40% of myocardial infarction patients come from 80% of our population without any high risk factor. But even in the asymptomatic patient in the high risk group, techniques such as exercise testing do not fulfill the requirements for community screening programs discussed by Cadman et al.[34] and shown in Table IV.

Table III
Evaluation of Value of Therapeutic and Preventive Measures in Reducing Sudden Death in Known and Unknown CAD Population

1. Determine incidence of sudden death in
   A) Known CAD population
   B) Unknown CAD population
2. Repeat the study 10 years later
3. Draw conclusions:
   A) Reduction in sudden death incidence in Group A suggests effect of therapy of CAD.
   B) Reduction in sudden death incidence in Group B suggests effect of preventive measures.

Table IV
Guidelines for Deciding on Community Screening Programs in Coronary Heart Disease According to Cadman et al.[34]

1. Has the program's effectiveness been demonstrated in a randomized trial?
2. Are efficacious treatments available and financially affordable?
3. Is there a good screening test?
4. Does the program reach those who could profit from it?
5. Can the health system cope and financially afford the screening program?
6. Will those with positive screening comply with subsequent advice and interventions?
7. Are psychological and socio-economic consequences of positive screening overcome by efficacious treatment?

Conclusions

Sudden cardiac death is a multifactorial problem. At the present time, only one-third of patients dying suddenly can be identified as likely candidates prior to the event. In patients with known coronary artery disease, every possible effort should be made to reduce myocardial damage during acute ischemia. In the patient who has suffered from myocardial damage, appropriate risk stratification should be performed and therapeutic measures taken. So far, only beta-blocking agents have been shown to be effective in preventing sudden death after survival from a myocardial infarction. Studies are urgently needed to establish the value of antiarrhythmic drugs in relation to risk. In those studies, value of the presently available tests to predict success or failure of drug therapy should be critically evaluated.

References

1. Roberts WC. Sudden cardiac death: Definition and causes. Am J Cardiol 1986;57: 1410–1413.
2. Doyle JT, Kannel WB, McNamara PM, Quickenton P, Gordon T. Factors related to suddenness of coronary death: combined Albany-Framingham studies. Am J Cardiol 1976;37:1073–1078.
3. Kulbertus HE, Wellens HJJ, eds. Sudden Death. The Hague, Martinus Nijhoff, 1980.
4. Greenberg HM, Dwyer EM, eds. Sudden Coronary Death. Ann NY Acad Sci 1982;382: 1–484.
5. Moss AJ, Bigger TJ, Case RB, Gillespie JA, Goldstein RE, Greenberg HM, Kronc R, Marcus FJ, Odoroff CL, Oliver GC. The Multicenter Postinfarction Research Group: Risk stratification and survival after myocardial infarction. N Engl J Med 1983;390: 331–336.
6. Ahnve S, Gilpin E, Henning H, Curtis G, Collins D, Ross J. Limitations and advantages of the ejection fraction for defining high risk after acute myocardial infarction. Am J Cardiol 1986;58:872–878.
7. Packer M. Sudden unexpected death in patients with congestive heart failure: a second frontier. Circulation 1985;72:681–685.
8. Dwyer EM, Greenberg H, Case RB, and the Multicenter Postinfarction Research Group. Association between transient pulmonary congestion during acute myocardial infarction and high incidence of death in six months. Am J Cardiol 1986;58:900–905.

9. Berthe C, Piérard LA, Hiernaux M, Trotteur G, Lempereur P, Carlier J, Kulbertus HE. Predicting the extent and location of coronary artery disease in acute myocardial infarction by echocardiography during dobutamine infusion. Am J Cardiol 1986;58: 1167–1172.
10. Fioretti P, Brower RW, Simoons ML, Bos RJ, Baardman T, Beelen A, Hugenholtz PG. Prediction of mortality during the first year after acute myocardial infarction from clinical variables and stress test at hospital discharge. Am J Cardiol 1985;55:1313–1318.
11. Akhras F, Upward J, Keates J, Jackson G. Early exercise testing and elective coronary artery surgery after uncomplicated myocardial infarction. Effect on morbidity and mortality. Br Heart J 1984;52:413–417.
12. Wellens HJJ, Brugada P, de Zwaan C, Bendermacher P, Bär FW. Clinical characteristics, prognostic significance and treatment of sustained ventricular tachycardia following acute myocardial infarction. In Kulbertus H, and Wellens HJJ, eds. Mount Kisco, NY, Futura Publishing Co., The First Year after a Myocardial Infarction. 1983;227–237.
13. Bigger JTh, Fleiss JL, Rolnitzky LM, and the Multicenter Post-infarction Research Group. Prevalence, characteristics and significance of ventricular tachycardia detected by 24 hour continuous electrocardiographic recordings in the late hospital phase of acute myocardial infarction. Am J Cardiol 1986;58:1151–1160.
14. Lichtlen PR, Bethge KP, Platiel H. Incidence of sudden death in relation to left ventricular anatomy and rhythm profile. Z Kardiol 1980;69:639–648.
15. Edlin DE, Morganroth J, Iskandrian AS, Spielman SR, Horowitz LN, Kay H. Ischemia at rest is independent of the extent of ventricular dysfunction and arrhythmias in patients with coronary artery disease. Am Heart J 1985;190:228–231.
16. Simoons ML, Van den Brand M, de Zwaan C, Verheugt RWA, Remme W, Serruys PW, Bär F, Res J, Krauss XH, Vermeer F. Improved survival after early thrombolysis in acute myocardial infarction. Lancet 1985;2:578–582.
17. Kersschot I, Brugada P, Ramentol M, Zehender M, Waldecker B, Geibel A, de Zwaan C, Wellens HJJ. Effects of early reperfusion in acute myocardial infarction on arrhythmias induced by programmed stimulation. A prospective randomized study. J Am Coll Cardiol 1986;7:1234–1242.
18. Madsen JK. Ischemic heart disease and prodromics of sudden cardiac death. Br Heart J 1985;54:27–32.
19. Goldstein S, Freidman L, Hutchinson R, Canner P, Romhilt D, Schlant R, Sobrino R, Verter J, Wasserman A, and The Aspirin Myocardial Infarction Study Research Group. Timing, mechanism and clinical setting of witnessed deaths in postmyocardial infarction patients. JACC 1984;3:1111–1117.
20. Mukharji J, Rude RE, Poole WK, Gustafson N, Thomas LJ, Strauss HW, Jaffe AS, Miller JE, Roberts R, Raabe DS, Croft CH, Passamani E, Braunwald E, Willerson JT and the MILIS Study Group. Risk factors for sudden death after acute myocardial infarction: two year follow-up. Am J Cardiol 1984;54:31–36.
21. Goldstein S, Vanderbrug Medendorp S, Landis JR, Wolfe RA, Leighton R, Ritter G, Vasu M, Acheson A. Analysis of cardiac symptoms preceding cardiac arrest. Am J Cardiol 1986;58:1195–1198.
22. Cobb LA, Hallstrom AP. Community-based cardiopulmonary resuscitation. What have we learned? N Engl J Med 1983;390:330–341.
23. Goldstein S, Landis JR, Leighton R, Ritter G, Vasu CM, Wolfe RA, Acheson A, Medendorp SV. Predictive survival models for resuscitated victims of out-of-hospital cardiac arrest with coronary heart disease. Circulation 1985;71:873–880.
24. de Zwaan C, Bär FW, Wellens HJJ. Characteristic electrocardiographic pattern indicating a critical stenosis high in the left anterior descending coronary artery in patients admitted because of impending myocardial infarction. Am Heart J 1982;103:730–35.
25. Holland Interuniversity Nifedipine/Metoprolol trial (HINT) research group. Early treatment of unstable angina in the coronary care unit: a randomized, double blind, placebo controlled comparison of recurrent ischemia in patients treated with Nifedipine or Metoprolol or both. Lancet 1986;56:400–413.

26. Vermeer F, Simoons ML, Bär FW, Tijssen JGP, Van Domburg RT, Serruys PW, Verheugt FWA, Res JCJ, de Zwaan C, Van der Laarse A, Krauss XH, Lubsen J, Hugenholtz PG. Which patients benefit most from early thrombolytic therapy with intracoronary streptokinase? Circulation 1986;74:1379–1389.
27. Bär FW, Vermeer F, de Zwaan C, Ramentol M, Braat S, Simoons ML, Hermens WT, Krauss XH, Wellens HJJ. Value of admission electrocardiogram in predicting outcome of thrombolytic therapy in acute myocardial infarction. Am J Cardiol 1987 (in press).
28. Passamani E, Davis KB, Gillespie MJ, Killip T, and the CASS principal investigators and their associates. A randomized trial of coronary artery bypass surgery. Survival of patients with a low ejection fraction. N Engl J Med 1985;312:1665–1671.
29. Holmes DR, Davis KB, Mack MB, Fisher LD, Gersh BJ, Killip T, Pettinger M. The effect of medical and surgical treatment on subsequent sudden cardiac death in patients with coronary artery disease: a report from the coronary artery surgery study. Circulation 1986;73:1254–1263.
30. May GS, Eberlein KA, Furberg CD, Passamani ER, Demets DL. Secondary prevention after myocardial infarction: a review of long term trials. Progr Cardiovasc Dis 1982;24:331–352.
31. Yusuf S, Peto R, Lewis J, Collins R, Sleight P. Betablockade during and after myocardial infarction: an overview of the randomized trials. Progr Cardiovasc Dis 1985;27:335–371.
32. Furberg CD, Morton-Hawkins C, Lichtstein E for the Beta-blocker Heart Attack Trial Study Group. Effect of propanolol in post-infarction patients with mechanical and electrical complications. Circulation 1984;69:761–767.
33. Pell S, Fayerweather WE. Trends in the incidence of myocardial infarction and in associated mortality and morbidity in a large employed population, 1957–1983. N Engl J Med 1985;312:1005–1011.
34. Cadman D, Chambers L, Feldman W, Sackett D. Assessing the effectiveness of community screening programs. JAMA 1984;251:1580–1580.

V

Strategies of Treatment of Ventricular Arrhythmias

25

Antiarrhythmic Therapy: Noninvasive Guided Strategy Versus Empirical or Invasive Strategies

Philippe Coumel
Jean-François Leclercq
Marc Zimmerman
Jean-Louis Funck-Brentano

Introduction

Empiricism is the traditional treatment strategy of tachyarrhythmias. In fact, it implies the absence of strategy. The trial and error method is still acceptable if the patient's outcome cannot be predicted with sufficient accuracy from invasive or noninvasive electrophysiological (EP) findings. On the other hand, empiricism should regress if increasing knowledge were provided by EP techniques.

Opposing the results of noninvasive EP to either empiricism or invasive EP is not the right challenge. The different strategies cannot be compared, because of important biases which are usually underestimated and explain persistent, sometimes acute controversies. The most common bias concerns the patient populations studied, the nature of the arrhythmias, which may differ considerably, as well as the etiology, the history, and the effects of previous treatments. The availability of drugs in the various countries and their more or less routine use may also generate considerable discrepancies: for example, how do we compare cohorts in whom "drug resistance" is defined after using quinidine, procainamide, or propranolol therapy with patients who have already used amiodarone, flecainide, propafenone, or nadolol? Generally speaking, any strategy will give good results in cases of short-history arrhythmias occurring in patients who are not severely diseased.[1] Not surprisingly, the success rate sharply decreases in patients with a long history of arrhythmias in the presence of depressed hearts. Especially in the latter situation, one should have better information regarding the treatment that should be selected.

Discussing the theoretical merits and drawbacks of the various strategies is more important than comparing their current practical value. The main limitation of empiricism is the impossibility to improve its performance. Clinical experience can be transmitted directly, but it is not quantifiable. At best results stagnate in a plateau phase, the level of which changes with the new drugs that become available. In this sense, empiricism depends in fact on the results of EP techniques which largely contribute to drug developments. The problem is different for EP investigations. One can conceive that even though they are currently imperfect, refining them can increase their practical value. Therefore, examining whether they are utilized to the fullest extent or whether their use can be optimized becomes an important issue. In our experience, however, less can be expected from invasive than from noninvasive techniques.

Do We Have to Expect Much More from Invasive Studies?

This book is aimed at celebrating the 20th birthday of programmed electrical stimulation, a technique that can now be considered as having reached maturity. However, serial drug testing still has an amount of uncertainty which may be incorrectable.[2-4] False responses of the provocative tests are characterized by the nonconsistency between the immediate result of the procedure and the clinical outcome. Testing that is too aggressive tends to give false positives by inducing nonclinical arrhythmias, whereas passive testing tends to generate false negatives. Some agreement has now been reached about the standards of the tests,[5] and the false responses reflect in fact the fundamental limitations of this procedure. The main aim of the "parallel approach"[6] is to provide an accurate evaluation of the false responses that cannot presently be recognized by using serial testing.

By definition, the application of programmed stimulation is restricted to inducible arrhythmias. Considerable limitations relate to the type of arrhythmia, the etiology, the type of patient, and the drugs used. While monomorphic sustained ventricular tachycardias (sVT) in healed myocardial infarction (MI) are almost always inducible, the list of cases that is beyond the field of application of EP testing is long:[7] ventricular fibrillation, polymorphic VT and nonsustained VT (nsVT) in chronic MI, and any of them in other diseases such as the acute phase of MI, hypertrophic or congestive cardiomyopathy, arrhythmogenic right ventricular dysplasia, mitral valve prolapse, not to mention "idiopathic" tachyarrhythmias, in which the proportion of inducible arrhythmias varies from 3/4 to less than 10%. This also applies to the various patterns of torsades de pointes.

Even when the largest cohort of candidates consists of patients with chronic MI and sVT, therapies that can be evaluated through this technique are limited to pure type I antiarrhythmic drugs. Even the supporters of serial testing admit that amiodarone and propafenone may lead to false results. This is probably due to their mode of action including some degree of beta-blockade. Actually the antiarrhythmic action of beta-blockers cannot be reliably checked with programmed stimulation.

To give an example, the proportion of inducible VT responding to propranolol may range from 21%[8] to 70%.[9] Notwithstanding the proportion of true or false responses in these "negatives," the difference between these two studies certainly relates to the proportion of post-MI VT in the cohorts: 86% and 16%, respectively.

In essence, programmed stimulation gives an artificial trigger to a patient with a potential arrhythmia substrate. EP testing ignores the spontaneous arrhythmia trigger: false positive tests (no spontaneous but an inducible arrhythmia) may result from the drug-related disappearance of the spontaneous initiating factor. More seriously, provocative tests can be falsely negative for various technical reasons[10,11] and because they ignore the important role of the sympathetic drive in ventricular arrhythmias. All the possible EP mechanisms of arrhythmias (reentry, triggered activity, automatism) are sensitive to the autonomic nervous system. This is not denied by clinicians but is not considered in EP testing. Adrenergic stimulation may generate the extrasystoles (ES) which are the most common initiating factor of tachyarrhythmias; it may modify their coupling interval thus changing them from potential into actual triggers. More importantly, adrenergic stimulation may make a substrate responsive which was quiescent, and Figure 1 is an example of it. In this patient, no VT could be induced by stimulation. However, an isoprenaline infusion consistently started VT when the sinus rate reached 125 beats per minute -1 thereby reflecting the necessity of a certain degree of sympathetic stimulation. When the infusion was maintained at lower rates, single electrically induced extrasystoles triggered longer and longer repetitive responses with higher and higher tachycardia rates. Although this case was illustrative, frequently the use of isoprenaline is not that rewarding: it probably is too simplistic an approach which mimics rather than really reproduces the complex interplay between several different determinants of arrhythmias. In particular, the predominant rate-dependency of ES cannot be clearly differentiated from the adrenergic-dependency of the substrate, thus explaining why the results of this test are not very dependable.

Which Patients are Amenable to the Noninvasive Approach?

A self-explanatory limitation of the Holter technique is the absence of a spontaneous arrhythmia. In contrast to what occurs with the invasive EP studies, the amount of spontaneous arrhythmias relates more to the myocardial status than to the etiology of the disease.[12] Paroxysmal idiopathic sVT is usually the most difficult to investigate and Figures 2 and 3 show what patience the physi-

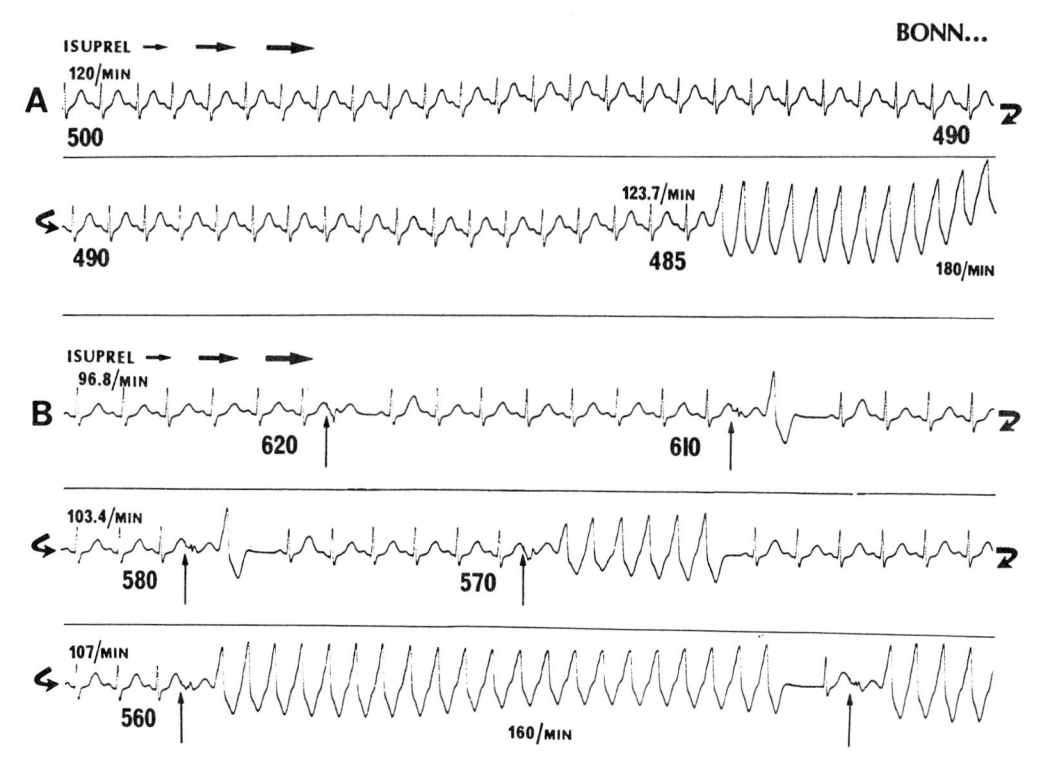

Figure 1: Isoprenaline infusion and arrhythmia inducibility. In panel A, an isoprenaline infusion provokes a VT which was not inducible with programmed stimulation. An indicator of the necessary amount of drug is given by the rate of the sinus tachycardia (123.7 beats/min -1), at the time of initiation of VT (the VT rate is 180 beats/min -1). In panel B, ventricular premature stimulations are inserted after the infusion is restarted. As the sinus cycle progressively shortens though not reaching the previous value of 485 ms, an electrical stimulus is not effective (at 620 ms), induces a single response (at 610 and 580 ms), a run of six beats (at 570 ms) and a nonsustained VT (at 650 ms). The rate of the VT is slower (160 beats/min -1) than the rate of the initial sustained, isoprenaline-induced episode of VT (panel A). In this case not only the inducibility of the arrhythmia but also its form depend on the amount of adrenergic stimulation. As shown, the arrhythmia can be classified as no arrhythmia or inducible sustained or nonsustained VT.

cian should have! From 1976 to 1982, several repeated Holter recordings were totally arrhythmia-free in this patient with a readily inducible sVT. In 1982, after 21 attacks in 7 years, the paroxysmal form progressively shifted to a repetitive, nonsustained but still inducible VT finally controlled by bepridil. Six different type 1 drugs (two forms of quinidine, procainamide, ajmaline, disopyramide, and flecainide), three beta-blockers (acebutolol, propranolol, and nadolol), and amiodarone had been used unsuccessfully according to the never false positive and ever false negative or true positive of repeated EP studies, bepridil itself finally giving a false positive result (inducible nsVT).

The choice between noninvasive (supposedly directed towards ES and nsVT) and invasive (directed towards sVT) techniques may in practice be dictated by the circumstances. It should not be based on theoretical beliefs. Patients with or without cardiac disease may have any form of ventricular arrhythmia, and oppos-

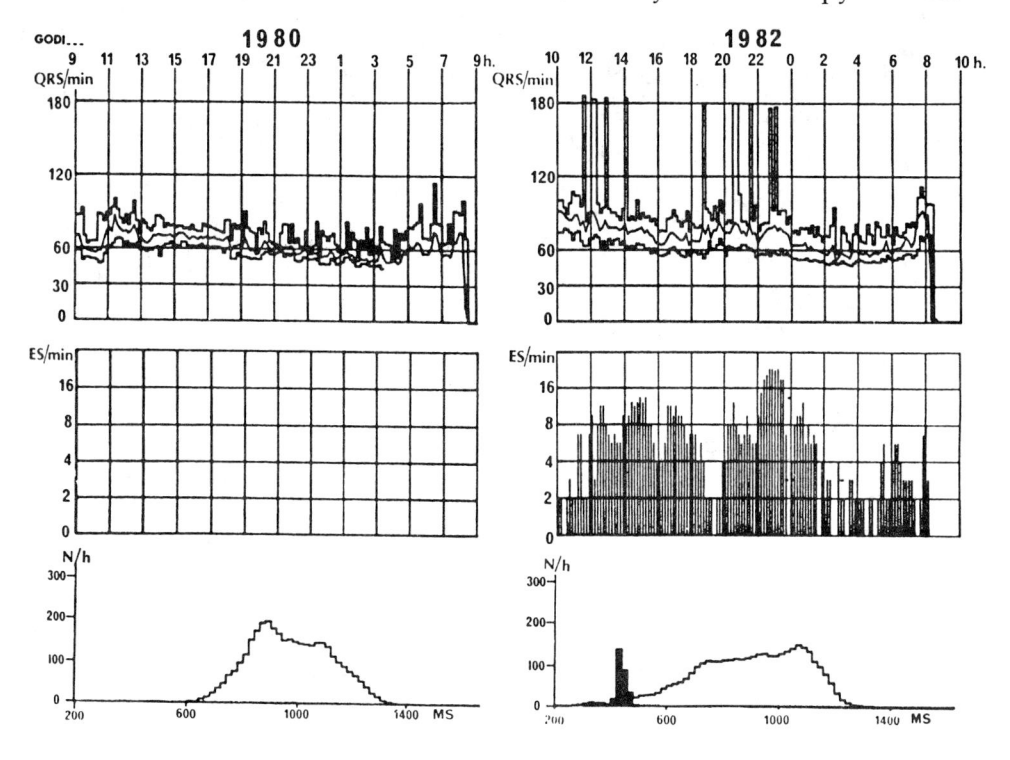

Figure 2: Different behavior of the same VT in the same patient. A patient with no apparent heart disease and a long history of paroxysmal and inducible sustained VT progressively developed an incessant nonsustained form; illustrative ambulatory monitorings are shown. In 1980, not a single extrasystole was recorded, whereas attacks and isolated extrasystoles were numerous in 1982. From top to bottom in both panels: the maximal, mean, and minimal trends of heart rate, the extrasystolic rate and histograms showing the two populations of large (solid area) and narrow QRS (open area). See also Figure 3.

ing the more common inducibility of sVT to the less frequent and less reliable provocability of nsVT[7,13] is not really justified. Neither is justified nor demonstrated any difference in terms of underlying mechanism, and evoking more frequently reentry in sVT or triggered activity or automatism in nsVT is totally inconsistent with the fact that they are observed in the same patients and with the same diseases. Experimentally, sustained arrhythmias tend to induce the conditions of their termination.[14] Clinically following the onset of an arrhythmia, the hemodynamic changes will engender sympathetic stimulation,[15] thereby favoring perpetuation of the arrhythmias. What should be opposed is not a shorter or longer duration of an arrhythmia but simply the presence or absence of repetitive activity following the initial ES. Even if an identical morphology suggests that both initiating ES and the subsequent tachycardia originate from the same myocardial area, this does not imply that their mechanisms are identical:[16] parasystole, reflection, or afterdepolarization may be the cause for ES, and start reentry, triggered activity, or abnormal automaticity leading to tachycardias.

Spontaneous arrhythmias are more regularly distributed throughout patients and diseases than inducible arrhythmias. The potential and practical impor-

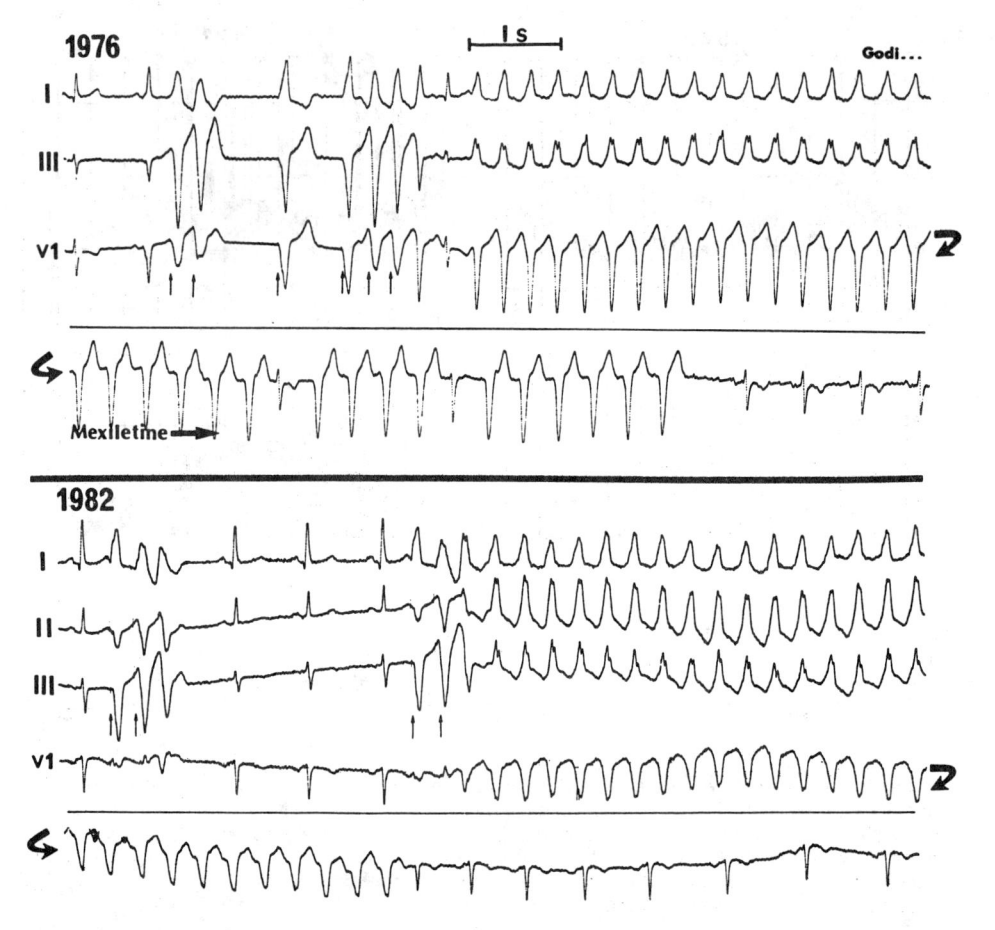

Figure 3: Inducible sustained and nonsustained VT. In the patient of Figure 2, the VT is inducible with a pair of ventricular stimuli. In 1976, the VT is sustained and has to be stopped by mexiletine, whereas it stops spontaneously in 1982, thus reproducing the spontaneous behavior of the arrhythmia.

tance of a guided strategy increases with the resistance of the arrhythmias which, as a consequence and almost by definition, becomes more frequent and thus amenable to Holter monitoring. The real problem is in fact to manage correctly the information provided by this technique.

The Commonly Used Classifications of Holter Data

Although many have been proposed, no classification of Holter data is really satisfactory. Schematically, two opposite ways can be followed: (1) to propose criteria based on importance or severity of arrhythmias on a priori basis; (2) to deduce from the patient's outcome the importance and the severity of arrhythmia on a posteriori basis.

A purely quantitative evaluation is appealing when a new technique providing numbers of events is proposed. This was initially done in the 1970s. It became rapidly apparent that the significance of arrhythmic events was more complex than their number alone. Lown's classification was a wise reaction against this initial trend. Actually, a single difference in morphology, repetitive activity, distribution, or coupling interval between two tracings containing a comparable amount of arrhythmias may be of crucial importance. On the other hand, if these variables are not correctly weighted, one may go too far in the other direction of an almost purely qualitative evaluation.

Numerous compromises were proposed between these two opposite trends, thus variously defining "simple" and "complex" arrhythmias. Reaching a common agreement in this matter would be as important as defining a standard protocol of programmed stimulation. This is still to be done and this state of things presently constitutes an important weakness of the noninvasive evaluation of arrhythmias. It would be equally important to combine the results of invasive and noninvasive EP. Rather than stressing their differences, we should look for their consistency. This was recently done by Gradman[17] who used a "repetition index" when he looked at results of ES in patients with or without repetitive activity on Holter. Now that much improvement has been achieved in the computerized analysis of Holter tracings, this technique becomes better adapted for comprehensive use. In addition to opposing nonrepetitive and repetitive arrhythmias, we think that the heart rate at which they occur should be considered as the third important parameter.[18]

Holter Monitoring and the Components of Arrhythmias

The real difficulty of managing the Holter data is to translate the information into terms of initiating factor, substrate, and autonomic nervous system (ANS) influence (Fig. 4). As long as this is not achieved, it is quite arbitrary to decide, for instance, that suppressing ES permits prediction of the prevention of VT, or that suppressing the repetitive activity is sufficient to prevent sudden death thereby neglecting in both instances that the main determinant of the therapeutic target may be its adrenergic-dependency. Evaluating separately these three components may be easy, for instance, in the case of ventricular fibrillation occurring at the end of an exercise test (Fig. 4), the arrhythmia substrate (VF) being triggered by the initiating factor (ES) in the setting of an increased sympathetic drive. Supposing that the patient was previously known to have an inducible VT and extrasystoles on Holter, the important consideration is to look for the reasons leading to VF. There is no chance of finding these either in the VF itself or in the initiating ES, but rather in the behavior of preceding rhythm.

The Experience of Recorded Sudden Death

In a recent cooperative study,[19] we examined 45 tapes of VF recorded during ambulatory monitoring. We found evidence of ischemia in only five cases, whereas it was present in 2/3 of 17 cases in which sudden death was due to cardiac

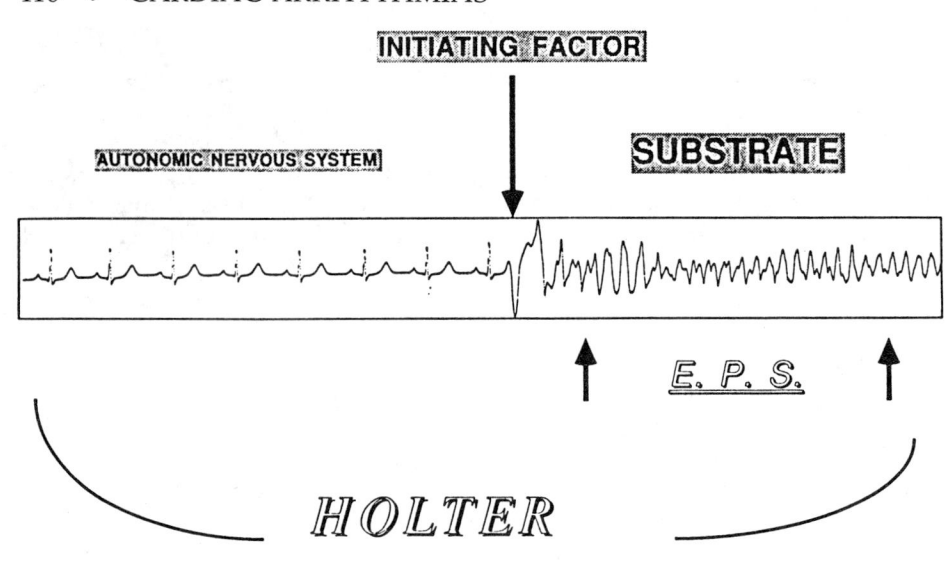

Figure 4: The three components of an arrhythmia and their analysis. Invasive EP study explores the arrhythmia substrate (with some limitations in the case of ventricular fibrillation) whereas Holter monitoring not only the tachyarrhythmia itself but also the initiating extrasystole and the background of the autonomic nervous system can be considered.

standstill or electromechanical dissociation. In contrast, the "environment" of VF cases in terms of heart rate revealed a significant trend of acceleration in the hour preceding VF, from 82 ± 22.8 beats per minute (mean ± SD) to 89.9 ± 24.8 ($p<0.001$), thus strongly suggesting an increasing sympathetic drive as a contributing factor. Eleven VF were primary and 34 were secondary to polymorphic (12 cases) or monomorphic VT (22 cases). Further markers of the role of adrenergic stimulation were also evidenced. A substantial number of ES preceded the terminal event in 35 cases, and in only 1/3 did their frequency increase by more than 50%, whereas the coupling interval dramatically shortened in the whole group from 446 ± 101 ms to 377 ± 77 ($p<0.001$). In 19 patients having previous nsVT, the duration of runs increased from 46 ± 22 beats to 453 ± 233 ($p<0.001$), and the nsVT rate accelerated from 219 ± 44 beats/min -1 to 236 ± 52 ($p<0.001$). Such observations shed some light on the mechanism of the demonstrated beneficial effect of beta-blockers in the prevention of sudden death. They also suggest how important it is to consider the relationship between the basic heart rate changes and parameters not restricted to the number of events.

Another important finding in this study was the frequent occurrence of a pause just preceding the lethal arrhythmia. It was present in 20 out of the 45 cases of VF, generally consecutive to ES, which were atrial or ventricular. Thus, an increased sympathetic drive and the existence of a cardiac pause appeared to be the two main determinants of sudden death in this study. It was logical to look after them in other arrhythmias; actually, they do not apply only to lethal, but also to life-threatening and even benign and more trivial arrhythmias (Fig. 5).

NO ARRHYHTMIA
(sinus rhythm)

ANS ± Long cycle ▶

▼

ISOLATED VPBs
("benign" arrhythmia)

ANS ± Long cycle ▶

▼▼

VENTRICULAR TACH.
("life-threatening" arrhythmia)

ANS ± Long cycle ▶

▼▼▼

VENTR. FIBRILLATION
(lethal arrhythmia)

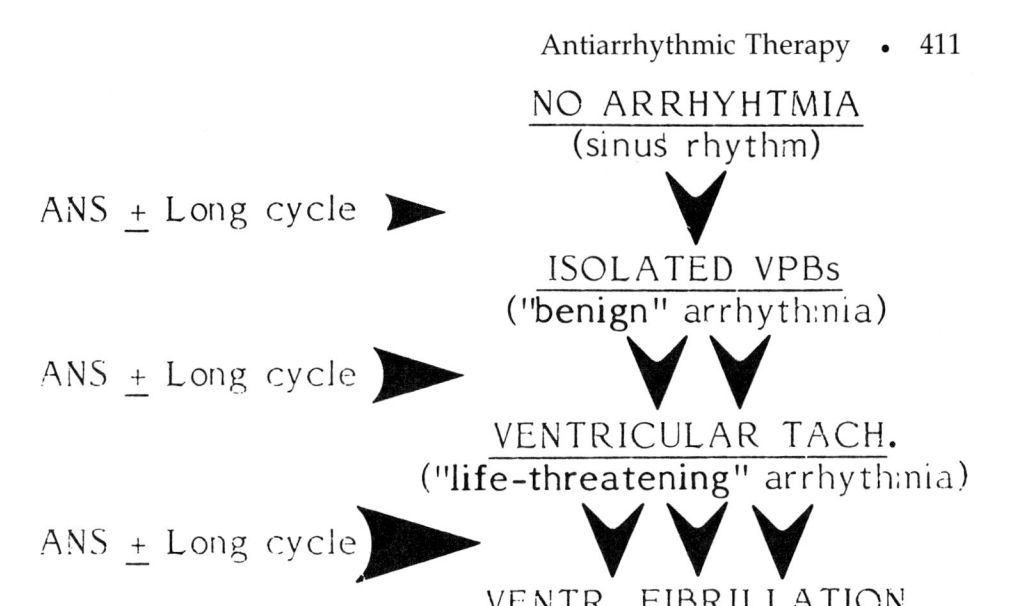

Figure 5: Common determinants of various arrhythmias. The role of the ANS and the presence of a long cycle just preceding the arrhythmia are the most common determinants of the various types of arrhythmias. From the benign to the lethal ones (see text).

A Continuous Spectrum from Benign to Lethal Arrhythmias: Their Common Determinants

We recently studied[20,21] the determinants of various forms of nsVT by analyzing the cycle length of the last preceding sinus beat and the mean heart rate during 3 minutes. Group A included 30 patients with recurrent monomorphic nsVT (86% with a left bundle branch block pattern and a normal or right axis deviation) without any evidence of heart disease. Group B also included 30 patients but with heart disease (18 coronary heart disease, 11 cardiomyopathies, 1 aortic stenosis) and various degrees of left ventricular dysfunction (mean ejection fraction of 41%). In this group, 18 patients had monomorphic VT (right bundle branch block pattern in 78% of the cases) and 12 had polymorphic nsVT.

Several thousands of events per patient per 24 hours were analyzed. The arrhythmias were classified as isolated ES (type 1), couplets (type 2), triplets (type 3), salvos of 4, 5, 6, to 10 and more than 10 beats of VT. The overall results concerning the mean RR interval during the 3 preceding minutes are displayed in Figure 6. In group A, correlation is highly significant ($r=0.98$, $p<0.001$) and reveals the strong relationship between the sympathetic tone and the type of arrhythmias. In group B, the relationship is still present but less marked ($r=0.58$, $p=0.16$).

In 65% of the cases (72% in group A and 57% in group B), a long cycle just preceded the repetitive phenomena. It was related either to a sudden sinus rate slowing or to a compensatory pause. A positive correlation was found between

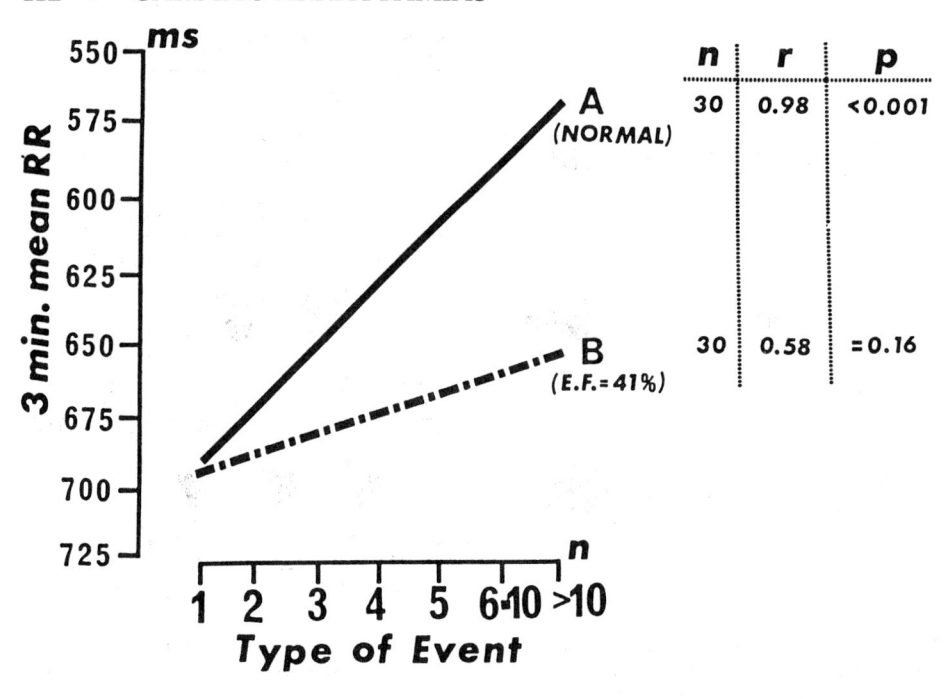

Figure 6: Relation between sympathetic drive and nonsustained VT. The mean RR interval during the 3 minutes before each arrhythmia is plotted against the type of arrhythmia: isolated ES (1), couplets (2), triplets (3), runs of 4 or 5, 6-to-10 (6-10) and more than 10 beats (> 10) of a nonsustained VT. The number of patients (n) in groups A and B is indicated on the right together with the correlation coefficient (r) of the regression line and the corresponding p value. Group A ("normal") consists of 30 cases without evidence of heart disease, and group B consists of 30 patients with a cardiopathy and heart failure with a mean ejection fraction (EF) of 41%. The less steep regression slope of group B does not reflect a lesser dependence on the sympathetic drive. On the contrary, it probably illustrates the adrenergic paradox phenomenon (see text).

this cycle length and the duration of the repetitive rhythm in both groups ($r=0.84$, $p<0.05$ in A, and $r=0.89$, $p<0.05$ in B). The value of this cycle was equivalent in the two groups (863 ± 36 ms in A, 883 ± 121 in B), but the phenomenon was less frequent in group B (8/30) than in group A (14/30), with less bigeminy or trigeminy resulting in cycle length oscillations (Fig. 7).

Finally, a comparison of the mean heart rate in patients with and without a pause preceding the initial ES showed that it was slower in the former than in the latter (Fig. 8). This reveals a balance between the two main determinants of the repetitive activity. A third, less contributive but frequent determinant of the repetitive activity was the coupling interval of the initial extrasystole: in 60% of group A patients and in 40% of group B patients a longer coupling interval clearly favored a more prolonged repetitive activity. However, this trend was not significant for the whole group because it was somewhat counterbalanced by the opposite trend of a shorter coupling interval at higher rates.

Antiarrhythmic Therapy • 413

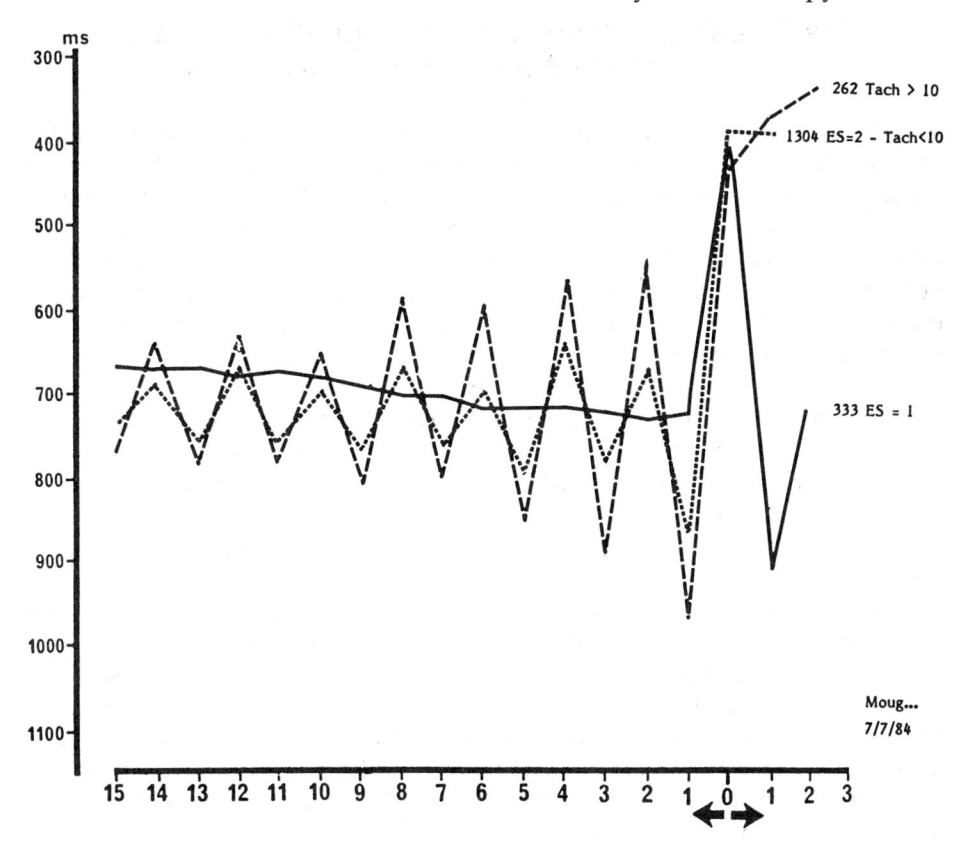

Figure 7: Long cycles and the repetitive response. Three types of ventricular arrhythmias have been collected in the 24-hour ambulatory monitoring and the 15 preceding and three following cycles have been systematically collected for the 333 isolated extrasystoles (ES) (solid curve), the 1304 runs of 2 to less than 10 beats (dotted line), and the 262 nonsustained VT of more than 10-beat duration (dashed line). The coupling interval (cycle 0) as well as the mean heart rate are not significantly different discriminants ($p<0.001$) of the events, with an oscillatory pattern reflecting a more or less prolonged bigeminy.

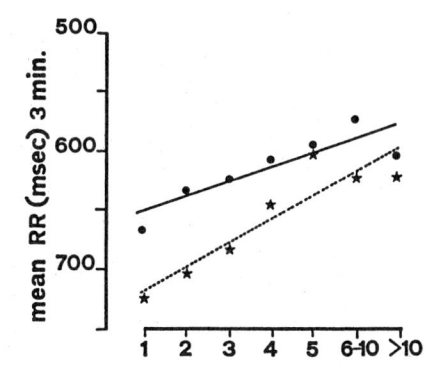

Figure 8: Interaction of the two determinants of the repetitive response: the sympathetic drive and the long cycle. Considering patients according to the presence (stars) or absence (circles) of a long cycle before the various types of repetitive response from 2 to more than 10 beats shows that the mean heart rate during the 3 minutes preceding each of the events is slower when a long cycle is present. The need for a greater sympathetic drive is clearly less marked in these patients than in those in whom this determinant is lacking.

The Rate-Dependency, the Adrenergic-Dependency, and the Adrenergic Paradox

The arrhythmia components depend differently on heart rate and on the sympathetic drive. Rate-dependency and adrenergic dependency are by no means synonyms in rhythmology. The rate-dependency of an EP mechanism is directly related to the length of the one or very few preceding cardiac cycles. The adrenergic-dependency relates to the level of sympathetic drive necessary for the EP phenomenon to occur, independent of heart rate. In the clinical setting, the difficulty is to dissociate these two concepts, as we are accustomed to take the heart rate as the marker of the sympathetic drive. Although this is generally true, there are important exceptions. At the end of exercise, a dramatic sinus rate slowing favoring ES coincides with a still elevated sympathetic drive leading to repetitive activity. This explains the frequent onset of tachyarrhythmias in such conditions. In practice, we have just seen that the most convenient way for distinguishing the two determinants is to consider separately the few last cycles preceding the arrhythmia, versus the heart rate environment over a longer scale of a few minutes.

The two arrhythmia components are usually not dependent to the same extent on rate and sympathetic drive. Isolated extrasystoles (the initiating factor) are essentially rate-dependent, a fact that can be studied by comparing the cycle length of sinus beats followed or not followed by an ES. As shown in Figure 9, a "window" of cardiac rate can thus be found with a lower and an upper rate limit. This is in fact a quantified evaluation of the rule of bigeminy,[22] but to realize how complex these phenomena are, one must also know that the thresholds themselves may vary a little with the sympathetic drive, and that within the limits of this window, the extrasystolic rate may be directly (Fig. 10) or inversely related to the heart rate. Conversely, we have just seen that repetitive activity, mainly related to the sympathetic drive, also partly depends on the last cycle length.

Finally, the dependence on the sympathetic drive may be difficult to evidence for a theoretical reason which probably explains why it is largely underestimated. If one accepts that an increasing heart rate preceding the arrhythmia onset indicates sympathetic drive as a contributing factor, one should realize that the more the arrhythmia is sensitive to the sympathetics, the smaller the necessary amount of adrenergic stimulation, hence the less apparent the sinus rate changes. This is what we call the "adrenergic paradox," which seems to apply particularly to diseased hearts.[12,21] It may be the explanation of the particularly beneficial effect of beta-blockers in the prevention of sudden death in patients with heart failure,[23] in the same way that the antiarrhythmic efficacy of these drugs is more evident in patients with diseased hearts than in idiopathic ventricular arrhythmias.[24]

Decision-Making Process in Noninvasive EP Investigation

A correct treatment strategy supposes that the arrhythmia components and their determinants have been identified. The symptomatic arrhythmia results from the combination of the initiating factor and the activated substrate, both of

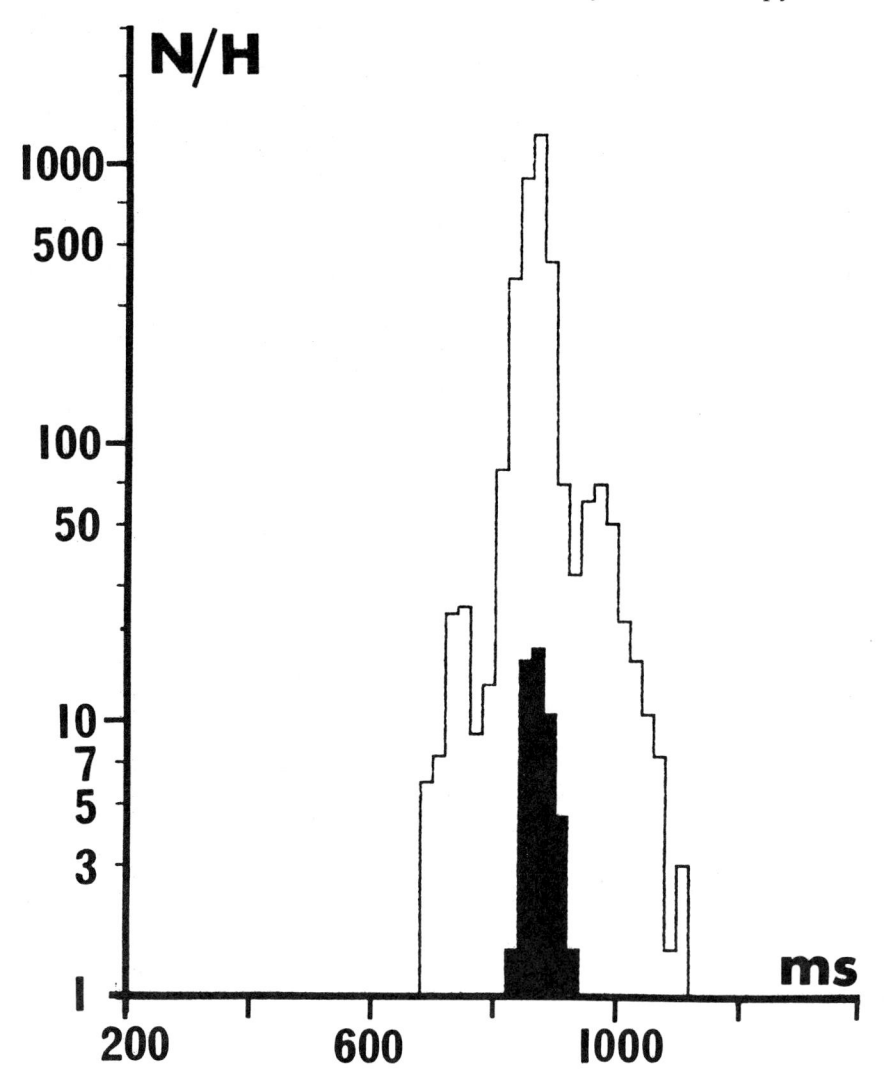

Figure 9: Histograms of the sinus cycle length and the rate-dependency phenomenon. The cycle length of the sinus beats immediately followed (black area) or not followed (open area) by a ventricular extrasystole were systematically collected and distributed in 20 ms classes. This figure clearly illustrates the sinus rate-dependency of ventricular extrasystoles.

them being subject to the ANS influence. Suppressing either component or all of them may result in controlling the arrhythmia itself, and identifying them may be more or less easy:

1. The initiating factor is usually formed by an isolated ES but it may well be that in a particular patient only a certain category of ES will trigger the substrate according to their morphology, or coupling interval, or occasional repetition.

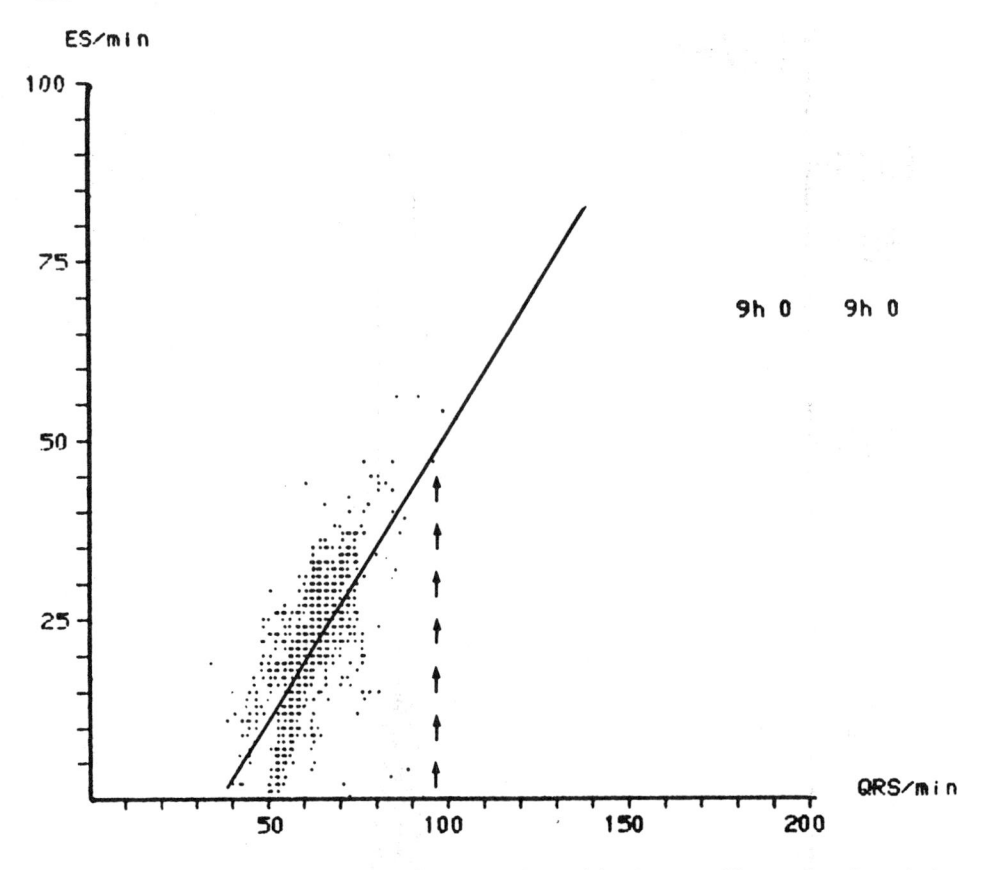

Figure 10: Relation between the number of extrasystoles and the sinus rate. The number of ventricular extrasystoles (ES/min) is plotted against the mean heart rate (QRS/min) during a 24-hour period starting at 9:00 am. The regression line clearly shows the positive correlation between the two parameters in this patient having a cardiopathy. In other situations, particularly in idiopathic arrhythmias, the number of extrasystoles decreases as the heart rate increases. The arrows point to the upper threshold where the extrasystolic decreases as the heart rate increases, and to the upper threshold where the extrasystolic phenomenon disappears.

2. The substrate usually consists of the repetitive activity, sustained or not.

3. Both of them depend on the ANS, directly or indirectly, and not necessarily to the same extent according to the nature and mechanism of the arrhythmia, the patient, the etiology of the disease, and the degree of heart failure. The arrhythmia variability depends on all these parameters.

Figure 11 is an attempt to schematize the prognostic and therapeutic decision-making progress, supposing that the three arrhythmia components are correctly evaluated. Some combinations are not compatible as they suppose opposite clinical outcomes: true negatives or false positives for one component with true positives or false negatives for the other. Areas 1 to 4 define the absence of arrhythmia in the follow-up of a treated patient after the initial evaluation, whereas areas 5 to 8 define the relapses. Considering the diagram, one realizes

Antiarrhythmic Therapy • 417

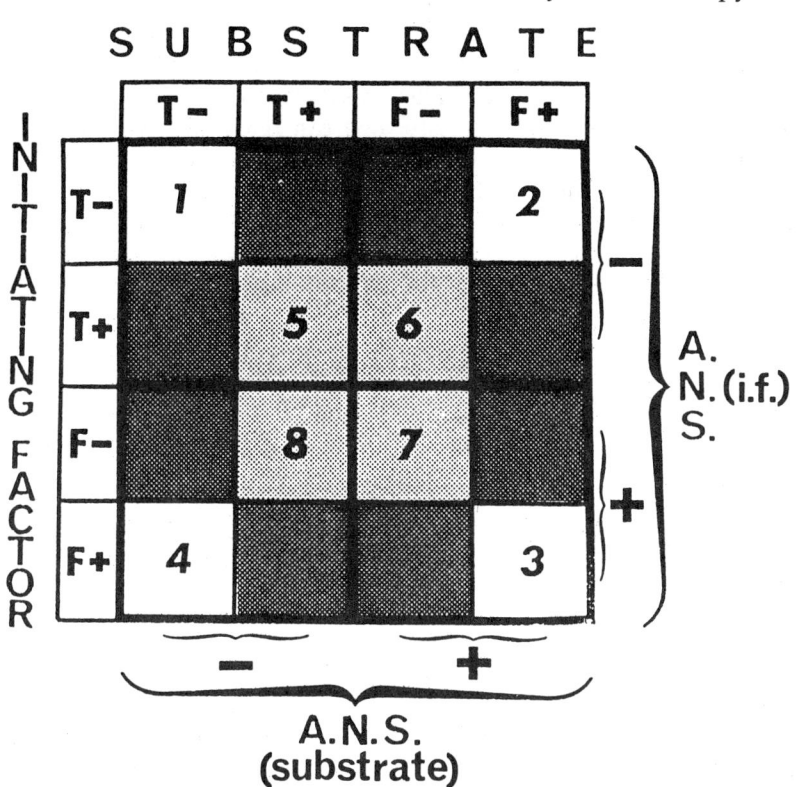

Figure 11: The process of prognostic and therapeutic decision making. Parameters concerning the substrate and the initiating factor have been collected. Their more (+) or less (-) marked sensitivity to the autonomic nervous system (ANS) of the substrate and of the initiating factor (i.f.) is supposed to be known as well as their chance to produce false negatives (F-) or false positives (F+), true negatives (T-), or true positives (T+), respectively. Black areas represent incompatible combinations as far as the follow-up is concerned, open areas (1,2,3,4) represent a free-of-arrhythmia outcome, and grey areas (5,6,7,8) indicate patients having arrhythmias during the follow-up. If the data concerning the three arrhythmia components are correct, it is theoretically possible to predict the prognosis or the therapeutic effect from the initial evaluation (see text for discussion).

that a good outcome may result from the true negatives, i.e., complete and permanent disappearance of ES forming the initiating factor (areas 1 and 2) or the true control of the repetitive activity forming the substrate (areas 1 and 4). At the same time one must admit that such a good outcome may be partly (areas 2 and 4) or even entirely (area 3) coincidental. The false positive response of either component consists of its transient or apparent presence at the time of control, but its disappearance or the absence of its combination with the other during the follow-up. Relapses (area 5 to 8) may also result from various combinations of true positives and false negatives. In other words, the real problem in predicting the outcome from the results of our initial test is not only to identify correctly the two components forming the arrhythmia, but also to have a good evaluation of the probability of true or false responses.[6]

A better identification of true and false responses can be approached rather simply by repeating the tests, and this is obviously easier with noninvasive than with invasive testing. If repeated Holter monitorings show the constant disappearances of ES and repetitive activity, one can reasonably conclude that the control is permanent rather than occasional. The statistical significance of ES reduction in drug evaluation has been largely debated. Studying their variability is presently the best way to resolve the permanent problem of the reliability of our tests. Another way to cope with this difficulty is to evaluate not the variability itself but its reasons. Among them, the importance of ANS can be assessed by ambulatory monitoring.

Assuming that the dependency of the initiating factor and the substrate on the sympathetic drive can be assessed correctly and that their variability is indeed related to this dependency, then the probability for true or false responses can be approached. This is what we have figured in the diagram (Fig. 10). Supposing that neither component is influenced by the sympathetic tone (-), the predictability of the tests is certainly much better (areas 1 and 5) than in the opposite situation (+) of a strong dependency (areas 3 and 7). Of course, intermediate situations can also be conceived (areas 2–6 and 4–8).

Conclusions

We agree that this discussion about the state of the art of ambulatory monitoring data analysis is for the time being rather theoretical. The use of invasive and noninvasive EP techniques have not yet definitely convinced the majority of cardiologists to abandon their traditionally empirical treatment habits. Simply put, the most important drawback of empiricism is that, as it collects no data, it will never allow us to increase our knowledge. The most important drawback of the invasive approach is that, although technically precise, it suffers from the fundamental limitation of addressing only one of the three components of arrhythmias: the substrate. Finally, the most important limitation of noninvasive EP is that the vast amount of information about the three arrhythmia components is complex and difficult to investigate, which explains why a large part of it is neglected. However, we believe that in the future it will probably be more rewarding in terms of comprehension and practical application in the management of clinical arrhythmias.

References

1. Swerdlow CD, Gong G, Echt DS, Winkle RA, Griffin JC, Ross DL, Mason JW. Clinical factors predicting successful electrophysiologic study in patients with ventricular tachycardia. JACC 1983;1:409–415.
2. Spielman SR, Schwartz S, McCarthy DM, Horowitz LN, Greenspan AM, Sadowsky LM, Josephson ME, Waxman ML. Predictors of the success or failure of medical therapy in patients with chronic recurrent sustained ventricular tachycardia: a discriminant analysis. JACC 1983;1:401–408.
3. Swiryn S, Bauernfeind RA, Strasberg B, Palileo E, Iverson N, Levy PS, Rosen KM. Predictors of response to class I anti-arrhythmic drugs during electrophysiologic study of ventricular tachycardia. Am Heart J 1982;104:43–50.

4. Breithardt G, Borgreffe M, Abendroth RR. Serial electrophysiologic testing of arrhythmic drug efficacy in patients with recurrent ventricular tachycardia. Eur Heart J 1980;1:11–20.
5. Brugada P, Wellens HJJ. Programmed electrical stimulation of the heart in ventricular arrhythmias. Am J Cardiol 1985;56:187–190.
6. Brugada P, Wellens HJJ. Need and design of a prospective study to assess the value of different strategic approaches for management of ventricular tachycardia or fibrillation. Am J Cardiol 1986;57:1180–1184.
7. Breithardt G, Borggreffe M, Podczeck A. Electrophysiology and Pharmacology of asymptomatic nonsustained ventricular tachycardia. Clin Prog Pacing Electrophysiol 1986;4:81–99.
8. Duff HJ, Mitchell LB, Wyse DG. Antiarrhythmic efficacy of propranolol: comparison of low and high serum concentration. JACC 1986;8:959–965.
9. Woosley RL, Kornhauser DK, Smith RL et al. Suppression of chronic ventricular arrhythmias with propanolol. Circulation 1979;60:819–827.
10. McPherson CA, Rosenfield LE, Batsford WP. Day-to-day reproducibility of responses of right ventricular programmed electrical stimulation: implications for serial drug testing. Am J Cardiol 1985;55:689–695.
11. Duff HJ, Mitchell LB, Wyse DG. Programmed electrical stimulation studies for ventricular tachycardia induction in humans. II. Comparison of indwelling electrode catheter and daily catheter replacement. JACC 1986;8:576–581.
12. Pratt CM, Slymen DJ, Wierman AM, Francis MJ, Seals AA, Quinones MA, Roberts R. Analysis of the spontaneous variability of ventricular arrhythmias: consecutive ambulatory electrocardiographic recordings of ventricular tachycardia. Am J Cardiol 1985; 56:67–72.
13. Platia EV, Reid PR. Nonsustained ventricular tachycardia during programmed ventricular stimulation: criteria for a positive test. Am J Cardiol 1985;56:79–83.
14. Wit AL, Cranefield P, Gadsby DC. Electrogenic sodium extrusion can stop triggered activity in the canine coronary sinus. Circ Res 1981;49:1029–1042.
15. Morady F, DiCarlo LA, Halter JB, de Buitler M, Krol RB, Baerman JM. The plasma catecholamine response to ventricular tachycardia induction and external countershock during electrophysiologic testing. JACC 1986;8:584–591.
16. Coumel Ph, Leclercq JF, Slama R. Repetitive monomorphic idiopathic ventricular tachycardia. In Zipes DP, Jalife J, eds. Cardiac Electrophysiology and Arrhythmias. NY, Grune & Stratton 1985;457–468.
17. Gradman AH, Batsford WP, Rieur EC, Leon L, Van Zetta AM. Ambulatory electrocardiographic correlates of ventricular inducibility during programmed electrical stimulation. JACC 1985;5:1087–1093.
18. Coumel Ph, Leclercq JF, Maisonblanche P, Attuel P, Cauchemez B. Computerized analysis of dynamic electrocardiograms: a tool for comprehensive electrophysiology. A description of the ATREC II system. Clin Progress 1985;3:181–201.
19. Leclercq JF, Coumel Ph, Maisonblanche P, Cauchemez B, Zimmerman M, Chouty F, Slama R. Mise en evidence des mecanismes determinants de la mort subite. Enquete cooperative portant sur 69 cas enregistres par la methode de Holter. Arch Mal Coeur 1986;79:1024–1036.
20. Zimmerman M, Maisonblanche P, Cauchemez B, Leclercq JF, Coumel Ph. Determinants of the spontaneous ectopic activity in repetitive monomorphic idiopathic ventricular tachycardia. JACC 1986;7:1219–1227.
21. Zimmerman M, Maisonblanche P, Cauchemez B, Leclercq JF, Coumel Ph. Determinants de l' activite repetitive dans les tachycardies ventriculaires en salves. Arch Mal Coeur 1986;79:1420–1428.
22. Langendorf R, Pick A, Winternitz MI. Appearance of ectopic beats dependent upon length of the ventricular cycle, the "ruel of bigeminy." Circulation 1955;11:422–430.
23. Chadda K, Goldstein S, Byington R, Curb JD. Effect of propranolol after acute myocardial infarction in patients with congestive heart failure. Circulation 1986;73:503–510.
24. Coumel Ph, Rosengarten MD, Leclercq JF, Attuel P. Role of sympathetic nervous system in non-ischemic ventricular arrhythmias. Br Heart J 1982;47:137–143.

26

The Preference of Programmed Stimulation-Guided Therapy for Sustained Ventricular Arrhythmias

Charles Gottlieb
Mark E. Josephson*

Potentially lethal ventricular tachycardias are a frequent complication of organic heart disease. Most commonly, these arrhythmias are encountered in patients with coronary artery disease and cardiomyopathies. Studies dating back to the 1930's have reported a high mortality rate in this population.[1-4] Because these arrhythmic events occur relatively infrequently and with unpredictable timing, empiric therapy often met with both failure and side effects. Therefore, therapeutic strategies based on potential markers of sustained arrhythmias were developed. Ambulatory electrocardiographic (Holter) monitoring and intracardiac electrophysiologic studies were two clinical techniques most commonly employed to guide antiarrhythmic therapy.[5-13] The former approach assumes that ventricular ectopic activity is a marker for sustained arrhythmias and that abolition of this ambient ectopy will prevent recurrences of sustained ventricular arrhythmias. On the other hand, inducibility of ventricular arrhythmias during programmed stimulation is felt to be a predictive marker for clinical recurrence. Patients who have a ventricular arrhythmia which is inducible in a drug-free state and which is subsequently noninducible after the institution of antiarrhythmic therapy are felt to have a good prognosis in the absence of intercurrent events.

The ability of programmed ventricular extrastimuli to provoke the presenting

---

From: Brugada P, Wellens HJJ. CARDIAC ARRHYTHMIAS: Where To Go From Here? Mount Kisco, NY, Futura Publishing Company, Inc., © 1987.

*Dr. Josephson is the Robinette Foundation Professor of Medicine (Cardiovascular Diseases).

arrhythmia in the baseline state is dependent upon the clinical arrhythmia that is being evaluated, the underlying cardiac disease, and the "aggressiveness" of the stimulation protocol.[14-16] The sensitivity for induction of ventricular arrhythmias during programmed stimulation is generally higher when the documented clinical arrhythmia is sustained uniform ventricular tachycardia than it is in patients presenting with cardiac arrest.[15] Factors intrinsic to the stimulation protocol that effect sensitivity include: (1) the number of extrastimuli delivered,[14-24] (2) the number of ventricular stimulation sites,[14,16,14-27] and (3) drive cycle lengths,[14,27,28] as well as (4) current strengths employed.[24,29]

Doherty et al.[26] evaluated the sensitivity of programmed ventricular stimulation at a second right ventricular site. Twenty-two of 38 patients (58%) with a history of documented sustained ventricular tachycardia or fibrillation, but without induction during right ventricular apical stimulation, had their arrhythmia induced with right ventricular outflow tract stimulation using a comparable number of extrastimuli. Morady et al.[20] found only a small yield from stimulation at a second right ventricular site after completion of a protocol which included triple ventricular stimulation at the right ventricular apex. However, given that specificity is compromised as the number of extrastimuli are increased and that the "ease" of induction during serial drug studies may be site-specific, we currently recommend stimulation at two areas within the right ventricle.

The sensitivity of programmed stimulation for induction of sustained ventricular tachycardia is critically dependent on the number of extrastimuli delivered.[14-24] The sensitivity for one ventricular extrastimuli is in the range of 20-50% while for double ventricular extrastimuli it appears to be 40% to 75%. With triple ventricular extrastimuli, the sensitivity of programmed electrical stimulation can approach 95% (Fig. 1). The stimulation protocol used to initiate sustained ventric-

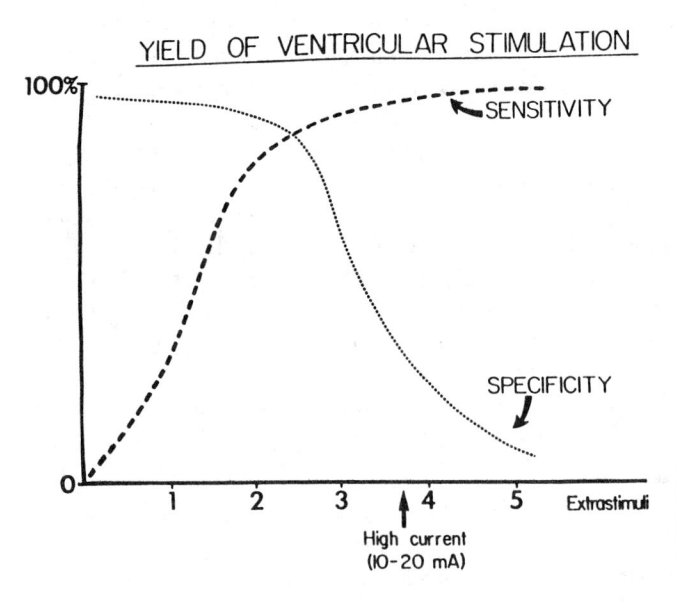

Figure 1: An idealized representation of the sensitivity and specificity of programmed electrical stimulation for ventricular tachycardia.

ular tachycardia in 461 patients who presented to our institution with this clinical arrhythmia was evaluated (Fig. 2). Including all stimulation modalities attempted, 433 patients (94%) had inducible sustained uniform ventricular tachycardia. Four hundred and six patients had their tachycardias initiated with right ventricular stimulation and 27 required access to the left ventricle for induction. One hundred and sixteen tachycardias (27%) were initiated with a single ventricular extrastimuli and 210 tachycardias (48%) were initiated with double ventricular extrastimuli. Rapid ventricular pacing had an additional yield of only 3% (11 patients) while 21% (89 patients) required triple ventricular extrastimuli for induction of sustained ventricular tachycardia. Of note, however, is that in 8/11 patients in whom rapid pacing was required to initiate ventricular tachycardia only double extrastimuli were used. Our experience since always employing three extrastimuli suggests almost all of those induced with rapid pacing would have been induced with triple extrastimuli. Had quadruple extrastimuli not been given, seven patients would have been considered noninducible. Thus, we have found that using a stimulation protocol that includes stimulation with up to three extrastimuli (and rapid ventricular pacing) at two pacing cycle lengths at two right ventricular sites will initiate sustained uniform ventricular tachycardia in 85–95% of patients who present with this clinical arrhythmia.[15] Four ventricular extrastimuli and left ventricular stimulation will have a small additional yield of 2–10%.[15,20,23,24]

The sensitivity of programmed electrical stimulation in patients who present with a cardiac arrest is markedly lower than in those who present with sustained monomorphic ventricular tachycardia.[15,20] Of 299 patients who presented at our institution up to January of 1986 with cardiac arrest, 226 (76%) had an arrhythmia induced with programmed stimulation. One hundred and eighty-one patients

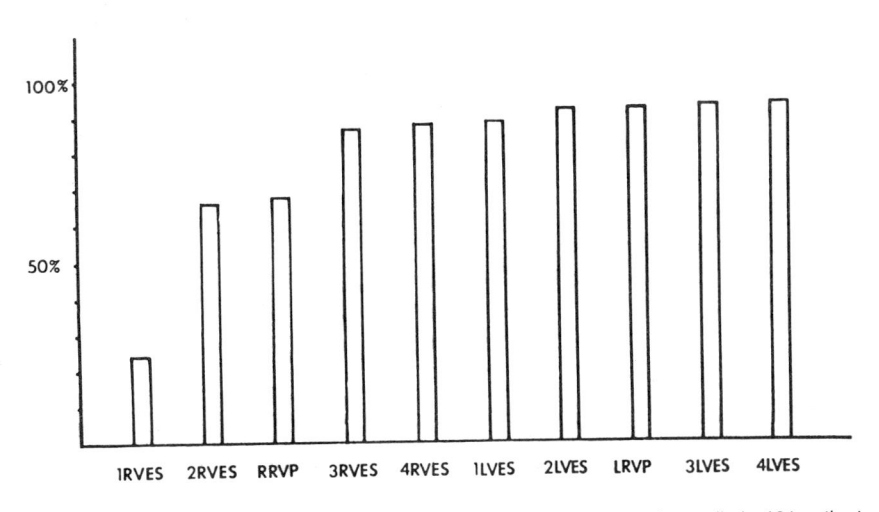

Figure 2: The cumulative percentage yield for induction of ventricular tachycardia in 461 patients who presented to the Hospital of the University of Pennsylvania for evaluation of ventricular tachycardia. RVES = right ventricular extrastimuli; RRVP = right ventricular rapid pacing; LRVP = left ventricular rapid pacing.

had sustained ventricular tachycardia or ventricular fibrillation induced, while 45 patients had a nonsustained ventricular tachycardia induced. If one analyzes only the last 4 years, our inducibility rate in patients presenting with cardiac arrest has been 83%, primarily due to consistent use of three extrastimuli.

The specificity of programmed electrical stimulation is more difficult to ascertain not only because of the limited number of patients who undergo programmed stimulation in the absence of malignant arrhythmias, but also because of its dependence on the presence of heart disease in the "control" population. With one ventricular extrastimuli, the specificity of programmed stimulation approaches 100%.[14,17,18,21,23,30-32] If all ventricular arrhythmias that are induced but have not been seen clinically are considered a false-positive response, the specificity with two ventricular extrastimuli remains high at approximately 90%.[14,17,18,21,23,30-32] There is a substantial decline in the specificity when three ventricular extrastimuli are used.[14,18,21,23,24,32] However, in patients without structural heart disease and no history or suspicion of ventricular arrhythmias, it is exceedingly rare to induce a sustained monomorphic ventricular tachycardia.[14,21,30,33] Patients with coronary artery disease and cardiac arrest are more likely to have a sustained arrhythmia induced than are those with no heart disease or cardiomyopathy.

While up to 25% of patients who present with cardiac arrest are noninducible in the baseline state and therefore not candidates for therapy guided by programmed stimulation, only 4-10% of patients with documented sustained monomorphic ventricular tachycardia cannot be evaluated by this strategy. Even the most ardent proponents of ambulatory electrocardiographic monitoring for control of malignant arrhythmias have found that 25% of patients with a history of sustained ventricular tachyarrhythmias lack sufficient ventricular ectopic activity in the baseline state upon which to base therapy.[34]

High degrees of ventricular ectopic activity can be found in patients without structural heart disease who are usually at a very low risk of sudden death due to malignant tachyarrhythmias.[35] Even those patients at high risk show marked variability in spontaneously occurring ectopy. Winkle[36] has shown that there is marked variability in ventricular premature depolarization frequency over half-hour time frames in individual patients, and Morganroth et al.[37] as well as Michelson et al.[38] have shown that this variability in both simple and complex ectopy is present from hour to hour, day to day, and month to month. Thus, the response to an antiarrhythmic agent that is interpreted as a drug effect may be mimicked by spontaneous variability. This is of particular importance if abolition of nonsustained ventricular tachycardia (which is often a low frequency spontaneous event) is the sole therapeutic end-point achieved on ambulatory electrocardiographic monitoring. In fact, if fewer than five episodes of nonsustained ventricular tachycardia occur in the baseline state over the recording period, then electrocardiographic monitoring utilizing abolition of nonsustained ventricular tachycardia as a therapeutic end-point should not be employed.[39]

The best therapeutic strategy is that which optimizes sensitivity and specificity and yields the highest predictive values. The sensitivity and specificity of programmed stimulation in predicting the clinical outcome of therapy for ventricular arrhythmias has been evaluated by a number of investigators.[5-7,40-44] The negative predictive value of programmed stimulation with classical antiarrhythmic agents (that is, the lack of clinical recurrence or sudden cardiac death if an antiarrhythmic agent is found which renders the arrhythmia noninducible) is excellent and ranges from 80–100% (see Table I). The ability of programmed stimulation to predict recurrence (the positive predictive accuracy) is variable from center to center and ranges from 30–100%. This variability may be explained on the basis of differences in stimulation protocol, definition of inducibility, therapeutic end-points, patient selection and referrals, and duration of clinical follow-up. Nevertheless, electropharmacologically guided therapy does allow for determination of a subset of patients who present with malignant ventricular arrhythmias who will have a good prognosis.

There is much less data available to allow evaluation of the sensitivity, specificity, and predictive values of noninvasive guided therapies with class I antiarrhythmic agents. Graboys et al.[11] followed 122 patients for an average of 32 months using ambulatory electrocardiographic monitoring and exercise stress testing to guide antiarrhythmic administration. Sixty-seven patients presented with ventricular fibrillation and 56 with hemodynamically compromising ventricular tachycardia. There were only six sudden deaths in the individuals who were "controlled" as compared with 17 sudden deaths in the 25 patients who were described as "uncontrolled." This would yield positive and negative predictive values of 68% and 73%, respectively, for this noninvasive approach. Unfortunately, these excellent results have not been well substantiated by other investigators.

If the noninvasive and invasive approaches yielded similar results, then it might be expected that there should be some concordance between the two methods. This has, in general, not been found to be the case. Herling et al.[45] found that although successful electropharmacologically guided therapy was often associated with a marked decrease in spontaneous ventricular ectopic activity, patients treated empirically who had clinical recurrences often (38%) had marked suppression of their arrhythmias on ambulatory electrocardiographic monitoring. Conversely, Holter monitoring after curative subendocardial resection for sustained ventricular tachycardia revealed that complex ectopy was

Table I
PES in Ventricular Arrhythmias

	Number of Patients Evaluated	Mean Follow-up Period (months)	REC and/or SCD NOT predicted By PES	REC and/or SCD predicted by PES	Sensitivity	Specificity	Positive Predictive Value	Negative Predictive Value
Swerdlow (1983)	239	15	12/100 (12%)	20/63 (32%)	63%	67%	32%	88%
Horowitz (1982)	111	18	4/65 (6%)	42/46 (91%)	91%	94%	91%	94%
Roy (1983)	119	17	4/24 (17%)	4/18 (22%)	50%	59%	22%	83%
Mason (1978)	33	8	1/14 (7%)	2/3 (67%)	67%	93%	67%	93%
Podrid (1983)	52	21	1/36 (3%)	5/9 (56%)	83%	89%	56%	97%
Ruskin (1980)	31	15	0/19 (0%)	3/6 (50%)	100%	86%	50%	100%
Skale (1986)	62	22	0/14 (0%)	10/25 (40%)	100%	48%	40%	100%
Horowitz (1978)	20	12	0/13 (0%)	7/7 (100%)	100%	100%	100%	100%
Kim (1986)	52	18	10/25 (40%)	8/27 (30%)	44%	44%	30%	60%

PES = programmed electrical stimulation; REC = recurrence; SCD = sudden cardiac death.

frequently present. Thus, Holter monitor recording did not predict the clinical response of antiarrhythmic therapy guided by electrophysiologic testing.

Kim et al.[46] similarly found a discordance between the results of electrophysiologic evaluation and the ambulatory electrocardiographic monitoring in patients treated with type 1A antiarrhythmic agents. In 54 patients referred for evaluation of recurrent sustained ventricular tachycardia or ventricular fibrillation, efficacy as predicted by programmed stimulation (i.e., noninducibility) and Holter monitoring (reduction of VPD frequency by 83% and abolition of ventricular tachycardia) showed concordance only 50% of the time. As noted by the authors, the source of this discordant result was therapy deemed to be efficacious by Holter monitoring but ineffective by programmed stimulation (Fig. 3). Unfortunately, because no information on clinical follow-up was presented, the predictive accuracy of each method could not be evaluated. We have similarly found that when discordance between these two therapeutic strategies exist with respect to predictive efficacies, the discordance is always in the subset of patients who would be predicted to respond to a particular antiarrhythmic agent by Holter criteria but not by programmed stimulation.

The negative predictive value of programmed stimulation is extremely high (that is, the ability of a noninducible electrophysiologic study to predict nonrecurrence) compared with the test's ability to predict recurrences (the positive predictive accuracy). Therefore, noninducibility during programmed stimulation may select a population that would not be likely to have recurrences in the absence of medication. This reasoning has recently been suggested by Platia et al.[47] to be incorrect. Thirty-three patients with recurrent sustained ventricular

	EPS PREDICTED	
HOLTER PREDICTED	EFFECTIVE	INEFFECTIVE
EFFECTIVE	11	32
INEFFECTIVE	10	31

Figure 3: Data presented by Kim et al.[46] showing the discordance between therapy predicted to be effective by programmed stimulation compared to that predicted effective by Holter monitoring criteria.

tachycardia all inducible in the baseline state and who subsequently became noninducible on antiarrhythmic therapy were followed for 11 to 33 months. All 33 patients either lowered the dose of their medication or discontinued it altogether. Twenty-eight patients (85%) had arrhythmia recurrence or sudden cardiac death.

As noted above, conventional antiarrhythmic therapy guided by noninvasive strategies would be predicted to be efficacious more frequently than antiarrhythmic therapy guided by programmed stimulation.[46] Since the majority of patients continue to remain inducible during programmed stimulation on antiarrhythmic therapy, it is therefore important to determine whether the invasive electrophysiologic test is nonspecific and therefore overpredicts failure of therapy or whether ambulatory electrocardiographic monitoring is insensitive and therefore overpredicting drug success. Although there has not been a large randomized study completed to answer this specific question, there are several series that compare the relative efficacies of these two therapeutic strategies (Table II).[44,46,48-50] The results of these studies with their inherent biases (which may favor programmed stimulation), strongly suggest that noninducibility during programmed electrical stimulation successfully predicts nonrecurrence (though the ability of this test to predict recurrences is not nearly as accurate) while a seemingly therapeutic response by Holter monitoring criteria tends to overpredict success. A notable exception to this trend is the data presented by Kim et al.[46] who had a not inconsequential number of recurrences in their noninducible patients. Since the recurrence of a sustained ventricular tachyarrhythmia is potentially a fatal event, it seems prudent, pending the results of a large randomized trial, to guide therapy with a strategy that errs in overpredicting drug failure.

Of the recently approved antiarrhythmic agents, flecainide appears to be a drug whose therapeutic efficacy in sustained ventricular arrhythmias may be evaluated by programmed stimulation. Webb et al.[51] recently reported on 24 patients with sustained ventricular tachyarrhythmias. Twenty-two percent of the patients became noninducible on flecainide. Five of the 10 patients who remained inducible on flecainide suffered from recurrence or sudden cardiac death as compared with no recurrences in the patients who were rendered noninducible. This would yield positive and negative predictive values for programmed stimulation with flecainide of 50% and 100%, respectively. Since only patients with a demonstrated Holter response were continued on flecainide, the predictive accuracy of ambulatory monitoring cannot be adequately assessed in this group.

Table II
PES vs. Holter Monitoring in Ventricular Arrhythmias

	Number of Patients Evaluated	Mean Follow-up Period (months)	REC and/or SCD if Therapy Efficacious by PES	REC and/or SCD if Therapy not Efficacious by PES	PES Positive Predictive Value	PES Negative Predictive Value	Holter Positive Predictive Value	Holter Negative Predictive Value
Mitchell (1986)	106	N/A	14%	43%	N/A	N/A	N/A	N/A
Chua (1983)	95	15	6%	27%	55%	94%	17%	73%
Platia (1984)	44	18	6%	50%	88%	94%	70%	50%
Skale (1986)	62	22	0%	44%	40%	100%	N/A	56%
Kim (1986)	65	19	40%	30%	30%	40%	N/A	70%

PES = programmed electrical stimulation; REC = recurrence; SCD= =sudden cardiac death.

Nevertheless, the recurrence rate was 50% in patients in whom flecainide was considered to be efficacious by Holter criteria.

The value of clinical electrophysiologic testing in evaluation of amiodarone for malignant ventricular arrhythmias has been controversial.[53-63] Because of its potential toxic side effects, this antiarrhythmic agent is often used only after type 1 agents have failed. It is therefore not surprising that the frequency of noninducibility during programmed stimulation in this population is relatively low. Also, because of the relatively long half-life of amiodarone, the clinical efficacy may not be achieved acutely. Controversy still exists as to whether the interval between the initiation of therapy and subsequent programmed stimulation affects the inducibility.[64,65,72,73] These limitations notwithstanding, there are several studies that have attempted to demonstrate the predictive values of ambulatory electrocardiographic monitoring (Table III)[61,66-71] and that of programmed stimulation (Table IV)[53-63] in patients taking amiodarone. As with type 1 agents, it appears that noninducibility during programmed stimulation portends an excellent clinical response with a negative predictive value in the 80–100% range.

Table III
Amiodarone Therapy Guided by Holter

	Number of Patients Evaluated	Mean Follow-up (months)	REC and/or SCD NOT Predicted by Holter	REC and/or SCD Predicted by Holter	Sensitivity	Specificity	Positive Predictive Value	Negative Predictive Value
Veltri (1986)	52	11	3/34	12/18	80%	84%	67%	91%
Marchlinski (1985)	74	11	6/34	11/21	65%	74%	52%	82%
Nademanee (1982)	13	12	0/13	—	—	—	—	—
Sokoloff (1986)	107	14	16/53	9/27	36%	67%	33%	70%
Kim (1987)	80	19	—	—	47%	75%	39%	80%
					31%	94%	71%	75%
					44%	88%	54%	82%
					42%	93%	67%	82%

REC = recurrence; SCD = sudden cardiac death.

Table IV
Amiodarone Therapy Guided by PES

	Patients Evaluated	Number of Pts IND on Amio (VT/VF ± NSVT)	Rec or SCD EPS Predicted Success	Rec or SCD EPS Predicted Failure	Mean Follow-up (months)	Sensitivity	Specificity	Positive Predictive Value	Negative Predictive Value
Hammer (1981)	9	7/8 (88%)	0/1	0/7	15	—	—	—	—
Nademanee (1982)	13	4/13 (33%)	0/8	0/4	12	—	67%	—	100%
Heger (1981)	45	12/13 (92%)	0/1	4/12	13	100%	11%	33%	100%
Morady (1983)	58	25/30 (83%)	1/5	6/25	25	87%	17%	24%	80%
McGovern (1984)	42	23/42 (55%)	1/19	10/23	10	91%	58%	43%	95%
Horowitz (1985)	100	80/100 (80%)	0/20	38/80	18	100%	32%	48%	100%
Veltri (1985)	13	12/13 (92%)	1/1	8/12	24	80%	—	33%	—
Haffajee (1986)	56	47/56 (83%)	0/9	25/47	23	100%	29%	53%	100%
Lavery (1986)	52	38/52 (73%)	0/14	11/38	15	100%	34%	29%	100%
Kim (1986)	50	7/34 (21%)	1/7	19/27	20	89%	24%	30%	86%

Amio = amiodarone; IND = inducible; PES = programmed electrical stimulation; REC = recurrence; SCD = sudden cardiac death.

However, continued inducibility while on amiodarone does not necessarily predict a poor clinical outcome (low positive predictive value).

We recently reviewed the results of 94 patients who presented with sustained ventricular tachycardia or cardiac arrest, were treated with amiodarone, and followed from 1980 to 1985.[74] All patients had a baseline electrophysiological study during which sustained ventricular tachycardia or fibrillation was induced except those patients who were having frequent episodes of ventricular tachycardia prior to the administration of amiodarone. Only 12 of the 94 patients (13%) were noninducible on amiodarone therapy. There were a total of 24 recurrences or sudden cardiac deaths during clinical follow-up. Twenty-two of these 24 patients remained inducible on amiodarone while two patients were considered noninducible having only nonsustained ventricular tachycardia initiated with programmed stimulation. This would yield positive and negative predictive values for programmed electrical stimulation on amiodarone of 27% and 83%, respectively. The negative predictive value of programmed stimulation in this patient population on amiodarone is of limited statistical significance because of the low noninducibility rate.

The utility of programmed electrical stimulation in patients treated with amiodarone, however, extends beyond the resultant inducibility status. Amiodarone often causes significant slowing of ventricular tachycardia and those patients who remain inducible but tolerate their tachycardia hemodynamically during electrophysiologic evaluation appear to have a more benign clinical course despite recurrences.[54,75]

The utility of ambulatory electrocardiographic monitoring to assess the antiarrhythmic efficacy of amiodarone in patients with refractory malignant ventricular arrhythmias has also been evaluated.[61,66-71] As with type 1 agents, the frequency of a response that would predict efficacy by Holter criteria occurs more frequently than with programmed stimulation. This is particularly relevant when also considering the less than adequate ability of programmed stimulation to accurately predict recurrence. Review of several reported series on the ability of ambulatory electrocardiographic monitoring to predict clinical outcome reveals that efficacy by Holter criteria has a negative predictive value that approaches that of programmed stimulation (Table III). Perhaps even of more significant importance is inefficacy as judged by Holter evaluation may be more predictive of recurrence than programmed stimulation (the positive predictive value for Holter monitoring is greater than that for programmed stimulation).

In conclusion, we preferentially use programmed electrical stimulation to guide pharmacological intervention for sustained ventricular tachycardia or sudden cardiac death. Patients who are noninducible in the drug-free (or baseline) state should strongly be considered as candidates for nonpharmacological intervention. Inducibility in the control study allows for evaluation of type 1 antiarrhythmic agent(s) alone or in combination. We do not rely on Holter monitoring to guide therapy with type 1 agents. Unfortunately, a majority of patients remain inducible and thus amiodarone, empiric therapy, or nonpharmacological intervention (subendocardial resection, catheter ablation, or the automatic implantable cardioverter/defibrillator) will, of necessity, have to be pursued. We feel that noninducibility on amiodarone is generally predictive of a good outcome. Induction of a hemodynamically poorly tolerated tachycardia with Holter results that would similarly predict inefficacy of amiodarone requires that additional therapy be instituted. The induction of a rapid tachycardia with a Holter response that predicts efficacy presents a clinical dilemma. Because recurrence in this population is life-threatening, additional therapy is probably warranted. This is said with the realization that many patients being treated with amiodarone may have a noneventful short-term clinical course in the absence of the subsequent intervention.

Acknowledgment: Supported in part by grants from the American Heart Association, Southeastern Pennsylvania Chapter, Philadelphia, PA and National Heart, Lung, and Blood Institute, Bethesda, MD (HL28093, HL24278, HL07346).

References

1. Lundy CJ, McLellan LL. Paroxysmal ventricular tachycardia: an etiological study with special reference to the type. Ann Int Med 1934;7:812–836.
2. Williams C, Ellis LB. Ventricular tachycardia: an analysis of thirty-six cases. Arch Int Med 1943;71:137–156.
3. Armbrust CA, Levine SA. Paroxysmal ventricular tachycardia: a study of one hundred and seven cases. Circulation 1950;1:28–40.
4. Herrmann GR, Park HM, Hejtmancik MR. Paroxysmal ventricular tachycardia: a clinical and electrocardiographic study. Am Heart J 1959;57:166–176.
5. Mason JW, Winkle RA. Electrode-catheter arrhythmia induction in the selection and assessment of antiarrhythmic drug therapy for recurrent ventricular tachycardia. Circulation 1978;58:971–985.
6. Horowitz LN, Josephson ME, Farshidi A, Spielman SR, Michelson EL, Greenspan AM. Recurrent sustained ventricular tachycardia. 3. Role of the electrophysiologic study in selection of antiarrhythmic regimens. Circulation 1978;58:986–997.
7. Ruskin JN, DiMarco JP, Garan H. Out-of-hospital cardiac arrest: Electrophysiologic observations and selection of long-term antiarrhythmic therapy. N Engl J Med 1980; 303:607–613.
8. Josephson ME, Horowitz LN. Electrophysiologic approach to therapy of recurrent sustained ventricular tachycardia. Am J Cardiol 1979;43:631–642.
9. Horowitz LN, Spielman SR, Greenspan AM, Josephson ME. Role of programmed stimulation in assessing vulnerability to ventricular arrhythmias. Am Heart J 1982;103: 604–610.
10. Lown B. Management of patients at high risk of sudden death. Am Heart J 1982;103: 689–697.
11. Graboys TB, Lown B, Podrid PJ, DeSilva R. Long-term survival of patients with malignant ventricular arrhythmia treated with antiarrhythmic drugs. Am J Cardiol 1982;50:438–443.
12. Lown B. Sudden cardiac death: The major challenge confronting contemporary cardiology. Am J Cardiol 1979;43:313–328.
13. Vlay SC, Kallman CH, Reid PR. Prognostic assessment of survivors of ventricular tachycardia and ventricular fibrillation with ambulatory monitoring. Am J Cardiol 1984;54:87–90.
14. Bigger JT Jr, Reiffel JA, Livelli FD Jr, Wang PJ. Sensitivity, specificity, and reproducibility of programmed ventricular stimulation. Circulation 1986;73(suppl II):II-73–II-78.
15. Buxton AE, Waxman HL, Marchlinski FE, Untereker WJ, Waspe LE, Josephson ME. Role of triple extrastimuli during electrophysiologic study of patients with documented sustained ventricular tachyarrhythmias. Circulation 1984;69:532–540.

16. Prystowsky EN, Miles WM, Evans JJ, Hubbard JE, Skale BT, Winkle JR, Heger JJ, Zipes DP. Induction of ventricular tachycardia during programmed electrical stimulation: analysis of pacing methods. Circulation 1986;73(suppl II):II-32–II-38.
17. Mann DE, Limacher MC, Luck JC, Magro SA, Griffin JC, Robertson NW, Wyndham CR. Induction of clinical ventricular tachycardia during electrophysiologic study: Value of third and fourth extrastimuli (abstr). Circulation 1982;66(suppl II):145.
18. Farré J, Grande A, Hernandez R, Comarti F, Rabago P, Diaz FJ. Sensitivity and specificity of inducing sustained ventricular tachycardia with up to three right ventricular extrastimuli (abstr). JACC 1984;3:609.
19. Lin H-T, Mann DE, Luck JC, Magro SA, Sakun V, Wyndham CRC. Prospective comparison of right and left ventricular stimulation in the induction of ventricular tachycardia (abstr). JACC 1986;7:72A.
20. Morady F, DiCarlo L, Winston S, Davis JC, Scheinman MM. A prospective comparison of triple extrastimuli and left ventricular stimulation in studies of ventricular tachycardia induction. Circulation 1984;70:52–57.
21. Brugada P, Green M, Abdollah H, Wellens HJJ. Significance of ventricular arrhythmias initiated by programmed ventricular stimulation: the importance of the type of ventricular arrhythmia induced and the number of premature stimuli required. Circulation 1984;69:87–92.
22. Herre JM, Mann DE, Luck JC, Magro SA, Wyndham CR. Effect of third and fourth extrastimuli and increased current on programmed ventricular stimulation: a prospective study (abstr). Circulation 1983;68:III–243.
23. Mann DE, Luck JC, Griffin JC, Herre JM, Limacher MC, Magro SA, Robertson NW, Wyndham CRC. Induction of clinical ventricular tachycardia using programmed stimulation: Value of third and fourth extrastimuli. Am J Cardiol 1983;52:501–506.
24. Herre JM, Mann DE, Luck JC, Magro SA, Figali S, Breen T, Wyndham CRC. Effect of increased current, multiple pacing sites and number of extrastimuli on induction of ventricular tachycardia. Am J Cardiol 1986;57:102–107.
25. Henthorn RW, Plumb VJ, Arciniegas JG, Zimmern SH, Waldo AL. Significance of the mode and site of ventricular tachycardia inducibility to assure adequate electrophysiologic study. (abstr) JACC 1983;1:594.
26. Doherty JU, Kienzle MG, Waxman HL, Buxton AE, Marchlinski FE, Josephson ME. Programmed ventricular stimulation at a second right ventricular site: An analysis of 100 patients, with special reference to sensitivity, specificity and characteristics of patients with induced ventricular tachycardia. Am J Cardiol 1983;52:1184–1189.
27. Brugada P, Wellens HJJ. Comparison in the same patient of two programmed ventricular stimulation protocols to induce ventricular tachycardia. Am J Cardiol 1985;55:380–383.
28. Estes NAM III, Garan H, McGovern B, Ruskin JN. Influence of drive cycle length during programmed stimulation on induction of ventricular arrhythmias: Analysis of 403 patients. Am J Cardiol 1986;57:108–112.
29. Morady F, DiCarlo LA Jr, Liem LB, Krol RB, Baerman JM. Effects of high stimulation current on the induction of ventricular tachycardia. Am J Cardiol 1985;56:73–78.
30. VandePol CJ, Farshidi A, Spielman SR, Greenspan AM, Horowitz LN, Josephson ME. Incidence and clinical significance of induced ventricular tachycardia. Am J Cardiol 1980:45:725–731.
31. Livelli FD, Bigger JT, Reiffel JA, Gang ES, Patton JN, Noethling PM, Rolnitzky LM, Glicklich JI. Response to programmed ventricular stimulation: sensitivity, specificity, and relationship to heart disease. Am J Cardiol 1982;50:452–458.
32. Brugada P, Abdollah H, Heddle B, Wellens HJJ. Results of a ventricular stimulation protocol using a maximum of 4 premature stimuli in patients without documented or suspected ventricular arrhythmias. Am J Cardiol 1983;52:1214–1218.
33. Morady F, Shapiro W, Shen E, Sung RJ, Scheinman MM. Programmed ventricular stimulation in patients without spontaneous ventricular tachycardia. Am Heart J 1984;107:875–882.

34. Podrid PJ, Lown B, Graboys TB, Lampert S. Use of short-term drug testing as part of a systematic approach for evaluation of antiarrhythmic drugs. Circulation 1986;73(suppl II):81–91.
35. Kennedy HL, Underhill SJ. Frequent or complex ventricular ectopy in apparently healthy subjects: A clinical study of 25 cases. Am J Cardiol 1976;38:141–148.
36. Winkle RA. Antiarrhythmic drug effect mimicked by spontaneous variability of ventricular ectopy. Circulation 1978;57:1116–1121.
37. Morganroth J, Michelson EL, Horowitz LN, Josephson ME, Pearlman AS, Dunkman WB. Limitations of routine long-term electrocardiographic monitoring to assess ventricular ectopic frequency. Circulation 1978;58:408–414.
38. Michelson EL, Morganroth J. Spontaneous variability of complex ventricular arrhythmias detected by long-term electrocardiographic recording. Circulation 1980;61:690–695.
39. Pratt CM, Slymen DJ, Wierman AM, Young JB, Francis MJ, Seals AA, Quinones MA, Roberts R. Analysis of the spontaneous variability of ventricular arrhythmias: Consecutive ambulatory electrocardiographic recordings of ventricular tachycardia. Am J Cardiol 1985;56:67–72.
40. Swerdlow CD, Winkle RA, Mason JW. Determinants of survival in patients with ventricular tachyarrhythmias. N Engl J Med 1983;308:1436–1442.
41. Kim SG, Seiden SW, Felder SD, Waspe LE, Fisher JD. Is programmed stimulation of value in predicting the long-term success of antiarrhythmic therapy for ventricular tachycardias? N Engl J Med 1986;315:356–362.
42. Podrid PJ, Schoeneberger A, Lown B, Lampert S, Matos J, Porterfield J, Raeder E, Corrigan E. Use of nonsustained ventricular tachycardia as a guide to antiarrhythmic drug therapy in patients with malignant ventricular arrhythmia. Am Heart J 1983;105:181–188.
43. Roy D, Waxman HL, Kienzle MG, Buxton AE, Marchlinski FE, Josephson ME. Clinical characteristics and long-term follow-up in 119 survivors of cardiac arrest: Relation to inducibility at electrophysiologic testing. Am J Cardiol 1983;52:969–974.
44. Skale BT, Miles WM, Heger JJ, Zipes DP, Prystowsky EN. Survivors of cardiac arrest: Prevention of recurrence by drug therapy as predicted by electrophysiologic testing or electrocardiographic monitoring. Am J Cardiol 1986;57:113–119.
45. Herling IM, Horowitz LN, Josephson ME. Ventricular ectopic activity after medical and surgical treatment for recurrent sustained ventricular tachycardia. Am J Cardiol 1980;45:633–639.
46. Kim SG, Seiden SW, Matos JA, Waspe LE, Fisher JD. Discordance between ambulatory monitoring and programmed stimulation in assessing efficacy of Class IA antiarrhythmic agents in patients with ventricular tachycardia. JACC 1985;6:539–544.
47. Platia EV. Programmed stimulation (PES)-directed drug therapy for sustained ventricular tachyarrhythmias: Long-term implications of altering therapy (abstr). Circulation 1986;74:II–313.
48. Mitchell LB, Duff HJ, Wyse DG. Randomized comparison of noninvasive and invasive approaches to drug therapy for sustained ventricular tachyarrhythmias (abstr). Circulation 1986;74:II–214.
49. Chua W, Roth H, Summers C, Zheutlin TA, Kehoe RF. Programmed stimulation versus ambulatory monitoring for therapy of malignant arrhythmias (abstr). Circulation 1983;67(suppl III):III–55.
50. Platia EV, Reid PR. Comparison of programmed electrical stimulation and ambulatory electrocardiographic (Holter) monitoring in the management of ventricular tachycardia and ventricular fibrillation. JACC 1984;4:493–500.
51. Webb CR, Morganroth J, Senior S, Spielman SR, Greenspan AM, Horowitz LN. Flecainide: Steady state electrophysiologic effects in patients with remote myocardial infarction and inducible sustained ventricular arrhythmia. JACC 1986;8:214–220.
52. Wellens HJJ, Brugada P, Stevenson WG. Programmed electrical stimulation: Its role in the management of ventricular arrhythmias in coronary heart disease. Prog Cardiovasc Dis 1986;29:165–180.

53. Waxman HL, Groh WC, Marchlinski FE, Buxton AE, Sadowski LM, Horowitz LN, Josephson ME, Kastor JA. Amiodarone for control of sustained ventricular tachyarrhythmia: Clinical and electrophysiologic effects in 51 patients. Am J Cardiol 1982; 50:1066–1074.
54. Horowitz LN, Greenspan AM, Spielman SR, Webb CR, Morganroth J, Rotmensch H, Sokoloff NM, Rae AP, Segal BL, Kay HR. Usefulness of electrophysiologic testing in evaluation of amiodarone therapy for sustained ventricular tachyarrhythmias associated with coronary heart disease. Am J Cardiol 1985;55:367–371.
55. Veltri EP, Reid PR, Platia EV, Griffith LSC. Results of late programmed electrical stimulation and long-term electrophysiologic effects of amiodarone therapy in patients with refractory ventricular tachycardia. Am J Cardiol 1985;55:375–379.
56. McGovern B, Garan H, Malacoff RF, DiMarco JP, Grant G, Sellers TD, Ruskin JN. Long-term clinical outcome of ventricular tachycardia or fibrillation treated with amiodarone. Am J Cardiol 1984;53:1558–1563.
57. Winkle RA. Amiodarone and the American way. JACC 1985;6:822–824.
58. Nademanee K, Singh BN, Cannom DS, Weiss J, Feld G, Stevenson WG. Control of sudden recurrent arrhythmic deaths: Role of amiodarone. Am Heart J 1983;106:895–901.
59. Naccarelli GV, Fineberg NS, Zipes DP, Heger JJ, Duncan G, Prystowsky EN. Amiodarone: Risk factors for recurrence of symptomatic ventricular tachycardia identified at electrophysiologic study. JACC 1985;6:814–821.
60. Heger JJ, Prystowsky EN, Jackman WM, Naccarelli GV, Warfel KA, Rinkenberger RL, Zipes DP. Amiodarone. Clinical efficacy and electrophysiology during long-term therapy for recurrent ventricular tachycardia or ventricular fibrillation. N Engl J Med 1981;305:539–545.
61. Nademanee K, Hendrickson J, Kannan R, Singh BN. Antiarrhythmic efficacy and electrophysiologic actions of amiodarone in patients with life-threatening ventricular arrhythmias: Potent suppression of spontaneously occurring tachyarrhythmias versus inconsistent abolition of induced ventricular tachycardia. Am Heart J 1982;103:950–959.
62. Hamer AW, Finerman WB, Peter T, Mandel WJ. Disparity between the clinical and electrophysiologic effects of amiodarone in the treatment of recurrent ventricular tachyarrhythmias. Am Heart J 1981;102:992–1000.
63. Morady F, Scheinman MM, Hess DS. Amiodarone in the management of patients with ventricular tachycardia and ventricular fibrillation. PACE 1983;6:609–615.
64. Ferrick KJ, Reiffel JA, Bigger JT, Livelli FD, Gang ES, Gliklich JI. Amiodarone therapy: time course of electrophysiologic effects (abstr). Clin Res 1983;31:182.
65. Kadish AH, Marchlinski FE, Josephson ME, Buxton AE. Amiodarone: Correlation of early and late electrophysiologic studies with outcome. Am Heart J 1986;112:1134–1140.
66. Kim SG, Felder SD, Figura I, Johnston DR, Waspe LE, Fisher JD. Value of Holter monitoring in predicting long-term efficacy and inefficacy of amiodarone used alone and in combination with Class IA antiarrhythmic agents in patients with ventricular tachycardia. JACC 1987;9:169–174.
67. Stamato NJ, Marchlinski FE. Role of Holter monitoring in the management of patients with ventricular tachycardia treated with amiodarone. Clin Prog Electrophysiol Pacing 1986;4:395–401.
68. Sokoloff NM, Spielman SR, Greenspan AM, Rae AP, Brady PM, Kay HR, Horowitz LN. Utility of ambulatory electrocardiographic monitoring for predicting recurrence of sustained ventricular tachyarrhythmias in patients receiving amiodarone. JACC 1986; 7:938–941.
69. Marchlinski FE, Buxton AE, Flores BT, Doherty JU, Waxman HL, Josephson ME. Value of Holter monitoring in identifying risk for sustained ventricular arrhythmia recurrence on amiodarone. Am J Cardiol 1985;55:709–712.
70. Veltri EP, Reid PR, Platia EV, Griffith LSC. Amiodarone in the treatment of life-threatening ventricular tachycardia: Role of Holter monitoring in predicting long-term clinical efficacy. JACC 1985;6:806–813.
71. Veltri EP, Griffith LSC, Platia EV, Guarnieri T, Reid PR. The use of ambulatory

monitoring in the prognostic evaluation of patients with sustained ventricular tachycardia treated with amiodarone. Circulation 1986;74:1054–1060.
72. Borggrefe M, Podczeck A, Breithardt G. Usefulness of early versus late electrophysiologic testing in patients with ventricular tachyarrhythmias treated with amiodarone. (abstr) Circulation 1986;74(suppl II):II–223.
73. Greenspon AJ, Volosin KJ, Greenberg RM, Vlasses PH, Rotmensch HH. Amiodarone therapy: Value of early and late electrophysiologic testing. Circulation 1986;74(suppl II):II–223.
74. Josephson ME. Unpublished data.
75. Haffajee CI, Gold RL, Yazaki Y, Sloan K, Alpert JS. Electrophysiologic predictors of long term outcome with amiodarone for refractory ventricular tachycardia (abstr). JACC 1986;7:109A.
76. Lavery D, Saksena S, Gordon S, Rothbart ST, Barr MJ. Long-term efficacy of amiodarone therapy in refractory sustained ventricular tachycardia: The role of electrophysiologic studies and ambulatory monitoring (abstr). JACC 1986;2:91A.
77. Kim SG, Felder SD, Figura I, Waspe LE, Fisher JD. Predictive accuracies of Holter monitoring and programmed stimulation in patients taking amiodarone (abstr). JACC 1986;7:143A.

27

Standardization of Noninvasive and Invasive Studies in the Assessment of Patients with Ventricular Arrhythmias

Manfred Zehender, Annette Geibel
Stefan Hohnloser, Thomas Meinertz
Hanjoerg Just

Introduction

Clinical tests and techniques are designed to evaluate diagnostic and therapeutic tools and preferentially to improve preexisting strategies. These techniques have to reach certain requirements of sensitivity and specificity, requirements that are sometimes difficult to meet in clinical practice because of the multiple variables that influence biological parameters. When analyzing a clinical problem, not only the technique but also the study design has to be tailored in relation to the patient population studied. The efficiency of the test and the criteria used for interpretation of the results have to be defined. Once an appropriate test is available, ideally it should be used in the same way by many institutions to allow comparison of results.

In the diagnostic and therapeutic evaluation of cardiac arrhythmias, different invasive and noninvasive techniques had been applied for many years. Long-term electrocardiographic monitoring developed in 1961 by Dr. Holter gained widespread use in the early 1970s.[35] Today, long-term electrocardiographic mon-

From: Brugada P, Wellens HJJ. CARDIAC ARRHYTHMIAS: Where To Go From Here? Mount Kisco, NY, Futura Publishing Company, Inc., © 1987.

itoring is a widely accepted method in the diagnostic evaluation of ventricular arrhythmias, such as to determine the frequency and severity of ventricular ectopies, to stratify the risk of a patient to develop malignant sustained ventricular arrhythmias, and to guide antiarrhythmic therapy. Unfortunately, there is no agreement about the exact methodology, such as duration of the recording, activity to which the patient is submitted during the recording, but most important, as discussed by Coumel et al. in another chapter of this book, about interpretation of results. Similar problems hold true for this technique of programmed electrical stimulation of the heart. This technique was first introduced in clinical cardiology by Durrer et al. and Coumel et al. in 1967.[17,25] Programmed electrical stimulation has markedly increased our understanding of cardiac arrhythmias. In the diagnostic evaluation, programmed electrical stimulation (PES) is especially important in patients with suspected or documented sustained ventricular tachycardia or ventricular fibrillation. In these patients, during 24, 48, or even 72 hour Holter monitoring, it is more or less a matter of chance whether or not an episode of fatal arrhythmia will be documented and a provocative test should be preferred. However, 20 years after its introduction in clinical cardiology, there is still no consent on stimulation protocols and on the significance given to arrhythmias that are initiated during programmed electrical stimulation. Some efforts in these directions have been undertaken recently.[13,82,83] On the basis of information obtained in recent years, we will discuss here the minimal requirements that should be applied to these techniques.

Holter Monitoring

Technical developments have improved our ability to record the electrocardiogram continuously in ambulatory patients during daily activities. Consequently, our knowledge on the prevalence (and prognostic significance) of chronic ventricular arrhythmias has increased. Because long-term ECG monitoring records spontaneous events, this technique has made it possible to investigate the relationship between symptoms reported by the patient and the observed arrhythmias. At the same time, however, new problems have been recognized, such as the spontaneous variability of arrhythmias or the differing significance of ventricular arrhythmias depending on the presence and type of underlying heart disease. These data have an important impact on the selection of patients considered for antiarrhythmic therapy and on the evaluation of the efficacy of treatment.

Methodical Considerations when Using Holter Monitoring

The American Heart Association has defined the technical requirements for appropriate long-term ECG monitoring.[74] It should be stressed that the majority of long-term ECG systems do not satisfy these technical standards.

No standard exists for the optimal duration of the recording, but several studies have examined the importance of the registration time to document the maximal severity of arrhythmias. Lown et al. indicated that 1 hour of registration detects about 70% of patients having premature ventricular beats, but only 25% of patients with "complex" ventricular arrhythmias.[44] When the recording is prolonged for 24 hours, Kennedy et al. detected high grade or frequent ventricular ectopy in 67–85% of patients with coronary artery disease. Further prolongation to 36 hours increased the incidence to 92–100% of patients. These authors also observed that in 55% of patients with arrhythmia complaints written in their diary, no significant arrhythmias occurred that time.[42] In a more recent study, Andresen et al.[2] analyzed the relation of registration time to severity of cardiac arrhythmias over 72 hours. The arrhythmias had been recognized in 70% of patients after 24 hours of registration. Prolongation of the registration to 48 hours increased the sensitivity to 93%. A further increase in registration time did not provide significant additional information. However, it should be emphasized that these data did not include patients with episodes of sustained ventricular arrhythmia, occurrences of which are sometimes separated by long time intervals. With respect to routine use of long-term ECG recording, it is now widely accepted that ambulatory ECG monitoring should have a minimal duration of 24 hours. In some patients, longer recording times may be necessary.

These studies bring us to another problem. Prolonging of the recording up to 48 or 72 hours only offers certain information on short-term variability of these arrhythmias. It does not provide information on the long-term variability of ventricular arrhythmias, which is actually the most important factor when assessing the prognostic value of findings during long-term ECG monitoring. When trying to assess the prognostic significance of arrhythmias recorded after myocardial infarction, data of predischarge long-term ECG monitoring are frequently compared to events (for instance, sudden death) occurring months after the recording was obtained. It is nowadays well known that the incidence and prognostic significance of ventricular arrhythmias after myocardial infarction decrease spontaneously in incidence and prognostic value with time[4,6,7,21,60,71] and the causes of sudden death are many.[61,62,66,68–71]

With respect to the spontaneous variability, in patients with frequent ventricular arrhythmias, Holter monitoring will give an idea of the density and severity of ventricular ectopy. In patients with suspected or documented sustained ventricular tachycardia or ventricular fibrillation, the diagnostic impact of Holter monitoring is frequently hampered by the occurrence of these fatal arrhythmias with widely separated intervals, sometimes months or years. Thus, documentation of a sustained arrhythmia in these patients during 24 hour Holter monitoring is more or less a matter of chance. Actually, the diagnostic value of long-term ECG monitoring to detect these last arrhythmias is close to nil. However, there had been some evidence to evaluate predictors of spontaneous occurrence of sustained arrhythmias during Holter monitoring to identify patients with increased risk for sudden cardiac death.

In the evaluation on the prognostic significance of ventricular arrhythmias during long-term ECG monitoring, Bigger and co-workers described in 1983 the mortality rate as a function of the frequency and complexity of ventricular premature beats.[3] They suggested a classification system of "malignant," "potentially malignant," and "benign" arrhythmias (Table I). However, it should be stressed that the so-called malignant arrhythmias are rare findings during routine 24 hour

Table I
Benign Versus Malignant Arrhythmias Defined by Bigger and Co-workers*

	Ventricular Arrhythmias	
Malignant	Potentially Malignant	Benign
• VF • sustained VT • QT-syndrom + VPB Recurrence rate: 25–40%	• frequent VPB • repetitive VPB	• VPB (Patients without HD)
No prognostic significance: Morphology, R-on-T-Phenomenon		

*Am J Cardiol 1983;52:47–54.
*VPB = ventricular premature beat; VT = ventricular tachycardia; VF = ventricular fibrillation; HD = organic heart disease.

Holter monitoring, even when the patient is known to suffer from this arrhythmia. In contrast, potentially malignant arrhythmias are a frequent finding in patients with severe heart disease; however, only a small group of these patients will experience sudden cardiac death.

In 27 of 30 patients who died from sudden cardiac death at the time of Holter monitoring, Panidis et al. and Pratt et al. described in all patients the occurrence of spontaneous ventricular tachycardia which initiates ventricular fibrillation and thus caused sudden cardiac death.[62,66] Panidis additionally demonstrated that in 9/15 patients, complex ventricular arrhythmias, and in 7/15 patients, frequent ventricular premature beats were present in the long-term ECG prior to the fatal event.[62] Many studies evaluated different parameters to predict an increased risk for sudden cardiac death, and agreed that additional clinical information such as the underlying heart disease and left ventricular function are required to evaluate a risk stratification.[1,3,4,6,15,20,46,59,60,71,73,88]

We studied by 24 hour Holter monitoring 267 patients with coronary artery disease and analyzed the incidence of ventricular arrhythmias before, 6 weeks to 3 months, 3–6 months, and more than 6 months after myocardial infarction.[15,28,58–60] Only 21% of all patients with coronary artery disease had no ventricular arrhythmias and 18% of the patients had complex ventricular arrhythmias. The incidence of complex arrhythmias was highest within 6 months after myocardial infarction. In 11 patients who died during a mean follow-up of 20 months, there was no significant relationship to the occurrence of complex ventricular arrhythmias. Since early studies described the occurrence of complex ventricular arrhythmias as an independent parameter worsening the prognosis of a patient,[59,73] other studies questioned this influence even when spontaneous ventricular tachycardia occurred.[1,4,21] Thus, Anderson described in 66 patients a 2 year mortality of 25% when ventricular tachycardia was present after myocardial infarction and of 13% when this was not the case.[1] Most recent findings suggest that not the occurrence of frequent and complex arrhythmias, but the occurrence of fast ventricular tachycardia in relation to depressed left ventricular function is of major importance in predicting an increased risk for sudden death in patients after myocardial infarction.

In 74 patients with dilated cardiomyopathy, we observed in 69% of patients complex ventricular arrhythmias of Lown class IV and only 4% of patients were free of ventricular ectopy.[34,50] We followed these patients for 4 years and demonstrated that the occurrence of frequent complex ventricular arrhythmias and the presence of a depressed left ventricular function identifies patients with an increased risk of sudden death.[34] In similar studies, when such complex ventricular arrhythmias were suppressed by antiarrhythmic medication, the prognosis of the patient improved.[19,36,65]

The decision to treat or not to treat a particular patient should be based on the incidence and severity of the arrhythmia and the patient's symptoms. This decision is, however, also markedly influenced by the underlying heart disease and the hemodynamic changes resulting from depressed left ventricular function caused by the disease. Table II summarizes some of the criteria proposed to reduce ventricular arrhythmias. However, these criteria are based on several assumptions which have not been proven. The first is that because of a course-to-effect relation between ectopic activity and sudden death, suppression of ectopic activity should prevent sudden death. The second is that suppression of ectopic activity as assessed from long-term ECG monitoring will be permanent. The third is that suppression of ventricular ectopy represents an effective treatment. There is much evidence accumulated up to now to suggest that none of these assumptions is valid. The problems concerning the course-to-effect aspect have already been discussed. In regard to the last two assumptions, the spontaneous variability in ectopic activity as discussed by the authors themselves who performed these treatment studies makes it impossible to think that a repeat 24 or 72 hour recording is sufficient to assess the permanent suppression of ectopic activity or the creation of new arrhythmias. Actually, there is only rare evidence thus far, with the exception of beta-blockers,[18] that suppression of ectopic activity improves prognosis. New studies designed to theoretically overcome those problems will still be facing the reality of treating a "marker" of a disease, but not the disease itself.[16,29]

Table II
Criteria Proposed to Prove Efficacy of Reduction
of Ventricular Arrhythmias

Investigator	Reduction in %		
	Single VPBs	Couplets	VT
Morganroth (1978)	> 83.4	> 75.3	> 64.8
Sami (1980)			
Incidence 2.2–3 VPB/h	> 90	—	—
> 20 VPB/h	> 65	—	—
Thomas A. Miller (1984)			
Incidence < 20 VPB/h	> 98	—	—
> 20 VPB/h	> 84	—	—
Lown (1985)	> 63–85	> 83–90	> 90–100

VPB = ventricular premature beats; VT = ventricular tachycardia.

Exercise-Induced Arrhythmias

A somewhat different situation occurs when data from exercise ECG are considered. The differences, however, only apply to exercise-induced sustained ventricular tachycardia or fibrillation. For asymptomatic ectopic activity, the same limitations as for long-term ECG monitoring apply. An exercise ECG may sometimes be helpful to reproduce exercise-induced ventricular tachycardia or ventricular fibrillation. However, if ischemia can be demonstrated to play a major role in the triggering of these arrhythmias during exercise, in patients with coronary artery disease there is no such place for antiarrhythmic drug treatment. These patients should receive antianginal medication or undergo coronary revascularization. These procedures should be considered for these patients even when no direct proof can be obtained for the role of overt ischemia (for instance, with reversible defect on thallium exercise at the time of occurrence of sustained ventricular tachycardia or ventricular fibrillation). In some cases, however, antiarrhythmic drugs may become an alternative together with antianginal medication. These considerations do not apply to exercise-induced ectopic activity.

An exercise ECG is extremely helpful in assessing the exercise capacity of patients with otherwise well-documented arrhythmias.[33,80] It is also helpful in assessing how treatment may influence (beneficially or not) the exercise capacity. The reproducibility of the test in that regard is good. The reproducibility of the results of an exercise ECG to induce sustained ventricular tachycardia or ventricular fibrillation is, on the contrary, poor.

Programmed Electrical Stimulation

The invasive assessment of cardiac arrhythmias by programmed electrical stimulation was first introduced by Durrer et al. and Coumel et al. in 1967.[17,25] Systematic evaluations in the early 1970s markedly improved our understanding of initiation and termination of supraventricular and ventricular arrhythmias.[84-86] Additionally, the influence of different antiarrhythmic agents on the electrophysiologic properties of cardiac structures further increased our understanding of the effects of these drugs on cardiac arrhythmias. Unfortunately, only two decades after the introduction of PES, some efforts have been made to try to reach certain agreements on the most appropriate stimulation protocol for the different types of tachycardias.[13,67,81] Programmed electrical stimulation of the heart has reached, however, a certain maturity much faster than noninvasive studies. If the physician performing these type of investigations is aware of the limitations of the method, very important information on the pathophysiology of the arrhythmias can be uncovered. One must realize that programmed stimulation, similar to long-term ECG monitoring and exercise ECG, offers only limited information about the arrhythmias being studied, and that programmed stimulation is also far from being a perfect method to assess the efficacy and particularly inefficacy of antiarrhythmic treatment. There are, as previously discussed,[5,13,82,83] many variables that influence results of programmed stimulation that cannot be controlled by the investigator, such as the autonomic tone, myocardial ischemia, and the cellular electrophysiologic and hemodynamic changes during pacing. Stimulation protocols also influence the results, but they can be closely controlled. The variables in a stimulation protocol are many, including the duration and strength of electrical stimuli, the number and rate of the basic stimuli, and number and intervals of premature stimuli, the type of current used, and the pacing site.[13]

While initially moderate stimulation protocols were used (one to two extrastimuli, one pacing site, three pacing rates), protocols have now been extended to include three or more extrastimuli, synchronized or asynchronized burst pacing, multiple pacing sites in the right and left ventricles, and different current strengths.[7,8–10,24,26,28,40,45,55,68,84–86] Introduction of these pacing modes has not always been accompanied by the necessary studies to analyze sensitivity, specificity, and efficiency of the stimulation protocol. However, most authors agree that diagnostic stimulation protocols for ventricular tachycardia should use an electrical stimulus of 1–2 ms duration, a current strength of two times diastolic threshold, and a minimum of either three pacing rates or two stimulation sites if three extrastimuli are not given. Use of three extrastimuli may make it unnecessary to use other stimulation sites.[12] Higher energies do not increase accuracy and safety of programmed electrical stimulation. They have a lower sensitivity and specificity than stimulation protocols using a strength of twice diastolic threshold and favor current leakage and catheter malfunction.[13]

Whatever the stimulation protocol used, whenever it fulfills the minimal standards determined by the North American Society of Pacing and Electrophysiology, that stimulation protocol should have clear known value in terms of sensitivity and specificity. It has been a matter of much concern to us to try to understand the variables that influence sensitivity and specificity of programmed electrical stimulation. For a long time, no consideration was given to the types of arrhythmias induced and their significance. At best, their duration was analyzed to classify them into nonsustained or sustained.[43,81] Thus, regular sustained monomorphic VT were analyzed together with sustained polymorphic ones or ventricular fibrillation. Recent results indicate, however, that the initiation of a sustained arrhythmia cannot be considered as a specific finding, unless the characteristics of the induced arrhythmia, the mode of initiation, and the clinical characteristics of the patient population under study have been carefully considered.[7,10,13,22,75,82,90,92] Additionally, we have demonstrated that an aggressive stimulation protocol induces sustained polymorphic ventricular arrhythmias also in the normal heart.[9] Recent studies have also demonstrated that even the initiation of a sustained monomorphic ventricular tachycardia per se is not a specific finding.[13,78,82,83,91,92] A sustained monomorphic ventricular tachycardia can be induced in up to 45% of patients after myocardial infarction who do not suffer from spontaneous episodes of that arrhythmia at the time of study or during the follow-up. Programmed electrical stimulation does have a high sensitivity in patients with documented sustained ventricular tachycardia after myocardial infarction. In this situation, careful documentation of the VT initiated during PES by 12-lead ECG is required, to compare it with the ventricular tachycardia which occurred clinically.

In a prospective study of more than 300 patients with and without a variety of ventricular arrhythmias, we have investigated the predictive accuracy of a standardized ventricular stimulation protocol using a maximum of three extrastimuli and three different pacing rates from the right ventricular apex.

The standardized stimulation protocol was designed after a series of preliminary studies[9,10,12] in patients with and without spontaneous ventricular arrhythmias. This protocol utilizes a maximum of three premature extrastimuli given during sinus rhythm and ventricular pacing at 100, 120, and 140 beats/min from the right ventricular apex. The stimuli are given bipolar and have a strength of twice diastolic threshold. The duration of the stimulus is 2 ms. The sequence of the different stimulation steps is shown in Figure 1. The end-points during programmed electrical stimulation have been: (1) repeat (at least five times) induction of a sustained monomorphic VT, when this was the clinical arrhythmia problem of the patient and did not require cardioversion, (2) induction of a ventricular arrhythmia requiring cardioversion twice in patients with spontaneous ventricular tachycardia or ventricular fibrillation, and (3) completion of the stimulation protocol.

In our Maastricht working group, we have analyzed results of this stimulation protocol by considering each stimulation step (a total of 12 steps) and the type of arrhythmias (Fig. 2) in relation to the clinical problem and the underlying heart disease.[92]

Old Myocardial Infarction

In patients with an old myocardial infarction, sensitivity of programmed electrical stimulation does not represent a major problem. Publications from many different laboratories have confirmed that in 90% or more of these patients a sustained monomorphic ventricular tachycardia can be induced when they suffer clinically from the arrhythmia[5,13,82,83,91] (Table III). This also minimizes the problem of reproducibility[5] in such a group of patients. The specificity of programmed stimulation is, however, much more controversial.[5,12,82,83]

In 111 patients studied within 1 year[77] after myocardial infarction, the induction of a sustained monomorphic VT by PES was closely related to the clinically documented arrhythmia and the mode of stimulation[92] (Table IV). In patients with spontaneous sustained monomorphic VT, the clinical arrhythmia was reproduced in 94% of patients (Fig. 3). Interestingly, 32–45% of patients without evidence of a sustained VT during a 2 year follow-up were induced during PES to a sustained monomorphic VT. Therefore, additional criteria are required to differentiate between patients with and without spontaneous sustained monomorphic VT. Our data indicate that the introduction of a rate limit of induced sustained monomorphic VT and reduction of the stimulation protocol of three extrastimuli during sinus rhythm (step 10) improved the specificity of PES to identify patients with spontaneous occurrence of sustained monomorphic VT to more than 90%, without marked loss of sensitivity. Both parameters are graphically displayed for each step during the stimulation protocol by the so-called "ROC" ("Receiver Operting Characteristics) curves (Fig. 4).[49]

(Stimulation in the right ventricular apex with 1-2 extrastimuli during sinus rhythm, SR, and at 100, 120 and 140 beats/min)

Basic pacing r.	SR		100		120		140		★SR	100	120	140 beats/min
Extrastimuli	1	2	1	2	1	2	1	2	3	3	3	3
Steps	1	2	3	4	5	6	7	8	9	10	11	12
	PART I								PART II			

(★ : Increasing rate in the atrium and ventricle, only in HCM-patients)

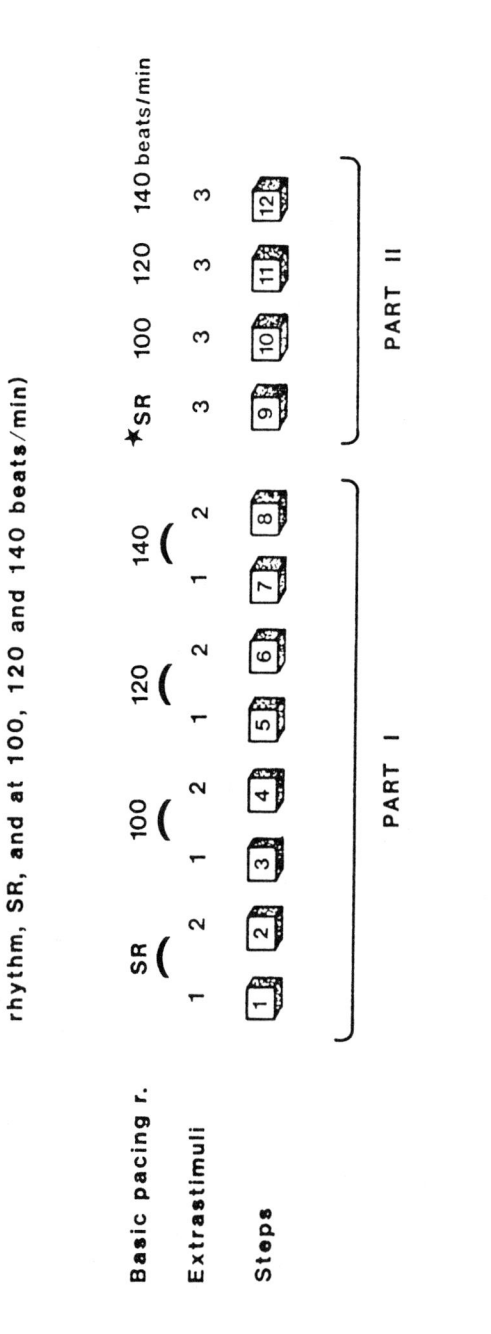

Figure 1: Standardized stimulation protocol.

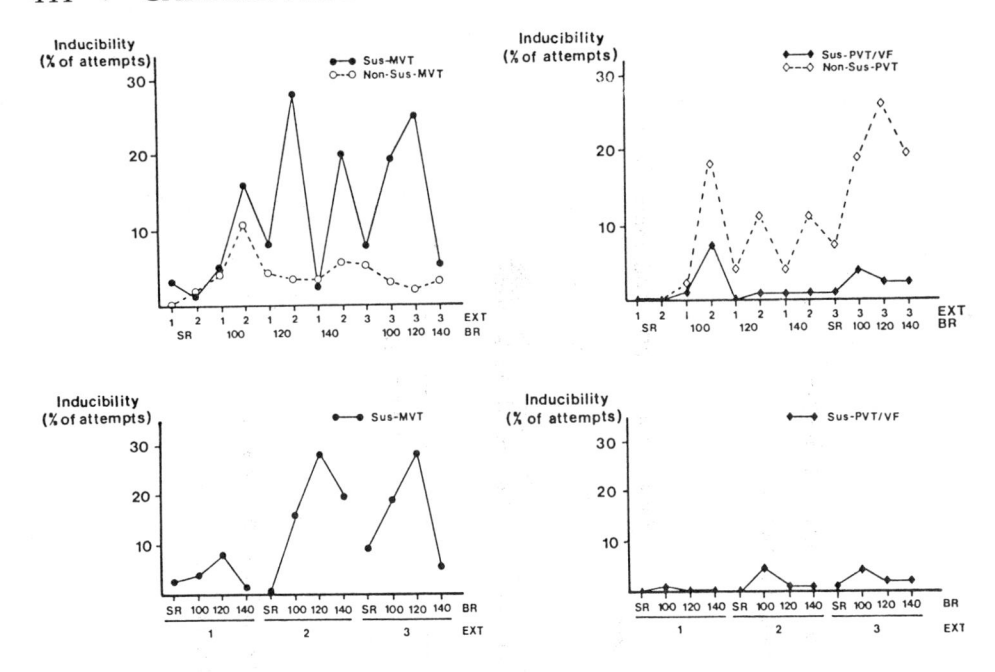

Figure 2: Inducibility of different types of ventricular tachycardia (VT) during the stimulation protocol (Parts I + II). The inducibility is calculated as percentage of successful attempts during each stimulation step. In the upper half, the ordinate gives the subsequent stimulation steps, in the lower half stimulation steps using one, two, and three extrastimuli are grouped together (SR = sinus rhythm, BR = basic pacing rate; EXT = extrastimulus.)

Table III
Sensitivity and Specificity of Programmed Electrical Stimulation

Study	No. of Patients	Spontaneous VT			Sensitivity	Specificity
		Sustained	Nonsustained	None		
Mason	33	33	0	0	82%	—
Ruskin	31	31	0	0	81%	—
Vandepol	529	57	29	443	84%	99%
Fisher	201	96	—	105	86%	95%
Livelli	100	31	18	51	65%	98%
Doherty	38	22	6	10	62%	100%
Zehender	111	32	50	29	94%	84%

Results of PES are also influenced by the location of myocardial infarction. While in patients with spontaneous sustained monomorphic VT the inducibility rate was 90–100%, the inducibility of sustained monomorphic VT in patients without such a history was higher when the infarction was located anteriorly (65%) compared to inferiorly (34%). These differences could not be explained on the basis of a larger infarction in patients with anterior infarction.

Table IV
Inducibility of Ventricular Tachycardia (VT) in Sudden Cardiac Survivors

Study	No. of Patients	CAD	Induced arrhythmia	
			Sustained VT	Nonsustained VT
Ruskin	31	71%	42%	32%
Roy	119	75%	61%	9%
Morady	45	78%	57%	17%
Benditt	31	65%	77%	4%
Zehender	32	100%	74%	14%

CAD = coronary artery disease.

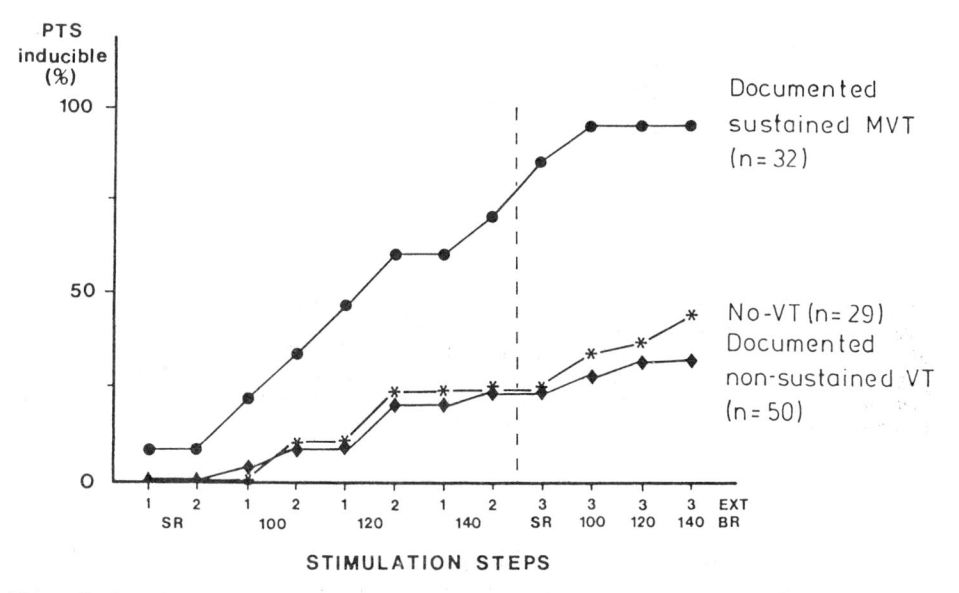

Figure 3: Cumulative inducibility of sustained monomorphic ventricular tachycardia (VT) during each step of the stimulation protocol in patients after myocardial infarction with different clinical arrhythmias (PTS = patients; SR = sinus rhythm; BR = basic pacing rate; EXT = extrastimulus.) Broken line separates Part I and II of the stimulation protocol in this figure.

Patients with Ventricular Fibrillation after MI

In patients with aborted sudden death, documentation by multiple ECG leads of the initial arrhythmia is usually not available. This contributes to the absence of unanimous opinion about the end-points and value of PES to identify patients at risk to die suddenly:[13] (1) induced nonsustained polymorphic VT were known to be an unspecific finding in all groups of patients,[11,75,85] (2) inducibility of a sustained monomorphic VT does not prove that this is the arrhythmia that happened clinically, and (3) VF initiated by PES might have a different mechanism than spontaneous VF. When assessing the specificity of PES to identify retrospec-

"ROC"-CURVES

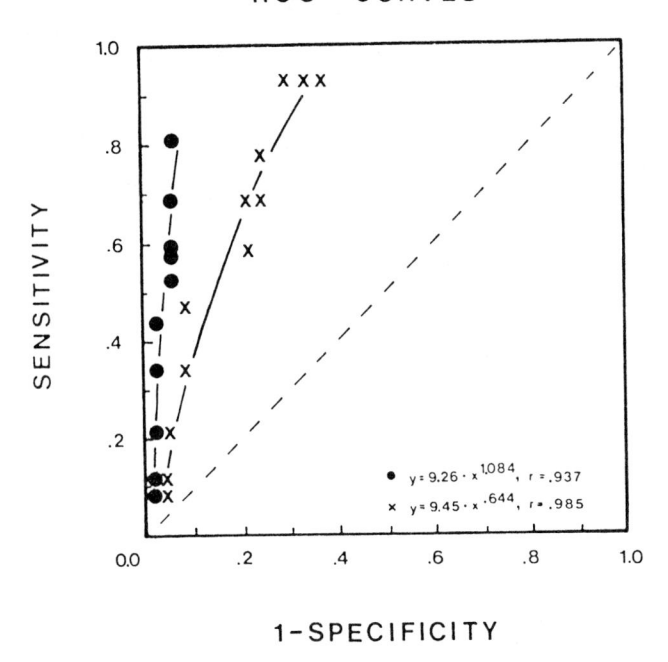

Figure 4: "Receiver Operating Characteristics" (ROC) curves of the stimulation protocol. The graphic display describes the relation of sensitivity (y-axis) and specificity (x-axis) at each of the 12 steps (x's) during the stimulation protocol and at each of the 10 steps during the limited stimulation protocol (black dots), when a rate limit of induced sustained monomorphic VT has been added. The limited protocol is characterized by a leftward shift of the curve, representing a higher efficiency of the test. The area above the broken line marks an efficiency of the method of .50.

Curve equations: $y = 9.26 \cdot x^{1.084}$, $r = .937$ (●); $y = 9.45 \cdot x^{.644}$, $r = .985$ (×)

tively and prospectively patients with sudden cardiac death, patients differing only in the presence of such a fatal event but who suffer from the same heart disease and from the same clinical arrhythmia documented previously to the fatal event should be analyzed for comparison.

Our data indicate that the induction of any sustained ventricular arrhythmia by PES in patients after myocardial infarction was not specific (Table IV). However, the incidence of induced ventricular arrhythmias was related to the clinical arrhythmia occurring before the fatal event in the patients surviving an episode of sudden death (Table IV). Patients with and without aborted sudden death differed in the rate of induced sustained monomorphic VT and the requirement of DC countershock for VT termination, as well as in the presence of a depressed left ventricular function.[11,14,89,91]

Previous studies in survivors of sudden cardiac death included different heart diseases (summarized in Table V); however, they all found a high inducibility of fast and frequently syncopal sustained VT in (45–61% of patients).[32,38,46,56,69,76]

Table V
Incidence of Different Types of Ventricular Tachycardia (VT) in Patients with and without Ventricular Fibrillation Late after Myocardial Infarction

Arrhythmias Documented	Group A (32 pts)			Group B (111 pts)		
	Sus-MVT 15 pts	Non-Sus-VT 12	No-VA 5	Sus-MVT 32	Non-Sus-VT 50	No-VA 29
induced to:						
Sus-VT/VF	93% (*)	67%	60%	94%	54%	29%
induced to (I/II):						
Sus-MVT	53/73%	25/50%	40/40%	68/94%	24/32%	24/45%
Non-Sus-MVT	20/27%	34/40%	0/0%	34/41%	14/20%	3/7%
Sus-PVT	7/7%	8/8%	0/0%	6/6%	10/16%	0/3%
Non-Sus-PVT	0/13%	17/17%	20/20%	13/22%	30/40%	14/72%
VF (directly)	13*/13*	8/8%	20*/20%	0/0%	2/10%	0/3%

Group A = patients with VF after MI; group B = patients without VF after MI; VF = ventricular fibrillation 72 hours after myocardial infarction; (Non)-Sus-MVT = (non-) sustained monomorphic ventricular tachycardia; No-VT = no VT and 10 ventricular premature complexes/hour, PVT = polymorphic VT, VF = ventricular fibrillation directly induced.
(I/II) = The first column always gives the inducibility during part I of the stimulation protocol, the second column the inducibility of part I + II.
pts = patients.
*p < 0.05 versus patients with the same diagnosis in the group B
(*)p < 0.05 versus patients with Doc-VF, but with Non-Sus-VT or No-VT documented previously.

Patients with Dilated Cardiomyopathy

In patients with dilated cardiomyopathy, PES initiates ventricular arrhythmias less frequently, as compared to patients with coronary artery disease (summarized in Table VI). Poll and co-workers induced 12/12 patients with idiopathic dilated cardiomyopathy and a history of sustained VT to the clinical VT by using an "aggressive" stimulation protocol.[64] We did not induce any sustained monomorphic ventricular tachycardia in 42 patients without sustained VT by using one to two extrastimuli.[51] Induced polymorphic VT was of no prognostic relevance in this study. In two recent publications, Das et al. and Poll et. al. confirmed their initial results suggesting inducibility of sustained monomorphic VT only in patients with such a history.[19,65] In both studies, the prognostic relevance of the induced arrhythmias was questionable, however. There was some evidence that effective suppression of induced arrhythmias could improve the prognosis of the patient.

In an ongoing study, we used a stimulation protocol with up to three extrastimuli in patients with dilated cardiomyopathy. The inducibility of a sustained monomorphic VT was low (Table VII) and mainly restricted to patients with a spontaneous history of this type of arrhythmia. Interestingly, there was also a lower incidence of polymorphic ventricular arrhythmias compared to patients with coronary artery disease.[92] All sustained ventricular arrhythmias induced in patients with dilated cardiomyopathy required cardioversion for termination. Until further data are available, the diagnostic and prognostic value of PES in

Table VI
Inducibility of Ventricular Tachycardia (VT) in Patients with Dilated Cardiomyopathy (VF = ventricular fibrillation, EX = number of extrastimuli)

Study	Pts	Spontaneous VT/VF	Induced Sustained VT	Induced Nonsustained VT	EX
Nacarelli	37	25	6	–	2
Poll	11	11	11	–	3
Meinertz	42	15	–	3	2
Morady	22	0	4	3	3
Poll	47	47	21	12	3
Das	24	11	3	5	3
Zehender	18	7	4	5	3

VF = ventricular fibrillation; EX = number of extrastimuli.

Table VII
Inducibility of Different Types of Ventricular Arrhythmias in Patients with Idiopathic Dilated Cardiomyopathy (IDC), Hypertrophic Cardiomyopathy (HCM), and Patients with Idiopathic Ventricular Tachycardia (IVT) Using 1–3 Extrastimuli during Sinus Rhythm and 3 Pacing

Disease →	IDC				HCM				IVT	
Arrhythmia →	SMVT	NSVT	No-VT	VF	SMVT	NSVT	No-VT	VT	SMVT	NSVT
Patients →	3	7	10	1	2	1	16	3	12	28
Induced arrhythmia:										
SMVT	2	1	–	–	2	–	2	–	7	2
NSMVT	–	–	–	–	1	–	1	–	5	4
SPVT	–	–	1	–	–	–	1	1	–	–
NSPVT	–	2	3	1	–	1	2	1	3	9
VF	–	–	–	–	–	–	4	2	–	1

In the first line, the underlying heart disease and the clinical arrhythmia problem of a patient is described. VF = ventricular fibrillation; (Non)-Sus-MVT = (non-) sustained monomorphic ventricular tachycardia; No-VT = no VT and 10 ventricular premature complexes/hour; PVT = polymorphic VT; VF = ventricular fibrillation directly induced.

patients with idiopathic dilated cardiomyopathy without a history of sustained monomorphic VT or prehospital cardiac arrest remains questionable.

Patients with Hypertrophic Cardiomyopathy

There are only limited data concerning the prognostic significance and inducibility of cardiac arrhythmias during PES in patients with hypertrophic cardiomyopathy.[37,41] Hypertrophic cardiomyopathy is, however, a disease with a well-known increased risk of sudden cardiac death.[47,48] In one-third of 22 patients with hypertrophic cardiomyopathy, we induced a ventricular arrhythmia during PES when using up to three extrastimuli from the right ventricular apex (Table VII). A sustained monomorphic VT was induced in four patients (18%), including the only two patients with spontaneous episodes of this arrhythmia. Induced polymorphic arrhythmias were not related to the clinical arrhythmia, nor to other clinical parameters. In total, the incidence of induction of polymorphic arrhythmias was three times higher as observed in patients after myocardial infarction studied by the same stimulation protocol.[92] In accordance with results reported recently by Kunze et al.[41] and also discussed by the same group in this book, a third extrastimulus does not increase the incidence of significant arrhythmias, but significantly increases the incidence of arrhythmias requiring DC cardioversion for VT termination.

Patients with Idiopathic Ventricular Tachycardia

In patients without any evidence of organic heart disease we have reported that the spontaneous occurrence of complex ventricular arrhythmias is a rare finding.[52] In such a group of patients without organic heart disease or spontaneous ventricular arrhythmias, we also described a very low incidence of inducible nonsustained or sustained VT when using one to two extrastimuli.[79] In a more recent study, we included 40 patients without organic heart disease who suffered from symptomatic nonsustained or sustained ventricular tachycardia. In these patients, PES with one to three extrastimuli reproduced the clinically documented sustained monomorphic VT in only 59% of the patients. In patients with nonsustained VT, the induction of a sustained VT was a rare finding (Table VII). A third extrastimulus was of no diagnostic help. It increased the incidence of polymorphic arrhythmias from 5 to 35% and DC cardioversion was required in two patients. When the spontaneous sustained VT was exercise-related, the ability to reproduce this arrhythmia by PES was 33%, when the VT was not exercise-related, the incidence of induction was 75%. Altogether, the sensitivity to identify patients with spontaneous sustained VT in the absence of an organic heart disease seems low.

Clinical Implications

In most patients with suspected or documented ventricular arrhythmias, Holter monitoring, exercise testing, and programmed electrical stimulation provide essential information for diagnostic evaluation and therapeutic guidance. Each of these techniques contributes to complete the diagnosis and to select effective treatment; however, each of these techniques has limitations. The experience from studies using invasive or noninvasive techniques supports the requirement of minimal standards for the study design, methods, and selection of patient populations. This reduces the risk of misinterpretation of results, and allows comparison of results obtained in different institutions. That would also allow much faster transfer of such results into consensual guidelines for further studies and clinical practice. Long-term monitoring provides information on the density of spontaneous ectopic activity, but is of limited value to determine the severity of cardiac arrhythmias in patients with paroxysmal sustained VT or with spontaneous ventricular fibrillation. Although our knowledge of the clinical significance of different types of cardiac arrhythmias in relation to the underlying heart disease has increased, we have to realize that in the treatment of so-called "malignant" arrhythmias, spontaneous short-term and long-term variability limit the possibilities to control our therapeutic efforts. Additionally, suppression of any ventricular arrhythmia by antiarrhythmic treatment alone will not improve the prognosis of the patient when an unstable or progressively worse underlying heart disease is not adequately treated at the same time.

Programmed electrical stimulation gives us data on the origin, localization, and characteristics of sustained ventricular arrhythmia. In clinical practice, the value of PES to guide antiarrhythmic medication is not yet established.

What can we expect from future studies on the three techniques? From the technical side, discontinuous long-term ECG will provide the possibility to extend the registration time to better document rare arrhythmic events. Simultaneous ST-segment analysis and arrhythmia detection will improve our knowledge about the possible role of ischemia. For programmed electrical stimulation, future aspects will concentrate on a better identification of patients at high risk for sudden death. With improved techniques for surgical and catheter-mediated antiarrhythmic therapy, the need for electrophysiologic data will increase. The role of PES to guide antiarrhythmic medication has to be established in further studies; however, if the results prove reliability, patients with rare spontaneous episodes of arrhythmias on noninvasive techniques will benefit most.

The prognostic significance of spontaneous or induced ventricular arrhythmia has to be further analyzed by means of these techniques. However, placebo-controlled studies with or without medication to determine the prognostic significance of cardiac arrhythmias have become difficult because of ethical reasons. During the "parallel study" recently introduced, independently from the results of the three techniques, patients with symptomatic sustained VT are treated for their symptoms caused by the recurrence of the VT. Thus, retrospective analysis will give us the possibility to prove for each technique different criteria considered for initiation and guidance of antiarrhythmic therapy in the different groups of patients. Whether conclusions from this strategy can be transferred also to patients with asymptomatic arrhythmias will require other types of studies.

References

1. Anderson JL, DeCamilla J, Mason JW. Clinical significance of ventricular tachycardia (3 beats or longer) detected during ambulatory monitoring after myocardial infarction. Circulation 1973;57:890–897.
2. Andresen D, Leitner VER, Wegscheider K, Schroeder R. Nachweis komplexer tachykarder ventrikulaerer Rhythmusstoerungen im Langzeit-EKG. Deut Med Wochr 1982;107:571–575.
3. Bigger T. Definition of benign versus malignant ventricular arrhythmias: Target for treatment. Am J Cardiol 1983;52:47C–54C.
4. Bigger JT, Heller CA, Wenger TL. Weld FM. Risk stratification after acute myocardial infarction. Am J Cardiol 1978;42:202–210.
5. Bigger JT, Reiffel JA, Livelli FD, Wang PJ. Sensitivity, specificity and reproducibility of programmed electrical stimulation. Circulation 1986;73(II):73–78.

6. Bluzhas J, Lukshiene D, Shlapikiene B, Ragaishis J. Relation between ventricular arrhythmia and sudden cardiac death in patients with acute myocardial infarction: The predictors of ventricular fibrillation. J Am Coll Cardiol 1986;8:69A–72A.
7. Buxton AE, Waxman HL, Marchlinski FE, Josephson ME. Electrophysiologic studies in nonsustained ventricular tachycardia: Relation to underlying heart disease. Am J Cardiol 1983;52:985–991.
8. Buxton AE, Waxman HL, Marchlinski FE, Untereker AJ, Waspe LE, Josephson ME. Role of triple extrastimuli during electrophysiologic study of patients with documented sustained ventricular tachycardia. Circulation 1984;69(3):532–540.
9. Brugada P, Abdollah H, Heddle B, Wellens HJJ. Results of ventricular stimulation protocol using a maximum of 4 premature stimuli in patients without documented or suspected ventricular arrhythmias. Am J Cardiol 1983;52:1214–1218.
10. Brugada P, Green M, Abdollah H, Wellens HJJ. Significance of ventricular arrhythmias initiated by programmed electrical stimulation: the importance of the type of ventricular arrhythmia induced and the number of premature stimuli required. Circulation 1984;69(1):87–92.
11. Brugada P, Waldecker B, Wellens HJJ. Characteristics of induced ventricular arrhythmias in four subgroups of patients with myocardial infarction. JACC (in press).
12. Brugada P, Wellens HJJ. Comparison in the same patient of two programmed ventricular stimulation protocols to induce ventricular tachycardia. Am J Cardiol 1985;55: 380–383.
13. Brugada P, Wellens HJJ. Standard diagnostic programmed electrical stimulation protocols in patients with paroxysmal recurrent tachycardia. PACE 1984;7:1121–1128.
14. Braat SH, Zwaan CD, Brugada P, Wellens HJJ. Values of left ventricular ejection fraction in extensive anterior infarction to predict development of ventricular tachycardia. Am J Cardiol 1983;52:686–692.
15. Califf RM, McKinnis, Burks J, Lee KL, Harell FE, Behar VS, Pryor DB, Wagner GS, Rosati RA. Prognostic implications of ventricular arrhythmias during 24 hour ambulatory monitoring in patients undergoing cardiac catheterization for coronary artery disease. Am J Cardiol 1982;50:23–31.
16. Chakko CS, Gheorghiade M. Ventricular arrhythmias in severe heart failure: incidence, significance and effectiveness of antiarrhythmic therapy. Am Heart J 1985;109 (3):497–504.
17. Coumel P, Cabrol C, Fabiato A. Tachycardie permanente par rhythme reciproque. Arch Mal Coeur Vaiss 1971;60:1830–1837.
18. Coumel P, Leclercq FJ, Zimmerman M. The clinical use of beta-blockers in the prevention of sudden death. Eur Heart J 1986;7:187–201.
19. Das SK, Morady F, DiCarlo L, Baerman J, Krol R, De Buitleir M, Crevey B. Prognostic usefulness of programmed ventricular stimulation in idiopathic dilated cardiomyopathy without symptomatic ventricular arrhythmias. Am J Cardiol 1986;58:998–1000.
20. Davis HT, DeCamilla J, Bayer LW, Moss AJ. Survivorship patterns in posthospital phase of myocardial infarction. Circulation 1979;60:1252.
21. DeBusk RF, Davidson DM, Houston N, Fitzgerald J. Serial ambulatory electrocardiography and treadmill exercise testing after myocardial infarction. Am J Cardiol 1980;45: 547–554.
22. Deniss AR, Cody DV, Russell PA, Young AA, Ross DL, Uther JB. Prognostic significance of inducible ventricular tachycardia after myocardial infarction. J Am Coll Cardiol 1984;3:610–617.
23. DiCarlo LA, Morady F, Schwartz AB, Shen EN, Baerman JM, Krol RB, Scheinman MM, Sung RJ. Clinical significance of ventricular fibrillation-flutter induced by ventricular programmed stimulation. Am Heart J 1985;5(1):959–963.
24. Doherty JU, Kienzle MG, Waxman HL, Buxton AE, Marchlinski FE, Josephson ME. Programmed electrical stimulation at a second right ventricular site: An analysis of 100 patients, with special reference to sensitivity, specificity and characteristics of patients with induced ventricular tachycardia. Am J Cardiol 1983;52:1184–1189.

25. Durrer D, Schoo L, Schuilenburg RM, Wellens HJJ. The role of premature beats in the initiation of supraventricular tachycardia in the Wolff-Parkinson-White syndrome. Circulation 1967;36:644–662.
26. Fisher JD, Mehra R, Furman S. Termination of ventricular tachycardia with bursts of rapid ventricular pacing. Am J Cardiol 1978;41:95–102.
27. Geibel A, Brugada P, Zehender M, Waldecker B, Kersschot I, Wellens HJJ. Programmed electrical stimulation in patients with hypertrophic cardiomyopathy. JACC 1986;7(2):195A.
28. Geibel A, Meinertz T, Tresse N, Kasper W, Pop T, Zehender M, Hofmann T, Just H. Incidence of spontaneous versus electrically induced ventricular arrhythmia in patients with coronary artery disease. Z Kardiol (in press).
29. Graboys TB, Lown B, Podrid PJ, DeSilva R. Longterm survival of patients with ventricular antiarrhythmic drugs. Am J Cardiol 1982;50:437–443.
30. Graboys TB, Almeida EC, Lown B. Recurrence of malignant ventricular arrhythmia after antiarrhythmic drug withdrawal. Am J Cardiol 1986;58:59–62.
31. Fisher L. Commentary: evaluation of antiarrhythmic drugs by sudden death trials. Circulation 1986;73(II):98–100.
32. Hamer A, Vohra J, Hunt D, Sloman G. Prediction of sudden death by electrophysiologic studies in high risk patients surviving acute myocardial infarction. Am J Cardiol 1982;50:223–229.
33. Helfant RH, Pine R, Kabde V. Exercise-related ventricular premature complexes in coronary heart disease. Correlations with ischemia and angiographic severity. Ann Intern Med 1974;80:589–592.
34. Hofmann T, Meinertz T, Kasper W, Geibel A, Zehender M, Hohnloser S, Stienen U, Treese N, Just HJ. 4-year-follow-up in idiopathic dilated cardiomyopathy: A multivariate analysis of prognostic factors. Am J Cardiol (in press).
35. Holter NJ. New method for heart studies. Science 1961;134:1214.
36. Huang SK, Messer JV, Denes P. Significance of ventricular tachycardia in idiopathic dilated cardiomyopathy: observations in 35 patients. Am J Cardiol 1983;51:507–512.
37. Ingham RE, Mason JW, Rosen RM, Goodman DJ, Harrison DC. Electrophysiologic findings in patients with idiopathic hypertrophic subaortic stenosis. Am J Cardiol 1978;41:811–816.
38. Josephson ME, Horowitz LN. Spielman SR, Greenspan AM. Electrophysiologic and hemodynamic studies in patients resuscitated from cardiac arrest. Am J Cardiol 1980;46:948–954.
39. Josephson ME, Horowitz LN. Electrophysiologic approach to therapy of recurrent sustained ventricular tachycardia. Am J Cardiol 1979;43:631–641.
40. Josephson ME, Marchlinski DE, Buxton AE, Waxman HL, Doherty JU, Kienzle MG, Falcone R. Electrophysiologic basis for sustained ventricular tachycardia. In: Josephson ME, Wellens HJJ (Eds). Tachycardias, Mechanisms, Diagnosis, Treatment. Philadelphia, Lea and Febiger, 1984;305–323.
41. Kunze KP, Kuck KH, Geiger M, Bleifeld W. Programmed electrical stimulation in hypertrophic cardiomyopathy-specificity and sensitivity of different stimulation protocols. JACC 1986;7(II):195A.
42. Kennedy HL, Chandra V, Sayther KL, Caralis DG. Effectiveness of increasing hours of continuous ambulatory electrocardiography in detecting maximal ventricular ectopy: Continous 48 hour study of patients with coronary artery disease and normal subjects. Am J Cardiol 1978;42:925–930.
43. Livelli FD, Bigger JT, Reiffel JA, Gang ES, Patton JN, Noethling PM, Rolnitzky LM, Gliklich JI. Response to programmed electrical stimulation: sensitivity, specificity and relation to heart disease. Am J Cardiol 1982;50:452–458.
44. Lown B, Wolf M. Approaches to sudden death from coronary heart disease. Circulation 1971;44:130–142.
45. Mann DE, Luck JC, Griffin JC, Herre JM, Limacher MC, Magro SA, Robertson NW, Wyndham CRC. Induction of clinical ventricular tachycardia using electrical stimulation. Value of third and fourth extrastimuli. Am J Cardiol 1983;52:501–506.

46. Marchlinski FE, Buxton AE, Waxman HL, Josephson ME. Identifying patients at risk of sudden death after myocardial infarction: Value of response to programmed stimulation, degree of ventricular ectopic activity and severity of left ventricular dysfunction. Am J Cardiol 1983;52:1190–1196.
47. Maron BJ, Savage DD, Wolfson JK, Epstein SE. Prognostic significance of 24h-ambulatory monitoring in patients with hypertrophic cardiomyopathy: A prospective study. Am J Cardiol 1981;48:252–257.
48. McKenna WJ, Deanfield J, Faruqui A, England D, Oakley CM, Goodwin JF. Prognosis in hypertrophic cardiomyopathy. Am J Cardiol 1981;47:532–538.
49. McNeil BJ, Keeler E, Adelstein SJ. Primer on certain elements of medical decision making. N Engl J Med 1975;293:211–217.
50. Meinertz T, Hoffmann T, Kasper W, Tresse N, Bechthold H, Steinen U, Pop T, Leitner EV, Andresen D, Meyer J. Significance of ventricular arrhythmias in idiopathic dilated cardiomyopathy. Am J Cardiol 1984;53:902–907.
51. Meinertz T, Treese N, Kasper W, Geibel A, Hoffmann T, Zehender M, Bohn D, Pop T, Just H. Determinants of prognosis in idiopathic dilated cardiomyopathy as determined by programmed electrical stimulation. Am J Cardiol 1985;56:337–341.
52. Meinertz T, Kasper W, Schmitt B, Treese N, Rueckel A, Zehender M, Hoffmann T, Pop T, Herzrhythmusstoerungen bei Herzgesunden. Dtsch Med Wochenschr 1983;108:527–531.
53. Michelson EL, Morganroth J. Spontaneous variability of complex ventricular arrhythmias detected by long-term electrocardiographic recording. Circulation 1980;61(4):690–695.
54. Misner JE, Imrey PB, Smith L. Secular variation in frequency of premature ventricular contractions in untreated individuals. J Lab Clin Med 1978;92:117–125.
55. Morady F, DiCarlo WS, Davis JC, Scheinman MM. A prospective comparison of the role of triple extrastimuli and left ventricular stimulation in studies of ventricular tachycardia induction. Circulation 1984;70:52–57.
56. Morady F, Scheinman MM, Hess DS, Sung RJ, Shen E, Shapiro W. Electrophysiologic testing in the management of survivors of out-of-hospital cardiac arrest. Am J Cardiol 1982;51:85–89.
57. Morganroth J, Michelson EL, Horowitz LN. Limitations of routine long-term electrocardiographic monitoring to assess ventricular ectopy. Circulation 1978;58:408–414.
58. Moss AJ. Clinical significance of ventricular arrhythmias in patients with and without coronary artery disease. Progr Cardiovasc Dis 1980;1:33–52.
59. Moss AJ, Davis HT, DeCamilla J, Bayer LW. Ventricular ectopic beats and their relation to sudden and nonsudden cardiac death after myocardial infarction. Circulation 1979;60:998–1003.
60. Moss AJ, DeCamilla JJ, Davis HP. Clinical significance of ventricular ectopic beats in the early posthospital phase of myocardial infarction. Am J Cardiol 1977;39:635–640, 1977.
61. Myerburg RJ, Conde C, Sheps DS, Appel RA, Kiem I, Sung RJ, Castellanos A. Antiarrhythmic drug therapy in survivors of prehospital cardiac arrest: Comparison of effects on chronic ventricular arrhythmias and recurrent cardiac arrest. Circulation 1979;59:855–863.
62. Panidis IP, Morganroth J. Sudden death in hospitalized patients: Cardiac rhythm disturbances detected by ambulatory electrocardiographic monitoring. JACC 1983;2:798–805.
63. Podrid PJ, Lown B, Graboys TB, Lampert S. Use of short-term drug testing as part of a systematic approach for evaluation of antiarrhythmic drugs. Circulation 1986;73(2):81–91.
64. Poll DS, Marchlinski FE, Buxton AE, Doherty JU, Waxman HL, Josephson ME. Sustained ventricular tachycardia in patients with idiopathic dilated cardiomyopathy: electrophysiologic testing and lack of response to antiarrhythmic drug therapy. Circulation 1984;70:451–456.

65. Poll DS, Marchlinski FE, Buxton AE, Josephson ME. Usefulness of programmed stimulation in idiopathic dilated cardiomyopathy. Am J Cardiol 1986;58:992–997.
66. Pratt CM, Francis MJ, Luck JC, Wyndham CR, Miller RR, Quinones MA. Analysis of ambulatory electrocardiograms in 15 patients during spontaneous ventricular fibrillation with special reference to preceding arrhythmia events. JACC 1983;2:789–797.
67. Prystowsky EN, Miles WM, Evans JJ, Hubbard JE, Skale BT, Windle JR, Heger JJ, Zipes DP. Induction of ventricular tachycardia during programmed electrical stimulation: analysis of pacing methods. Circulation 1986;73(II):32–38.
68. Richards DA, Cody DV, Deniss AR, Russell PA, Young AA, Uther JB. A new protocol of programmed electrical stimulation for assessment of predisposition to spontaneous ventricular arrhythmias. Eur Heart J 1983;4:376–382.
69. Ruskin JN, DiMarco JP, Garan H. Out-of-hospital cardiac arrest. Electrophysiologic observations and selection of long-term antiarrhythmic therapy. N Engl J Med 1980;303:607–613.
70. Roy D, Waxman HL, Kienzle MG, Buxton AE, Marchilinski FE, Josephson ME. Clinical characteristics and long-term follow-up in 119 survivors of cardiac arrest: Relation to inducibility at electrophysiologic testing. Am J Cardiol 1983;52:969–974.
71. Ruberman W, Weinblatt E, Goldberg J. Ventricular premature beats and mortality after myocardial infarction. N Engl J Med 1977;297:750–757.
72. Sami M, Kraemer H, Harrison DD, Houston N, Shimasaki C, DeBusk R. A new method for evaluating antiarrhythmic drug efficacy. Circulation 1980;62:1172–1179.
73. Schulze RA, Strauss HW, Pitt B. Sudden death in the year following myocardial infarction. Am J Med 1977;62:192–199.
74. Sheffield LT, Berson A, Bragg-Remschel D, Gillette PC, Hermes RE, Hinkle L, Kennedy H, Mirvis DM, Oliver CH. Recommendations for standards of instrumentation and practice in the use of ambulatory electrocardiography. Circulation 1985;72:824–829.
75. Stevenson WG, Brugada P, Waldecker B, Zehender M, Wellens HJJ. Can potentially significant polymorphic ventricular arrhythmias initiated by programmed stimulation be distinguished from those that are non-specific? Am Heart J 1986;111:1073.
76. Stevenson WG, Brugada P, Waldecker B, Zehender M, Wellens HJJ. Clinical angiographic, and electrophysiologic findings in patients with aborted sudden death as compared to patients with sustained ventricular tachycardia after myocardial infarction. Circulation 1985;6:1146–1152.
77. Stevenson WG, Brugada P, Waldecker B, Zehender M, Geibel A, Wellens HJJ. Electrophysiologic characteristics of patients with ventricular tachycardia or fibrillation in relation to the age of myocardial infarction. Am J Cardiol 1985;57:387–391.
78. Treese N, Pop T, Meinertz T, Kasper W, Geibel A, Stienen U, Meyer J. Prognostic significance of repetitive ventricular response in chronic coronary artery disease. Eur Heart J 1985;6:594–601.
79. Treese N, Geibel A, Kasper W, Meinertz T, Pop T, Meyer J. Incidence and significance of repetitive ventricular response in patient without identifiable organic heart disease. Int J Cardiol 1984;6:489–499.
80. Udall JA, Ellestad MH. Predictive implications of ventricular premature contractions associated with treadmill stress testing. Circulation 1977;56:985–989.
81. Vandepol CJ, Farshidi A, Spielman SR, Greenspan AM, Horowitz LN, Josephson ME. Incidence and clinical significance of induced ventricular tachycardia. Am J Cardiol 1980;45:725–731.
82. Wellens HJJ, Brugada P, Stevenson WG. Programmed electrical stimulation of the heart in life-threatening ventricular arrhythmias. What is the significance of induced arrhythmias and what is the correct stimulation protocol? Circulation 1985;72(1):1–7.
83. Wellens HJJ, Brugada P, Stevenson WG. Programmed electrical stimulation: Its role in management of ventricular arrhythmias in coronary artery disease.
84. Wellens HJJ, Durrer DR, Lie KI. Observations on mechanisms of ventricular tachycardia in man. Circulation 1976;54:237–244.
85. Wellens HJJ, Lie KI, Durrer D. Further observations on ventricular tachycardia studied by electrical stimulation of the heart. Chronic recurrent ventricular tachycardia and ventricular tachycardia during acute myocardial infarction. Circulation 1974;49:647–653.

86. Wellens HJJ, Schuilenburg RM, Durrer D. Electrical stimulation of the heart in patients with ventricular tachycardia. Circulation 1972;46:216–226.
87. Winkle RA. Antiarrhythmic drug effect mimicked by spontaneous variability of ventricular ectopy. Circulation 1978;57:1116.
88. Winkel RA. Ambulatory electrocardiography and diagnosis, evaluation and treatment of chronic ventricular arrhythmias. Progr Cardiovasc Dis 1980;2:99–128.
89. Zehender M, Brugada P, Geibel A, Waldecker B, Kersshot I, Wellens HJJ. Programmed electrical stimulation in patients with ventricular fibrillation late after myocardial infarction. PACE 1986;9:281.
90. Zehender M, Brugada P, Geibel A, Waldecker B, Kersshot I, Wellens HJJ. Significance of non-sustained monomorphic ventricular tachycardia during programmed electrical stimulation. PACE 1986;9:281.
91. Zehender M, Brugada P, Geibel A, Waldecker B, Kersshot I, Wellens HJJ. Sensitivity and specificity of a standardized ventricular stimulation protocol in patients with sustained ventricular tachycardia after myocardial infarction. Circulation 1985;72(III):359.
92. Zehender M, Brugada P, Geibel A, Waldecker B, Kersshot I, Wellens HJJ. Programmed electrical stimulation using a standardized stimulation protocol in patients after healed myocardial infarction. Am J Cardiol (in press).
93. Zehender M, Brugada P, Waldecker B, Stevenson W, Geibel A, Kersschot I, Bartolucci J, Wellens HJJ. Programmed electrical stimulation in patients with myocardial infarction versus idiopathic ventricular tachycardia. PACE 1985;8:316.

28

Treatment of Patients with Ventricular Tachycardia or Ventricular Fibrillation: First Lessons from the "Parallel Study"

Pedro Brugada, Robert Lemery
Mario Talajic, Paolo Della Bella
Hein J.J. Wellens

Introduction

Treatment of patients suffering from recurrent ventricular tachycardia and survivors of ventricular fibrillation remains a difficult problem. Empirical treatment with antiarrhythmic drugs in these patients results in high rates of recurrent arrhythmic events and a high mortality. New, more rational ways to approach the management of these arrhythmias have been developed in recent years.

In the early 1970s, several techniques were available for the study of arrhythmias. Long-term electrocardiographic monitoring is a valuable tool to detect symptomatic or asymptomatic ventricular arrhythmias. Exercise electrocardiography is helpful to reproduce exercise-related ventricular arrhythmias. Programmed electrical stimulation of the heart has been used since 1967[1,2] to reproduce a large variety of supraventricular arrhythmias occurring in the human heart. Combined with recordings of endocardial electrical activation and administration of antiarrhythmic drugs, programmed electrical stimulation of the heart proved valuable in the study of the mechanisms of not only supraventricular but

---

From: Brugada P, Wellens HJJ. CARDIAC ARRHYTHMIAS: Where To Go From Here? Mount Kisco, NY, Futura Publishing Company, Inc., © 1987.

also ventricular arrhythmias and to study the effects of antiarrhythmic drugs on the tachycardia mechanisms.[3-9] Many studies were initiated to assess the value of these techniques in the management of cardiac arrhythmias and to overcome the problems encountered with empirical treatment.[10]

These noninvasive and invasive techniques have certain limitations. Long-term ECG monitoring looks at spontaneously occurring events. However, the spontaneous paroxysm of a sustained ventricular tachycardia or fibrillation is rarely recorded by that method. Ectopic activity and short runs of ventricular tachycardia can be observed in about 50% of patients suffering from documented sustained paroxysmal ventricular tachycardia, but the incidence of these arrhythmias during long-term ECG monitoring is very low in patients suffering from paroxysmal ventricular fibrillation. The relation between ectopic activity and the spontaneous paroxystic sustained arrhythmias is unknown.

During programmed electrical stimulation of the heart, the arrhythmias are forced to occur by providing the triggers (premature stimuli). The ability to provoke an arrhythmia by programmed electrical stimuli, however, does not necessarily mean that the arrhythmia will occur spontaneously. Programmed electrical stimulation does not look at the spontaneous triggers of arrhythmias.

Exercise electrocardiography can reproduce exercise-related arrhythmias, but exercise-related arrhythmias represent only a small proportion of all clinically occurring arrhythmias.

In the early 1970s, thus, three different techniques were available that look at three different aspects of arrhythmias. A logical step would have been to combine them in a large, prospective study to learn the indications and value of each technique in the management of the different types of human arrhythmias. Most investigators, however, dedicated their efforts to the study of the value of either invasive or noninvasive techniques. Several strategies of treatment of arrhythmias were born in that way.

The problems with these strategies of treatment of ventricular arrhythmias (noninvasive guided strategies, serial electropharmacologic testing of antiarrhythmic drugs) have been discussed elsewhere.[11] The main problem is that they do not allow probabilistic analysis of results. No assessment of the true value of noninvasive and invasive techniques to predict results of treatment is possible: (1) The empirical strategy of treatment not only lacks standardization in data collection and analysis, but also in the steps of the decision-making process (how to select an antiarrhythmic agent, when to change the dose, when to discontinue a drug). (2) The approach using the so-called "serial testing of antiarrhythmic agents,"[12] whether using noninvasive or invasive studies, does not allow probabilistic analysis of results because false and true positives cannot be recognized. During serial testing of antiarrhythmic drugs, potentially helpful drugs are discontinued on the basis of preselected criteria of uncertain significance. (3) The approach using plasma levels of antiarrhythmic drugs is difficult to use in clinical practice not only because of the retrospective nature of the measurement, but also because the "therapeutic" plasma level (the level preventing recurrences of the arrhythmia) cannot be determined beforehand for the individual patient. Also each patient has different electrophysiological properties of the tissues involved in the spontaneous initiation and perpetuation of arrhythmias, and it cannot be expected that the same effect will be obtained in all patients with the same plasma level of a drug. (4) Finally, combinations of the above strategies confuse the probabilistic analysis of results rather than facilitate understanding of the value of the different techniques in the management of cardiac arrhythmias because of the negative additive effects of limitations.

With these considerations in mind, we decided to undertake a prospective study to assess the value of long-term ECG monitoring, exercise ECG, programmed stimulation of the heart, plasma levels of antiarrhythmic drugs, and other techniques, such as signal averaging of the ECG in the management of patients suffering from ventricular tachycardia and/or ventricular fibrillation. The study was designed in such a way that : (1) it would allow probabilistic analysis of the value of any of the techniques employed without using preselected criteria of efficacy or inefficacy, and (2) it would be prospective, using standardized methodology.

The decision to use this approach was facilitated by the fact that we had been using exercise electrocardiography, long-term ECG monitoring, and programmed electrical stimulation of the heart more as *tools to understand* mechanisms of arrhythmias rather than to *guide antiarrhythmic treatment*. Selecting standardized methodology was more difficult. The Bruce protocol on a treadmill was selected for exercise ECG. We also decided to continuously monitor the patient with ventricular tachycardia or ventricular fibrillation from the time of admission to the hospital until discharge. Both qualitative and quantitative analysis of the results of long-term ECG monitoring and exercise ECG could be performed. Standardizing programmed electrical stimulation of the heart required a critical review of previous studies followed by additional investigations.

At the time we were considering starting our "parallel" testing (1982), many different definitions and stimulation protocols were being used. Many pacing modes had been introduced to initiate and terminate arrhythmias, such as burst pacing, use of more than three premature stimuli, stimulation at sites other than the right ventricular apex (right ventricular outflow tract, left ventricle), current strength above twice diastolic threshold (10 or 20 mA), administration of isoproterenol, and use of alternating current.[13-17] For the majority of these protocols, sensitivity and specificity were not known. There were also problems with the definitions used to classify spontaneous and induced arrhythmias (monomorphic versus polymorphic, sustained versus nonsustained). It was also unclear whether all induced arrhythmias had the same clinical significance.[18,19] Before standardizing our stimulation protocol, we performed several studies directed to answer these questions. The first series[20,21] addressed the problem of the significance of arrhythmias induced by programmed ventricular stimulation. Using a stimulation protocol from the right ventricular apex at twice diastolic threshold and a maximum of four premature stimuli given during sinus rhythm and pacing at three different rates, we observed that both the type of arrhythmia induced (polymorphic versus monomorphic, sustained versus nonsustained) and the mode of induction (number of premature stimuli) had to be considered before giving an arrhythmia clinical significance. The second set of studies compared that stimulation protocol with the number of premature stimuli limited to three to a protocol using increased current strength, one single pacing rate, and two stimulation sites in the right ventricle.[22] That study demonstrated better sensitivity of a stimulation protocol using three premature stimuli at twice diastolic threshold from the right ventricular apex during sinus rhythm and three pacing rates than one using a maximum of two premature stimuli (at twice diastolic threshold and 20 mA) from two right ventricular sites at a single pacing rate.

The next series of studies consisted of the prospective use of a standardized stimulation protocol (Table I) in patients with clinically documented ventricular tachycardia,[23] ventricular fibrillation late after myocardial infarction,[24] patients with idiopathic ventricular tachycardia,[25] right ventricular dysplasia, hypertrophic cardiomyopathy,[26] and also in patients without spontaneous ventricular arrhythmias after myocardial infarction.[27,28] These studies demonstrated a good sensitivity (94%) of the stimulation protocol in patients with ventricular tachycardia after myocardial infarction but also showed its limitations. The limitations were not only related to the type of ventricular arrhythmia but also to its etiology and electrophysiologic mechanisms. The main limitation of the protocol, however, was its specificity.[23,28] In approximately 45% of patients with a recent myocardial infarction not suffering clinically from ventricular arrhythmias, we could initiate a sustained monomorphic ventricular tachycardia. Initiation of that arrhythmia had no prognostic significance.

We then carefully compared the characteristics of the ventricular tachycardia initiated by the same stimulation protocol in patients after myocardial infarction with and without spontaneous episodes of ventricular tachycardia or ventricular fibrillation. Clear-cut differences appeared: monomorphic ventricular tachycardia initiated in patients not clinically suffering from the arrhythmia were faster and required more premature stimuli to be initiated than the monomorphic ventricular tachycardia initiated in patients having clinical documentation of the arrhythmia. This finding suggested to us that in approximately half of the patients after myocardial infarction, the substrate for a sustained ventricular tachycardia is

Table I
The Standardized Minimal Programmed
Stimulation Protocol Developed at Our Institution

Step	
1.	1 extrastimulus during sinus rhythm.
2.	2 extrastimuli during sinus rhythm.
3.	1 extrastimulus during pacing at 100 beats/min.
4.	2 extrastimuli during pacing at 100 beats/min.
5.	1 extrastimulus during pacing at 120 beats/min.
6.	2 extrastimuli during pacing at 120 beats/min.
7.	1 extrastimulus during pacing at 140 beats/min.
8.	2 extrastimuli during pacing at 140 beats/min.
9.	3 extrastimuli during sinus rhythm.
10.	3 extrastimuli during pacing at 100 beats/min.
11.	3 extrastimuli during pacing at 120 beats/min.
12.	3 extrastimuli during pacing at 140 beats/min.

All stimulation from the right ventricular apex using a current strength of twice diastolic threshold and a 2 ms duration of pulses.

present. The electrophysiologic properties of the reentry circuit, however, are not appropriate for the clinical spontaneous occurrence of the arrhythmia. The reentry circuits of these patients seem to have short refractory periods and short revolution times preventing spontaneous episodes of sustained ventricular tachycardia. Patients who after myocardial infarction spontaneously suffer from ventricular tachycardia or ventricular fibrillation have reentry circuits with longer refractory periods and longer revolution times, facilitating the spontaneous initiation and perpetuation of the arrhythmia.

Therefore, in any type of ventricular arrhythmia which is initiated by programmed electrical stimulation, the characteristics of the induced arrhythmia, the mode of induction, and the clinical characteristics of the patient have to be considered before giving the arrhythmia clinical significance.

Design of the "Parallel Study"

The study on "parallel" testing of antiarrhythmic treatment was designed as illustrated in Figure 1.

The patient with documented ventricular tachycardia or ventricular fibrillation or surviving an episode of cardiac arrest is admitted to a unit where cardiac rhythm is continuously monitored. This is done until discharge of the patient. A washout period may be necessary if the patient is on antiarrhythmic drugs at the time of admission. In the basal state, when the patient is not receiving any antiarrhythmic drug an exercise ECG, programmed electrical stimulation of the heart, coronary angiography, and left ventricular angiography are performed. The left ventricular (and when indicated right ventricular) ejection fraction is also measured by noninvasive techniques (bidimensional echocardiography, or nuclear angiogram) to allow comparison by noninvasive methods during follow-up. During the electrophysiologic study, effects of an intravenously given antiarrhythmic drug may be assessed and a plasma level measured. Irrespective from the results of these studies, the patient is thereafter loaded with an orally given antiarrhythmic drug which has been selected empirically on the basis of the type of spontaneous arrhythmia, etiology, previous antiarrhythmic drug history, and possible side effects (cardiac and extracardiac). Exceptions are patients who are direct surgical candidates because of left main coronary artery disease or severe angina or severe valvular dysfunction.

During the loading phase, the antiarrhythmic agent recurrences of the arrhythmia, if they occur, are treated with an intravenous drug, pacing, or cardioversion, but the dose of the oral drug is not changed. The initial dose of the antiarrhythmic drug is the minimally recommended one. We do not increase the dose to the maximally tolerated one for the following reasons. Antiarrhythmic drugs may prevent arrhythmias at a certain dose but might worsen them at a higher dose, or result in the occurrence of other types of arrhythmias ("torsade de pointes") and/or other side effects. When the patient is loaded with the antiarrhythmic drug and no spontaneous sustained arrhythmias or very frequent and symptomatic nonsustained arrhythmias occur spontaneously or during the exercise ECG, the same studies as made before drug administration are repeated.

Irrespective of the results of these studies, the patient is discharged on the drug and followed-up at the outpatient clinic.

When spontaneous arrhythmias recur after the steady state has been reached, the next step is to increase the dose and repeat the studies. In that way, probabilistic analysis of any desired criteria can be done if the the follow-up is long enough (to be determined for the individual patient) or if recurrences of the arrhythmia occur.

No preselected criteria of efficacy or inefficacy are used. Only the recurrence of the clinical arrhythmia (spontaneous ventricular tachycardia or ventricular fibrillation) is a reason to change the dose of a drug or the type of drug. The different techniques are used "in parallel," their results not modifying the clinically selected treatment. That is why we called this strategy "parallel testing" of antiarrhythmic treatment.

The typical duration of admission of a patient with ventricular tachycardia or fibrillation responding to the first selected antiarrhythmic drug is 1 week, with the exception of amiodarone because of the long loading time required for this drug.

Feasibility of "Parallel Testing"

We analyzed data from a retrospective and a pilot prospective series of patients in whom the "parallel" strategy had been followed at our institution before the definite "parallel study" was initiated. Both the incidence of sudden arrhythmic death (6% after 14 months follow-up) and total mortality (30% by actuarial analysis of 240 patients at 10 years follow-up) were low.[29] After approval by the ethical committee, the prospective study was initiated in Maastricht in February 1983. As of January 1987, a multicenter prospective evaluation of the "parallel study" has been started in the Netherlands. The following is a discussion of some of our initial findings.

Antiarrhythmic Drugs are Helpful to Prevent Recurrences of Ventricular Tachycardia or Ventricular Fibrillation

Several studies have demonstrated that antiarrhythmic agents when given intravenously can acutely terminate arrhythmias. Many other studies have also demonstrated that antiarrhythmic drugs suppress ectopic activity or ventricular tachycardia on electrocardiographic monitoring. Demonstration of prevention of paroxysmal sustained recurrent arrhythmias by antiarrhythmic drugs is, however, much more difficult. The difficulty arises because of the absence of information on the natural history of sustained ventricular tachycardia and ventricular fibrillation in relation to its etiology. Patients with sustained ventricular tachycardia or ventricular fibrillation have been systematically treated with antiarrhythmic drugs or other forms of antiarrhythmic treatment in order to prevent recurrences. Demonstrating that antiarrhythmic drugs have a beneficial effect on the natural history of these arrhythmias requires a randomized study with a control group not receiving any form of antiarrhythmic treatment. Given the possible lethal

PARALLEL TESTING OF AAD

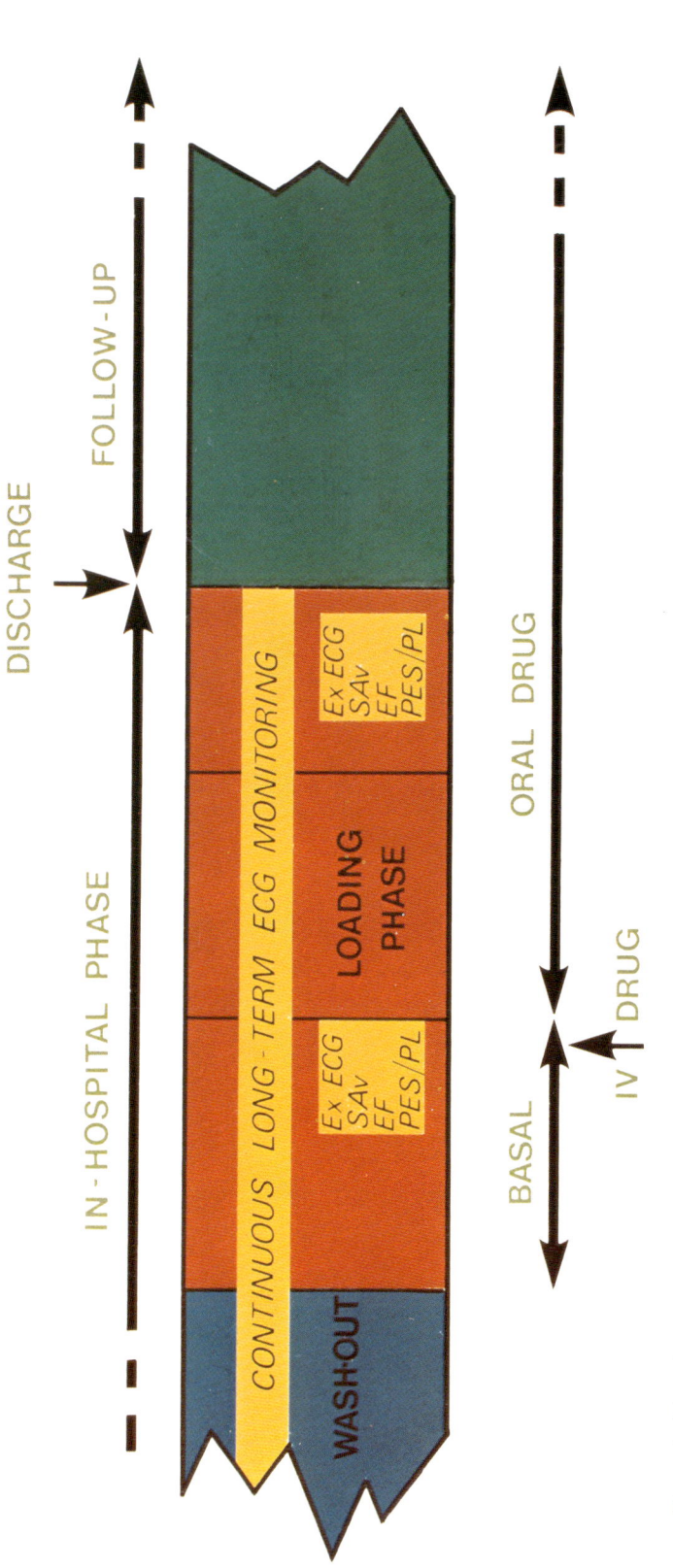

Figure 1: Flow chart of the "parallel study." See text for details. Abbreviations: EF = ejection fraction; Ex ECG = exercise electrocardiogram; IV = intravenous; PES = programmed electrical stimulation; PL = plasma level; SAv = averaged electrocardiogram.

consequences of ventricular tachycardia and ventricular fibrillation, such a study has always been considered unethical. The availability of the implantable cardioverter-defibrillator might make it possible to undertake such a study. At the present time, however, one has to analyze the effects of antiarrhythmic drugs on recurrences of these arrhythmias in a different way, each patient serving as his own control.

The incidence of recurrences of ventricular tachycardia or ventricular fibrillation was 90% before antiarrhythmic treatment and 30% once patients were treated with antiarrhythmic drugs.[29] Considered as a group, therefore, antiarrhythmic drugs did prevent recurrences of tachycardias.

Recurrent Ventricular Tachycardia Does not Equate with Sudden Death

The incidence of sudden death in our patients is low if one considers the "high risk" patients thus far included in the parallel study. We have analyzed data from 35 patients prospectively included in the parallel study who had a myocardial infarction (in 75% located anteriorly) and the spontaneous development of sustained monomorphic ventricular tachycardia late after the event. These patients had a left ventricular ejection fraction of less than 40% (mean 29%) and remained inducible to a sustained monomorphic ventricular tachycardia during treatment with an empirically selected antiarrhythmic drug. The recurrence rate of ventricular tachycardia was 30% at a mean follow-up of 20 months, but only 11% of this high-risk group developed sudden death during the follow-up. Thus, in severely ill patients with monomorphic ventricular tachycardia included in the parallel study, empirical treatment with an antiarrhythmic drug did not result in sudden death rates of 30–40%, which have been reported in previous studies. While ventricular tachycardia did recur in 30% of these patients, the arrhythmia was generally slow in rate and well tolerated. This allowed the patient to seek medical help in our clinic. These data support that there is no need to continue to look for noninducibility during programmed electrical stimulation studies as done during serial testing of antiarrhythmic drugs. It raises the question of why in the serial testing studies the death rate is so high in patients who continue to be inducible. This may be related to differences in counseling of the patient or the compliance of the referring physician and patient to continue to take the assigned treatment. In our environment, ventricular tachycardia does not equate with death. The same results have been obtained in patients treated because of spontaneous ventricular fibrillation and cardiac arrest after myocardial infarction.

Idiopathic Ventricular Tachycardia and the Right Ventricular Dysplasia Syndrome Have an Excellent Prognosis when Treated Medically

In a series of 54 patients with ventricular tachycardia in a structurally normal heart, not a single patient died from an arrhythmia during a mean follow-up of 7 years after the first episode of ventricular tachycardia. Recurrence of the arrhythmia occurred, however, in 50% of patients. The only patient who died in this series died of cancer. Of the six patients with idiopathic ventricular fibrillation included in the parallel study, only one had a recurrence after antiarrhythmic drugs were given. All patients are alive. In one of these patients, a defibrillator has been implanted. No shocks were needed, however, during a follow-up of 1 year.

Five of the 10 patients with the syndrome of right ventricular dysplasia included in the parallel study had recurrences of ventricular tachycardia on antiarrhythmic drugs. However, no patient treated with antiarrhythmic drugs has died despite recurrences. The only patient who was treated surgically by right ventricular disconnection died of a low-output state after surgery.

These data indicate that ventricular tachycardia occurring in the structurally normal heart (idiopathic ventricular tachycardia) and in patients with right ventricular dysplasia (with normal left ventricular function) has an excellent prognosis when treated medically. Also in these patients, a recurrence of the arrhythmia does not equal death.

Proarrhythmic Effects Observed During Programmed Electrical Stimulation Have no Prognostic Significance

It has been reported that 10 to 30% of patients develop proarrhythmic effects when given an antiarrhythmic drug.[30,31] This information comes from studies where the clinical significance of criteria of "arrhythmogenesis" were not assessed prospectively. When "proarrhythmic" effects (variously defined) were observed, the patient never received the drug on a long-term basis thereby making it impossible to assess the clinical significance of these observations. As in the "parallel study," results of programmed electrical stimulation are not used to modify treatment, and we could retrospectively analyze the significance of criteria of arrhythmogenesis in 65 patients prospectively included in our study. Seventy-five percent of these patients had an old myocardial infarction. Fifty-two patients had documented sustained monomorphic ventricular tachycardia, and 13 patients documented ventricular fibrillation. Propafenone was given to 22 patients, amiodarone to eight, sotalol to another eight, and bepridil to eight patients. Class 1a antiarrhythmic drugs were given in five and combinations in 14 patients. When results of programmed stimulation were compared before and after treatment with the oral drug, "proarrhythmic" effects were observed in 14 patients (an incidence of 22%). These "proarrhythmic" effects consisted of a change from induced nonsustained to sustained ventricular tachycardia in two patients, induction of the same ventricular tachycardia with a lesser number of premature beats in eight patients, while a faster rate of induced ventricular tachycardia was observed in four patients. As already discussed, patients were discharged on the same antiarrhythmic drug irrespective from the results of programmed stimulation. During a mean follow-up period of 24 months, the 14 patients who showed "proarrhythmic" effects had the same recurrence rate (43%) and incidence of sudden death (one patient) as patients not showing "proarrhythmic" effects during programmed simulation. These data suggest that "proarrhythmic" effects of antiarrhythmic drugs are common during programmed stimulation (22%), but have no prognostic significance and should not be used as an indication to discontinue a drug that may potentially be helpful.

Efficiency of Programmed Electrical Stimulation of the Heart and Long-Term ECG Monitoring

Data from 84 patients prospectively included in the "parallel study" have been analyzed to assess efficiency of programmed electrical stimulation and long-term ECG monitoring. Sixty-four patients had documented sustained monomorphic ventricular tachycardia and 20 patients documented ventricular fibrillation. All these patients had an old myocardial infarction. Programmed stimulation and continuous long-term ECG monitoring were performed before treatment and after loading with an oral antiarrhythmic drug. All 84 patients were inducible to a sustained monomorphic ventricular tachycardia or ventricular fibrillation before treatment. However, only 29 of these 84 patients showed Lown 4b ventricular arrhythmias on long-term ECG monitoring before any drug was given. Thus, long-term ECG monitoring showed possible "markers" of paroxysmal sustained arrhythmias in only 34% of these patients with well-documented sustained ventricular arrhythmias. In other words, 66% of patients had a false negative long-term ECG monitoring before drugs. When antiarrhythmic drugs were given, 68/84 (80%) patients remained inducible to a sustained monomorphic ventricular tachycardia or ventricular fibrillation, while Lown 4b arrhythmias persisted in 8/29 (27%) patients having these arrhythmias on long-term ECG monitoring before drugs. Patients were discharged on the same drug they received at the time of study and followed up for a mean of 16 months. A recurrence of ventricular tachycardia occurred in 25/68 inducible patients and in 2/16 noninducible patients ($p < 0.05$). Sudden death occurred in 3/68 inducible patients and in 1/16 noninducible patients (p=ns). Ventricular tachycardia recurred in 4/8 patients having no Lown 4b ventricular arrhythmias after antiarrhythmic drugs were given and in 9/21 patients with Lown 4b arrhythmias on long-term ECG monitoring at discharge (p=ns). The positive predictive value of programmed stimulation was low (37%) because 63% of patients discharged on a drug on which they remained inducible did not have recurrences of their arrhythmia. The negative predictive value of programmed stimulation was good (87%) although 13% of patients noninducible at discharge did have a recurrence of their arrhythmia. Overall, the efficiency of programmed stimulation (a measure of overall agreement of results and follow-up) was low (46%). A value of 46% indicates that from results of programmed stimulation (inducibility versus inducibility while on oral antiarrhythmic drugs), a wrong prediction of arrhythmic events during follow-up will be made in half of the patients. Patients who become noninducible after antiarrhythmic drugs, however, have a lower incidence of recurrent ventricular tachycardia than those patients in whom the arrhythmia remains inducible, although the incidence of sudden death is similar in the two groups.

These data do not support continuation of programmed stimulation until noninducibility by performing serial studies with different agents because: (1) not only in our experience but also in the experience of other authors,[32] noninducibility will be attained in only a minority of patients; (2) most inducible patients will do well at follow-up; (3) as previously stated, a recurrence of ventricular tachycardia on antiarrhythmic drugs does not equal death of the patient; (4) incidence of sudden death was similar in noninducible and inducible patients; and (5) the cost-to-benefit ratio of serial testing, given the low number of patients who become noninducible and results of follow-up, is not appropriate.

Programmed Electrical Stimulation of the Heart, Exercise ECG, and Long-Term ECG Monitoring Underestimate True Clinical Efficacy of Antiarrhythmic Drugs

Using the design of the "parallel study," it is possible to look at any desired criterion applied to these tests to predict results of treatment. The true clinical efficacy of the drug (ability to prevent recurrences of *spontaneous* arrhythmias) can be compared to the efficacy of the drug as defined from results of noninvasive or invasive studies.

We have analyzed the efficacy of propafenone as defined from noninvasive and invasive studies and compared this "efficacy" to the true clinical efficacy of propafenone in a series of 48 patients with symptomatic nonsustained ventricular tachycardia (n=11), sustained monomorphic ventricular tachycardia (n=30), or ventricular fibrillation (n=7). Efficacy of propafenone as defined by its ability to prevent induction of a sustained ventricular tachycardia was 20% in patients with spontaneous nonsustained ventricular tachycardia, 17% in patients with spontaneous sustained ventricular tachycardia, and 0% in patients with spontaneous ventricular fibrillation. The percentage of efficacy of propafenone as defined by ability to suppress Lown's 4b arrhythmias during exercise ECG was 100%, 50%, and 0% for the three groups, respectively. For long-term ECG monitoring, using the same definition, it was 70%, 52%, and 33% for the three groups. These results were in contrast with the true clinical efficacy of propafenone defined as survival and arrhythmia-free survival during a mean of 18 months. After that period of time, 91% of patients with spontaneous nonsustained ventricular tachycardia, 60% of patients with sustained monomorphic ventricular tachycardia, and 71% of patients with spontaneous ventricular fibrillation were alive and free from recurrences of arrhythmias. Interestingly, 50% of these 48 patients were treated with the minimally recommended dose of propafenone (450 mg/day).

These data indicate that, should results of programmed electrical stimulation have been used to guide treatment, less than 20% of patients would have received propafenone long-term. Because, and as previously discussed, many patients did not have Lown's 4b arrhythmias on noninvasive studies before propafenone, less than 25% of patients would have received propafenone on the basis of data from noninvasive studies, should they have been used to guide treatment.

Noninvasive and invasive studies underestimate the true clinical efficacy of propafenone. Using the design of the "parallel study," we have learned that the same holds true for flecainide, bepridil, amiodarone, sotalol, d-sotalol, and also some classic antiarrhythmic drugs such as procainamide and disopyramide.

Identification of High-Risk Groups from Clinical Data

The "parallel study" offers some unique opportunities to reassess not only the value of sophisticated methods of study of arrhythmias but also the value of very simple clinical means such as the clinical history. Predicting the results of antiarrhythmic treatment is not an easy endeavor. While in the future this might become easier, our present methods of study of arrhythmias have limited value.

We have recently analyzed the value of an episode of syncope in patients with spontaneous ventricular tachycardia or ventricular fibrillation during treatment with antiarrhythmic drugs to predict the subsequent risk of sudden death. Like many other observations in clinical medicine, this study was not based on a previously consciously designed strategy to study that phenomenon, but rather on empirical observations at the outpatient clinic while following-up patients with ventricular tachycardia or ventricular fibrillation. We had observed that patients with spontaneously occurring ventricular tachycardia or ventricular fibrillation suffering from an episode of syncope during treatment with antiarrhythmic drugs seemed to have a high incidence of sudden death later on. With a few exceptions, all these patients were readmitted to the hospital and/or the antiarrhythmic drug treatment was modified at the time the syncopal episode occurred. In spite of this, many of these patients died suddenly during follow-up. Whether a brady- or a tachyarrhythmia was responsible for the patient's demise is unknown to us at the present time. When data were retrospectively analyzed, 22 patients with a syncopal episode during treatment with antiarrhythmic drugs were identified in the "parallel study" out of a series of 100 patients with ventricular tachycardia ($n=69$) or ventricular fibrillation ($n=31$) after myocardial infarction. The sensitivity, specificity, and positive predictive value of a history of syncope during treatment with antiarrhythmic drugs for later sudden death was 80%, 89%, and 49%, respectively. This was higher than inducibility by programmed stimulation on the same drug (80%, 25%, and 11%, respectively) or a left ventricular ejection fraction of less than 40% (sensitivity 70%, specificity 25%, positive predictive value 10%). While one cannot obviously predict beforehand which patient will develop syncopal episodes during treatment with antiarrhythmic drugs, these data clearly suggest that patients developing these symptoms at follow-up deserve special attention and readmission to the hospital to assess what has been responsible for syncope. As discussed, in-hospital monitoring was not helpful and our present policy includes implantation of a VVI pacemaker with monitoring facilities in these patients in order to prevent bradyarrhythmias but also to recognize tachyarrhythmias. These patients may be candidates for implantation of an automatic defibrillator if the tachyarrhythmic nature of the syncopal episode can be proven. Further treatment has to be carefully individualized in these patients.

Discussion

The "parallel study" is not a strategy of treatment of patients with ventricular tachycardia or ventricular fibrillation. The "parallel study" is a scientific approach designed to understand the value of presently available methods of study of arrhythmias in the management of patients with ventricular tachycardia or ventricular fibrillation. The treatment which is given to a particularly patient is selected clinically by considering a multitude of factors. Treatment is highly individualized. The results obtained with this approach are acceptable, particular when one compares our results with results obtained using the strategies discussed in the beginning of this chapter. The clinical experience on which selection of treatment is based is difficult to transmit at the present time. There is, however, no magic formula that can be applied to the patients. This magic formula will never come, because patients are individuals who have individual characteristics.

These first lessons from the "parallel study" to test the value of present methods of study in the management of patients suffering from arrhythmias are of interest. There still remain many gaps in our knowledge on the natural course and prognosis of ventricular arrhythmias and coronary artery disease in man. It is also clear that the presently available noninvasive and invasive techniques have only a limited value in predicting the subsequent course of our patients. As discussed by Coumel and co-workers in another chapter of this book, no single technique (long-term ECG monitoring, exercise ECG, or programmed electrical stimulation) allows simultaneous information on the triggers, substrate, and modulating factors of ventricular tachycardia or ventricular fibrillation. No technique gives us sufficient information on the balance among these three factors, a balance which is necessary for a spontaneous arrhythmia to initiate and perpetuate, and that also explains the paroxysmal, apparently unpredictable behavior of sustained ventricular tachycardia or fibrillation.

Our antiarrhythmic armentarium allows us at the present time acceptable treatment in a remarkable number of patients with spontaneously occurring ventricular tachycardia or ventricular fibrillation. In the coming years, however, we still have a lot to learn in order to solve the problems which remain in the management of these arrhythmias.

As discussed by Stevenson et al. in another chapter of this book, we may have been too naive when considering the causes of sudden death late after myocardial infarction. We have accepted without much hesitation that most of these sudden deaths were caused by a recurrent arrhythmia similar to the one previously documented or not in a particular patient. In patients with coronary artery disease, recurrent ischemia is as frequently the cause of sudden death as a pure electrical event. We know that the degree of left ventricular dysfunction is also a major determinant of prognosis in patients with a variety of cardiac diseases. Sudden death finds itself in the middle of a triangle which is discussed in another chapter of this book.

Reduction of infarct size is accompanied by a reduction in inducible[27] and spontaneous[33] ventricular arrhythmias. These observations are in accordance with studies indicating the importance of the degree of left ventricular dysfunction on inducibility[27,28,32] and spontaneous occurrence of ventricular arrhythmias and sudden death.

The challenge for arrhythmology in the near future goes far beyond the recognition and treatment of cardiac arrhythmias, but should be directed towards recognition and prevention of the arrhythmia substrates. For some diseases, such as idiopathic ventricular tachycardia, recognition of the real cause will take a long time or may even never be recognized. For others, like ventricular tachycardia after myocardial infarction, the causes are clear and solutions at least partially available. When a substrate for an arrhythmia does not exist, no arrhythmia can develop. Prevention of coronary artery disease and reduction of infarct size (if myocardial infarction cannot be avoided) are therefore our targets in the prevention of ventricular tachycardia after myocardial infarction. A reduction in the incidence of this arrhythmia may have already taken place in centers using thrombolytic therapy in patients with impending or evolving myocardial infarction.[33]

References

1. Durrer D, Schoo L, Schuilenburg RM, Wellens HJJ. The role of premature beats in the initiation and the termination of supraventricular tachycardia in the Wolff-Parkinson-White syndrome. Circulation 1967;36:644–662.
2. Coumel Ph, Cabrol P, Fabiato A, Gourgon R, Slama R: Tachycardie permanente par rhythme reciproque. Arch Mal Coeur 1967;60:1830–1834.
3. Wellens HJJ. Electrical stimulation of the heart in the study and treatment of tachycardias. Baltimore, University Park Press, 1971.
4. Wellens HJJ. Schuilenburg RM, Durrer D. Electrical stimulation of the heart in patients with ventricular tachycardia. Circulation 1972;46:216–226.
5. Wellens HJJ, Bar FWHM, Lie KI. Effect of procainamide, propranolol and verapamil on mechanism of recurrent ventricular tachycardias. Am J Cardiol 1977;40:579–585.
6. Mason JW, Winkle RA. Electrode-catheter arrhythmia induction in the selection and assessment of anti-arrhythmic drug therapy for recurrent ventricular tachycardia. Circulation 1978;58:971–985.
7. Horowitz LN, Josephson ME, Farshidi A, et al. Recurrent sustained ventricular tachycardia. 3. Role of the electrophysiologic study in selection of anti-arrhythmic regimens. Circulation 1978;58:986–996.
8. Josephson ME, Horowitz LN, Farshidi A et al. Recurrent sustained ventricular tachycardia. 2. Endocardial mapping. Circulation 1978;57:470–477.
9. Josephson ME, Horowitz LN, Spielman SR, et al. Comparison of endocardial catheter mapping with intraoperative mapping of ventricular tachycardia. Circulation 1980; 61:395–404.
10. Wellens HJJ. Value and limitations of programmed electrical stimulation of the heart in the study and treatment of tachycardias. Circulation 1978;57:845–853.
11. Brugada P, Wellens HJJ: Need and design of a prospective study to assess the value of different strategic approaches for management of ventricular tachycardia or fibrillation. Am J Cardiol 1986;57:1180–1184.
12. Wu D, Wyndham CR, Denes P, et al. Chronic electrophysiologic study in patients with recurrent paroxysmal tachycardia. In Kulbertus HE, ed. Re-entrant Arrhythmias. MTP, Lancaster, 1977;294–311.
13. Richards DA, Cody DV, Denniss AR, et al. Ventricular electrical instability: A predictor of death after myocardial infarction. Am J Cardiol 1983;51:75–80.
14. Buxton AE, Waxman HL, Marschlinski FE, et al. Role of triple extrastimuli during electrophysiologic study of patients with documented sustained ventricular tachyarrhythmias. Circulation 1984;69:532–540.
15. Morady F, DiCarlo L, Winston S, et al. A prospective comparison of triple extrastimuli and left ventricular stimulation in studies of ventricular tachycardia induction. Circulation 1984;70:52–57.
16. Morady F, Shapiro W, Shen E, et al. Programmed ventricular stimulation in patients without spontaneous ventricular tachycardia. Am Heart J 1984;107:875–882.

17. Mann DE, Luck JC, Griffin JC, et al. Induction of clinical ventricular tachycardia using programmed stimulation: Value of a third and fourth extrastimuli. Am J Cardiol 1983;53:501–506.
18. Wellens HJJ, Brugada P, Stevenson W. Programmed electrical stimulation of the heart in life-threatening ventricular arrhythmias. What is the significance of induced arrhythmias and what is the correct stimulation protocol? Circulation 1985;72;1–5.
19. Wellens HJJ, Brugada P, Stevenson W. Programmed electrical stimulation: Its role in the management of ventricular arrhythmias in coronary heart disease. Progr Cardiovasc Dis 1986;23:165–180.
20. Brugada P, Green M, Abdollah H, Wellens HJJ: Significance of ventricular arrhythmias initiated by programmed ventricular stimulation. Circulation 1984;69:87–92.
21. Brugada P, Abdollah H, Heddle B, Wellens HJJ. Results of a ventricular stimulation protocol using a maximum of 4 premature stimuli in patients without documented or suspected ventricular arrhythmias. Am J Cardiol 1983;52:1214–1218.
22. Brugada P, Wellens HJJ. Comparison in the same patient on 2 programmed ventricular stimulation protocols to induce ventricular tachycardia. Am J Cardiol 1985;55:380–383.
23. Zehender M, Brugada P, Geibel A, Waldecker B, Kersschot I, Wellens HJJ. Sensitivity and specificity of a standardized ventricular stimulation protocol in patients with sustained ventricular tachycardia after myocardial infarction. Circulation 1985;72(III)359.
24. Zehender M, Brugada P, Geibel A, Waldecker B, Kersschot I, Wellens HJJ: Programmed stimulation in patients with ventricular fibrillation later after myocardial infarction (abstr). PACE 1985;9:281.
25. Zehender M, Brugada P, Waldecker B, Stevenson W, Geibel A, Kersschot I, Bartolucci J, Wellens HJJ. Programmed electrical stimulation in patients with myocardial infarction versus idiopathic ventricular tachycardia (abstr). PACE 1985;8:316.
26. Geibel A, Brugada P, Zehender M, Kersschot I, Wellens HJJ. Results of standardized ventricular stimulation protocol in patients with hypertrophic cardiomyopathy (abstr). J Am Coll Cardiol 1986;7:195.
27. Kersschot I, Brugada P, Ramentol M, Zehender M, Waldecker B, Geibel A, de Zwaan C, Wellens HJJ. Effects of early reperfusion in acute myocardial infarction on arrhythmias induced by programmed stimulation. A prospective, randomized study. J Am Coll Cardiol 1986;7:1234–1242.
28. Brugada P, Waldecker B, Kersschot I, Zehender M, Wellens HJJ. Ventricular arrhythmias initiated in 4 groups of patients with myocardial infarction. J Am Coll Cardiol 1986;8:1035–1041.
29. Brugada P, Wellens HJJ. "Parallel" testing to evaluate efficacy of antiarrhythmic therapy in patients with ventricular tachycardia or fibrillation. Circulation 1985;72(III):477.
30. Velebit V, Podrid P, Lown B, Cohen BH, Graboys TB. Aggravation and provocation of ventricular arrhythmias by antiarrhythmic drugs. Circulation 1982;65:868–872.
31. Poser RF, Podrid PJ, Loma B, Cohen BH, Graboys TB. Aggravation of arrhythmia induced with antiarrhythmic drugs during electrophysiologic testing. Am Heart J 1985;110:9–15.
32. Swerdlow CD, Winkle RA, Mason JW. Determinants of survival in patients with ventricular arrhythmias. New Engl J Med 1983;308:143–145.
33. Simoons ML, Serruyes PW, Brand M van der, et al. Improved survival after early thrombolysis in acute myocardial infraction. Lancet 1985;578–582.

29

Prospective Criteria for the Selection of Therapy for Ventricular Tachycardia and Ventricular Fibrillation

John D. Fisher
Anthony D. Mercando
Soo G. Kim

Introduction

While ventricular fibrillation (VF) is an immediate life-threatening event, ventricular tachycardia (VT) ranges from slow, well tolerated, and infrequent, to incessant and catastrophic with consequences akin to those of VF. Pharmacologic therapy of VT/VF has advanced through the use of prospective randomized trials, in which results using a new agent are compared with those of a standard agent and/or a placebo. The same antiarrhythmic drugs may be effective against the whole range of benign and serious ventricular arrhythmias. Other therapeutic modalities are applicable only to a portion of the range of ventricular arrhythmias. Patients with slow, well-tolerated, and infrequent VT are not ordinarily subjected to the considerable risk of antitachycardia surgery. Similarly, such patients are not candidates for early generations of implantable cardioverter/defibrillators (ICDs), since these devices are able to detect only relatively rapid tachycardias, as well as VF.

The process of determining therapy for individual patients has often been

From: Brugada P, Wellens HJJ. CARDIAC ARRHYTHMIAS: Where To Go From Here? Mount Kisco, NY, Futura Publishing Company, Inc., © 1987.

time-consuming, involving trial and error.[1] Criteria were therefore established to increase the efficiency of the therapeutic selection process. This paper reports the selection criteria used, the difficulties encountered, and the follow-up of patients treated for VT/VF.

Methods

Development of Treatment Selection Criteria

Therapeutic Options

Five major therapeutic modalities are currently available in the antiarrhythmia arsenal. These are: (1) medications, (2) surgery, (3) nonsurgical ablation, (4) antitachycardia pacers, and (5) implantable cardioverter/defibrillators (ICDs). A sixth modality, cardiac transplant, may be appropriate in certain instances.

Patient Population

All patients in this study had sustained spontaneous ventricular tachycardia or fibrillation, not associated with an acute myocardial infarction, drug toxicity, or remediable metabolic or related abnormalities. All these patients also underwent programmed electrical stimulation (PES) during electrophysiologic testing (EPS). This study begins with the first patient to be treated at our own institution using the most recently introduced modality, i.e., ablation.

Random Allocation (Fig. 1)

The possibility of random allocation of patients to each of the five therapeutic modalities was considered, but rejected. As outlined in the introduction, random allocation would lead to anomalous or inappropriate therapy that could not possibly work. For example, slow VT will not meet the fixed diagnostic rate criteria of early generation ICDs.

Modified Random Allocation (Fig. 2)

Using this scheme, patients would be divided after initial screening into those with rapid and those with slower arrhythmias. Those with rapid VT or VF would be randomly allocated to surgery, ICD, or medications. Patients with slower tachycardias would be randomized to ablation, pacer therapy, or medications. Once again, realities imposed themselves to thwart this scheme. Patients in whom pacing regularly induced an acceleration of the arrhythmia would have to

Selection of Therapy for VT/VF • 473

RANDOM ALLOCATION

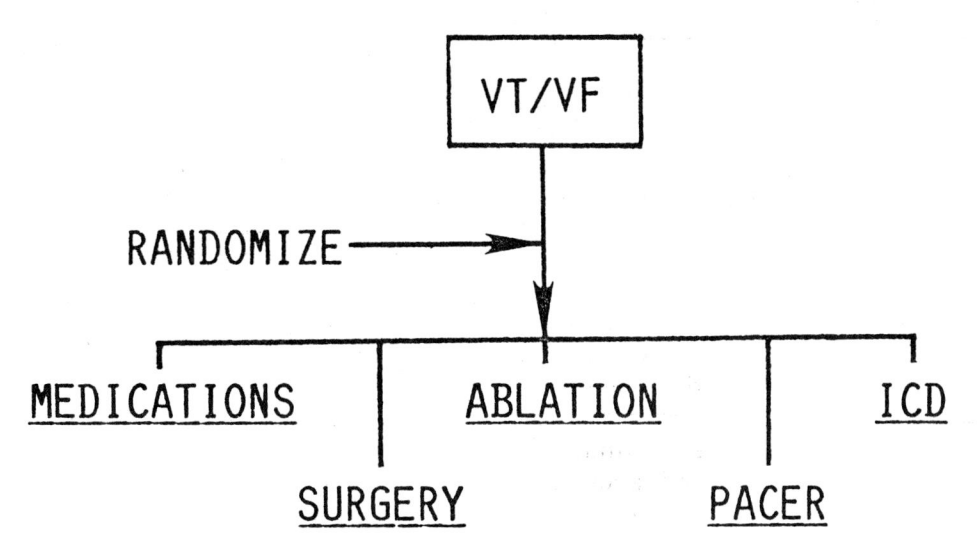

Figure 1: Selection of therapy by random allocation. VT = ventricular tachycardia; VF = ventricular fibrillation; ICD = Implantable cardioverter/defibrillator. See text for details.

MODIFIED RANDOM ALLOCATION

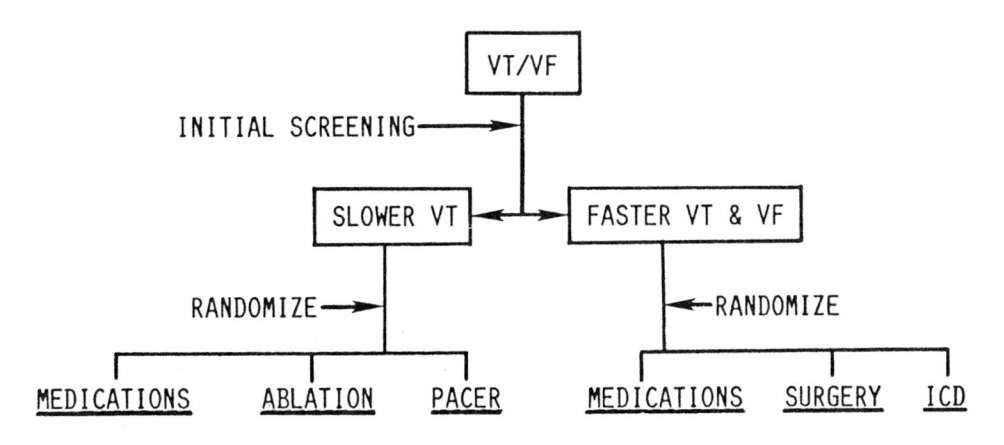

Figure 2: Modified random allocation. Abbreviations as in Figure 1.

be deleted from that group. Such considerations made it clear that there were several necessary points of decision prior to establishing the final therapy. Criteria could be established initially, but an unacceptable response to the initial modality would lead to a mid-course change in direction.

Allocation By Inclusion and Exclusion Criteria (Fig. 3)

Selection criteria for immediate consideration of each therapeutic modality have been established in sequence at our institution, and adjusted as new options have evolved. Soon after admission to our program, an initial screening series of evaluations categorized patients by eight variables designated as determinants in formulating the immediate therapeutic plan for each patient. Some of these variables were dichotomous, so that a total of 14 variables could be identified (Table I). Inclusion and exclusion criteria were based on groupings of the eight variables. These criteria are outlined in Table II. After an initial history, physical, cardiac catheterization and/or nuclear ejection fraction and initial electrophysiologic and noninvasive arrhythmia testing, the data was screened for inclusion or exclusion criteria for indication of therapeutic modality.

Patients remaining after subtraction of those treated according to inclusion

SEQUENTIAL USE OF INCLUSION/EXCLUSION CRITERIA
PLUS MODIFYING FACTORS

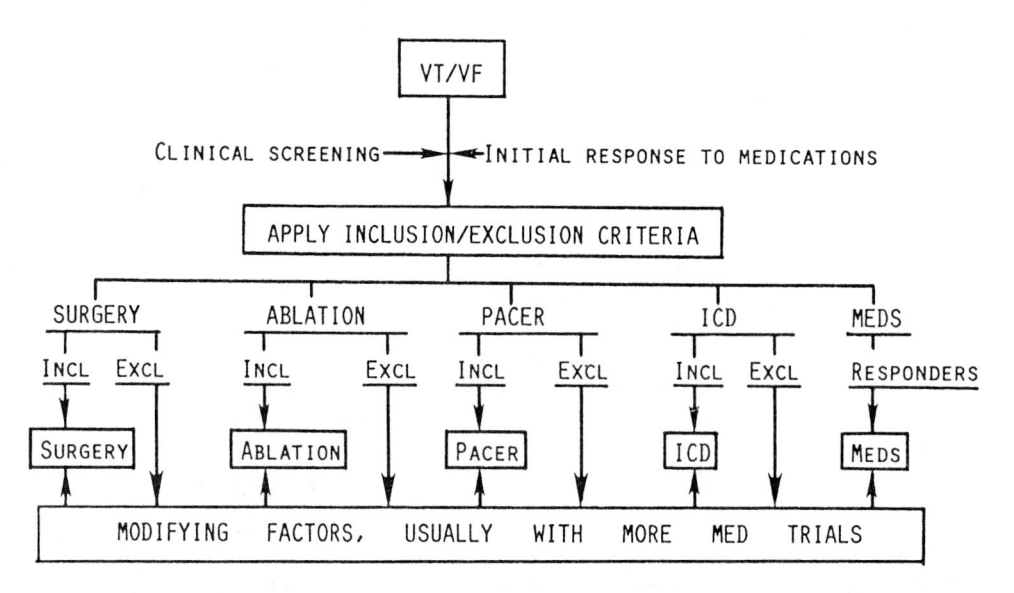

Figure 3: Selection of therapy by sequential use of inclusion/exclusion criteria plus modifying factors. Incl = patients meeting inclusion criteria; Excl = patients meeting exclusion criteria; Meds = treatment by medications. Other abbreviations as in Figures 1 and 2. Patients excluded from various therapies after initial screening may receive any of the various therapeutic modalities later during their hospital course, after consideration of modifying factors. See text for details.

Table I
Selection of Therapy: Variables Used for Initial Inclusion/Exclusion Criteria

1. VT morphologies (spontaneously or with PES): 1–2 vs ≥ 3
2. CAD vs other heart disease
3. Need for other heart surgery
4. Incessant VT/VF
5. Arrhythmia severity: VF, CPR vs well-tolerated VT
6. Number MIs: 1 vs multiple
7. Age: < 70 vs ≥ 70
8. EF: < 30 vs ≥ 30

CAD = Coronary artery disease.
CPR = Cardiopulmonary resuscitation.
EF = Ejection fraction.
MI = Myocardial infarction.

Table II
Selection of Therapy: Inclusion and Exclusion Criteria after Initial Screening

Therapy	Inclusion	Exclusion
Surgery	Incessant VT/VF, or Need other OHS	Age ≥ 70 Non-CAD heart disease Well-tolerated VT Multiple MIs
Ablation	1–2 VT morphs, and Age < 70, and Well-tolerated VT	≥ 3 VT morphologies
Antitachy Pacer	Well-tolerated VT, and No acceleration of VT	Acceleration of VT
Implantable cardioverter/defibrillator	Age ≥ 70, and EF < 30, and ≥ 3 VT morphologies and CPR/VF	Well-tolerated VT
Medications	Responders at screen	(Patients meeting other inclusion criteria)

CAD = Coronary artery disease.
CPR = Cardiopulmonary resuscitation.
EF = Ejection fraction.
Morph = Morphologies.

criteria were given additional medication trials, while other modifying factors were considered. The 10 basic factors, involving a weighted point system that might differ considerably among institutions, have been reported in detail.[2] Three additional factors are also of major importance in this process: (1) patient toleration of testing procedures, (2) patient acceptance of therapeutic recommendations, and (3) response to additional therapeutic trials. These factors are outlined in Table III. Of primary importance is the risk/benefit ratio. Our objective

Table III
Modifying Factors in the Choice of Antiarrhythmic Therapy

1.	Long-term efficacy	7.	Comfort
2.	Risks	8.	Compliance
3.	Success rate of entry	9.	Side effects
4.	Cure/suppressant/rescue	10.	Convenience
5.	Cost	11.	Patient acceptance of recommendation
6.	Availability (general vs. specialized center, device availability	12.	Patient tolerance of testing
		13.	Responses to therapeutic trials

was to maximize the number of live, functional patients at the end of the follow-up period, based on the present state of knowledge. Thus we would decline to perform aggressive and high risk therapeutic procedures if the known and perceived risk of these procedures in our institution were substantially greater than those of an alternative that was felt likely to provide substantial efficacy with less risk. "Exit criteria" for patients with VF and life-threatening VT requiring CPR were (1) noninducibility by PES or (2) implantation of an ICD. Other patients were expected to have noninducibility or evidence of improvement by PES, or a device, or to meet criteria for a "Holter cure."[3]

Follow-Up

We followed patients both in the hospital and after discharge. The objectives were to access whether predetermined inclusion/exclusion criteria would lead to prompt selection of the indicated therapy; to determine the relative importance of the selection criteria vs the modifying factors; and to observe the actuarial mortality at 1 year of patients in each of the therapeutic groups.

Results

Patient Population (Table IV)

Since the first nonsurgical ablation procedure for ventricular tachycardia at our institution in November 1983, 148 patients were entered into the protocol through January 1987. These included 108 men and 40 women, with a mean age of 58. All had spontaneous sustained VT or VF and had been referred for electrophysiologic studies combined with Holter and exercise testing as described elsewhere.[4,5] Coronary artery disease was present in 103, and 84 (57%) of the entire group had ejection fractions of under 30%.

Table IV
Demographics of the 148 Patients in This Study

		N	%
1.	VT morphologies		
	• 1–2	64	43
	• ≥ 3	84	57
2.	Heart disease		
	• CAD	103	70
	• Other	45	30
3.	Need other surgery	13	9
4.	Incessant VT/VF	10	7
5.	Severity		
	• Well tolerated	30	20
	• Poorly tolerated	118	80
	• CPR	84	57
6.	Number MIs		
	• One	62	42
	• Multiple	31	21
7.	Age		
	• ≥ 70	21	14
	• < 70	127	86
8.	Ejection fraction		
	• ≥ 30	64	43
	• < 30	84	57

Limited Effectiveness of Inclusion/Exclusion Criteria

Antitachycardia Surgery

Seven patients met the inclusion criteria for immediate surgery, and this was performed on four patients. Of the others, one died prior to intended surgery, and two underwent nonsurgical ablation procedures for which they also qualified. Antitachycardia surgery was also performed on an additional five patients after further drug trials, and consideration of modifying factors.

Nonsurgical Ablation

During this period, six patients met criteria for ablation. Two of these accepted the recommendation and underwent an ablation procedure. Three refused, preferring to undergo further drug trials; one of these ultimately underwent an ablation procedure. The sixth patient underwent surgical therapy, since this appeared to offer a better risk/benefit ratio after considering all the modifying factors.

Altogether, ten patients underwent ablation procedures, seven of whom did not meet initial inclusion criteria. In these cases, ablations were performed after medications were identified that reduced the rate of their VT to tolerable ranges, and eliminated all but 1-2 morphologies, except in one patient. In the latter subject, attempts were made to ablate the most frequently recurring of his many morphologies.

Antitachycardia Pacemaker

Only two patients received anti-VT pacemakers. Following the initial screen, all patients with well-tolerated VT were considered, but only one patient fulfilled the additional inclusion criteria of passing a rigorous series of pre-implant pacing trials.[6] Another patient qualified after medications resulted in a more manageable tachycardia.

Implantable Cardioverter/Defibrillator (ICD)

During the study period, 17 patients received ICDs. Only one of these met the inclusion criteria after the initial screening. Of the remaining 16, 15 were too young, 12 had ejection fractions above the criteria, three had two or fewer VT morphologies, and two had never had CPR or VF. However, after failure of multiple drug trials and application of the modifying factors, devices were ultimately implanted.

Medical Therapy

One hundred and thirty-three patients did not meet the inclusion criteria for other forms of therapy, and thus were treated initially with serial drug testing. After consideration of the modifying factors, some of these patients went on to receive other treatment modalities, while patients who met criteria for other therapy but refused or for other reasons were treated medically.

Overall Results of Inclusion/Exclusion Criteria and Modifying Factors

Only 15 of the 148 patients (10%) met inclusion criteria after initial screening for treatment categories other than medications. Of these 15, only eight were actually treated initially as indicated by inclusion and exclusion criteria. In spite of continuing efforts, it proved impossible to avoid an early and major impact of the modifying factors (Fig. 4).

Follow-Up

Patients discharged from the hospital through February 1986 were included in the follow-up, to provide an estimate of the number of patients dying in the first year, together with at least 1 year follow-up on the survivors. The total number of

**ACTUAL INTERPLAY OF
INCLUSION/EXCLUSION CRITERIA AND MODIFYING FACTORS**

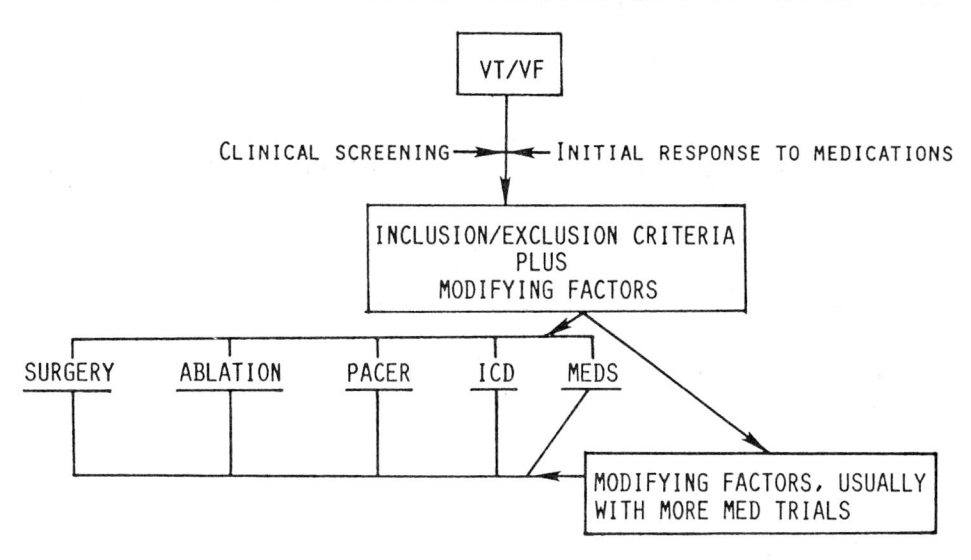

```
                        ┌───────┐
                        │ VT/VF │
                        └───┬───┘
 CLINICAL SCREENING ──────► │ ◄────── INITIAL RESPONSE TO MEDICATIONS
                        ┌───▼──────────────────────┐
                        │ INCLUSION/EXCLUSION CRITERIA │
                        │          PLUS             │
                        │     MODIFYING FACTORS     │
                        └──────────────────────────┘
  │        │        │       │      │
SURGERY  ABLATION  PACER   ICD   MEDS
  │        │        │       │      │
                                   ┌──────────────────────────────┐
                                   │ MODIFYING FACTORS, USUALLY   │
                                   │ WITH MORE MED TRIALS         │
                                   └──────────────────────────────┘
```

Figure 4: Actual interplay of inclusion/exclusion criteria and modifying factors in the selection of therapy. Abbreviations as in previous figures. Modifying factors were found to play an important role in the selection of therapy very early in the hospital course. If a decision could not be made after initial screening, further medical trials were carried out, influenced again by the modifying factors. These modifying factors also led to the development of exit criteria which had to met prior to discharge from the hospital, as described in the text.

patients in each of the therapeutic groups therefore may be less than the overall group described previously, since patients entered after February 1986 are excluded. The total number of patients discussed below adds up to 122, since one patient received ablation, surgery, and an ICD. The overall 1 year sudden death rate was 1.7% (2 of 119 patients).

Surgical Patients

Among the eight surgical patients includes in the follow-up study, five were "cured," i.e., not inducible during electrophysiologic study (PES) at the time of discharge. There were no deaths among these patients; this includes those who were not cured, but were discharged on the best medical regimen determined after further PES and noninvasive evaluations.

VT Ablation

Six patients underwent ablation procedures during the follow-up group period. None of these patients were cured by the ablation procedure, and they were subsequently treated with the best medical regimen as assessed by PES and noninvasive evaluations. There were no deaths among these patients.

Antitachycardia Pacer Patients

There were two patients in this group, and none died during the follow-up period.

ICD Patients

Thirteen patients received ICDs during the time period allowing them to enter the follow-up group. There were three deaths among these patients, none of them sudden.

Medical Therapy

Ninety-three patients were treated with medications at a time qualifying them for entry into the follow-up group. There were 18 deaths among these patients, eight of them sudden. Forty of the 93 patients (43%) were considered cured on the basis of PES. Among these, two (5%) died suddenly; both had severe coronary disease with heart failure, and one had historically been noncompliant with therapy.

Discussion

Several questions are raised by our experience with attempts to establish prospective arrhythmia therapy selection criteria. As these issues are raised below, it should be kept in mind that the 1 year sudden death mortality rate was less than 2%, far better than would ordinarily be expected in such a group of patients.[7,8]

Were the Inclusion Criteria Too Exclusive?

Only 15 patients (10%) met inclusion criteria after initial screening. There is no question that the inclusion criteria reflect the combination of our prejudices, together with (even here!) the influence of modifying factors. For example, although it may be true that ICDs are the most effective way to prevent sudden death,[9,10] limited device availability would have precluded the establishment of a less restricted set of inclusion criteria.

Could Modifying Factors Have Been Suppressed?

Some of these factors (Table III) are subject to manipulation or variation. Estimates of risk, the importance of convenience to the patient, and similar factors may be specific to individual physicians or institutions. Many factors affect patient acceptance of recommendations and toleration of procedures. These include the approach of the physician, individual patient characteristics, and cultural background. Factors such as device availability, costs, and reimbursement policies may also vary with both time and place, but are often beyond the influence of the patient or physician. Indeed, it is clear that the inclusion and exclusion criteria are themselves dependent to a large extent on the modifying factors they may individually or in combination determine the ultimate therapy.

Is the Actual Process (Fig. 4) Adequate?

Follow-up data from patients entered in this protocol were gratifying. These patients represent a microcosm of our overall experience (updated from ref. 3) but the results were comparable. In the present study, all of the sudden deaths occurred in the medically treated group. In our overall experience, the likelihood of sudden death in patients felt to be "cured" on the basis of PES was comparable to that of patients treated with the ICD, a group which also suffered instances of sudden death.

Are Exit Criteria More Important than Inclusion/Exclusion Criteria?

Most of the sudden deaths in our patient group are due to progressive disease, or noncompliance with the prescribed treatment. For patients with the ICD, "noncompliance" would include patients with malfunctioning or depleted devices. Our present policy has been to insist upon a very high degree of protection for patients with a history of VF or need for cardiopulmonary resuscitation. This implies either noninducibility by PES, or the implantation of an ICD. Through extensive medical trials, combined with surgery, ablation, and in some cases the implantation of an ICD, these criteria are now achieved in virtually all patients prior to discharge. The low sudden death rate in these high risk patients implies that satisfying these exit criteria provides an excellent prognosis. Most of the deaths in our patient group are due to nonarrhythmic complications of progressive heart disease. For patients who fail to meet the exit criteria in our overall series of similar patients, the 1-year sudden death rate is about 20%.

Do Scientific Benefits Justify Randomized Approaches?

The results with patients enrolled in the present study were excellent, with therapy based on a multi-tiered approach using inclusion criteria, modifying factors, and exit criteria. It could be argued that our patients constitute a special group, and that results with randomized allocation would have been just as good, or even better. The serious reasons for doubting this are outlined in the Introduction and Methods sections. The demographics of the group in this study are typical of high risk patients. Perhaps the patients described above who fail to meet exit criteria and suffered a high 1-year sudden death rate constituted a significantly different group. We are presently examining this possibility using multivariate analysis.

Conclusions

The desirability of early selection of the discharge treatment modality remains. However, the objective of shortening the hospital course, with its attendant costs and inconveniences for all concerned, must be balanced against the ultimate objective of maximizing the number of live and functional patients at the end of any given follow-up period. Thus far, we have not found prospective criteria for early selection of the final therapy that have met all these objectives.

Acknowledgments: The authors appreciate the efforts of Margaret Criscuolo, Debra R. Johnston, Diane Acosta, and other members of the Arrhythmia Service in the work leading to completion of this manuscript.

References

1. Fisher JD, Mercando AM, Kim SG. Antitachycardia strategies. PACE 1986;9:1309–1311.
2. Fisher JD. Arguments in favor of electrical antitachycardia techniques (pacing, endocardial cardioversion, intracardiac defibrillation). In: Breithardt G, Borggrefe M, Zipes DP, eds. Non-pharmacological Therapy of Tachyarrhythmias. Mt. Kisco, NY, Futura Publishing Co. (in press).
3. Fisher JD, Fink D, Matos JA, Kim SG, Waspe LE. Programmed stimulation and ventricular tachycardia therapy: Benefits of partial as well as complete "cures" (abstr). PACE 1982;6:A139.
4. Kim SG. The management of patients with life-threatening ventricular tachyarrhythmias: Programmed stimlulation or Holter monitoring? Either or both? Circulation (in press).
5. Kim SG, Felder SD, Figura I, Johnston DR, Waspe LE, Fisher JD. Comparison of programmed stimulation and Holter monitoring for predicting long-term efficacy and inefficacy of amiodarone used alone or in combination with a class 1A antiarrhythmic agent in patients with ventricular tachyarrhythmia. J Am Coll Cardiol 1987;9:398–404.
6. Fisher JD, Kim SG, Furman S, Matos JA. Role of implantable pacemakers in control of recurrent ventricular tachycardia. Am J Cardiol 1982;49:194–206.
7. Cobb LA, Baum RS, Alvarez H III, et al. Resuscitation from out-of-hospital ventricular fibrillation: 4 years follow-up. Circulation 1975;51&52:(Suppl 3):III-223–228.
8. Swerdlow C, Winkle RA, Mason JW. Determinants of Survival In Patients with Ventricular Tachyarrhythmias. New Engl J Med 1983;308:1436–1442.
9. Echt DS, Armstrong K, Schmidt P, Oyer PE, Stinson EB, Winkle RA. Clinical experience, complications, and survival in 70 patients with the automatic implantable cardioverter defibrillator. Circulation 1985;71:289–296.
10. Fisher JD, Kim SG, Mercando AM. Electrical devices for treatment of arrhythmias. Am J Cardiol (in press).

VI

ANTIARRHYTHMIC DRUGS

30

A Clinical Classification of Antiarrhythmic Drugs

Paul Puech
Josep Brugada

General Considerations

Relatively simple classifications of antiarrhythmic agents based upon their effects on the electrophysiologic properties of isolated cells[1-3] and intact human heart[4] or on the transmembrane ionic currents (Na, Ca, and K channel blockers) and the autonomic nervous system (beta-blockers, vagomimetic substances) have been proposed in recent years. A clinical classification of antiarrhythmic drugs, however, is by necessity complex, due to the multiple factors involved in therapeutic choices and subsequent results.

The knowledge of the electrophysiologic effects of a given antiarrhythmic agent is a necessary prerequisite. This permits the allocation of new and investigational substances into the well-known therapeutic classes. The limitation of such a reference system is that only the chief effect of the drug is taken into consideration, while many drugs belong to more than one category. Also, drugs may have different effects on normal or damaged tissues. From electrophysiologic studies, certain conclusions are drawn as to its expected antiarrhythmic action which may or may not be confirmed during clinical application. In some cases, the electrophysiologic effects lead to an opposite effect such as the exacerbation of the treated arrhythmia or the provocation of a new rhythmic disorder. Both complications are known as the so-called proarrhythmic effect of antiarrhythmic drugs.

From: Brugada P, Wellens HJJ. CARDIAC ARRHYTHMIAS: Where To Go From Here? Mount Kisco, NY, Futura Publishing Company, Inc., © 1987.

A clinical classification of antiarrhythmic drugs must consider the characteristics of the arrhythmic which has to be treated, such as its atrial, junctional, or ventricular origin, its paroxysmal or permanent form, its hemodynamic consequences, the age of the patient, etc. The arrhythmia mechanism is very often speculative. Only in paroxysmal supraventricular tachycardias has the mechanism (reentry in the AV node or involving an accessory pathway) been precisely defined.

Therapeutic objectives differ according to the cases and can be divided into three categories:

1. Suppression of a sustained arrhythmia in order to restore sinus rhythm, or at least the previous rhythm, if it was well tolerated.
2. Improvement of the hemodynamic setting by slowing the ventricular rate. This palliative effect is obtained by lengthening the atrioventricular conduction in case of atrial arrhythmias (atrial fibrillation, flutter, tachycardia) and by decreasing the rate of junctional and ventricular tachycardias.
3. Elimination of extrasystoles when their treatment is justified by the presence of symptoms and/or if they play a role in the occurrence of more severe arrhythmias, sustained or nonsustained.

Knowledge about the triggering factors may have practical consequences for treatment, such as variations of the autonomic balance (arrhythmias induced by catecholergic discharge or by enhancement of the vagal tone) and acute ischemic episodes (for instance, arrhythmias occurring during spastic angina).

Other factors of importance for the clinical classification of antiarrhythmic drugs include pharmacokinetic and metabolic data, modes of administration (oral or parenteral), and side effects which can reduce to second place a drug having a very potent antiarrhythmic action (for instance, amiodarone).

Some substances not incorporated in the traditional classifications of antiarrhythmic drugs have to be included in a clinical classification because they have curative, palliative, or preventive effects. Examples are digitalis, purinergic substances, and ions such as potassium and magnesium.

Expected Responses to Antiarrhythmic Drugs

The fast Na channel blockers (class I) prolong refractoriness and for some of them conduction velocity in atria, ventricles, and the His-Purkinje system and also raise the threshold of the propagated responses. They can be effective in suppressing atrial and ventricular arrhythmias. This effect is probably based upon change from uni- to bidirectional block in reentrant circuits, leading to termination of circus movement excitation. The termination of a paroxysmal reentrant supraventricular tachycardia using an accessory pathway is made possible via depression of the Kent bundle by class IA and IC antiarrhythmic agents.

Slowing in rate of an ectopic rhythm is one of the effects of the fast Na channel blockers. In case of a rapid atrial rhythm, the decreased rate may be deleterious if atrioventricular conduction is not depressed also. The decreased ectopic atrial activity will be more easily transmitted to the ventricles and a 2-to-1 AV relation can be changed into a 1-to-1 response, as in the case of atrial flutter.

Lengthening of ventricular repolarization by class IA antiarrhythmic agents may contribute to the induction of torsade de pointes, as found in the classical "quinidine syncope." The clinical experience with class IC antiarrhythmic drugs (flecainide, propafenone, encainide) which electively depress intraventricular conduction, has shown that these drugs can induce incessant patterns of ventricular tachycardias.

Class IB antiarrhythmic drugs (lidocaine, mexiletine, tocainide) have little electrophysiologic effects on normal fibers but exert marked depressive effects on ischemic, partially depolarized cells. That explains the infrahisian conduction defects occurring sometimes after administration of these substances in the acute stage of myocardial infarction.

The supplementary actions of some Na channel antagonists (e.g., vagolytic effect, mainly observed with disopyramide and partial block of beta-receptors with propafenone) can explain the variable effect of these agents when the autonomic nervous system plays a role in the initiation of the tachycardia, as in vagal or catecholergic paroxysmal atrial fibrillation.

The Ca channel blockers effectively slow conduction and prolong refractoriness of the slow response fibers of the AV node. These drugs have demonstrated their efficacy on arrhythmias involving the AV node such as paroxysmal reentrant intranodal tachycardia or supraventricular tachycardia involving the AV node as part of a reentry circuit (Wolff-Parkinson-White syndrome, among others). The intra-AV nodal conduction delay obtained by the Ca channel blockers explains the decrease in ventricular rate in case of atrial fibrillation and the use of digitalis in association with Ca channel blockers to obtain a further depression of AV conduction. Termination of peculiar ventricular tachycardias by verapamil has been an empirical discovery suggesting the intervention of the Ca channel and mechanisms other than reentry (triggered activity?). No electrophysiologic proof has been obtained, however. The same holds true for exercise-related ventricular arrhythmias which are prevented by Ca channel blockers.

Arrhythmias depending on an acute ischemic episode of variant angina are sensitive to Ca channel blockers, but they are used in that particular situation because of their antispastic properties rather than because of their electrophysiologic effects.

Beta-blockers do not have significant cellular electrophysiologic effects in therapeutic doses, even if they have membrane-stabilizing properties. The only exception known at the present time is sotalol, which prolongs membrane repolarization.

The antiarrhythmic action of beta-blockers seems to exclusively depend on their beta-adrenolytic effect, resulting in slowing of sinoatrial discharge, delaying of conduction in the AV node, and opposition to catecholinergic arrhythmias. Clinical experience has demonstrated that beta-blockers and Na channel blockers have synergistic effects in the prevention of atrial fibrillation and some ventricular tachycardias. Beta-blockers are the only drugs that have reduced mortality in the post-myocardial infarction period, probably by reducing catecholinergic-induced lethal arrhythmias. Beta-blockers can facilitate the occurrence of vagal paroxysmal atrial fibrillation[5] and may increase the number of ventricular extrasystoles by lowering the sinoatrial rate. In the absence of cardiac failure, the depression of AV nodal conduction can be used, usually in association with digitalis, to decrease the ventricular rate in atrial fibrillation. Hyperthyroid patients have a special advantage of beta-blockers for either sinus tachycardia or atrial fibrillation.

Amiodarone lengthens the action potential duration and refractoriness by interfering with the K outward current during the fast phase of membrane repolarization. A depressive effect on conduction in the fast response fibers, much less marked than the Na channel blockers, particularly those of IC class, may play a role in the powerful antiarrhythmic properties of this drug. Other effects of amiodarone are a slowing in sinus rate, delay in AV nodal conduction, partial alpha- and beta-adrenolytic activity, and an improvement of myocardial perfusion. Clinical experience has shown that prolongation of repolarization under amiodarone does not predispose to torsade de pointes, a finding which could be explained by the diffuse and homogenous delay in recovery of myocardial excitability, avoiding the risk of desynchronization.

Classification According to Therapeutic Objectives

Antiarrhythmic Drugs for Suppression of Sustained Tachycardias

The chamber in which the arrhythmia arises and the type of disorder are important to consider.

Atrial Arrhythmias (Atrial Tachycardia, Flutter, and Fibrillation)

The attempt to suppress chronic forms of atrial arrhythmias using antiarrhythmic drugs is practically abandoned, considering the limited percentage of success to restore sinus rhythm, but also the need for careful clinical supervision and the duration of hospitalization. In these patients, class IA and IC antiarrhythmic drugs may have unwanted effects like acceleration of the ventricular rate, torsade de pointes, and intraventricular conduction disturbances. Electrotherapy (external cardioversion, transesophageal, or endocardial stimulation) is usually more effective.

When these arrhythmias are of recent onset (within a few days or weeks), an attempt to suppress them under cardiological supervision is possible with a class IA or IC antiarrhythmic drug or amiodarone. For the latter drug, a loading oral dose, which is preferred to intravenous administration, permits the reduction in delay of the therapeutic effect.

Tachycardias at Junctional Level

The paroxysmal supraventricular tachycardias based upon intra-AV nodal reentry or a loop incorporating an accessory pathway can rapidly be terminated by Ca channel blockers or purinergic substances.

A Clinical Classification of Antiarrhythmic Drugs • 489

The Ca channel antagonists (verapamil, diltiazem, bepridil) are efficacious when a rapid intravenous injection (within 1–2 minutes) is given and they are generally well tolerated. Restoration of sinus rhythm is more often obtained with verapamil and diltiazem (75–100% success rate) than with bepridil (30 to 75% success rate).

The purinergic substances (ATP, adenosine) represent another way to obtain the immediate arrest of paroxysmal supraventricular tachycardias. ATP has been used for the longest time and is considered as the first choice of treatment of an acute episode of paroxysmal junctional tachycardia in France for nearly two decades. The injection as a bolus of ATP (Striadyne®) leads in more than 90% of the cases of termination of the tachycardia in less than 1 minute. The discovery of the efficacy of ATP was purely empirical and its action has since been attributed to a vagal effect which is clinically noted after a rapid injection. Recently, the two components, purinergic and cholinergic, of the ATP action have been demonstrated in animals and humans.[6,7]

Adenosine, whose purinergic effect is dominant and for some authors exclusive,[8] has also proven very effective in acutely terminating reentrant paroxysmal supraventricular tachycardias, with or without incorporation of an accessory pathway. The side effects seem to be fewer than those observed with ATP. Purinergic substances probably exert their electrophysiological impact by blocking the slow inward Ca current.

Digitalis, whose predominant action is the depression of intra-AV nodal conduction and prolongation of refractoriness, is effective on paroxysmal junctional tachycardias. The drug has some delay in its action, however, even after an intravenous injection. Supraventricular tachycardias occurring in the newborn and in young infants are the preferential indications for the use of digitalis.

Giving class IA or IC Na channel blockers intravenously is justified only when an accessory pathway of the Kent type is involved in the reentry circuit and when the refractory period of the accessory pathway is relatively long. This information is often ignored by the clinician.

Tachycardias at Ventricular Level

The antiarrhythmic drugs effective in arresting the common forms of ventricular tachycardia are the Na channel blockers and amiodarone. The use of these agents is legitimate only when the hemodynamic situation does not require immediate cardioversion. Of the class I antiarrhythmic agents, substances belonging to class IB (lidocaine, mexiletine, lorcainide, tocainide) are used in preference to class IA (procainamide, disopyramide, quinidine) or the IC (propafenone, flecainide, encainide) or cibenzoline because of a lower risk of myocardial depression and unwanted electrophysiologic effects. The intravenous injection is given slowly while the ECG and arterial pressure are monitored in order to stop administration of the drug as soon as maltolerance occurs.

Amiodarone slowly infused has an antiarrhythmic effect that is less rapid than that of the Na channel blockers, but its hemodynamic tolerance is generally better.

The Ca channel blockers are effective in the peculiar variety of ventricular tachycardia occurring in young patients without structural heart disease. In these patients, the QRS complexes usually show a right bundle branch block pattern with left axis deviation in the frontal plane. The arrhythmia is often inducible by atrial stimulation.[9,10] More experience is needed to be informed about the efficacy of adenosine in these cases.[11]

Antiarrhythmic Drugs Depressing Atrioventricular Conduction

These drugs are indicated in atrial arrhythmias with a fast ventricular response. They act by increasing concealed conduction in the AV node or, in the case of ventricular preexcitation, by a depressing effect on the accessory pathway. When the hemodynamic situation does not require immediate electrical cardioversion, the Na channel blockers of IA and IC categories intravenously or amiodarone in infusion may slow the ventricular rate. These drugs may reduce or even suppress ventricular responses resulting from conduction over the Kent bundle if the anterograde refractory period is not too short.

Antiarrhythmic Drugs Effective on Extrasystoles and Used in the Prevention of Nonsustained and Sustained Recurrent Tachycardias

The fast Na channel blockers are the drugs of first choice. All substances belonging to the class I antiarrhythmic drugs (IA, IB, IC) can be useful in case of ventricular ectopy, while only the IA and IC agents are effective on atrial arrhythmias. The antiarrhythmic drugs active on the AV node (digitalis, beta-blockers, Ca blockers) can be used to prevent paroxysmal supraventricular tachycardias by modifying the electrophysiological properties of the reentrant circuit, even though their impact on the trigger (extrasystoles) is weak or nil.

Amiodarone is currently the most efficient antiarrhythmic drug for preventing recurrent atrial, junctional, and ventricular tachycardias. It is usually prescribed after failure of other antiarrhythmic drugs, alone or in combination, because of fear of its side effects.

Antiarrhythmic Drugs for Peculiar Malignant Ventricular Tachyarrhythmias

Ionic therapy is indispensable when an ionic deficit is demonstrated, chiefly in case of hypokalemia-induced torsade de pointes. Apart from compensatory treatment, magnesium ion has shown its efficacy during intravenous administration for suppressing torsade de pointes complicating various situations in which the QT interval is prolonged.[13]

Bretylium tosylate is the only known antiarrhythmic drug capable of raising the ventricular fibrillation threshold significantly in experimental conditions. It also has very real antifibrillatory properties in humans. The infusion of bretylium is effective in recurrent ventricular tachycardias which degenerate easily into ventricular flutter or fibrillation in the acute stage of myocardial infarction.[14] The clinical administration of bretylium, orally, is strongly limited by important side effects.[15]

Antiarrhythmic Drugs for Some Triggering Factors

Catecholinergic Arrhythmias

The onset of an arrhythmia during exercise, stress conditions, or after acceleration of the sinoatrial rate suggests a catecholinergic triggering factor. The beta-blockers are indicated in such a situation. Among the Na channel blockers, propafenone may be useful because apart from its class IC effects, it also has beta-blocking effects. Ca channel blockers (verapamil) have been successfully prescribed in some ventricular tachycardias occurring on exercise, in patients without structural heart disease; these arrhythmias are probably Ca current-dependent.

Ischemic Arrhythmias

The beta-blockers have been shown to be effective in ventricular arrhythmias occurring in acute myocardial infarction but their use has remained limited by the risk of hemodynamic complications due to their negative inotropic effect. After the acute episode, beta-blockers are the only drugs whose benefit on the reduction of cardiac death (probably by decreasing the incidence of lethal arrhythmias) is demonstrated. The Ca channel blockers, including nifedipine, have a preventive effect on arrhythmias in acute ischemia, in the setting of Prinzmetal's angina, because of their coronary antispastic and vasodilator action. Amiodarone has the advantage of combining coronary vasodilating properties with its antiarrhythmic effects.

Digitalis Arrhythmias

Diphenylhydantoine, a class IB antiarrhythmic drug, is used for this indication. Recent path-clamp studies on single isolated guinea pig ventricular cells have shown that the drug blocks not only Na channels but also Ca channels and binds to the dihydropyridine receptor.

Conclusion

The clinical classification of the antiarrhythmic drugs is summarized in Tables I, II, and III. They refer to the three goals of treatment: (1) curative effect by arresting the sustained atrial, junctional, and ventricular arrhythmias; (2) palliative effect by slowing the ventricular rate in atrial arrhythmias by their effects on the normal AV conduction system of the accessory pathway; and (3) preventive

Table I
Drugs for Termination of Sustained Tachycardias

Atrial Arrhythmias (A. fibrillation, flutter, tachycardia)		Junctional Arrhythmias (Re-entrant paroxysmal SVT)		Ventricular Arrhythmias common VT	uncomm
• Na channel blockers (classes IA and IC) • Amiodarone	} Arrhythmias of recent onset	• Ca channel blockers • Purinergic substances (ATP, Adenosine)	} immediate suppression	• Na channel blockers (classes IA, IB and IC) • Amiodarone	• Ca channel blockers • Adenosin
		• Digitalis } Pediatric population • Na channel blockers (classes IA and IC)	} Kent bundle incorporated		

VT = ventricular tachycardia; SVT = supraventricular tachycardia

Table II
Drugs for Slowing of Ventricular Rate in Atrial Tachyarrhythmias

Normal AV Conduction Pathway		AV Accessory Pathway	
• Digitalis • Ca channel blockers Beta-blockers Amiodarone	} usually to complement the effect of Digitalis	• Na channel blockers (classes IA and IC)	} Kent bundle with long antegrade R. P.

Table III
Drugs for Extrasystoles. Prevention of Recurrent Sustained and Nonsustained Tachycardias

Common Forms of Atrial, Junctional and Ventricular Arrhythmias	Peculiar Arrhythmias				
	Catecholinergic	Ischemic	Malignant VT	Torsades de Pointe (TP)	Digitalis Intoxication
• Na channel blockers IA and IC: all levels + IB: ventricular level	• Beta-blockers (all levels)	• Ca channel blockers	• Bretylium (Acute MI)	• Mg	• Diphenylhydantoine
	• Ca channel blockers	(spastic angina)	• Beta-blockers (Acute MI Post MI)	• Isoprenaline (nonischemic TP)	
• Amiodarone	(exercise-induced VT)				

MI = myocardial infarction; VT = ventricular tachycardia

effect by suppressing extrasystoles and factors triggering recurrent nonsustained and sustained tachycardia.

This classification is obviously open to criticism and represents the authors' long clinical experience in treating arrhythmias with drugs available in Europe. It will probably be obsolete in the coming years with the expected arrival of drugs at least as powerful as amiodarone but free from similar long-term side effects. It will also be affected by the increasing number of nonpharmacological interventions, including various forms of electrotherapy and the direct approach to arrhythmia ablation, such as fulguration or cardiac surgery.

References

1. Vaughan-Williams EM. The classification of antiarrhythmic drugs. In Sandoe E, Flenstedt-Jensen F, Olesen KH, eds. Symposium on Cardiac Arrhythmias. A.B. Astra, Södertälje, Sweden, 1970;449–468.
2. Vaughan-Williams EM. A classification of antiarrhythmic actions reassessed after a decade of new drugs. J Clin Pharmacol 1984;24:129.
3. Harrison DC. Antiarrhythmic drug classification: new science and practical applications. Am J Cardiol 1985;56:185–190.
4. Touboul P, Attalah G, Gressard A, Michelon G, Chatelain MT, Delahaye JP. Effets électrophysiologiques des agents antiarythmiques chez l' homme. Tentative de classification. Arch Mal Coeur 1980;72:72–81.
5. Coumel Ph, Attuel P, Lavallée J, Flammang D, Leclercq JF, Slama R. Syndrome d'arythmie auriculaire d'origine vagale. Arch Mal Coeur 1979;71:645–656.
6. Munoz A, Sassine A, Lehujeur C, Koliopoulos N, Puech P. Mode d'action des substances purinergiques dérivées de l'adénine sur la conduction auriculo-ventriculaire. Etude expérimentale chez le chien. Arch Mal Coeur 1984;76:143–150.
7. Puech P, Sassine A, Munoz A, Masse C, Zettelmeier F, Leenhardt A, Yoshimura H. Electrophysiologic effects of purines: Clinical applications. In Zipes DP, Jalife J, eds. Cardiac Electrophysiology and Arrhythmias. NY, Grune and Stratton, 1985;443–450.
8. DiMarco JP, Sellers TD, Lerman BB, Greenberg LM, Berne RM, Belardinelli L. Diagnostic and therapeutic use of adenosine in patients with supraventricular tachycardias. J Am Coll Cardiol 1985;6:417–425.
9. Belhassen B, Rotmensch HH, Laniado S. Response of recurrent sustained ventricular tachycardia to verapamil. Br Heart J 1981;46:679–682.
10. Ward DE, Nathan AW, Camm AJ. Fascicular tachycardia sensitive to calcium antagonists. European Heart J 1984;5:896–905.
11. Lerman B, Bellardini L, West A, Berne R, DiMarco JP. Adenosine-sensitive ventricular tachycardia: Evidence suggesting cyclic AMP-mediated triggered activity. Circulation 1986;74:270–280.
12. Roth A, Harrison E, Mitani G, Cohen J, Rahimtoola SH, Elkayam U. Efficacy and safety of medium- and high-dose diltiazem alone and in combination with digoxin for control of heart rate at rest and during exercise in patients with chronic atrial fibrillation. Circulation 1986;73:316–324.
13. Tzivoni D, Keren A, Cohen A, Loebel H, Zahavi I, Chenzbraun A, Stern S. Magnesium therapy for torsades de pointe. Am J Cardiol 1984;53:528–530.
14. Torresani J. Bretylium tosylate in patients with acute myocardial infarction. In Symposium on the management of ventricular dysrrhythmias. Am J Cardiol 1984;54:20–25 A.
15. Benditt DG, Benson W Jr, Dunnigan A, Kriett JM, Pritzker MR, Bacaner NB. Antirrhythmic and electrophysiologic actions of bethanidine sulfate in primary ventricular fibrillation or life-threatening ventricular tachycardia. Am J Cardiol 1984;53:1268–1274.

31

A Comparison of Electrophysiologic Effects of Antiarrhythmic Agents in Humans

Eric N. Prystowsky, Elwyn A. Lloyd
Naomi Fineberg, Douglas P. Zipes
Elizabeth Darling, James J. Heger

Introduction

Antiarrhythmic agents are usually segregated into various classes, mainly based on the electrophysiologic effects of drugs on normal Purkinje fibers.[1] In this system, class I consists of drugs that primarily reduce V_{max}, for example quinidine; class II drugs inhibit sympathetic activity, for example propranolol; class III drugs have a major effect to prolong action potential duration, for example amiodarone; and class IV drugs block the slow inward current, for example verapamil. Recently it has been suggested that class I agents be subgrouped into IA, IB and IC.[2] Drugs in class IA compared with those in class IC have a more marked effect on prolonging refractoriness and less of an effect on slowing cardiac conduction. Although this classification scheme has gained widespread popularity, there are many potential drawbacks to its use. For example, all drugs in a particular group do not have identical physiologic properties, and several agents

From: Brugada P, Wellens HJJ. CARDIAC ARRHYTHMIAS: Where To Go From Here? Mount Kisco, NY, Futura Publishing Company, Inc., © 1987.

have characteristics of more than one class. Further, since the classification scheme depends on the effects of antiarrhythmic agents on normal Purkinje fibers, it does not take into account the multitude of factors in humans, fixed or evanescent, that may alter the role of a drug in the initiation, maintenance, or termination of an arrhythmia. Some of these factors include autonomic tone, ischemia, metabolic and acid-base status, electrolyte levels, as well as the effects of drugs on damaged tissue. Newer information on use-dependent characteristics of drugs further complicates matters.[3,4]

The problems of classifying antiarrhythmic agents are exemplified by amiodarone, a drug that affects cardiac tissues directly and also by interacting with multiple physiologic systems.[5-7] The purpose of this study was twofold: (1) to investigate whether antiarrhythmic agents of various classes cause different electrophysiologic effects in humans, and (2) to compare alterations of electrophysiologic properties between amiodarone and class IA and IC agents.

Methods

Patients with ventricular tachyarrhythmias were admitted to a cardiac care unit where their heart rhythms were continuously monitored by telemetry. All antiarrhythmic agents, including digitalis, were withdrawn. Heart disease was diagnosed by history and physical examination, echocardiography, electrocardiography, and coronary angiography.

All patients underwent an electrophysiologic study in the drug-free control state after giving informed, written consent. If a patient had been receiving an antiarrhythmic agent, at least five half-lives were allowed to elapse prior to the control electrophysiologic study. Two to four multipolar electrode catheters were introduced percutaneously into the femoral, antecubital, internal jugular, or subclavian veins and positioned under fluoroscopic guidance at the high right atrium, across the tricuspid valve in the region of the His bundle, and at the right ventricular apex. Intracardiac recordings filtered at 30 to 500 Hz and standard electrocardiographic leads I, II, III, and VI filtered at 0.1 to 20 Hz were displayed simultaneously on a multiple-channel oscilloscope (Electronics for Medicine VR-12) and recorded at paper speeds of 50 to 150 mm/sec. Pacing was performed with a custom-built programmable stimulator using 2.0 ms rectangular pulses at twice late diastolic threshold. Repeat studies during drug therapy were performed with the catheters in approximately the same intracardiac positions and refractory period measurements were done at identical pacing cycle lengths.

Our pacing protocol to study cardiac electrophysiologic properties and to initiate ventricular tachycardia has been described in detail.[8,9] In brief, programmed right ventricular stimulation was performed during sinus rhythm and during ventricular pacing at three cycle lengths (600, 500, and 400 ms) using one to three extrastimuli. If ventricular tachycardia was not induced at the first right ventricular endocardial site tested, then a second right ventricular site, usually the outflow tract, was tested.

Electrophysiologic testing during drug therapy was accomplished during a time when steady-state plasma drug levels were expected, except for amiodarone therapy in which retesting was performed after 14 days of therapy at 800 mg/day.

Dosage regimens for the various drug trials were: quinidine, 1600 to 2400 mg/day; procainamide (oral), 3000 to 6000 mg/day, (IV), ≥ 1000 mg; disopyramide, 600 to 1000 mg/day; encainide, 200 to 300 mg/day; and aprindine, 100 to 150 mg/day.

Statistical Methods

Data are given as mean ± standard deviation. Comparisons of control and drug studies within treatment groups are performed with a paired t-test or Wilcoxon rank test depending on the distribution of the data. Differences between treatment groups for continuous variables were analyzed with an analysis of variance. If the analysis of variance was significant, comparisons to amiodarone were made with a group t-test. Significant levels were interpreted taking into account the multiple tests performed. For discrete variables, differences between treatment groups were assessed using a chi-square test for contingency tables.[10]

Results

Patient Characteristics

All patients were referred for treatment of symptomatic ventricular tachyarrhythmias (Table I). Patients received quinidine (n = 24), procainamide (n = 20), disopyramide (n = 9), encainide (n = 17), aprindine (n = 12), and amiodarone (n = 46). Although some patients underwent more than one antiarrhythmic drug trial, for each drug group there was no significant difference in age, gender, underlying heart disease, or presenting ventricular arrhythmia (Table I).

Electrophysiologic Effects of Antiarrhythmic Agents

Spontaneous Sinus Cycle Length

The effects of the various antiarrhythmic drugs on sinus cycle length are noted in Figure 1. It is noteworthy that only amiodarone showed a significant increase in sinus cycle length, from 793 ± 142 ms to 899 ± 172 ms ($p < 0.001$). In contrast, a decrease in sinus cycle length was noted with quinidine (888 ± 104 ms to 829 ± 130 ms, $p < 0.05$) and procainamide (792 ± 148 to 733 ± 120 ms, $p < 0.02$). Changes noted during amiodarone therapy differed from all drugs except aprindine.

Atrioventriuclar (AV) Nodal Conduction

The AH interval was measured during spontaneous sinus cycle length (Fig. 2). Significant increases in AH interval occurred with amiodarone (89 ± 22 to 105 ± 24 ms, $p < 0.001$) and encainide (74 ± 15 to 97 ± 19 ms, $p < 0.001$)

Table I
Patient Data

	Quinidine	Procainamide	Disopyramide	Encainide	Aprindine	Amiodarone	p value
Number of Patients	24	20	9	17	12	46	
Mean Age	54 ± 12	54 ± 14	44 ± 16	53 ± 13	56 ± 9	55 ± 12	NS
Male/Female	18/16	19/1	8/1	15/2	11/1	38/8	NS
Underlying heart disease							NS
CAD	13	16	4	12	10	32	
Other	11	4	5	5	2	14	
Presenting arrhythmia							
VF	15	14	5	9	4	21	NS
VT-S	5	5	3	3	0	13	NS
VT-NS	4	1	1	5	8	12	

Comparative Effects of Antiarrhythmic Drugs

EFFECT OF DRUGS ON SPONTANEOUS CYCLE LENGTH

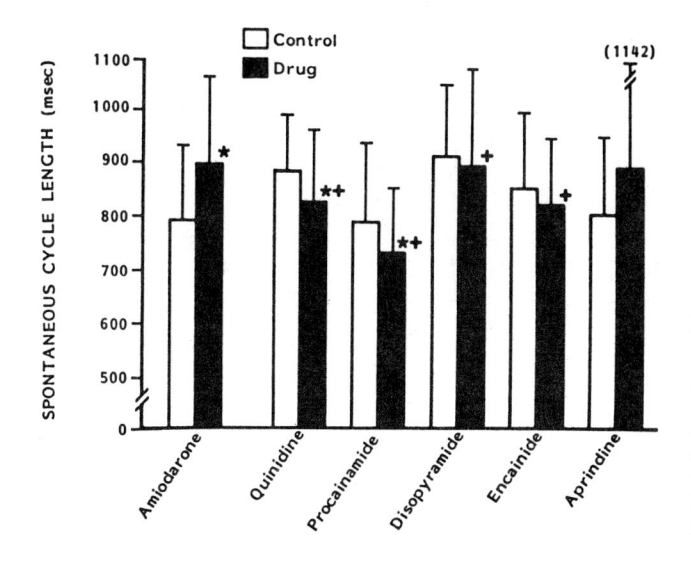

Figure 1: Effect of drugs on spontaneous cycle length. For this and all subsequent figures, * = a statistically significant change from control values during drug therapy and + = a significant difference in the change produced by a drug other than amiodarone when compared with the change noted during amiodarone treatment.

EFFECT OF DRUGS ON A H INTERVAL

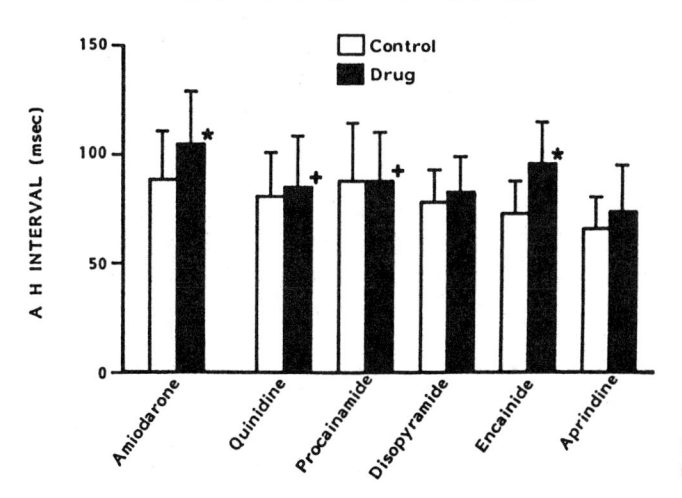

Figure 2: Effect of drugs on AV nodal conduction.

therapy. Although changes in AH interval differed for amiodarone compared with quinidine or procainamide, there was no significant difference between amiodarone and disopyramide, encainide, or aprindine.

His-Purkinje Conduction

Drug effects of HV interval are seen in Figure 3. The HV interval significantly ($p < 0.001$) increased with all drugs except disopyramide. Marked HV prolonga-

EFFECT OF DRUGS ON H V INTERVAL

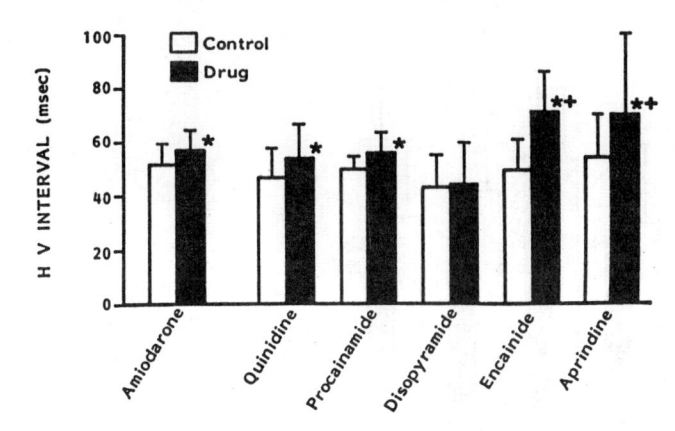

Figure 3: Effect of drugs on His-Purkinje conduction.

tion occurred with both encainide (21 ms) and aprindine (16 ms), and these were the only drugs with changes that differed from amiodarone.

Right Ventricular Effective Refractory Period

The effect of drugs on right ventricular effective refractory period measured at pacing cycle length 500 ms is illustrated in Figure 4. The effective refractory period was significantly prolonged with all drugs except aprindine, which increased but did not reach statistical significance. Of interest, the effective refractory period significantly increased from 232 ± 31 to 272 ± 24 ms ($p < 0.01$) in a subgroup of five patients treated with aprindine in whom refractoriness was determined at pacing cycle length 400 ms at control and drug study. The most marked prolongation of refractoriness occurred with quinidine, and except for this drug, the increase in ventricular refractoriness noted with amiodarone was similar to that observed for the other drugs tested.

Ventricular Tachycardia Cycle Length

All drugs except disopyramide significantly increased induced ventricular tachycardia cycle length (Fig. 5). The mean increases in ventricular tachycardia cycle length did not differ among the drugs tested and were 54, 84, 52, 34, 58, and 95, for amiodarone, quinidine, procainamide, disopyramide, encainide, and aprindine, respectively.

Electrophysiologic Changes during Therapy with Amiodarone Compared with Other Drugs

Table II is a summary of the comparison of changes in electrophysiologic parameters observed between therapy with amiodarone and other drugs. Only

EFFECT OF DRUGS ON RIGHT VENTRICULAR ERP

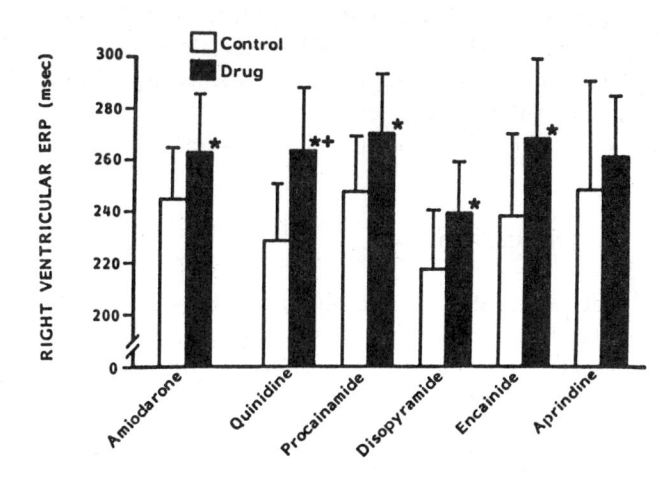

Figure 4: Effect of drugs on right ventricular effective refractory period. Significant levels for changes from control to drug effect were $p < 0.001$ for amiodarone and quinidine, $p < 0.005$ for procainamide, $p < 0.03$ for disopyramide, and $p < 0.01$ for encainide. The change in effective refractory period noted with quinidine versus amiodarone was $p < 0.05$.

EFFECT OF DRUGS ON VT CYCLE LENGTH

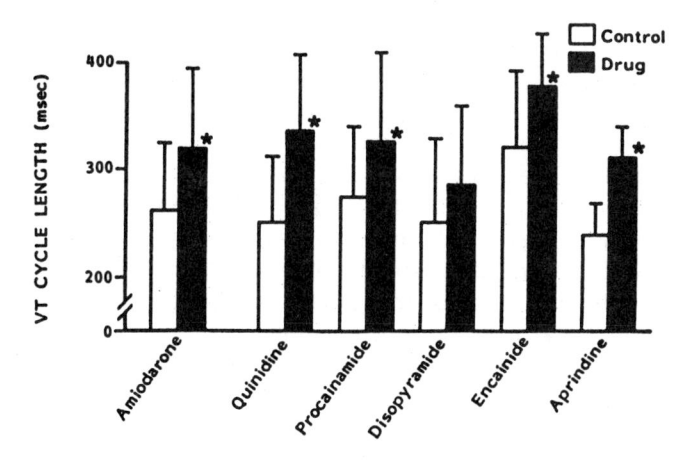

Figure 5: Effect of drugs on ventricular trachycardia cycle length induced at electrophysiologic study. Changes from control during drug therapy were significant to $p < 0.001$ for amiodarone, quinidine, and procainamide, $p < 0.03$ for encainide, and $p < 0.01$ for aprindine.

Table II
Changes in Electrophysiologic Parameters During Drug Therapy
Amiodarone versus Other Drugs

Variable	Quinidine	Procainide	Disopyramide	Encainide	Aprindine
SCL	< .001	< .001	< .02	< .002	NS
AH	< .01	< .001	NS	NS	NS
HV	NS	NS	NS	< .001	< .01
RV$_{ERP}$	< .05	NS	NS	NS	NS
VT$_{CL}$	NS	NS	NS	NS	NS

NS = nonsignificant; RV$_{ERP}$ = right ventricular effective refractory period; SCL = sinus cycle length; VT$_{CL}$ = ventricular tachycardia cycle length.

depression of sinus nodal automaticity clearly separated amiodarone from most of the other drugs tested. As expected, prolongation of the HV interval was more marked with encainide and aprindine,[2,11] but the changes associated with amiodarone were similar to those that occurred with quinidine, procainamide, and disopyramide. Alterations of ventricular refractoriness or the induced ventricular tachycardia cycle length were essentially the same for all drugs tested.

Discussion

The results of this study demonstrate the inadequacies of the presently employed antiarrhythmic drug classification system. This is noted most strikingly by the observation that drugs in class IA, IC, and III show almost no differences in their ability to prolong right ventricular refractoriness and induced ventricular tachycardia cycle length in humans. Although certain "class actions" occurred as expected, e.g., encainide, a class IC drug, had a more marked effect to increase HV interval,[2,11] the effect of amiodarone on HV interval was similar to the class IA agents. Previous data demonstrated that amiodarone increased His-Purkinje conduction time, and in vitro studies showed that amiodarone decreased the inward sodium current.[12-15] Thus, amiodarone shares at least some of the properties of class IA drugs.

Most of the observed differences in electrophysiologic changes among the drugs tested were on the sinus and AV nodes. This is interesting since the classification scheme does not directly address the effect of antiarrhythmic agents on these structures. Amiodarone was the only drug to suppress substantially sinus nodal automaticity, as has been noted previously.[12] It is probable that depression of sinus nodal automaticity was due both to a direct effect of amiodarone on the sinus node and to an indirect effect of amiodarone, for example, antagonism of sympathetic activity.[16-19] Similarly, prolongation of AV nodal conduction time during amiodarone therapy could be multifactorial. Encainide was the only other drug that prolonged AV nodal conduction time. Although this has been demonstrated previously,[11] the mechanism by which encainide increases the AH interval is not clear since it does not appear to have a substantial effect on the slow inward current. It is interesting that encainide also has a potent effect to block accessory pathway conduction,[20] and it is conceivable that drugs that markedly depress conduction may have a pronounced effect on tissues with anisotropic fiber orientation or possibly few intercellular connections.[21,22] How these effects can be translated to a classification scheme is presently unclear.

Several limitations are evident in our study. First, serial electrophysiologic studies performed on separate days or possibly even at a different time on the same day will not always yield similar results, even without the addition of antiarrhythmic drugs. One usually does not control for the level of autonomic tone or other potentially significant factors such as electrolyte levels. Although these factors may vary little in some patients, in other patients, substantial changes may occur and affect the results of serial drug testing. It is more likely that alterations in autonomic tone will affect primarily sinus nodal and AV nodal function rather than His-Purkinje or ventricular function,[8] although autonomic effects on diseased tissue may be prominent.[23,24] Another problem is that patient tolerance to drugs precludes all individuals from receiving identical doses of the different antiarrhythmic agents, and variations in pharmacokinetic properties between patients will yield a wide spectrum of plasma drug levels. This will obviously affect the drug-induced changes in electrophysiologic properties that are dose-related. Further, some of the nonsignificant changes observed by some agents in this study may have been due to analysis of small sample sizes.

Amiodarone presents a specific problem since it was not tested during steady-state conditions. This cannot be accomplished unless one is willing to wait many months before repeat testing is performed.[25] We[26] showed that electrophysiologic changes evaluated after 2 weeks of amiodarone treatment were similar with loading doses of 800 mg versus 1600 mg daily. Others demonstrated that ventricular refractoriness did not change from 1 week to 2 months of therapy, although there was a further prolongation of induced ventricular tachycardia cycle length.[27] However, none of these studies were done at steady-state.

In essence, many of the limitations of this investigation are the "real-life" applications of drug therapy for the treatment of arrhythmias. It is not surprising that there is such a marked patient to patient variability in response to antiarrhythmic agents, in different or even within the same class. One should not conclude that the similar electrophysiologic changes during therapy observed in our study in humans implies that the effect of a drug in one class will always equal the effect of a drug in another class. On the contrary, a modification of the anatomic/autonomic/electrophysiologic milieu could alter this entire situation.

Conclusion

Electrophysiologic data during drug therapy in humans demonstrate that the presently employed antiarrhythmic drug classification scheme is inadequate. Although it may have a place to help physicians understand certain broad categories of drugs, future studies on the effects of antiarrhythmic agents under several pathophysiologic states hopefully will provide a more meaningful classification of these agents.

Acknowledgment: This study was supported in part by the Herman C. Krannert Fund, Indianapolis, Indiana, by Grants HL-06308, HL-07182 and HL-18795 from the National Heart, Lung and Blood Institute, National Institutes of Health, Bethesda, Maryland and by the American Heart Association, Indiana Affiliate, Inc., Indianapolis, Indiana.

References

1. Vaughan Williams EM. Classification of antiarrhythmic drugs. In Sandoe, et al, eds. Symposium on Cardiac Arrhythmias. Sodertalji, Sweden, A.B. Astra, 1970.
2. Keefe DL, Kates RE, Harrison DC. New antiarrhythmic drugs: Their place in therapy. Drugs 1981;22:363–400.
3. Hondeghem LM, Katzung BG. Time and voltage dependent interactions of antiarrhythmic drugs with cardiac sodium channels. Biochem Biophys Acta 1977;472:373.
4. Starmer CF, Grant AO, Strauss HC. Mechanisms of use-dependent block of sodium channels in excitable membranes by local anesthetics. Biophys J 1984;46:15–27.
5. Zipes DP, Prystowsky EN, Heger JJ. Amiodarone: electrophysiologic actions, pharmacokinetics and clinical effects. J Am Coll Cardiol 1984;3(4):1059–1071.

CARDIAC ARRHYTHMIAS

6. Beck-Peccoz P, Volpi A, Maggioni AP, Cattaneo MG, Piscitelli G, Giani P, Landolina M, Tognoni G, Faglia G. Evidence for an inhibition of thyroid hormone effects during chronic treatment with amiodarone. Horm Metab Res 1986;18(6):411–414.
7. Heath MF, Costa-Jussà FR, Jacobs JM, Jacobson W. The induction of pulmonary phospholipidosis and the inhibition of lysosomal phospholipases by amiodarone. Br J Exp Pathol 1985;66(4):391–397.
8. Prystowsky EN, Jackman WM, Rinkenberger RL, Heger JJ, Zipes DP. Effect of autonomic blockade on ventricular refractoriness and atrioventricular nodal conduction in humans: Evidence supporting a direct cholinergic action on ventricular muscle refractoriness. Circ Res 1981;49:511–518.
9. Prystowsky EN, Miles WM, Evans JJ, Hubbard JE, Skale BT, Windle JR, Heger JJ, Zipes DP. Induction of ventricular tachycardia during programmed electrical stimulation: Analysis of pacing methods. Circ 1986;73(2):32–38.
10. Snedecor GW, Cochran WG. Statistical Methods. Ames, Iowa, Iowa State University Press, 1967.
11. Jackman WM, Zipes DP, Naccarelli GV, Rinkenberger RL, Heger JJ, Prystowsky EN. Electrophysiology of oral encainide. Am J Cardiol 1982;49:1270–1278.
12. Heger JJ, Prystowsky EN, Jackman WM, Naccarelli GV, Warfel KA, Rinkenberger RL, Zipes DP. Amiodarone: Clinical efficacy and electrophysiology during long-term therapy for recurrent ventricular tachycardia or ventricular fibrillation. N Engl J Med 1981;305:539–545.
13. Waxman HL, Groh WC, Marchlinski FE, et al. Amiodarone for control of sustained ventricular tachyarrhythmia: Clinical and electrophysiologic effects in 51 patients. Am J Cardiol 1982;50:1066–1074.
14. Mason JW, Hondeghem LM, Katzung BG. Amiodarone blocks inactivated cardiac sodium channels. Pflügers Arch 1983;396:79–81.
15. Varro A, Nakaya Y, Elharrar V, Surawicz B. Use-dependent effects of amiodarone on $\dot{V}_{max}$ in cardiac purkinje and ventricular muscle fibers. Eur J Pharmacol 1985;112:419–422.
16. Charlier R, Deltour G, Baudine A. Pharmacology of amiodarone, an antianginal drug with a new biological profile. Arzneimittelforsch 1968;18:1408–1418.
17. Polster P, Broekhuysen J. The adrenergic antagonism of amiodarone. Biochem Pharmacol 1976;25:131–134.
18. Heger JJ, Moran M, Prystowsky EN. Effects of amiodarone on sympathetic and parasympathetic control of heart rate in man. Clin Res 1986;34(4):999A.
19. Heger JJ, Prystowsky EN, Miles WM, Zipes DP. Clinical use and pharmacology of amiodarone. Med Clin N Am 1984;68(5):1339–1366.
20. Prystowsky EN, Klein GJ, Rinkenberger RL, Heger JJ, Naccarelli GV, Zipes DP. Clinical efficacy and electrophysiologic effects of encainide in patients with the Wolff-Parkinson-White syndrome. Circ 1984;69:278–287.
21. Spach MS, Kootsey JM. The nature of electrical propagation in cardiac muscle. Am J Physiol 1983;244(13):H3-H22.
22. Kadish AH, Spear JF, Levine JH, Moore EN. The effects of procainamide on conduction in anisotropic canine ventricular myocardium. Circulation 1986;74(3):616–625.
23. Markel ML, Miles WM, Zipes DP, Prystowsky EN. The effects of autonomic blockade on Mobitz II heart block. Circulation 74:IV–31.
24. Dhingra RC, Winslow E, Pouget JM, Rahimtoola SH, Rosen KM. The effect of isoproterenol on atrioventricular and intraventricular conduction. Am J Cardiol 1973;32:629–636.
25. Holt DW, Tucker GT, Jackson PR et al. Amiodarone pharmacokinetics. Am Heart J 1983;106:840–847.
26. Prystowsky EN, Heger JJ, Miles WM, Zipes DP. Amiodarone: Interrelationship of dose and time on electrophysiologic and antiarrhythmic effects. Circulation 1984;70(2):II–3.
27. Kennedy EE, Rosenfeld LE, McPherson CA, Batsford WP. Evaluation by serial electrophysiologic studies of an abbreviated oral loading regimen of amiodarone. Am J Cardiol 1985;56:867–871.

32

Factors Leading to Decreasing Mortality Among Patients Resuscitated From Out-of-Hospital Cardiac Arrest

Robert J. Myerburg, Kenneth M. Kessler
Liaqat Zaman, Richard G. Trohman
Pedro Fernandez, Agustin Castellanos

Introduction

The development of effective community-based emergency rescue systems in the early 1970's was followed by the observation that survivors of out-of-hospital cardiac arrest remain at high risk for sudden cardiac death during follow-up.[1,2] This prompted attempts to identify interventions that would reduce the high recurrence rates. Recent reports indicate that recurrent cardiac arrest rates as much as 67% lower than those originally reported can be achieved,[3-6] but the extent to which this is due to interventions designed to control potentially lethal arrhythmias, as opposed to changes resulting from other factors, is not easily determined. This dilemma is a direct result of the fact that there are no studies using true concurrent controls in a randomized study design to evaluate methods of management of survivors of out-of-hospital cardiac arrest.

From: Brugada P, Wellens HJJ. CARDIAC ARRHYTHMIAS: Where To Go From Here? Mount Kisco, NY, Futura Publishing Company, Inc., © 1987.

Natural History of Cardiac Arrest Survivors

The data on neutral history of survivors of out-of-hospital cardiac arrest is difficult to interpret. From the very earliest studies,[1,2,7] therapeutic interventions were used, albeit in an uncontrolled fashion, and in the absence of approaches to therapy and efficacy criteria that would be used at present. The earliest experience with survivors of out-of-hospital cardiac arrest demonstrated very high recurrence rates during follow-up: approximately 30% at 1 year, and 45% at 2 years[1,2] (Fig. 1); but many interventions that are more broadly used today, or have become available since the early studies, did not play a role in the long-term management of these patients. With specific reference to antiarrhythmic drugs, no early studies uniformly used, or controlled for the use of antiarrhythmic drugs during long-term follow-up.[1,2,7] In both Miami[1] and Seattle,[2,7] a large fraction of patients were not on long-term antiarrhythmic drugs, and those who were, received dosages different from those considered therapeutic today. *Thus, the recurrence rates observed in the early 1970s provide the best approximation of natural history available, but these early data only indicate the risk for recurrence extant at that time.* Many factors, in addition to the better use of conventional antiarrhythmic drugs and the development of new ones, have changed since the original studies: e.g., improved prehospital intervention, an unexplained decline in coro-

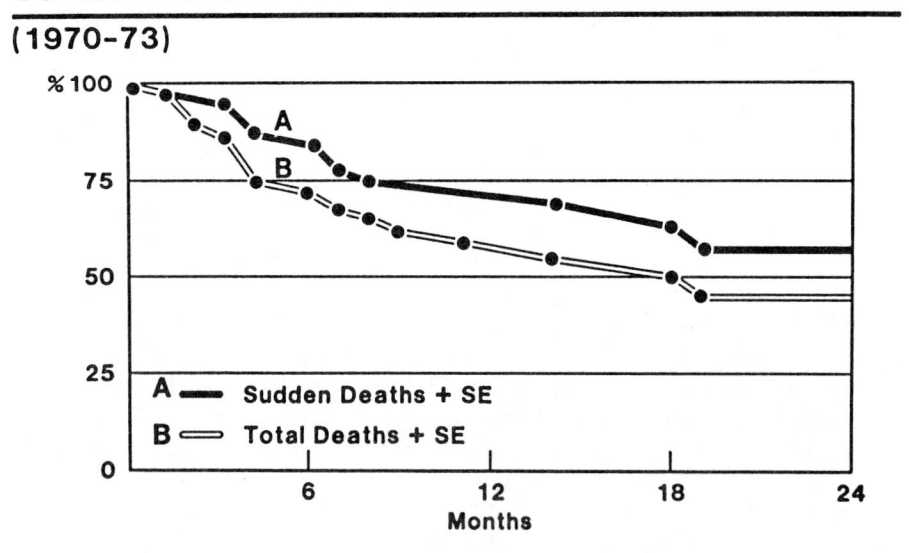

Figure 1: Long-term follow-up of survivors of out-of-hospital cardiac arrest from the 1970–73 Miami study. The 1-year recurrent cardiac arrest rate (curve A-sudden death) was 30% and the 2-year recurrence rate was 45%. The 2-year total mortality rate (curve B-total deaths) was nearly 60%. (From Myerburg RJ. Sudden Cardiac Death and the Management of Potentially Lethal Arrhythmias [Miles Laboratories Cardiovascular Resource Series], published by Gardiner-Caldwell Synermed, 1986.)

nary disease death rates, community and professional education for blood pressure control, widespread use of β-blocking drugs, Ca^{++}-entry blockers, antiplatelet prophylaxis, and coronary artery surgery, to name only the most obvious. *Thus, the risk of recurrent cardiac arrest in survivors not receiving controlled antiarrhythmic interventions today cannot be presumed to be the same as it was in the early 1970s, and this fact must be considered in the interpretation of any data on interventions.*

Study design factors may influence the expected recurrent cardiac arrest rate, and serve to confound further the observed data. It is likely that sources of patient populations, unintended selection processes, and direct versus indirect control of antiarrhythmic and other therapy, may have powerful influences upon observed outcome. Primary entrants versus referral populations, the relative frequency of cardiac arrest by the mechanism of ventricular fibrillation versus ventricular tachycardia, absence of stratification on the basis of the characteristics of chronic PVCs or measures of LV function, populations dominated by transient ischemia versus structural substrates, and populations in whom general care is provided by the study team which is also controlling antiarrhythmic care, all may influence the outcome in individual studies. For example, in the report from our institution based upon follow-up from 1975 to 1983,[3] study patients were restricted to those who were primary entrants at the time of an out-of-hospital cardiac arrest, were dominated by the mechanism of ventricular fibrillation rather than ventricular tachycardia, were unselected for chronic ventricular ectopic activity or for etiology, and had both general care and specific antiarrhythmic management continuously controlled by our study team. The strength of this approach is protection from selection processes that would bias outcome observations to the characteristics of a single group, and the absence of uncontrolled management factors in patients who have multiple sources of medical care; the weakness is the limited numbers, mixing of outcome risk according to specific etiology, and the inability to control prospectively for the influence of chronic PVCs on outcome. Analysis of any of the other major intervention studies during the past 10 years also yields patterns of counter-balancing strengths and weaknesses, differing only in specific factors confounding each study. Few, if any, of these studies are comparable with one another.

Influence of Prehospital Care and Early In-Hospital Risk on Outcome

There is a compelling body of information suggesting that two factors in prehospital care have had an impact on initial survival and entry into long-term follow-up: (1) immediate defibrillation by emergency rescue personnel at the scene of cardiac arrest,[8] and (2) the effect of bystander CPR prior to the arrival of emergency rescue personnel.[9] The former has led to clearly improved outcome, measured in terms of both initial resuscitation (53% vs. 23%, $p<.05$) and of survival to entry into long-term follow-up (26% vs. 7%, $p<.05$). Bystander CPR has had little influence on initial resuscitation, but significantly improved the chances of patients entering long-term follow-up (43% with bystander CPR vs.

22% without) because of protection of the central nervous system (CNS) function. Data on causes of in-hospital death after initial successful resuscitation indicate that CNS injury or infectious complications of respirator dependence are the major determinants of early mortality (approximately 60% of in-hospital deaths), and that recurrent arrhythmias are only a minor cause (10% of in-hospital deaths).[10,11] Low output states and cardiogenic shock account for the remaining 30% of early deaths.[10] The extent to which these factors influence risk of recurrent cardiac arrest during long-term follow-up is unknown. It is possible, though unproved, that better prehospital care might result in better myocardial preservation, in parallel with the already documented improvement in CNS function; but its influence on long-term risk of recurrent cardiac arrest is unknown. The absence of data on the effect of improved prehospital care on long-term post-hospital outcome serves only to confound the interpretation of data on expected risk after survival, and is an area requiring further study.

Etiologic and Pathophysiologic Determinants of Risk of Recurrent Cardiac Arrest

The accumulation of information on the clinical characteristics of survivors of out-of-hospital cardiac arrest has led to the identification of low- and high-risk subgroups, whose management is dictated by the etiology and pathophysiologic mechanisms responsible for the index event. The goals of evaluation during convalescene include: (1) identification of specific etiology and mechanism of the cardiac arrest, (2) assessment of the functional status of the patient, (3) the development of plans for long-term general care and specific antiarrhythmic therapy, and (4) determining end-points for estimating predicted efficacy of the plan of therapy.

The extent of the work-up for identifying etiology, functional status, and a plan for long-term management depends largely upon CNS recovery, and upon factors already known to have contributed to the cardiac arrest. Patients whose cardiac arrests were initiated by a new transmural myocardial infarction have a long-term risk which is similar to other patients with new transmural acute myocardial infarctions,[12] and their clinical evaluation is not much different from that of the general pool of patients with acute myocardial infarction. Those patients who have limited return of CNS function do not generally undergo extensive diagnostic evaluations, and those whose cardiac arrests are due to identifiable pro-arrhythmic drug effects or electrolyte disturbances usually do not require extensive work-up.[13] Long-term management of the latter group is usually based upon avoidance of agents or conditions that predispose to the initiating event. In contrast, for the large majority of patients whose underlying etiology of out-of-hospital cardiac arrest is coronary atherosclerosis *not* associated with acute transmural myocardial infarction, cardiac catheterization and angiography, an estimation of functional significance of coronary lesions by stress imaging techniques, and an evaluation of susceptibility to life-threatening arrhythmia are generally carried out.[13]

General Management of Survivors: Potential Impact on Long-Term Outcome

The general management of survivors of out-of-hospital cardiac arrest includes identification of the specific underlying etiology and attention to its interaction with other transient pathophysiologic factors, control of episodes of myocardial ischemia, optimization of therapy for left ventricular dysfunction, and control of general medical problems. All are addressed simultaneously.

Causes and Contributing Factors

Coronary atherosclerosis is by far the most common cause of out-of-hospital cardiac arrest, accounting for approximately 80% of unselected victims.[10,14] Pathologic studies have demonstrated that at least 75% of cardiac arrest victims have two or more coronary arteries with >75% stenosis.[15,16] No more than 20–30% have pathologic evidence of acute myocardial infarction as a precipitating cause,[15–17] and clinical studies in survivors of out-of-hospital cardiac arrest suggest a similar proportion of acute transmural myocardial infarction as a precipitating event.[1,2,10] The various cardiomyopathies as a group constitute the second most frequent cause of out-of-hospital cardiac arrest (approximately 10%), and the many other primary causes contribute progressively fewer cases to the total pool (Table I).[14] While these numerous but infrequent specific etiologies for sudden cardiac death must be considered in evaluating individual patients, a more important concept is the *interaction between the primary underlying disease and chronic or transient contributing factors*. In Figure 2, a schematic demonstration of the most important factors that contribute to the transition of chronic ischemic heart disease to the sudden cardiac death syndrome is provided as an example. The recognition of interplay between basic underlying etiology and contributing factors is conceptually and practically important. General clinical care commonly controls for many of these factors (e.g., blood pressure, electrolyte status, autonomic activity, metabolic states, heart failure), may influence outcome, and at the same time confounds the interpretation of antiarrhythmic intervention data in all but the most carefully controlled studies.

Anti-Ischemic Therapy

In those patients in whom a transient ischemic mechanism is clearly documented to be the pathophysiologic cause of transition from chronic atherosclerotic heart disease to cardiac arrest, an anti-ischemic approach to management provides an important element of therapy. Unfortunately, transient ischemia may be unrecognized in many instances of out-of-hospital cardiac arrest; and, therefore, chronic anti-ischemic therapy is commonly used in conjunction with antiarrhythmic therapy. This again serves to confound data on the results of antiarrhythmic therapy in many studies. Either medical or surgical anti-ischemic therapy may be

Table I
Causes and Contributing Factors in Sudden Cardiac Death

Common Causes and/or Contributing Factors	Less Common Causes

• Coronary Artery Disease
  -With acute MI
  -Without acute MI
  -Ventricular aneurysm
  -Plaque fissuring; platelet aggregation
	• Myocarditis, infiltrative, inflammatory, and restrictive diseases
	
	• Specific anatomic abnormalities
	  -Congenital heart disease
	    • With plumonary hypertension
	    • After corrective surgery

• Cardiomyopathies
  -Congestive
  -Hypertrophic
    • Obstructive
    • Non-obstructive
	-Mitral valve prolapse
	-Arrhythmogenic right ventricular dysplasia
	-Wolff-Parkinson-White syndrome

• Hypertension; LV hypertrophy
 	
• Heart Failure
  -Acute
  -Chronic
	• Functional Abnormalities
	  -Long Q-T interval syndrome
	    • Congenital
	    • Acquired
	  -Autonomic nervous system influences
	  -Acute metabolic, electrolyte, toxic disturbances

• Valvular Heart Disease • Conducting System Disease	• VT/VF with no identifiable heart disease -Idiopathic VT/VF

advised, depending upon the anatomy and physiology of the disease process. Cobb and co-workers[18] reported limited data suggesting that coronary bypass surgery may improve the recurrent cardiac arrest rate and total mortality rate after survival from out-of-hospital cardiac arrest, but there have been no properly controlled prospective studies on the topic. A report from the Coronary Artery Surgery Study (CASS) provides nonrandomized observational data suggesting that sudden death during follow-up was significantly less frequent in the surgical than in the medically treated group.[19] The differences were greatest in the subgroup with triple-vessel disease and a history of heart failure (Fig. 3), a combination that correlates well with risk for sudden death.[14] Despite these impressive differences, the study design limits interpretation, and *provides no more than suggestive data for cardiac arrest survivors*. Therefore, indications for coronary bypass surgery should be limited to two groups of patients: (1) those who have conventional indications based on symptoms (e.g., uncontrolled angina pectoris) or anatomy (e.g., left main coronary artery disease or its equivalent), and (2) those who have a clearly defined ischemic mechanism for cardiac arrest and appropriate surgical anatomy.[20] Specialized antiarrhythmic surgery will be discussed later.

Medical anti-ischemic therapy is commonly used in survivors of out-of-hospital cardiac arrest who have chronic ischemic heart disease. Beta-adrenergic blocking agents have both an antianginal effect and may limit the influence of sympathetic activity on the genesis of potentially lethal arrhythmias. The separation of these effects from each other, and from conventional antiarrhythmic

Out-of-Hospital Cardiac Arrest • 511

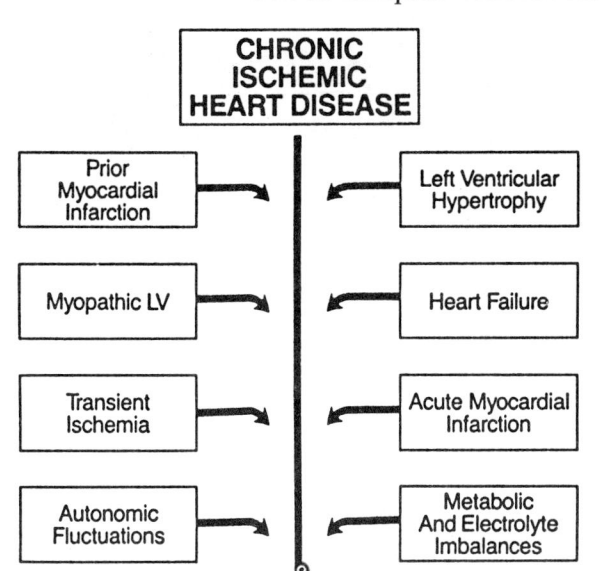

Figure 2: Contributing factors to the initiation of cardiac arrest in chronic ischemic heart disease. The transition from chronic ischemic heart disease, as a primary underlying etiology, to the sudden cardiac death syndrome, cannot be viewed independently of other factors which interact between the underlying etiology and the terminal event. These include the prior pathologic state of the myocardium (e.g., prior myocardial infarction, left ventricular hypertrophy or myopathy), acute or subacute alterations of the functional status of the heart (e.g., heart failure, transient ischemia, acute myocardial infarction), and fluctuations in neurohumoral, metabolic, and/or electrolyte state of the myocardium (see text for details).

effects, is difficult. Studies to date have not been able to discriminate a specific role for beta-adrenergic blocking agents in out-of-hospital cardiac arrest survivors; and in our studies, the use of beta-adrenergic blocking agents was not different in long-term survivors compared to a subgroup who had recurrent cardiac arrest.[3] However, Morady et al.[21] suggested that anti-ischemic therapy may be useful for those out-of-hospital cardiac arrest survivors in whom transient myocardial ischemia appeared to be the precipitating factor. Categories of anti-ischemic drugs other than beta-blockers, including C^{++}-entry blocking agents and aspirin, could also be effective, but there is even less data for the role of these agents in cardiac arrest survivors.

Therapy Directed at Improving Cardiovascular Function

Survivors of out-of-hospital cardiac arrest as a group have significantly impaired left ventricular function as measured by ejection fraction data, but there is a broad range of observed values with as many as 1/3 to 1/2 of the survivors having normal or only mildly impaired left ventricular function.[10,22] Most studies report

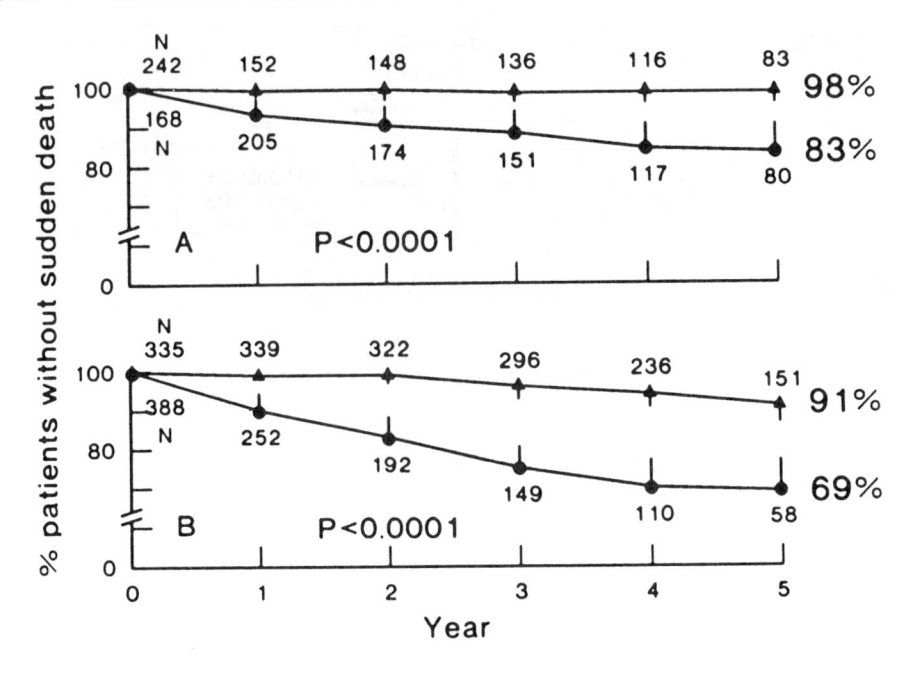

Figure 3: Sudden cardiac death in the medical and surgical groups of the CASS study. Percent of patients without sudden cardiac death in the surgically treated group (triangles) compared with that in the medically treated group (circles). All of these patients had a history of congestive heart failure. The patients in panel A had two-vessel disease, and those in panel B had three-vessel disease. The actual numbers of patients are given for each survival curve at each point in time. There was a significantly lower risk of sudden death during follow-up with surgical treatment in both groups, and the differences were greatest in patients with three-vessel disease. (From Holmes et al.,[19] reproduced with the permission of the authors and the American Heart Association, Inc.)

mean values in the range of 35–40%, and Packer[23] has recently emphasized the importance of cardiac arrest as a cause of death in chronic heart failure patients. Whether improvement of left ventricular function by careful pharmacologic management alters this risk is unknown. Data from our studies, however, demonstrate that the severity of ejection fraction abnormalities correlates beter with non-sudden death during long-term follow-up than it does with recurrent cardiac arrest[3] (Fig. 4).

Long-term management of left ventricular dysfunction by the routine use of digitalis and diuretic preparations has recently been the subject of debate. Data from the Multiple Risk Factor Intervention Trial (MRFIT) suggests a higher mortality rate in the special intervention group,[24] presumably related to diuretic use and potassium depletion. This and other data regarding the relationship between potassium depletion and arrhythmias have raised questions about the proper use of such drugs. Although the clinical impact is far from conclusive at present,[25] diuretics must be used with care and accompanied by careful monitoring of electrolyte status.

Similar issues have been raised about the use of digitalis in high-risk patients.

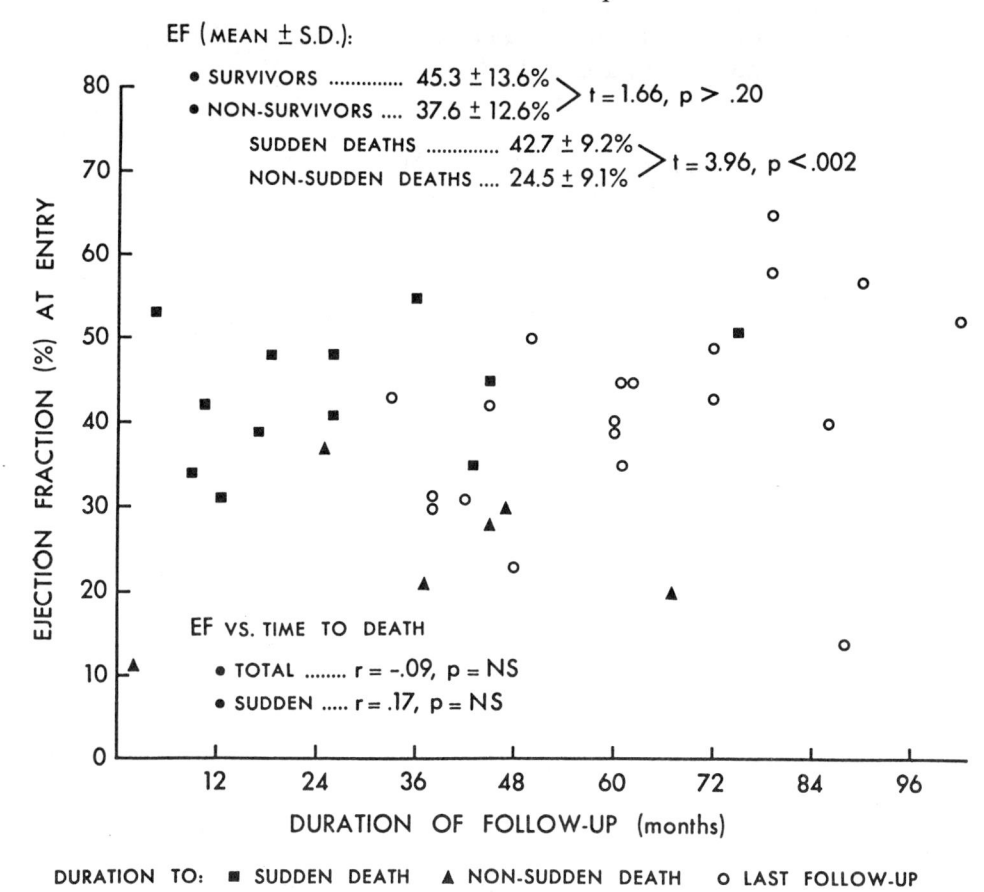

Figure 4: Left ventricular ejection fractions at entry to long-term follow-up in survivors of out-of-hospital cardiac arrest. Left ventricular ejection fractions on cineangiograms at entry into the study are plotted as a function of duration of follow-up to sudden death (closed squares), non-sudden death (closed triangles), and to the time of last follow-up in survivors (open circles). The mean (±SD) ejection fraction (EF) among long-term survivors was 45.3 ± 13.6% compared to 37.6 ± 12.6% in nonsurvivors. These differences did not achieve statistical significance because of the wide range of EFs in both groups (p=ns). Among the patients who had fatal terminating events, there was a significant difference between the ejection fractions in those who had recurrent cardiac arrest (42.7 ± 9.2%) compared to those who had non-sudden deaths (24.5 ± 9.1%) (p<.002). There was no relationship between ejection fraction at entry and duration of follow-up to death, either sudden or total. (From Myerburg et al.,[3] reproduced with permission of the American Heart Association, Inc.)

Two studies[26,27] reported higher than expected mortality rates in digoxin-treated post-myocardial infarction patients, and two others[28,29] concluded that excess mortality was explained by differences in baseline characteristics of the patients. In a fifth study, Mueller et al.[30] reported no excess moralilty, but cautioned that the question can be properly answered only by a prospective randomized study. Until such information is available, digoxin use in survivors of out-of-hospital cardiac arrest should be tailored to specific indications for left ventricular dysfunction; however, this will still serve as another confounding influence on the interpretation of antiarrhythmic efficacy data.

Antiarrhythmic Drugs in Survivors of Out-of-Hospital Cardiac Arrest

The difficulty in interpreting antiarrhythmic drug data in survivors of out-of-hospital cardiac arrest, resulting from the absence of a current natural history denominator, and from the other co-factors listed, is further compounded by the fact that several different therapeutic strategies intended to prevent recurrent cardiac arrest have been evaluated.[13]

Noninvasive Management Techniques

Antiarrhythmic therapy for long-term management of survivors of out-of-hospital cardiac arrest have been prompted by two hypotheses: (1) that the high frequency of chronic ventricular ectopic activity (PVCs) identified in many survivors of cardiac arrest constitutes a triggering mechanism for the recurrence of potentially lethal arrhythmias (VT/VF), and (2) that the electrophysiologic instability of the myocardium predisposing to potentially lethal arrhythmias can be modified by antiarrhythmic drugs.[31,32] Some strategies are also based on the hypothesis that PVC suppression and prevention of potentially lethal arrhythmias are independent variables.[31]

In an 8-year follow-up study of 61 survivors of out-of-hospital cardiac arrest managed by dose titration of antiarrhythmic drugs to achieve stable high plasma concentrations, regardless of effect on PVCs or laboratory-induced VT/VF, the 1-year recurrent cardiac arrest rate was 10%, and the 2-year cumulative rate was 15% (Fig. 5).[3] Survival was independent of suppression of PVCs, but 31% of the recurrences occurred in patients whose drugs had been stopped or changed without monitoring levels of the new drug.[3] This approach to antiarrhythmic management of survivors of out-of-hospital cardiac arrest was begun in the mid-1970s,[33] before ambulatory monitoring techniques had flourished[34] and before programmed electrical stimulation had been generally applied to such patients. Our initial apparent success, compared to the earlier recurrence statistics, encouraged us to continue this approach in order to acquire long-term data. In the early 1980s, however, more specific and individualized noninvasive end-points for evaluating drug therapy, such as suppression of complex forms of PVCs on ambulatory monitoring, were reported. Graboys and co-workers[4] reported the outcome in a group of 123 patients with prior VT/VF who had survived one or more cardiac arrests. The ability of single or multiple drug regimens to suppress specific forms of PVCs (salvos ≥ 3 PVCs, early cycle PVCs) identified on ambulatory monitoring or exercise testing, resulted in a 90% survival rate at 3 years, compared to a mortality rate >80% in those patients in whom complex forms could not be suppressed. The interpretation of these data is limited by the highly selected nature of this tertiary referral population, and absence of control of other factors which could influence outcome.

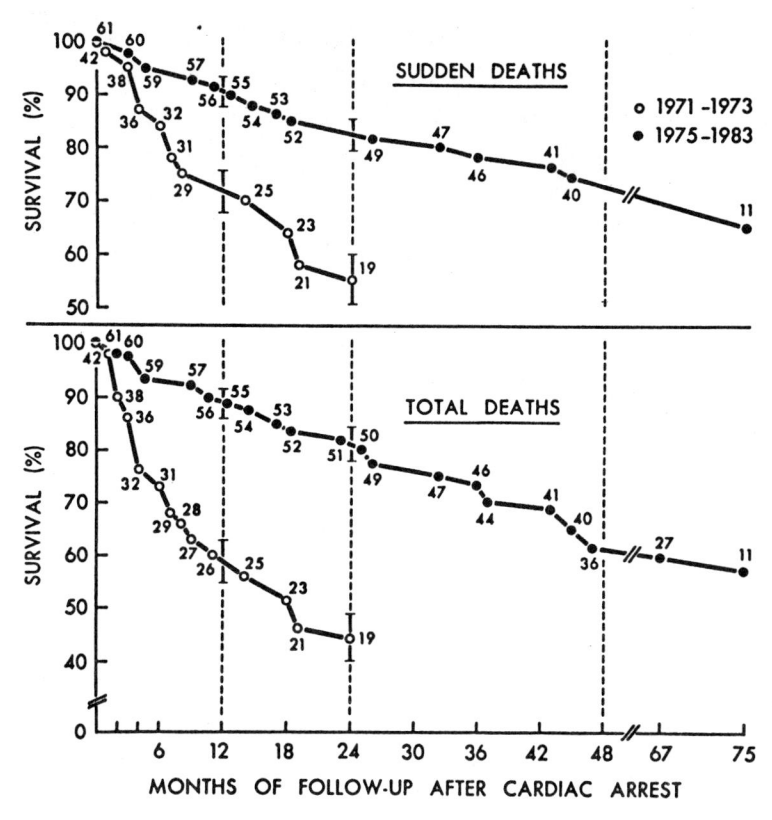

Figure 5: Sudden deaths and total deaths in survivors of prehospital cardiac arrest during an 8-Year follow-up period (closed circles), compared to 1970–73 historic experience during the initial Miami studies (open circles). The 1975–1983 follow-up data indicate a 67% reduction in recurrent cardiac arrest rate during the first year of follow-up. Whether this was due to aggressive antiarrhythmic therapy or other factors in the patient populations or their management cannot be determined from comparison to historic controls. However, the 10% 1-year mortality rate is similar to outcome with other end-points of antiarrhythmic intervention in recent years. See text for details. (From Myerburg and Kessler,[13] with the permission of the American Heart Association, Inc.)

Management Based on Programmed Electrical Stimulation Studies

This approach is highly individualized and has demonstrated encouraging results when used within the limits of our current knowledge.[13,35–37] In survivors of out-of-hospital cardiac arrest, its use is confounded in part by the problems related to sensitivity and specificity of the various pacing protocols, uncertainty about the validity of end-points of suppressed induction, and concerns about whether the myocardial status at the time of electrophysiologic testing is comparable to that at the time of the clinical cardiac arrest (Fig. 6).[37] However, among five studies,[38–42] induction of sustained VT or VF at baseline study ranged from 31–58%, and successful suppression of inducibility ranged from 18–78%. The mortality rate during follow-up of those patients who had inducibility suppressed by antiarrhythmic therapy ranged from 0–22% (mean =9%), compared to a range of 22–78% (mean=43%) in those patients who

PATHOPHYSIOLOGY OF INITIATION OF POTENTIALLY LETHAL ARRHYTHMIAS

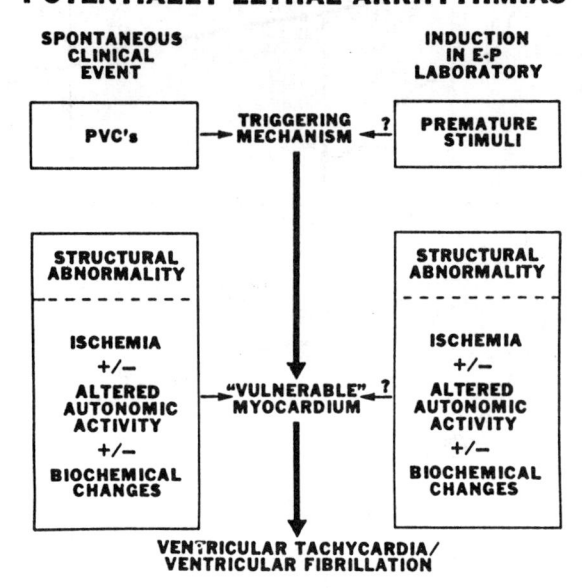

Figure 6: Pathophysiology of initiation of potentially lethal arrhythmias. The rationale for EPS testing for VT/VF patients assumes parallels between the spontaneous clinical event and the laboratory-induced event. These assumptions are as yet unproven. Is the PVC induced by premature stimuli equivalent to spontaneous PVCs? Are ischemia, autonomic status, and metabolic/biochemical status electrophysiologically equivalent in the two settings? Are structural pathways fundamentally stable? (From Myerburg and Zaman,[37] reproduced with the permission of the American Heart Association, Inc.)

remained inducible (see Table II). In the report by Ruskin and co-workers,[38] only 31% of prehospital cardiac arrest survivors were inducible into *sustained* VT or VF, 40% into nonsustained arrhythmias, and another 30% were noninducible. In contrast, Roy and colleagues[39] reported that 72 of 119 patients (61%) were inducible into sustained VT or VF, 11 (9%) were inducible into nonsustained VT, and 36 (30%) were not inducible. Morady et al.[40] reported that 26 of 45 survivors (58%) were inducible into sustained arrhythmias, and eight (18%) into nonsustained tachycardia. In most studies, the fraction of patients who are *noninducible* fall within the narrow range of 25–30%. The fractions who were inducible into nonsustained arrhythmias were more variable, possibly because of different stimulation protocols, anatomy, and definitions of inducibility.[35] Until future studies clarify these issues, one can anticipate that approximately 30–40% of *unselected* survivors of cardiac arrest will be inducible into sustained arrhythmias at baseline study. For that subgroup with discrete ventricular aneurysms, as many as 70–80% may be inducible.

While it is generally agreed that *sustained VT* or *VT degenerating to VF* induced at baseline study provides an indication of risk, and prevention of its induction on therapy is a valid end-point, the significance of induction of *nonsustained* forms is

Table II
Data from Five Studies of Electrophysiologic Testing in Survivors of Cardiac Arrest

Inducible at baseline study:	
-sustained VT	31%–58%
-sustained or nonsustained VT, VF	60%–87%
Inducibility suppressed by antiarrhythmic therapy	18%–78%
-recurrent cardiac arrest	0–22% (mean = 9%)
Inducibility not suppressed by antiarrhythmic therapy	22%–82%
-recurrent cardiac arrest	22%–78% (mean = 43%)
Noninducible at baseline-mortality, extrapolated to 24 month F/U	3%–38%

(From Myerburg and Kessler,[13] reproduced with permission of the American Heart Association, Inc.)

more controversial. Induction of nonsustained forms may indicate risk, depending in part upon the aggressiveness of the protocol used,[35] but their use as a baseline against which to evaluate drug therapy is not clear at this time.

The significance of *noninducibility* at baseline electrophysiologic testing is a controversial issue. Opinions range from the assumption that noninducible patients are at risk only because of ischemia and require no long-term antiarrhythmic therapy,[21] to the conclusion that such patients may still be electrically unstable and therefore must be treated by complex form suppression or empirically.[13] Undoubtedly some patients in this group have had cardiac arrest based upon transient ischemia, but the difficulty of identifying patients who could be managed by anti-ischemic therapy alone is considerable; most patients in this category now receive *both* anti-ischemic and antiarrhythmic therapy.

The Role of Implantable Devices

The development of reliable implantable antitachycardia/defibrillatory devices has added a new dimension to the management of patients at high risk for cardiac arrest.[43] Mirowski and co-workers[44] reported outcome in 52 patients who had survived an arrhythmic arrest, with at least one recurrence not associated with acute myocardial infarction. All of these patients had failed other forms of preventive therapy, and the group had a mean of 3.9 cardiac arrests/patient. The analysis is complicated by the fact that concomitant cardiovascular surgical procedures were carried out in 15 patients, and approximately the same number had had prior surgery; nine had also had pacemaker implantation. Although 12 of these 52 very high risk patients died during a 14-month follow-up period (23% 1-year total mortality rate), the 1-year *sudden death* rate was 8.5%. Moreover, devices were triggered 62 times in 17 patients, and if death had followed in these patients in the absence of the device, the total 1-year mortality rate would have been 48%. In a subsequent study. Echt and colleagues[45] reported their experience in 70 patients. Since 35 of their patients (50%) had had no prior cardiac arrest (14 patients who had VT uncontrolled on treatment) or only one prior cardiac arrest (21 patients), this population may have been less unstable than the patients in Mirowski's study. During a mean follow-up of 8.9 months (range = 1–33 months), 37 patients (53%) received one or more shocks. The 1-year total death rate was 10%, and the sudden death rate <2%, with an acceptably low complication rate. Finally, Platia et al.[46] evaluated concomitant use of the implantable defibrillator with ventricular endocardial resection for recurrent VT/VF. During a mean 25-month follow-up, four of 25 patients (16%) had recurrent VT/VF which was successfully reverted by the device; one patient died because the defibrillator malfunctioned. While these devices appear effective for automatic interventions, concurrent antiarrhythmic therapy is commonly used to limit the number of shocks delivered.

An Approach to Management of Survivors of Out-of-Hospital Cardiac Arrest and Possible Influence on Long-Term Outcome

Because of the complexities inherent in options for management of survivors of out-of-hospital cardiac arrest, and the numerous confounding influences outlined above, we developed a system which takes into account problems unique to each method of management based upon current knowledge and limitations. This is a two-tiered algorithm, the first stage of which (Fig. 7) addresses diagnosis and general management, and the second (Fig. 8) addresses advanced antiarrhythmic strategies. Those patients in whom prehospital cardiac arrest is precipitated by a new transmural myocardial infarction, those who have certain forms of noncoronary heart disease (e.g., critical aortic stenosis or acquired prolonged Q-T interval syndrome), those with life-threatening co-morbid states, and those who have significant residual CNS dysfunction reach their management end-points in the first stage of management (Fig. 7). Among the remainder, who constitute the majority of survivors and most commonly have chronic ischemic heart disease, programmed electrical stimulation is performed (see Fig. 8, stage 2). In that subgroup of patients in whom sustained VT is inducible, with or without degeneration to VF, the preferred end-point of therapy is prevention of inducibility by an appropriate antiarrhythmic agent or drug combination (pathway A). Once identified, the plasma concentration required to achieve noninducibility should be measured and monitored periodically during long-term follow-up.[13] In those patients in whom this approach is not feasible because of noninducibility into sustained VT or VF at baseline, another objective approach should be applied—specifically, the evaluation of response of complex PVCs to antiarrhythmic agents on ambulatory monitoring (AM in pathway B). Kim et al.[47] have proposed this approach for patients who fail to have inducibility suppressed during EPS drug studies, but have suppressible PVCs on ambulatory monitoring. Those patients who have salvos or nonsustained VT on baseline AM are titrated with antiarrhythmic drugs, singly or in combination, in order to suppress these repetitive forms.[34] If this is successful, it is used as an end-point of therapy. In those

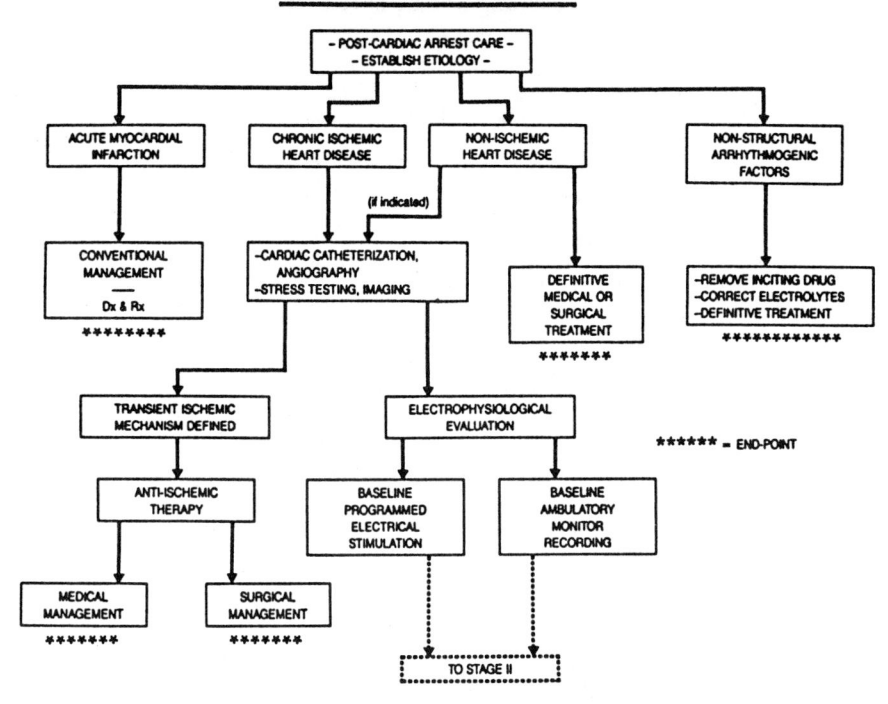

Figure 7: Management algorithm—stage I. Flow diagram for initial management and diagnostic activities in survivors of out-of-hospital cardiac arrest. Patients whose arrests were associated with new acute transmural myocardial infarction or nonstructural arrhythmogenic factors are managed by conventional techniques. All patients with chronic ischemic heart disease, and many with nonischemic heart disease, enter a pathway which leads to advanced electrophysiologic study and management (From Myerburg and Kessler,[13] reproduced with the permission of the American Heart Association, Inc.)

patients who have neither inducibility on EPS nor complex forms on baseline AM, we use empiric antiarrhythmic therapy titrated to the upper half of normalized therapeutic plasma concentrations[3] (Fig. 9). We have also used the latter successfully in some patients whose baseline inducibility in the electrophysiology laboratory failed drug trials, or whose ambulatory monitor repetitive forms were not suppressible,[3,33,48] but the promising statistics on surgical procedures and implantable devices (pathway C) now warrant their use in lieu of empiric therapy in appropriate patients in this category.[43-45] Antiarrhythmic surgical intervention[49,50] is the method of choice for patients who have suitable anatomy (especially discrete ventricular aneurysms) and are inducible into sustained VT/VF which cannot be prevented by antiarrhythmic drugs. The results in such patients are encouraging,[49,50] even though antiarrhythmic therapy is still needed postoperatively in some.[51] The antitachycardia/defibrillatory devices are the evolving method of choice for patients who have survived a recurrence on apparently adequate therapy, and in many of those who fail the algorithm and have high-risk indicators.

A review of the most recent outcome data for each of the approaches outlined

MANAGEMENT STAGE II

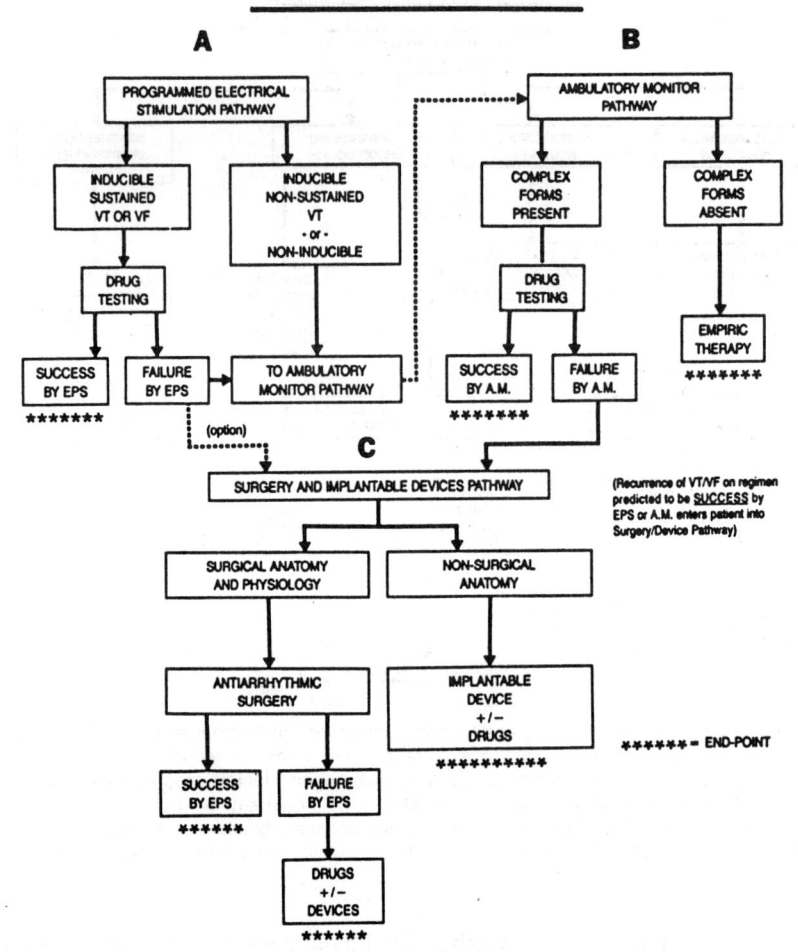

Figure 8: Management algorithm—stage II. Advanced electrophysiologic evaluation of survivors of prehospital cardiac arrest. Patients generally enter pathway A–programmed electrical stimulation (EPS), and if inducible into sustained VT or VT/VF, they are managed by drug testing using this technique. If successful, this becomes the end-point. If the patient fails EPS, or if patients are inducible into nonsustained VT or are non-inducible at baseline study, they enter the ambulatory monitor (A.M.) pathway (pathway B). Some patients who fail EPS, if unstable, might enter directly to pathway C–surgery or implantable devices. The route through pathways B and C is explained in the text. (From Myerburg and Kessler,[13] reproduced with the permission of the American Heart Association, Inc.)

above is enlightening. With each method, patients who achieve successful end-points have recurrent cardiac arrest rates of no more than 10–15% during the first year of follow-up, compared to the 30% rate previously reported. Whether this means that each of the methods is equally effective in those in whom it is applicable, that other uncontrolled factors such as anti-ischemic therapy is influencing outcome, or even that the intrinsic risk of recurrence has undergone

PANEL A

NORMALIZED PLASMA LEVELS OF ANTIARRHYTHMIC DRUGS IN SURVIVORS OF PREHOSPITAL CARDIAC ARREST

SCORE	PLASMA LEVEL RANGE
0	NIL
1	Below Standard
2	Lower Half of Standard
3	Upper Half of Standard
4	Above Standard

GROUP	SCORE	
. Recurrent Cardiac Arrest (n = 16)	1.33 ± 1.23	
. Total Deaths (n = 24)	1.63 ± 1.20	
. Survivors at 24-27 Months of Follow-Up (n = 24)	$*2.63 \pm 0.94$	[*p < 0.01 vs Recurrent Cardiac Arrest]
. Survivors at Last Follow-Up (n = 35)	$*2.56 \pm 0.94$	

PANEL B

DRUG STATUS PRIOR TO RECURRENT CARDIAC ARREST

. Drug Stopped (n = 3) or Changed for Reasons Other Than
 Drug Failure (n = 2) $\leq$ 4 Months Before Recurrence 5/16 (31%)

. Status of Therapy at Time of Recurrent Arrest
 – Last Plasma Level NIL or Below Target Range 14/16 (87%)
 – Last Plasma Level Within Target Range 2/16 (13%)

. Matched Therapeutic Status In Long-Term Survivors
 – Plasma Levels NIL or Below Target Range 10/34 (29%)
 – Plasma Levels Within Target Range 24/34 (71%)

Figure 9.

significant reduction independent of specific antiarrhythmic or anti-ischmic interventions, has not been clarified. However, there does appear to be a risk attendant upon indiscriminate changes in antiarrhythmic therapy which has been determined to be effective by any of the end-point criteria used. Swerdlow et al.[51] and Myerburg et al.,[3] using very different end-points of therapy, have both observed that arbitrary cessation or changes in therapy, without re-testing for the end-point used to establish initial therapy, is accompanied by a high risk of recurrent cardiac arrest.

Conclusion

The 1-year recurrent cardiac arrest rate in survivors of out-of-hospital cardiac arrest in 1970–73 was 30%; the 1-year recurrent cardiac arrest rate in survivors of out-of-hospital cardiac arrest in the 1980s is 10–15% in most studies, and <10% in some. However, it is not possible to identify with certainty which one or combination of antiarrhythmic or general medical factors applied since 1970 is responsible for this decline. Since it is ethically impossible to carry out concurrently controlled studies in such high-risk patients, except possibly in those who have an implantable defibrillator, it is not likely that we will know the reason for the decreased mortality rate among survivors of out-of-hospital cardiac arrest in the foreseeable future. It *is* clear that we have identified a few subgroups at low risk for recurrences, and a large body of patients who appear to remain at high risk. The scientific and practical desirability of dissecting out the variables responsible for better outcome will have to yield to the pragmatic imperative of using the available data for the best care of these patients, until we have a better understanding of the impact of individual intervention factors on outcome. To this end, our management algorithm incorporates much of the available information, but it too must be viewed with flexibility, in recognition of the fact that its guidelines were developed in the absence of important elements of definitive information.

Acknowledgment: Supported in part by research grants from the NHLBI, Grant No. HL28130, and NHLBI Training Grant No. HL07436 (Pedro Fernandez, M.D.), and from a Grant-in-Aid from the Florida Heart Association (Kenneth M. Kessler). We are grateful to Mrs. Thelma L. Gottlieb for administrative and secretarial support.

References

1. Liberthson RR, Nagel EL, Hirschman JC, Nussenfeld SR. Prehospital ventricular fibrillation: Prognosis and follow-up course. N Engl J Med 1974;291:317–321.
2. Baum RS, Alvarez H, Cobb LA. Survival after resuscitation from out-of-hospital ventricular fibrillation. Circulation 1974;50:1231–1235.
3. Myerburg RJ, Kessler KM, Estes D, Conde CA, Luceri RM, Zaman L, Kozlovskis PL, Castellanos A. Long-term survival after prehospital cardiac arrest: Analysis of outcome during an 8-year study. Circulation 1984;70:538–546.
4. Graboys TB, Lown B, Podrid PJ, DeSilva R. Long-term survival of patients with malignant ventricular arrhythmias treated with antiarrhythmic drugs. Am J Cardiol 1982;50:437–443.
5. Vlay SC, Kallman CH, Reid PR. Prognostic assessment of survivors of ventricular tachycardia and ventricular fibrillation with ambulatory monitoring. Am J Cardiol 1984;54:87–90.
6. Wilber DJ, Garan H, Kelly E, McGovern B, Newell J, Ruskin JN: Out-of-hospital cardiac arrest: Role of electrophysiologic testing in prediction of long-term outcome (abstr). Circulation 1986;74(Suppl II):482.
7. Schaeffer WA, Cobb LA. Recurrent ventricular fibrillation and modes of death in survivors of out-of-hospital ventricular fibrillation. New Engl J Med 1975;293:259–262.
8. Eisenberg MS, Copass MK, Hallstrom AP, Blake B, Bergner L, Short FA, Cobb LA. Treatment of out-of-hospital cardiac arrests with rapid defibrillation by emergency medical technicians. New Engl J Med 1980;302:1379–1383.
9. Thompson RG, Hallstrom AP, Cobb LA. Bystander-initiated cardiopulmonary resuscitation in the management of ventricular fibrillation. Ann Int Med 1979;90:737–740.

10. Myerburg RJ, Conde CA, Sung RJ, Mayorga-Cortes A, Mallon SM, Sheps DS, Appel RA, Castellanos A. Clinical, electrophysiologic, and hemodynamic profile of patients resuscitated from prehospital cardiac arrest. Am J Med 1980;68:568–576.
11. Cobb LA, Weiner JA, Trobaugh GB. Sudden cardiac death. II. Outcome of resuscitation; management and future directions. Mod Concepts Cardiovasc Dis 1980;49: 37–42.
12. Cobb LA, Baum RS, Alvarez H, Schaffer WA. Resuscitation from out-of-hospital ventricular fibrillation: 4 year follow-up. Circulation 1975;52(suppl III):223–228.
13. Myerburg RJ, Kessler KM. Management of patients who survive cardiac arrest. Mod Concepts Cardiovasc Dis (in press).
14. Myerburg RJ, Castellanos A. Cardiac arrest and sudden cardiac death. In Braunwald E, ed. Heart Disease, 3rd edition. Philadelphia, W.B. Saunders, 1987 (in press).
15. Perper JA, Kuller LH, Cooper M. Arteriosclerosis of coronary arteries in sudden, unexpected deaths. Circulation 1975;52(suppl III):27–33.
16. Liberthson RR, Nagel EL, Hirschman JC, Nussenfeld SR, Blackbourn BD, Davis JR. Pathophysiologic observations in prehospital ventricular fibrillation and sudden cardiac death. Circulation 1974;49:790–798.
17. Davis MJ. Pathological view of sudden cardiac death. Br Heart J 1981;45:88–96.
18. Cobb LA, Hallstrom AP, Zia M, Trobaugh GB, Greene HL, Weaver WD. Influence of coronary revascularization on recurrent sudden cardiac death syndrome (abstr). J Am Coll Cardiol 1983;1:688.
19. Holmes DR, Davis KB, Mock MB, Fisher LB, Gersh RJ, Killip T, Pettinger M, and Participants in the Coronary Artery Surgery Study. The effect of medical and surgical treatment on subsequent sudden cardiac death in patients with coronary artery disease: A report from the Coronary Artery Surgery Study. Circulation 1986;73: 1254–1263.
20. Harken AH, Wetstein L, Josephson ME. Mechanisms and surgical management of ventricular tachyarrhythmias. In Josephson ME, ed. Sudden Cardiac Death. Philadelphia, F.A. Davis, 1985;287–300.
21. Morady F, DiCarlo L, Winston S, Davis JC, Scheinman MM. Clinical features and prognosis of patients with out-of-hospital cardiac arrest and a normal electrophysiologic study. J Am Coll Cardiol 1984;4:39–44.
22. Ritchie JL, Hallstrom AP, Troubaugh GB, Caldwell JH, Cobb LA. Out-of-hospital sudden coronary death: Rest and exercise radionuclide left ventricular function in survivors. Am J Cardiol 1985;55:645–651.
23. Packer M. Sudden unexpected death in patients with congestive heart failure: A second frontier. Circulation 1985;72:681.
24. Multiple Risk Factor Intervention Trial Research Group. Baseline rest electrocardiographic abnormalities, antihypertensive treatment, and mortality in the Multiple Risk Factor Intervention Trial. Am J Cardiol 1985;55:1–15.
25. Kuller LH, Hulley SB, Cohen JD, Neaton J. Unexpected effects of treating hypertension in men with electrocardiographic abnormalities: A critical analysis. Circulation 1986;73:114–123.
26. Moss AJ, Davis HT, Conard DL, deCamilla JJ, Odioroff CL. Digitalis-associated cardiac mortality after myocardial infarction. Circulation 1981;64:1150–1156.
27. Bigger JT, Fleiss JL, Rolnitzky LM, Merab JP, Ferrick KL. Effect of digitalis treatment on survival after acute myocardial infarction. Am J Cardiol 1985;55:623–630.
28. Ryan TJ, Bailey KR, McCabe CH, Luk S, Fisher LD, Mock BM, Killip T. The effects of digitalis on survival in high risk patients with coronary artery disease: The Coronary Artery Surgery Study (CASS). Circulation 1983;67:735–742.
29. Madsen EB, Gilpin E, Henning H, Ahnve S, LeWinter M, Mazur J, Shabetal R, Collins D, Ross J. Prognostic importance of digitalis after acute myocardial infarction. J Am Coll Cardiol 1984;3:681–689.
30. Muller JE, Turi ZG, Stone PH, Rude RE, Raabe DS, Jaffe AS, Gold HK, Gustafson N, Poole WK, Passamani E, Smith TM, Braunwald E, and the MILIS Study Group. Digoxin therapy and mortality after myocardial infarction: Experience in the MILIS study. New Engl J Med 1986;314:265–271.

31. Myerburg RJ, Kessler KM, Kiem I, Pefkaros KC, Conde CA, Cooper D, Castellanos A. The relationship between plasma levels of procainamide, suppression of premature ventricular contractions, and prevention of recurrent ventricular tachycardia. Circulation 1981;64:280–290.
32. Myerburg RJ, Bassett AL, Epstein K, Gaide MS, Kozlovskis P, Wong SS, Castellanos A, Gelband H. Electrophysiologic effects of procainamide in acute and healed experimental ischemic injury of cat myocardium. Circ Res 1982;50:386–393.
33. Myerburg RJ, Conde CA, Sheps DS, Appel RA, Kiem I, Sung RJ, Castellanos A. Antiarrhythmic drug therapy in survivors of prehospital cardiac arrest: Comparison of effects on chronic ventricular arrhythmias and on recurrent cardiac arrest. Circulation 1979;59:855–863.
34. Lown B, Graboys TB. Management of patients with malignant ventricular arrhythmias. Am J Cardiol 1977;39:910–919.
35. Wellens HJJ, Brugada P, Stevenson WG. Programmed electrical stimulation of the heart in patients with life-threatening ventricular arrhythmias: What is the significance of induced arrhythmias and what is the correct stimulation protocol? Circulation 1985;72:1–7.
36. Rahimtoola S, Zipes DP, Akhtar M, Burchell H, Mason J, Myerburg RJ, O'Rourke R, Ruskin J, Schlant R, Surawicz B. Consensus statement of the conference on the state of the art of electrophysiological testing in the diagnosis and treatment of patients with cardiac arrhythmias. Circulation (in press).
37. Myerburg RJ, Zaman L. Discussion of indications for intracardiac electrophysiologic studies in survivors of prehospital cardiac arrest. Circulation (suppl) (in press).
38. Ruskin JN, DiMarco JP, Garan H. Out-of-hospital cardiac arrest: Electrophysiologic observations and selection of long-term antiarrhythmic therapy. New Engl J Med 1980;303:607–613.
39. Roy D, Waxman HL, Kienzie MG, Buxton AF, Marchlinski FE, Josephson ME. Clinical characteristics and long-term follow-up in 119 survivors of cardiac arrest: Relation to inducibility at electrophysiologic testing. Am J Cardiol 1983;52:969–974.
40. Benditt DG, Benson DW Jr, Klein GJ, Pritzker MC, Kriett JM, Anderson RW. Prevention of recurrent sudden cardiac arrest: Role of provocative electropharmacologic testing. J Am Coll Cardiol 1983;2:418–425.
41. Morady F, Scheinman MM, Hess DS, Sung RJ, Shen E, Shapiro W. Electrophysiologic testing in the management of survivors of out-of-hospital cardiac arrest. Am J Cardiol 1983;51:85–89.
42. Skale BT, Miles WM, Heger JJ, Zipes DP, Prystowsky EN. Survivors of cardiac arrest: Prevention of recurrence by drug therapy as predicted by electrophysiologic testing or electrocardiographic monitoring. Am J Cardiol 1986;57:113–119.
43. Mirowski M, Reid PR, Mower MM, Watkins L, Gott VL, Schauble JF, Langer A, Heilman MS, Kolenik SA, Fischell RE, Weisfeldt ML. Termination of malignant ventricular arrhythmias with an implanted automatic defibrillator in human beings. New Engl J Med 1980;303:322–324.
44. Mirowski M, Reid PR, Winkle RA, Mower MM, Watkins L, Steinson GB, Griffith LSC, Kallman CH, Weisfeldt ML. Mortality in patients with implanted automatic defibrillators. Ann Int Med 1983;98:585–588.
45. Echt DS, Armstrong K, Schmidt P, Oyer PE, Stinson EB, Winkle RA. Clinical experience, complications, and survival in 70 patients with the automatic implantable converter/defibrillator. Circulation 1985;71:289–296.
46. Platia EV, Griffith LSC, Watkins L, Mower MM, Guarnieri T, Mirowski M, Reid PR. Treatment of malignant ventricular arrhythmias with endocardial resection and implantation of the automatic cardioverter-defibrillator. New Engl J Med 1986;314:213–216.
47. Kim SG, Seiden SW, Felder SD, Waspe LE, Fisher JD. Is programmed stimulation valid in predicting long-term success of antiarrhythmic therapy for ventricular tachycardias? New Engl J Med 1986;315:356–362.

48. Myerburg RJ, Kessler KM, Zaman L, Conde CA, Castellanos A: Survivors of prehospital cardiac arrest. J Am Med Assoc 1982;247:1485–1490.
49. Josephson ME, Hauken AH, Horowitz LN. Endocardial excision: A new surgical technique for the treatment of recurrent ventricular tachycardia. Circulation 1979;60:1430–1439.
50. Guiradon G, Fontaine G, Frank R, Escarde G, Etievant P. Encircling endocardial ventriculotomy: A new surgical treatment for life-threatening ventricular tachycardias resistant to medical treatment following myocardial infarction. Am Thor Surg 1978;26:438–444.
51. Swerdlow CR, Winkle RA, Mason JW. Determinants of survival in patients with ventricular tachycardia. New Engl J Med 1983;308:1436–1442.

VII

PERCUTANEOUS ABLATION

33

Catheter Electrical Ablation of Cardiac Arrhythmias: A Summary Report of the Percutaneous Cardiac Mapping and Ablation Registry*

Melvin M. Scheinman
G. Thomas Evans, Jr.

Introduction

In 1982, a worldwide voluntary registry was formed to collect data for patients undergoing catheter ablative procedures for control of cardiac arrhythmias. Taking the cue from cardiosurgical procedures, a variety of closed-chest catheter techniques have been introduced which allow for ablation of atrial[1] or ventricular tachycardia[2] foci as well as accessory pathways[3] or the atrioventricular junction[4] for control of drug-refractory cardiac arrhythmias in man. To date, only those procedures involving high energy direct current shocks have been

---

From: Brugada P, Wellens HJJ. CARDIAC ARRHYTHMIAS: Where To Go From Here? Mount Kisco, NY, Futura Publishing Company, Inc., © 1987.
*The authors listed are members of the Executive Committee of the Percutaneous Cardiac Mapping and Ablation Registry; M.M. Scheinman and D.P. Zipes, co-chairmen; D. Benditt, G. Breithardt, A.J. Camm, N. El-Sherif, J. Fisher, G. Fontaine, L. German, M. Josephson, S. Levy, F. Morady, J. Ruskin.

reported to the registry. The purpose of this review is to summarize the available data submitted to the registry with regard to atrioventricular junctional ablation or ablation of the ventricular tachycardia foci. Only a limited number of atrial or accessory pathway ablative procedures have been reported and are deemed to be too few to allow for meaningful conclusions.

Catheter Ablation of the Atrioventricular Junction

Catheter ablation of the atrioventricular junction may be used for any supraventricular arrhythmia in which the atrioventricular junction is used to funnel impulses into the ventricle. In the absence of an accessory pathway, ablation of the atrioventricular junction results in complete atrioventricular block and a pacemaker dependency state ensues. The procedure has also been applied in patients with tachyarrhythmias incorporating either extranodal or nodoventricular bypass tracts. As long as the atrioventricular junction forms a critical component of the reentrant circuit, destruction of this pathway should result in arrhythmia control. Obviously, those patients with short effective refractory periods of the accessory pathway are not candidates for atrioventricular junctional ablation alone since they are not protected from very rapid ventricular responses should atrial fibrillation or flutter occur. In addition, while patients with accessory pathways are not pacemaker-dependent, a backup pacemaker is deemed desirable since the long-term natural history of conduction over these pathways are not known.

Results of Atrioventricular Junctional Ablation Registry

To date, data from 475 patients who underwent catheter ablation of the atrioventricular junction have been submitted. In this report, data from the first 367 patients are analyzed. The clinical descriptors for this patient cohort is summarized in Table I. The patients were described as being very symptomatic from their arrhythmias, with presyncope (36%) or frank syncope (25%) being the most common presenting complaint. Nine patients suffered a cardiac arrest and 61 required at least one external direct-current countershock for arrhythmia control. Over half the patients had organic cardiac disease with coronary artery disease, the most common diagnosis.

Patients failed or proved intolerant to a mean of 3.5 antiarrhythmic drugs. A majority failed digitalis (82% of patients), beta-blockers (72%), calcium channel blockers (71%), type I antiarrhythmic drugs (77%), and 56% failed chronic amiodarone therapy. The primary rhythm disturbance requiring ablation was paroxysmal or chronic atrial fibrillation or flutter, which occurred in 60% of the reported cases. Other major arrhythmias included atrioventricular nodal reentry tachycardia (22%), atrioventricular tachycardia (11%), atrial tachycardia (13%), and a lesser number of patients with the permanent form of junctional reentrant tachycardia, junctional ectopic tachycardia, and sinus node reentrant tachycardia.

Table I
Clinical Findings in Patients with Drug and/or Pacemaker-Resistant Supraventricular Tachycardia

Heart Disease (type/% of patients)	Arrhythmia (type/% of patients)	Symptoms (type/% of patients)	Prior Treatment (type/% of patients)
No organic disease/48	Atrial fibrillation/flutter/60	Palpitations/70	Digitalis/82
Coronary artery disease/16	Atrioventricular node reentry/22	Dizziness/36	Type I/77
Cardiomyopathy/14	Atrial tachycardia/13	Dyspnea/40	Beta-blockers/72
Valvular heart disease/12	Accessory pathway/11	Syncope/25	Calcium channel blockers/71
Hypertensive cardiovascular disease/8	Permanent JRT/2	Chest pain/17	Amiodarone/56
Cor pulmonale/2	Other/4	Fatigue/17	Other experimental drugs/24
Other/6		Angina/11 Other/6	Antitachycardia pacemaker/7

The percentages total more than 100% since more than one parameter may have been present in a given patient.
JRT = junctional reciprocating tachycardia, Type I = type I antiarrhythmic agents.

Procedural Data

A single ablative session was used for 80% of patients while 2 or more sessions were used in the remainder. The stored energy per shock ranged from 50–500 joules but was usually in the range of 200–300 joules. The mean stored cumulative energy used was 603 ± 453 joules. There was no significant difference in stored energy between those in whom complete atrioventricular block was achieved compared to those who showed resumption of atrioventricular conduction. Data were available in 113 patients relative to the maximal unipolar His bundle and atrial deflections. The mean maximal recorded unipolar His bundle deflection was 0.38 ± 0.29 mV and the atrial deflection was 0.87 ± 0.83 mV. There was no significant difference in the recorded amplitudes of these deflections between responders (third-degree atrioventricular block) and nonresponders.

Clinical Response

Immediately after delivery of the shock(s), 90% of patients showed either complete atrioventricular block (or maximal preexcitation in those with accessory pathways). The average rate of the escape pacemaker was 45 ± beats/minute. The escape pacemaker was infrahisian in 58%, suprahisian in 32%, and indeterminate in the remainder. Patients were followed over a mean of 11 ± 10 months and 63% maintained chronic stable third-degree atrioventricular block and required no antiarrhythmic drugs. The remaining patients showed resumption of atrioventricular conduction with a mean of 6 ± 18 days after the procedure. Ten percent of patients who had resumption of atrioventricular conduction were asymptomatic without drug therapy, while another 12% had arrhythmia control but required resumption of antiarrhythmic drug therapy. The procedure was judged unsatisfactory in 15% of patients.

Complications of the Atrioventricular Junctional Ablation

Immediate Complications

The most frequent acute complications occurring after delivery of the electrical shocks were arrhythmic in nature. Six patients developed ventricular tachycardia or fibrillation after application of the shock and required external direct-current cardioversion. Two additional patients developed ventricular tachycardia within 24 hours of the procedure. Transient sinus arrest, atrial tachycardia, atrial flutter, or nonsustained ventricular tachycardia (17 patients) were reported but no specific therapy was required. Hypotension, post-shock, was reported in six patients, three of whom required pressor support. The hypotensive episode was transient in five and persisted for 72 hours in one. No deaths have been reported in the immediate post-shock period. Thromboembolic complications included a pulmonary embolus in one, thrombosis of the left subclavian vein in one, and thrombophlebitis in four patients. One patient developed a large right atrial thrombus despite prior anticoagulant therapy. In addition, infectious complications all related to pacemaker insertion were recorded in four patients. One patient with a presumed immunodeficient state died of overwhelming sepsis. One patient had diaphragmatic pacing and ventricular tachycardia which resolved on repositioning of the temporary pacing electrode.

Late Complications

Late complications included a cerebrovascular accident 17 months after ablation in a patient with atrial fibrillation; another had a probable arterial embolus after the procedure. Long-term pacemaker complications included a pacemaker-mediated tachycardia in three, pacemaker tracking of supraventricular tachycardia in two, pacemaker inhibition due to myopotential sensing in one, and two patients had symptoms due to acute pacemaker failure. A slow underlying pacemaker emerged in the latter two patients.

Follow-Up Mortality Statistics After Atrioventricular Junctional Ablation

A total of 19 patients died in the follow-up period. The death was sudden and of natural causes in eight and occurred from 3 days to 13 months after ablation.

Seven of these patients had underlying organic cardiac disease and one was free of known heart disease. Four patients died of severe congestive heart failure which was present prior to the ablative procedure, one died 2 years after the procedure from infective endocarditis, and one from surgery after attempted accessory pathway division. Noncardiac deaths were recorded due to sepsis (after pacemaker revision in one), severe chronic lung disease in one, and cerebral hemorrhage in one patient. The cause of death was unknown in one.

Ventricular Tachycardia Ablation

Clinical Studies

As of December 1986, a total of 141 patients who underwent attempted electrical ablation of ventricular tachycardia foci has been reported to the registry. The clinical data are summarized in Table II. The mean age was 53 ± 15 years and there was a large predominance of males (86% of the group). The most frequent cardiac diagnosis included coronary artery disease (63%), cardiomyopathy (17%), and arrhythmogenic right ventricular dysplasia (12%). The most frequent symptoms included palpitations (68%), syncope or presyncope (66%), and 26% suffered one or more episodes of cardiac arrest. Patients proved unresponsive or intolerant to a variety of treatments including type I antiarrhythmic drugs (94%), amiodarone (80%), cardiac electrosurgery (5%), automatic internal defibrillator (2%), or antitachycardia pacing (2%). A total of 85 patients required one or more external direct-current shocks for arrhythmia control.

Table II
Clinical Findings in Patients with Drug and/or Pacemaker-Resistant Ventricular Tachycardia*

Heart Disease (type/% of patients)	Symptoms (type/% of patients)	Prior Treatment (type/% of patients)
Coronary artery disease/63	Palpitations/74	Type I/95
Cardiomyopathy/16	Dizziness/41	Amiodarone/78
Arrhythmogenic right ventricular dysplasia/10	Syncope/36	Other experimental drugs/55
Valvular heart disease/6	Dyspnea/34	Digitalis/36
Others/6	Cardiac arrest/25	Beta-blockers/33
Hypertensive cardiovascular disease/2	Fatigue/18	Calcium channel blockers/29
No organic disease/6	Angina/18	Cardiac electrosurgery/6
	Chest pain/10	Antitachycardia pacemaker/4
	Other/7	Automatic internal cardioverter defibrillator/2

The percentages total more than 100% since more than one parameter may have been present in a given patient.
Type I = Type I antiarrhythmic drug.
*Used with permission from Evans et al. Catheter ablation for control of ventricular tachycardia: A report of the percutaneous cardiac mapping and ablation registry. PACE 9 (Part II):1392, 1986.

Characteristics of Spontaneous and Induced Ventricular Tachycardia

A single ventricular tachycardia morphology was found in 70% of patients while the remainder had multiple unimorphic morphologies (22%) or sustained polymorphic ventricular tachycardia, ventricular flutter or fibrillation (8%). The mean cycle length of spontaneous ventricular tachycardia was 383 ± 81 ms. The induced ventricular tachycardia morphology showed a right bundle branch block morphology in 63 patients and a left bundle branch block in 42. An indeterminate bundle branch block pattern was induced in the remainder. The inducible ventricular tachycardia morphology was identical or similar to that of the spontaneous ventricular tachycardia in 94% and was usually inducible from the right ventricular apex (84%). In 8% of patients, the tachycardia was induced from the right ventricular outflow tract and in 8% from the left ventricle.

Procedural Data

One ablative session was used in 78% of patients while the remainder underwent two to four separate ablative procedures. Sixty-five patients received one or two direct-current shocks while the remainder received more than two shocks. The mean cumulative stored energy used was 923 ± 680 joules, range 160–5200 joules. For clarity of data analysis, only those patients (109) receiving shocks to a single ventricular site were analyzed. For these patients, the ventricular tachycardia was localized to the right ventricle in 35%, to the ventricular septum in 29%, and to the left ventricle in 36%. The time from earliest endocardial activation to onset of the surface QRS was −43 ± 27 ms. Data for ventricular pace-mapping was available in 26 patients and was judged to be excellent (correspondence of paced and spontaneous ventricular tachycardia morphology in all 12 leads) in 13, good (correspondence in nine of 12 leads) in 8, and poor (correspondence in less than nine leads) in five.

Clinical Response

The patients were followed for a mean of 12 ± 10 months and their response to catheter ablation was divided into three groups. Group I consisted of 34 patients (24%) who are currently asymptomatic without antiarrhythmic drugs. Group II consists of 59 patients (42%) who have arrhythmia control but require antiarrhythmic agents, while 48 patients (34%) failed to respond. There was no significant difference in clinical outcome between groups and the earliest endocardial activation found (group I −46 ± 27 ms, group II −35 ± 24 ms, group III −50 ± 32 ms). Similarly, there was no correlation between clinical outcome and whether one (109 patients) or more ventricular sites (33 patients) were shocked. There was a higher incidence of excellent pacemaps (8 of 12) for group I compared with the other groups (group II, 2 of 7, group III, 3 of 7) but the differences among the groups were not significant. Post-ablation ventricular tachycardia induction data was available in 118 patients and was correlated with the clinical outcome. The same ventricular tachycardia morphology was induced in 49 patients, a different morphology was induced in 25, and tachycardia was not inducible in 43. There was a significantly higher incidence of an excellent clinical response for those whose tachycardia was not inducible after the ablative procedure (Table III).

Complications

A procedure-related death was defined as any death occurring within 24 hours of the ablative shocks. Seven procedure-related deaths were reported in Table IV and consisted of electromechanical dissociation in four, intractable ventricular fibrillation in one and severe low output state leading to death in two. New sustained ventricular arrhythmias occurred in eight patients after shock. One patient had ventricular fibrillation 5 days after the ablative procedure. Other in-hospital complications included hypotension in 12 patients, pericarditis in four, systemic embolization in three, myocardial infarction in two, ventricular perforation in one, and sepsis in two.

Mortality

Over a mean follow-up of 12 months, 31 patients died. Seven patients had procedure-related deaths (as described), 14 died suddenly, and documented ventricular tachycardia was found in nine of these 14. The sudden deaths occurred from 2 weeks to 23 months after ablation. Seven patients died of congestive heart failure and three noncardiac deaths (gastrointestinal hemorrhage in one, cerebrovascular accident in one, suicide in one).

Discussion

The available data from the registry suggest that catheter ablation of the atrioventricular junction is associated with an excellent response in 74% of pa-

Table III
Post-Ablation Ventricular Tachycardia Induction and Clinical Outcome

Group	I	II	III
Inducible:			
Same morphology	7	21	21
Different morphology	4	13	8
Noninducible	22*	15	6
	N = 118	p = <.001	

*Incidence of noninducible arrhythmias higher for group I compared with groups II or III.

Table IV
Procedure-Related Deaths

Diagnosis of Heart Disease	Ejection Fraction	Total Energy	Number of Shocks	Hospital Course
Arrhythmogenic right ventricular dysplasia	NA	1140	5	Electromechanical dissociation
Coronary artery disease	11	300	1	Electromechanical dissociation
Cardiomyopathy	NA	240	1	Electromechanical dissociation
Arrhythmogenic right ventricular dysplasia	NA	340	2	Ventricular fibrillation
Coronary artery disease	NA	480	2	Electromechanical dissociation
Coronary artery disease/ cardiomyopathy	20	300	1	Hypotension, intraaortic balloon assist
Coronary artery disease	11	900	3	4 hours post-shock, ventricular tachycardia recurred, died of pump failure during anesthesia for ventricular tachycardia surgery

tients. A somewhat higher success rate has been reported by others.[5-7] Resumption of atrioventricular conduction was noted to occur early after ablation. For example, approximately 70% of those showing return of atrioventricular conduction did so within 36 hours of the ablation. It should be noted that very late resumption of atrioventricular conduction (up to 1 year after ablation was noted in one) has been reported. Similarly, late onset of complete atrioventricular block after resumption of atrioventricular conduction has been reported as late as 6 months after the ablation. Late onset of complete atrioventricular block may be predicted in some by exercise or pacing-induced infranodal block.[8] Thus, patients undergoing ablative procedures should be carefully monitored for both late onset resumption of atrioventricular conduction or, more importantly, late development of atrioventricular block.

The available data does not allow for prediction of patients likely to have a successful result after ablation. For example, there was no significant difference between either the number of shocks or mean stored energy used between responders and nonresponders. Similarly, there was no significant difference in type of arrhythmia or magnitude of His bundle or atrial deflection found between responders and nonresponders. These findings suggest that technical factors are related either to ability to manipulate the catheter in close proximity to the atrioventricular junction and/or differences in delivered energy because of differing characteristics of the defibrillator/catheter electrical discharge.

Although significant post-shock complications including ventricular arrhythmias, hypotension, and myocardial perforation have been reported, no acute procedure-related deaths have been reported. Of concern is the 1.9% incidence of sudden death which occurred from 3 days to 13 months after the ablative procedure. Seven of the eight patients with sudden death had associated organic cardiac disease but one had no obvious cardiac disease. Even if the sudden deaths

Ventricular Tachycardia Ablation

The available published data relative to ventricular tachycardia ablation is sparse.[2,10,11] This report is the largest reported series. In contrast to electrical ablation of the atrioventricular junction, ventricular tachycardia ablation was associated with significant procedure-related deaths and complications. There was no significant difference in number of shocks or amount of stored energy used for those with procedure-related deaths compared to those who survived the ablative procedure. Three of the seven who died did so after delivery of one shock which ranged from 140 to 300 joules. Systemic embolization occurred in three patients after attempted left ventricular ablation. The most severe was a dense hemispheric cerebrovascular accident. Embolization may occur as a result of bubbles generated or clots occurring after the ablative procedure. New sustained ventricular arrhythmias requiring emergent interruption has also been reported as well as depression of left ventricular function after delivery of shocks to the ventricle. These complications have been extensively described in animals.[12]

A beneficial response to catheter ablation was not associated with the type of cardiac disease, location of the ventricular tachycardia focus, or to differences in the endocardial activation times. The paucity of data available relative to pace-mapping precludes any definitive statement with regard to its predictive power relative to arrhythmia response. The lack of correlation between clinical outcome and earliest endocardial area may be related to technical factors making it impossible to truly identify the exit site of the ventricular tachycardia focus. In addition, in the presence of a relatively large macroreentrant circuit, the finding of an "early area" may be of limited value.

The only variable that significantly predicted a beneficial response was inability to induce a ventricular arrhythmia in the post-ablative ventricular tachycardia induction study. This study was performed 3 to 7 days after the ablation. Induction of "nonclinical" ventricular arrhythmias was not predictive of a beneficial response. On the basis of available data, it would appear to be prudent to repeat ventricular tachycardia induction studies in all patients undergoing ventricular tachycardia ablation. If no arrhythmia is induced, then a follow-up trial without antiarrhythmic drugs would appear to be reasonable. If a ventricular arrhythmia is induced, then repeat drug testing or ablative procedures would appear to be indicated.

In summary, electrical catheter ablation of the atrioventricular junction has supplanted the need for cardiac surgical procedures previously utilized to disrupt atrioventricular conduction. This procedure will remain of limited applicability since a pacemaker-dependency state is produced and because of the small but real risk of sudden death which may be related to the procedure. Catheter ablation of ventricular tachycardia foci should at present be limited to patients with symptomatic ventricular arrhythmias who are not candidates for surgical intervention or for an automatic internal cardioverter defibrillator.

References

1. Silka MJ, Gillette PC, Garson A, Zinner A. Transvenous catheter ablation of a right atrial automatic ectopic tachycardia. J Am Coll Cardiol 1985;5:999–1001.
2. Fontaine G, Tonet JL, Frank R, Gallais Y, Farenq G, Grosgogeat Y. La fulguration endocavitaire. Une nouvelle methode de traitement des troubles du rythme? Ann Cardiol Angeiol 1984;33:543–561.
3. Morady F, Scheinman MM, Winston SA, DiCarlo LA, Davis JC, Griffin JC, Ruder M, Abbott JA, Eldar M. Efficacy and safety of transcatheter ablation of posteroseptal accessory pathways. Circulation 1985;72:170–177.
4. Scheinman MM, Morady F, Hess DS, Gonzalez R. Catheter-induced ablation of the atrioventricular junction to control refractory supraventricular arrhythmias. JAMA 1982;248:851–855.
5. Davis MJE, Mews GC, Cope GD. Transvenous ablation of atrioventricular conduction for refractory or malignant supraventricular arrhythmias. Aust NZ J Med 1984;14:479–486.
6. Gallagher JJ, Svenson RH, Kasell JH, German LD, Bardy GH, Broughton A, Critelli G. Catheter technique for closed-chest ablation of the atrioventricular conduction system: A therapeutic alternative for the treatment of refractory supraventricular tachycardia. N Engl J Med 1982;306:194–200.
7. Nathan AW, Bennett DH, Ward DE, Bexton RS, Camm AJ. Catheter ablation of atrioventricular conduction. Lancet 1984;1:1280–1284.
8. Personal communication, Dr. Samuel Levy.
9. German LD, Pressley J, Smith JS, O'Callaghan WG, Ellebogen KA. Comparison of cryoblati of the atrioventricular node versus catheter ablation of the His bundle (abstr). Circulation 1984;70:II–412.
10. Winston SA, Davis JC, Morady F, DiCarlo LA, Matsubara T, Wexman MP, Scheinman MM. A new approach to electrode catheter ablation for ventricular tachycardia arising from the interventricular septum (abstr). Circulation 1984;70:II–412.
11. Hartzler GO: Electrode catheter ablation of refractory focal ventricular tachycardia. J Am Coll Cardiol 1983;2:1107–1113.
12. Lerman BB, Weiss JL, Bulkley BH, Becker LC, Weisfeldt ML. Myocardial injury and induction of arrhythmia by direct current shock delivered via endocardial catheters in dogs. Circulation 1984;69:1006–1012.

34

Electrode Catheter Ablation of Resistant Ventricular Tachycardia by Endocavitary Fulguration Associated with Antiarrhythmic Therapy: Experience of 38 Patients with a Mean Follow-up of 23 Months

G. Fontaine, J.L. Tonet
R. Frank, Y. Gallais
I. Touzet, S. Kounde
G. Farenq, M. Baraka
Y. Grosgogeat

Introduction

Fulguration (electrode catheter ablation) and antiarrhythmic surgery are two methods used for the radical treatment of ventricular tachycardia. These approaches may alter permanently the arrhythmogenic substrate preventing arrhythmia relapses. The last one is, however, a definitely aggressive form of therapy considered when none of the palliative methods of treatment including drugs, antitachycardia pacemakers,[1] the cardioverter,[2] and the implantable defibrillator[3] are appropriate. However, surgery was an excellent teacher, in particular at the beginning when simple ventriculotomy proved successful in some patients.[4] The interesting concept suggested by this technique was that a limited surgical procedure precisely directed by epicardial mapping modified enough myocardium to prevent relapse of life threatening VT. Later on other approaches were developed and also proved successful. Significant series have been reported recently.[5-7] However the main limitation of surgery is its restriction to patients with a cardiac function good enough to enable them to withstand the procedure.

Therefore, we investigated other surgical methods for modification of conduction in a limited area of myocardium. These techniques which use physical agents have been referred to as "ablative techniques."[8] Many physical agents were considered: cryosurgery,[9] radiofrequency waves,[10] microwaves,[11] laser irradiation,[12] and high energy ultrasounds.

Endocardial catheter fulguration, which uses the effects of a strong electrical shock delivered at the tip of an endocardial catheter positioned in the area to be modified, is also an ablative technique whose usefulness for interruption of normal AV conduction has been extensively explored for the indirect treatment of supraventricular tachycardia.[13,14] The same electrical energy applied directly on the site of origin of abnormal ventricular activation as determined by endocardial mapping in the treatment of chronic ventricular tachycardia, because of its potential for the reduction of the risk of sudden death, is a more recent and promising development.[15-17] It was used for the first time in the treatment of VT by Hartzler in 1982[15] and by Puech in a case of arrhythmogenic right ventricular dysplasia.[16] We have been involved in the evaluation of this new form of therapy with a series of 44 cases.

Clinical Series

We report an analysis of our experience concerning the first 38 fulgurated cases with a follow-up period extending from 12 to 43 months starting in May 1983. To present our results in perspective, this group is taken from a larger cohort of 117 consecutive cases constituting the totality of major ventricular arrhythmias observed at Jean Rostand Hospital during the same period. The series consists of six cases of ventricular fibrillation and 111 cases of chronic recurrent sustained ventricular tachycardia. Almost all of these patients were referred from other institutions where they were considered resistant cases. All of them were restudied and only those patients who were resistant to drug reevaluation including amiodarone alone or in combination with class I antiarrhythmic drugs and/or beta-blocking agents were considered candidates for the fulguration procedure. The cases are consecutive, there was no exclusion due to age, cardiac, or clinical condition or other factors. The series of fulgurated patients consists of 38 patients (33 men and 5 women) with an age range of 14 to 74 years (mean age, 44 ± 18 SD).

Ventricular tachycardia etiologies include 12 cases of arrhythmogenic right ventricular disease, 13 cases of VT after an old myocardial infarction (range, minimum 3 months, maximum 10 years), seven cases of VT complicating an idiopathic dilated cardiomyopathy and five cases of idiopathic ventricular tachycardia, including three patients with right bundle branch block—left axis ventricular tachycardia, two patients with infundibular idiopathic ventricular tachycardia, and one case of ventricular tachycardia occurring 7 years after infundibular resection in a congenital anomaly. Their main clinical features are summarized in Table I.

In this series of fulguration cases, we did not have to use forms of therapy other than fulguration alone or in association with drug treatment.

Materials

The techniques developed in our department were based primarily on clinical research that profitted from a background provided by previous studies in antiarrhythmic surgery in a center dedicated to the treatment of cardiac arrhythmias and cardiac pacing. The equipment available is therefore important, and only some specific aspects will be presented in this report.

Catheter Technology and Selection

The first step of an endocardial catheter fulguration procedure is the localization by endocardial mapping of the area to be fulgurated. Catheter selection should stress the ability of the catheters to be appropriately positioned inside the cavities. An important prerequisite for this ability is the property of torque control. In our experience, the USCI catheters are the most suitable probably because of their unique woven Dacron structure. The problems concerning their steering properties, however, have not been completely solved at the present time. Their standard length is not sufficient when a femoral approach to the left ventricle is necessary, for example, for mapping in cases of a large aneurysm or in older patients with a dilated aortic arch.

The schematic description of the USCI catheter internal structure is related to the number of electrodes. In bipolars, the structure is "coaxial," like a television cable. The conductor connected to the electrode tip consists of a cable of low resistance. The other conductor is a shield composed of an interwoven mesh of wires separated and isolated from the cable by the woven Dacron and covered by a coat of plastic. In multipolars, the conductors going to the nondistal electrodes are made of discrete wires which form a long spiral around the woven Dacron axis. Given these designs, it is possible to understand why the steering properties of the different models are not the same. In addition, these design features strongly affect the catheter insulation properties. It has been demonstrated in our own laboratory and in those of others that the regular catheters that have been developed for endocardial recording or pacing are for the most part unable to withstand the high peak voltage and/or current used in the fulguration procedure.[18,19] The differences in the catheter internal structures also explain why the insulation properties of multipolar catheters are generally better than those of bipolars (Figs. 1–3). These insulation properties have also changed with time as modifications

Table I
Summary of Clinical Data on 41 Patients

No.	Age	Sex	Dx	LOC	FC	EF	TI	NM	NE	LI	SI	INC	Nb	ENERG	RIP	AR	MT	10D	FOL
1	35	M	ARVD	DIAPH	1	—	>20	1	<2	M	M	—	II	240*1	RM	—	—	NP	DC0D
2	62	F		DIAPH	2	—	36	2	>20	M	W	—	I	160*5	RM	O	O	RM	38M
3	74	M		INFUN	2	52%	12	1	3	M	M	—	—	160*1	M	AMIO	PRO	NI	37M
4	37	M		DIAPH	1	58%	6	1	3	M	<D	—	II	240*6	RM	O	O	NI	33M
5	27	M		DIAPH	4	25%	120	4	6	Y	—	+	—	160*17	RM	O	O	NP	DC8D
6	56	M		LV	1	45%	84	5	>20	Y	M	—	III	240*4	R	A+Pr	TH	IN	24M
7	40	F		INFUN	1	59%	48	2	16	M	M	—	—	240*1	TL	O	O	RM	27M
8	32	M		INFUN	1	—	4	1	2	W	<D	—	—	210*4	NI	AMIO	PRO	NI	31M
9	30	M		F.W.	1	56%	12	2	2	M	M	—	—	240*3	TL	A+Fl	TH	IN	31M
10	38	M		INFUN		—			>20	<Y	D	+	—	240*3	NP	—	—	—	DC0D
11	37	M		INFUN	2	50%	408	3	>20	M	—	+	II	240*9	TL	A+Fl	TH	NC	DC7M
12	27	M		RV FW	2	59%	120	3	>20	—	—	—	—	240*4	M	Bb+QD	TH	NC	10M
13	26	M		SEPTRV	2	59%	96	1	12	Y	M	—	II	240*1	—	O	—	NI	4M
14	60	M		ANTSEP	2	12%	1	2	>20	W	D	+	II	260*1	NI	AMIO	PRO	NP	43M
15	29	M	MI	INF	1	42%	24	3	4	M	M	—	II	260*7	RM	A+Pr	TH	NP	31M
16	73	M		ANTSEP	2	22%	1	2	>20	M	—	+	—	160*1	NP	AMIO	PRO	NP	36M
17	65	M		ANTSEP	2	—	—	3	2	W	<D	—	—	160*5	NI	O	O	NI	34M
18	55	M		INF	1	—	12	1	10	M	M	—	IV	240*2	NP	AMIO	PRO	NI	29M
19	60	M		ANTSEP	3	<25%	24	3	10	M	M	—	—	240*2	NP	—	—	—	DC4D
20	67	M		ANTSEP	3	<25%	1	1	2	D	D	—	—	240*2	NP	AMIO	PRO	NP	DC1M
21	74	M		ANTSEP		<30%	—	2	10	M	D	—	—	240*2	NI	AMIO	TH	NI	28M
22	64	M		ANTSEP	2	46%	2	2	14	M	D	—	—	240*2	NC	AMIO	TH	IN	DC22M
23	62	F		ANTSEP	3	26%	4	6	>20	M	—	—	IV	240*3	R	A+Bb	TH	NP	DC9M
24	53	M		ANTPOST	1	—	3	2	7	W	M	—	—	240*2	NC	AMIO	TH	IN	DC4M
25	64	M		INF	3	25%	16	2	>20	Y	D	—	—	240*2	NC	A+PM	TH	NP	24M
26	55	M		INF	1	<30%	2	3	7	W	D	—	—	280*3	NI	AMIO	PRO	NI	23M
27	52	M		ANTPOST	2	—	12	2	>20	Y	M	—	—	240*3	NI	AMIO	PRO	NI	7M
28	18	M	IDCM	ANTSEP	2	<30%	12	1	>20	M	—	+	—	260*5	O	AMIO	TH	NI	DC14M
29	14	F		SEPTLV	3	<20%	168	1	>20	—	—	+	—	160*3	O	O	O	NP	DC2M
30	56	M		LV	2	20%	36	1	6	Y	M	—	—	240*3	NI	AMIO	PRO	NI	DC16M

#	Age	Sex	Dx	LOC	EF	TI	NM	NE	LI/SI	INC	D	FC	ENERG	RIP	MT	AR	NP	FOL
31	28	M		RV	48%	—	3	>20	<Y	D	+	III	240*1	NI		FLEC	TH	IN	27M
32	58	M		RV+LV	—	120	2	>20	M	D	—	III	280*3	NC		QD	TH	IN	23M
33	21	M		RV APX	—	3	1	4	M	D	—	I	240*1	NC		A+Fl	TH	IN	18M
34	16	M		SEPTRV	—	24	1	>20	—	D	+	I	240*1	O		—	—	NP	DC1D
35	23	F		SEPTRV	51%	24	1	>20	I	—	+	II	240*3	NI		R+Dis	TH	NI	4M
36	22	M	IDIO	POSTSEP	—	60	1	>20	M	W	—	II	240*2	NI		O	TH	NP	7M
37	53	F		INFUN	59%	96	1	>20	M	D	+	II	240*2	NI		O	O	NI	32M
38	17	M		SEPTLV	70%	40	1	6	Y	D	—	II	240*4	NI		O	O	NI	12M
39	38	M		SEPTLV	47%	252	1	>20	W	D	—	I	240*1	NI		O	O	NI	13M
40	26	F		SEPTLV	50%	48	1	>20	Y	D	—	I	240*6	TL		QD	TH	NP	13M
41	21	M	CONG	INFUN	61%	120	4	10	M	D	—	I	240*4	NI		AMIO	PRO	NP	36M

Dx = Cardiac diagnosis.
ARVD = arrhythmogenic right ventricular dysplasia; MI = myocardial infarction; IDCM = idiopathic dilated cardiomyopathy; IDIO = idiopathic VT (no structural heart disease); CONG = congenital malformation.
LOC = Location of abnormality.
DIAPH = diaphragmatic; INFUN = infundibulum; LV = left ventricle; F.W. = free wall; ANTSEP = anteroseptal; ANTPOST = anterior and posterior; INF = inferior; SEPTLV = left ventricular septum; RV = right ventricle; POSTSEP = posteroseptal.
FC = Functional class (NYHA).
EF = Ejection fraction (echography, angiography, scintigraphy).
TI = Time interval since the first attack of VT (months).
NM = Number of clinical morphologies of VT.
NE = Total number of VT episodes prior to fulguration.
LI, SI = Longest and shortest interval between two episodes of VT. I = incessant, day, week, month or year.
INC = Incessant VT in the electrophysiological laboratory.
Nb = Number of fulguration sessions.
ENERG = Joules delivered : 160*5 = 5 discharges of 160 joules (value concerning the last procedure).
RIP = Reasons for interrupting the procedure.
R = changes in rate; M = changes in morphology; NP = programmed pacing not performed; TL = time limit; NC = nonclinical VT; NI = VT not inducible.
AR = Antiarrhythmic prescription upon hospital discharge.
AMIO = amiodarone; A+Pr = amiodarone + propafenone; A+Fl = amiodarone + flecainide; FLEC = flecainide; A+Bb = amiodarone + beta-blockers; A+PM = amiodarone + pacemaker; QD = quinidine.
MT = Mode of treatment. PRO = prophylactic or therapeutic treatment.
10D = Provocative test performed 10 days after fulguration.
NP = provocative test not performed; NI = VT not inducible; IN = inducible by programmed stimulation; RM = change in rate and morphology of VT morphology.
FOL = Follow-up. DC = death.

544 • CARDIAC ARRHYTHMIAS

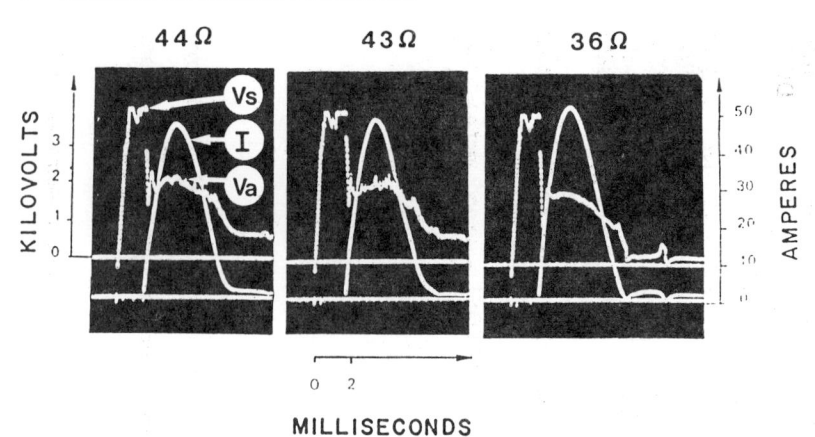

Figure 1: Progressive deterioration of the insulation properties of a USCI quadripolar catheter after several shocks of 280 joules. The waveforms of voltage and current and corresponding impedance at the peak of current are indicated. The amount of current delivered to the catheter is progressively increasing. The impedance is decreasing suggesting a progressive electrical deterioration of the catheter insulation properties. Vs = stored voltage; Va = applied voltage; I = intensity.

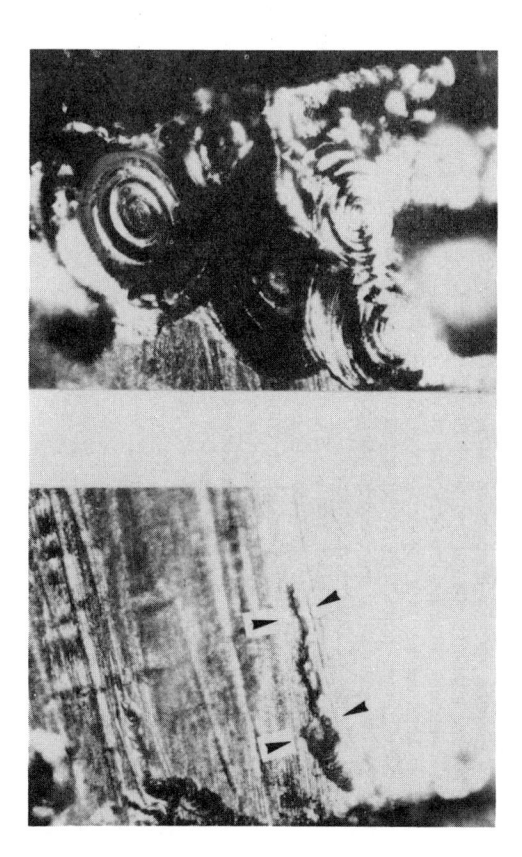

Figure 2: Same catheter as in Figure 1. **A:** Macrophotograph of the tip after several shocks of fulguration at 280 joules showing the typical "pitting" observed on the active electrode (anodal shocks). The platinum has been melted due to the high temperature of the electrical arc. **B:** The electrode #3 of the same quadripolar catheter shows a less pronounced pitting (arrows). This suggests the occurence of another electrical arc at this electrode. This abnormal data demonstrate a catheter insulation problem which could be only observed by microscopic examination.

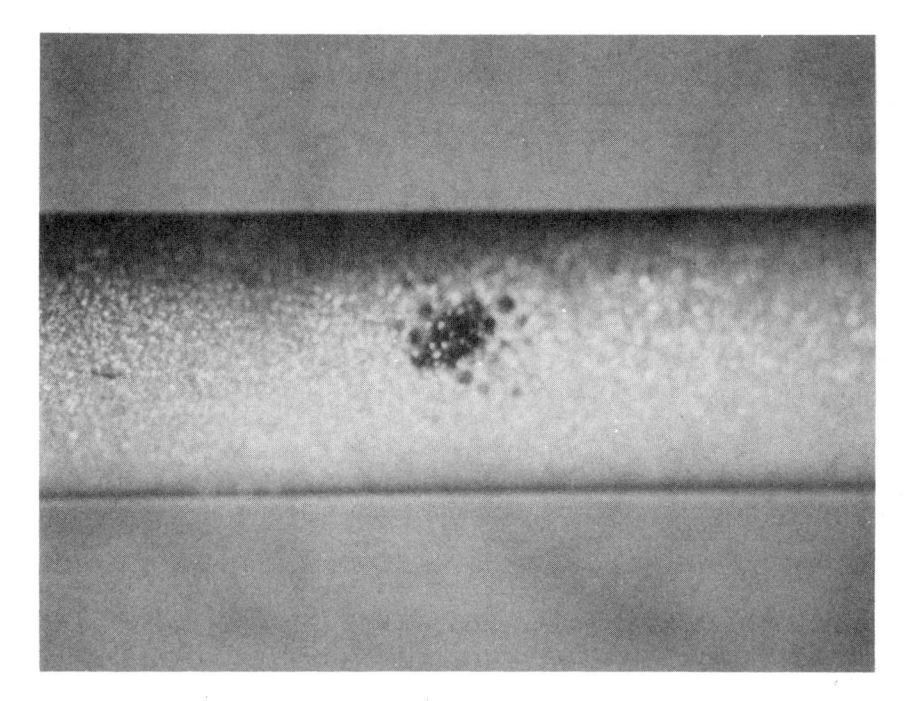

Figure 3: Macrophotograph of a different catheter in a case of arching under the sheath. This aspect was only seen by microscopic examination.

have been made in manufacturing. Therefore, we had to develop a method to select catheters prior to their sterilization.[20] The industry is now aware of these problems and more specific equipment will be released quite soon.

Since fulguration shocks are always delivered through the distal electrode to ensure close contact with the endocardium, the number of electrodes is not crucial. In practice we use either tri- or quadripolar catheters. The catheters which were used for mapping are also subsequently used for shock delivery. In the case of a right-sided VT, catheters are introduced through the femoral vein. Two catheters positioned in the infundibulum and apex, are introduced for endocavitary recording and pacing in addition to a catheter in the coronary sinus or the atrial wall. For left-sided VT, the catheter used for fulguration and mapping is introduced by a femoral or axillary artery puncture. The use of a guiding tube pushed beyond the aortic cusps facilitates catheter positioning within the left ventricle and prevents inadvertent entry into the ostium of the coronary arteries.

Fulgurator

The preselected discharge energy varied from 160 to 320 joules with the actual value set at an amount equal to 3 joules per Kg of bodyweight. This equation was determined from animal experiments that suggested it was appropriate with our equipment.[21,22] The shock is provided by a piece of equipment developed specifically for this application (Fulgucor ODAM, Wissembourg, France). This equipment incorporates a capacitor of 45μF and an inductor of 45 mH with the internal resistance of this latter component being around 10 ohms. This equipment also includes an electric circuit that measures both the current and voltage applied to the fulgurating catheter.[23] Voltage and current curves are displayed on a 5115 Tektronix oscilloscope with 5A18 vertical amplifier and 5B12N time base plug-in units. Polaroid pictures of the screen are taken after each shock. This protocol assumes that the catheter has been able to withstand the energy used for each fulguration. It is not impossible that a catheter which has passed the test prior to sterilization becomes defective during the next clinical procedure, or during successive shocks delivered in a given session (Fig. 2). Moreover, the high voltage electromechanical relay system developed for our first His bundle ablation procedure[17] automatically switches the catheter from the recording of the endocardial signals to the capacitor containing the fulgurating energy. Therefore, review of recordings assumes that when the endocardial electrogram remains the same, the fulgurating electrode tip has not changed its position until the shock is released.

An electrically completely independent defibrillator is located in the same piece of equipment. It is left in a waiting position charged at 40 joules connected to an anterior patch defibrillating electrode (R2 Corporation, Morton Grove, USA) made with an adhesive ring positioned on the precordial region. Its other electrode is the indifferent electrode used for the fulguration shock provided that the indifferent electrode is located on the left side of the patient's back. A back-up independent defibrillator with regular paddles is left in the waiting position ready to be charged at 400 joules.

Fluoroscopy and Videotape Recordings

A custom-made video system records either the signal from a camera focused on the areas of catheter entry in the femoral vessels or the video signal generated by the fluoroscopic equipment. Alpha-numeric data concerning the patient name, the date, and the characteristics of the shocks are superimposed on the video images.

A video tape recorder is connected to the fluoroscopic equipment to store the data from the video system. During the time when the fluoroscope is off, a separate solid state memory is used to store and display the final image obtained. An electronic arrow provides a manually controlled indication for each point to be mapped. In our recently modified protocol, video recording is done on a JVC U-matic Video cassette recorder during the entire procedure except for two vital periods: the catheters' final position descriptions just prior to the shock, and the end of the fulguration countdown. These important data are stored on a permanent independent tape kept in the file. The other tape is erased during the next procedure but played back when special investigation is required. Fulguration video recording is frequently played back during the session to study the catheter behavior during the shock. In addition, polaroid pictures are taken in both the anterior and left anterior oblique views to ascertain catheter position before the shock. A specially developed computer program "Chronos" stores the timing of important events throughout the procedure.

Hemodynamic Monitoring

Radial arterial pressure and pulmonary capillary wedge pressure are continuously monitored using a Swan-Ganz catheter. The cardiac output is also studied by thermodilution. These measurements are taken by the anesthesia team. In addition, in cases of patients with poor cardiac contractility, permanent watch of the radial artery blood pressure is done by a dedicated team member located in the technical room. Blood pressure signal is displayed on a 5115 storage Tektronix oscilloscope with a 5A14N vertical amplifier and a 5B12N time base plug in units, the sweep being adjusted at a slow speed (5 s/Div.).

Equipment for Activation Time Measurements

ECG leads D_1, VF, V_1, V_6 or D_1, D_2, D_3, V_1 are recorded with an Electronics for Medicine machine (VR 12). Activation times are measured on the 12-channel ink jet paper recorder Siemens Mingograph (Solna, Sweden). Comparison is made with a digital measurement from a 5116 Tektronix oscilloscope with a 2D10 signal sampling and storage unit. We store two channels on the screen. The first one is the endocardial mapping signal and the second is derived from the analogic summation of the absolute value of one to four orthogonal surface leads. Prematurity is easily determined on the oscilloscope screen by moving two cursors positioned on the signals' relevant points. Each mapped area is indicated on a schematic representation of the inside of the heart.

ECG and endocardial signals are also amplified by a custom made piece of equipment incorporating analogic low-pass and high-pass filters adapted for both surface ECG and endocardial signals (Odam, Wissembourg, France). In the same equipment, two markers indicate QRS detection and positioning of the shock in the cardiac cycle. An automatic calibrating signal for both amplitude and filtering is delivered every 5 to 30 seconds, and is interrupted just before the shock. Triggering of the shock can be linked either to the ECG or an endocardial signal when the surface recording of the QRS complexes during VT shows a smooth rise time. Surface and endocardial signals are recorded with an EMI SE 7000, 14-channel magnetic tape recorder.

Five of the ten people involved in the procedure, three in the technical room and two in the sterile room, wear microphones and headsets; multiplexing allows recording of all the comments on the same voice recording channel. These comments have proven to be of the utmost importance in the event of major complications.

Precise comparison between documented arrhythmias and pacemapping is performed with a 12-lead ECG by an independent battery-operated three-channel microprocessor-based recorder.

METHODS

Prior to the procedure, class I antiarrhythmic drug therapy is interrupted for a period equivalent to five half-lives. When present, amiodarone therapy is not discontinued (about 60% of the cases). Protracted general anesthesia is used because of the duration of the procedure and the frequent need to deliver more than one shock in a single procedure.

Endocardial Mapping

In cases where VT is not incessant, programmed stimulation is used to induce the arrhythmia. In our equipment, remote controlled electric relays switch catheters from signal recording amplifiers to a Savita programmed stimulation unit. The protocol includes the introduction of progressively more premature stimuli ranging from 1 to 3 delivered as a paced basic stimulation at a progressively increasing rate. In some cases, isoproterenol is injected to facilitate VT induction. VT induction was not possible during the procedure in only two cases. When unstable VT or VF is induced during the pacing protocol, the session is interrupted or postponed and drugs are prescribed to make the arrhythmia easier to handle.

Endocavitary mapping is used to localize the presumed area of the VT origin.[24] Confirmation is sought by trying to reproduce the morphology of the VT[25] with ventricular pacing during sinus rhythm or VT.[26] Three methods of ventricular pacemapping are used: continuous pacing in sinus rhythm at a rate identical to the tachycardia rate, slight overdrive of ventricular tachycardia, and introduction of a premature stimulus during ventricular tachycardia. Comparison of QRS morphologies is performed using the independent portable 12-lead recorder. In the most recent studies, special attention was paid to identification of the area of slow conduction and investigation of its role as a necessary link of ventricular tachycardia (Fig. 4). An interesting marker could be the recording of perfect reproduction of VT morphology after either pacing in sinus rhythm or VT, provided that ventricular activation is obtained after a delay which is similar to the interval between presystolic endocardial potential and onset of the ventricular QRS complex during VT[27] (see also Chapter 10).

Fulguration

Fulguration is delivered at the conclusion of a check list protocol which is followed by a countdown during which every piece of relevant equipment is put into action. The shock is synchronized with the surface QRS complexes during either VT or sinus rhythm.[28] This latter method is now preferred. As a last resort, a nonsynchronized shock is automatically delivered after 2 seconds. The shock is applied between the distal electrode of the fulgurating catheter used as an anode and an indifferent electrode which functions as a cathode and is positioned in the patient's back. From one to eight shocks are delivered during each session.

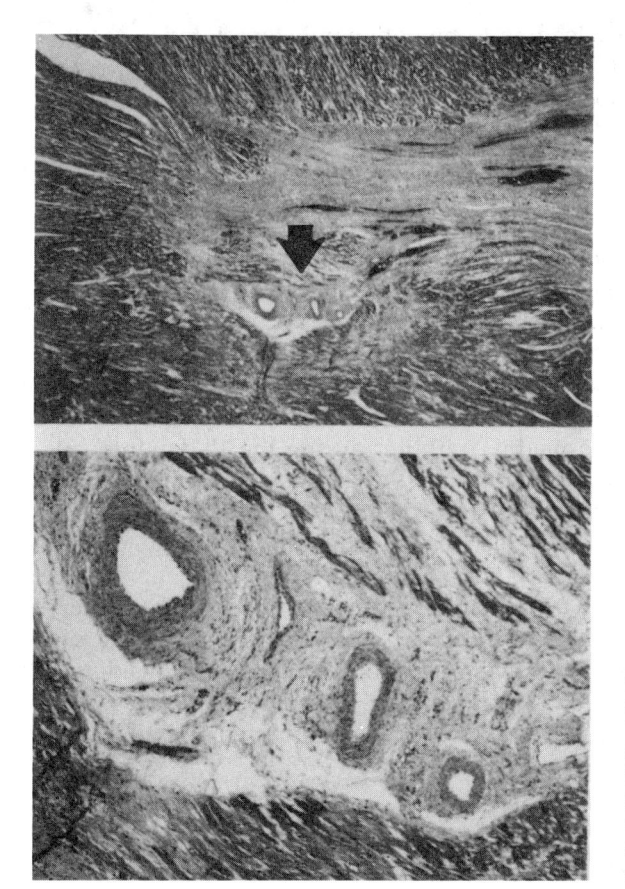

Figure 4: Effect of delivering several shocks of high energy on a pig heart. The animal has been sacrificed after 1 month. Fibrous tissue is oriented from the active electrode toward the indifferent electrode, suggesting a preferential direction of current. Small vessels are imbedded in fibrosis but alteration of their media is not shown.

In case of atrioventricular block, ventricular pacing is performed. In case of acceleration of ventricular tachycardia or its degradation to ventricular fibrillation, a defibrillating external shock is immediately delivered.[29] Within a few minutes after fulguration, provided that the catheter has not moved, the pacing threshold returns to a level compatible with stimulation. After completion of the fulguration shock, provided stability of the fulgurating electrode is maintained, it is possible to record flattening of the endocardial potential.[23] After a 10-minute rest period to permit electrical and haemodynamic stabilization, programmed stimulation is resumed.

The main end-points of the session are:

- Failure to induce a stable, monomorphic VT by a programmed pacing protocol equivalent to or more aggressive than that employed for initiating the VT required for mapping.
- Spontaneous interruption in less than 1 minute of a previously sustained VT.
- Induction of repeated episodes of acceleration of VT or VF after fulguration.

550 • CARDIAC ARRHYTHMIAS

- Repeated induction of VT leading to hemodynamic deterioration.
- Time limitation due to technical considerations (procedure listing more than 8 hours or eight shocks).

Postoperative Surveillance

The patient radial artery and venous blood pressures are monitored for 24 hours. A left subclavicular catheter is left at the apex of the right ventricle in order to permit reassessment of bedside VT reinduction which is done at or within 10 days after fulguration provided that no recurrence has occurred spontaneously. This reassessment is done using a programmed pacing protocol incorporating up to three extrastimuli on basic pacing cycles of 600 to 400 ms.

Regular ECG monitoring is done by computer during the 10-day interval, either by cable or telemetrics (Hewlett-Packard HP 78225 system associated with the NADIA software). All alarm signals are recorded. Graphs indicating trends in cardiac rhythm, extrasystole frequency, tachycardia, etc., can be printed out, and the data can be corrected when necessary by using the "recall" function.

When ventricular tachycardia comparable to previous attacks either occurs spontaneously or is inducible, antiarrhythmic drug therapy is attempted again (Fig. 5). When the latter proves ineffective, fulguration therapy is reconsidered. Amiodarone is generally continued preventively (50% of the cases, dosage ≤ 400 mg/day) in cases where the previous attacks of VT were life-threatening. This is

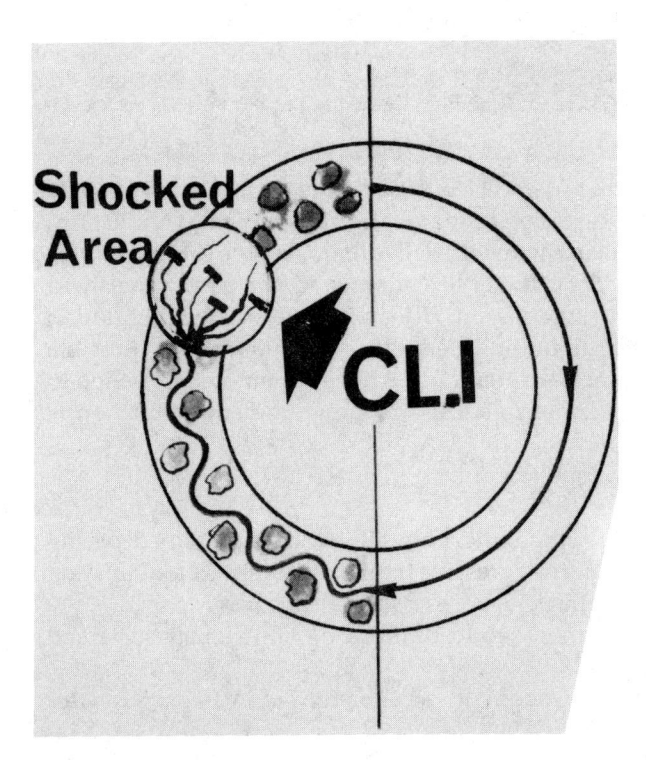

Figure 5: Possible explanation of the effect of drug combined with the fulguration procedure. The fulguration destroyed a part of the arrhythmogenic substrate in the area of slow conduction. Arrhythmia is brought under control by class Ic antiarrhythmic therapy which could produce a decrease in the activation propagation safety factor.

called "prophylactic" antiarrhythmic treatment (Table I). This category also includes patients who are taking amiodarone for treatment of extrasystoles. When drugs are necessary to prevent spontaneous or programmed pacing induced VT, the treatment is called "therapeutic" antiarrhythmic treatment. Table I lists the antiarrhythmic drugs administered, whether therapeutically or prophylactically.

Effectiveness of fulguration is reassessed before patient discharge by use of 24-hour Holter recording, stress testing on a stationary bicycle, and programmed stimulation.

Follow-Up

Total coverage of the outcome of this series of patients is based on the general computer data bank of our department. A specialized application program has been developed to facilitate the follow-up. Patient information given by the patient's physician, cardiologist, or family member is permanently updated in the computer system. In case of an absence of information, direct phone calls to the patient's home or a family member has proven to be the most effective form of follow-up. Despite the fact that one-third of our patients were referred from other countries, no patient has been lost to follow-up. Follow-up time was computed from the difference between the last fulguration procedure and the current date. Each death was investigated in order to determine if it met the definition of "sudden death," which according to our standard is an unexpected death occurring within 1 hour after the first symptom.

Results

The follow-up periods for the 38 patients expressed in months range from 1 (no. 19) to a maximum of 43 (no. 13) (mean value, 23 ± 10). In view of the fact that five (nos. 5, 13, 15, 22, 24) of the candidates for fulguration therapy were moribund, and 2 (nos. 5, 15) were already unconscious, the results were surprisingly favorable. Five (nos. 1, 5, 10, 18, 32) early deaths occurred, however, but none of the deaths seemed to be related to arrhythmia or perforation or to have occurred as a direct result of the fulguration itself. For reasons explained later, we choose to assess the success rate at 3 months after hospital discharge.

Description of Success Rate of VT

Of the 38 patients on whom a first fulguration procedure was performed, two (nos. 18, 32) died within a few days following the procedure. The follow-up study group is therefore limited to 36 cases. During reevaluation of the rhythm disorder after the first fulguration procedure, including the hospital stay and the follow-up period of up to 3 months, no VT relapse was observed in 12 patients. Therefore, a single session without the need for drug therapy was able to prevent arrhythmia in 12 out of 36 survivors 33% (in this percentage we have included as a success of

VT fulguration patient no. 5 who died after 8 days of a noncardiac cause; this short follow-up was nevertheless considered a success based on the fact that this patient was referred in incessant VT and no arrhythmia recurred before death). Spontaneous or induced ventricular tachycardia occurred in 24 patients. Drug therapy which was not effective before the fulguration procedure became effective in eight patients. As a result, the success rate increased to 20 cases (56%) when eight cases (nos. 9, 20, 21, 23, 24, 26, 31, 33) of therapeutic drug therapy after the first fulguration procedure were added.

The remaining population of of 16 resistant cases was submitted for a new attempt. Two patients (nos. 1, 10) died during the second fulguration procedure. The study group in which the second fulguration procedure was used was therefore reduced to 16 cases and the study population to 34 cases. After the second fulguration procedure, six more patients of the 14 survivors were brought under control without therapeutic drugs. At that point the success rate became 76%. Three more patients were controlled by drug therapy. Therefore the combination of two fulguration procedures plus drug therapy led to the control of 29 patients, for a success rate of 85%. Spontaneous or induced ventricular tachycardia recurred in five patients.

A third fulguration procedure was attempted but in no case was this third fulguration procedure effective alone. However, drug therapy was effective in three patients. At this point in this analysis, 32 out of the study population of 34 cases are considered treated which gives a success rate of 94%. Only two patients were not controlled. A fourth fulguration attempt was performed in these two last cases. Antiarrhythmic treatment was necessary, however, in both to achieve complete in-hospital prevention of VT. We then reach a success rate for VT of 100%. However, recurrences of ventricular tachycardia after discharge, although better tolerated, were observed on several occasions in three patients (nos. 6, 9, 17).

These three last cases experienced relapses which were more rare and better tolerated. These cases were originally considered as fulguration failures. However, after 3 months these three patients experienced no further episodes of VT despite progressive reduction of their antiarrhythmic treatment, with one now being classified as prophylactic (no. 17).

In summary, of 34 patients surviving the perioperative period, single or multiple VT was brought under control in all of them by means of one or more fulguration sessions, with 16 (47%) requiring the help of therapeutic antiarrhythmic treatment following the fulguration therapy.

Mortality

During the overall period of this study which extended up to 43 months, 13 deaths were observed, none of which were attributable to fulguration itself.

Early Death

Five deaths were early (less than 1 month after the procedure).

Cardiac Deaths: Two technically related deaths, leading to low cardiac output, occurred during the procedure. The first of these (no. 1) was a case of arrhythmogenic right ventricular dysplasia, successfully operated on 7 years previously but with recent recurrent episodes of life-threatening VT. Death was probably the consequence of a lack of hemodynamic monitoring (at the beginning of our experience) during the procedure. The second patient (no. 10) succumbed from an irreversible low cardiac output associated with a progressive decline of myocardial contractility. A few minutes before the patient died, external heart massage was administered following a single external defibrillation shock for VT acceleration.

Noncardiac Deaths: The first case (no. 5), referred after multiple episodes of VT following angiography, was unconscious and in a state of incessant VT upon arrival. A series of low-energy (160 joules) shocks led to a reduction in the rate of VT, which stopped spontaneously a few hours later without the need of antiarrhythmic therapy. The patient nevertheless succumbed 8 days later from refractory hypoxemia due to preexisting extensive pulmonary infection. No recurrence of VT was observed until death.

A second case of death was observed in a patient (no. 18) with a low ejection fraction following an old myocardial infarction. He had been rejected as a candidate for surgical treatment. Delay in the resuscitation procedures resulted in irreversible brain damage and death 4 days after fulguration.

The third case (no. 32) had very poor cardiac function due to idiopathic dilated cardiomyopathy and was in permanent VT for two years: he went into hemodynamic distress during the procedure before fulguration. Despite the fact that this complication was partially under control, the patient died one day after the procedure.

Anatomical and histological examinations were performed for cases nos. 1, 5, 10. They revealed myocardial modifications which, when superimposed on the particular histologic structure of the underlying pathology were similar to histological lesions found in experimental animals[30] following the application of endocavitary shock therapy.

Late Mortality

Eight late deaths were observed.

Cardiac Death:

Sudden Death: Three cases (nos. 21, 23, 26) met the criteria for sudden death 4, 14, and 22 months after the fulguration procedure. These deaths were considered the consequence of VT relapses and will be presented in detail later.

Congestive Heart Failure: Case no. 19 died 1 month following discharge from acute pulmonary edema without recurrence of VT. The patient, suffering from severe triple vessel coronary artery disease with poor distal vessels, a low ejection fraction cardiomegaly and left-sided ventricular failure, was not a surgical candidate. Case no. 27 was diagnosed as idiopathic dilated cardiomyopathy; death resulted from pulmonary edema 3 months following fulguration, with no recurrence of major rhythm disturbance. Case no. 22 died of cardiac failure 10 months after the fulguration procedure while on effective therapeutic antiarrhythmic drug treatment.

Noncardiac Death: Two cases (nos. 11, 28) died of noncardiac causes. All the preceding late deaths occurred outside of the hospital, therefore, autopsy was not possible.

Complications

Acute pulmonary edema was observed in two cases (nos. 13, 15) during the first 10 minutes following fulguration. The problem was however manageable using standard therapy.

In one case (no. 6) during the second fulguration session, the patient experienced chest pain associated with modification of the ST segment and transient right bundle branch block. The rise in the CPK and particularly the CPK MB fraction was 140 IU, greater than that observed in the other patients treated (37 ± 15 SD).

Transient complete atrioventricular block was frequently observed in the course of the procedure, and occurred immediately after the shocks (17% for 167 shocks). In two cases (nos. 13, 15), only it persisted after the session and resolved in a maximum of 2 hours (no. 15). Intraventricular conduction anomalies of short duration were also noted (8% LBBB and 5% RBBB for 167 shocks).

Ventricular tachycardia acceleration and ventricular fibrillation were observed equally in 15% of the shocks immediately following the initial electrical discharge. They were easily defibrillated,[29] except in two cases (nos. 18, 32), one of which was in acute hemodynamic cardiac failure (no. 18) and the other of which was in hypoxia. However, no malignant arrhythmia resistant to defibrillation was observed following fulguration.

One pacemaker patient (no. 19) in whom the fulguration shocks were delivered close to the ventricular pacing electrode needed generator replacement.

Long-Term Relapse of VT

These relapses could be classified in the following categories.

Relapses Better Tolerated and Disregarded

This situation was observed in three patients (nos. 21, 23, 26) of whom one (no. 23) was asymptomatic. Case no. 26 died suddenly 14 months after fulguration, when he was in a major phase of heart failure, due to the terminal stage of an idiopathic dilated cardiomyopathy. Patient no. 23 had two forms of sustained VT elicited during programmed pacing. A fulguration procedure was performed and seemed to be effective for one form. The nonfulgurated VT was still inducible at the time of discharge but the attacks were slower and better tolerated. Nondocumented sudden death occurred 4 months after the procedure and it is unknown if this was due to recurrence of the fulgurated VT, degradation of the *non*fulgurated VT, or a different complication. Case no. 21 was in incessant VT when the fulguration procedure was performed. Relapse was observed a few hours later and at that time VT could be terminated by pacing. It was reproducibly demonstrated that class Ic antiarrhythmic drug was than able to prevent VT. This drug had not been effective prior to the procedure. One year later, the patient was reevaluated by programmed pacing 1 week after class Ic discontinuation and was found noninducible. The patients took amiodarone only. Holter monitoring exhibited nonsymptomatic VT at 110 bpm. Class Ic drug therapy was resumed without reinvestigation at Jean Rostand Hospital. The patient experienced sudden death 4 months later.

Relapses Controlled by Drugs

This was obtained in one case (no. 31) in which a modification in drug therapy led to the control of the arrhythmia. This patient had a first relapse 12 months after fulguration during an attempt at reduction of the two drugs given as therapeutic treatment. Two more episodes were later observed after resumption of the original therapy; finally replacement of class Ic antiarrhythmic therapy by a beta-blocking agent continues to appear to be preventing relapses.

Relapses Controlled by Refulguration

This approach was used in two cases with success of the second procedure, although in case no. 12 some additional episodes were observed and finally disappeared. This behavior suggests the previously mentioned evolution of some of our early relapses. Patient no. 33 experienced a syncopal relapse of VT 14 months after the fulguration. He denied this event for 10 months for professional reasons. Later relapses became more frequent and this patient has recently undergone a second fulguration procedure. Follow-up seems to indicate that the patient benefited from the second attempt.

Discussion

Our results confirm in a larger series and with a longer follow-up the favorable results reported both by Hartzler[15,31] in coronary artery disease patients and Puech[16] in a case of arrhythmogenic right ventricular dysplasia. These authors reported the first cases of fulguration in the treatment of VT, adapting to this form of cardiac arrhythmia a technique derived from the His bundle fulguration technique for the indirect treatment of supraventricular tachycardia.[14,32–35]

Other investigators have reported irregular results in the management of VT with this technique.[36-43] In view of the very poor cardiac condition of most of our cases, we do not think that differences in patient population explain why we observed better results. We think rather that it could be explained by a difference in the selection of the equipment and methods. We observed at the beginning of our experience (no. 13, second patient in the VT series) that the vast majority of the regular USCI catheters were not able to withstand the high peak of current and voltage necessary to obtain a sufficient effect on the endocardium. As no alternative equipment was available despite a screening of commercial catheters, we developed a technique for selection of USCI tri- or quadripolar catheters by a nondestructive high voltage test.[20,44] As a result, we were able to demonstrate in some cases that a successful outcome could be obtained using a relatively low fulgurating energy delivered in a single shock.[45]

A second difference is based on the fact that we originally decided to use the active electrode as an anode instead of a cathode because in vitro studies of the effect of shocks demonstrated that anodal shocks provided a stronger mechanical effect. We also observed with acute electron microscopy, rupture of myofibrilles at a distance of 1 cm from the fulguration site. Since it is well known that the stretch of myocardial fibers modifies cardiac conduction,[46] we choose to incorporate this parameter in our protocol. Recently we have observed that the variation in waveforms generated by different types of defibrillators should also be taken into account. Limited in vitro experiments have shown that anodal shocks with fast rise times lead to stronger mechanical effects and tissue damage.

These three points (catheter selection, anodal shocks, shock impulse waveform) therefore make difficult any comparison between our group and others concerning the results obtained in animal experiments or in the clinical field.

Electrophysiology

Ventricular Tachycardia Morphologies

The induction of ventricular tachycardia by programmed pacing may lead to varied results. It is now well accepted that some forms of nonsustained or polymorphic VT induced by programmed pacing may not have clinical significance.[47] Therefore only sustained monomorphic VT has been considered. However, programmed pacing can also induce episodes of types of VT not previously documented, the so-called "nonclinical" VTs. As all the class I antiarrhythmic treatments are interrupted several days before the fulguration procedure, it is unlikely that they would alter the morphology of VT induced during the fulguration procedure.[48] We have learned from experience that in most cases both clinical as well as nonclinical VT should be considered for fulguration treatment.[49,50] In general, a correlation was observed between the number of VT morphologies and the number of sessions (or the number of shocks per session). On the other hand, we have also observed cases in whom a single shock was able to ablate more than one VT morphology.

Some cases have shown that so-called resistant and almost incessant VT was not the result of ineffectiveness of drug therapy but rather the proarrhythmic effect of the drugs. In one patient studied with the arrhythmia monitoring computer system, a direct relationship was observed between the amount of a class Ic antiarrhythmic agent and the amount of nonsustained episodes of VT and/or extrasystoles.

Endocardial Catheter Mapping

Evaluation of the endocavitary potential as a marker for determination of the fulguration site was bleak. However, we came to the conclusion that the absence of presystolic activity led invariably to failures. On the other hand, our results indicate that success was generally greater in cases where high amplitude presystolic VT potential had a definite prematurity.[23] The briefly discussed concept of VT prevention through the delivery of one or more "blind" shocks within the cavity was never substantiated.

Manipulation of the catheter all over the large area of the endocardium, although theoretically possible, requires expertise and appropriate training. Thorough investigation of the endocardium in preparation for the fulguration procedure seems to be more critical than the endocardial mapping needed prior to an open heart surgical attempt. In this latter situation, the direct view of the lesions provides an additional marker. Also, surgical action of any type is in fact never restricted to the limited area of endocardium determined by mapping.[51] The area of resection is extended by the resection of an amount of scar tissue based on anatomic criteria. Therefore, endocardial resection is larger than the area determined by either the preoperative or the peroperative mapping. This is probably a part of the explanation of questionable long-term results reported recently.[52]

Mortality

Three patients (nos. 5, 13, 15) were moribund when effective fulguration was performed. At least 11 cases (nos. 5, 10, 13, 15, 18, 19, 22, 24, 26, 27, 32) involved prohibitive surgical risks. None died of the immediate effect of the endocardial electrical shocks.

It is possible that two deaths early in the study could have been avoided: the first (no. 1) by hemodynamic monitoring, and the second (no. 18) by avoiding a real-time modification of an anesthetic protocol which was not properly reviewed. The six deaths (nos. 5, 10, 19, 22, 27, 32) have been interpreted as consequences of the evolution of preexistent pathological processes. In the first (no. 5) and second (no. 10) cases, death was foreseen as inevitable in view of precarious hemodynamic situation. It should be recalled that the cases included in the series were consecutive. No patient was excluded. In the four cases (nos. 19, 22, 27, 32), clinical evidence of deterioration of myocardial function apart from the rhythm disorder had been observed during the period preceding fulguration.

The three last cases (nos. 21, 23, 26) died suddenly. The death of patient (no.

23) was critical. In this patient, the nonfulgurated less rapid VT was still inducible at the time of discharge; recurrences did occur but were better tolerated. In retrospect, this patient, who was not in definite cardiac failure, would have been a candidate for other investigational methods of therapy (implantable defibrillator or another fulguration procedure). The sudden death of patient no. 21 is also critical; this patient had an ejection fraction of 46% and the cardiac failure observed at the time of nonsymptomatic VT was probably related more to the arrhythmia rather than to intrinsic cardiac contractility. The question of out-of-hospital patient surveillance must be raised; some form of continuous Holter monitoring with an implantable device is mandatory. In any case, this patient should have had his arrhythmia completely reevaluated when the nonsymptomatic VT was discovered. Here again an implantable defibrillator or a new fulguration procedure could have been considered. In case no. 26, sudden death was observed 14 months after the procedure. Despite documented episodes of VT, preterminal deterioration of cardiac function did not prompt us to attempt a repeat fulguration; again a new fulguration or the implantation of an implantable defibrillator could have been considered.

Recurrences

In some cases, recurrences are easily ascribed to technical difficulties involving the catheter[44] leading to insufficient energy output (no. 13) on the one hand and fulguration situated too far from the zone of origin of the VT on the other (nos. 15, 17). Other recurrences are less easily accounted for and allow only the formulation of hypotheses: inadequate mapping, arrhythmogenic area extending beyond the zone benefiting from fulguration, thus partially inhibiting abnormal activation, and increasing sensitivity to antiarrhythmics. The implications of a favorable spontaneous evolution of the disease remain to be evaluated. On the other hand, the fact that some cases were able to be cured after a transient period of relapses led us to postulate the possibility of delayed effects of fulguration. Several investigators have seen the late development of AV conduction impairment several weeks or months after a seemingly inadequate fulguration procedure aimed at His bundle ablation.

Experience gained during follow-up prompted us to realize the need for an implantable device both for arrhythmia detection and possible temporary treatment.

The Fulguration Process

The technique of VT fulguration is still in a discovery phase and many of its most basic aspects are at the present time only partially understood.[53-56]

This very complex physical phenomenon involves different sciences: fluid dynamics, thermodynamics, electricity, electrochemistry, and biology. At the risk of oversimplification, fulguration can be reduced in our view to two principal mechanisms: (1) a flow of electric current crossing the myocardium in the area between the active electrode and the indifferent one (Fig. 6), and (2) the formation

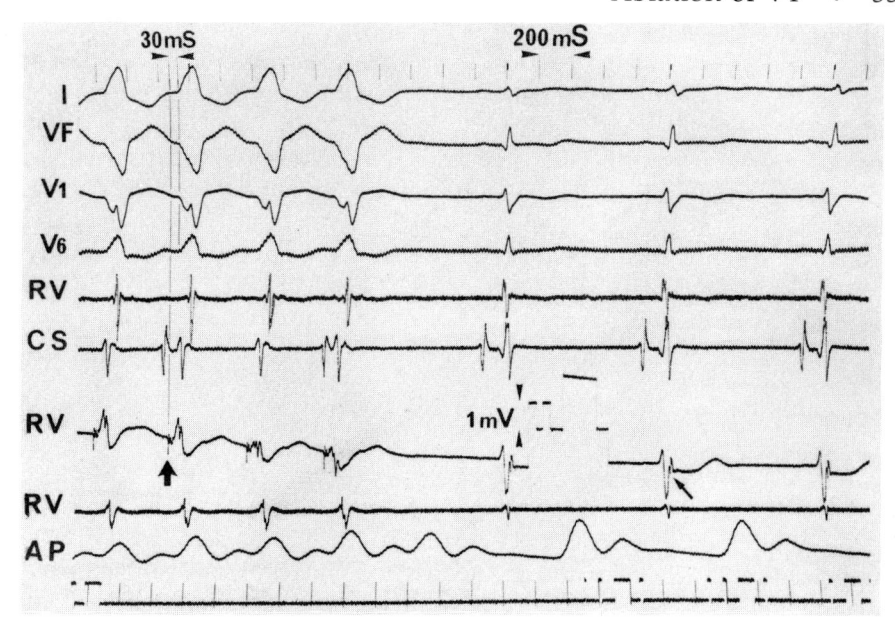

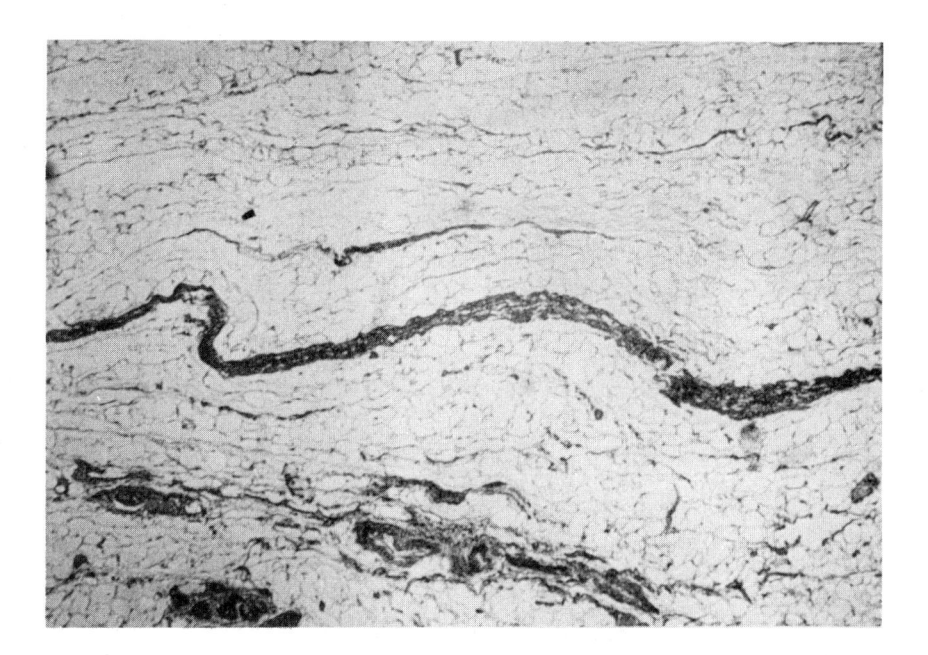

Figure 6: Endocardial potential observed during VT and after return in sinus rhythm in a patient with an arrhythmogenic right ventricular dysplasia. A presystolic activity occurs 30 ms before the onset of the QRS complex on the surface tracing during VT. A sharp deflexion which looks like His Purkinje system potential is recorded at the right side of the heart, far from the right branch, and is probably related to the phenomenon of slow conduction occurring in partially degenerated myocardial fibers.

of at least two shock waves (Fig. 7). The first shock wave is produced by the abrupt surge of vapor generated by the creation of ionized plasma around the active electrode tip within the liquid environment, and the second when the vapor globe collapses after the end of the delivery of current.[57] This mechanical result of the electrical discharge is propagated in all directions. However, collapse of the vapor globe against the wall of the myocardium could cause a particularly violent impact.[58] While the effect of electrical current on the myocardium has been extensively discussed with respect to external defibrillation,[59-63] the same is not true for its endocavitary application.[30] The respective parts played by both electrical and mechanical agents in the process of fulguration remain to be clarified.

Secondary Effects

Cardiac Output

In some cases, as assessment of cardiac function was performed 7 days after the procedure by 2D echo and yielded normal valves. However, the results of hemodynamic studies demonstrate that there is a temporary drop in cardiac output after the procedure which reverts to its control values within 10 to 15

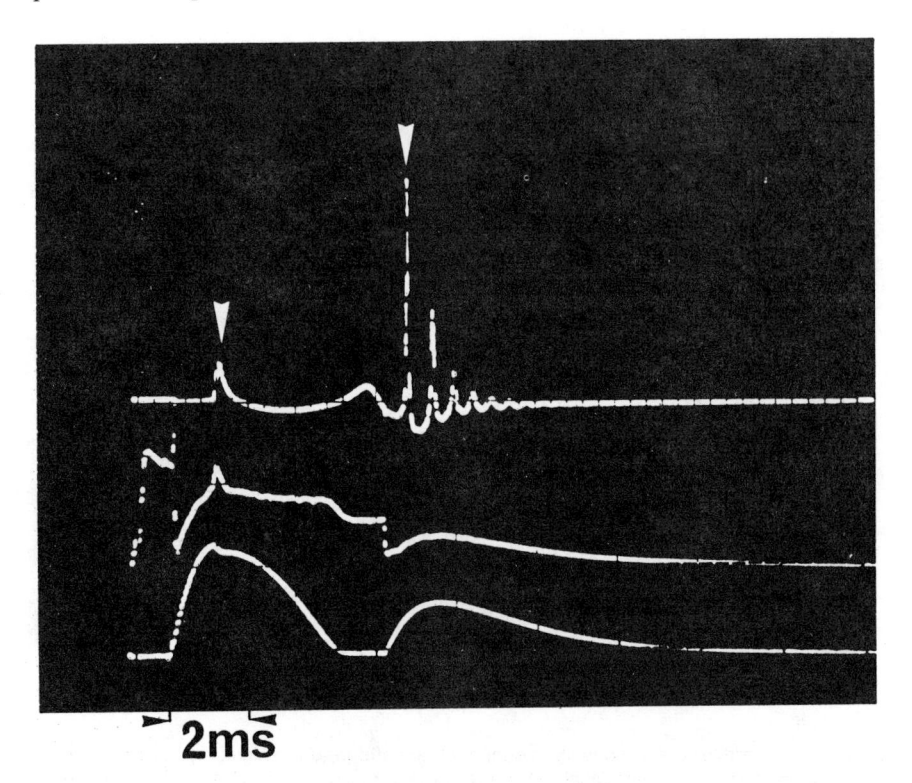

Figure 7: Upper trace represents the shock waves observed during a fulguration shock delivered in saline. The first deflection corresponds to the growth of the vapor globe, the second is due to the collapse of the globe and is followed by several rebounds of smaller amplitude. Voltage and current curves are also represented for appropriate timing.

minutes after the shocks.[28] In addition, the small amount of CPK-MB fraction obtained after the shocks made this concern less important. This was also in agreement with some experimental data from our laboratory which indicates that following endocavitary fulguration delivered to a healthy endocardium (pig weighing 80 kilos), the left ventricular cardiac output decreases by 10 to 15% for approximately 10 minutes. One of the acute pulmonary edema (no. 13) cases in our series was, however, probably related to the fulguration of nearly normal myocardium distant to the area of infarction.

Arrhythmias

Episodes of ventricular tachycardia acceleration or fibrillation brought on by fulguration or occurring during programmed VT activation were occasionally observed, and all of these arrhythmias represented minor electrophysiological events and were immediately brought under control by instant defibrillation.[29] Such episodes further demonstrate the necessity of prepositioning the defibrillating electrode in an anterior position in order to avoid emergency removal of sterile surgical fields and fluoroscopic equipment.

No malignant ventricular arrhythmia was observed after the procedure; however, extrasystoles were frequent and new forms of sustained ventricular tachycardia were even observed in some patients, especially in those without coronary artery disease, but these arrhythmias disappeared after a few days and did not look like the creation of a new arrhythmogenic substrate.

Myocardial Infarction

The case of myocardial infarction (no. 6) observed during the fulguration procedure was the consequence of difficulty encountered during manipulation of the catheter in the root of the aorta in an attempt to reenter the ventricle after inadvertant withdrawal. Subsequent review of the magnetic tapes revealed that during the left-sided catheter insertion, the patient, who was not yet asleep, complained of chest pain which was rapidly followed by progressive ST segment modification and right bundle branch block. At the same time, voice channel data from the magnetic tape recorder indicated that the catheter tip appeared to be blocked in the root of the aorta. Myocardial ischemia resulting in a definite increase of CPK isoenzyme MB fraction was therefore produced. Modification of the technique employed subsequently eliminated this risk, which could be critical. Our experimental studies have shown that a discharge of 240 joules in the coronary artery of a pig of 80 Kg resulted in instantaneous irreversible hemodynamic failure due to rupture of this vessel and subsequent tamponade.

Effect on a Permanent Pacemaker and Implantable Defibrillator

A defect in the functioning of one patient's pacemaker (no. 19) at the time of fulguration required replacement of the generator. This risk is higher in case of a unipolar device and malfunctioning might not be obvious after the shock. Thorough evaluation of pacemaker pacing safety margin, sensing, and programming functions are mandatory before as compared to after the fulguration procedure.[64,65]

Despite the fact that no systematic study has been made, it is probable that an implantable defibrillator could be rendered completely ineffective. Since any patient who has an implantable defibrillator could present with subentrant episodes needing a more radical approach because of repeated episodes of ventricular tachycardia/fibrillation, it may be necessary to temporarily disconnect the implantable defibrillator before delivering the fulgurating shocks.

Alternative Therapy and Patient Selection

To put our results in perspective, we compared the overall results in terms of global mortality and relapse from the original cohort of 117 consecutive patients with chronic stable VTs. Almost all of these so-called resistant cases were reevaluated in terms of antiarrhythmic treatment. It appeared that only one-third needed the fulguration procedure. This suggests that two-thirds were controlled by drug therapy (only one patient was referred for surgery). This study has already been presented in part[66] and was done from review of the outcome of the nonfulgurated patients available in April 1986. Therefore this comparison is valid vis-à-vis the results of 31 fulguration cases in the same time period.

The global mortality in the group of the nonfulgurated patients was 15 cases (21%) with six cases of sudden death (8%). Relapses were observed in five patients who survived and six patients who died, yielding a relapse rate of 15%.

In the fulgurated population, a suitable comparison should omit the patients who died because of inappropriate protocols (three cases: nos. 1, 18, 32). The global mortality was seven calculated from 35 survivors (20%), and sudden death was observed in three cases (8%). Long-term relapses were observed in four cases out of 35 survivors (11%).

Finally, despite the *small* number of patients in each series and the relatively short follow-up, it was possible to conclude in April 1986 that the fulguration procedure associated with drug therapy yields results comparable to those from drug treatment alone. However, as fulguration was performed only in patients resistant to drug therapy and in particularly poor condition, it is suggested that this form of treatment provides a definite adjunct in the management of ventricular arrhythmias. It is also concluded that refulguration should be definitely considered when a previously fulgurated patient presents with relapses.

Effectiveness of the Technique

Fulguration appears to be a new milestone in the treatment of chronic stable VT in humans. We have seen that a success rate for VT of 100% was finally achieved. This confirmed, with a *significant* patient series, our former views concerning the effectiveness of limited physical action for the long-term prevention of arrhythmia.

In addition, in seven cases (nos. 3, 7, 13, 15, 29, 31, 36), a single fulguration shock of an amplitude varying between 160 and 240 joules was sufficient to prevent recurrence of VT without the need for therapeutic antiarrhythmic treatment. This suggests that the injury produced by a single shock is at least in some cases able to modify the pathologic substrate which was the basis of a life-threatening arrhythmia. This important remark confirms a previously reported similar result when we observed that a minor surgical action (simple ventriculotomy) was able to prevent recurrence of resistant VT.[4,67] However, due to the limited endocardial surface modified by the shock, we have to stress that precise endocardial mapping is probably a crucial prerequisite for the success of the procedure. From a theoretical basis, it should be more appropriate to deliver the fulgurating shock to the area of slow conduction provided that this area is indeed a necessary link for the perpetuation of the arrhythmia, rather than the "site of origin" of VT which is in any case located near normal myocardium. Recent data suggest that this goal could be achieved successfully in at least some cases.

However, three patients died suddenly during the follow-up, 17 patients (45%) required two or more sessions, and 15 patients (44%) needed antiarrhythmic therapy. This suggests that fulguration is not for the time being an "ideal" form of therapy. Two points should be mentioned:

1. The current precision of mapping is probably not sufficient, this is suggested by the need for several shock sessions and antiarrhythmic therapy in most cases.
2. The amount of modified tissue is probably too restricted. The behavior of myocardial contractility after the shock and the small amount of the CK MB fraction suggest that a more aggressive physical agent could be employed.

From a practical standpoint the present techniques require general anesthesia, a large number of personnel and are long and difficult, therefore this technique is limited to dedicated centers. Despite the fact that fulguration itself could be perfected other ablative techniques could be considered.

Limitations of the Study

This report tends to conclude that the fulguration procedure is a safe and effective form of therapy for ventricular tachycardia. Nevertheless, many points could be criticized. A limited number will be mentioned here:

- There is a bias in patient population. For instance, since our population was a second or third generation of so-called resistant cases, it does not provide a valuable sampling of the population at large and represents only a high risk group.

Because of the unpredictable outcome of the fulguration procedure as suggested by some clinical reports[15,68-72] and laboratory experiments,[53,73-77] patient preselection was particularly restricted at the beginning of our experience. The technique was used as a last resort procedure and its use was restricted to the most resistant and difficult cases which were beyond operability; some patients were even moribund when the fulguration procedure was performed.[45]

On the other hand, observing how well the procedure was tolerated, we extended its indications to high risk cases in order to learn about the possible limits of this method.

- Our patient referral corresponds to a particular entity of patient with ventricular tachycardia in whom other indications of cardiac surgery were not present (rather, we had to treat some patients who had VT after surgery for cardiac revascularization or even antiarrhythmic surgery).

- The experience accumulated over years with surgical procedures tends to bring to our centers patients with VT related to noncoronary diseases such as arrhythmogenic right ventricular disease and RBBB + left axis ventricular tachycardia in young adults.[78] In other countries and especially in the United States, patients with post-myocardial infarction VT are primarily considered. This could also reflect the prevalence of the basic disease which is different in different countries. In addition, it is evident that the arrhythmogenic substrate is different if we compare the borderline zone of an old myocardial infarction and the right ventricular wall of a case of arrhythmogenic right ventricular dysplasia. Therefore, it may be appropriate to adapt the endocardial shock procedure to the underlying pathology.

- Some bias could also be introduced in each step of our study which does not follow the same antiarrhythmic protocol. It could be that a combination of drugs which was effective after fulguration could have been effective before the procedure if the same combination had been used.

- The learning phase has introduced some variations concerning both the protocols and the equipment.

- A limitation in the evaluation of the control of arrhythmia is due also to the fact that after treatment, a previously symptomatic patient could become asymptomatic due to a slower rate of tachycardia, negative inotropic effect of antiarrhythmic treatment, or spontaneous degradation of cardiac function. Later re-evaluation by invasive methods was performed in one case (no. 21), and rehospitalization and monitoring in another case (no. 30) 1 year after the procedure. In one case (no. 2), attempts to reinduce VT was done with burst pacing through a radiofrequency pacemaker connected to a catheter located at the right ventricular apex during the few months following the procedure.

- When a patient enters the electrophysiological laboratory in incessant VT, complete disappearance of the arrhythmia is a clear-cut effect of the treatment. This situation is in fact quite rare. An algorithm to determine when a VT should be considered ablated is not available at the present time. For instance, case no. 9 could be argued. This patient had only two episodes of VT tolerated badly, with a time interval between attacks of 6 months. One documented relapse of VT with the same morphology occurred within 3 months after discharge and then disappeared. Recently, a new relapse was observed 25 months after the last episode. In the same episode, two morphologies were observed. One was similar to the previous documented episode; the other happened to exhibit a new morphology. Was this a new VT due to the evolution of an unstable myocardium (arrhythmogenic right ventricular disease) or the relapse of the fulgurated VT?

- The fact that antiarrhythmic treatment is frequently needed is not in our view a sign of failure but a sign of incomplete effectiveness of the procedure, similar to the fact that several shocks are frequently needed in the same session or that several sessions are needed for a particular patient.

Many questions concerning the treatment of VT by fulguration remain to be answered. Little is known about the cellular modification of the arrhythmogenic substrate resulting from the electrical discharge. The various mechanical factors involved need clarification: how important is the positioning of the indifferent electrode? Which electrical parameters are the most reliable? What should be the size and shape of fulguration electrodes? What are the best criteria for choosing the fulguration target?[70]

Despite the fact that the pace mapping technique needs to be fully perfected, it nevertheless has proved to be highly valuable in some cases when VT could not be induced during the session. Guided exclusively by this method, it was possible to deliver discharges which proved to be effective in some patients.

The predictive value of VT reinduction during sessions is relatively unreliable. From a general standpoint, it seemed at first view that 50% of recurrences took place in cases where it was not possible to reinduce VT at the end of the session. However, a more thorough analysis of VT morphology demonstrated that the recurrences were observed mainly in the nonfulgurated VTs[49] suggesting that in all of the patients who remained inducible, a spontaneous recurrence was observed. Better results were obtained, however, 10 days following fulguration, although this indication completely failed in one case (no. 17). Nor can the protocol of reevaluation on the 10th day account for modifications apt to develop over a longer period. It might be too early for long-term evaluation, since stabilization of lesion on myocardium generally needs a longer time. Also the possible modifications induced inside the fibrous tissues created by the procedure may need an even longer time which could be extended to several months before the stage of stable retractile fibrosis is reached. As usual, it is difficult to extrapolate to humans results obtained in animal experiments. In this latter situation, shocks have generally been delivered to normal myocardium.

Measurement of the myocardial isoenzyme of the creatine kinases revealed low values (38 ± 15 international units), confirming what we noted in experimental studies: the myocardial area altered by the endocavitary shock is limited.[30] Consequently, fulguration may be performed without danger one or more times in the absence of an adequate result on the first attempt, before the procedure is determined to be ineffective. In our experience, another attempt at fulguration was preferred by the patients over its cardiovascular surgical counterpart.

Acknowledgments: Supported in part by grants from: Centre de Recherche sur les Maladies Cardiovasculaires de l'Association Claude Bernard; La Fondation de Cardiologie; L'Institut National de la Santé et de la Recherche Médicale (INSERM Contrat N°865005).

We are indebted to Ms. Heidi R. Wyle, Ph.D., from Bard Electrophysiology for her invaluable assistance in the styling of most parts of the manuscript and to Mrs. N. Proust for her secretarial support.

References

1. Dulk KD, Bertholet M, Brugada P. Clinical experience with implantable devices for control of tachyarrhythmias. PACE 1984;7:548.
2. Zipes DP, Heger JJ, Miles WM, Prystowsky EN. Synchronous intracardiac cardioversion. PACE 1984;7:522.
3. Mirowski M, Reid PR, Mower MM, Watkins L, Platia EV, Griffith LSC, Juanteguy JM. The automatic implantable cardioverter-defibrillator. PACE 1984;7:534.
4. Fontaine G, Guiraudon G, Frank R, Gerbaux A, Cousteau JP, Barillon A, Gay RJ, Cabrol C, Facquet J. La cartographie epicardique et le traitement chirurgical par simple ventriculotomie de certaines tachycardies ventriculaires rebelles par reentree. Arch Mal Coeur 1975;68:113–124.
5. Garan H, Nguyen K, McGovern BA, Buckley MJ, Ruskin JN. Perioperative and long-term results after electrophysiologically directed ventricular surgery for recurrent ventricular tachycardia. J Am Coll Cardiol 1986;8:201–209.
6. Ostermeyer J, Breithardt G, Kolvenbach R, Borggrefe M, Seipel L, Schulte HD, Bircks W. The surgical treatment of ventricular tachycardias: simple aneurysmectomy versus electrophysiologically guided procedures. J Thorac Cardiovasc Surg 1982;84:704–715.
7. Miller JM. Presented for the collaborative report of antitachycardic surgery. In: Non-Pharmacological Therapy of Tachyarrhythmias Borggrefe M, Breithardt G, Ostermeyer J, Dusseldorf 1987 (In press).
8. Fontaine G. Les methodes ablatives. Arch Mal Coeur 1984;77:1299–1300.
9. Gallagher JJ, Anderson RW, Kasell JH, Rice JR, Pritchett ELC, Gault JH, Harrison LA, Wallace AG. Cryoablation of drug-resistant ventricular tachycardia in a patient with a variant of scleroderma. Circulation 1978;57:190.
10. Fontaine G, Guiraudon G, Frank R, Tereau Y, Pavie A, Cabrol C, Chomette G, Grosgogeat Y. Surgical management of ventricular tachycardia not related to myocardial ischemia. In: ME Josephson, HJJ Wellens, eds. Tachycardias: Mechanisms, Diagnosis and Treatment. Philadelphia, Lea & Febiger, 1984;451–473.
11. Fontaine G, Lechat Ph, Cansell A, Guiraudon G, Linares-Cruz E, Koulibaly M, Chomette G, Auriol M, Grosgogeat Y. Advances in the treatment of cardiac arrhythmias in the last decade: Definition and role of ablative techniques. In: G Fontaine, MM Scheinman, eds. Ablation in Cardiac Arrhythmias. Mount Kisco, NY, Futura Publishing Co., 1987 (In press).
12. Mesnildrey P, Laborde F, Beloucif S, Mayolini P, Piwnica A. Tachycardies ventriculaires d'origine ischemique: Traitement chirurgical par thermo-exclusion circonferentielle au laser Nd-Yag. Presse Med 1986;15:531–534.
13. Scheinman MM, Evans-Bell T. Catheter ablation of the atrioventricular junction: A report of the percutaneous mapping and ablation registry. Circulation 1984;70:1024–1029.
14. Gallagher JJ, Svenson RH, Kasell JH, German LD, Bardy GH, Broughton A, Critelli G. Catheter technique for closed-chest ablation of the atrioventricular conduction system. N Engl J Med 1982;306:194–200.
15. Hartzler GO. Electrode catheter ablation of refractory focal ventricular tachycardia. J Am Coll Cardiol 1983;2:1107–1113.
16. Puech P, Gallay P, Grolleau R, Koliopoulos N. Traitement par electrofulguration endocavitaire d'une tachycardie ventriculaire recidivante par dysplasie ventriculaire droite. Arch Mal Coeur 1984;77:826–835.

17. Fontaine G, Tonet JL, Frank R, Gallais Y, Farenq G, Grosgogeat Y. La fulguration endocavitaire: Une nouvelle methode de traitement des troubles du rythme? Ann Cardiol Angiol 1984;33:543–561.
18. Bardy GH, Coltorti F, Ivey TD, Yerkovich D, Greene HL. Effect of damped sine-wave shocks of catheter dielectric strength. Am J Cardiol 1985;56:769–772.
19. Fisher JD, Brodman R, Johnson D, Waspe LE, Kim SG, Matos JA, Scavin G. Nonsurgical electrical ablation of tachycardia: Importance of in vitro testing of catheter leads. PACE 1984;7:74–81.
20. Fontaine G, Cansell A, Lechat Ph, Frank R, Grosgogeat Y. Method of selecting catheters for endocavitary fulguration. Stimucoeur 1984;12:285–289.
21. Fontaine G, Lechat Ph, Cansell A, Linares-Cruz E, Chomette G, Grosgogeat Y. Anatomical and histological effects of endocardial catheter fulguration: An experimental study. In: MM Scheinman, ed. Catheter Ablation in Cardiac Arrhythmias. Hingham, Martinus Nijhoff Pub, 1987 (In press).
22. Tonet JL, Fontaine G, Frank R, Grosgogeat Y. Treatment of refractory ventricular tachycardias by endocardial fulguration (abstr). Circulation 1985;72(III):388.
23. Fontaine G, Tonet JL, Frank R, Touzet I, Farenq G, Dubois-Rande JL, Baraka M, Abdelali S, Grosgogeat Y. Traitement des tachycardies ventriculaires rebelles par fulguration endocavitaire associee aux anti-arhythmiques. Arch Mal Coeur 1986; 79:1152–1162.
24. Frank R, Fontaine G, Baraka M, Kounde S, Farenq G, Grosgogeat Y. Catheter endocardial mapping in fulguration. In: Ventricular Tachycardia: From Mechanism to Therapy. Vittel, 1986 (In press).
25. O'Keefe DB, Curry PVL, Prior AL, Yates JK, Deverall PB, Sowton E. Surgery for ventricular tachycardia using operative pace mapping. Br Heart J 1980;43:116.
26. Holt PM, Smallpeice C, Deverall PB, Yates AK, Curry PVL. Ventricular arrhythmias: A guide to their localisation. Br Heart J 1985;53:417–430.
27. Fontaine G. Prevention of sudden arrhythmic death: Catheter ablation. In: Proceedings of the 1985 Sydney Opera House Symposium, Telectronics Vectors Pub., Sydney, October 1986;18–21.
28. Gallais Y, Touzet M, Gateau O, Maneglia R, Frank R, Fontaine G, Cousin M. Th. Anesthesie et surveillance dans la fulguration endocavitaire pour le traitement radical des tachycardies ventriculaires. Ann Cardiol Angiol 1986;35:539–549.
29. Tonet JL, Baraka M, Fontaine G, Abdelali S, Frank R, Menezes-Falcao L, Funck-Brentano C, Grosgogeat Y. Ventricular arrhythmias during endocardial catheter fulguration of ventricular tachycardias (abstr). J Am Coll Cardiol 1986;7(No. 2):236A.
30. Lechat Ph, Fontaine G, Cansell A, Grosgogeat Y. Epicardial and endocardial myocardial damage related to catheter ablation techniques (abstr). Eur Heart J 1984;5:258.
31. Hartzler GO, Giorgi LV. Electrode catheter ablation of refractory ventricular tachycardia: Continued experience. J Am Coll Cardiol 1984;3:512.
32. Gonzalez R, Scheinman MM, Margaretten W, Rubinstein M. Closed chest electrode-catheter technique for His bundle ablation in dogs. Am J Physiol 1981;241:H283–H287.
33. Scheinman MM, Morady F, Shen EN. Interventional electrophysiology: Catheter ablation technique. Clin Prog Pacing Electrophysiol 1983;1:375–381.
34. Scheinman MM, Morady F, Hess DS, Gonzalez R. Catheter-induced ablation of the atrioventricular junction to control refractory supraventricular arrhythmias. JAMA 1982;248:851–855.
35. Scheinman MM, Morady F, Hess DS, Gonzalez R. Transvenous catheter technique for induction of damage to the atrioventricular junction in man (abstr). Am J Cardiol 1982;49:1013.
36. Winston SA, Morady F, Davis JC, DiCarlo LA Jr, Wexman MP, Scheinman MM. Catheter ablation of ventricular tachycardia. Circulation 1984;70 (Suppl II):412.
37. Steinhaus D, Whitford E, Stavens C, Schneller S, McComb J, Carr J, McGovern BA, Garan H, Ruskin JN. Percutaneous transcatheter electrical ablation for recurrent sustained ventricular tachycardia. Circulation 1984;70(Suppl II):100.
38. Scheinman MM. Electrical ventricular endocardial ablation: A tomato ripe or rotted? J Am Coll Cardiol 1985;5:961–962.

39. Huang SK, Marcus FI, Ewy GA. Clinical experience with endocardial catheter ablation for refractory ventricular tachycardia. J Am Coll Cardiol 1985;5:473.
40. Henthorn RW, Cohen M, Anderson PG, Epstein AE, Plumb VJ, Olshansky B, Waldo AL. Pathological and clinical observations after catheter fulguration in man (abstr). J Am Coll Cardiol 1986;7:236.
41. Downar E, Parson I, Cameron DA, Waxman MB, Yao L, Easty A. Unipolar and bipolar catheter ablation techniques for management of ventricular tachycardia: Initial experience. J Am Coll Cardiol 1985;5:472.
42. Belhassen B, Miller HI, Geller E, Laniado S. Transcatheter electrical shock ablation of ventricular tachycardia. J Am Coll Cardiol 1986;7:1347-1355.
43. Evans GT, Scheinman MM. Catheter ablation of ventricular tachycardia foci: A report of the percutaneous cardiac mapping and ablation registry (abstr). Circulation 1986; 74:460.
44. Fontaine G, Cansell A, Lechat Ph, Frank R, Tonet JL, Grosgogeat Y. Les chocs electriques endocavitaires: Problemes lies au materiel. Arch Mal Coeur 1984;77: 1307-1314.
45. Fontaine G, Tonet JL, Frank R, Lacroix H, Farenq Q, Gallais Y, Drobinski G, Grosgogeat Y. Traitement d'urgence de la tachycardie ventriculaire chronique apres infarctus du myocarde par la fulguration endocavitaire. Arch Mal Coeur 1985;78:1037-1043.
46. Hoffman BF, Cranefield PF. Electrophysiology of the Heart. Mount Kisco, NY, Futura Publishing Co., 1976.
47. Brugada P, Green M, Abdollah H, Wellens HJJ. Significance of ventricular arrhythmias initiated by programmed ventricular stimulation: The importance of the type of ventricular arrhythmia induced and the number of premature stimuli required. Circulation 1984;69:87-92.
48. Horowitz LN, Vetter VL, Harken AH, Josephson ME. Electrophysiologic characteristics of sustained ventricular tachycardia occurring after repair of tetralogy of Fallot. Am J Cardiol 1980;46:446-452.
49. Tonet JL, Baraka M, Frank R, Fontaine G, Gallais Y, Abdelali S, Grosgogeat Y. Endocardial catheter fulguration of ventricular tachycardias: Pitfalls of the clinical and nonclinical approach (abstr). Circulation 1985;72(Suppl III):388.
50. Miller JM, Kienzle MG, Harken AH, Josephson ME. Morphologically distinct sustained ventricular tachycardias in coronary artery disease: Significance and surgical results. J Am Coll Cardiol 1984;4:1073-1079.
51. Mason JW, Stinson EB, Winkel RA, Oyer PE, Griffin JC, Ross DL. Relative efficacy of blind left ventricular aneurysm resection for the treatment of recurrent ventricular tachycardia. Am J Cardiol 1982;49:241-248.
52. McGiffin DC, Kirklin JK, Plumb VJ, Waldo AL, Blackstone EH, Kirklin JW. Survival and relief of life-threatening ventricular tachycardia after direct operatons (abstr). Circulation 1986;74(Suppl. II):460.
53. Holt, PM, Boyd, E.G.C.A. Hematologic effects of the high energy endocardial ablation technique. Circulation 1986:73:1029-1036.
54. Fontaine, G, Volmer W, Nienaltowska E, Aaddaj S, Cansell A, Grosgogeat Y. Approach to the physics of fulguration. In: GG Fontaine, MM Scheinman, eds. Ablation in Cardiac Arrhythmias. Mount Kisco, NY, Futura Publishing Co., (In press).
55. Levine JH, Spear JF, Weisman HF, Kadish AA, Prood C, Siu CO, Moore EN. The cellular electrophysiologic changes induces by high-energy electrical ablation in canine myocardium. Circulation 1986;73:818-329.
56. Lee BI, Rodriguez ER, Notargiacomo A, Ferrans VJ, Chen YW, Fletcher RD. Thermal effects of laser and electrical discharge on cardiovascular tissue: Implications for coronary artery recanalization and endocardial ablation. J Am Coll Cardiol 1986: 8:193-200.
57. Tidd MJ, Webster J, Cameron Wroght H, Harrison IR. Mode of action of a surgical electronic lithoclast high speed pressure, cinematographic and Schlieren recordings following an ultrashort underwater electronic discharge. Biomed Engin 1976;1:5-11.

58. Chahine GL. Etude locale du phenomene de cavitation. Analyse des facteurs regissant la dynamique des interfaces. These de Doctorat es Sciences, Paris. 1979.
59. Van Vleet, JF, Tacker WA, Geddes LA, Ferrans VF. Acute cardiac damage in dogs given multiple transthoracic shocks with a trapezoidal wave form defibrillator. Am J Vet Res 1977;38:617–626.
60. Dahl CF, Ewy GA, Warner ED, Thomas ED. Myocardial necrosis from direct current countershock: Effect of paddle electrode size and time interval between discharges. Circulation 1974;50:956–961.
61. Ehsani A, Ewy GA, Sobel BE. Effects of electrical countershock on serum creatine phosphokinase (CPK) isoenzyme activity. Am J Cardiol 1976;37:12–18.
62. Slodki SJ, Falicov RE, Katz MJ, West M, Zimmerman HJ. Serum enzyme changes following external direct current shock therapy for cardiac arrhythmias. Am J Cardiol 1966;17:792–797.
63. Mandecki T, Giec L, Kargal W. Serum enzyme activities after cardioversion. Br Heart J 1970; 32:600–602.
64. Fontaine G, Touil F, Frank R, Cansell A, Gorins D, Tonet JL, Grosgogeat Y. Defibrillation, fulguration et cardioversion: Effets sur les pacemakers. Stimucoeur 1984;12:91.
65. Bowes RJ, Bennet DH. Effect of transvenous atrioventricular nodal ablation on the function of implanted pacemakers. PACE 1985;8:811–814.
66. Fontaine G, Frank R, Tonet JL, Gallais Y, Touzet I, Todorova M, Baraka M, Grosgogeat Y. Treatment of resistant ventricular tachycardia by endocavitary fulguration associated with antiarrhythmic therapy as compared to antiarrhythmic therapy alone: Experience of 111 consecutive patients with a mean follow-up of 18 months. In: Non-Pharmacological Therapy of Tachyarrhythmias. Dusseldorf, 1986 (In press)
67. Fontaine G, Frank R, Bonnet M, Cabrol C, Guiraudon G. Methode d'etude experimentale et clinique des syndromes de Wolff-Parkinson-White et d'ischemie myocardique par cartographic de la depolarisation ventriculaire epicardique. Coeur Med Interne 1973:12:105.
68. Hartzler GO, Giorgi LV, Diehl AM, Hamaker WR. Right coronary spasm complicating electrode catheter ablation of a right lateral accessory pathway. J Am Coll Cardiol 1985;6:250–253.
69. Gallagher JJ. Ablation by transcatheter shock: Current status. Chest 1985;88:804–806.
70. Josephson ME. Catheter ablation of arrhythmias. Ann Intern Med 1984;101:234–237.
71. Bharati S, Scheinman MM, Morady F, Hess DS, Lev M. Sudden death after catheter-induced atrioventricular junctional ablation. Chest 1985;88:883–889.
72. Fisher JD, Kim SG, Matos JA, Waspe LE, Brodman R, Merav A. Complications of catheter ablation of tachyarrhythmias: Occurence, protection, prevention. Clin Prog Pacing Electrophysiol 1985;3:292–298.
73. Lerman BB, Weiss JL, Bulkley BH, Becker LC, Weisfeldt ML. Myocardial injury and induction of arrhythmia by direct current shock delivered via endocardial catheters in dogs. Circulation 1984:69:1006–1012.
74. Bardy GH, Coltorti F, Ivey TD, Alferness C, Rackson M, Hansen K, Stewart R, Greene HL. Some factors affecting bubble formation with catheter-mediated defibrillator pulses. Circulation 1986;73:525–538.
75. Kempf F, Falcone RA, Waxman HL, Marchlinski FE, Josephson ME. Anatomic and hemodynamic effects of electrical discharges in the ventricle (abstr). Circulation 1983;68:696.
76. Westveer DC, Nelson T, Stewart JR, Thornton EP, Gordon S, Timmis GC. Sequelae of left ventricular electrical endocardial ablation. J Am Coll Cardiol 1985;5:956–960.
77. Hauer RH, Robles de Medina EO, Tweel IVD, Borst C. Incidence and course of ventricular tachycardia induced by electrical catheter ablation in the ventricular wall (abstr). Circulation 1985;72(Suppl.III):390.
78. Tonet JL, Frank R, Fontaine G, Grosgogeat Y. Ventricular tachycardia responsive to verapamil: Treatment by catheter fulguration (abstr). Circulation 1986;74(Suppl. II):461.

VIII

SURGICAL TREATMENT OF ARRHYTHMIAS

35

Surgical Treatment of the Wolff-Parkinson-White Syndrome: Current Indications, Techniques, and Results

Olaf C. Penn

Introduction

In patients with the Wolff-Parkinson-White (WPW) syndrome, the presence of an accessory pathway connecting atrium and ventricle can cause troublesome and sometimes life-threatening arrhythmias. After the presence of these accessory pathways was demonstrated by results of epicardial mapping[1] and programmed electrical stimulation of the heart,[2] a logical step was to attempt to divide these structures surgically. The first successful operation was performed at Duke University in 1968.[3] Shortly thereafter, other institutions also reported successful surgical interruption of accessory atrioventricular pathways.[4,5] One can state that some 20 years later, surgical treatment of the WPW syndrome has become a reality and a fully accepted form of treatment of this disease, and for some patients, the treatment of choice. The indications for surgical interruption of preexcitation are clearly related to the results and complications of the operation which, in turn, are dependent of the techniques used.

From: Brugada P, Wellens HJJ. CARDIAC ARRHYTHMIAS: Where To Go From Here? Mount Kisco, NY, Futura Publishing Company, Inc., © 1987.

Indications for Surgery of the Wolff-Parkinson-White Syndrome

Surgical treatment of the Wolff-Parkinson-White syndrome, as will be discussed later, can be performed nowadays with a high success rate and a low operative risk. This is the result of multiple factors including, among others, the refinement in cardiac surgery techniques in general, improvement of cardiac preservation during cardio-pulmonary bypass, better pre- and postoperative cardiological support, improved anesthesia techniques, but also, a better understanding of the pathophysiology of the disease, possibility of associated conditions and better localization of the accessory pathway due to improved pre- and postoperative electrical stimulation and mapping studies.

Unlike treatment with antiarrhythmic drugs or antitachycardia pacemakers, surgical interruption of an accessory pathway offers a curative (and not palliative) solution to the problem. This, and the above-mentioned factors, have resulted in a widening of the spectrum of indications for surgical treatment of patients with the Wolff-Parkinson-White syndrome. While the indication for surgical interruption of an accessory pathway is presently made individually and very carefully, we may not be far from an era where the Wolff-Parkinson-White syndrome will be considered a "surgical disease."

A multitude of factors play a role in the indications for surgery.

1. *The complaints of the patient.* The Wolff-Parkinson-White patient can present clinically with a wide spectrum of problems: from the asymptomatic patient with preexcitation discovered on a screening electrocardiogram to the patient suffering sudden arrhythmic death because of atrial fibrillation causing very rapid ventricular rates and ventricular fibrillation. While the incidence of asymptomatic preexcitation is not fully known, the incidence of sudden death in this syndrome has to be considered as low. Most patients seen by physicians suffer from paroxysmal circus movement tachycardia and atrial fibrillation. The variations in conduction properties of the heart determine that some patients present with rare episodes of a well-tolerated arrhythmia, while others present with very frequent (sometimes permanent or "incessant") episodes of circus movement tachycardia, causing more or less severe symptoms. Other patients may suffer from very rare, but severe episodes of fast circus movement tachycardia or atrial fibrillation. While traditionally only patients with very severe symptoms in spite of treatment with antiarrhythmic drugs have been considered candidates for surgical treatment, in the light of the presently available results, it has become clear that in patients with severe symptoms one should not necessarily wait for recurrence of symptoms to consider the possibility of surgery.

2. *Need and results of other forms of treatment.* Surgical interruption of the accessory pathway can be indicated when considering results of other previous forms of treatment in a particular patient. While surgical treatment should be considered in any patient who does require treatment for this condition, in some patients it may be the last resort, either because they do not satisfactorily respond to drugs and/or an antitachycardia pacemaker or because these forms of treatment

cannot be used or are not desired by the patient. In the decision to select one or another form of treatment, many other factors play an important role. To be submitted to life-long antiarrhythmic drug treatment or antitachycardia pacing is no longer acceptable for a patient who may be offered a definite, curative procedure, particularly in young patients or females with childbearing potential. The patient should have a detailed explanation of the expected results of the different forms of treatment and should actively participate in the decision regarding surgery. In patients with severe symptoms, the physician's preference (when present) for a surgical procedure should be made clear to the patient.

3. *The localization of the accessory pathway* also plays a role in the indication for surgical treatment, but more important in this respect is the experience of the surgeon, electrophysiologist, and other members of the arrythmia surgery unit. Right and left-sided accessory pathways can be successfully operated in almost 100% of cases. The initially lower percentage of success with septally located accessory pathways is increasing and now approximating the success rate of other localizations. Because of the possible risk of atrioventricular block when operating on a septally located accessory pathway, one may remain more conservative in these patients if complaints are not too severe. In patients with severe symptoms who can be operated on by an experienced team, the localization of the accessory pathway should not be considered a limiting factor.

4. *The presence of other cardiac diseases* requiring or amenable to successful surgical treatment (coronary bypass surgery, for instance) may be of influence in the indication for surgical treatment. If the two problems can be successfully solved with a single operation, it should be strongly recommended. That is not the case when the presence of other cardiac disease increases the surgical risk. If the theoretical risk surpasses the possible benefits (something very difficult to assess in practice), the operation should not be recommended.

5. For *extracardiac diseases*, similar guidelines apply. If the extracardiac disease increases the risk of the operation or is fatal in the short term, the operation should not be performed.

6. Many other factors influence the decision. As discussed, *age* and *sex* have to be considered, but also the *social* and *psychological consequences* of both the arrhythmias and the operation itself. A very difficult point to consider is also the *cost-to-benefit* ratio of the possible treatment that can be offered to the patient. Medication, pacemakers, and surgery cost money, but so does the disease. In some patients surgical interruption of the accessory pathway may be the only way to return them to a fully productive and problem-free active professional life (i.e., airline pilots). The disease brings also costs and inconveniences because of recurrences of the arrhythmias with sometimes frequent admissions to hospital, loss of productivity, or simply lack of confidence from the employer. The same holds true for insurance, school results, and the attitude toward day-to-day regular or unusual problems. In financial terms, it can be easily calculated that a single operative procedure curing the disease and avoiding limitations in quality of life

has a better cost-to-benefit ratio than palliative treatments requiring, at least, frequent controls at the out-patient clinic, if not repeated admissions because of recurrences of the arrhythmia.

As previously stated, the decision to operate has to be taken for the individual patient. However, it is helpful to have general guidelines. In an attempt to standardize the way indications for surgery are taken at our institution and referring hospitals, we have developed a scoring system (Table I). That system is based on our experience in medical and surgical treatment of the Wolff-Parkinson-White syndrome and is being tested prospectively. The assumptions behind it are as follows:

- Patients with a surgically easily accessible accessory pathway requiring any

Table I
A Scoring System for Recognition of Patients With an Accessory Pathway Who Are Surgical Candidates

	Score
1. Sex	
Male	0
Female, no children desired or possible	0
Female, childbearing potential	+10
2. Age (years)	
0–1	0
2–10	+5
11–40	+10
41–65	+5
> 65	0
3. Does the patient require treatment?	
Yes	+10
No	0
4. Did the patient suffer from syncope or aborted sudden death caused by the accessory pathway?	
Yes	+25
No	0
5. Possibilities of treatment	
Not possible with antiarrhythmic drugs	+10
Not possible with antitachycardia pacing	+10
Not possible with antiarrhythmic drugs or antitachycardia pacing	+20
Possible with antiarrhythmic drugs or antitachycardia pacing	0
6. The complaints of the patient cause psychological and/or social problems	
Yes	+10
No	0
7. Extracardiac disease(s)	
No	0
Yes	
• No consequences for surgery	0
• Increase surgical risk	−10
• Fatal within 1 year	−45

Table I *(Continued)*

	Score
8. *Other cardiac disease(s)*	
No	0
Yes	
• Can be operated on without increasing surgical risk	+10
• No influcence on surgical risk	0
• Increase, surgical risk	−10
9. *Does the patient prefer surgery to other forms of treatment?*	
Yes	+10
No	0
10. *Do you prefer surgery for your patient?*	
Yes	+ 5
No	0
11. *Localization accessory pathway*	
Left	+10
Right	+10
Septal	0
Multiple	0
12. *The ECG during tachycardia shows:*	
• Atrial fibrillation with mean ventricular rates above 180/min.	+20
• Circus movement tachycardia with a rate above 180/min.	+10
• Both	+25

SCORE:
    Less than 25 points = No surgical candidate
    25–65 points = Surgical candidate
    > 65 points = Direct surgical candidate

form of treatment for that condition are surgical "candidates" unless contraindications for surgery exist. That decision is positively influenced by physician's and/or patient's preference for the operation, severe symptoms (syncope or sudden death, very fast tachycardias), negative results with other forms of treatment or inability to use them, need for other cardiac surgery not increasing the surgical risk, young age, or female sex with childbearing potential. The decision is negatively influenced by associated conditions (cardiac or extracardiac) that are either fatal on the short term or markedly increase the surgical risk. A "candidate" does not indicate need for the operation, but simply that surgery should be considered as strongly as other forms of treatment when they can be still used. However, if a score above 65 is reached, surgical treatment deserves preference ("direct surgical candidate").

• Patients with severe symptoms are "direct surgical candidates" unless contraindications as described above exist.

• A patient with the Wolff-Parkinson-White syndrome who does not require any form of treatment is not a "surgical candidate" nor a "direct surgical candidate" unless other cardiac surgery will be performed or the patient's and/or physician's preference exists (for instance because of job or insurance situation).

Two additional problems that require consideration are the *asymptomatic patient with preexcitation* and the patient with an accessory pathway who may be *at risk* but who has not yet suffered from those problems to which he (she) is considered at risk of (for instance, ventricular fibrillation). In the asymptomatic patient with preexcitation, the accessory pathway may have a long or a short anterograde effective refractory period. Using the ajmaline or procainanide test,[6,7] one can noninvasively obtain an idea of the duration of that parameter. That can also be done by using endocavitary or esophageal pacing.[8] Patients who have been resuscitated from sudden death or who suffer syncopal episodes because of their arrhythmias characteristically have a very short anterograde effective refractory period of the accessory pathway allowing fast ventricular rates during atrial fibrillation, sometimes degenerating into ventricular fibrillation.[9,10] The contrary, however, is not true. The specificity of this finding is very low. The large majority of patients with a short anterograde effective refractory period of the accessory pathway do not suffer from sudden arrhythmic death.[9,11] Therefore, one has to be conservative at the present time when indicating surgical treatment or treatment at all in asymptomatic patients with preexcitation. As previously discussed, exceptions may be patients who cannot run a normal life (because of job or other problems) after discovery of that theoretical risk. When these problems are not present, surgery should not be indicated on the basis of the duration of the anterograde refractory period of the accessory pathway alone.

On the basis of the above discussion, one can categorize the present indications for surgical interruption of accessory pathways as detailed in Table II.

Table II
Categories of Indications for Surgical Treatment of Preexcitation

Strictly indicated
- Severe symptoms (syncope, sudden death)
- Failure of medical treatment and pacemaker treatment or impossibility to use these treatments

Indicated
- Any patient requring treatment at all
- Patient's preference and physician's preference

Not indicated
- Asymptomatic preexcitation

Contraindicated
- Assocaited cardiac or extracardiac conditions with a fatal short-term outcome or markedly increasing surgical risk

Surgical Treatment of WPW Syndrome

Techniques

The first successful surgical division of an accessory atrioventricular connection (accessory pathway) for the treatment of the WPW syndrome was accomplished by Sealy at Duke University on May 28, 1968.[3] Since that time, he and Gallagher have provided us with many extremely accurate, beautifully illustrated, and extensive descriptions of the clinical, anatomical, and surgical management of the WPW syndrome. Their work played an important role in our understanding of the complexity and vagaries of this syndrome. As a result of their work, a variety of surgical approaches have evolved, most of which are quite successful.

The surgical technique described by Sealy is the result of a carefully executed study of the anatomical manifestations of the atrioventricular bundles, as described by Stanley Kent in the *Journal of Physiology* in 1914.[12] The accessory pathways are anomalous atrioventricular connections which cross from atrium to ventricular wall and are neither palpable nor visible.

The procedure for interruption of the pathways consists of two steps. The epicardial activation sequences of the atria and ventricles are determined and used to locate the crossing points of the pathways. This is then used as a guide for a systematic step-by-step dissection for interruption of the accessory pathway. A successful operation for interruption of the accessory pathways is based upon electrophysiological data which define the localization of the anatomic area harboring the pathway. This information should be translated into the different possibilities of the pathway's route from atrium to ventricle.

The operative procedure therefore includes epicardial mapping during normothermic perfusion followed by total body hypothermia to 28°C, cross-clamping of the ascending aorta, and the use of cold cardioplegia. After closure of the atrium and rewarming of the heart, the electrocardiogram is checked for the presence of preexcitation. Incremental pacing of the atria and ventricles is done to demonstrate the Wenckebach phenomenon, its presence indicating that the accessory pathway has been interrupted.

For the left free wall accessory pathways, the left atrium is opened wide, similar to the exposure for mitral valve replacement. Exposure can be very difficult because of the normal size of the left atrium.

In both right free wall and left free wall accessory pathways, the atrial end of the pathway is marked by passing a suture from the epicardium to the atrial cavity. An atrial endocardial incision is then made above the annulus of the AV valve, leaving only enough atrium to permit closure of the incision. For the left atrial incisions, this avoids injury to the circumflex artery or the coronary sinus. The incision is extended up to 2 cm on each side of the marker. The fat in the sulcus is separated from the external aspect of the upper lip of the atrial incision. The sulcus fat is separated from the superior aspect of the ventricle almost to the attachment of the epicardium to the ventricle. The superficial fibers of the ventricular myocardium as they enter the annulus fibrosus are interrupted.

The surgical approach to the anterior and posterior divisions of the septal area is definitely more difficult than for the lateral wall accessory pathways and requires more anatomical insight and surgical experience. This is because of the complicated anatomy of the region and because of the fact that the septal area of the heart contains the critical elements of the normal conduction system. Sealy's descriptions of the anatomical and surgical considerations are the most extensive and elaborate studies in this field and it is clear how much he has dedicated himself to find the surgical solution for arrhythmias using the accessory pathway(s).

Sealy gives a very precise description for the location of Kent bundles in the septal area. The posterior septal accessory pathways were found to course with the His bundle, between the right fibrous trigone and the coronary sinus, underneath the coronary sinus, from the left atrium to the posterior superior process of the left ventricle. They may arise from the atrial muscle around the coronary sinus and insert into the top of the muscular ventricular septum or the posterior superior process of the left ventricle.

The pathways in the anterior septal area can course from the atrium to the ventricle adjacent to the right fibrous trigone and the membranous ventricular septum or somewhat anterior to this point.[13]

The surgical approach to the septal area of the heart is a planned and systematic dissection of the most likely crossing point of the pathway from the atrium to the ventricle at the annulus fibrosus. In these cases it is also very practical to perform electrophysiological mapping on the inside of the right atrium. Special care must also be given to venous cannulation in order to keep a clear view into the right atrium. At Duke University, it was routine to cannulate the superior caval vein and the right femoral vein during these operations.

For the posterior septal pathways, the pyramidal space is dissected free through a right atrial endocardial atriotomy and through an epicardial incision beneath the coronary sinus. Right atrium, right ventricle, left atrium, and left ventricle are all cleared of the fat that can contain possible accessory pathways. The most difficult point in this dissection is the clearing of the undersurface and medial surface of the coronary sinus. If these maneuvers fail to interrupt the pathway, then the left atrium is opened and a posterior dissection is carried out.

The anterior septal pathways are dealt with by an incision located anterior to the right fibrous trigone after which the anterior space is being dissected free.[13]

The permanent or recurring form of junctional reciprocating tachycardia (PJRT), which is an incessant tachycardia based upon slow VA conduction over an accessory pathway, characteristically refractory to medical therapy, can surgically be regarded as a posteroseptal accessory pathway and divided as described for dissection of the posterior septum.[14,15] In 1985, Cox described the modifications to Sealy's technique in a series of 118 consecutive patients. These included the use of 2.5 power optical magnification, the exclusive use of the endocardial approach under cardioplegic arrest, wider margins of surgical dissection, sharp dissection of the involved valve annulus, division of only the ventricular insertion of the accessory pathway, and internal identification of the ventricular endocardial peel in all regions of dissection.[16]

In 1981 Guiraudon started to develop a new technique. Initially he was also using Sealy's open-heart technique for the surgery of the WPW syndrome and applied cardiopulmonary bypass and cross-clamping of the aorta associated with cold cardioplegia. A minor change he made was leaving no cuff of atrium at the atrioventricular annulus during dissection. Using his innovative and artistic way of thinking, and together with Klein,[17] a former pupil of Gallagher,[18] he began to give cryoablation an important role in the surgical treatment of the WPW syndrome. A decrease in mortality and morbidity rates by avoiding cross-clamping of the aorta and cardiopulmonary bypass was the main reason for this change in technique.[19,23]

Guiraudon's technique involves mobilization of the atrioventricular fat pad with exposure and cryoablation of the atrioventricular junction at the site of the accessory pathway. The operations were performed at a normothermic beating heart and in most of the cases (97%) with normothermic cardiopulmonary bypass.[19,23] He also described in one patient the exposure of the left atrioventricular sulcus via a left thoracotomy.[20] It is obvious that for right ventricular free wall accessory pathways, extracorporeal circulation is not required. His description of the disappearance of accessory pathway conduction during the course of dissection is very appealing.[19,23]

In the beginning, he used his technique only for the right and left lateral located accessory pathways but later he extended his technique to the posteroseptally located accessory pathways,[19] the main reason being the possibility of inadvertent permanent AV block using the conventional technique for posterior septal accessory pathways. As he is using a normothermic beating heart, continuous monitoring of AV conduction is possible.

Regarding the anatomical considerations for the location of posteroseptal pathways, the description of Guiraudon is much more simple than Sealy's. Guiraudon argues that posterior septal accessory pathways attach on the posterior superior process of the left ventricle. But for him, as for Sealy, coronary sinus mobilization is the key to the mobilization of the whole atrioventricular fat pad in the posteroseptal region.

Apart from the pathways coursing with the His bundle, Sealy gives four other possible locations of posterior septal Kent bundles. They can be located between the right fibrous trigone and the coronary sinus, underneath the coronary sinus, from the left atrium to the posterior superior process of the left ventricle, and they might arise from the atrial muscle around the coronary sinus.

It is clear then that in both approaches, coronary sinus mobilization and dissection of the posterior superior process of the left ventricle are important steps in the treatment of posteroseptal bypasses.

In his latest review about further experience and potential limitations for his closed heart technique, Guiraudon introduced the concept of true endocardial or intracavitary accessory pathways.[23] These have to be regarded as a potential problem when using his technique and would need transmural cryonecrosis.

In 1985 Bredikis proposed a new surgical technique for right parietal and septal accessory atrioventricular connections.[24] For the right parietal connections, his technique did not differ from the one described by Guiraudon, except for the fact that he used an ultrasonic scalpel for dissection. The septal connections were ablated by applying a cryoprobe to the mouth of the coronary sinus in a closed heart. It might be clear that by this technique only an accessory bypass with the atrial site located near the coronary sinus can be ablated and not all the other ones as described by Sealy. The cases reported by Bredikis seem also to be the ones that could be suitable for catheter ablation at the time of the electrophysiologic investigation.

The surgical technique the author has been using is based on the technique originally described by Sealy, supplemented by the modifications of Cox and Guiraudon.

For the surgical treatment of the left free wall accessory pathways, the original technique of Sealy is used as the basis for the dissection, and in most cases this technique is sufficient. Extensive mobilization of the caval veins is performed to improve exposure of the mitral valve annulus. Venous cannulation is done through the right atrium.

One must always realize that some accessory pathways can follow a more treacherous course. Pathways can be so close to the left fibrous trigone that the superficial fibers of the trigone have to be interrupted. Also the coronary sinus can contain atrial myocardium in its wall and they can be the origin of the pathway. The pathways can run over the outer aspect of the mitral valve annulus but can also run epicardially. Therefore sometimes electrocautery has to be applied to the outer aspect of the mitral valve annulus or a cryoprobe must be put over the AV connection. There is a 15–20% incidence of a second accessory pathway and the pathway can spread like a fan or web over a broad distance of a few centimeters.

Sealy's technique also forms the basis for surgery of the accessory pathways in the septal area. The cryoprobe, however, is frequently applied to the posterior superior process of the left ventricle or for diagnostic purposes. Temporary cooling of the pathway can cause disappearance of conduction which can be very helpful in the process of localizing the bundle of Kent. In reoperations, the cryoprobe can be used successfully in eliminating accessory pathways by application to the posterior superior process of the left ventricle from the outside only. However, we do not think this method to be the prime objective. The aim of the surgical intervention should always be the interruption of the accessory pathway, and isolation techniques are secondary. It must be stressed that during the operation, the exact location of the accessory pathway should be established and the possibility of other accessory pathways excluded or determined. Optimal cooperation between cardiac surgeon and cardiologist is an absolute necessity.

Results

The Duke Experience

On the surgical treatment of left free wall accessory pathways, Sealy reported in 1981 an overall success rate of 90% in a group of 79 patients. Three patients died at operation or in the immediate postoperative period. In a series of 45 patients with Kent bundles in the septal area, he reported 20 successful interruptions in 31 patients with posterior septal Kent bundles and 11 successful dissections in 14 patients with anterior septal Kent bundles. A review on the first 200 consecutive patients undergoing operation for the WPW syndrome at Duke University by Gallagher showed an overall success rate of 86%, a reoperation rate of 15%, and an incidence of postoperative heart block of 10.5%[25] (Table III).

Table III
Results of Surgical Treatment of the WPW Syndrome: Duke University series[16]

Accessory Pathways	No. of Patients	Successful Interruption
LFW	101	93
PS	58	42
RFW	41	39
AS	21	17
Total	221	191 (86%)

The St. Louis Experience

In his latest review of 118 patients, Cox claims that his modifications of the surgical technique have resulted in successful division of 100% of all accessory pathways. Although his mortality remains at 5% for all patients, it was 0.8% for patients without associated anomalies undergoing elective operation.[16] There were no reoperations and a 0.8% incidence of complete heart block (Table IV).

The London Experience

Guiraudon claims to have had one recurrence of conduction via an accessory pathway in a series of 105 patients (0.9%).[23] There was no mortality and there were no postoperative complications. Four patients required a second operation (3.8%) and one patient required a third operation (0.9%) (Table V).

Our Results

Our own experience started 3 years ago and the present communication reports the experience with 50 consecutive patients operated upon for the WPW syndrome by the author either at the University Hospital of Groningen (3 patients), the University Hospital of Utrecht (17 patients), or at the University Hospital of Maastricht (30 patients) between June 1983 and January 1987.

The ages of the patients ranged from 8 to 64 years with a mean of 31 years. There were 40 males (80%) and 10 females (20%). A total of 59 accessory pathways were present in the 50 patients, 41 patients having single and 9 patients having multiple accessory pathways. The locations of the accessory pathways were as follows: 36 left free wall (74%), 11 posterior septal (22%), two anterior septal (4%), and one right lateral (2%).

Forty-five of the accessory pathways were conducting antegrade from atrium to ventricle, causing ventricular preexcitation and a delta wave on the electrocardiogram during normal sinus rhythm. All patients suffered from circus movement tachycardias or atrial fibrillation with rapid conduction over the accessory pathway. The other five accessory pathways were "concealed" and conducted

Table IV
Result of Surgical Treatment of the WPW Sydrome: St. Louis University Series[16]

Accessory Pathways	No. of Patients	Successful Interruption
LFW	79	79
PS	33	33
RFW	17	17
AS	8	8
Total	137	137 (100%)

Table V
Results of Surgical Treatment of the WPW Syndrome: London Series[23]

Accessory Pathways	No. of Patients	Successful Interruption
LFW	74	74
PS	23	22
RFW	11	11
AS	—	—
Total	108	107 (99%)

only retrogradely from ventricle to atrium, therefore no preexcitation was present on the electrocardiogram. In one of them, the accessory pathway was of the slowly conducting type.

Six patients had other cardiac abnormalities in addition to the WPW syndrome. Two patients had Ebstein's anomaly and one of these also had Mahaim fibers and associated AV node reentry tachycardias. Coronary artery disease was present in one of the patients. This patient was having a nonsymptomatic WPW-syndrome which became symptomatic after a coronary bypass operation. One patient presented with a cardiomyopathy after having suffered for at least 20 years from the permanent or incessant form of circus movement tachycardia using a slowly conducting accessory pathway for ventriculo-atrial conduction.[14,15] Fifty-six percent of the patients were using amiodarone before the operation.

All patients in this series underwent endocardial catheter electrophysiological study before the operation. These studies were performed by Van Wijk in Groningen, Van Hoogenhuyze in Rotterdam, Hauer in Utrecht, and Brugada in Maastricht and not only confirmed the diagnosis of the WPW syndrome but were accurate in identifying the location of 54 of the 59 accessory pathways preoperatively (90%).

A total of 50 of the 59 accessory pathways were successfully divided at the initial operation. Reoperations were required in eight patients (16%) for early or late recurrences. In one patient, the accessory pathway was successfully eliminated by catheter ablation after an early recurrence. At the moment, two patients are having recurrences of both delta waves and circus movement tachycardias (4%), leaving an overall success rate of 96% (Table VI). One of these patients developed preexcitation 4 days after an operation for a left-sided posteroseptal accessory pathway. Since his pericardium had been closed and he showed signs of tamponade, cryoablation of the posterior superior process of the left ventricle was performed at resternotomy and reopening of the pericardium. This was done because he refused a complete reoperation at that time. A postoperative electrophysiologic investigation before discharge showed no signs of conduction over an accessory pathway but a few weeks later preexcitation reappeared followed by circus movement tachycardias.

The second patient was known to have an asymptomatic WPW syndrome at the time of coronary bypass surgery. After this operation, he became symptomatic with circus movement tachycardias, and when his grafts became occluded, he developed angina during the arrhythmia. As he was known to have a left lateral accessory bypass, it was thought that it could be easily dissected during his operation for revascularization. After repeat bypass grafting and endocardial dissection, preexcitation was still present and after the dissection was extended, it became evident that a second posteroseptal accessory pathway was present. As the total cross-clamping time had already been very long, it was decided to stop further attempts to divide the Kent bundle. The patient developed extracorporeal circulation and suffered from circus movement tachycardias in the postoperative period. Two patients developed a soft apical systolic murmur after the operation for a left lateral accessory pathway, suggesting the possibility of mild mitral incompetence.

All patients had an electrophysiological investigation before discharge. Evidence of preexcitation at that time or the possibility to detect ante- or retrograde conduction over an accessory pathway in our experience always leads to recurrences of circus movement tachycardia or high ventricular rates during atrial fibrillation.

There was no surgical mortality in this group of patients operated for a WPW syndrome, nor did any patient die later. Surgical complications were temporary right ventricular dysfunction in one patient, chronic cardiac tamponade after closure of the pericardium in one patient, and postoperative hemorrhage in three patients. No long-term sequelae developed from any of these complications.

Table VI
Results of Surgical Treatment of the WPW Syndrome: Author's Results

Accessory Pathways	No. of Patients	Successful Interruption
LFW	36	35
PS	11	10
RFW	1	1
AS	2	2
Total	50	48 (96%)

Two patients developed AV nodal conduction abnormalities postoperatively, necessitating the insertion of a permanent pacemaker (4%). In one patient this had been a calculated risk as he was known to have a posteroseptal parahisian accessory pathway. In the other patient, a continuous circus movement tachycardia using two posteroseptal pathways did mask normal AV conduction during cryoablation which resulted in damage to the AV node. Both patients developed a high junctional rhythm immediately after relief of cross-clamping.

Discussion

Surgical treatment for patients with the Wolff-Parkinson-White syndrome can be performed with a high success rate and a low operative risk. This has influenced indications for surgery resulting in a gradual shift from an operation performed only in patients who do not respond to medical treatment to an attractive option for patients who have to be treated medically for the rest of their lives.

Several surgical techniques have been developed in recent years but they have all been based on the outstanding descriptions of the surgical anatomy by Sealy. In this light, one should look at the modifications introduced by Cox and Guiraudon. Both started with Sealy's technique but improved the results of surgical treatment significantly by using their modifications.

At present, therefore, two schools have developed in the field of surgery for the Wolff-Parkinson-White syndrome. The school of Sealy-Cox using extensive anatomical dissection and open-heart surgery, and that of Guiraudon using minimal dissection, cryoablation, and closed-heart surgery.

Generally speaking, one may say that extensive or minimal dissection is of no use when the accessory pathway is missed. Therefore, the value of peroperative mapping is critical. This requires the utmost cooperation between cardiac surgeon and cardiologist. Looking at the history of surgical treatment for the surgical treatment of the Wolff-Parkinson-White syndrome, the name of the cardiac surgeon has always been connected with the name of the cardiologist. It has been Sealy and Gallagher, Cox and Cain, Guiraudon and Klein.

Sealy's method, or the conventional endocardial approach, was designed to divide both the atrial and the ventricular end of the accessory pathway during cardiopulmonary bypass and cardioplegic arrest. The use of cardiopulmonary bypass makes the patient prone to a certain number of complications. Cardiopulmonary bypass has a mortality rate of 0.1%, a 0.2% rate of serious invalidating complications, and a 1% incidence of minor complications. Safety of cardiopulmonary bypass, however, has improved tremendously in recent years and is one of the main topics of our institution.

Presence or absence of amiodarone medication has not led to any differences in the postoperative course, including the need for inotropic support.

Guiraudon directed himself to the atrial end of the accessory pathway. He created some confusion by referring to his technique as a "closed-heart technique," which is generally understood as a cardiac operation without the use of cardiopulmonary bypass. It is the intention with his technique, however, to avoid cardiopulmonary bypass as much as possible in order to avoid its associated complications.

The advantages of Guiraudon's technique are obvious. The possibility of continuous monitoring of conduction over the AV and accessory pathway during dissection is an extremely useful guide during this type of surgery. It helps to protect normal AV conduction and it is fascinating to see preexcitation disappear in the course of dissection. As shown in five of Guiraudon's patients, however, disappearance of preexcitation during dissection does not always prove that conduction over the accessory pathway has been definitely interrupted. Traction must have been the cause for temporary dysfunction of the pathway in these patients.

It is indeed questionable whether a closed heart technique is necessary to decrease mortality and morbidity. A carefully executed extracorporeal circulation and well-conducted perfusion reduces these risks to a minimum.

The danger of causing an inadvertent permanent AV block during the operation for a posteroseptal pathway is present in both techniques. It is related to the dissection of the mouth of the coronary sinus. Here it is possible to injure the AV node, which is located at the cranial site of the coronary sinus.

Disadvantages of Guiraudon's technique are that in some patients, especially in the left lateral pathways, the AV groove is extremely difficult to visualize, even with venting of the heart and extracorporeal circulation. A left lateral thoracotomy improves exposure of the left AV groove but limits the surgeon's mobility when a second, more difficultly located, accessory pathway is involved.

Some patients have concealed accessory pathways and disappearance of preexcitation cannot be used to guide the dissection, although it can be performed during circus movement tachycardia. The patient can also temporarily lose conduction properties over the accessory pathways during the operation. This can be caused by many factors including a decrease in circulating catecholamines, changes in body temperature, or manipulation. Lifting the heart can cause accessory pathways to lose their conducting properties.

Contrary to Sealy's technique, Guiraudon relies on a minimum of dissection. Cryoablation is then necessary to ablate or isolate deeper or broader extending accessory pathways. A further minor detail is that Guiraudon's technique for dissection of posteroseptal accessory pathways requires a median sternotomy incision that is extended further inferiorly than normal, up to 5 cm above the umbilicus.

Looking at the history and the development of different operative techniques, I believe it to be very important that the surgeon be familiar with the possibilities and disadvantages of each of the techniques. Depending upon information from pre- and intraoperative mapping, he should be able to decide at the right time whether to choose an endocardial, an epicardial, or even a combined approach, and to apply cryoablation when needed.

The ability to adapt one's technique to the circumstances will, in our opinion, result in the best possible results in the surgical treatment of the Wolff-Parkinson-White syndrome.

Acknowledgments: I am much indebted to Hein Wellens and Pedro Brugada in our combined search for the best treatment for patients with rhythm disturbances. I would also like to thank Joep Smeets, Pim Dassen, Jan Jonkers, en Bert v.d. Stelt for considerable technical support; my fellow associates Erik Jansen and Henry van Swieten for their cooperation; and our team of cardioanesthesiologists Chris Lawrence, Paul Roekaerts, Riet Smets, Ruud Timmer, and clinical perfusionists Dick de Jong, Ellen Retera, and Gijs Bastianen for their patience and expertise. Thanks also to our secretarial staff Anna Lemmens, Caroline Muurmans, and Helma Poesen for preparing the manuscript, and to the staff of our whole cardiothoracic unit for caring for the patients. The cooperation with Richard Hauer, J.F. Hitchcock (Utrecht), Diederik van Hoogenhuyze (Rotterdam), Leen van Wijk, Harry Crijns, and Tjark Ebels (Groningen) always was greatly appreciated. Finally, I would like to thank Jaques den Bakker, Frans van Capelle, and Michiel Janse, from the laboratory of experimental cardiology in Amsterdam, who took care for the peroperative mapping in Utrecht and Groningen.

References

1. Durrer D, Roos JP. Epicardial excitation of the ventricles in a patient with Wolff-Parkinson-White syndrome (type B). Circulation 1967;35:15–21.
2. Durrer D, Schoo L, Schuilenburg RM, Wellens HJJ. The role of premature beats in the initiation and the termination of supraventricular tachycardia in the Wolff-Parkinson-White syndrome. Circulation 1967;36:644–662.
3. Cobb FR, Blumenschein SD, Sealy WC, Boineau JP, Wagner GS, Wallace AG. Successful surgical interruption of the bundle of Kent in a patient with Wolff-Parkinson-White syndrome. Circulation 1968;38:1018–1029.
4. Fontaine GC, Guiraudon G, Bonnet M, Bernard JP, Potier JC, Grosgogeat J, Cabrol A, Cobrol C. Section d'un faisceau de Kent dans un cas de syndrome de Wolff-Parkinson-White de type AB. Arch Mal Coeur 1972;85:925–941.
5. Wellens HJJ, Janse MJ, van Dam RTh, van Capelle FJC, Meyne WG, Mellink HM, Durrer D. Epicardial mapping and surgical treatment in Wolff-Parkinson-White syndrome type A. Am Heart J 1974;88:69–78.
6. Wellens HJJ, Bär FWHM, Dassen WRM, Brugada P, Vanagt EJ, Farre J. Effects of drugs in the Wolff-Parkinson-White syndrome. Importance of initial length of effective refractory period of the accessory pathway. Am J Cardiol 1980;46:665–669.
7. Wellens HJJ, Braat S, Brugada P, Gorgels APM, Bär FWHM. Use of procainamide in patients with the Wolff-Parkinson-White syndrome to disclose a short refractory period of the accessory pathway. Am J Cardiol 1982;50:1087–1089.
8. Wellens HJJ. Value and limitations of programmed electrical stimulation of the heart in the study and treatment of tachycardias. Circulation 1978;57:845–853.
9. Wellens HJJ, Durrer D. Wolff-Parkinson-White syndrome and atrial fibrillation: Relation between refractory period of accessory pathway and ventricular rate during atrial fibrillation. Am J Cardiol 1974;777–782.
10. Klein GJ, Bashore TM, Sellers TD. Ventricular fibrillation in the Wolff-Parkinson-White syndrome. N Engl J Med 1979;301:1080–1085.
11. Registry on Sudden Death in the Wolff-Parkinson-White syndrome. Sudden death in the Wolff-Parkinson-White syndrome. (In preparation.)
12. Kent AFS. A conducting path between the right atrium and the external wall of the right ventricle in the heart of the mammal. J Physiol 1914:48,lvii.
13. Sealy WC, Gallagher JJ. The surgical approach to the septal area of the heart based on experiences with 45 patients with Kent bundles. J Thorac Cardiovasc Surg 1980;79:542–551.
14. Guarnieri T, Sealy WC, Kasell JH, German LD, Gallagher JJ. The non pharmacologic management of the permanent form of junctional reciprocating tachycardia. Circulation 1984;69(2):269–277.
15. Farré J, Ross D, Wiener J, Bär FW, Vanagt EJ, Wellens HJJ. Reciprocal tachycardias using accessory pathways with long conduction times. Am J Cardiol 1979;44:1099–1109.

16. Cox JL, Gallagher JJ, Cain ME. Experience with 118 consecutive patients undergoing operation for the Wolff-Parkinson-White Syndrome. J Thorac Cardiovasc Surg 1985;90: 490–501.
17. Klein GJ, Guiraudon GM, Perkins DG, Jones DL, Yee R, Jarvis E. Surgical correction of the Wolff-Parkinson-White Syndrome in the closed heart using cryosurgery. J Am Coll Cardiol 1984;3:405–409.
18. Klein GJ, Sealy WC, Pritchett EL, Harrison L, Hackel DB, Davis D, Kasell J, Wallace AG, Gallagher JJ. Cyrosurgical ablation of the atrioventricular node-His bundle: long-term follow-up and properties of the junctional pacemaker. Circulation 1980;61:8–15.
19. Guiraudon GM, Klein GJ, Sharma AD, Jones DL, McLellan DG. Surgical ablation of posterior septal accessory pathways in the Wolff-Parkinson-White Syndrome by a closed heart technique. J Thorac Cardiovasc Surg 1986;92:406–413.
20. Guiraudon GM, Klein GJ, Sharma AD, Jones DL, McLellan DG. Surgery for Wolff-Parkinson-White Syndrome: Further experience with an epicardial approach. Circulation 1986;74(3):525–529.
21. Guiraudon GM, Klein GJ. Closed heart surgery for Wolff-Parkinson-White Syndrome. Int J Cardiol 1984;5:387–391.
22. Guiraudon GM, Klein GJ, Jones DL, Kerr CR. Surgical treatment of Wolff-Parkinson-White syndrome. Can J Surg 1983;26(2):147–149.
23. Guiraudon GM, Klein GJ, Sharma AD, Milstein S, McLellan DG. Closed-heart technique for Wolff-Parkinson-White Syndrome: further experience and potential limitations. Ann Thorac Surg 1986;42:651–657.
24. Bredikis J, Bukauskas F, Zebraskaus R, Sakalauskas J, Loschilov V, Nevsky V, Bredikis A, Liakas R. Cryosurgical ablation of right parietal and septal accessory atrioventricular connections without the use of extracorporeal circulation. J Thorac Cardiovasc Surg 1985;90:206–211.
25. Gallagher JJ, Sealy WC, Cox JL, Kasell JH. Results of surgery for preexcitation in 200 cases. Circulation 1981;64(suppl. 4):146.

36

Surgical Treatment of Supraventricular Tachycardia Without the WPW Syndrome: Current Indications, Techniques, and Results

David L. Ross, David C. Johnson
Chee Choong Koo, Peter Mortensen
Mark J. Cooper, A. Robert Denniss
David A. Richards, John B. Uther

Introduction

Since Cobb, Sealy, and colleagues first described a successful operation in 1968,[1] curative surgery for supraventricular tachycardia has usually been limited to patients with Wolff-Parkinson-White (WPW) syndrome. This latter term is taken to include both classical WPW syndrome and those patients with concealed ventriculoatrial pathways. Curative surgery was not considered feasible for most other forms of supraventricular tachycardia and palliative ablation of the AV node-His bundle was usually performed if medical therapy failed. However, 56% of paroxysmal supraventricular tachycardias are not due to WPW syndrome,[2] and cardiologists found it frustrating to be unable to offer curative surgery to this majority. Beginning in the early 1980s, we[3] and others[4–12] therefore explored new curative surgical approaches for this latter group. Almost all of these arrhythmias now have surgical cure rates equal to the WPW syndrome. The types of arrhythmias which will be considered in this paper and their incidence in terms of cases presenting for electrophysiological study for supraventricular tachycardia[2] are: (1) AV junctional ("AV nodal") reentrant tachycardia (41% of cases), (2) atrial tachycardias, including inappropriate sinus tachycardia (7% of cases), (3) "nodo-ventricular fiber" tachycardias (2% of cases), and (4) atrial flutter and fibrillation (5% of cases).

Current Indications for Surgery

Supraventricular tachycardias not due to WPW syndrome are rarely fatal, although occasional deaths do occur due to the arrhythmia. Thus, risk of death is not an indication for surgery in this group. Failed medical therapy is a common indication for surgery. This is because extensive trials of several antiarrhythmic drugs do not prevent further recurrences of tachycardia in over 50% of cases, similar to clinical experience with WPW syndrome.

Patients undergoing cardiac surgery for other reasons can also be offered concomitant surgical cure of their arrhythmia without significant increase in operative risk. However, the most common current indication for surgery is patient preference for an attempt at surgical cure. This is based on the management strategy described in more detail below. This approach was developed because:

1. An erroneous diagnosis of anxiety is often made because the arrhythmia terminated before examination by a physician, and physical examination, ECG, and Holter monitors are usually normal.

2. Patients often do not complain of palpitations, but of chest pain, dyspnea, dizzy spells, or syncope instead. Often a paroxysmal arrhythmia is not even considered in the differential diagnosis of these symptoms.

3. Many physicians do not perceive just how troubled patients are by their "benign" arrhythmia. Years of wrong diagnosis, ineffective treatment, and diagnosis of "nerves" may have a profound effect on personality and approach to life. Certain occupations (pilots, train drivers, etc.) are not available to patients with paroxysmal tachycardias. Often employment is hard to obtain once a medical problem with recurrent tachycardias is mentioned. Life and health insurance may be difficult to obtain or more expensive. Certain sporting activities may become dangerous with paroxysmal tachycardias—rock climbing, diving, hang gliding, etc. These patients therefore end up with tunnel vision of the opportunities open to them in life.

4. Antiarrhythmic drug therapy is ineffective or causes significant side effects in over 50% of patients.

5. Most patients are young (teenagers or in their twenties) at the time of diagnosis and will require life-long therapy.

6. A majority of patients with AV junctional reentry are young women who wish to have further pregnancies. They are keen to avoid antiarrhythmic drugs.

7. Current surgical cure rates for non-WPW syndrome are very high and the

operative risk is very low and similar to closure of an uncomplicated secundum atrial septal defect.

8. Most physicians do not even mention the possibility of curative surgery to patients when long term treatment is first discussed.

9. Many physicians are very conservative in recommending curative surgery for supraventricular tachycardia and tend to wait too long, until the patient is desperate.

We therefore recommend the following strategy for management:

1. Perform an electrophysiological study early in all patients who feel significantly troubled by their symptoms and who either have documented supraventricular tachycardia or a history suggestive of a paroxysmal sustained arrhythmia.

2. Make an accurate electrophysiological diagnosis of the type(s) of tachycardia present and the locations of the tissues involved.

3. Present all the available options of therapy to the patient including no treatment, antiarrhythmic drugs, surgery, antitachycardia pacemaker, and catheter ablation. All the relevant risks and benefits pertaining to each mode of therapy should be explained in detail.

4. Let the patient weigh the severity of his/her symptoms and their wider effects on life against the risks and benefits of therapy and decide what general type of therapy he/she would prefer. The doctor's role is as an expert adviser, but it is the patient who chooses his/her sequence of therapy.

Approximately half of patients approached in this way choose surgery as an early option of therapy, fully accepting the small operative risk involved.

Techniques

Palliative techniques such as AV node-His bundle section will not be discussed since they are now either obsolete due to newer curative surgical techniques or superseded by catheter ablation of the conduction system.

Preoperative Investigation

Preoperative work-up includes electrophysiological study[2,13] with catheter mapping to make an accurate diagnosis, identification of the tissues of the arrhythmia circuit, and determination as accurately as possible of their locations. We stop all antiarrhythmic drugs 7 days before surgery. Amiodarone should be stopped 2–3 months before surgery.

Anesthesia

Routine premedication for surgery is omnopon or morphine (0.3 mg/kg). Anticholinergics are avoided because they may either cause increased arrhythmias or sometimes inhibit arrhythmia induction for mapping. It is important to withhold anticholinergics in cases with atrial or sinus node tachycardias because the resultant sinus tachycardia can be confused with the pathological arrhythmia.

Venous and arterial lines are inserted under local anesthesia. A triple-lumen CVP line is inserted via the internal jugular vein and Swan-Ganz catheters are avoided since they cross the operative field. Anesthesia is induced with thiopentone (2-3 mg/kg) and maintained with fentanyl (10-20 micrograms/kg initially with repeats as necessary) and halothane (0.5%, avoiding higher concentrations which tend to make arrhythmias harder to induce). Over the last 6 months, halothane has been replaced by isofluorane 1%, and arrhythmias seem easier to induce for mapping. Pancuronium (0.15-0.20 mg/kg) is used as a relaxant.

Perfusion

It is vitally important to maintain normothermia for mapping. Heating and space blankets may be required. We aim for a temperature of 37.5° to 38°C.

Two separate right-angled cannulae are placed in the superior and inferior venae cavae to give maximum exposure within the right atrium. With right atrial or sinus node tachycardias, it is wise to perform mapping before caval cannulation since atrial manipulation may make the arrhythmia noninducible. Otherwise, bypass is instituted before induction of tachycardia in all other types because tachycardia is not well tolerated hemodynamically under general anesthesia.

The pump priming solution should have physiological concentrations of potassium and high potassium solutions should be avoided. At the conclusion of mapping, the patient is cooled to 28°C, and St. Thomas cardioplegic solution administered (potassium 16 mmol/l, magnesium 16 mmol/l, and procaine 1 mmol/l) in a dose of 10-12 mls/kg. Pump flows are maintained at 2-2.4 l/m²/min but may be cautiously reduced to ¾ or even ½ flow if the return to the heart is too high and obscures the surgical field.

Mapping

We place reference electrodes on the left atrial appendage using a modified vascular clamp which serves as a clip electrode, and the right ventricular free wall using a plaque electrode sutured to the wall. The reference electrodes are used for recording and pacing. Surface ECG leads are placed on all four limbs and a back electrode is used for the V lead. A hand-held malleable probe with bipolar electrodes 1 mm apart is used for mapping.

Signals are passed via a junction box to a custom-made mapping system whose details (for a slightly modified system) have been described.[14] Direct cardiac signals are filtered with a band pass of 50-500 Hz. Signals are displayed on a storage oscilloscope with a graticuled screen. Any signal may be used to trigger the scope. A marker blip is generated 50 ms after triggering. The cardiac signals can be delayed by a variable delay bucket brigade circuit so that the blip may be positioned at will at onset of QRS or J junction, etc. The blip activates the counter. Counting is stopped when the probe signal is sensed, and the time is displayed in milliseconds on a beat to beat basis. The probe signal generates a second blip on the screen when it triggers so that the triggering point can be edited by altering the gain of the probe signal to ensure that triggering occurs on the appropriate part of the electrogram. All electrograms are simultaneously recorded on paper at 250 mm/sec on a Siemens Mingograf 804 to enable measurements to be checked and for long-term storage. Mapping is performed during the induced tachycardia by moving the probe to predetermined mapping sites (Fig 1.). When the area of interest has been localized, more detailed mapping is then performed. In AV junctional reentry, only endocardial sites adjacent to the tricuspid annulus are mapped, with detailed mapping from just anterior to the central fibrous body backwards to the mouth of the coronary sinus. There is no point in mapping other atrial sites more distant from the circuit in this type of arrhythmia.

For atrial tachycardias, epicardial mapping of both atria is performed then endocardial mapping of the appropriate atrium. Most atrial tachycardias originate from the right atrium in our experience. With nodoventricular fiber tachycardias, the ventricles are mapped to confirm that earliest activation during preexcitation is over the termination of the right bundle branch and not adjacent to the AV ring as in WPW syndrome. Atrial mapping during tachycardia shows earliest activation in the region of the AV node or in the region of concomitant accessory ventriculoatrial pathway(s). Stimulus to delta maps with atrial pacing have not been useful in our experience in determining where the proximal end of the anomalous pathway is located.

Tachycardia may be difficult to induce under general anesthesia. After attempts in the baseline state, isoprenaline in 5−10 mcg aliquots is given, and if that fails to facilitate induction, atropine 0.5−1.0 mg is given. Occasionally, no arrhythmia is inducible and the surgery must be based on the preoperative data from the electrophysiological study.

Usually mapping takes 5−20 minutes of normothermic bypass time. We arbitrarily set a maximum limit of 30 minutes since normothermic bypass, rapid pacing, tachycardia, and cardiac manipulation produce significant although potentially reversible mitochondrial changes and therefore should not be unduly prolonged.

Surgery

AV Junctional Reentry

There are two main types of AV junctional reentry which we designate types A and B.[3] In type A, the classical type, the VA interval in tachycardia is short (Fig. 2) and the earliest site of atrial activation in tachycardia is anterior to the AV node (Fig. 3). In this type, the right atrial wall is incised (from an endocardial approach) 2 mm above the tricuspid annulus starting just lateral to the mouth of the coronary sinus. The incision is carried medially to the apex of the triangle of Koch. The coronary sinus end is dissected down to the right ventricular free wall to ensure that the correct plane has been identified. The delicate atrium overlying the

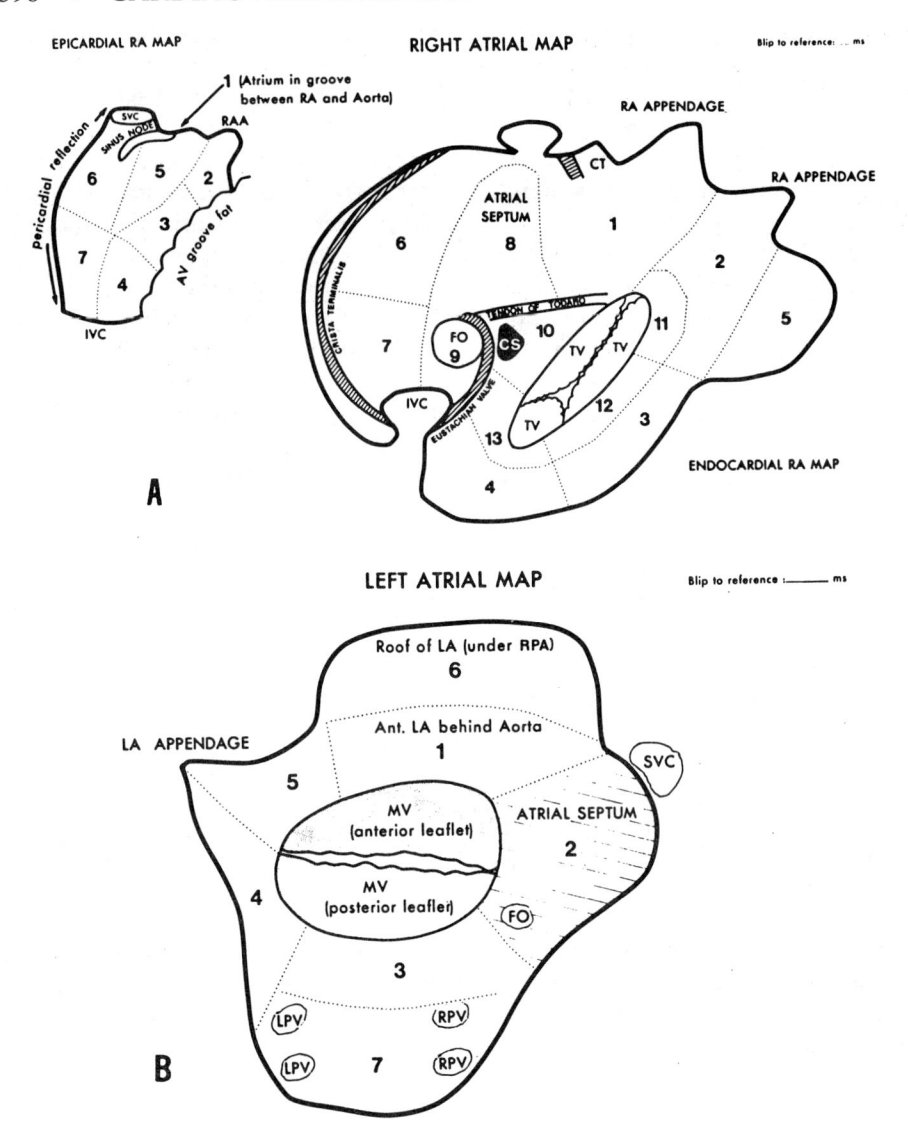

Figure 1 A,B: Schematic right and left atrial maps. Note that some regions adjacent to the AV groove are covered by epicardial fat and can only be mapped from the endocardium. Note also that the atrial septum is relatively small, and that the aorta lies behind area 1 in the right atrium. The AV node is located at the apex of the triangle of Koch designated as area 10. RA = right atrium; LA = left atrium, SVC = superior vena cava; IVC = inferior vena cava, CS = coronary sinus; FO = foramen ovale; TV = tricuspid valve; MV = mitral valve, PV = pulmonary vein; RPA = right pulmonary artery.

posterior space is then dissected free from the underlying fat, gradually exposing the AV nodal artery and vein, the tendon of Todaro, the left atrial septum, and the central fibrous body (Fig. 4). The AV node lies at the apex of the triangle of Koch and is usually visible as a slightly greyish-yellow tissue.

All atrial muscular connections overlying the central fibrous body and the medial border of the AV node are dissected free, gradually exposing the submu-

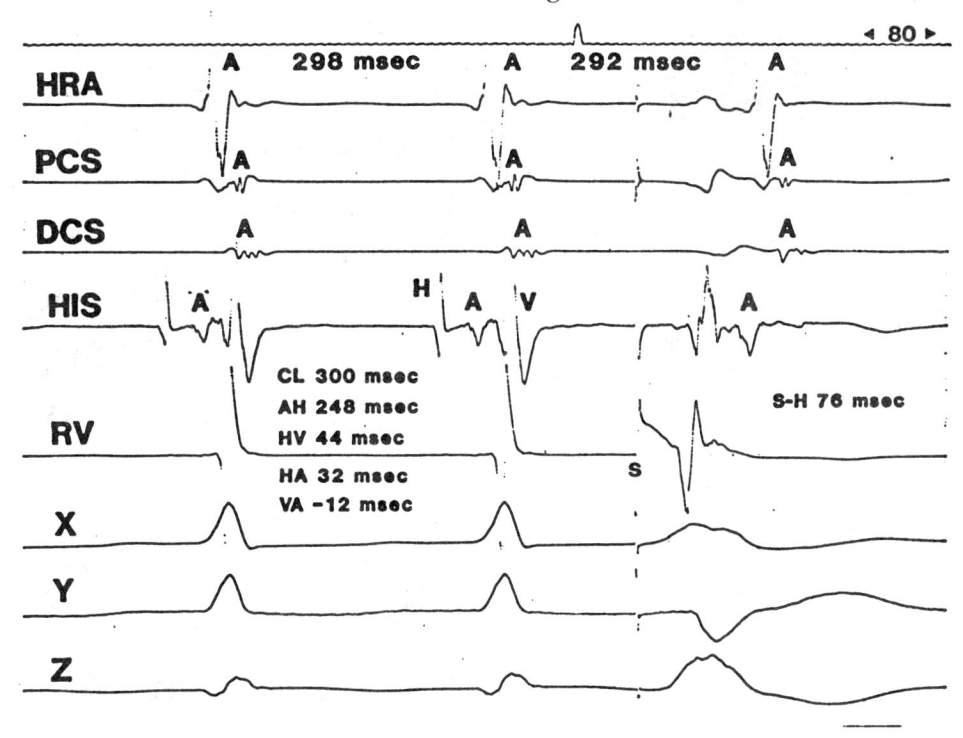

Figure 2: Electrophysiological tracings in a case of type A AV junctional reentry. Note that atrial activity precedes onset of ventricular activation, and that high right atrial (RA appendage) and atrial activation in the His bundle lead precede atrial activation in the coronary sinus electrograms. VA intervals in this type of tachycardia are usually less than 40 ms. Note that early ventricular extrastimuli (last complex) may advance atrial activation during tachycardia, but stimuli more than 50 ms before the His bundle electrogram are required. HRA = high right atrium; P (proximal) and D (distal) coronary sinus (CS); His = His bundle lead; RV = right ventricle; orthogonal surface Frank electrocardiographic leads X, Y and Z; A = atrial electrogram; H = His bundle electrogram; V = ventricular electrogram; S = extrastimulus.

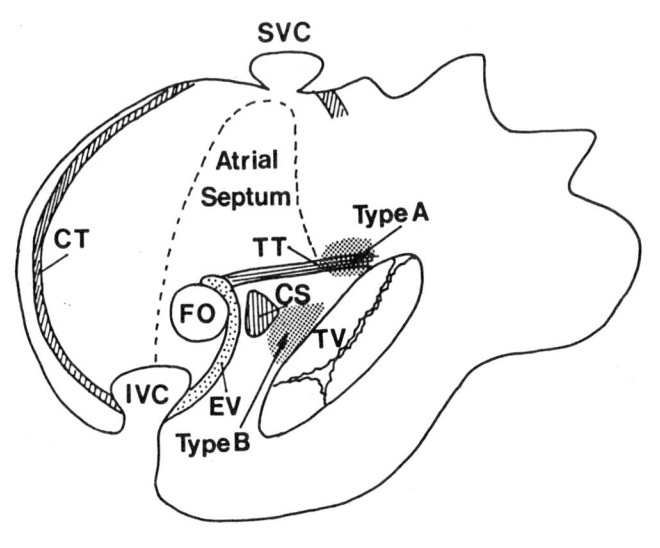

Figure 3: The regions of earliest activation during tachycardia on endocardial mapping are shown by the closely stippled areas. Activation in type A AV junctional reentrant tachycardia is anteromedial to the AV node, whereas in type B it is posterior to the AV node. TT = tendon of Todaro; CT = crista terminalis; other abbreviations are the same as in Figs. 1 and 2.

598 • CARDIAC ARRHYTHMIAS

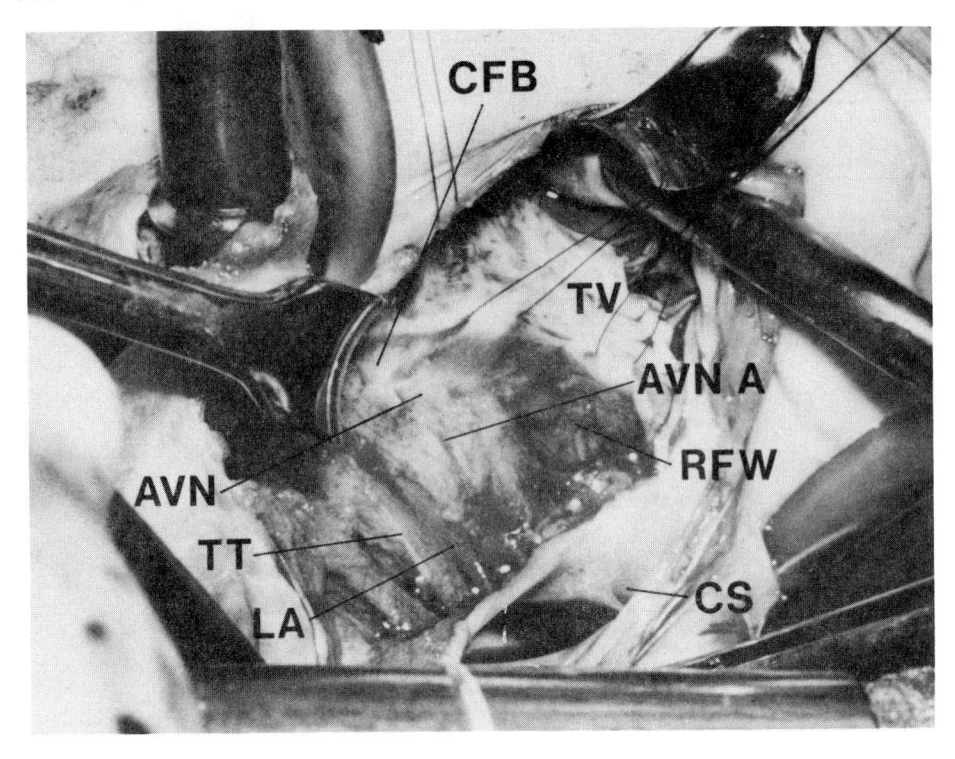

Figure 4: Operative photograph. The atrium overlying the posterior septal space has been reflected to display the tendon of Todaro (TT), left atrial septum (LA), AV node (AVN), the white gritty central fibrous body (CFB), posterior leaflet of the tricuspid valve (TV) pulled anteriorly by stay sutures, the AV nodal artery (AVNA), the right ventricular free wall (RFW) below the tricuspid annulus, and the orifice of the coronary sinus (CS).

cosa of the left atrium and sometimes the mitral annulus. The dissection is carried back along the medial border of the posterior space as far as the coronary sinus. The fat of the posterior space, which also contains atrial muscle and the posterior border of the space adjacent to the coronary sinus are left untouched so as to preserve atrium-to-AV node continuity. The incision is then closed with 4–0 prolene to minimize hematoma and prevent embolism. In the region of the central fibrous body, care should be taken to avoid damage to the conduction system.

In type B AV junctional reentry, the VA interval is longer than in type A (Fig. 5) and earliest atrial activation in tachycardia is recorded posterior to the AV node (Fig. 3). In the type B dissection, the posterior space is opened as above. However, the dissection down to the right ventricular free wall is carried under the vascular pedicle to the AV node, stripping fat and muscle off the ventricular surface just as in a posterior septal dissection for an atrioventricular pathway. In addition, the coronary sinus is dissected free from its attachments to posterior space tissue along the anterior and inferior surfaces of the coronary sinus from its orifice to opposite the left atrial septum. This dissection divides the posterior inputs to the AV node but preserves the medial and anterior septal inputs.

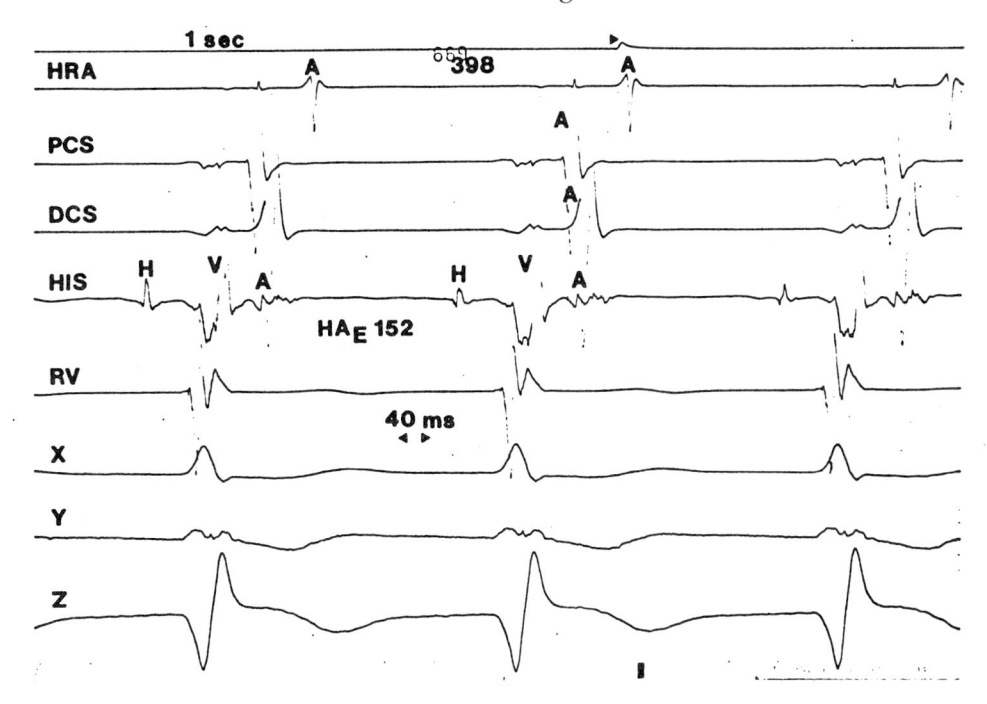

Figure 5: Electrophysiological tracings in a case of type B AV junctional reentry. Note that the VA interval is long, and that atrial activation occurs *after* ventricular activation. Earliest atrial activation is recorded in the region of the proximal coronary sinus. Abbreviations as used previously.

Atrial Tachycardias

Atrial tachycardias usually arise from the lateral wall of the right atrium, but may occur anywhere. A wide excision of the affected area is performed with repair by a pericardial patch. A wide excision, more than one would expect, is also necessary to excise the sinus node, again with repair by a pericardial patch to preserve the shape and volume of the atrium.

Nodoventricular Fibers

The exact anatomy comprising the tachycardia circuit in "nodoventricular fiber" tachycardia is unknown. The distal end of the fiber appears to insert into the right bundle branch. The name implies that the proximal end inserts into the AV node, but we and others[12] believe it is usually a totally separate AV pathway, possibly incorporating accessory AV nodal tissue. In many cases there are additional accessory pathways of standard WPW type. These are sectioned in the usual way.[15,16] A dissection from anterior to the central fibrous body along the anterior tricuspid annulus, identical to that performed for anterior right free wall atrioventricular accessory pathways, is performed for the "nodoventricular fiber."

Uncontrolled Atrial Fibrillation or Flutter

The traditional operation for this problem is His-bundle section. However, Holman et al. have developed a cryosurgical technique to modify AV nodal transmission,[17,18] and human trials have begun. It seems quite likely that this will prove to be clinically effective.

Results

AV Junctional Reentry

We designed and performed our first curative operation for AV junctional reentry in October 1983, and found excellent results in the first 10 patients.[3] To date, we have performed 48 operations in 47 patients with AV junctional reentry, 39 patients having type A tachycardia and eight having type B tachycardia. Ages ranged from 10 to 73 years. All had symptoms at least every few months, and the majority had at least weekly episodes of tachycardia. Median follow-up is 13 months. Recurrences of tachycardia have not occurred in 46 patients (96%), none of whom were taking antiarrhythmic drugs. Only one patient was inducible at a limited electrophysiological study prior to discharge, and she was a redo operation after a previous failed attempt at curative surgery.

We routinely schedule all patients for a comprehensive electrophysiological study 6 months after surgery to assess the final result. If the baseline study is negative, attempts at induction are repeated after isoprenaline and then atropine. To date, 34 patients have had 6 month studies. Both patients with symptoms suggestive of recurrence of supraventricular tachycardia were inducible. An additional two asymptomatic patients had inducible sustained AV junctional reentry. The arrhythmia was harder to induce in both these patients. Thus the electrophysiological failure rate is 12%. All four failures occurred in the third decade of our series where a less extensive dissection was being used because the initial results were so uniformly good. We have subsequently returned to the original method with a more vigorous dissection of the left atrial approaches to the AV node. One patient with recurrent symptoms underwent a second operation but this was also unsuccessful. However, we believe that it should be feasible to reoperate successfully and await further experience. All recurrences so far have been in type A tachycardias. There has been no operative mortality. Complete heart block occurred in one patient (2%). This patient has therefore had no recurrence of tachycardia, and with implantation of an Activitrax pacemaker has felt extremely well and is delighted with the clinical result. Significant perioperative complications have included pulmonary embolism (two patients), pericardial effusion (one patient), and major wound infection (two patients). The total incidence of a significant perioperative complication was 8% (one patient having both pulmonary embolism and pericardial effusion), similar to our findings with surgery for WPW syndrome.[16] An additional four patients had a postpericardiotomy syndrome some weeks after surgery which gradually resolved.

The overall clinical result has been excellent. Almost all patients report a marked improvement in well-being, often due to cessation of antiarrhythmic drug therapy as well as abolition of tachycardia. Cox has also reported long-term success in four patients using a cryosurgical procedure for AV junctional reentry.[4]

Atrial Tachycardia

We have operated on eight patients with atrial tachycardias. Median follow-up has been 5 years. Tachycardia has not recurred in seven (88%) patients who were not taking antiarrhythmic drugs. Tachycardia recurred in one patient. An additional five patients had surgery for inappropriate paroxysmal sinus tachycardia with no evidence for an extracardiac cause. Median follow-up has been 2 years. Symptoms were abolished in four (80%) patients. One patient had continued episodes of paroxysmal atrial tachycardia and required His-bundle ablation. There were no significant perioperative complications in these 13 patients. Two early patients had permanent pacemakers inserted as a precautionary measure. All patients have had a stable low atrial escape rhythm and the latter patients have not received prophylactic pacemakers and have had no problems.

Other workers have reported a variety of successful surgical approaches[4-11] for true atrial tachycardias in a small number of cases. Patients with atrial arrhythmias due to diffuse atrial disease should be expected to have lower surgical cure rates. We have observed that ablation of one focus may result in alternative foci being the cause of subsequent arrhythmias.

"Nodoventricular" Fiber Tachycardias

We have operated on three patients. One patient early in our experience had surgical AV node-His bundle ablation with preservation of conduction over the anomalous pathway. A permanent pacemaker was inserted as a precautionary measure because the durability of AV conduction over the anomalous pathway was unknown. The other two patients had successful section of the anomalous pathway with preservation of normal AV conduction. One patient also had a coexistent posterior septal accessory atrioventricular connection which was also successfully sectioned. All patients have been cured of their arrhythmia on long-term follow-up of 1 to 6 years without antiarrhythmic drugs. There have been no significant perioperative complications.

Gillette et al. have operated successfully on three patients with this type of tachycardia.[12] Their opinions about the anatomy of this pathway are similar to ours.

Uncontrolled Atrial Fibrillation or Flutter

These studies are in progress and no detailed reports of surgical outcomes have been published yet.

Conclusions

Surgery for supraventricular tachycardia without the WPW syndrome is as safe and as effective as AV accessory pathway surgery. We believe that the indications for surgery should be expanded for these patients, and that they should be offered surgery as one of the options of treatment when long-term therapy is first discussed in patients significantly troubled by their symptoms.

References

1. Cobb FR, Blumenschein SD, Sealy WC, Boineau JP, Wagner GS, Wallace AG. Successful surgical interruption of the bundle of Kent in a patient with Wolff-Parkinson-White syndrome. Circulation 1968;38:1018–1029.
2. Ross DL, Denniss AR, Uther JB. Electrophysiological study in supraventricular arrhythmias. In Schroeder JS, Brest AN, eds. Invasive Cardiology Cardiovascular Clinics. Philadelphia, FA Davis, 1985;187–213.
3. Ross DL, Johnson DC, Denniss AR, Cooper MJ, Richards DA, Uther JB. Curative surgery for atrioventricular junctional ("AV nodal") reentrant tachycardia. JACC 1985;6:1383–1392.
4. Cox JL. The status of surgery for cardiac arrhythmias. Circulation 1985;71:413–417.
5. Coumel PH, Aigueperse J, Perrault MA, Fantoni A, Slama R, Bouvrain Y. Reparge et tentative d'exerese chirugical d'un foyer ectopique auriculaire gauche avec tachycardie rebelle: Evolution favorable. Ann Cardiol Angeiol 1973;22:189–199.
6. Wyndham CRC, Arnsdorf MF, Levitsky S, Smith TC, Dhingra RC, Denes P, Rosen KM. Successful surgical excision of focal paroxysmal atrial tachycardia: Observations in vivo and in vitro. Circulation 1980;62:1365–1372.
7. Gillette PC, Garson A, Hesslein PS, Karpawich PP, Tierney RC, Cooley DA, McNamara DG. Successful surgical treatment of atrial, junctional and ventricular tachycardia unassociated with accessory connections in infants and children. Am Heart J 1981;102:984–991.
8. Anderson KP, Stinson EB, Mason JW. Surgical exclusion of focal paroxysmal atrial tachycardia. Am J Cardiol 1982;49:869–874.
9. Josephson ME, Spear JF, Harken AH, Horowitz LN, Dorio RJ. Surgical excision of automatic atrial tachycardia: Anatomic and electrophysiologic correlates. Am Heart J 1982;104:1076–1085.
10. Olsson SB, Blomstrom P, Sabel K, William-Olsson G. Incessant ectopic atrial tachycardia: Successful surgical treatment with regression of dilated cardiomyopathy picture. Am J Cardiol 1984;53:1465–1466.
11. Iwa T, Ichihashi T, Hashizume Y, Ishida K, Okada R. Successful surgical treatment of left atrial tachycardia. Am Heart J 1985;109:160–162.
12. Gillette PC, Garson A, Cooley DA, McNamara DG. Prolonged and decremental antegrade conduction properties in right anterior accessory connections: Wide QRS antidromic tachycardia of left bundle branch block pattern without Wolff-Parkinson-White configuration in sinus rhythm. Am Heart J 1982;103:66–74.
13. Ross DL, Uther JB. Diagnosis of concealed accessory pathways in supraventricular tachycardia. PACE 1984;7:1069–1085.
14. Rosenfeldt FL, Harper RW, Wall RE, Uther JB, Hilder R, Shardey GC. A digital timing and display unit for intraoperative mapping of cardiac arrhythmias. PACE 1984;7:985–992.
15. Johnson DC, Nunn GR, Richards DA, Uther JB, Ross DL. Surgery for supraventricular tachycardia, a potentially curable disorder. J Thorac Cardiovasc Surgery (in press, 1987).

16. Sealy WC, Gallagher JJ. Surgical treatment of left free wall accessory pathways of atrioventricular conduction of the Kent type. J Thorac Cardiovasc Surg 1981;81:698–706.
17. Holman WL, Ikeshita M, Lease JG, Smith PK, Ferguson TB, Cox JL. Elective prolongation of atrioventricular conduction by multiple discrete cryolesions: A new technique for the treatment of paroxysmal supraventricular tachycardia. J Thorac Cardiovasc Surg 1982;84:554–559.
18. Holman WL, Ikeshita M, Lease JG, Ferguson TB, Lofland GK, Cox JL. Alteration of antegrade atrioventricular conduction by cryoablation of periatrioventricular nodal tissue. J Thorac Cardiovasc Surg 1984;88:67–75.

37

Preoperative and Intraoperative Mapping of Ventricular Tachycardia: Is it Necessary for the Success of Surgical Treatment?

Isaac Wiener

Introduction

Ventricular tachycardia is a life-threatening manifestation of coronary artery disease. Chronic recurrent ventricular arrhythmias are associated with areas of post-infarction ventricular scar. A direct attack on the offending myocardium has great intellectual appeal and becomes clinically necessary when conventional therapies are unsuccessful. A variety of approaches are currently employed for the operative treatment of ventricular tachycardia associated with myocardial scar. We will examine these approaches and evaluate the importance of preoperative and intraoperative mapping.

In 1959, Couch reported the successful surgical removal of aneurysmal ventricular scar. Numerous other case reports followed. However, when Ostermeyer et al. reviewed the cases reported in the literature, they reported a 39% success rate in 160 patients.[1] Although these studies are retrospective and do not allow for improvements in surgery, simple aneurysmectomy appears to be an unacceptable approach to surgery for ventricular tachycardia.

A more sophisticated approach to surgery for ventricular tachycardia was possible only after major advances in our understanding of the mechanism of the

From: Brugada P, Wellens HJJ. CARDIAC ARRHYTHMIAS: Where To Go From Here? Mount Kisco, NY, Futura Publishing Company, Inc., © 1987.

arrhythmia. The pioneering work of Professor Wellens using techniques of electrical stimulation suggested that the mechanism of chronic, recurrent sustained ventricular tachycardia was reentrant.[2] Subsequent studies using both left ventricular catheter recordings[3] and intraoperative recordings[4] suggested that the site of reentry was the border zone between aneurysmal tissue and normal tissues, frequently along the interventricular septum. The poor results of simple aneurysmectomy were ascribed to failure to excise the border zone of the aneurysm, particularly when it involved the septum. A variety of operations for ventricular tachycardia were developed. The operations can be classified as visually guided (encircling endocardial ventriculotomy, extensive endocardial resection), and electrically guided (activation sequence mapping, pace mapping, and sinus rhythm mapping).

Visually Guided Operations

The encircling endocardial ventriculotomy employs an incision at the visually identified border between the endocardial fibrosis and surrounding myocardium with normal appearance. The incision is made around the entire circumference of the aneurysm up to the subepicardium on the left ventricular free wall and 1 cm deep on the septum. Initially the incision was performed perpendicular to the endocardial plane but this was subsequently modified to an oblique incision attempting to follow the plane between normal and abnormal myocardium. After completion, the incision is repaired. Encircling endocardial ventriculotomy may exert its beneficial effect by isolating the arrhythmogenic area or by interrupting reentrant pathways in the border zone. In a series of 27 patients with refractory ventricular tachycardia who underwent encircling endocardial ventriculotomy, there was an 18% operative mortality. Of the survivors, over a 1 to 2 year follow-up, 95% had no ventricular tachycardia (72% surgery alone, 23% surgery plus antiarrhythmic drugs).[5]

Moran et al. introduced the technique of visually directed extensive endocardial excision. In this operation, all areas of white endocardial scar are resected from the underlying myocardium. Mitral valve replacement was performed in 13% of patients in whom dense scarring involved papillary muscles.[6] In 79 patients (51 sustained ventricular tachycardia and 28 ventricular fibrillation), there was a 13% operative mortality. Of the survivors, over a 27 ± 15 months follow-up, 84% (including some treated with medication) remained free of ventricular tachycardia.[7]

Map Guided Operations

Electrically guided operations use preoperative and intraoperative electrical recordings in an attempt to guide the surgeon to those areas of the ventricle where tachycardia originates. The most widely employed approach is activation sequence mapping. In this approach, a roving probe is introduced through the ventriculotomy and electrograms are recorded from multiple endocardial sites during induced ventricular tachycardia. Particular attention is directed to the endocardial border zone of the aneurysm. The earliest site of activation is presumed to be the focus of origin of the tachycardia and that site, with a margin of 1 to 1½ cm on each side and 1 to 2 mm thick, is excised. As some tachycardias may not be inducible in the operating room, preoperative catheter mapping is essential. In a series of 100 patients, there was a 9% operative mortality. Of the survivors, over a 28 ± 19 months follow-up, 91% were free of ventricular tachycardia (66% surgery alone, 25% surgery plus antiarrhythmic medications).[8] Other electrically guided approaches include pace mapping which defines the site of origin of the tachycardia by the site where the morphology of paced beats matches the tachycardia.[9] Sinus rhythm mapping directs attention to areas that demonstrate fractionated electrograms in sinus rhythm.[10,11] These methods appear to resect larger areas of myocardium than activation sequence mapping. A sufficient number of patients has not been studied to allow conclusions.

Comparison of Visually and Map Guided Approaches

At the current time, a direct comparison, ensuring comparable patient populations, of visually guided and map guided surgery is not possible. Moreover, it seems unlikely that a prospective randomized trial will be performed. It is possible, however, to define unique advantages and disadvantages of each approach.

Advantages and Disadvantages of Visually Guided Operations

The visual approaches have an acceptable success rate and obviate the need for preoperative and intraoperative mapping. A major concern with visually guided surgery is whether excessive amounts of myocardium are being sacrificed. Experimental studies of encircling endocardial ventriculotomy have demonstrated a marked decrease in regional blood flow and concomitant depression of regional myocardial function of any nonfibrosed tissue that is encircled.[12] Detailed pre- and postoperative hemodynamic studies are not available for encircling endocardial ventriculotomy, but damage to myocardium may result in an increased mortality from pump failure and progressive postoperative left ventricular failure.[13] An advantage of encircling endocardial ventriculotomy is that the posterior papillary muscle may be safely encircled without compromising mitral valve function. However, the ventriculotomy cannot be safely extended to the mitral or aortic annulus to complete the encirclement. Completion of the encirclement with cryolesions adjacent to the annulus has been described.[14] Encircling endocardial cryoablation may eventually be an alternative to encircling endocardial ventriculotomy with less adverse effects on myocardial function. In a preliminary report of 16 patients, there was one operative death, 14 patients cured with surgery alone, and one patient cured with surgery and antiarrhythmic medication. Average ejection fraction increased from .36 to .45.[15]

Despite the extent of the operation, extensive endocardial resection is generally well tolerated hemodynamically, presumably because only abnormal myocardium is removed. In one series, mean ejection fraction increased from 29% preoperatively to 35% postoperatively.[16] A concern with extensive endocardial excision is that fibrosis frequently involves the papillary muscle. Mitral valve replacement may be performed in some patients undergoing extensive excision despite the fact that the apparatus may not have been involved in the arrhythmia.

Advantages and Disadvantages of Map Guided Surgery

Map guided surgery allows operations to be performed in patients whose visual landmarks are unclear and allows excision of a smaller amount of myocardium than visually directed surgery. A concern is that the prolonged period (30 to 55 minutes)[8] on bypass at normothermia required for mapping might be injurious for some patients. The hemodynamics of subendocardial resection have been well studied, and in a series of 62 patients, ejection fraction increased from $28 \pm 9\%$ preoperatively to $39 \pm 10\%$ postoperatively.[17]

However, activation sequence mapping has important limitations. Mapping requires the ability to induce stable sustained ventricular tachycardia. In some patients, this may not be possible in the operating room under general anesthesia or may be possible initially but become impossible after the ventriculotomy is performed. In these patients, surgery must be based on the results of preoperative catheter mapping. While the earliest site of activation determined by catheter mapping falls within 4–8 cm^2 of intraoperative findings, the catheter technique does result in some loss of precision.[18] In other patients, ventricular tachycardia may be induced in the operating room but is so rapid that it degenerates to ventricular fibrillation making mapping impossible. Pleomorphic ventricular tachycardia has constantly changing activation patterns and cannot be mapped with conventional techniques. For some ventricular tachycardias, the onset of QRS may not be distinct and it may be difficult to define earliest sites. Activation sequence mapping data may not be obtainable in up to 36% of tachycardias.[19]

Moreover, up to 81% of patients with sustained ventricular tachycardia have multiple clinical and nonclinical morphologies. It is important to realize that sustained ventricular tachycardias that are induced in the laboratory or operating room but not documented clinically recur after surgery as often as clinical tachycardias.[20] Mapping and excision of the earliest site of each tachycardia is necessary and not all morphologies may be induced at a given time. While some different morphologies may originate from the same site, as many as 47% may have different sites of origin.[19,21] It has been demonstrated that failure of subendocardial resection correlates with the presence of multiple morphologies of tachycardia.[8]

Subendocardial resection is also less successful for patients with inferior wall infarctions. The endocardium of this region is highly trabeculated and may make peeling a homogeneous layer of tissue more difficult. The proximity of the mitral valve apparatus may limit the size of the resection. Cryothermy, by destroying electrically active tissue while leaving structural elements intact, may be helpful in this location.[22]

Perhaps most important, the concept that the earliest site of activation represents the micro-reentrant origin of tachycardia probably does not apply to all patients. In some patients, the site of origin may be in fibrotic tissue from which electrograms cannot be recorded. In a sizable percentage of patients, VT may represent a macro-reentrant circuit without identifiable earliest site.[23,24]

Combined Approaches

At the current time it seems that an eclectic approach combining different modalities and selecting the operation based on the anatomy and electrical findings in the individual patient would be most appropriate.[14,25,26] Preoperative catheter mapping should be done whenever possible to aid in this selection. Patients who appear to be poor surgical candidates based on preoperative hemodynamic and electrical studies should be considered for alternative therapy, i.e., automatic implantable defibrillator. For patients in whom all morphologies of ventricular tachycardia can be induced and mapped and have an earliest activation site in an accessible location, endocardial resection seems preferable. Cryoablation should be considered for patients with clearcut early sites in surgically inaccessible locations, i.e., papillary muscles. For patients who cannot be adequately mapped, a visually guided procedure is used. For large anterior aneurysms, this would probably be an extensive endocardial resection, while for patients with posterior aneurysms, this might be an encircling endocardial ventriculotomy or variation thereof.

Another example of a combined approach is the map-directed regional approach. Krafchek et al.[27] performed activation sequence mapping of each morphology of ventricular tachycardia (90% of morphologies mapped, 76% of morphologies with preoperative catheter maps, 28% of morphologies with intraoperative maps). In addition to resecting the earliest site of activation of each morphology, all sites with activation before QRS were excised, resulting in a wide excision including up to 40 cm^2 of endocardium. Supplemental cryothermy was used for foci found in papillary muscles, near valve annuli or outside of scar areas, or when full-thickness ablation of the septum was required. The earliest site of activation was outside visible scar in 10 of 35 patients. (However, in view of difficulties interpreting earliest sites, this finding does not prove that resection of all scarred areas would have been unsuccessful.) With the regional approach in 25 patients, there was a 4% operative mortality. Of survivors, with a follow-up of 17 ± 10 months, 100% of patients are free of arrhythmia (96% surgery alone, 4% surgery plus medication). Results were not affected by the presence of multiple morphologies, disparate sites of origin, or inferior wall foci.

Newer Types of Mapping

Several technical improvements are likely to enhance the usefulness of mapping. Mapping using a balloon with multiple electrodes to allow simultaneous recordings from multiple sites will yield more accurate information about activation patterns and will greatly speed the time required.[27] Introduction of the mapping balloon through the left atrium allows mapping before the ventriculotomy and may increase the ability to induce tachycardias.[29] A mathematical analysis of catheter mapping has been described which develops a wire skeleton representation of arrhythmogenic sites. This wire skeleton is inserted into the left ventricle at the time of surgery to identify arrhythmogenic sites. This technique may substantially increase the accuracy of catheter mapping and lead to better surgical results for those tachycardias that are not induced in the operating room.[30]

All of the current approaches were developed following the recognition of the importance of the border zone in the origin of ventricular arrhythmias. Further advances in surgical therapy will result from further advances in our understanding of the mechanism of ventricular tachycardia.

As discussed above, some tachycardias have been shown to represent large reentrant circuits without a clearcut earliest site. Identifying the tissue which forms a crucial part of such a circuit may represent an important theoretical and practical advance. Gallagher et al. studied patients with induced sustained ventricular tachycardia and identified the site where cooling with a cryoprobe reproducibly terminated ventricular tachycardia.[31] The cryo termination site was associated with diastolic activity during ventricular tachycardia and late potentials during normal sinus rhythm but differed from the site of earliest activation in five of seven patients. In most patients, both the earliest site and the cryo termination site were excised. However, in one operative survivor, only the cryo termination site was excised and ventricular tachycardia was not inducible postoperatively. This type of mapping offers physiologic information beyond timing of electrograms. Findings in patients with multiple morphologies will be of particular interest.

Another impetus to refinement of mapping techniques is the development of catheter ablative techniques to treat refractory ventricular tachycardia. As endocardial visual landmarks do not exist in the catheterization laboratory, electrical guidance becomes even more crucial. Most ablation studies have used activation sequence mapping to identify sites of earliest activation. We have recently identified left ventricular sites with abnormal electrograms where extrastimuli entrained the tachycardia with marked conduction delay without changing the morphology of the QRS or right ventricular electrograms. These findings may indicate that stimulation is occurring in close proximity to the tachycardia circuit and may aid in localizing sites for surgical or catheter ablation.[32]

Summary

In summary, while surgery for ventricular arrhythmias can be accomplished without mapping, mapping may improve the success rate and is likely to result in conservation of myocardium. Patients undergoing surgery for ventricular tachycardia should have preoperative and intraoperative mapping performed whenever possible, although the most appropriate type of mapping and the proper application of mapping findings are not fully defined. Visual techniques will continue to be important as an adjunct to mapping.

References

1. Ostermeyer J, Breithardt G, Kolvenbach R, Borggrete M, Seipel L, Schulte H, Bircks W. The surgical treatment of ventricular tachycardias. J Thorac Cardiovasc Surg 1982;84:704–715.
2. Wellens HJ, Schuilenberg RM, Durrer D. Electrical stimulation of the heart in patients with ventricular tachycardia. Circulation 1972;46:216–230.
3. Josephson ME, Horowitz LN, Farshidi A, Spear JF, Kastor JA, Moore GV. Recurrent sustained ventricular tachycardia: 2. Endocardial mapping. Circulation 1978;57:440–7.
4. Wiener I, Mindich B, Pitchon R. Determinants of ventricular tachycardia in patients with ventricular aneurysms: Results of intraoperative epicardial and endocardial mapping. Circulation 1982;65:856–862.
5. Guiraudon G, Fontaine G, Frank R, Cabral C, Grosgozent Y. Apport de la ventriculomie circulaere d'exclusion: dans le traitment de la tachycardie ventriculaire recidivante apres infarctus du myocarde. Arch Mol Coeur 1982;75:1013–1020.
6. Moran J, Kehoe R, Loeb J, Fredrickson J, Zheutlin T, Sanders J, Michaelis L. The role of papillary muscle resection and mitral valve replacement in the control of refractory ventricular arrhythmia. Circulation 1983;68:II–154.
7. Kehoe R, Zheutlin T, Finkelmeier B, Steinman R, Loeb J, Michaelis L, Moran J. Visually directed endocardial resection for ventricular arrhythmia: long term outcome and functional status (abstr). JACC 1985;5:497.
8. Miller J, Kienzle M, Harken A, Josephson M. Subendocardial resection for ventricular tachycardia: Predictors of surgical success. Circulation 1984;70:624–631.
9. Josephson ME, Waxman HL, Cain ME, Gardner M, Buxton AE. Ventricular activation during ventricular endocardial pacing II. Role of pace-mapping to localize origin of ventricular tachycardia. Am J Cardiol 1982;50:11–22.
10. Wiener I, Mindich B, Pitchon R. Fragmented endocardial electrical activity in patients with ventricular tachycardia: A new guide to surgical therapy. Am Heart J 1984;107:86–90.
11. Kienzle M, Miller J, Falcone R, Harken A, Josephson ME. Intraoperative endocardial mapping during sinus rhythm: Relationship to site of origin of ventricular tachycardia. Circulation 1984;70:957–965.
12. Ungerleider RM, Holman WL, Calcagno D, Williams JM, Lofland GK, Smith PK, Stanley TE III, Quick G, Cox JL. Encircling endocardial ventriculotomy for refractory ischemic ventricular tachycardia III: Effects on regional left ventricular function. J Thorac Cardiovasc Surg 1982;83:857–864.
13. Ostermeyer J, Breithardt G, Borggrete M, Godehart E, Seigel L, Bircks W. Surgical treatment of ventricular tachycardias. J Thorac Cardiovasc Surg 1984;87:517–525.
14. Cox JL, Gallagher JJ, Ungerleider R. Encircling ventriculotomy for refractory ischemic ventricular tachycardia. J Thorac Cardiovasc Surg 1982;83:865–872.
15. Guiraudon G, Klein G, Jones D, McLellan D. Encircling endocardial cryoablation for ventricular arrhythmias after myocardial infarction: Further experience (abstr). Circulation 1985;72:III–222.
16. Gardner M, Landymore R, Johnstone D, Kinley CE. Visually directed endocardial resection for recurrent ventricular tachycardia: Long-term results and effects on LV function (abstr). Circulation 1985;72:III–221.
17. Martin J, Untereker W, Harken A, Horowitz L, Josephson M. Aneurysmectomy and endocardial resection for ventricular tachycardia: Favorable hemodynamics and antiarrhythmic results in patients with global left ventricular dysfunction. Am Heart J 1982;103:960–966.
18. Josephson ME, Horowitz LN, Farshidi A, Spielman SR, Michelson EL, Greenspan AM. Comparison of endocardial catheter mapping with intraoperative mapping of ventricular tachycardia. Circulation 1980;61:395–404.
19. Waspe LE, Bradman R, Kim SG, Matos JA, Johnston D, Scavin G, Fisher JD. Activation mapping in patients with coronary artery disease with multiple ventricular tachycardia configurations: Occurrence and therapeutic implications of widely separate apparent sites of origin. JACC 1985;5:1075.

20. Miller J, Kienzle M, Harken A, Josephson ME. Morphologically distinct sustained ventricular tachycardias in coronary artery disease: Significance and surgical results. JACC 1984;4:1073.
21. Beckman K, Cheirif J, Krafchek J, Lin H, Lawrie G, Magro S, Wyndham C. Multiple QRS morphologies of ventricular tachycardia imply multiple sites of origin (abstr). Circulation 1986;74:II−186.
22. Klein GJ, Harrison L, Ideker RF, Smith WM, Kosell J, Wallace AG, Gallagher JJ. Reaction of myocardium in cryosurgery: Electrophysiology and arrhythmagenic potential. Circulation 1979;59:364−372.
23. Mason J, Stimson E, Oyer P, Winkle R, Anderson KP. Arrhythmia mechanisms and outcome in surgery for recurrent ventricular tachycardia (abstr). Circulation 1983;68: III−176.
24. Miller J, Harken AH, Hargrove C, Josephson M. Pattern of endocardial activation during sustained ventricular tachycardia. JACC 1985;6:1280−1287.
25. Anderson KP, Mason JW. Surgical management of ventricular tachyarrhythmias. Clin Cardiol 1983;6:415−425.
26. Kron I, Lerman B, Dimarco J. Extended subendocardial resection: A surgical approach to ventricular tachyarrhythmias that cannot be mapped intraoperatively. J Thorac Cardiovasc Surg 1985;90:586−591.
27. Krafchek J, Lawrie G, Roberts R, Magro S, Wyndham C. Surgical ablation of ventricular tachycardia: improved results with a map-directed regional approach. Circulation 1986;73:1239−1247.
28. Harris L, Downar E, Mickleborough L, Parson J. Activation sequence in human ventricular tachycardia (abstr). Circulation 1985;72:III−476.
29. Mickleborough L, Harris L, Downer E, Parson I, Gray G. A new approach for mapping ventricular tachycardia (abstr). Circulation 1985;72:III−222.
30. Hauer R, De Zwart M, Bakker J, Hitchcock J, Penn O, Nysen-Karelse M, Robles de Medina E. Endocardial catheter mapping: Wire skeleton technique for representation of computed arrhythmogenic sites compared with intraoperative mapping. Circulation 1986;74:1346−1354.
31. Gallagher JD, Del Ross A, Fernandez J, Maranho V, Strong M, White M, Gessman L. Cryothermal mapping of recurrent ventricular tachycardia in man. Circulation 1985;72: 733−739.
32. Stevenson W. Weiss J, Wiener I, Nademonec K, Wohl-gelerter D, Yeatman L, Josephson M. Entrainment as a guide for localizing the site of ventricular tachycardia for catheter ablation (abstr). JACC, in press.

38

Intraoperative Computerized Mapping Techniques: Do They Help Us to Treat Our Patients Better Surgically?

James L. Cox

Introduction

The early work of Dirk Durrer, Hein Wellens, John Boineau, Madison Spach, Andrew Wallace, and many others made it possible to use intraoperative epicardial mapping techniques to characterize the activation patterns in normal and abnormal human hearts. One of our first clinical applications of intraoperative electrophysiology was to show the surgeon where to bury the end of the internal mammary artery in the myocardium of the left ventricle when performing a Vineberg procedure.[1,2] The year was 1968, coronary bypass surgery was not yet being performed clinically, and certainly not many surgeons would contemplate operating on the heart for *arrhythmia* control! How could a responsible surgeon consider operating on something that he could not see? Thus, the two-point intraoperative mapping system, consisting of one fixed and one roving epicardial electrode, was a clinical oddity and the operating room was a hostile environment for any cardiologist who dared to enter the inner sanctum of the surgeon's turf. On a bright spring day that year, however, the once-inviolable iron curtain of the operating theater was irrevocably shattered by a single operation—the first successful surgical correction of the Wolff-Parkinson-White syndrome by Dr. Will Sealy on May 28, 1968.[3] Not only was an invisible cardiac abnormality surgically

From: Brugada P, Wellens HJJ. CARDIAC ARRHYTHMIAS: Where To Go From Here? Mount Kisco, NY, Futura Publishing Company, Inc., © 1987.

614 • CARDIAC ARRHYTHMIAS

corrected that day, but the absolute necessity for a team approach to the surgical treatment of cardiac arrhythmias was established. For the first time, a cardiac surgeon had found it necessary to depend on eyes other than his own and the era of arrhythmia surgery guided by intraoperative electrophysiologic mapping was born.

Single-Point Intraoperative Mapping Systems

A schematic representation of the basic system we originally used for the intraoperative mapping is shown in Figure 1.[4] The system employed one fixed and one roving electrode. The recorded epicardial data were related to the surface of the heart by using an arbitrary grid composed of 53 points.[5] Local activation was determined on a point-by-point basis with the roving, hand-held electrode and the difference in activation times recorded by this electrode and the fixed reference electrode was recorded. The first time-saving modification of the system was to add the digital activation timer which allowed a preliminary scan of the

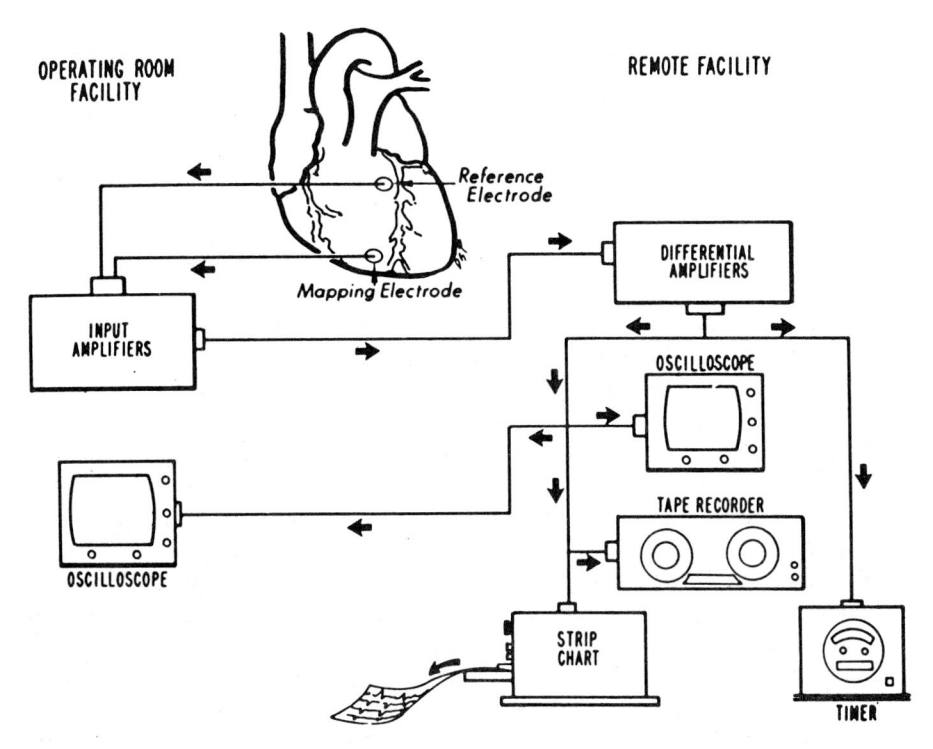

Figure 1: A typical single-point intraoperative mapping system used in the operating theater is depicted. Data recorded from a reference and a roving electrode are relayed by buffer amplifiers in the operating room to a remote facility. The activation data are then relayed by differential amplifiers to a digital timer with simultaneous display on an oscilloscope operating in parallel with an oscilloscope in the operating room. All analog data are permanently stored on a magnetic tape and can be intermittently displayed in graphic form by a strip chart recorder (reproduced from Gallagher et al.[4] with permission of the American Heart Association, Inc.).

heart to be made so that the area of most interest could then be mapped in greater detail. This basic system has been used for intraoperative mapping in patients with the Wolff-Parkinson-White (WPW) syndrome for nearly two decades and is still used by most centers for all types of arrhythmia surgery.

Although the single-point system was adequate in most patients with the WPW syndrome, several limitations were noted over the years as progressively more complex cases presented for surgery. It was frequently impossible, for example, to identify the site of ventricular preexcitation in patients with only intermittent antegrade conduction across the accessory pathway. In such patients, one frequently had to depend entirely on the retrograde atrial map recorded during induced reciprocating tachycardia or ventricular pacing. The problem was compounded if the patient had atrial fibrillation with only intermittent antegrade preexcitation because the retrograde map could not be performed. Intraoperative mapping with a single-point system in such a patient is virtually impossible. Another problem inherent with this mapping system was the necessity for excessive cardiac manipulation and retraction of the apex of the heart out of the pericardium in order to map the posterior surface of the heart where most accessory pathways are located. This frequently resulted in conduction block across the accessory pathway, thereby precluding further mapping until conduction returned. The retraction and manipulation of the heart also dictated that cardiopulmonary bypass be employed to accomplish satisfactory mapping in most instances. It was also frequently difficult to identify multiple accessory pathways in patients with this type of mapping system, especially if one or more of the pathways were concealed. This was no minor consideration since 20% of our patients undergoing surgery for WPW syndrome have multiple accessory pathways.[6]

When surgery for ventricular tachycardia became feasible, it was even more apparent that the single-point mapping system was inadequate because these arrhythmias often last for only a few cardiac cycles intraoperatively and they may be multifocal in origin. The desirability of a mapping system capable of recording electrograms from multiple sites simultaneously was obvious. Since such a system lent itself to computerization, several groups designed various electrode arrays and started to develop computerized systems for rapid data acquisition and display. The major problem, however, was user interaction with the system in an on-line fashion. As a result, the earliest clinically applicable multipoint mapping systems were not computer-based but rather were analog systems that took advantage of either multichannel analog tape recorders or high-speed, high-frequency analog ink writers such as the ubiquitous Mingograf.

Multipoint Intraoperative Mapping Systems

The first multielectrode array to become clinically feasible for mapping ventricular tachycardia intraoperatively was the so-called "sock electrode" (Fig. 2). Our sock electrode consisted of 32 bipolar electrodes imbedded in silastic buttons that were held in place on the epicardial surface of the heart by an elastic mesh stocking material. The electrograms were recorded on a 32-channel analog tape

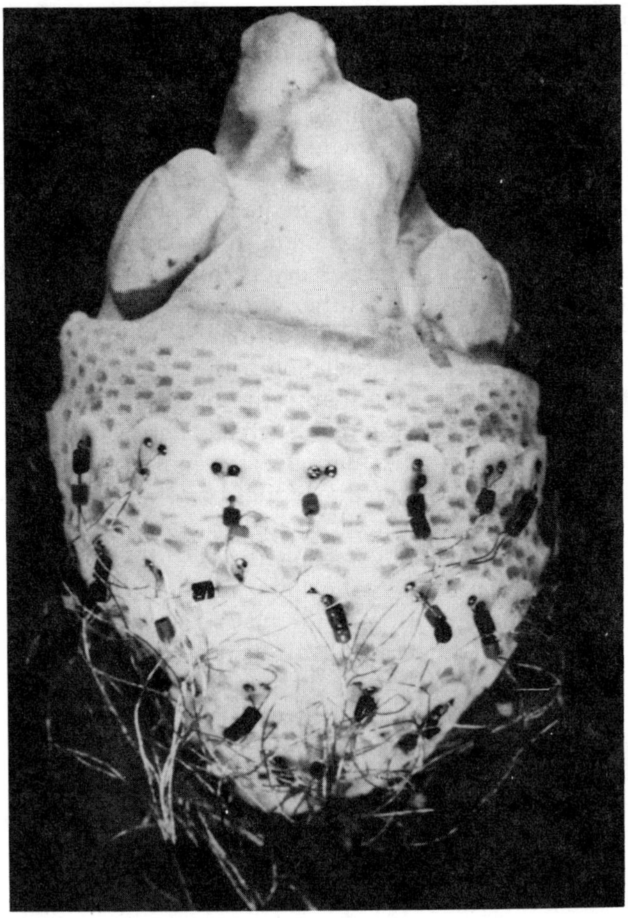

Figure 2: A "sock electrode" shown in position over a clay model of a canine heart. The material used is a flexible nylon mesh that is contoured to fit the heart and can be slipped over the ventricles and positioned in a matter of seconds. Within the nylon mesh, we presently embed 96 pairs of electrodes such that the global epicardial activation sequence can be obtained from a single beat (reproduced from Cox JL[22]).

recorder. Sixteen channels could be played back simultaneously on the Mingograf in the operating room and with appropriate referencing, the channel showing the earliest activation during ventricular tachycardia could be identified. The major limitation of the sock electrode was that only epicardial data could be obtained. Since ventricular tachycardia usually arises from either the endocardium or intramurally and since the most common anatomic site of origin is the ventricular septum, the value of the epicardial data recorded with the sock electrode was limited.

Because of the limitations of the sock electrode and the necessity to obtain endocardial data in patients with ventricular tachycardia, virtually all endocardial maps were initially recorded with single-point mapping systems. As already mentioned, these systems suffered major disadvantages in ventricular tachycardia mapping because of the frequent difficulty in inducing a stable tachycardia that was sustained long enough to allow a complete map to be performed. Our first attempt at obtaining endocardial data from multiple points simultaneously was to place multi-point plunge needle electrodes circumferentially around the

Intraoperative Computerized Mapping Techniques

base of the aneurysm or infarct and then record data from only the endocardial electrode on each needle shaft. While this method was helpful in determining the "quadrant" of the aneurysm base giving rise to the tachycardia, the amount of endocardial data was limited, the endocardial electrode was frequently difficult to identify, and the septum remained largely inaccessible. As a result, a rather simple device was developed, the so-called "egg electrode" (Fig. 3). A plastic toy egg was divided in its middle, its end was amputated to allow left ventricular venting, and 12 bipolar strip-electrodes were fixed to its external surface. The egg shape allowed the electrode array to fit into both large and small ventricular aneurysms and the strip-electrode arrangement assured good tissue contact with the endocardium. The 12 electrograms recorded simultaneously from the endocardium were displayed in real-time on a 12-channel recorder in the operating room (Fig. 4). Localized subendocardial resection procedures and endocardial cryoablation procedures were then performed at appropriate sites based on the data obtained from the egg electrode.

Advanced Multipoint Systems Including Computerized Mapping Systems

The development of a computerized intraoperative mapping system was begun at Duke in 1976 by Dr. Ray Ideker and associates.[7,8] Although it was

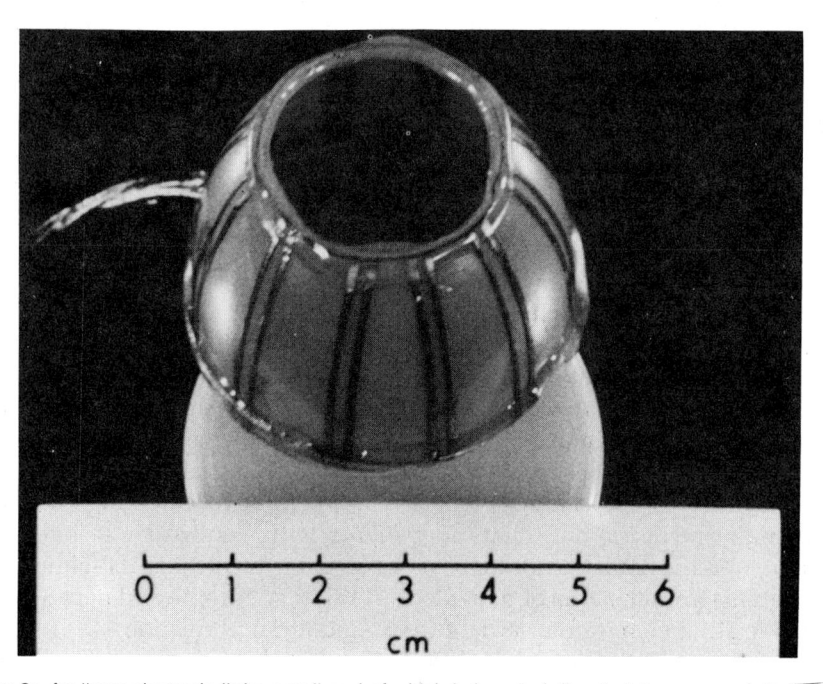

Figure 3: An "egg electrode," the small end of which is inserted directly into an open left ventricular aneurysm for purposes of recording simultaneous data from 12 different endocardial sites around the circumference of the aneurysm. The analog data recorded from the 12 pairs of strip electrodes were recorded directly on a 12-channel strip chart recorder in the operating theater for immediate analysis.

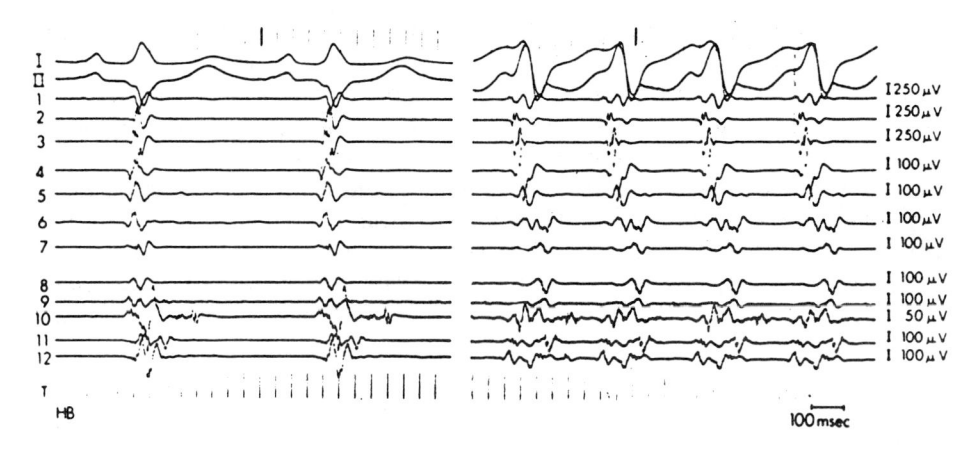

Figure 4: Endocardial data recorded from 12 endocardial sites and synchronized to peripheral ECG leads during normal sinus rhythm (left panel), and during induced ventricular tachycardia (right panel). Note that the electrograms showing the greatest degree of fragmentation and continuous electrical activity during normal sinus rhythm also exhibited at the earliest endocardial activation during ventricular tachycardia.

eventually possible to display local epicardial activation times recorded from the sock electrode with this system and to draw isochrones manually (Fig. 5), the ability to record intraoperative computerized maps in time to base an operative approach on them was not possible. In 1984, three separate mapping systems that were "user interactive" intraoperatively were described.[9-11] As expected, the Amsterdam group was on the leading edge of this technology.[9] They placed inflatable balloons uniformly covered with electrode terminals directly into the left ventricular cavity to record 16 endocardial electrograms simultaneously during ventricular tachycardia. After gross localization of the apparent site of origin of the arrhythmia, a rectangular grid with up to 64 electrode terminals was placed over the region of arrhythmogenesis for refined resolution. Witkowski and Corr from our group described an automated transmural cardiac mapping system that could record a virtually unlimited number of electrograms simultaneously and could analyze and display the data within 120 seconds.[10] Experimentally, the system recorded 240 channels simultaneously from 60 plunge needle electrodes with four bipolar terminals located along the shaft of each needle from endocardium to epicardium. Clinically, 16 channels of the 48-channel system were first used for mapping patients with WPW syndrome.[12] The clinical system has now been expanded to 160 channels and is employed for constructing endocardial, intramural, and epicardial maps in patients with ventricular tachycardia. In addition, for the past 6 months, we have been recording 160 simultaneous electrograms from the atria of patients with WPW syndrome and in patients with automatic atrial tachycardia, atrial flutter, and atrial fibrillation.

Parson and Downar took a different approach to the need for an on-line intraoperative mapping system capable of recording data from multiple sites simultaneously. Their noncomputerized, battery-operated multiplexed system analyzes analog data and incorporates a marker-matrix visual display of the

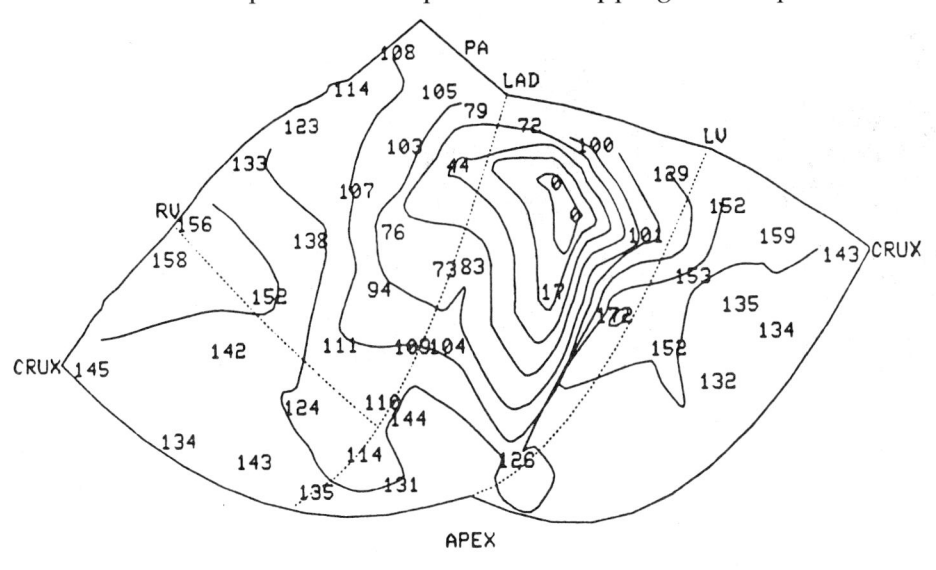

```
PROCEDURE GARRET.PRE        ACTIVATION TIME MAP
BEAT NUMBER   1
TIME ZERO IS EARLIEST LAT IN BEAT
ISOCHRONE INTERVAL = 20 MSEC
```

Figure 5: An epicardial electrophysiologic map recorded intraoperatively from a patient who had sustained blunt injury to the chest resulting in total occlusion of the left anterior descending coronary artery with subsequent development of a large anterior septal left ventricular aneurysm and intractable ventricular tachycardia. This epicardial map was recorded during ventricular tachycardia and demonstrates that the earliest site of epicardial breakthrough of the tachycardia is just left of the left anterior descending coronary artery at the base of the anterior left ventricular aneurysm. This map was recorded in August 9, 1979 and was drawn several days later (reproduced by permission from Cox JL[22]).

epicardial activation sequence recorded from an epicardial sock electrode array.[11] They have recently used the same system to display endocardial activation data recorded from inflatable cavitary balloons similar to those employed by the Amsterdam group.

Present Technique of Intraoperative Mapping

Computerized Mapping System

The intraoperative mapping system currently used in our operating theater was developed and reported by Drs. Witkowski and Corr in 1984.[10] The system is presently capable of recording 160 bipolar electrograms simultaneously, analyzing the data, and displaying it in various forms within 2 minutes after data acquisition. Analog data recorded from the heart enter the front-end system located in the operating theater (Fig. 6) where each electrogram is individually filtered and digitized (Fig. 7). The digitized data are then transferred across a fiberoptic cable

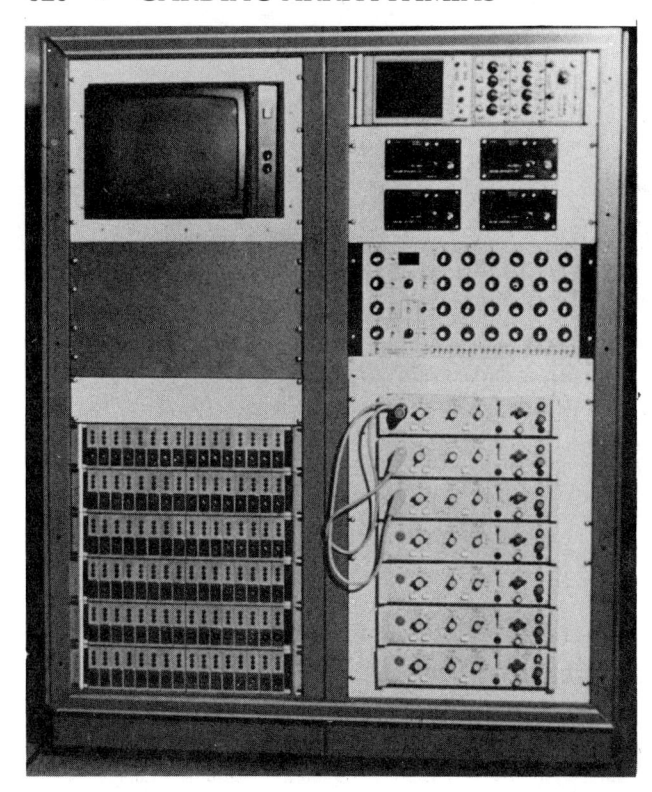

Figure 6: The front-end hardware of the 48-channel computerized mapping system used until recently at Barnes Hospital. The system has now been expanded to 160 channels.

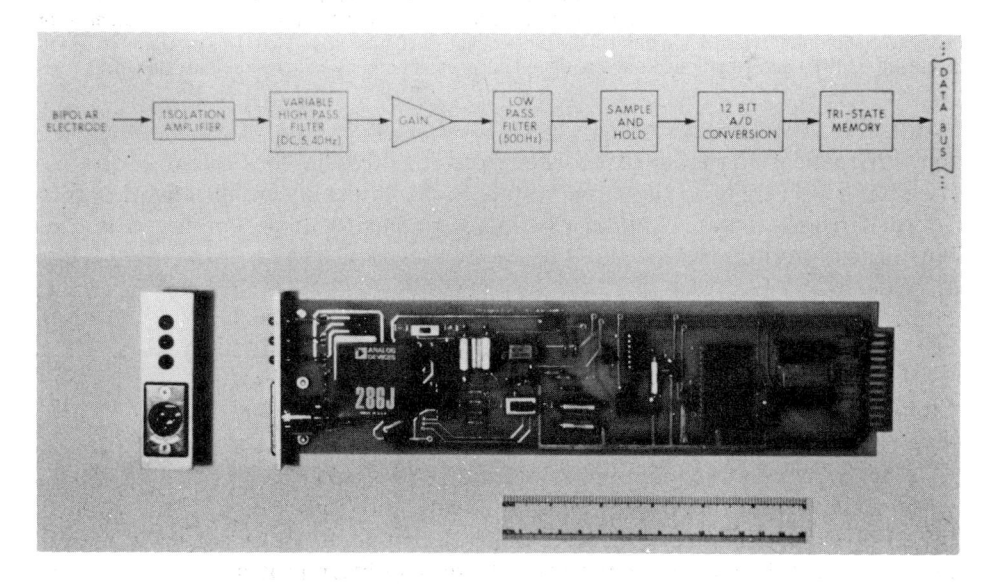

Figure 7: Electrogram amplifier block diagram and physical appearance. Standard double-sided epoxy-printed circuit card construction is used throughout. Each analog electrogram enters one such amplifier on the left and is then filtered and converted to digital form before being transferred via a fiberoptic cable to the computer facility (reproduced by permission from Witkowski and Corr[10]).

to a remote computer facility located approximately 1500 meters away (Fig. 8). The personnel in the operating theater and those in the computer facility are connected by both an audio system (headphones) and a video camera and display system for constant communication during the mapping procedure. Only 16 channels of the mapping system are used for patients undergoing surgery for WPW syndrome, but all 160 channels are used to map atrial flutter, atrial fibrillation, ectopic atrial tachycardias, and ventricular tachyarrhythmias.

WPW Syndrome

The computerized mapping system has obviated the need to use cardiopulmonary bypass for the intraoperative mapping of patients with WPW syndrome. Epicardial pacing and sensing electrodes are sutured onto the atrium and ventricle near the suspected site of the accessory pathway. The band electrode (Fig. 9)[12] is placed around the ventricular side of the AV groove (Fig. 10) and electrograms are recorded simultaneously from the 16 bipolar electrodes during normal sinus rhythm and during atrial pacing. Two minutes later, three digitized tracings from the standard ECG are displayed simultaneously on the color graphics terminals in the operating theater and in the computer facility. The adjustable window is

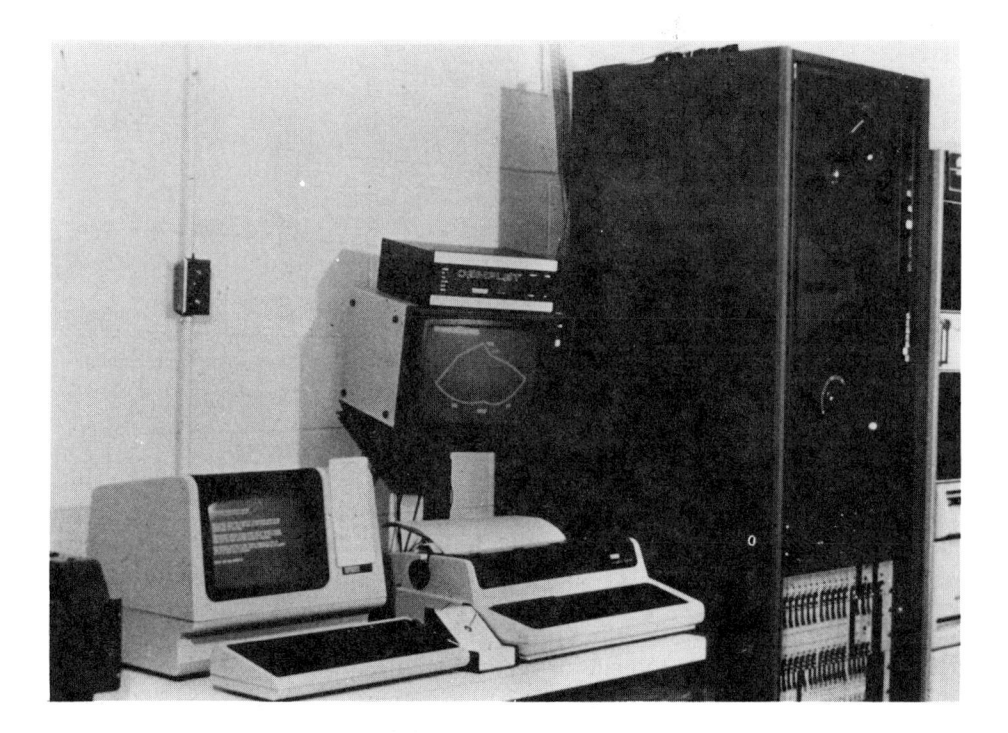

Figure 8: Computer facility used for intraoperative electrophysiologic mapping. The fiberoptic cable (which is approximately 1500 meters long) can be seen entering the room through the ceiling. Data are first recorded on a digital tape recorder and then are played back into the computer at a slower speed for analysis.

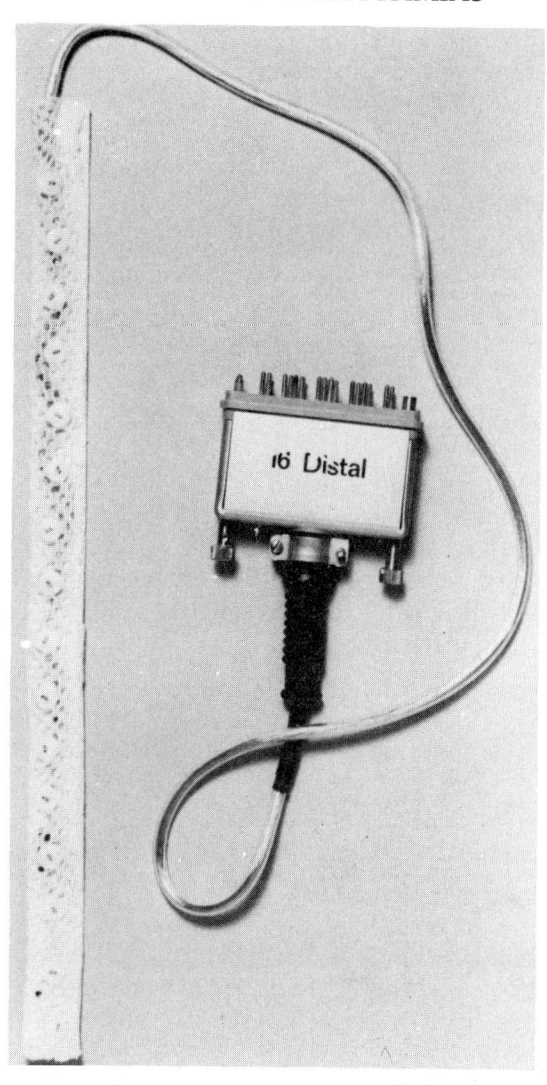

Figure 9: Epicardial band containing 16 bipolar button electrodes (reproduced by permission from Kramer et al.[12]).

positioned over the preexcited QRS complex (Fig. 11) and the computer is commanded to display the activation sequence of the 16 electrodes during the time interval encompassed by the window. The 16 digitized electrograms are then automatically displayed on the graphics terminals (eight channels at a time) and the point of rapid deflection (local activation time) is automatically marked by a vertical cursor on each electrogram (Fig. 12). The electrogram recorded from the electrode located nearest the site of the ventricular insertion of the accessory pathway shows the earliest activation. The computer then displays the digital data on a schematic drawing of the base of the heart and automatically encompasses the earliest point in a box (Fig. 13). This method of graphics display is particularly helpful in detecting the presence of multiple accessory pathways that are capable of conducting in the antegrade direction.

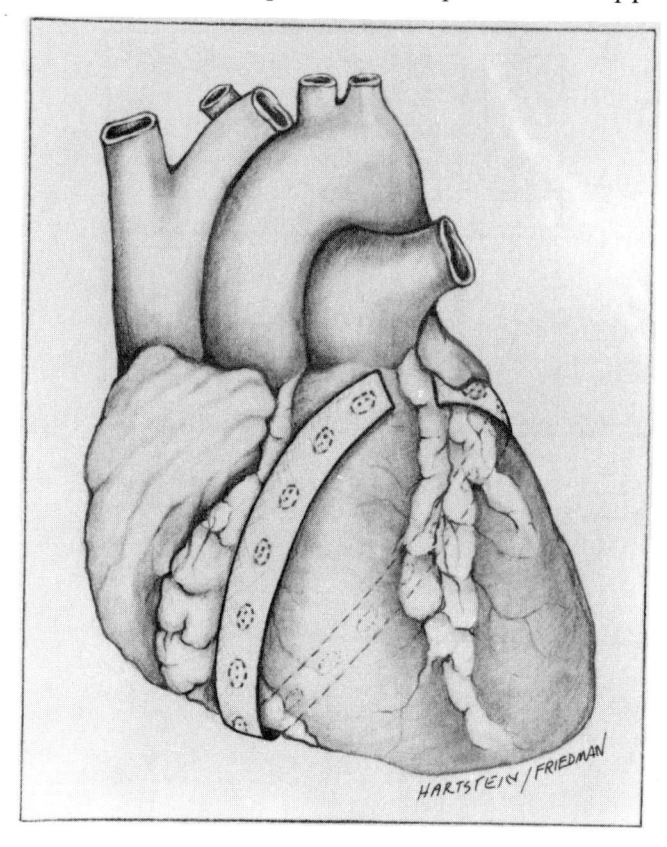

Figure 10: Diagrammatic sketch showing the placement of the band electrode around the ventricular side of the AV groove in a patient with WPW syndrome during stable antegrade preexcitation.

The band electrode is then moved to the atrial side of the AV groove and reciprocating tachycardia is induced with programmed electrical stimulation (Fig. 14). Only a few cycles of tachycardia are allowed to occur since hemodynamic compromise is common and the patients are not on cardiopulmonary bypass. Atrial electrograms are recorded from the bipolar electrodes on the band and again the digitized ECG tracings are displayed. Since only the retrograde atrial data are of interest, the window is positioned over that portion of the ECG tracing that contains the retrograde P-wave (Fig. 15). The computer then displays the activation sequence of the atrial electrograms recorded during reciprocating tachycardia (Fig. 16). Since the band electrode is usually too long for the atrial aspect of the AV groove, the distal three to five electrodes on the band are usually not in contact with the atria and are, therefore, ignored. The computer also displays the digital atrial data on the schematic drawing of the base of the heart (Fig. 17). This display of the atrial data is especially important because it demonstrates unsuspected concealed accessory pathways that would have gone undetected until this point in the mapping procedure. When reciprocating tachycardia cannot be induced, the retrograde atrial map is performed during ventricular pacing.

The antegrade and retrograde mapping techniques described above are capable of detecting not only free wall pathways but also anterior septal and posterior

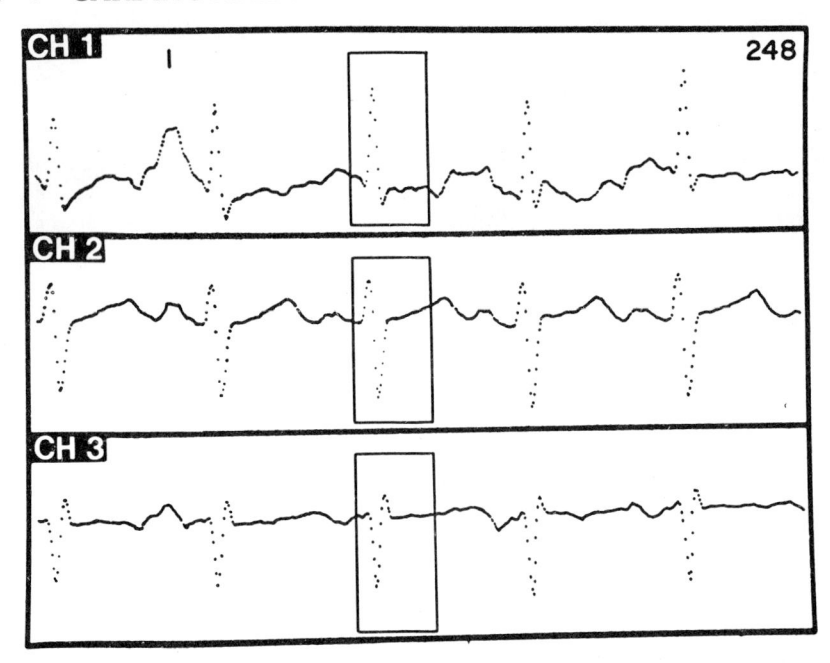

Figure 11: Hard copy of the color graphics terminal display of three digitized standard ECG leads used to select the desired preexcited QRS complex (inside window). The window can be narrowed or enlarged and it can be moved to any portion of the QRS complex.

septal accessory pathways. However, if either is detected during the computerized mapping procedure, the patient is placed on cardiopulmonary bypass, a right atriotomy is performed, and endocardial mapping of the right atrium and atrial septum is completed using the hand-held single-point mapping system prior to proceeding with surgical dissection.

Ventricular Tachycardia

As mentioned above, all 160 channels of the computerized system are used to map the heart in patients with ventricular tachycardia. The sock electrode is first used to determine the epicardial activation sequence during sinus rhythm and during induced ventricular tachycardia (Fig. 18). The sock electrode presently employed contains 96 electrodes. The earliest site of epicardial breakthrough is automatically cursored in red by the computer for rapid detection of the region of most interest (Fig. 19). It should be emphasized that the epicardial data are not used to guide the surgeon in selecting the site to be ablated but rather the data are used to guide the subsequent placement of plunge needle electrodes to further delineate the specific site of arrhythmogenesis. The epicardial map is helpful not only as an initial screening device that can be obtained in 2 to 3 minutes, but it is also most useful in characterizing nonclinical arrhythmias that may be induced during programmed electrical stimulation.

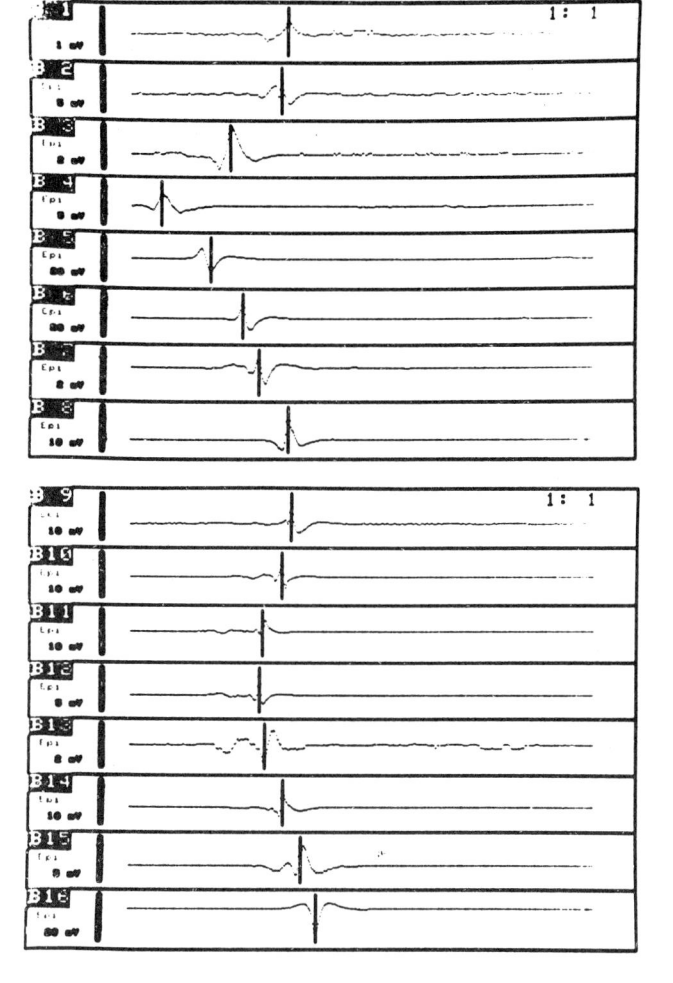

Figure 12: Hard copy of the color graphics terminal display showing the activation sequence of the 16 electrodes contained in the band. Since this is an antegrade ventricular preexcitation map and the band has been placed on the ventricular side of the AV groove, the electrode showing the earliest activation (electrode number 4) is located at the site of the ventricular insertion of the accessory pathway.

Once the epicardial activation sequence during ventricular tachycardia has been established, multiple plunge needle electrodes containing four bipolar pairs of contacts along the needle shaft are inserted into the ventricle in the region of earliest epicardial activation. If the epicardial map has suggested that the tachycardia is arising from the ventricular septum, a right atriotomy is performed and up to 15 right-angle needle electrodes are inserted into the ventricular septum from the right side, access being gained across the tricuspid valve. This provides up to 60 transmural data points from the ventricular septum without the necessity for performing a ventriculotomy. As many as 25 other needle electrodes can be placed in or near the arrhythmogenic region, yielding a total of 160 endocardial, intramural, and epicardial data points simultaneously from the septum and free wall without performing a ventriculotomy. It has been demonstrated on many occasions by a variety of authors that a ventriculotomy frequently alters the electrophysiologic milieu sufficiently to prevent further inducibility of the ventric-

Day 2

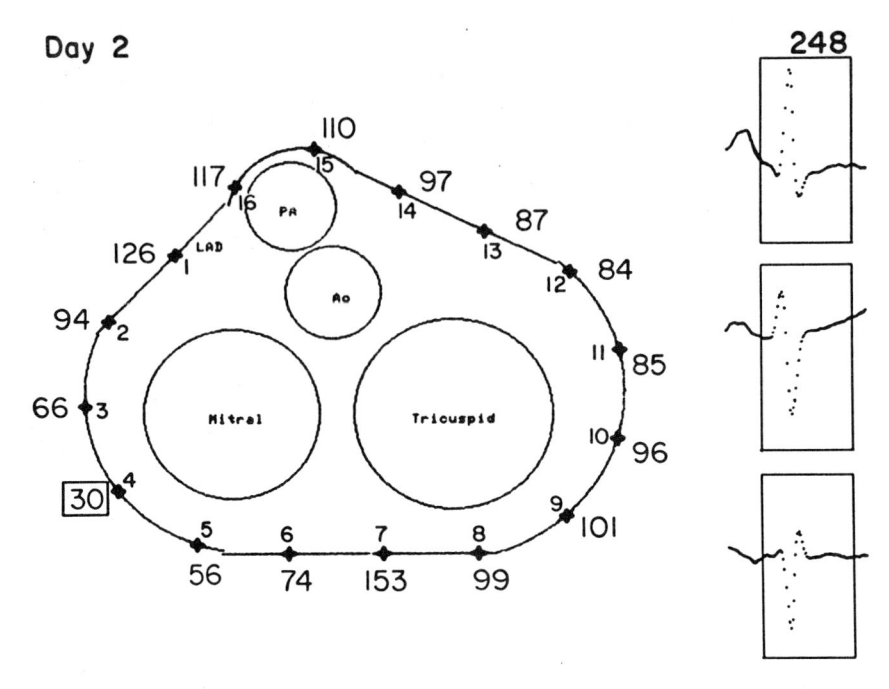

Figure 13: Hard copy of the color graphics terminal display showing the activation sequence of the base of the ventricles during stable antegrade preexcitation. The designated window is displayed on the right side of the screen and the activation sequence is related to a diagrammatic sketch of the base of the heart with the earliest site of ventricular activity during stable antegrade preexcitation being enclosed in a box.

ular tachycardia, thereby preventing further mapping and necessitating a non-guided operation to be performed.

Does Computerized Mapping Make A Difference?

WPW Syndrome

Since only 16 channels of our computerized mapping system are used to map patients with WPW syndrome, we do not believe that a computerized system per se is necessary to obtain optimal surgical results in these patients. However, we feel strongly that a *multipoint* intraoperative mapping system significantly improves the surgical results. The multipoint system may be analog or digital but the essential feature is the capability of recording electrograms from several sites simultaneously.

As mentioned previously, although single-point mapping systems are satisfactory for most cases of WPW syndrome, several limitations exist and essentially all of these limitations are circumvented with a multipoint system. Perhaps the most common problem encountered is in patients with only intermittent ventricular preexcitation. With the single-point system, it may be virtually impossible to

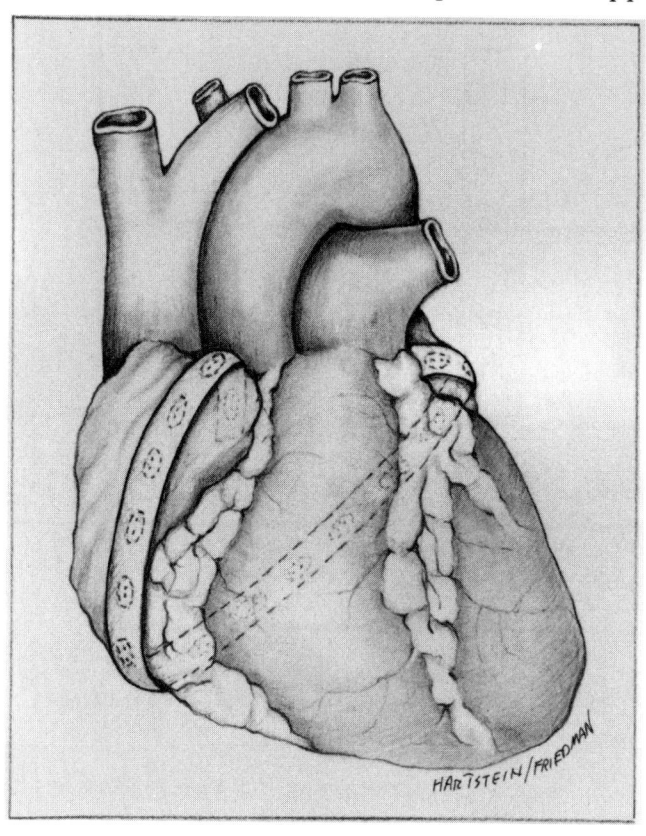

Figure 14: Once the band electrode has been moved to the atrial side of the AV groove as demonstrated in this diagrammatic sketch, reciprocating tachycardia is induced and a retrograde atrial map is performed.

determine the precise location of the site of preexcitation because the entire AV groove must be mapped on a point-by-point basis and if the preexcitation is fleeting, the groove simply cannot be mapped for preexcited beats only. This problem is obviated with a multipoint system since only one beat is necessary for complete mapping of the AV groove (Fig. 20). Moreover, the previously insurmountable problem of mapping intermittently preexcited beats in the presence of chronic atrial fibrillation is of no concern with multipoint mapping systems. Another potentially important problem is intermittent retrograde conduction across a concealed accessory pathway. This is the type of complex electrophysiologic abnormality that can result in surgical failure not because of an inadequate surgical procedure, but because of the inability to map the patient's problem accurately and completely. The computerized mapping system reduces this potentially serious problem to one of little consequence (Fig. 21).

Another common problem is that of multiple accessory pathways, a condition that occurs in 20% of our patients.[6] Although most of these patients can be mapped satisfactorily with a single-point system in experienced hands, the simplicity of mapping these patients with the computerized system (Fig. 22), the time saved by doing so, and the frequency of multiplicity of pathways would seem

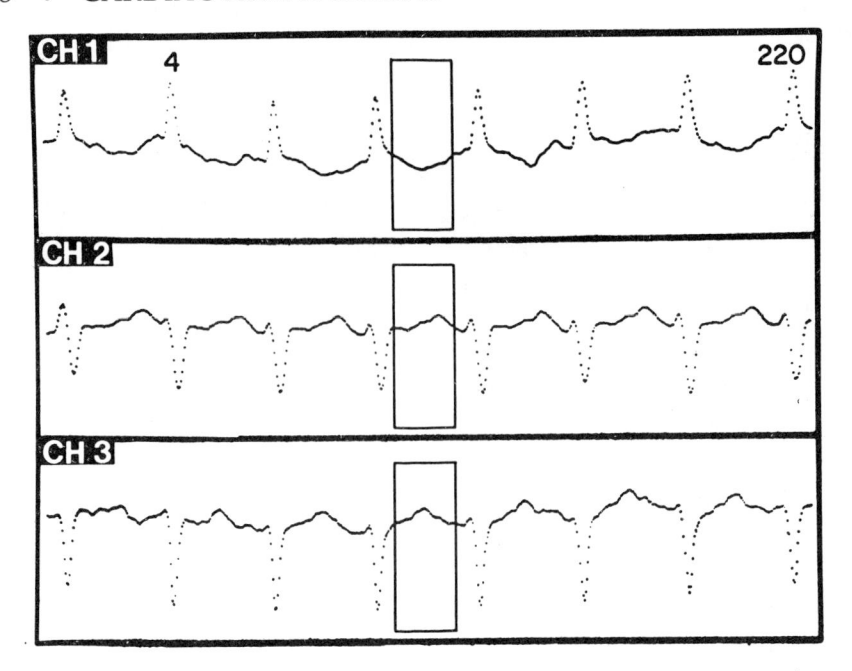

Figure 15: Hard copy of the color graphics terminal display showing the window centered over the suspected site of the retrograde P-wave (following QRS complex) during reciprocating tachycardia.

justification enough to develop some type of multipoint mapping system in all centers performing WPW surgery.

Finally, placement of the band electrode used in our institution requires almost no cardiac manipulation. This factor greatly reduces the likelihood that either a suspected or unsuspected manifest or concealed accessory pathway will be blocked by excessive torsion or traction on the heart during the mapping procedure. Therefore, the inadvertent masking of an accessory pathway during surgery that reappears postoperatively because it was not detected and mapped intraoperatively is now a problem of historical interest only.

In summary, multipoint intraoperative mapping systems are clearly superior to single-point systems in patients undergoing surgery for WPW syndrome. Because of the availability of our computerized system that was developed for use in ventricular tachycardia surgery, we adapted it so that it could also be used in patients with WPW syndrome. The band electrode technique offers accurate and rapid identification of accessory pathways and obviates the need for cardiopulmonary bypass during cardiac mapping. Both the ventricular and atrial insertion sites can be identified rapidly using antegrade and retrograde maps. This approach promotes stable pathway conduction by reducing the need for extensive cardiac manipulation during mapping and accurate data can be obtained during intermittent conduction over the accessory pathway. In cases of multiple accessory pathways, distinct pathways can be discerned from a single beat or when multiple pacing sites are required to elicit conduction over alternate pathways, several maps can be obtained rapidly.

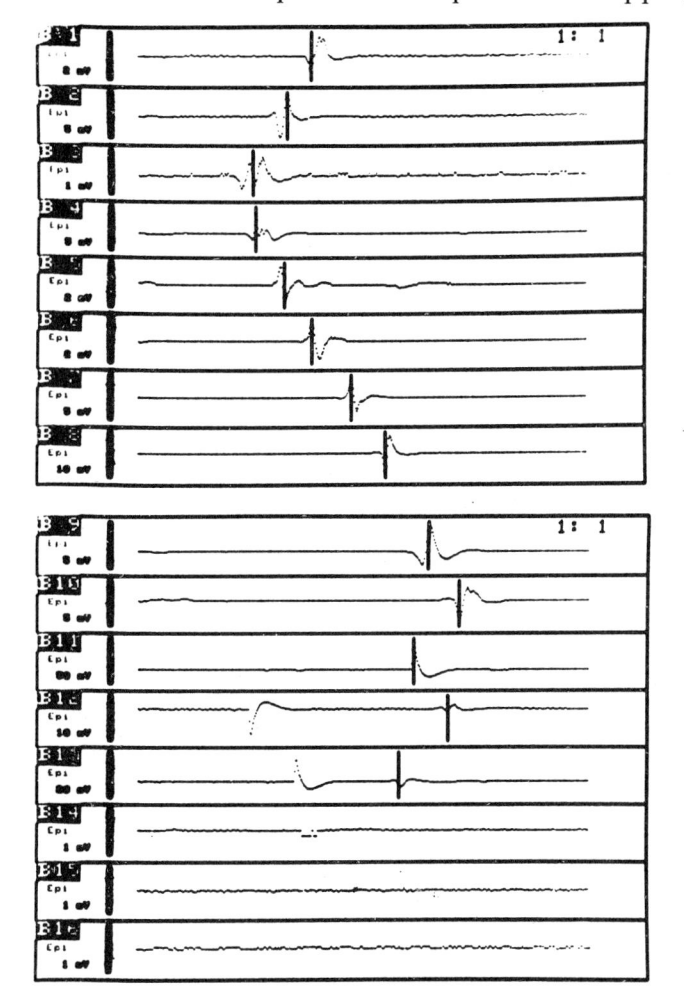

Figure 16: Hard copy of the color graphics terminal display showing the activation sequence of the base of the atrium during reciprocating tachycardia as determined by the band electrode array. The distal three electrograms were not in contact with the heart and are, therefore, to be ignored.

Supraventricular Tachyarrhythmias other than WPW Syndrome

The incidence of tachycardia due to WPW syndrome is extremely low in comparison to other types of supraventricular arrhythmias. However, the spatial separation of the reentrant components and the temporal relationships involved make the reciprocating tachycardia of WPW syndrome the ideal arrhythmia to study. These two characteristics undoubtedly account for the fact that WPW syndrome was the first clinical arrhythmia that could be mapped accurately in the operating theater.

Ectopic atrial tachycardias can also be mapped intraoperatively with a single-point system if the arrhythmia persists long enough to complete the point-by-point mapping process. Unfortunately, these tachycardias are usually automatic in nature and if they are not continuous, they are frequently difficult to induce intraoperatively. AV node reentry tachycardia is a common arrhythmia that can

630 • CARDIAC ARRHYTHMIAS

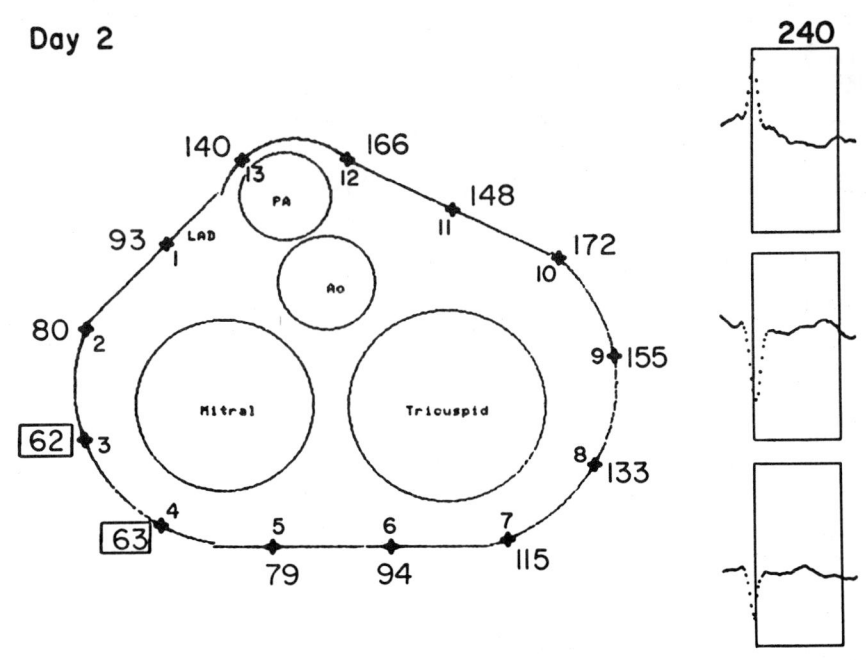

Figure 17: Hard copy of the color graphics terminal display showing the retrograde atrial activation sequence of the base of the atrium during reciprocating tachycardia superimposed on a diagrammatic sketch of the base of the heart. Electrodes 3 and 4 activate almost simultaneously, indicating that the insertion of the atrial end of the accessory pathway is located midway between these two electrodes.

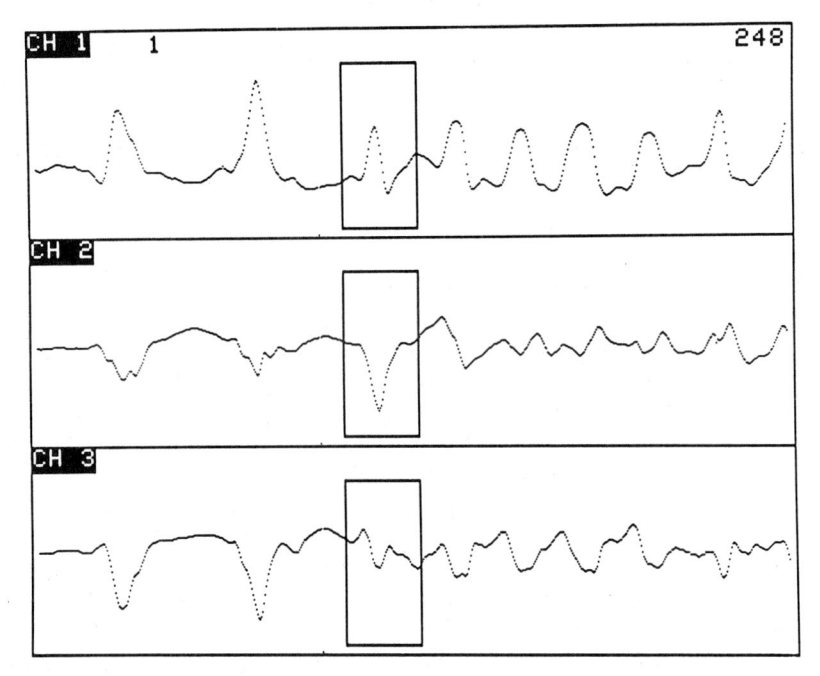

Figure 18: Hard copy of the color graphics terminal display of three digitized standard ECG leads during the induction of ventricular tachycardia by programmed electrical stimulation. The window encompasses the first beat of ventricular tachycardia.

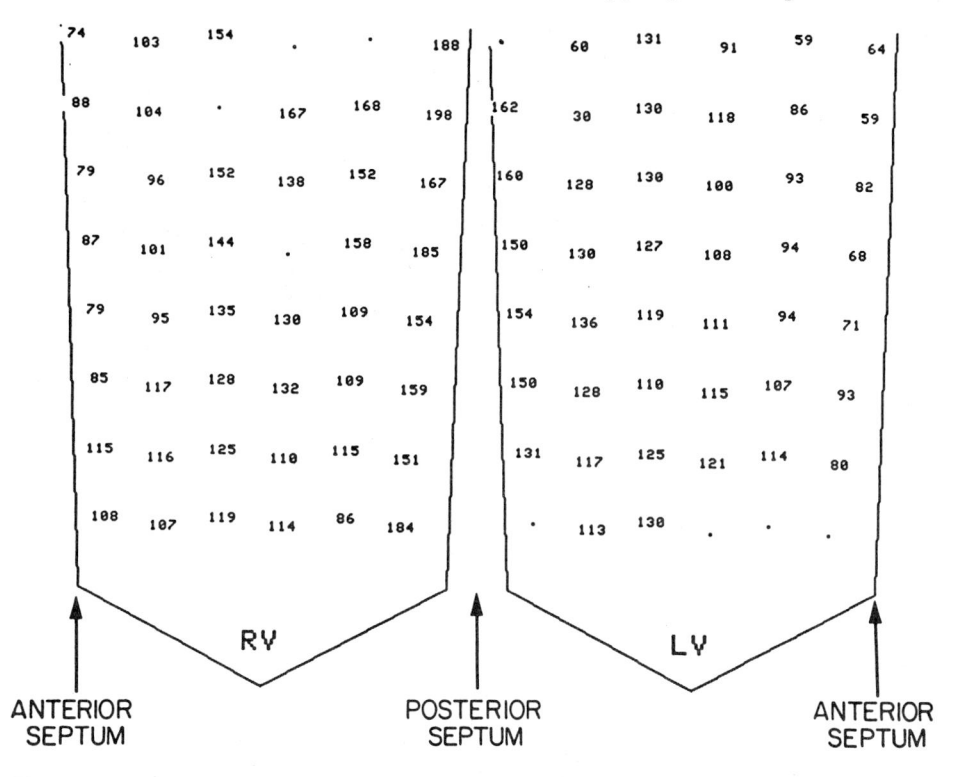

74	103	154	.	.	188	.	60	131	91	59	64
88	104	.	167	168	198	162	30	130	118	86	59
79	96	152	138	152	167	160	128	130	100	93	82
87	101	144	.	150	185	150	130	127	108	94	68
79	95	135	130	109	154	154	136	119	111	94	71
85	117	128	132	109	159	150	128	110	115	107	93
115	116	125	110	115	151	131	117	125	121	114	80
108	107	119	114	86	184	.	113	130	.	.	.

RV   LV

ANTERIOR SEPTUM   POSTERIOR SEPTUM   ANTERIOR SEPTUM

Figure 19: Hard copy of the color graphics terminal display of data recorded from the 96 epicardial electrodes in the sock electrode array during induced ventricular tachycardia. The epicardial data show that the earliest area of epicardial breakthrough is over the upper anterior ventricular septum. These data were used to guide the subsequent placement of multiple plunge needle electrodes in the ventricular septum and anterior right and left ventricular free wall to obtain data from 160 endocardial, intramural and epicardial sites in and around this region of early epicardial breakthrough.

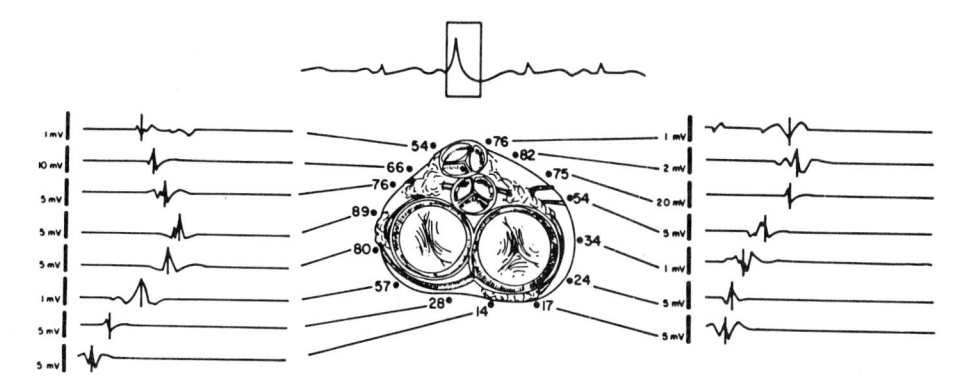

Figure 20: Antegrade ventricular epicardial activation times during intermittent ventricular preexcitation in a patient with WPW syndrome. The electrocardiogram shows a single preexcited beat. The activation map indicates the presence of a right-sided paraseptal bypass tract (reproduced by permission from Kramer et al.[12]).

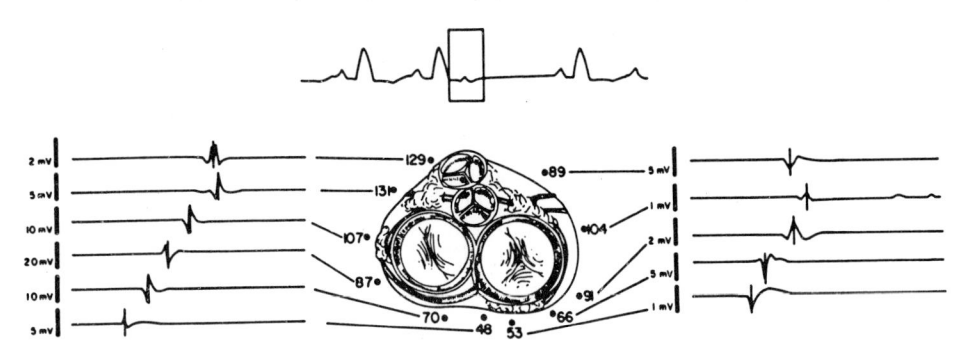

Figure 21: Retrograde atrial epicardial activation times during a single atrioventricular echo beat. The accessory pathway was located in the posterior septum (reproduced by permission from Kramer et al.[12]).

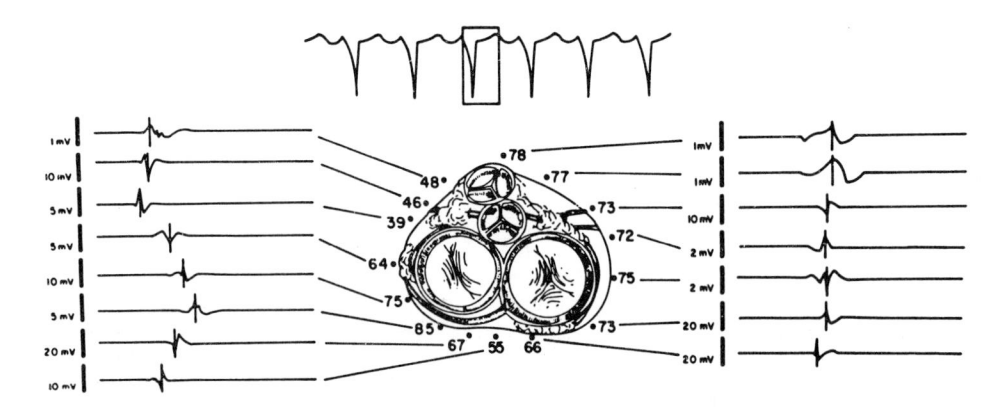

Figure 22: Antegrade ventricular epicardial activation showing two distinct accessory pathways, one located in the left anterior lateral position and one in the posterior septal position (reproduced by permission from Kramer et al.[12]).

now be treated surgically with uniform success,[13] but intraoperative mapping is not essential and is not routinely employed as a part of the surgical procedure. Since essentially the same operative technique is used to ablate other types of paranodal bypass tracts such as Mahaim fibers,[14] little interest has been shown in developing more sophisticated mapping techniques for atrial arrhythmias.

This apparent apathy has resulted in our having ignored the potential role of surgery in the most common and lethal of all supraventricular arrhythmias, atrial fibrillation. Large screening studies sugggest that 0.4% of the general population has atrial fibrillation[15] and pathological studies have shown that the number of autopsied patients who had atrial fibrillation before death is 17–19%.[16] The incidence of cerebral embolism due to atrial fibrillation is approximately 5% per patient year[17] and 10% of all strokes are due to atrial fibrillation.[18] These figures suggest that roughly 50,000 Americans experience cerebral embolism due to atrial fibrillation each year. In order to appreciate the magnitude of this problem, we as cardiologists and cardiac surgeons have only to talk with our neurology colleagues who deal with the complications of this "benign" arrhythmia.[18] With the development of computerized intraoperative mapping systems, the potential exists for mapping atrial flutter and atrial fibrillation in patients. Just as in the case of WPW syndrome and ventricular tachycardia, if an arrhythmia can be mapped, a surgical technique can be developed to ablate it. We have recently adapted our computerized mapping system so that 160 sites on the atria can be mapped simultaneously. An example of a normal sinus beat recorded in this manner from a patient undergoing WPW surgery is shown in Figures 23 and 24. These data were displayed on the computer graphics terminal in the operating theater within 2 minutes of the time of recording. The ability to obtain this type of data accurately and rapidly provides the opportunity to map more complex atrial arrhythmias such as flutter and fibrillation. Thus, there would seem to be great potential for computer mapping systems to improve the care of this group of patients.

Ventricular Tachycardia

One of the major problems that has persisted since the direct surgical approaches to ventricular tachycardia were introduced in the late 1970s is the frequent difficulty in inducing a stable sustained tachycardia intraoperatively. Several factors may suppress the inducibility and stability of ventricular tachycar-

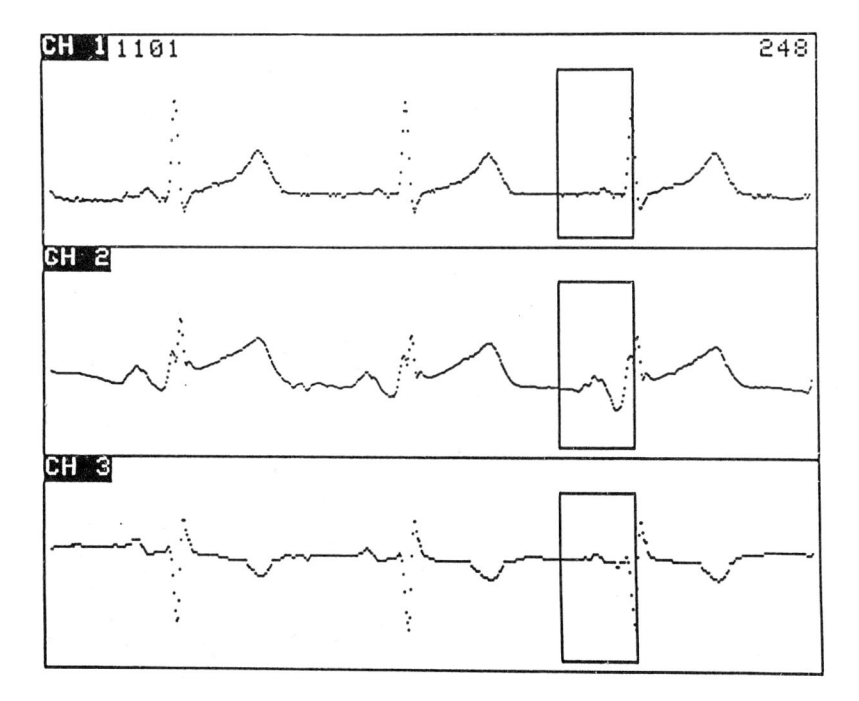

Figure 23: Hard copy of the color graphics terminal display showing the P-wave of the digitized ECG tracing encompassed in the window to be mapped during normal sinus rhythm.

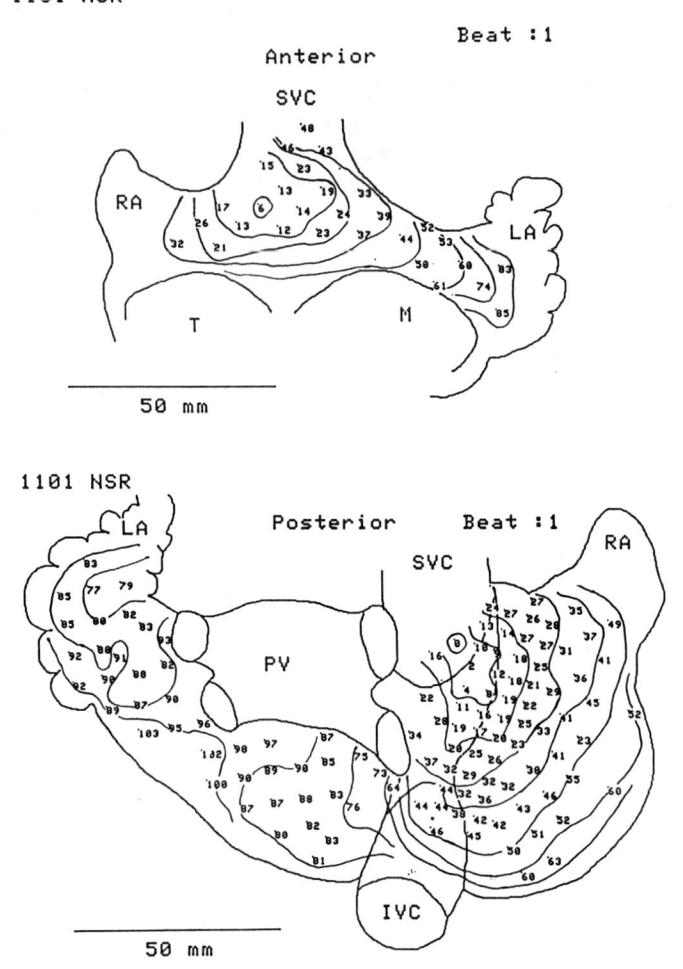

Figure 24: Hard copy of the color graphics terminal display showing a comuterized map of the human atrium recorded from 160 data points during a single beat of sinus rhythm. The lower portion of the figure shows the posterior view of the atria and demonstrates that the sinus beat is originating at the junction of the superior vena cava and right atrium. The upper portion of the figure is an anterior view of the two atria. SVC = superior vena cava; IVC = inferior vena cava; LA = left atrium; RA = right atrium; PV = pulmonary veins; T = tricuspid valve orifice; M = mitral valve orifice.

dia intraoperatively, including general anesthesia, cardiac manipulation, myocardial hypothermia, electrolyte imbalance, varying serum catecholamine levels, and alterations in ventricular wall tension accompanying cardiopulmonary bypass. In addition, the ventriculotomy required to gain access to the endocardium for mapping frequently interrupts or alters the reentrant circuit responsible for the arrhythmia, thereby precluding further data collection. Thus, the ideal intraoperative mapping system would incorporate the ability to record data from multiple sites simultaneously and to record endocardial data without opening the ventricle.

Such a system could overcome the problems of trying to map a nonsustained tachycardia arising at or near the endocardial level and the avoidance of a ventriculotomy would enhance the likelihood of arrhythmia induction.

The endocardial balloon electrode array described above satisfies both of these requirements if it is introduced transatrially into the ventricle. We have chosen instead to use the combination of an epicardial sock electrode array and multiple plunge needle electrodes because of the ease of using them and the added benefit of being able to obtain transmural as well as endocardial and epicardial data. The entire intraoperative mapping sequence normally takes approximately 10 minutes, the majority of that time being consumed by attempts at tachycardia induction. If polymorphic tachycardia is present, each of the different morphologic types of tachycardia is mapped in a similar manner.

A considerable controversy has existed in the past as to whether or not intraoperative mapping actually improves the results of surgery for ventricular tachycardia. Many authorities feel that since the surgical techniques used to treat ventricular tachycardia are directed at an obvious visible anatomic substrate (endocardial fibrosis), it is only necessary to remove, encircle, or cryoablate this substrate and intraoperative mapping is not only unnecessary but it is also time-consuming and expensive. It now seems clear that the results with electrophysiologically guided surgery are superior to those of "visually guided" surgery.[19] However, even though electrophysiologically guided surgery is superior, it should be kept in mind that most comparisons have been made between single-point mapping systems and no mapping at all. This is analogous to discussing the differences in rapid transportation with the horse (no mapping system) and the horseless carriage (single-point mapping system) when the first airplanes (computerized mapping systems) were being developed. It is clearly still too early to demonstrate that the use of computerized intraoperative mapping systems will decrease the operative mortality rate, decrease the failure rate, and increase the surgery alone success rate, but it would seem almost inevitable that striking improvements are on the horizon. It is perhaps worth recalling that the overall success rate for WPW surgery during the first 13 years was only 86%.[20] The success rate for ventricular tachycardia surgery in institutions where extensive intraoperative mapping is employed is already over 90%, even though multipoint mapping systems were not available in their patients.[19,21] Thus, it would seem reasonable to expect that with the newer mapping systems and more experience, the results of surgery for ventricular tachycardia will approach those of surgery for WPW syndrome at the 100% level.

Summary and Conclusions

Multipoint and/or computerized intraoperative mapping systems improve the results of surgery for WPW syndrome and show tremendous potential for opening an entirely new era of surgical intervention for the more common and lethal types of supraventricular tachyarrhythmias such as atrial flutter and atrial fibrillation. In addition, the ability to map and ablate the sometimes fleeting automatic atrial tachycardias is greatly enhanced by computerized mapping systems. On the other hand, the success of surgical intervention for AV node reentry tachycardia and arrhythmias due to Mahaim fibers does not depend on sophisticated intraoperative mapping systems and, therefore, a computerized system offers no advantages over standard systems.

Because of the paucity of functioning, user-interactive computerized mapping systems presently in use, it is too early to document their impact on the overall results of ventricular tachycardia surgery. However, the history of arrhythmia surgery would strongly suggest that such systems will simplify the operative procedures and improve the results of surgery for ventricular tachycardia. "Do they help us to treat our patients better surgically?" Yes.

References

1. Daniel TM, Cox JL, Sabiston DC Jr, Boineau JP. Epicardial and intramural mapping activation of the human heart. A technique for localizing infarction and ischemia of the myocardium (abstr). Circulation 1969;40:(Suppl)III:III-66.
2. Daniel IM, Boineau JP, Cox JL, Sabiston DC Jr. Mapping of epicardial and intramural activation of the heart. J Thoracic Cardiovasc Surg 1970;60:704-709.
3. Cobb FR, Blumenschein SD, Sealy WC, Boineau JP, Wagner GS, Wallace AG. Successful surgical interruption of the bundle of Kent in a patient with Wolff-Parkinson-White syndrome. Circulation 1968;38:1018-1029.
4. Gallagher JJ, Kasell J, Sealy WC, Pritchett ELC, Wallace AG. Epicardial mapping in the Wolff-Parkinson-White syndrome. Circulation 57:854-866, 1978.
5. Gallagher JL, Kasell JH, Cox JL, Smith WM, Ideker RE, Smith WM: Techniques of intraoperative electrophysiologic mapping. Am J Cardiol 1982;49:221-240.
6. Cox JL, Gallagher JJ, Cain ME. Experience with 118 consecutive patients undergoing surgery for the Wolff-Parkinson-White syndrome. J Thoracic Cardiovasc Surg 1985;90:490-501.
7. Ideker RE, Smith WM, Wallace AG, Kasell J, Harrison LA, Klein GJ, Kinicki RE, Gallagher JJ. A computerized method for the rapid display of ventricular activation during the intraoperative study of arrhythmias. Circulation 1979;59:449-458.
8. Smith WM, Ideker RE, Kinicki RE, Harrison L. A computer system for the intraoperative mapping of ventricular arrhythmias. Comput Biomed Res 1980;13:61-72.
9. deBakker JMT, Janse MJ, van Capelle FJL, Durrer D. An interactive computer system for guiding the surgical treatment of life-threatening ventricular tachycardias. IEEE Trans Biomed Eng 1984;BME-31:362-368.
10. Witkowski FX, Corr PB. An automated simultaneous transmural cardiac mapping system. Am J Physiol 1984;247:H661-H668.
11. Parson I, Downar E. Clinical instrumentation for the intra-operative mapping of ventricular arrhythmias. PACE 1984;7:683-692.
12. Kramer JB, Corr PB, Cox JL, Witkowski FX, Cain ME. Arrhythmia and conduction disturbances: simultaneous computer mapping to facilitate intraoperative localization of accessory pathways in patients with Wolff-Parkinson-White syndrome. Am J Cardiol 1985;56:571-576.
13. Cox JL: Surgery for cardiac arrhythmias. Current Problems in Cardiology, Chicago, Yearbook Medical Publishers, VIII, No. 4, 1983.
14. Cox JL: Current status of cardiac arrhythmia surgery. Circulation 1985;71:413.
15. Godtfredsen J: Atrial fibrillation: course and prognosis: A follow-up study of 1,212 cases. In Kulbertus HE, Olsson SB, Schlepper M, eds. Atrial Fibrillation. Molndal, Sweden, AB Hassle Publishing Co., 1982;134-147.
16. Aberg H: Atrial fibrillation. 1. A study of atrial thrombosis and systemic embolism in a necropsy material. Acta Med Scand 1969;185:373-379.

17. Szekely P: Systemic embolism and anticoagulant prophylaxis in rheumatic heart disease. Br Med J 1964;1:1209–1212.
18. Fisher CM: Embolism in atrial fibrillation. In Kulbertus HE, Olsson SB, Schlepper M, eds. Atrial Fibrillation. Molndal, Sweden, AB Hassle Publishing Co., 1982;192–207.
19. Krafchek J, Lawrie GM, Roberts R, Magro SA, Wyndham CRC. Surgical ablation of ventricular tachycardia: improved results with a map-directed regional approach. Circulation 1986;73:1239–1247.
20. Gallagher JJ, Sealy WC, Cox JL, Kasell JH. Results of surgery for preexcitation in 200 cases (abstr). Circulation 1981;(Suppl)64:545.
21. Ostermeyer J, Breithardt G, Borggrefe M, Godehardt E, Seipel L, Bircks W. Surgical treatment of ventricular tachycardias: Complete versus partial encircling endocardial ventriculotomy. J Thoracic Cardiovasc Surg 1984;87:517–525.
22. Cox JL. Surgical management of cardiac arrhythmias. In Sabiston DC Jr, Spencer FC, eds. Gibbon's Surgery of the Chest, 4th edition. Philadelphia, WB Saunders Company, 1983;1552–1584.

39

Use of Old and New Anatomic, Electrophysiologic, and Technical Knowledge to Develop Operative Approaches to Tachycardia

Gerard M. Guiraudon
George J. Klein
Arjun D. Sharma
Raymond Yee

Introduction

In 1967, W. C. Sealy and his colleagues at Duke University Medical Center successfully ablated the atrioventricular accessory pathway in a fisherman with incessant reentrant atrioventricular tachycardia associated with the Wolff-Parkinson-White syndrome.[1] This was the first map-guided direct surgery for arrhythmia. Since then, intensive efforts have been made to design surgical therapies for all varieties of cardiac arrhythmias. Although this goal has been greatly advanced, surgery for Wolff-Parkinson-White syndrome remains the ideal model. It established that the surgical rationale should take into account: (1) the mechanism of the tachycardia, (2) mapping data, (3) pathology, (4) cardiac anatomy, and (5) surgical concepts. The surgeon's task is to translate basic science knowledge pertaining to arrhythmia into practical surgical strategies. Currently, the supraventricular tachycardias are better understood but surgical therapy requires con-

From: Brugada P, Wellens HJJ. CARDIAC ARRHYTHMIAS: Where To Go From Here? Mount Kisco, NY, Futura Publishing Company, Inc., © 1987.

siderable expertise while ventricular tachycardia is poorly understood but amenable to technically less demanding surgical techniques.

Supraventricular Tachycardias

The Wolff-Parkinson-White Syndrome

The Wolff-Parkinson-White syndrome is associated with a discrete surgical end-point, the accessory AV pathway. The ablation of the accessory pathway prevents AV reentrant tachycardia and atrial fibrillation. The accessory pathway is a congenital myocardial bundle coursing across the coronary sulcus or endocardium within the septum. The accessory pathway can be ablated using either an endocardial[2] or an epicardial approach.[3]

Endocardial Approach

The first accessory pathway ablated at Duke University was a right ventricular free wall accessory pathway which could be divided using an epicardial dissection combined with an endocardial approach. The ventricular attachment of the accessory pathway was severed using a para-annular right ventriculotomy.[1] This approach was unsuitable to the more common left ventricular free wall accessory pathways when ventriculotomy could be complicated by bleeding and repair hazardous. This prompted Sealy and his colleagues to approach the left coronary sulcus using an endocardial approach.[4] The tricuspid and mitral valve annuli were exposed as for mitral valve or tricuspid valve surgery. The atrial wall was incised along the atrioventricular annulus without any potential injury to the valvular apparatus and the AV fat pad was dissected in situ along the ventricular wall. The major coronary arteries and/or veins were spared. The epicardium and the subepicardial fat pad were not opened to contain the postoperative oozing secondary to blunt dissection. The mitral valve approach via a normal-sized heart was cumbersome but was made easier by the development of the cold cardioplegic cardiac arrest which allowed safe, prolonged aortic cross-clamping. The approach to septal accessory pathways was to be the last frontier for the endocardial approach.[5,6] Sealy documented that the AV node–His bundle region could be approached safely when the accessory pathway was para-Hisian. He designed a specific approach for the accessory pathway in the anterior septal or posterior septal portion of the coronary sulcus. The posterior septal region was described as a toppled pyramidal space. After a few years, accessory pathways in all locations, i.e., left ventricular free wall, posterior septal, right ventricular free wall, and anterior septal regions, could be ablated with high efficacy and low surgical risk.[7]

Epicardial Approach

In 1981, we embarked on designing an alternative epicardial approach.[3] The aim was to avoid aortic cross-clamping associated with cold cardioplegic myocardial preservation. Aortic cross-clamping is still associated with postoperative left ventricular dysfunction and increased surgical morbidity and mortality,[8] especially when prolonged or repetitive aortic cross-clamping is used. In addition, aortic cross-clamping prevents electrophysiological testing during the rewarming period and increases the risk of "delayed" undetected post-dissection recurrence. Another goal was to be able to operate on the normothermic beating heart preferably without cardiopulmonary bypass. Electrophysiological testing before, during, and after the ablative procedure would be possible. The feasibility of the epicardial approach was based on pathology and anatomy. Pathology shows that the vast majority of accessory pathways course within the AV sulcus (epicardial accessory pathways).[9] They are mostly para-annular but may course everywhere in the depth of the fat pad. A minority of accessory pathways courses across the AV junction within the subendocardium or within an intracavitary bundle[10,11] (subendocardial accessory pathways). Subendocardial accessory pathways have been described essentially in the right ventricular free wall region. Some subendocardial accessory pathways are true septal accessory pathways near the membranous septum in the para-Hisian region. Pathology suggested that most accessory pathways can be ablated by epicardial dissection of the coronary sinus. Mobilization en block of the AV fat pad and its vascular contents, associated with careful cleaning of the adjacent atrial wall, the AV annulus, and the neighboring ventricular wall should ablate most accessory pathways except the subendocardial accessory pathways. The subendocardial accessory pathway should be ablated using discrete endocardial dissection when they are located in the para-Hisian region[12] or by transmural cryoablation if they are located in the right ventricular free wall region or posterior septal and left ventricular free wall region. Consequently, an approach was designed which involved two steps: (1) dissection and mobilization of the accessory pathway fat pad and exposure of the coronary sulcus and the AV junction, and (2) cryoablation of the AV junction.

The feasibility of AV fat pad mobilization was documented by anatomical (13) data and experimental study in the dog (14). The coronary arteries can be mobilized without injury to their ventricular branches, after division of their atrial branches. The coronary arteries can be intramural and course within the right and left atrial wall. Our clinical experience proved that anticipated potential limitations were manageable. Greater concern was raised regarding the coronary sinus dissection and mobilization but the coronary sinus proved to handle similar to any other vein. The last concern was the potential deleterious effects of dividing the sinus node artery which can originate from the proximal right coronary artery or from the circumflex coronary artery. There was experimental evidence that the artery can be divided without impairing the sinus node function.[15] The endocardial approach had already proved that the AV nodal artery can be divided without any effect on the AV node. Mobilization of the AV fat pad was carried out on human heart specimens in the left ventricular free wall, posterior septal, right ventricular free wall, and anterior septal region. Experimental surgery in the dog showed that the dissection was feasible on the beating heart without cardiopulmonary bypass.[14] In addition, a clean dissection was achieved which alleviated the fear of bleeding based on previous experience with others.[16] Pathologic examination suggested that transmural atrial cryoablation was achieved and that endocardial accessory pathways could be ablated using epicardial cryoablation on the beating heart. At that point, we felt that we had enough information and experimental training to commence our clinical experience.

We started in July 1982 in patients with left ventricular free wall accessory pathways.[3] The heart was exposed via a median sternotomy to obtain complete intraoperative mapping. The left ventricular AV fat pad was exposed by dislocating the heart under normothermic cardiopulmonary bypass. Since then, our experience has proven that the epicardial approach is feasible with high efficacy and low surgical risk.[17-19] We have gained better insight into the anatomy of the accessory pathway. The possibility of continuous on-line testing allowed us to obtain electrophysiological testing before and after mobilization of the AV fat pad and after cryoablation as well. The presence of accessory pathway conduction after exposure of the sulcus suggested an endocardial accessory pathway. Based on the experimental study, it was hypothesized that the endocardial accessory pathway could be ablated by epicardial cryoablation. Our clinical experience did not confirm that hypothesis and we currently use combined endocardial and epicardial cryoablation for infrequently occurring endocardial accessory pathways. Our clinical experience shows that endocardial accessory pathways are essentially limited to the right ventricular free wall but can be found in the posterior septal and left ventricular free wall region. The epicardial approach for the anterior septal accessory pathway has documented that most so-called anterior septal accessory pathways are true septal accessory pathways in the para-Hisian region.[20] The latter usually still requires an endocardial approach.

In summary, the epicardial approach has proved to be feasible with high efficacy and low surgical risk. The epicardial approach is a valid alternative to endocardial approach.

The Atrial Flutter

Atrial flutter is the second best model of macro-reentrant tachycardia amenable to surgery. Atrial flutter is defined as a rapid and regular atrial rhythm with a rate close to 300 beats per minute. The "common" type of flutter is characterized by a cephalad activation sequence of the atrium with negative flutter waves in the inferior leads. Thomas Lewis in 1921[21] first suggested that the atrial flutter was due to macro-reentry in the right atrium. We have learned much about atrial flutter from Puech and colleagues.[22] He showed us that the common atrial flutter was due to a macro-reentrant circuit traveling cephalad into the interatrial septum, anterior to the fossa ovale, then caudally within the crista terminalis and then entering a zone of slow conduction in the coronary sinus region to reenter the anterior atrial septum and recycle. These findings have been corroborated by other researchers—Boineau,[23] Waldo,[24] Allessie,[25] and Wellens.[26] Atrial flutter is characterized by a continuous activation encircling the fossa ovale. Activation revolves around an anatomical obstacle via two identified internodal pathways, i.e., the anterior internodal pathway and the posterior internodal pathway (crista terminalis) connecting cranially within the sinus node region and caudally via the slow conduction area in the coronary sinus region.

Consequently, we thought that there were two distinct surgical approaches: (1) transection of the fossa ovale and the two adjacent "critical" bundles (right atrial transection), and (2) ablation of the critical zone of slow conduction and one-way block using cryoablation.

In June 1978, we (Guiraudon, Fontaine, and Frank) carried out a right atrial transection in a patient with recurrent atrial flutter associated with a concealed left ventricular free wall accessory pathway. Postoperative electrophysiological study showed no evidence of an accessory pathway and no inducible atrial flutter. The patient has been subsequently free of tachycardia. Since then, few patients have been successfully operated on using this technique. Later in 1984, we (Guiraudon, Klein, and Sharma) operated on two patients with chronic recurrent common atrial flutter. The surgery was carried out on the beating heart using epicardial cryoablation of the slow conduction area in the pericoronary sinus region.[27] Our experience shows that the two distinct approaches are valid, although cryoablation of the slow conduction area is simpler and does not require cardiopulmonary bypass.

AV Nodal Reentrant Tachycardia

AV nodal reentrant tachycardia is very common. There are stringent electrophysiological criteria to define AV nodal reentrant tachycardia which suggests that neither the atria nor the ventricles participate in the genesis of the tachycardia. The striking feature is the presence of "dual" AV nodal conduction.[28] The electrophysiological properties of the two pathways are more in favor of anatomically separated pathways than functionally separated pathways. The key question as to the surgical approach is to document if the "accessory" pathway is intranodal or extranodal. Pathological data are scarce. In a patient with AV nodal reentrant tachycardia, Lev could not identify extranodal or intranodal structures compatible with an accessory pathway.[29] Consequently, AV nodal reentrant tachycardia has been considered "nonsurgical." The atrionodal fibers described by James[30] in all hearts may account for extranodal pathways. Brechenmacher described atrio-Hisian fibers.[31] Multiple James fibers or Brechenmacher fibers may constitute extranodal nodo-nodal, or nodo-Hissian fibers. Under certain circumstances, these accessory pathways can produce tachycardias which satisfy the criteria for AV nodal reentrant tachycardia. It must be remembered that the presence of an AV accessory pathway is not necessarily associated with arrhythmia (asymptomatic Wolff-Parkinson-White syndrome). His, Jr., identified the His bundle in 1893 and he clearly showed that the AV node-His bundle tract is a macroscopic structure that can be surgically exposed. Serendipitous cure of an AV nodal reentrant tachycardia[32] demonstrated the possibility of interrupting the tachycardia with preservation of AV conduction.

It was to the credit of Ross and Johnson in Sidney, Australia,[33] to surgically approach the AV node to ablate potential extranodal accessory pathways. Ross published an initial series of 10 patients successfully operated on using discrete dissection around the AV node. Their uniform success is strongly in favor of discrete extranodal pathway(s). We have recently operated successfully on six patients with AV nodal reentrant tachycardia using similar discrete AV node dissection on the beating heart. The surgical approach to AV nodal reentrant tachycardia is a unique case where successful surgical approach confirms the mechanism and documents the presence of associated extranodal pathways.

Atrial Fibrillation

In this chapter, we will deal with idiopathic atrial fibrillation without structural heart disease. The mechanism of such atrial fibrillation is controversial, but the surgical approach can be based on one electrophysiological concept: atrial fibrillation is due to chaotic reentrant activity that requires a critical atrial area to sustain. This concept is in accordance with the wavelet model of Moe[34] and recent work of Allessie.[35] We designed two surgical concepts: (1) the concept of fragmentation, and (2) the concept of reduction of mass. The concept of fragmentation consists of multiple atrial incisions aimed at preventing the permanence of continuous activation and at preserving the atrial synchrony and subsequently the mechanical atrial function.

We have clinically used the concept of reduction of mass with preservation of chronotropic sinus node function but not the mechanical atrial function. We first established the feasibility of a sinus node–AV node insulation in the dog.[37] The sinus node–AV node insulation (corridor) comprises a cuff of right atrium that harbors the sinus node, the triangle of Koch which harbors the AV node, and a strip of atrial septum which connects the sinus node and AV node. The "corridor" operation is aimed at insulating the sinus node from the rest of the fibrillating atria and at preventing the corridor from fibrillating because of its small area. Three patients with chronic atrial fibrillation have undergone a "corridor" procedure at our institution. Insight has been gained after this limited experience. (1) The selection of patients is paramount. Patients with sick sinus syndrome should be identified. Sinus node dysfunction and/or potential AV nodal conduction disturbances are surgical contraindications. (2) The left atrium was fibrillating in all three patients after concomitant exclusion of the left atrial free wall. This suggests that the left atrial free wall is still large enough to sustain the reentrant chaotic process and/or another mechanism located in the left atrial free wall was associated. Consequently, if we were to use the fragmentation concept in a surgical procedure designed for chronic fibrillation, the left atrium should be fragmented in at least two to three fragments.

Chronic atrial fibrillation associated with mitral valve dysfunction may be surgically approached using exclusion of the left atrium where the atrial fibrillation is likely to originate.[38]

Atrial Tachycardia

Atrial tachycardias can be due to intra-atrial reentry or enhanced automaticity. Their surgical approach seemed relatively easy because (1) extensive atrial mapping can be carried out preoperatively, and (2) large segments of the atrial wall can be resected, excluded, or cryoablated. A "pin-point" localization is not required and extensive treatment of the region of interest can be performed, and long-term efficacy could be expected.

We (Guiraudon, Fontaine, Frank) started our experience in 1975 with two patients with "ectopic" atrial tachycardia. One was localized in the right atrial free wall, the other into the superior left atrial free wall. Both sites of origin were treated using a 4 cm diameter circular resection. Both patients had recurrence of atrial tachycardia at a distant site of origin. In 1982, three patients with so-called paroxysmal sinus node tachycardia were treated with subtotal exclusion of the right atrium.[39] All patients had good early operative results after uncomplicated subtotal right atrial exclusion (extensive exclusion of sinus node region). However, long-term results were disappointing.[40] During a mean follow-up of 21 months, two patients had paroxysmal atrial fibrillation and two patients had symptomatic bradycardias requiring permanent pacemaker implantation. One patient developed exercise-induced ectopic left atrial tachycardia. All three patients are on drug therapy.

Other investigators, particularly those with pediatric experience,[41] had better results. However, we believe that many of these patients may have diffuse atrial electrical instability and that direct surgical treatment cannot be recommended as a valid alternative to medical therapy. If used, surgical therapy should be extensive. We operated on two patients with intra-atrial reentrant tachycardia using extensive cryoablation who remain free of tachycardia after a mean follow-up of 3 months. The mechanism of tachycardia is an essential prognostical factor and "ectopic" tachycardia is, in our experience, likely to be associated with diffuse electrical abnormality. Preferably, conservative or noninvasive intervention should be attempted.

Ventricular Tachycardia

Ventricular Tachycardia in the Absence of Coronary Artery Disease

Our conception of surgical approaches to ventricular arrhythmias stems from our experience with ventricular tachycardia in patients without coronary disease. The absence of a reliable animal model for cardiac arrhythmia has precluded the development of any surgical technique in the experimental laboratory. The translation of fundamentals pertaining to arrhythmogenesis into the surgical procedure was to be done in the operating room. Electrophysiological fundamentals to be used were: (1) The concept of reentry—the inducibility of the tachycardia should lead to successful intraoperative assessment and ablation. (2) The concept of arrhythmogenic substrate—the substrate is often associated with macroscopic diffuse or discrete lesions, where slow conduction and delayed late or fractionated activation are recorded. The arrhythmogenic anatomical substrate harbors the critical slow conducting part of the circuit. The "exit" of the circuit which activates the rest of the heart is a critical site as well, mostly at the junction between the slow conducting pathway and the excitable gap.

We applied our experience with cardiac mapping acquired in patients with Wolff-Parkinson-White syndrome. We believed that cardiac mapping should determine the site of earliest activation, which we thought would be located in the proximity of the "critical" area.

Our first patient was a 33-year-old man with dilated cardiomyopathy associated with congestive heart failure and complicated by recurrent resistant ventricular tachycardia, with two distinct morphologies. At surgery, in May 1973, the left ventricle was dilated and hypokinetic. Epicardial mapping during sinus rhythm was normal, although delayed abnormal activation was identified in the aftermath. The two morphologies of ventricular tachycardia were induced. One tachycardia originated from the apex, the other tachycardia originated in the obtuse margin region of the left ventricle. It was impossible to map the obtuse margin region because the tachycardia stopped everytime the probe was applied onto that region. Any pressure on the apex reproducibly terminated the apical tachycardia. This finding strongly suggested that the site of apparent origin was a critical area. It was decided to perform a transmural ventriculotomy at each site of origin, 5 cm at the apex and 2 cm at the obtuse margin region. The patient remained free of ventricular arrhythmia but died of congestive heart failure 9 months after surgery.[42,43] This patient's outcome convinced us that cardiac mapping was a unique surgical guide in dealing with diffuse lesions. In the following months, two patients with what we were to later identify as arrhythmogenic right ventricular dysplasia were referred to us. Both patients had a slightly dilated right ventricular free wall. One had a typical ectatic pulmonary infundibulum where the tachycardia originated and where delayed and late potentials were recorded. One patient had more diffuse right ventricular free wall dilation with a tachycardia originating on the inferior right ventricular wall. The infundibulum was resected and a "simple ventriculotomy" was performed over the inferior right ventricular wall. These two patients were to remain free of tachycardia.

At that point, we had developed a surgical approach guided by epicardial mapping: (1) a simple ventriculotomy was performed at the site of origin of the tachycardia; (2) a wall resection was carried out in areas where slow conduction or delayed or fractionated activation were recorded. These areas were labeled arrhythmogenic. They either were in close proximity to the origin of the tachycardia and were considered the site of the mechanism of the actual tachycardia or they could be observed at a distance of the actual tachycardia and were considered potentially arrhythmogenic and a potential cause of relapse. They were either resected or incised, depending on their location.

Further experience showed important limitations to that approach. (1) Epicardial mapping did not explore the septum adequately. Due to the thickness of the left ventricular wall, left ventricular epicardial mapping did not have the same value as right ventricular free wall epicardial mapping. (2) Left ventriculotomies or septal approaches in patients with cardiomyopathies were difficult to repair and deleterious to left ventricular function.[44] A "noninvasive" approach to the left ventricular cavity had to be designed.

The surgical experience with ventricular tachycardia in the absence of coronary artery disease prompted us to describe a new electrophysiological pathological entity: arrhythmogenic right ventricular dysplasia.[45] Two other lessons were learned were: (1) The long-term prognosis of these patients is as much determined by the eradication of the tachycardia as by left ventricular function. (2) The long-term result in terms of arrhythmia is determined by an adequate map-guided extensive surgical procedure, and by the nature of the lesions: discrete or diffuse, quiescent or progressive. Left ventricular idiopathic aneurysm associated with ventricular tachycardia can be definitively eradicated while the diffuse possibly progressive lesions of arrhythmogenic right ventricular dysplasia could not be definitively neutralized and associated ventricular tachycardia were prone to relapse. The incidence of long-term relapses (50%) in patients with arrhythmogenic ventricular dysplasia prompted us to design a more extensive operation, total exclusion of the right ventricular free wall. The right ventricular free wall disconnetion.[46,47] is hemodynamically tolerated and confines all abnormal activity within the excluded right ventricular free wall.

Recently, we (Guiraudon, Vermeulen, and van Hemel) have used better tactics to ablate the arrhythmogenic substrate in patients with left ventricular tachycardia. In three patients, the left ventriculotomy was avoided by approaching the left ventricular cavity via the aortic orifice on the beating heart, after the aorta had been cross-clamped and intracoronary artery perfusion instituted. Endocardial mapping was obtained using simultaneous recordings of an array of 30 unipolar electrodes attached onto an inflatable balloon introduced into the left ventricle via the aortic root.[48] Subsequent cryoablation was carried out using epicardial cryoablation combined with endocardial cryoablation via the aortic orifice. This technique avoids left ventriculotomy and reduces postoperative left ventricular dysfunction. Cryoablation produced discrete measurable lesions. It can be applied everywhere to the left ventricular walls. We have recently shown that the posterior papillary muscle can be extensively cryoablated in the dog without subsequent long-term mitral valve or ventricular dysfunction.[49]

Ventricular Tachycardias Associated with Coronary Artery Disease

Parallel to our experience with ventricular tachycardia in the absence of coronary artery disease, we were mapping patients with ventricular tachycardias associated with a left ventricular aneurysm or an infarct scar. This experience was aimed at developing a better surgical approach than blind aneurysmectomy. Our initial experience was disappointing. Epicardial mapping was not as informative as in patients without coronary artery disease. An endocardial approach on the beating heart was used in few patients but ventricular tachycardia could not be induced after ventriculotomy. At that time deep concern was raised about injury to the myocardium by prolonged normothermic cardiopulmonary bypass. Cardiac mapping was considered harmful in patients with coronary artery disease and was censored. Consequently, we had to design a direct approach based on the pathophysiology of the scar and on anatomical landmarks. It was well established that the arrhythmogenic substrate of the chronic inducible ventricular tachycardia was in the border zone and that the entire border zone was actually or potentially arrhythmogenic.[50] The border zone circumscribes the central transmural necrotic zone and is essentially subendocardial.[51] Thick endocardial fibrosis develops opposite to the entire ischemic area. Therefore, the limits of the endocardial fibrosis corresponds to the limits of the border zone. The endocardial fibrosis was the anatomical guide that we were looking for. It made the assessment of the pathology of the aneurysm clear and easy via endocavitary exploration while the epicardial exploration remained misleading. We were concerned that the resection of the border zone would excessively reduce the ventricular wall and the ventricular closure would be technically difficult and result in a small left ventricular cavity associated with low cardiac output failure. We were in a quandary when a patient came up with a solution.[52] This patient presented with ventricular tachycardia associated with a small left ventricular apical scar after myocardial infarction. The ventricular tachycardia was well tolerated and the three morphologies of ventricular tachycardia were mapped using epicardial mapping. The three early sites of activation were located along the left anterior descending coronary artery. The epicardial activation time preceded the onset of QRS and suggested three "superficial" sites of origin in the anterior septum, which was contracting, and where no scar was visible. A ventriculotomy along the left anterior descending coronary artery was likely to injure the left anterior descending artery. The repair of the ventriculotomy was likely to be difficult and associated with significant loss of contractile myocardium. I consequently elected to approach the left ventricle via a short apical incision and to carry out an endocardial incision deep, but not transmural, along the anterior septum. The ventriculotomy was easily repaired and the ventricle was closed. Good left ventricular function was present and no bleeding or local ischemia were observed. This experience suggested that an endocardial incision has many advantages: (1) it can be done anywhere without regard to the large epicardial coronary arteries, (2) it involves the subendocardium where the ischemic arrhythmogenic substrate is frequently situated, and (3) it is easy and safe to repair under the protection of the subepicardial layers which prevent bleeding. We concluded at that time that the border zone should not be resected but excluded by an endocardial ventriculotomy encircling the border zone and carried out along but within the limits of the endocardial fibrosis. The incision would be deep but not transmural and slightly oblique to follow the oblique limit of the border zone. The encircling endocardial ventriculotomy[52-54] was aimed at (1) excluding the border zone to confine the abnormal electrical activation with the infarct scar, but also at (2) acting as a simple ventriculotomy as in a patient without coronary artery disease. The encircling endocardial ventriculotomy was to follow the loci where the endocardial origins of ventricular tachycardia are most likely to arise. Consequently, the encircling endocardial ventriculotomy would act as a simple ventriculotomy at the "site of origin" of the tachycardia.

On November 10th, 1975, we carried out the first encircling endocardial ventriculotomy in a patient 1 month after anterior myocardial infarction with ventricular tachycardias associated with low output failure. The second patient a few months later presented with a posterior left ventricular aneurysm. The encircling endocardial ventriculotomy would "exclude" the posterior papillary muscle without secondary mitral valve dysfunction. Despite there early promising results, we failed to convince our colleagues that the encircling endocardial ventriculotomy was a better surgical alternative than the obsolete aneurysmectomy. In 1978, we reported only a series of five patients.[53] In 1981, one series amounted to 30 patients after a 6-year experience.[54] In the interval, Josephson had developed a most successful surgical approach using map-guided endocardial resection.[55] The concept of exclusion of the encircling endocardial ventriculotomy was to be partially documented by Cox et al.[56] The encircling endocardial ventriculotomy was adopted and perfected in other centers.[57] The encircling endocardial ventriculotomy was thought to be associated with postoperative left ventricular dysfunction. This was mostly associated with encircling endocardial ventriculotomy performed at the periphery of the endocardial fibrosis, across the normal myocardium. A recent experimental study documented that the encircling endocardial ventriculotomy and the endocardial resection are not associated with left ventricular dysfunction.[58] In 1982, we used extensive encircling endocardial cryoablation of the "border zone" to replace the encircling endocardial ventriculotomy.[59] The cryosurgical scar is discrete, well delineated and does not need any subsequent surgical repair. We thought that cryoablation can neutralize the arrhythmogenic substrate within the border zone without impairing the surrounding contracting myocardium. Nineteen patients have been operated on using the encircling endocardial ventriculotomy. Only one patient had recurrence of ventricular arrhythmia after surgery.

In conclusion, we still favor extensive surgery everytime it is safely feasible. We strongly believe that the ultimate goal of surgery for arrhythmia should be the entire neutralization of the potentially arrhythmogenic areas where these areas are not contractile. Discrete map-guided procedures are selected with the arrhythmogenic substrate is located within contracting myocardium.

Acknowledgment: This research was funded in part by the Ontario Heart Foundation, the University Hospital Pooled Research Fund, and the J.P. Bicknell Foundation. We wish to affectionately thank Charlene Paquette for her secretarial assistance.

References

1. Sealy WC, Hattler BG, Blumenschein SC, Cobb FR. Surgical treatment of Wolff-Parkinson-White sydrome. Ann Thorac Surg 1968;8:1–11.
2. Sealy WC, Wallace AJ, Ramming KP, Gallagher JJ, Svenson RH. An improved operation for the definitive treatment of the Wolff-Parkinson-White sydrome. Ann Thorac Surg 1974;2:107–113.
3. Guiraudon GM, Klein GJ, Gulamhusein S, Jones DL, Yee R, Perkins DG, Jarvis E. Surgical repair of Wolff-Parkinson-White syndrome: A new closed-heart technique. Ann Thorac Surg 1984;37(1):67–71.
4. Sealy WC, Gallagher JJ, Wallace AG. The surgical treatment of Wolff-Parkinson-White Syndrome: Evolution of improved methods for identification and interruption of the Kent bundle. Ann Thorac Surg 1976;22(5):443–457.
5. Sealy WC, Mikat EM. Anatomical problems with identification and interruption of posterior septal Kent bundles. Ann Thorac Surg 1983;36,5:584–595.
6. Sealy WC. Kent bundles in the anterior septal space. Ann Thorac Surg 1983;36(2):180–186.
7. Gallagher JJ, Sealy WC, Cox JL, German LD, Kasell JH, Bardy GH, Packer DL. Results of surgery for preexcitation caused by accessory atrioventricular pathways in 267 consecutive cases. In Josephson ME, Wellens HJJ, ed. Tachycardias: Mechanisms, diagnosis, treatment. Philadelphia, Lea & Febiger, 1984;259.

8. Buckberg GD. A proposed "solution" to the cardioplegic controversy. J Thorac Cardiovasc Surg 1979;77:803–815.
9. Anderson RH, Becker AE. Stanley Kent and accessory atrio-ventricular connections. J Thorac Cardiovasc Surg 1981;81:649–658.
10. Bharati S, Strasberg B, Bilitch M, Salibi H, Mandel W, Rosen KM, Lev M. Anatomic substrate for preexcitation in idiopathic myocardial hypertrophy with fibroelastosis of the left ventricle. Am J Cardiol 1981;48:47–58.
11. Lev M, Sodi-Pallares D, Friedland C. A histopathologic study of the atrio-ventricular communications in a case of WPW with incomplete left bundle branch block. Am Heart J 1963;66:399–404.
12. Guiraudon GM, Klein GJ, Sharma AD, Jones DL. Surgical Treatment of Wolff-Parkinson-White Syndrome: The Epicardial Approach. In Benditt DG, Benson DW, eds. Cardiac Preexcitation Syndromes. Boston, Martinus Nijhoff Publishing, 1986; 535–541.
13. McAlpine WA. Heart and Coronary Arteries. New York, Springer-Verlag, 1975.
14. Klein GJ, Guiraudon GM, Perkins DG, Jones DL, Yee R, Jarvis E. Surgical Correction of the Wolff-Parkinson-White syndrome in the closed heart using cryosurgery: A simplified approach. JACC 1984;3:405–409.
15. Sealy WC, Bache RJ, Seaber AV. The atrial pacemaking site after surgical exclusion of the sinoatrial node. J Thorac Cardiovasc Surg 1973;65:841–850.
16. Cox JL. The status of surgery for cardiac arrhythmias. Circulation 1985;71:413–417.
17. Guiraudon GM, Klein GJ, Sharma AD, Jones DL, McLellan DG. Surgery for Wolff-Parkinson-White sydrome: Further experience with an epicardial approach. Circulation 1986;74:525–529.
18. Guiraudon GM, Klein GJ, Sharma AD, Jones DL, McLellan DG. Surgical ablation of posterior septal accessory pathways in the Wolff-Parkinson-White syndrome by a closed-heart technique. J Thorac Cardiovasc Surg 1986;92:406–413.
19. Guiraudon GM, Klein GJ, Sharma AD, Milstein S, McLellan DG. Closed-heart technique for Wolff-Parkinson-White syndrome: Further experience and potential limitations. Ann Thorac Surg 1986;42:651–657.
20. Guiraudon GM, Klein GJ, Sharma AD, Jones DL. Anteroseptal AV pathways are true septal, para-hisian structures: verification by ice mapping (abstr). Circulation 1984; 70(II):338.
21. Lewis T, Drury AN, Iliescu CC. A demonstration of circus movement in clinical flutter of the auricles. Heart 1921;8:341–345.
22. Puech P, Latour M, Grolleau R. Le flutter et ses limites. Arch Mal Coeur 1970;63: 116–120.
23. Boineau JP, Mooney CR, Hudson RD, Hughes DG, Erchin RA Jr, Wylds AC. Observations on re-entrant excitation pathways and refractory period distributions in spontaneous and experimental atrial flutter in the dog. In Kulbertus HE, ed. Re-entrant Arrhythmias: Mechanisms and Treatment. Baltimore, University Park Press, 1977; 72–98.
24. Waldo AL, Some observations concerning atrial flutter in man. PACE 1983;6:1181–1189.
25. Allessie MA, Lammers WJEP, Bonke IM, Hollen J. Intra-atrial reentry as a mechanism for atrial flutter induced by acetylcholine and rapid pacing in the dog. Circulation 1984;70:123–135.
26. Wellens HJJ, Janse MJ, van Dam RT, Durrer D. Epicardial excitation of the atria in a patient with atrial flutter. Br Heart J 1971;33:233–237.
27. Klein GJ, Guiraudon GM, Sharma AD, Milstein S. Demonstration of macroreentry and feasibility of operative therapy in the common type of atrial flutter. Am J Cardiol 1986;57:587–591.
28. Denes P, Wu D, Dhingra RC, Chuquimia R, Rosen KM. Demonstration of dual AV nodal pathways in patients with paroxysmal supraventricular tachycardia. Circulation 1973;48:549–555.
29. Sheinman MM, Gonzalez R, Thomas A, Ullyot D, Bharati S, Lev M. Reentry confined to the atrioventricular node: Electrophysiologic and anatomic findings. Am J Cardiol 1982;49:1814–1818.

30. James TN. Morphology of the human atrioventricular node, with remarks pertinent to its electrophysiology. Am Heart J 1961;62:756–771.
31. Brechenmacher C, Laham L, Iris L, Gerbaux A, Lenegre J. Etude histologique des voies anormales de conduction dans un syndrome de Wolff-Parkinson-White et dans un syndrome de Lown-Ganong-Levine. Arch Mal Coeur 1974;67,5:507–520.
32. Pritchett ELC, Anderson RW, Benditt DG, Kasell J, Harrison L, Wallace AG, Sealy WC, Gallagher JJ. Reentry within the atrioventricular node: Surgical cure with preservation of atrioventricular conduction. Circulation 1979;60:440–446.
33. Ross DL, Johnson DC, Denniss AR, Cooper MJ, Richards DA, Uther JB. Curative surgery for atrioventricular junctional ("AV nodal") reentrant tachycardia. JACC 1985; 6:1383–1392.
34. Moe GK. On the multiple wavelet hypothesis of atrial fibrillation. Arch Int Pharmacodyn Ther 1962;140:183–188.
35. Allessie MA, Bonke FIM, Schopman FJG. Circus movement in rabbit atrial muscle as a mechanism of tachycardia. III. The "leading circle" concept: a new model of circus movement in cardiac tissue without the involvement of an anatomic obstacle. Circ Res 1977;41:9–18.
36. Garrey WE. The nature of fibrillary contraction of the heart. Its relation to tissue mass and form. Am J Physiol 1914;33:397–414.
37. Guiraudon GM, Campbell CS, Jones DL, McLellan DG, MacDonald JL. Combined sino-atrial node atrio-ventricular isolation: A surgical alternative to His bundle ablation in patients with atrial fibrillation (abstr). Circulation 1985;72(III):220.
38. Williams JM, Ungerleider RM, Lofland GK, Cox JL. Left atrial isolation. New technique for the treatment of supraventricular arrhythmias. J Thorac Cardiovasc Surg 1980;80: 373–380.
39. Yee R, Guiraudon GM, Gardner MJ, Gulamhusein SS, Klein GJ. Refractory paroxysmal sinus tachycardia: Management by subtotal right atrial exclusion. JACC 1984;3:400–404.
40. Sharma AD, Klein GJ, Guiraudon GM, Gardner MJ. Paroxysmal sinus tachycardia: Further experience with subtotal right atrial exclusion suggesting diffuse atrial disease (abstr). JACC 1986;7:128.
41. Ott DA, Gillette PC, Garson A, Cooley DA, Reul GJ, McNamara DG. Surgical management of refractory supraventricular tachycardia in infants and children. JACC 1985;5: 124–129.
42. Guiraudon G, Frank R, Fontaine G. Interet des cartographies dans le traitement chirurgical des tachycardies ventriculaires rebelles recidivantes. Nouv Presse Med 1974;3:321.
43. Fontaine G, Guiraudon G, Frank R, Gerbaux A, Cousteau JP, Barrillon A, Gay J, Cabrol C, Facquet J. La cartographie epicardique et le traitement chirurgical par simple ventriculotomie de certaines tachycardies ventriculaires rebelles par reentree. Arch Mal Coeur 1975;68,2:113–124.
44. Guiraudon G, Fontaine G, Frank R, Leandri R, Barra J, Cabrol C. Surgical treatment of ventricular tachycardia guided by ventricular mapping in 23 patients without coronary artery disease. Ann Thorac Surg 1981;32:439–450.
45. Marcus FI, Fontaine GH, Guiraudon G, Frank R, Laurenceau JL, Malergue C, Grosgogeat Y. Right ventricular dysplasia: A report of 24 adult cases. Circulation 1982;60: 384–398.
46. Guiraudon GM, Klein GJ, Gulamhusein S, Painvin GA, Del Campo C, Gonzales JC, Ko PT. Total disconnection of the right ventricular free wall: Surgical treatment of right ventricular tachycardia associated with right ventricular dysplasia. Circulation 1983; 67:463–470.
47. Jones DL, Guiraudon GM, Klein GJ. Total disconnection of the right ventricular free wall: Physiological consequences in the dog. Am Heart J 1984;107:1169–1177.
48. de Bakker JMT, Janse MJ, Van Capelle FJL, Durrer D. Endocardial mapping by simultaneous recording of endocardial electrograms during cardiac surgery for ventricular aneurysm. JACC 1983;2:947–953.

49. Guiraudon GM, Jones DL, Klein GJ, Kostuk WJ, Jablonsky G, McLellan DG, MacDonald JLM. Feasibility of cryoablation of the posterior papillary muscle in the dog (abstr). JACC 1986;7:236.
50. Wittig JH, Boineau JP. Surgical treatment of ventricular arrhythmias using epicardial, transmural, and endocardial mapping. Ann Thorac Surg 1975;20:117–126.
51. Mallory GK, White PD, Salcedo-Salgar J. The speed of healing of myocardial infarction: A study of the pathologic anatomy in seventy-two cases. Am Heart J 1939;18:647–671.
52. Guiraudon G, Fontaine G, Frank R, Vedel J, Escande G, Cabrol C. New concepts in the surgical treatment of ventricular tachycardia. In Kelly DT, ed. Advances in the Management of Arrhythmias. Australia, Telectronics Pty. Limited, 1978;225–238.
53. Guiraudon G, Fontaine G, Frank R, Escande G, Étievent P, Cabrol C. Encircling endocardial ventriculotomy: A new surgical treatment for life-threatening ventricular tachycardias resistant to medical treatment following myocardial infarction. Ann Thorac Surg 1978;26:438–444.
54. Guiraudon G, Fontaine G, Frank R, Caborl C, Grosgogeat Y. Apports de la ventriculotomie circulaire d'exclusion dans le traitement de la tachycardie ventriculaire recidivante apres infarctus du myocarde. Arch Mal Coeur 1982;75:1013–1021.
55. Josephson ME, Harken AH, Horowitz LN. Endocardial Excision: A new surgical technique for the treatment of recurrent ventricular tachycardia. Circulation 1979;60:1430–1439.
56. Ungerleider RM, Holman WL, Stanley TE, Lofland GK, Williams JM, Ideker RE, Smith PK, Quick G, Cox JL. Encircling endocardial ventriculotomy for refractory ischemic ventricular tachycardia. J Thorac Cardiovasc Surg 1982;83:840–849.
57. Ostermeyer J, Breithardt G, Borggrefe M, Godehardt E, Seipel L, Bircks W. Surgical treatment of ventricular tachycardias: Complete versus partial encircling endocardial ventriculotomy. J Thorac Cardiovasc Surg 1984;87:517–525.
58. Mickleborough LL, Wilson GJ, Weisel RD, Mackay CA, Ivanov J, Takagi M, Akagawa H, McLaughlin PR, Baird RJ. Endocardial excision versus encircling endocardial ventriculotomy: A Comparison of effects on ventricular structure and function. J Thorac Cardiovasc Surg 1986;91:779–787.
59. Guiraudon GM, Klein GJ, Jones DL, McLellan DG. Encircling endocardial cryoablation for ventricular arrhythmias after myocardial infarction: Further experience (abstr). Circulation 1985;72:III–222.

# IX

THE IMPLANTABLE
DEFIBRILLATOR

40

The Automatic Implantable Defibrillator: Some Historical Notes

M. Mirowski
Morton M. Mower

During the past several years, the efficacy of the automatic implantable cardioverter-defibrillator (AICD) in preventing sudden cardiac death has been clearly demonstrated. Extensive evidence is now available to indicate that this device significantly reduces the mortality of patients with malignant ventricular tachyarrhythmias.[1-5] While the clinical results with the use of the AICD in the United States and Europe are presented elsewhere, the purpose of this paper is to place this new therapeutic modality in its historical context.

The concept of a fully implantable automatic system for recognition and treatment of ventricular fibrillation was first proposed in the late 1960s.[6,7] This period in the history of cardiology saw numerous advances in our understanding of the epidemiologic, electrophysiologic, and clinical aspects of ventricular arrhythmias and was most propitious for new ideas. From a personal vantage point, a number of observations provided particular impetus for the development of such a device.

The first observation concerned the magnitude of the sudden cardiac death syndrome. The figures which became available indicated that approximately 450,000 people were dying suddenly each year in the United States alone. Sudden cardiac death was thus exposed, for the first time, as a major, if not *the* major, public health problem in the developed countries of the world. The second

From: Brugada P, Wellens HJJ. CARDIAC ARRHYTHMIAS: Where To Go From Here? Mount Kisco, NY, Futura Publishing Company, Inc., © 1987.

observation stemmed from the newly acquired coronary care unit experience that implicated ventricular fibrillation as the arrhythmia responsible for the sudden cardiac death syndrome.

A third group of observations dealt with therapeutic issues. Although it was well established that ventricular fibrillation can be a reversible condition, usually responding to the delivery to the heart of a sufficiently strong electrical countershock, it also became evident that the effectiveness of this maneuver is entirely dependent upon prompt availability of specialized personnel and equipment. Since no alternatives were available for the required personnel and equipment, efforts were made to minimize the role of the time factor through the establishment of mobile coronary care unit networks and other community-based rescue systems. But even under the best of circumstances, these efforts could only be partially successful because the great majority of cardiac arrest victims could not be reached in time for effective defibrillation and because those who were revived remained at continuing high risk of sudden death due to their residual propensity for recurrent malignant arrhythmias.

These apparently unsurmountable constraints, inherent in the conventional out-of-hospital resuscitation, underscored a need for new approaches. Although there was clearly no short-term solution to the problem, it occurred to us that the basic challenge was to create a system assuring successful defibrillation wherever and whenever needed, while simultaneously obviating the need for medical personnel and equipment. The next step in this line of thought was to envision an automatic implanted device capable of continuously monitoring the heart, recognizing ventricular fibrillation, and then delivering the corrective electrical countershock to restore normal rhythm. We became convinced that, for high-risk patients, such standby automatic defibrillation could provide at least a partial answer to the awesome challenge of sudden arrhythmic death.

It goes without saying that the development of an implantable medical device and its introduction into the clinical arena is never a simple matter. This truism is particularly obvious during periods of economic constriction and stringent regulatory constraints, so characteristic of the past two decades. Thus, even before the developmental process actually begins, it is highly desirable to ensure that a number of preconditions are met. The most crucial one is the perceived need for the device and the soundness of the underlying concept. Another area of concern is the availability of technology required for its implementation. If the necessary technology does not exist, one would certainly require some evidence suggesting that such could be developed. The need to identify and secure adequate funding sources is self-evident. Last but not least, governmental and/or institutional backing, extending beyond purely financial support, is extremely helpful in creating a propitious social and scientific climate for the project.

It is now of only historical interest to note that at the inception of our work none of these basic preconditions were met. In fact, the very idea of an automatic implantable defibrillator was poorly received by both the engineering and the cardiological communities. The need for such a device was not recognized and, for reasons that are even today not entirely clear, the validity of the assumptions underlying this concept was vigorously questioned. However, there certainly must have been something intriguing about the entire idea, because the criticism was at times vociferous, reaching the editorial pages of specialty journals.[8] Even those who appeared to be more objective maintained that an automatic implantable defibrillating device was beyond the capabilities of contemporary technology.

This generally negative reaction was quite unexpected because the automatic implantable defibrillator concept, when first conceived, hardly appeared to us as a likely source of controversy. In fact, we looked upon this device, in a very broad sense, as similar to the generally accepted implantable demand pacemaker, except that ventricular fibrillation instead of asystole would be sensed and that the electrical discharges would have defibrillating magnitude. Under the circumstances, therefore, we were less surprised when public and private funding organizations were unwilling to underwrite the developmental costs of the device.

Admittedly, the technological difficulties inherent in the development of the automatic implantable defibrillator were far from negligible. To name only a few, there were no ready solutions as to how to miniaturize the bulky external defibrillator, how to design a safe and reliable algorithm for arrhythmia detection, or how to develop the required power sources comprised of batteries with high-energy density and high-power rating and of capacitors characterized by extremely low leakage. No clear directions were seen suggesting the proper defibrillating waveform or the optimal electrode configuration. The energy requirements for internal defibrillation of closed-chest patients were unknown and no methods for non-invasive testing of implanted defibrillators were available. Even more importantly, serious concerns had been raised as to the safety of such a system. Such apparently esoteric problems as the maintenance of extremely high voltage in an implanted device with components in close proximity were not even considered during the early stages of this work. It soon became evident, however, that answers to many of these and other questions and problems required an extensive amount of fundamental research, a great deal of effort and time and, not infrequently, a completely new technological foundation.

Significantly enough, the obstacles we found most difficult and frustrating were not technological in nature. The skepticism regarding the engineering and biological feasibility of the automatic implantable defibrillator concept was pervasive, with the critics challenging not only its rationale but also requiring answers to all questions and solutions to all problems even before there was an opportunity to approach and study the issues. The old saying that "nothing can ever be accomplished if all possible objections must first be overcome" had been forgotten. It was only small consolation to be reminded that, in the history of medical research, opposition to new concepts is not a new phenomenon. Many years ago, Rushmer had already observed that "at times scientific progress depends less upon the acquisition of new knowledge than upon the removal of conceptual obstacles."[9]

It was soon realized that the skeptics would be very little influenced, if at all, by any amount of intellectual discourse or persuasion and that the only way to demonstrate the validity of the automatic implantable defibrilltor concept was to actually implement it, despite the general view that such an attempt was bound to fail. Thus, guided more by intuition than by hard data, we felt that the goal of developing the automatic implantable defibrillator was worth pursuing.

The initial work was carried out in the basement of Sinai Hospital in Baltimore where our first experimental model of the device was built and successfully tested in dogs in 1969. Although Sinai was only a community hospital, it had an enlightened Chief of Medicine, namely Dr. Albert I. Mendeloff. Also, it was well suited to our needs as it had not only a somewhat underutilized experimental animal laboratory but also a clinical engineering department under the direction of Mr. William S. Staewen. In absence of grants, we could hardly afford the exorbitant costs of conditioned research animals, but the problem was solved by devising an unconventional way of securing them directly from the pound for $2 per dog. The various components needed for the construction of the early prototypes were also purchased with strictly personal funds. In 1973, we were fortunate to team up with Dr. Marlin S. Heilman, a physician whose medical instrumentation company, Intec Systems, subsequently played a decisive role in transforming the early experimental models into a reliable and sophisticated clinical device. The "incubation" period of the project, defined as the time which elapsed from the inception of the idea until its first clinical application extended over some 13 years. Figure 1 lists a few of the major milestones in this long developmental process.[6,10-18]

While each of these milestones has its own story, there is one that might be of some special interest to this audience. In 1976, our work had reached a stage in which the first chronic animal implants of the device became possible. The main objective of these implants was to demonstrate that the implanted difibrillator performed as initially intended and that, at least in the experimental setting, sudden arrhythmic death could indeed be prevented. The nature of the experiments required repeated inductions of ventricular fibrillation in active, conscious animals, a procedure which, to the best of our knowledge, had never been performed before. In order to accomplish this, an implantable fibrillator, in the form of a magnetically triggered alternating current generator, was designed. By placing a magnet over the implanted fibrillator, the fibrillating current was trans-

THE AUTOMATIC IMPLANTABLE DEFIBRILLATOR
Historical Perspective

1967   1969   1970   1976   1980   1982   1985
- Conception
  - First Experimental Model
    - Transvenous Catheter Defibrillation
      - First Animal Implant
        - First Human Implant
          - Addition of Cardioverting Capability
            - F.D.A. Approval

Figure 1: A few of the milestones in the development of the automatic implantable defibrillator. FDA = United States Food and Drug Administration.

mitted to the animal's heart through a right ventricular catheter (Fig. 2) and ventricular fibrillation could be initiated at will without interfering with the dog's activity; the chronically implanted automatic defibrillator then promptly diagnosed and terminated the malignant arrhythmia within seconds. Thus, a convenient and reliable experimental model of sudden arrhythmic death in active animals had been created.[19]

Many of our colleagues, however, still had great difficulties visualizing how the two implanted devices, the fibrillator and the defibrillator, could actually perform the functions we were describing. With a picture being worth a thousand words, we thought that a movie, rather than another paper, would more vividly explain the described experimental sequence. Several fibrillation-defibrillation episodes in alert, nonanesthetized dogs chronically implanted with fibrillators and defibrillators were thus filmed. The impact of this movie on changing the audience's perception of the automatic defibrillator was rather striking. For the first time one could actually witness experimental sudden cardiac death due to ventricular fibrillation, with the arrhythmia being automatically diagnosed and terminated not just once but over and over again, and with the dog cheerfully playing with us only moments after each resuscitation (Fig. 3)!

The role of this movie in convincing many of the skeptics as to the feasibility of this approach to prevention of sudden cardiac death cannot be overestimated; but even at that time, very few could predict that in the not-too-distant future

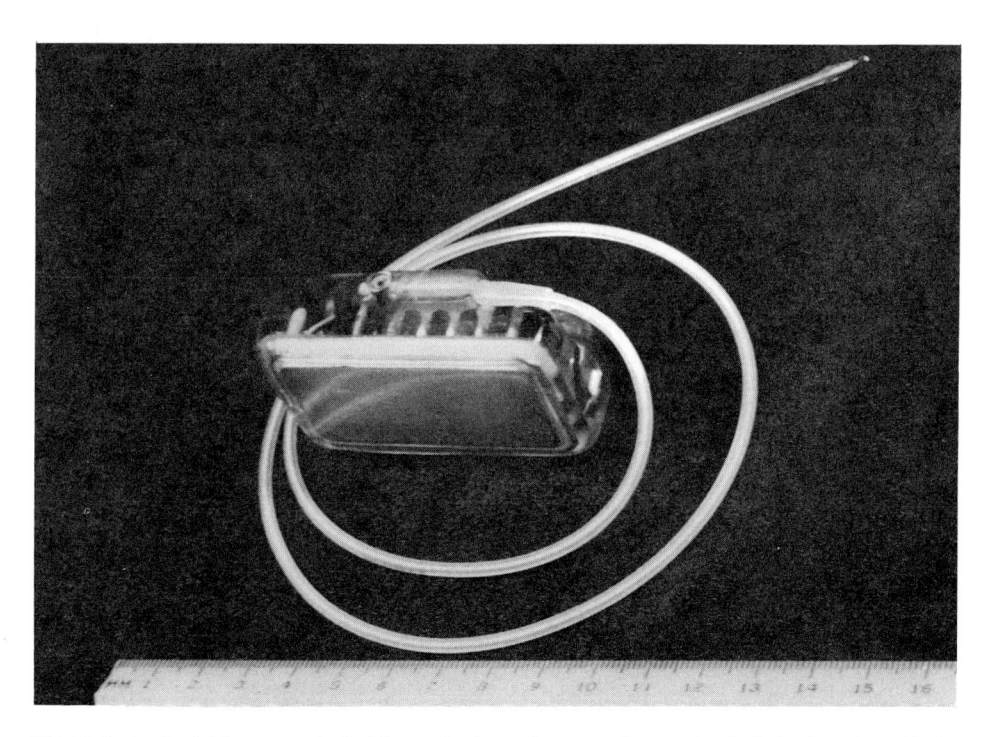

Figure 2: Implantable, magnetically triggered, alternating current generator for induction of ventricular fibrillation in the active experimental animal. The fibrillating current is delivered to the heart through a right ventricular endocardial catheter.

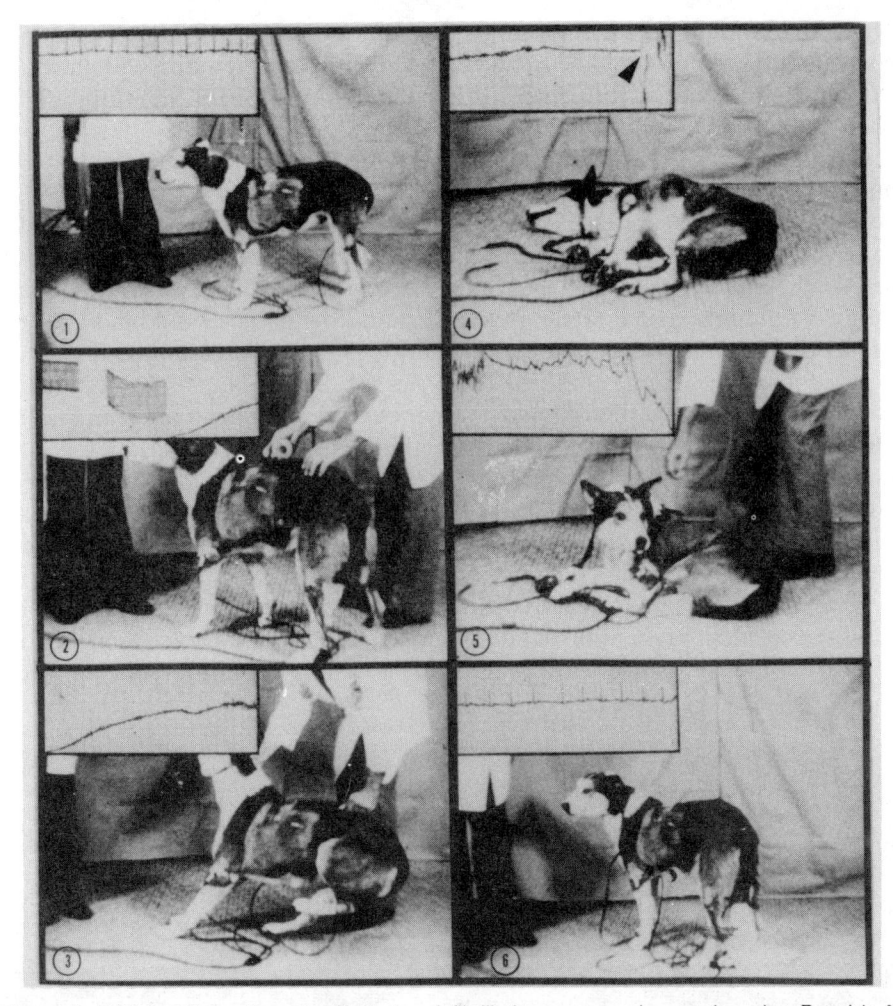

Figure 3: ECG monitoring through a fibrillation-defibrillation sequence in conscious dog. Panel 1: Normal sinus rhythm. Panel 2: Induction of ventricular fibrillation with a magnet placed over the implanted fibrillator. Panel 3: Resultant syncope. Panel 4: Fifteen seconds following induction of ventricular fibrillation automatic internal countershock is delivered (black triangle) by the implanted defibrillator. Panels 5 and 6: The animal is seen at 3 seconds and 15 seconds after defibrillation.

similar fibrillation-defibrillation sequences would become a routine event during a clinical electrophysiological study.

Of course, the full story of how the automatic implantable defibrillator was developed still needs to be told. It might be of interest to describe some day the details of how the specific problems had been solved, how the functional and structural characteristics of the device were finally determined, how the numerous clinical, technological, financial, and even legal hurdles have been overcome, etc. The basic atmosphere, however, in which these problems were approached bears some striking similarities to that described by Frank Wilson in a paper written some 35 years ago.[20] When discussing the advances made during the previous three decades in the field of electrocardiography, he emphasized that these advances came about "not as the result of organized attacks aimed at the solution of specific problems, nor by the expenditure of large sums of money for elaborate apparatus, technical assistants, fellowships and the like, but by individual men who have been permitted to work on problems of their own choosing in their own way, under no pressure to make progress reports or to justify the expenditures of the small sums at their disposal, or to present or publish the results of their efforts before they are ready."

As the saga of the automatic implantable defibrillator enters its third decade, it seems only fair to conclude that this new therapeutic modality has withstood the test of time. The earlier doubts about the feasibility and usefulness of such an approach have clearly been dispelled. Even though our initial hopes have been fulfilled, a great deal of work still remains to be done, work which one day may contribute to the virtual elimination of the sudden cardiac death syndrome as a major public health problem.

References

1. Mirowski M, Reid PR, Winkle RA, Mower MM, Watkins Jr L, Stinson EB, Griffith LSC, Kallman CH, Weisfeldt ML. Mortality in patients with implanted automatic defibrillators. Ann Intern Med 1983;98:585–588.
2. Echt DS, Armstrong K, Schmidt P, Oyer PE, Stinson EB, Winkle RA. Clinical experience: complications and survival in 70 patients with the automatic implantable cardioverter-defibrillator. Circulation 1985;71:289–296.
3. Reid PR, Mower MM, Griffith LSC, Platia EV, Watkins Jr L, Juanteguy J, Guarnieri T, Mirowski M. Comparative effects on mortality of the first and second generation implantable defibrillators (abstr). Circulation 1984;70:II–401.
4. Mirowski M. The automatic implantable cardioverter-defibrillator: An overview. J Am Coll Cardiol 1985;6:461–466.
5. Marchlinski FE, Flores BT, Buxton AE, Hargrove III WC, Addonizio VP, Stephenson LW, Harken AH, Doherty JU, Grogan Jr, EW, Josephson ME. The automatic implantable cardioverter-defibrillator: Efficacy, complications, and device failures. Ann Intern Med 1986;104:481–488.
6. Mirowski M, Mower MM, Staewen WS, Tabatznik B, Mendeloff, AI. Standby automatic defibrillator. An approach to prevention of sudden coronary death. Arch Intern Med 1970;126:158–161.
7. Schuder JC, Stoeckle H, Gold JH, West JA, Keskar PY. Experimental ventricular defibrillation with an automatic and completely implanted system. Trans Am Soc Artif Organs 1970;16:207–212.
8. Lown B, Axelrod P. Implanted standby defibrillators (editorial). Circulation 1972;46:637–639.
9. Rushmer RF, Van Citters RL, Franklin DL. Some axions, popular notions, and misconceptions regarding cardiovascular control. Circulation 1963;27:118–141.
10. Mirowski M, Mower MM, Staewen WS, Denniston RH, Mendeloff AI. The development of the transvenous automatic defibrillator. Arch Intern Med 1972;129:773–779.
11. Mirowski M, Mower MM, Staewen WS, Denniston RH, Tabatznik B, Mendeloff AI. Ventricular defibrillation through a single intravascular catheter electrode system (abstr). Clin Res 1971;19:328.
12. Mirowski M, Mower MM, Gott VL, Brawley RK, Denniston RH. Transvenous automatic defibrillator: Preliminary clinical tests of the defibrillating subsystem. Trans Amer Soc Artif Intern Organs 1972;18:520–524.

13. Mirowski M, Mower MM, Gott VL, Brawley RK. Feasibility and effectiveness of low-energy cathether defibrillation in man. Circulation 1973;47:79–85.
14. Heilman MS, Langer A, Mower MM, Mirowski M. Analysis of four implantable electrode systems for automatic defibrillator (abstr). Circulation 1975;52:II–205.
15. Mower MM, Mirowski M, Spear JR, Moore EN. Patterns of ventricular activity during catheter defibrillation. Circulation 1974;49:858–861.
16. Langer A, Heilman MS, Mower MM, Mirowski M. Considerations in the development of the automatic implantable defibrillator. Med Instrum 1976;10:163–167.
17. Mirowski M, Mower MM, Langer A, Heilman MS. Schreibman J. A chronically implanted system for automatic defibrillation in active conscious dogs. Experimental model for treatment of sudden death from ventricular fibrillation. Circulation 1978;58:90–94.
18. Mirowski M, Mower MM, Bhagavan BS, Langer A, Kolenik SA, Fischell RE, Heilman MS. Chronic animal and bench testing of the implantable automatic defibrillator. In Meere C, ed: Proceedings of the VIth World Symposium on Cardiac Pacing, Montreal, Canada, Pacesymp 1980, Chap. 27–2.
19. Mirowski M, Reid PR, Mower MM, Watkins L, Gott VL, Schauble JF, Langer A, Heilman MS, Kolenik SA, Fischell RD, Weisfeldt ML. Termination of malignant ventricular arrhythmias with an implanted automatic defibrillator in human beings. N Engl J Med 1980;303:322–324.
20. Wilson, FN. The origin and nature of the progress made in our understanding of the electrocardiogram during the last three decades. In Johnston FD, Lepeschkin E, eds: Selected Papers of Dr. Frank N. Wilson. Ann Arbor, JW Edwards, Publisher, Inc. 1954;20.

41

The Automatic Implantable Cardioverter Defibrillator: The U.S. Experience

Roger A. Winkle
Andra Thomas

Introduction

After more than 10 years of research and development,[1-5] Mirowski and colleagues performed the first automatic defibrillator implantation in the United States at The Johns Hopkins University Medical Center on February 4, 1980.[6] For the first year, defibrillator implantation was performed only at The Johns Hopkins Hospital with expansion to Stanford University Medical Center in March 1981. Beginning in 1982, with the introduction of the automatic implantable cardioverter defibrillator, expansion continued to a total of 42 centers in the United States. A total of 37 patients received the initial automatic implantable defibrillator (AID®) device, and as of August 1986, a total of 949 patients had received the current automatic implantable cardioverter defibrillator (AICD®). A comprehensive, independent cardioverter defibrillator implantation registry has not existed in the United States, and data tracking remains possible because there is only a single device manufacturer at the present time. As for any new therapy, even within a single country, there is a broad spectrum of opinion regarding the indications for implantation, the most appropriate implantation technique,[7-9] measurements of device efficacy, and acceptable complications rates.[10,11] It is therefore difficult to present a single paper properly reflecting "the U.S. experience" with the

From: Brugada P, Wellens HJJ. CARDIAC ARRHYTHMIAS: Where To Go From Here? Mount Kisco, NY, Futura Publishing Company, Inc., © 1987.

664 • CARDIAC ARRHYTHMIAS

automatic implantable cardioverter defibrillator. This chapter, therefore, of necessity represents the authors' best judgment concerning many areas where no objective data exist. Whenever possible, data from the CPI clinical computer data base will be presented to accurately reflect the total United States experience with regard to patient selection, patient and generator survival rates, and device failure modes.

Patient Selection

The very first patients undergoing automatic defibrillator implantation were required to have drug refractory recurrent ventricular tachyarrhythmias despite having survived at least two episodes of cardiac arrest. Early in this clinical trial, this strict criterion was liberalized to permit inclusion of patients surviving only a single episode of cardiac arrest or hemodynamically compromising sustained ventricular tachyarrhythmias. Patients whose arrhythmias were associated with acute myocardial infarction, severe electrolyte imbalance, or drug toxicity were excluded. The original AID® device relied solely on the probability density function for sensing and could only reliably recognize very rapid and/or sinusoidal episodes of ventricular tachycardia, flutter, or fibrillation. It was not until the introduction of the automatic implantable cardioverter defibrillator (AICD®) generation of devices in April 1982 that patients with slower and more organized ventricular tachycardias became good candidates for the device. The relatively limited availability of devices which has continued until the present time has caused most implanting physicians to reserve this device primarily for those patients with prior cardiac arrests or very poorly hemodynamically tolerated ventricular tachycardias. In the United States there has been a long-standing effort to train lay persons in cardiopulmonary resuscitation and large sums of public and private money have been spent to provide excellent paramedic services in most urban and rural areas of the country. This has resulted in a large pool of patients with extremely rapid and poorly tolerated ventricular tachyarrhythmias who are ideal candidates for these devices.

To date, almost all automatic cardioverter defibrillator implants in the United States have been performed at centers with a major interest in electrophysiology. Virtually all patients receiving one of these devices has undergone electrophysiologic and usually angiographic study, and those with ventricular tachycardia or fibrillation inducible at baseline electrophysiologic studies have failed serial antiarrhythmic drug testing. Most implanting centers are also experienced in techniques of endocardial mapping and resection and, as a result, this option has been considered as an alternative treatment choice for most patients receiving the implantable cardioverter defibrillator. There is fairly uniform agreement among implantation centers that patients with primary ventricular fibrillation are not good candidates for endocardial mapping and resection and that the implantable cardioverter defibrillator is the preferred treatment when drug therapy is not an option or has been shown ineffective. Likewise, patients with extraordinarily frequent episodes of sustained ventricular tachycardia uncontrolled by pharmacologic means are not generally considered candidates for an automatic implantable cardioverter defibrillator because of the likelihood of extremely frequent device discharges. There is moderate disagreement among implanting centers as to the proper ranking of therapeutic choices for those patients having failed drug therapy with only occasional episodes of sustained hypotensive ventricular tachycardia. Centers with excellent surgical results including a low operative mortality and a high "cure" rate tend to favor endocardial mapping and resection in such patients. Other centers quoting higher mortality figures and lower overall "cure" rates tend to favor implantation of an automatic implantable cardioverter defibrillator as the initial choice and proceed to endocardial mapping and resection or ablative therapy only if patients received excessively frequent defibrillator discharges despite drug therapy. Most centers seem to follow an intermediate course with endocardial mapping and resection performed in "ideal" candidates and AICD system implantation chosen for the remainder. There is also a difference of opinion regarding the advisability of leaving defibrillator patch leads in patients undergoing endocardial mapping and resection. Many physicians would prefer to leave two patches in the event that the endocardial mapping proved unsuccessful. Other centers do not routinely leave defibrillator patches in place in such patients. Considerable controversy exists regarding the advisability of placing a cardioverter defibrillator generator in those patients undergoing apparently successful endocardial mapping and resection. At most centers, those patients who have no ventricular tachycardia or fibrillation induced at a postoperative electrophysiologic study do not undergo implantation of automatic cardioverter defibrillator generators. Some physicians, however, citing relatively high ventricular tachycardia and sudden death recurrence rates over the subsequent years, favor placing an automatic cardioverter defibrillator in all patients undergoing endocardial mapping and resection, regardless of the outcome of the postoperative electrophysiologic study.[12]

Opinion in the United States is divided on the proper management of patients with a single cardiac arrest who have no ventricular tachyarrhythmia inducible at electrophysiologic study. Some centers believe that such patients have a relatively low risk for subsequent cardiac arrest while others feel such patients have an intermediate to high risk of experiencing a subsequent cardiac arrest. Most centers handle this problem on an individual case by case basis and there seems to be no uniform policy even at a single implant center. It is the authors' personal bias to favor device implantation in such patients, especially those with left ventricular dysfunction and complex ventricular ectopy which may place them in a higher risk group for subsequent recurrence.

During the first several years of the use of automatic implantable cardioverter defibrillation in the United States, many investigators considered amiodarone as adequate therapy for preventing sudden cardiac death,[13] and viewed the implanted device as a competitive or alternative therapy. Increasing use and longer term follow-up of patients treated with amiodarone has indicated a high rate of side effects and subsequent sudden cardiac death.[14] Most implanting physicians now consider the AICD as preferable to amiodarone or, in cases where amiodarone is required to control frequent arrhythmia recurrences, use an implantable cardioverter defibrillator as a backup device. This is especially true for those patients who continue to have a poorly tolerated ventricular tachyarrhythmia induced at electrophysiologic study after a brief period of amiodarone loading since recent studies have shown that such findings predict clinical failures with the drug.[15,16] Based on data reported to the CPI clinical database, 66.4% of patients with the automatic implantable cardioverter defibrillator are treated concomitantly with drug therapy. Of those treated with drugs, 74.4% were treated with antiarrhythmic drugs; amiodarone was the drug used in 39.4% of antiarrhythmic drug-treated patients. Beta-blocking drugs were used in 7.8% of cases, and in the remaining 17.8% of cases, a variety of other drugs were used (e.g., digoxin, calcium channel blockers, antihypertensive agents, etc.).

Device System Components

Pulse Generators

The initial implantable defibrillator (AID®) had no cardioverting capability and no heart rate cut-off as part of its sensing circuitry. Arrhythmias were sensed using a transcardiac (superior vena caval spring to apical epicardial patch) bipolar electrocardiographic signal using the probability density function (PDF) for arrhythmia sensing. The probability density function evaluates the amount of time this transcardiac ECG signal spends away from the baseline with sinus rhythm spending most of the time near the isoelectric line and sinusoidal rhythms spending a high percentage of time away from the baseline. The threshold chosen for the PDF markedly alters arrhythmia sensing. Initially the probability density function was adjusted to be sensitive to sinusoidal ventricular tachycardia and ventricular fibrillation, and rarely to detect supraventricular or sinus tachycardias, but at this threshold it failed to detect some rapid and many slower ventricular tachycardias. In some instances when it did sense tachycardia, the detection times were inappropriately long; however, further adjustment of the PDF "window" or threshold improved ventricular tachycardia detection but resulted in false positive shocks for sinus and supraventricular tachycardias especially in patients with intraventricular conduction delays. Initial attempts at rate counting using the signals from the transcardiac defibrillation leads were unsuccessful resulting in episodes of double counting of the P wave and QRS complex in patients with large atrial electrograms. The addition of a local bipolar ventricular sensing lead and detection circuitry which gave accurate rate determination, an automatic gain control circuit, and a refractory period of approximately 150 ms permitted reliable detection of ventricular tachycardia as well as ventricular fibrillation.[17] With the threshold for satisfying the probability density function lowered considerably, the nondetection of ventricular tachyarrhythmias (as long as the tachyarrhythmia rate exceeded the rate cut-off of the device) virtually disappeared. Nondetection of ventricular tachyarrhythmias was replaced by clinically inappropriate shocks (false positive shocks) for sinus and supraventricular tachycardias whose rate exceeded the cut-off of the device. Although such shocks occurred by definition in the device utilizing rate cut-off only (model AID®-BR), they can also occur in the model of the device requiring satisfaction of both the rate criterion and the probability density function (model AID®-B). False positive device response remains a clinical management problem with both models of the current devices. The delivery of AICD® shocks synchronized to the R wave during supraventricular tachycardia has proven relatively safe, but the shocks are nonetheless unpleasant for the patient due to the conscious state and generally asymptomatic state at the time of the shock.

The very early days of the implantable defibrillator were filled with all of the problems and challenges that occur in the development of any new technology. The very first AID® device to be implanted was inadvertently dropped on the operating room floor because the packaging was inadequate for such a heavy pulse generator. The first AID® defibrillator devices were shipped unsterile to the investigators and required gas sterilization at the implant center. Occasionally they were overheated and rendered nonfunctional. The early generators also required warming to body temperature and were placed in isolettes in the newborn nursery for 24 hours prior to implantation. Since the AID® and the currently utilized AICD® devices were composed of discrete electronic components stacked on printed circuit boards, it was possible in the early days to make rapid design changes, and this greatly shortened the iteration time for device improvements; however, this discrete component design made the device quite difficult to manufacture.

After the introduction of the AICD®, new innovations have been slow to reach the clinical investigation phase. In the fall of 1986, CPI introduced a new version of the AICD®, the Ventak™ AICD, which improves the ease of manufacturing of the devices but which fails to make any major advances with regard to programmability, back-up bradycardia pacing, antitachycardia pacing, or other more sophisticated features.

Lead Systems

The intention of Dr. Mirowski and colleagues was to utilize a transvenous superior vena caval spring electrode and an epicardial cup-like electrode placed over the cardiac apex for the initial human implants. This electrode configuration was the primary one utilized during the preclinical chronic animal testing. However, at the time of initial human implantation, it was recognized that the dilated, diseased human heart did not have a discrete cardiac apex and consequently a flat patch electrode was substituted for the apical cup for the first human implant. This patch lead became the standard and, in fact, the apical cup was only utilized in a single patient. Both the original superior vena caval and patch lead wires were made of a silver tinsel conductor which had an extremely high failure rate. Silver tinsel leads were only utilized until December 1981 when DBS wire became the standard lead conducting material. The titanium superior vena caval spring and patch mesh have remained unchanged throughout this period.

At the very first defibrillator implants, no intraoperative electrophysiologic testing was performed and the only testing was done at a postoperative electrophysiologic study. Subsequently in late 1980, limited intraoperative testing of the device was performed by the elective induction of ventricular tachycardia or fibrillation using programmed stimulation, and permitting the implanted device to terminate the episode. No equipment existed for formal defibrillation threshold testing, and so the margin of safety of the implanted devices could not be evaluated. After approximately 2 years of implantation of devices, in September 1982 the External Cardioverter Defibrillator (ECD) testing device was introduced and extensive intraoperative defibrillation threshold testing became possible. It quickly became apparent that cardioversion thresholds for stable ventricular tachycardia were considerably lower than the thresholds for termination of ventricular fibrillation and testing for the ability of the device to terminate ventricular fibrillation became routine even when the clinical arrhythmia was ventricular tachycardia.[18] In the early implantation experience it became readily apparent that not all patients could be successfully defibrillated by the 25 to 32 joule device utilizing the spring-patch lead configuration, and in one instance, a 42 joule energy device was constructed and implanted. However, design limitations precluded the development of devices that routinely delivered 35–40 joules. Problems with unacceptably high defibrillation thresholds were largely resolved with the replacement of the superior vena caval spring lead with a second patch, i.e., a "double patch" configuration, the first such implant being done in September 1982. Shortly thereafter "large" patches with surface area (twice the area of the standard patches) were introduced that also facilitated defibrillation in high threshold patients. With the introduction of routine defibrillation threshold testing with the External Cardioverter Defibrillator box, it became apparent that the two patch lead configuration was superior to the spring-patch lead configuration for defibrillating most patients.[19] Improved defibrillation efficacy, coupled with the early problems of spring lead migration, insulation damage, and lead fracture, and the fact that there have been few reported patch lead fractures in the United States, have resulted in the shift of most centers to the use of two patches as the standard lead configuration. Patch leads placed in the United States have generally been sutured in place in contrast to some centers in Europe which utilize fibrin glue for placement. The majority of leads have been placed intrapericardially although approximately 40% are implanted extrapericardially. As of August 1986, 40.6% of patients in the U.S. had the spring-patch lead configuration and 57.0% of patients had the patch-patch lead configuration. Configuration was unreported for 2.4%.

The original AID® unit did not require bipolar sensing leads as it had no rate detection parameter. However, as the models AID®-B and AICD®-BR devices have such rate detection parameters, they require a bipolar ventricular sensing lead system which has been either a pair of closely spaced epicardial screw-in leads or a specially designed transvenous bipolar endocardial sensing lead. A standard bipolar endocardial pacing lead is not suitable for use with the AICD system.

Clinical Results in the United States

Not all of the data one would desire to know about the patients undergoing defibrillator implantation in the United States is available for review. This lack of data availability has occurred for several reasons. Because of the rapidly evolving implant techniques, clinical variables found to be relevant to patient/device interaction, and clinical problems, the initially designed and periodically updated manufacturer case report forms did not include all information which, in retrospect, would have been desirable to collect. Additionally, some implanting centers failed to collect and/or provide these types of information in all or even a majority of their patients, especially after the device was no longer investigational. These data may therefore underestimate the actual occurrences of reported events. Despite these limitations, a remarkable amount of information is available about the United States experience with the automatic defibrillator and cardioverter defibrillator from the CPI clinical computer data base. This section summarizes these data.

Patient Population

As of August 1986, 949 patients (748 males, 201 females) had undergone automatic implantable cardioverter defibrillator generator implantation. Excluded from data analysis were 37 patients undergoing the original AID generator unless they subsequently received a model AID®-B or AID®-BR pulse generator generator. These 949 patients range in age from 11 to 80 years (see Table I) with an average age of 58 years. The most frequent primary diagnosis was coronary artery disease present in 71.8% of patients with nonischemic cardiomyopathy accounting for another 18.9% of patients (see Table II). A secondary diagnosis was reported in 400 patients and was listed as congestive heart failure in 53% of those reported. Ejection fraction was reported for 448 patients and averaged 32.9%. The primary rhythm disturbance was ventricular tachycardia in 46.4%, ventricular fibrillation in 16.3%, and both ventricular tachycardia and fibrillation in 37.0%. Primary rhythm disturbance was not specified in three patients (0.3%). Information regarding the outcome of electrophysiologic studies and prior anitarrhythmic therapy is unavailable.

Table I
Age Distribution of Patients Receiving the AICD® in the United States

Age	Number
< 20	13 (1.4%)
20–29	20 (2.1%)
30–39	41 (4.3%)
40–49	111 (11.7%)
50–59	252 (26.6%)
60–69	336 (35.4%)
70–79	122 (12.8%)
> 80	1 (0.1%)
Not specified	53 (5.6%)
Total	949 (100.0%)

Table II
Primary Diagnosis of Patients Receiving the AICD® in the United States

Diagnosis	Number
Coronary artery disease	681 (71.8%)
Cardiomyopathy	179 (18.9%)
Other (valve disease 3, mitral prolapse 8, long QT 4, idiopathic ventricular arrhythmias 9, coronary spasm 1)	25 (2.6%)
Not specified	64 (6.7%)
Total	949 (100.0%)

Operative Mortality

Surgical intervention was reported to have been performed concomitantly in 280 (20.3%) of AICD® system implantations. Coronary artery bypass grafting was performed in 174 implantations (62.1%), combination procedures for specific treatment of arrhythmia disturbance were performed in 80 implantations (28.6%), and other surgical procedures, e.g., heart valve replacement, pacemaker insertion, etc., were performed in 26 of the implantations (9.3%). Two hundred and seventeen patients underwent staged procedures with lead implants at one operation and subsequent placement of a cardioverter defibrillator generator. The percentages of patients undergoing left thoracotomy, median sternotomy, and subcostal or subxiphoid implantation approaches were not available. Eight patients died within 24 hours of new generator implantation and one patient died on the same day as generator exchange. Thirty-one other patients died within 1 month of a new generator implant or replacement. Thus, for new implants, the total 1 month operative mortality was 3.9%. Nine of the 40 patients who died within 1 month of implant also underwent other concomitant surgical procedures. Causes of the 1 month operative mortality were classified by reporting physicians as follows: sudden death (9), of which in three patients the AICD® device was *deactivated* at time of death, cardiac deaths (22), noncardiac deaths (9). In two cases the device had been removed before the patients expired.

Although not included in the above analysis, two patients who did not receive pulse generators died during intraoperative testing of the implanted lead system. One patient, whose primary diagnosis was hypertrophic cardiomyopathy complicated by ventricular arrhythmias, was converted out of induced ventricular arrhythmias on three occasions but ultimately could not be converted out of ventricular fibrillation despite multiple shocks from an External Cardioverter Defibrillator (ECD), and additional defibrillatory shocks—both internal and external—from a standard defibrillator. Infusion of drugs and cardiopulmonary bypass were also not effective. The second patient, who had been unresponsive to ventricular fibrillation conversion attempts through the implanted lead system, was undergoing patch lead reconfiguration (with concomitant bypass surgery) when he developed spontaneous ventricular fibrillation during manipulation of his heart. Despite reinstitution of cardiopulmonary bypass and drug infusion, the patient could not be resuscitated.

Long-Term Patient Survival

The longest implant time for the models AID®-B and BR generators was 52 months with an average implant time of 16.0 months. The longest cumulative implant for any patient, including patients receiving the original AID® unit, is 72 months. Table III summarizes the long-term annual survival figures for the patients receiving the AICD® series of generators including operative mortality. The 1 year sudden death rate was 2.0% and increased only 7.7% by 4 years. Nonsudden cardiac mortality was 6.7% at 1 year and increased to 15.4% at 4 years. Total cardiac and sudden mortality at 1 year was 8.7% and increased to 23.1% at 4 years.

Infections, Lead Fractures, and Lead Migration

Thirty of the 949 patients experienced infection, erosion, or extrusion. In those patients who developed AICD system or pocket infections,[21] early infections (≤ 30 days) occurred in nine patients and late infections (> 30 days) occurred in 12 patients. Seventeen of these 21 infections occurred following the initial implant and four occurred after replacement. Five of the patients with infections reportedly had identifiable circumstances which were presumed to make them more susceptible to the occurrence of infection: one diabetic patient traumatized his pulse generator pocket during a fall, one had his pulse generator pocket contaminated during an abdominal surgical procedure, one patient was a documented drug addict, one was on immunosuppression following renal transplant, and one was known to have cancer in the terminal phases with attendant debilitation. One patient experienced infection of his pulse generator pocket while a "simulator" was implanted and two patients experienced infection of the site of SVC lead insertion near the clavicle. In fifteen of these 21, the device was explanted; in the remaining six cases the patients were treated medically. Six

Table III
Life Table Analysis of Mortality in Patients Receiving the AICD® in the United States (Includes Operative Deaths)

	Sudden	Cardiac, Nonsudden	Total Cardiac	Noncardiac	Total
12 months	2.01%	6.70%	8.71	2.83%	11.54%
24 months	3.59%	10.73%	14.32	4.15%	18.47%
36 months	6.16%	14.13%	20.29	4.15%	24.44%
48 months	7.70%	15.36%	23.06	4.15%	27.21%
52 months	7.70%	15.36%	23.06	4.15%	27.21%

patients reportedly experienced device explantation secondary to erosion or extrusion of their pulse generator without infection. Five of the six patients experiencing erosion/extrusion did so after a pulse generator replacement procedure.

Lead fractures occurred in 12 cases when the original lead material, silver tinsel wire, was being used for early AID® defibrillator implantation (four SVC lead fractures and eight patch lead fractures). Since the introduction of DBS wire for the manufacturing of the SVC and patch defibrillation leads, there have been only five SVC lead fractures and no patch lead fractures reported to date. Lead fractures have occurred with two bipolar endocardial leads and three epicardial leads of which two epicardial leads were those of another manufacturer. Four cases of lead fractures reported occurred in patients for which implant forms were not received specifying type of rate sensing lead system being used.

Insulation breaks occurred in 10 cases: two patches which were repaired and left implanted, six bipolar endocardial leads, and two epicardial leads. Lead migration/dislodgements occurred in 30 cases: 16 SVC leads prior to the use of a lead anchor to secure its position and in 14 bipolar endocardial leads. Most bipolar endocardial lead dislodgements occurred in the early postop period usually as the result of the AICD shocks.

Defibrillation Shocks

Of the 949 patients receiving AICD® pulse generators, 481 (50.7%) have received spontaneous pulse generator shocks. One hundred and fifty-nine of these 481 patients received in-hospital shocks and 410 patients received out-of-hospital shocks. Eighty-eight patients received both in and out-of-hospital shocks.

A total of 3432 shocks have been reported representing 7.1 per patient, averaged over those patients receiving a shock. For all patients, the average was 3.6 shocks and its was 2.5 for each device implanted. Twenty-eight patients (5.8%) received ⩾ 20 shocks. Eleven of these patients had VT/VF storms requiring medication adjustment, two experienced multiple shocks during terminal death events, four had a combination of atrial arrhythmias and VT/VF, and five had shocks for atrial arrhythmias. In six patients the ⩾ 20 shocks were cumulative over the entire implant time of their device, i.e., a few shocks at various intervals.

Pulse Generator Performance

Including both new implants and generator changes, a total of 1381 AICD units have been implanted (see Table IV). Seventy-five percent were AID®-B and 25% were AID®-BR rate only units. Six hundred and seventy-eight units have been high energy. A much higher percentage of the rate-only units have been high energy reflecting the fact that one large implantation center (the Stanford-Sequoia series) has used almost exclusively rate only/high energy units. Pulse generator performance is summarized in Table V. The median generator survival time has been 19.1 months and 96 units (7.0%) have failed prematurely. The largest single failure mode was for battery glass corrosion which accounted for

Table IV
AICD® Pulse Generator Data for United States Implants

Model	Total	High Energy	Standard Energy	Implant Months
AICD-B	1036	371	655	11,446
AICD-BR	345	307	38	3,789

Total presently implanted = 763.
Mean implant months = 11.0.
Median actual survival of explanted units = 19.1 months.

Table V
United States Experience with AICD® Generator Failures

Nonfailed generators = 1285 (93.0%)
Failed generator = 96 (7.0%)
Failure modes
   glass corrosion   61
   electronic component   13
   argon   2
   hermeticity   5
   mechanical (set screws)   6
   misdirect   9

approximately two-thirds of all generator failures. This failure mode has not recurred since Teflon battery coating was implemented shortly after its discovery.

Recently, a component failure mode that could result secondary to a defect in the load resistor utilized for internal magnet test discharges has been identified. This failure mode was discovered after the data cut-off of patients reported in this series. Although to date only two such secondary failures have been reported, the impact of this failure mode is not currently known and is not reflected in the data given. No significant differences were noted for failure modes between models AID®-B and BR. Actuarial pulse generator reliability figures are summarized in Table VI.

Table VI
United States AICD® Implants: Actuarial Analysis of Generator Reliability

	12 months	18 months	24 months
Total	94.9%	87.2%	86.6%
glass corrosion only	97.8%	90.3%	90.3%
nonglass corrosion	97.1%	96.6%	96.0%
component	98.9%	98.4%	98.4%
mechanical	99.6%	99.6%	99.6%

Elective Replacement/End of Life

The initial engineering projections for the automatic implantable cardioverter defibrillator was that periodic magnet tests (capacitor charge-internal discharge cycles) would yield slowly increasing charge times resulting in elective pulse generator replacement when the charge time exceeded a certain value of "plots of charge time vs. implant time" showed a steep ascending curve. Initial generator life was projected to be $2\frac{1}{2}$ to 3 years or 100 shocks. This was in fact the pattern seen for the very first implanted AID® devices. The addition of the bipolar sensing circuitry in the AICD® device model increased the current drain during routine monitoring and in actual practice only a small number of AICD generators have gone beyond 24 months. Subsequent and as yet not well understood, changes in the capacitor manufacturing process have yielded capacitors with increased and variable leakage currents secondary to capacitor deformation which occurs during periods of disuse. This resulted in many pulse generators with excessively prolonged first charge times, requiring second and, at times, third charge times to be checked during post-implant magnet testing in order to obtain a reliable indication of battery status rather than the degree of capacitor deformation. Over the course of the past 6 years, there have been several changes in the manufacturer's recommendations for determining elective replacement indicators and end of life including the performance of more than one magnet test on each outpatient visit, permitting 10 minutes to elapse between magnet tests, and modified follow-up intervals for patients whose first charge time is excessively prolonged. The differences in capacitor performance from generator to generator as well as changing recommendations about follow-up have made predicting end of life difficult. The first Elective Replacement Indicator (ERI) widely publicized as part of the device's market approval was based on primarily engineering specifications, and with analysis of a sample of explanted pulse generators, proved too conservative. This ERI indicator would have resulted in device explantation in many instances with only half of the battery energy having been utilized. Fortunately, information spread quickly by word of mouth among implanting physicians that this recommendation was too conservative in most cases and relatively few generators were removed prematurely despite physician concerns about the medical–legal aspects of failing to follow the manufacturer's ERI recommendations. Recently new elective replacement indicators have been proposed based on retrospective analysis of actual generator *end of life* charge time behavior. Although this elective replacement indicator seems much improved over the previous indicator, its long-term usefulness has not yet been proven in prospective patient follow-up.

Difficulties with Patient Follow-Up

In the United States there have been a number of issues related to the long-term follow-up of patients receiving the automatic implantable cardioverter defibrillator. Initially there were only a few widely scattered implantation centers. Patients often traveled thousands of miles to undergo an implant. They returned home to physicians either inexperienced in the intricacies of the device or who because of limited manufacturing capabilities could not be provided with AID-Check® devices to perform post-implant magnet tests. Even with increased availability of AIDCheck® devices, many patients are of necessity followed by physicians who know little about the function of the device. The possibility of occasional (there have been 20 since the beginning of device use) misdirects during magnet testing with energy being delivered to the patient rather than dumped internally creates a need for immediate access to an external defibrillator in the event a misdirect precipitates a lethal ventricular tachyarrhythmia. This rare though potential occurrence heightens the anxiety of both the patients and inexperienced physicians at the time of magnet test procedure. Patients who have had a number of magnet tests performed at experienced implanting centers frequently tell stories about physicians performing their first magnet test who seem apprehensive and on occasion refuse to perform the test despite the availability of the proper equipment. Variability of individual cardioverter defibrillator generators such as long first charge times and different handling characteristics (such as the need to turn the newer integrated circuit Ventak units off and on after each magnet test) further complicate follow-up. Although follow-up guidelines are available in the Manufacturer's Instructions for Use, no single set of follow-up instructions is applicable to all cardioverter defibrillator patients. Many following physicians are either slow or fail to forward magnet test results or other important information to the implanting center or the manufacturer. When units that have apparently malfunctioned have been returned for analysis to the manufacturer, failure analysis reports have taken long periods of time to be returned to the physician, although this has improved in recent months. At times clearly clinically malfunctioning generators have been reported as meeting manufacturer's specifications, due to the manufacturer's inability to reproduce exactly the clinical scenario resulting in the malfunction. On other occasions, devices have been returned to the manufacturer as malfunctioning when in reality the implanting physician simply did not fully understand proper device function or did not carefully follow the instructions for use in the Physicians' Manual.

Device Availability

Limited supplies of implantable defibrillator generators have caused major problems since the beginning of the defibrillator program. In the earliest years, even the few centers doing implants did not have enough generators to meet their needs. On occasions difficult decisions would need to be made as to whether a patient should remain in the hospital for weeks to months awaiting a generator or to be sent home with the risk of sudden cardiac death. New investigational implant centers were recruited far in advance of the manufacturer's capacity to supply them with devices. Even though device availability has improved considerably since market approval and a fair rationing schedule developed, device availability continues to remain a major problem. From the beginning this supply versus demand problem reflects as much the phenomenal increase of interest in and demand for the device as it does the manufacturer's ability to produce them.

Introduction of the newly approved and more easily manufactured Ventak AICD device with integrated circuitry was to have eliminated this problem; however, demand continues to outstrip available devices.

Unrealistic Promises and Expectations

In addition to overly optimistic production estimates, formerly Intec and those new manufacturers working to develop an automatic cardioverter defibrillator have alluded to the early arrival of sophisticated devices with backup bradycardia pacing, antitachycardia pacing, memory to store ECG strips before and after defibrillator shocks, patient alert mechanisms and multi-programmability. These devices have been slow in coming and this has enhanced the physicians' frustration levels in the U.S. Physicians, on the other hand, have had unrealistic expectations of the manufacturers. The sophistication, availability and reliability of today's dual chamber pacemakers has given physicians in the United States unrealistic expectations with regard to implantable cardioverter defibrillators. The past 6 years have in fact been very similar to the early days of bradycardia pacing with large devices, short battery life, lead fractures, and requirements for major surgical procedures for implantation. The development of sophisticated implantable cardioverter defibrillators requires expertise not immediately available throughout the pacing industry as well as millions of dollars of capital investment and years of work. The failure of any manufacturers other than CIP/Intec to complete clinical trials on these early devices reflects these facts and reinforces the magnitude of Dr. Mirowski's vision and the accomplishments of his colleagues at the former Intec. The pacing industry, which is currently facing generally flat sales and declining profits, must of necessity move cautiously into the cardioverter defibrillator field. Even under ideal circumstances development of a new model implantable cardioverter defibrillator or antitachycardia-defibrillator devices can cost tens of millions of dollars with extensive time required for electrical and mechanical design, integrated circuit production and the extensive animal and human testing currently required by regulatory agencies. Thus, the improvements desired by physicians are for good reason slow to come causing inappropriate and/or unfair criticism of the manufacturers from segments of the medical community.

Costs

The current manufacturer's price for a cardioverter defibrillator pulse generator and leads is approximately $14,000.00, depending upon the lead configuration utilized. The average cost of an initial cardioverter defibrillator implant in the United States is $51,000.00, and the average cost of a generator replacement is $18,000.00. Unfortunately, for most patients, the device implantation often comes at the end of a rather lengthy hospitalization during which patients have often recovered from cardiac arrest and undergone serial electrophysiologic tests. Reimbursement from third-party payers for cardioverter defibrillator implantation cost has been generally good since approval was obtained from the Food and Drug Administration and it is no longer considered investigational. There have, however, been regional exceptions. The largest number of complaints from physicians about reimbursement comes from Massachusetts, New York, and New Jersey. Although Medicare DRG codes were recently allocated for AICD implantation and attempt to take into account the long hospitalization before an actual implant is considered, in many instances, hospitals continue to lose considerable amounts of money on Medicare patients receiving initial implant of an automatic implantable cardioverter defibrillator. The greatest problem comes with AICD pulse generator replacements which are reimbursed by Medicare as a pacemaker generator replacement. This does not reflect adequate reimbursement to hospitals by Medicare, a fact which the proper government agencies are being made aware of.

Future Directions

A number of obvious technological changes will occur in the devices utilized in the United States and the rest of the world. These will include incorporation of flexible programming capabilities, backup bradycardia pacing support, antitachycardia pacing, low energy cardioversion capabilities,[20] as well as incorporation of hemodynamic sensors into the devices. The devices will become more easily manufactured, and should be available in plentiful supply from several manufacturers. While these are all desirable changes, with them will undoubtedly come a number of new problems, some of which may be unique to the United States. These new devices will require increased levels of sophistication on the part of the implanting surgeons and electrophysiologists for patient selection, device implantation, and long-term follow-up and reprogramming. In countries having more socialized delivery of medical care, the implantation of these expensive devices will undoubtedly be strictly controlled and limited to selected centers. In the United States, pressure to maintain patient volume at individual hospitals as well as marketing efforts by the manufacturers will result in a rapid expansion in the number of centers performing cardioverter defibrillator implants. Patient selection and quality control of implant procedures will be difficult to monitor. Other therapeutic options for patients receiving these devices such as endocardial mapping and catheter ablation may not be readily available and these factors may influence the selection of patients receiving these devices. Using current patient selection criteria, the total number of patients seen needing an automatic cardioverter defibrillator at smaller nontertiary care hospitals will be small and it will be difficult for such centers to maintain a team experienced in implantation of these complicated devices.

Given the efficacy of these devices to prevent sudden death,[21,22] there may be increased pressure to implant automatic cardioverter defibrillators in high risk patients who have not yet experienced a life-threatening arrhythmia such as patients surviving an acute infarction with poor left ventricular function and complex ventricular ectopy. While this may in fact be appropriate in many instances, it will cause controversies and require controlled clinical trials. Unfortunately, such trials will almost certainly be too expensive for either government or industry to fund independently.

If health care reimbursement in the United States moves more toward a capitation or fixed budget system similar to that used in many other countries, cardioverter defibrillator implantation will consume a disproportionate share of available medical resources and potentially deprive a patient or other patients of other required types of medical care. This could result in implementation of strict controls regarding device implantation similar to those seen in some other countries.

Conclusions

The automatic defibrillator and cardioverter defibrillator has now undergone 7 years of clinical use in nearly 1200 patients in the United States as of February 1987. The early phases of the defibrillator program were associated with frequent device modifications and improvements and a steep learning curve with respect to proper patient selection, implantation techniques, intraoperative and postoperative testing, and long-term follow-up. The device has been recognized as life-saving in a high risk patient population with as much as a tenfold reduction in the expected sudden death rates. It has been generally well accepted by both patients and physicians. Although compared to current generation permanent pacemakers, there have been a number of technical device-related problems and limited device availability, for a first generation discrete component device, the reliability and success of the AICD has been remarkably good. In retrospect, the decision on the part of the early investigators and manufacturer to build a discrete component device was a wise one. If they had waited to develop a complex multiprogrammable integrated circuit device, many errors would have been made and the necessary delay of device introduction would have deprived the medical community of a large number of valuable years of experience with this remarkable technology. A number of problems such as long-term capacitor behavior, problems related to intravascular spring leads, etc., have been identified only through this extensive clinical use. The experience gained in the United States and other countries should form a substantial base on which to build in future years.

Acknowledgments: The authors would like to thank all of the numerous investigators, implanting physicians, and their associates throughout the United States who have contributed to the data contained in the CPI data base; Mark Smutka, CPI Biostatistics; and Glenda Rhodes for her assistance in manuscript preparation.

References

1. Mirowski M, Mower MM, Staewen WS, Tabatznik B, Mendeloff AI. Standby automatic defibrillator: An approach to prevention of sudden coronary death. Arch Intern Med 1970;126:158–161.
2. Langer A, Heilman MS, Mower MM, Mirowski M. Considerations in the development of the automatic implantable defibrillator. Med Instrum 1976;10:163–167.

3. Mirowski M, Mower MM, Langer A, Heilman MS, Schreibman J. A chronically implanted system for automatic defibrillation in active conscious dogs. Circulation 1978;58:90–94.
4. Mirowski M, Mower MM, Bhagavan BS, Langer A, Kolenik SA, Fischell RE, Heilman MS. Chronic animal and bench testing of the implantable automatic defibrillator. Proceedings of the VIth World Symposium on Cardiac Pacing, Montreal, Canada, October 2–5, 1979.
5. Mirowski M. The automatic implantable cardioverter-defibrillator: An overview. J Am Coll Cardiol 1985;6:461–466.
6. Mirowski M, Reid PR, Mower MM, Watkins L, Gott VL, Schauble JF, Langer A, Heilman MS, Kolenik SA, Fischell RE, Weisfeldt ML. Termination of malignant ventricular arrhythmias with an implanted automatic defibrillator in human beings. N Engl J Med 1980;303:322–333.
7. Watkins L Jr, Mirowski M, Mower MM, Reid PR, Freund P, Thomas A, Weisfeldt ML, Gott VL. Implantation of the automatic defibrillator: The subxiphoid approach. Ann Thorac Surg 1982;34:515–520.
8. Watkins L Jr, Mower MM, Reid PR, Platia EV, Griffith LSC, Mirowski M. Surgical techniques for implanting the automatic implantable defibrillator. PACE 1984;7:1357–1362.
9. Winkle RA, Stinson EB, Echt DS, Mead RH, Schmidt P. Practical aspects of automatic cardioverter/defibrillator implantation. Am Heart J 1984;108:1335–1346.
10. Marchlinski FE, Flores BT, Buxton AE, Hargrove WC, III, Addonizio VP, Stephenson LW, Harken AH, Doherty JU, Grogan EW Jr, Josephson ME. The automatic implantable cardioverter-defibrillator: Efficacy, complications, and device failures. Ann Intern Med 1986;104:481–488.
11. Winkle RA, Mead RH, Ruder MA, Schmidt P, Stinson E, Buch WS, Gaudiani V. Five year experience with the automatic implantable defibrillator in 157 patients (abstr). J Am Coll Cardiol 1987;9:167A.
12. Platia EV, Griffith LSC, Watkins L Jr, Mower MM, Guarnieri T, Mirowski M, Reid PR. Treatment of malignant ventricular arrhythmias with endocardial resection and implantation of the automatic cardioverter-defibrillator. N Engl J Med 1986;314:213–216.
13. Nademanee K, Singh BN, Hendrickson J, Intarachot V, Lopez B, Feld G, Cannom DS, Weiss JL. Amiodarone in refractory life-threatening ventricular arrhythmias. Ann Intern Med 1983;98:577–584.
14. Dicarlo LA Jr, Morady F, Sauve J, Malone P, Davis JC, Evans-Bell T, Winston SA, Scheinman MM. Cardiac arrest and sudden death in patients treated with amiodarone for sustained ventricular tachycardia or ventricular fibrillation: Risk stratification based on clinical variables. Am J Cardiol 1985;55:372–374.
15. Horowitz LN, Greenspan AM, Spielman SR, Weeb CR, Morganroth J, Rotmensch H, Sokoloff NM, Rae AP, Segal BL, Kay HR. Usefulness of electrophysiologic testing in evaluation of amiodarone therapy for sustained ventricular tachyarrhythmias associated with coronary heart disease. Am J Cardiol 1985;55:367–371.
16. McGovern B, Garan H, Malacoff RF, DiMarco JP, Grant G, Sellers D, Ruskin JN. Long-term clinical outcome of ventricular tachycardia or fibrillation treated with amiodarone. Am J Cardiol 1984;53:1558–1563.
17. Winkle RA, Bach SM, Echt DS, Swerdlow CD, Imran M, Mason JW, Oyer PE, Stinson EB. The automatic implantable defibrillator: Local ventricular bipolar sensing to detect ventricular tachycardia and fibrillation. Am J Cardiol 1983;52:265–270.
18. Winkle RA, Stinson EB, Bach SM Jr, Echt DS, Oyer P, Armstrong K. Measurement of cardioversion/defibrillation thresholds in man by a truncated exponential waveform and an apical patch-superior vena caval spring electrode configuration. Circulation 1984;69:766–771.
19. Troup PJ, Chapman PD, Olinger GN, Kleinman LH. The implanted defibrillator: Relation of defibrillating lead configuration and clinical variables to defibrillation threshold. J Am Coll Cardiol 1985;6:1315–1321.

20. Ciccone JM, Saksena S, Shah Y, Pantopoulos D. A prospective randomized study of the clinical efficacy and safety of transvenous cardioversion for termination of ventricular tachycardia. Circulation 1985;71:571–578.
21. Echt DS, Armstrong K, Schmidt P, Oyer PE, Stinson EB, Winkle RA. Clinical experience, complications, and survival in 70 patients with the automatic implantable cardioverter/defibrillator. Circulation 1985;71:289–296.
22. Mirowski M, Reid PR, Winkle RA, Mower MM, Watkins L Jr, Stinson EB, Griffith LSC, Kallman CH, Weisfeldt ML. Mortality in patients with implanted automatic defibrillators. Ann Intern Med 1983;98:585–588.

42

The Implantable Defibrillator AICD: European Clinical Experience

Henri E. Kulbertus
Seah Nisam

Introduction

The first European AICD implantation was performed at the Hospital Lariboisière, in Paris, in December 1982, nearly 3 years after Dr. Mirowski's own institution, the Johns Hopkins University School of Medicine, had initiated this new therapeutical approach. Up to September 1986, 127 systems were implanted in Europe. The purpose of this presentation is to describe the European experience.

Description of Patients and Techniques

Of the 127 patients, 107 (84%) were male. They ranged in age from 11 to 76 years with an average of 51.5. Sixty-six percent (84) suffered from coronary heart disease and 28% (36) from a dilated cardiomyopathy. The remaining 6% included diagnoses such as the long QT syndrome, mitral valve prolapse, or "primary electrical disease."

The average ejection fraction of the total population was 35% (8 to 75%). Although the exact figure could not be obtained, one can estimate that some 20% of the patients had additional cardiovascular surgery at some time of their treatment. Furthermore, nine patients (7%) received antitachycardia pacemakers in addition to the AICD with a view toward avoiding delivery of too many high energy shocks when episodes of sustained ventricular tachycardia were too frequent.

From: Brugada P, Wellens HJJ. CARDIAC ARRHYTHMIAS: Where To Go From Here? Mount Kisco, NY, Futura Publishing Company, Inc., © 1987.

Initially a few centers used the spring-patch electrode system (seven cases), although more recently the patch-system was almost exclusively used (120 cases), and one large patch was used in 115 subjects (90%). The exact description of lead configuration is given in Table I.

In the majority of cases, the system was placed through a median sternotomy, but more recently several centers have changed to a left subcostal approach which was used in 14 cases. (11%).

Table II gives a list of the various European centers in which at least one AICD unit has been implanted. The majority of all European implantations were performed in five institutions: Hôpital Lariboisière, Paris, Medizinische Hochschule Hannover, Universitätsklinik Bonn, Universitätsklinik Köln, and Fundacion Jimenez Diaz, Madrid. These five centers all have an experience of more than 2 years. Each has implanted between nine and 32 systems: their total number is 79. The average follow-up is 16 ± 12 months. These five centers were contacted and kindly agreed to provide their results which have been pooled and will be later described.

Results in 79 Patients from the Five Most Active Centers

Mortality

There were three perioperative deaths: one due to pneumonia, one due to cardiac failure, and one to pulmonary embolism. Nine patients died during their first year follow-up. There was no arrhythmia death. Five cardiac deaths were due to heart failure and four were noncardiac deaths. Four additional deaths were recorded, all of which occurred during the second year of follow-up: one was arrhythmic and occurred in a patient with battery depletion; another two were cardiac, and the last noncardiac. This, again, shows the low sudden cardiac death rate in patients treated by AICD in spite of their high initial risk.

Complications

Nearly all patients had a pericardial friction rub which subsided after a few days. Four patients suffered complications which were directly related to the surgery or anesthesia: two local infections and two cases of atrial fibrillation. Eight patients suffered complications directly related to the AICD system: three cases of extrusion of battery, three cases of need for early battery replacement,

Table I
Electrode System

Spring-patch: 7 cases	Patch-patch: 120 cases
4 small patches	5 small-small
3 large patches	82 small-large
	33 large-large

Table II
Institutions Who Have Implanted AICD Systems to Date (1986)

AUSTRIA	Wilhelminenspital	Vienna
	Allgemeines Krankenhaus	Linz
BELGIUM	Akademisch Ziekenhuis	Gent
	Hôpital de Bavière	Liège
CZECHOSLOVAKIA	IK + EM	Prague
ENGLAND	St. Guy's Hospital	London
	St. Bartholomew Hospital	London
	St. George's Hospital	London
FRANCE	Hôpital Lariboisière	Paris
	Centre Cantini	Marseille
GERMANY	Universitätsklinik	Düsseldorf
	Medizinische Hochschule	Hannover
	Universitätsklinik	Bonn
	Universitätsklinik	Münster
	Klinikum Grosshadern	München
	Med. Universitätsklinik	Köln
	Uni-Krankenhaus Eppendorf	Hamburg
	Universitätsklinik	Heidelberg
	Charité	Berlin
	Reha Zentrum	Bad Krozingen
HOLLAND	Akademisch Ziekenhuis	Utrecht
	St. Antonius Hospital	Nieuwegein
	Akademisch Ziekenhuis	Maastricht
ITALY	Polyclinico	Naples
	Ospedale S. Chiara	Trento
	Catholic University	Roma
NORWAY	Ulleval Sykehus	Oslo
	Haukeland Sykehus	Bergen
SPAIN	Hospital San Pablo	Barcelona
	Fundacion Jimenez Diaz	Madrid
	Centro Ramon y Cajal	Madrid
	Hôpital Provincial	Madrid
SWEDEN	Sahlgrenska Hospital	Göteborg
	Lasarettet Thoraxkliniken	Lund
SWITZERLAND	Universitätspital	Zürich
	Centre Universitaire	Lausanne
YUGOSLAVIA	Institute of Surgery	Belgrade

and two cases of shocks received for atrial fibrillation. One patient suffered from a complication related to inhibition of sensing by a unipolar pacemaker which had been simultaneously implanted.

Discussion

The first striking feature of the European experience is the relatively small number of patients who were treated by the device. An easy answer would be to say that this is due to the availability of a larger number of potent antiarrhythmic drugs in Europe. This cannot be true. Potent antiarrhythmics have always been available in the US and many of the drugs that can be readily prescribed in Europe are also under investigation in the US, especially in those centers where the AICD was first used. We believe that several other factors account for the smaller number of cases implanted in Europe.

First of all, although we have no sound epidemiological data to support this hypothesis, it is our general feeling that European hospitals admit fewer patients resuscitated from an out-of-hospital cardiac arrest than do American hospitals. One can speculate that the crowded cities and relatively narrow streets in the "Old World" make rapid ambulance access more difficult. In addition, most of our communities do not have an excellent rescue system, such as those developed in Seattle and several US cities.

Secondly, social security systems are different and vary from country to country. In some, the AICD may be implanted at no cost to the patient whenever the cardiologist deems the system is indicated. These are the exception. In other countries, the patient will be reimbursed only if he or she is properly covered by private insurance. In some countries, the number of units that may be implanted per year is strictly limited and only some centers are permitted to exercise this therapy. Finally, there are countries (i.e., Belgium) where no reimbursement can, as yet, be obtained.

The limited availability of devices from the manufacturer is a third factor that may also have played a role. We believe that these various constraints account for the difference in the number of implantations between Europe and the United States. There is no objective reason to believe that European cardiologists are more conservative than their US counterparts; there are conservative and aggressive therapists on both sides of the ocean.

Another difference in comparison with the US experience lies in the fact that most US centers have at least initially used the spring-patch system whereas European centers almost exclusively use the patch-patch system generally via medium sternotomy. Lower defibrillation thresholds were demonstrated with the patch-patch configuration as compared to the spring-patch configuration.[1] Several proposals to improve the technique originated from Europe. Thus, the Laribosière group[2] showed a marked reduction in the incidence of local problems and easier postoperative course by use of a single subcostal incision, an approach already proposed by Lawrie et al.[3] The Hannover group reduced their operation time and obtained a consistently lower defibrillation threshold by using fibrin glue for patch fixation.[4] They also showed that the patch does not impair left ventricular function.[5] Manz et al.[6] showed the advantages of using antitachycardia pacemakers in conjunction with the AICD to avoid delivering too many high energy shocks in patients with frequent episodes of sustained ventricular tachycardia.

There has been a general feeling that patients implanted in Europe were somewhat less sick than those implanted in the US. This is difficult to demonstrate. A representative subset of the American implantees has been previously described by one of us (SN). Their clinical profile, sex ratio, and the proportion of patients with coronary heart disease or cardiomyopathy are not significantly different from the European implantees. The mean ejection fraction is strikingly similar in both groups (35% in Europe vs 36% in the US). The European group, however, is on the average 4 years younger. It is possible and likely that the constraints imposed by the difficulties linked to reimbursement have forced cardiologists at least in some countries to use very stringent selection criteria and to reserve this therapy to cases that were very severe because of their tachycardia but otherwise had an acceptable prognosis. The overall low mortality by sudden death among patients implanted in Europe is, however, of the same order of magnitude as that observed in the US.

The complications rate was strikingly low in the European series. We have surely profited from the initial experience made in the United States. The various complications, whether surgery-related, device-related or due to drug or pacer interactions, were already known when most centers started. For example, it had been observed that if a patient was given amiodarone after implantation, it could be deleterious either by rising the defibrillation threshold[1] or by reducing the tachycardia rate below cut-off point.[8]

Problems occurred in patients who received unnecessary shocks triggered by bouts of unsustained ventricular tachycardia, by supraventricular tachycardia, or even by excessive sinus tachycardia linked to exercise.[8] Inhibition of sensing by unipolar pacemakers was seen.[9] For all these reasons, all European cardiologists who wished to implant an AICD in a patient had a checklist (Table III) that allowed them, with the help of the company coordinator, to delineate clearly the areas of potential difficulties and thus to try to resolve them or else to refuse the indication. This probably played a role in reducing the overall incidence of complications.

Table III
Check-List Used for the Discussion with the Company Coordinator Prior to Any AICD Implantation

Doctor:
Date:
AID PATIENT PROFILE

Age:
Disease: ASHD Cardiomyop. Other
MI's:
Cardiac arrests:
Highest Vent. Rate (e.g. under exercise) without VT:
VT rate: Characteristics:
Frequency of VT/VF episodes:
Any AF or SVT?
Results of EP Tests:
Any nonsustained runs of VT?
Will patient's antiarrhythmic regimen be altered post-op?:
Heart Block?   PM?
EF: Heart size:
Other operation: CABG: Endo-resection PM: Other:
Device for inducing VT/VF intra-op:
Fluoroscopy in OR in case SVC preferred:
Myocardial screw-in Electrodes:
                Date/Time for pre-op discussion:
                Date/Time for operation:

Thus, the European experience, like the American one, has demonstrated the value of AICD for the treatment of some patients with life-threatening arrhythmias. Even if no randomized trial has ever been performed with the system, it is clear that in the very high risk groups in which the device is used, the AICD has saved many lives.

It is sad to note that the system is not yet available to all Europeans with the same conditions. The system is no more in its experimental stage, even if it can still be considerably improved. The time has come for European cardiologists to reach a consensus on the indications for implantation and then try to force their governmental agencies to give the problem the required attention, so as to avoid what will soon appear as a medico-social injustice.

References

1. Troup P, Chapman P, Olinger G, Kleinman, L. The implanted defibrillator: relation of defibrillating lead configuration and clincal variables to defibrillation threshold. J Am Coll Cardiol 1985;6:1315.
2. Laborde F, Mesnildrey P, Menasche P, Piwnica A. Surgical alternatives for implantation of the automatic implantable defibrillator. Clin Prog Electrophysiol Pacing (Suppl) 1986;4:31.
3. Lawrie G, Griffin J, Wyndham C. Epicardial implantation of automatic implantable defibrillator by left subcostal thoracotomy. PACE 1984;7:1370.
4. Frank G, Wahlers T, Klein H, Trappe H, Lichtlen P, Borst H. Implantable defibrillator-alternative treatment for recurrent ventricular fibrillation and ventricular tachycardia. Clin Prog Electrophysiol Pacing (Suppl) 1986;4:31
5. Trappe H, Werner D, Klein H, Frank G. Do patch electrodes of the implantable defibrillator impair left ventricular function? Circulation 1986;74:II-III.
6. Manz M, Gerckens, U, Funke H, Kirchoff P, Luderitz B. Combination of antitachycardia pacemaker and automatic implantable cardioverter/defibrillator for ventricular tachycardia. PACE 1986;9:676.
7. Nisam S. The automatic implantable cardioverter/defibrillator (AICD). Update on clinical results. 1987 (in press).
8. Marchilinski FE, et al. The automatic implantable cardioverter-defibrillator: efficacy, complications and device failures. Ann Intern Med 1986;104:481.
9. Bach SM. AID-B cardioverter-defibrillator: possible interactions with pacemakers. Intec Systems Technical Communication. Aug. 1983.

SCIENTIFIC RESEARCH

X

43

Control of Scientific Research

Shahbudin H. Rahimtoola

*Sow hundreds of thousands of seeds and
hundreds of excellent flowers may bloom.*
—Adapted from an Old Chinese Saying

Introduction

The mechanisms that can be or should be used to: (1) eliminate fraud in research, and (2) control scientific research will be discussed in this chapter. The hypothesis is that data collected is increasing exponentially to the detriment of the quality of the data, and is also stimulating an increase of fraud; therefore, there is a need to control research. The potential difficulty with this approach is that if we exercise control, it is likely to be imperfect, and even worse, it may stifle innovative, creative research that does not appeal to those entrusted to control research. Moreover, the major cause of fraud is likely not related to the problem. Some of the problems that confront us and possible solutions will be discussed in the following sections.

Problems of Fraud and Plagiarism

Rapid, effective methods of dissemination of news have ensured that knowledge of instances of fraud and plagiarism in science are widely disseminated. However, there is no hard data to show that this problem was not present in earlier times and that it has increased in frequency relative to the number of investigators in science. A related problem is that of fictitious claims of fraud and plagiarism.

Fraud, plagiarism, and fictitious claims are, in my view, not necessarily an indication of the failure of or a problem of research, but rather of people who likely have a personality problem. As long as we have a sufficient number of people

From: Brugada P, Wellens HJJ. CARDIAC ARRHYTHMIAS: Where To Go From Here? Mount Kisco, NY, Futura Publishing Company, Inc., © 1987.

doing science and people in science are not too dissimilar from people in the rest of society, we will have a certain percentage who will practice fraud and plagiarism and a certain percentage who will make fictitious claims of fraud and plagiarism.

I believe there is no way to stop either. However, we can and should have increased vigilance and supervision to deter them or detect them early and should exercise appropriate punitive measures once these transgressions are proven. At present, we have measures for dealing with those shown to practice fraud and plagiarism but have no well-developed punitive measures for those shown to make fictitious claims. The latter are needed or else it is possible we will see an increasing number of inadequate personalities who will try to bask in undeserved glory and/or try to denigrate established investigators.

In our Section of Cardiology, we have established a policy since April, 1984, that requires two forms to be filled out prior to a manuscript being submitted for publication (Figs. 1A, B); for abstracts, the forms have to be filled prior to or within 2 weeks of submission. The forms are intended to: (1) identify the individual who accepts responsibility for veracity of the data; (2) ensure that all authors have read and agree with the contents of the manuscript and authorship; and (3) provide an administrative oversight to ensure that the policy is followed. The forms cannot eliminate fraud, plagiarism, or fictitious claims but are intended to try and ensure acceptance of responsibility and concurrence with the published work.

Areas of Concern with Randomized and Nonrandomized Comparative Studies

Some of the concerns and problems with randomized and nonrandomized clinical trials[1-7] are listed in Tables I and II; many problems are common to both. The major problems common to both include: (1) errors of study design (for example, bias of patient entry into study, bias in changing therapy, bias in data analysis, and evaluation of outcomes between groups that were not identical in most if not all major and relevant characteristics); (2) belief that errors of study design can be corrected by complex statistical adjustments; (3) poor training for doing research; and (4) inappropriate conclusions and extrapolations.

In addition, multicenter clinical trials are not scientifically innovative and usually provide no real "new" information. They have only stirred more controversy rather than provided clinically meaningful answers. Clinical trials are slow, ponderous, and expensive. Frequently, rapid evolution leads to obsolescence of treatments and of hypotheses that are being tested; moreover, a declining incidence of morbidity and mortality often precludes the ability to prove or disprove the hypotheses that are being tested.

The problem with randomized clinical trials is not with the concept or principle of randomization or of clinical trials but with the difficulty human beings are having in designing and executing them perfectly. Nevertheless, large multicenter randomized clinical trials are very useful and have provided important informa-

A
PAGE 1

LOS ANGELES COUNTY-UNIVERSITY OF SOUTHERN CALIFORNIA MEDICAL CENTER

SECTION OF CARDIOLOGY

TO: Shahbudin H. Rahimtoola, M.D.
     Chief, Section of Cardiology
     General Hospital, Room 7131

TITLE OF MANUSCRIPT

LIST OF AUTHORS IN ORDER

WILL BE SUBMITTED FOR PUBLICATION TO

I have checked and certify that the data in the manuscript listed above is true and correct.

SIGNATURE* _____

NAME _____

DATE _____

* Faculty member who has done the research or was responsible for supervising it.

Figure 1A, B: Forms used at LAC-USC Medical Center, Los Angeles, California, U.S.A. These forms are an example of methods that can be utilized to control one problem.

B
PAGE 2

TITLE OF MANUSCRIPT

We have reviewed the above and agree with the contents of the manuscript.

SIGNATURES OF AUTHORS

1. _____	9. _____
2. _____	10. _____
3. _____	11. _____
4. _____	12. _____
5. _____	13. _____
6. _____	14. _____
7. _____	15. _____
8. _____	16. _____

===

I approve the manuscript for publication   _____

I do not approve the manuscript for publication   _____

Shahbudin H. Rahimtoola, M.D.
Chief, Section of Cardiology

Table I
Areas of Concern of Randomized Trials

1. Nonuniformity of patients, data acquisition and analysis, and treatment between various centers
2. Method of screening for patients
3. Delay between screening and randomization, and between randomization and administration of therapy
4. Very small numbers of patients from any individual institution
5. Problems of bias:
   a. Nonrandomization of eligible patients
   b. Crossover between therapeutic groups
   c. Small numbers of patients in various subgroups
   d. Methods of data analysis
   e. Alteration of methods of data analysis and of goals as study progresses
   f. Presentation of data
6. Unproven biostatistical tenets
7. Arbitrariness of p values
8. Patients heterogeneous and frequently at low risk
9. Quality of therapy administered less than ideal
10. Trail obsolete because of technological and other developments
11. Inappropriate conclusions and extrapolation

Table II
Areas of Concern of Nonrandomized Comparative Studies

1. Comparisons are not current with regard to therapy
2. Patients are not comparable because of failure to use similar admission criteria
3. Different criteria for judging effectiveness and ineffectiveness
4. Inadequate numbers of patients
5. Problems of bias:
   a. In selection of therapy
   b. Small numbers of patients in various subgroups
   c. Methods of data analysis
   d. Alteration of methods of data analysis and of goals of study
   e. Presentation of data
6. Unproven biostatistical tenets
7. Arbitrariness in p values
8. Quality of therapy administered less than ideal
9. Inappropriate conclusions and extrapolation

tion. They are most easily applied to assessing efficacy of short-term "curative" therapy, particularly of pharmacological agents.

Funding Agencies

It is important to remember that industry, governmental, and other agencies are made up of people, and therefore similar to people in science, they have their fair share of individuals who may like to ensure that results of the studies they are conducting or sponsoring will conform to their own beliefs. Industry has an additional problem, namely, its marketing section which is largely concerned with increasing sales; there is nothing inherently wrong with this goal. However, they have large amounts of monies available to them which in some unscrupulous hands may be used to manipulate and seduce some investigators.

Like science, most of industry is totally honest and ethical. Nevertheless, I believe that industry should not have exclusive control of the data or data analysis even though their support of research is important and essential.

Control of research by health agencies and by government will also be very deleterious. Their proper role is in the realm of fair and proper peer review of the proposed research.

Multinational Research

Several of the multinational clinical trials have been very successful, for example, the European Coronary Artery Surgery Study.[8] On the other hand, over 40,000 patients were randomized in seven different trials of mild systemic hypertension conducted in many different countries;[9] is so much duplication of work and effort necessary and affordable in the late 1980s? Some consideration should be given to organizing well-designed and properly executed multinational clinical trials on topics that really need to be studied.

Is There a Problem and What Are the Solutions?

In my view, it is unlikely there will ever be too much research.

A problem is "bad" research or what is being passed off as research. The natural outcome of this kind of work should be an inability to have it published, and frequently, that is what happens. For example, it is estimated that the overwhelming majority of studies presented at large scientific meetings in the United States are never published as full-length, peer-reviewed articles in high-quality scientific journals. The reasons for this are many and include the following: the research is poor or inadequate, the data is repetitive or has been split into nonviable fragments, or the investigators are too busy and/or too lazy to write it up. If there were not too many journals being published, then a form of control would be exercised.

We must not stifle inquiry. Therefore, one way to deal with the problem of "bad" research is to cut off its access to publication, that is, to limit the number of journals that are published. In the U.S., there is an increasing number of journals devoted exclusively to one of the many diagnostic techniques in use in cardiology or to a very narrow topic in cardiovascular medicine. Could these journals be safely eliminated without a major loss to the profession? If we were to discourage new journals from being published and were to encourage dissolution of several or all of the journals currently being published that are of poor quality, then it is possible and indeed likely that control of "bad" research would be exercised by the best possible means, that is, by peer review in the surviving high-quality "broad-based" cardiology journals. An inevitable result would be publication of high-quality and worthwhile work. However, since peer review is conducted by humans who have weaknesses, it is inevitable that some poor-quality work will be published and also that some high-quality work may not be published.

Fewer journals would inevitably mean more power and influence for the remaining journals; and thus, two important issues need to be discussed:

1. Who should control the journals? and
2. Who should appoint editors, and what is the appropriate term of office for an editor?

The journals should be controlled by scientists. There are usually well-established procedures of control by scientists when the journals are owned by scientific and professional societies and when the journals are owned by commercial companies but operated by scientific and professional societies. Journals that are owned and operated by commercial companies could consider having an "independent scientific board of trustees" that supervises the scientific part of the publications. Part-time editors should have a limited, fixed one term of office. Full-time talented editors should undergo an "academic" type of review by scientists every 5 to 10 years.

In summary, I believe that *if* a need to control research is accepted as a goal, then one way to proceed is to control research indirectly by having fewer journals and by establishing rigorous standards for journals and editors.

Personal Initial Thoughts and Suggestions

If we are to get the just benefits of research, that is, the flowers, I firmly believe that there should be more clinical research rather than less; that is, we must sow many more seeds. How, then, should we go about organizing clinical research and taking care of some of our problems? I suggest the following:

1. We need to identify problems that need resolution (Fig. 2). We should dissect out questions of interest. High-quality original investigators (i.e., talented young investigators and proven scientific leaders who continue to be innovative and productive) should come up with innovative ideas and design protocols to study the problem. They should perform many (hundreds of thousands, the "seeds") "small" research studies. These studies should form the bulk, and be the backbone, of our research efforts. From these studies will arise the need for a modest number of small, short-lived, randomized clinical trials and small prospective, specific, goal-oriented registries. Given the above knowledge base and effort, occasionally large multicenter randomized trials, and rarely, "epidemiological" multicenter randomized trials may be needed. These could be done by "old" investigators and burnt-out leaders; since none of us wishes to think of ourselves in this manner, the enthusiasm for these "mega" trials may abate. The "mega" studies are occasionally needed;

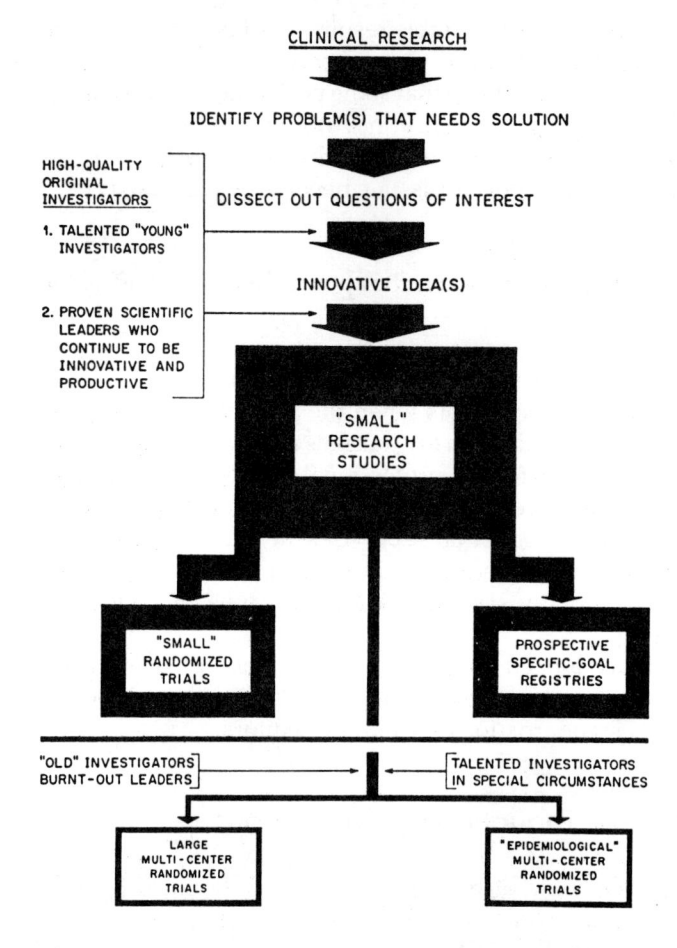

Figure 2: One format for organizing clinical research.

therefore, in special circumstances, talented investigators should participate in and conduct these trials.

2. Some thought and consideration should be given to undertaking more well-designed, well-executed, *multinational* clinical trials in order to avoid duplication of effort and to conserve resources and utilize to the maximum the strengths of each of the participating centers.

3. Industry support of research is essential and important. However, exclusive industrial control of data and of data analysis from clinical trials should be discouraged, or preferably, eliminated. These should be controlled by the investigators, or preferably, by an independent group of scientists who have no inherent bias in the outcome of the clinical trial.

4. Governmental and other health agencies should obtain and provide funds for research and provide peer review of research grant applications. They should not control the data which is the prerogative of investigators. They should also not do the research.

5. All investigators must maintain an extraordinary high standard of the quality and ethics of research. They must not allow themselves to be manipulated.

6. We probably need fewer journals in cardiovascular medicine; these should preferably be "broad-based," high-quality, cardiology journals. Journals devoted to techniques, devoted to a small group of workers, and controlled by few individuals and/or industry should be critically examined and severely curtailed, or possibly eliminated. How can we achieve this? Publications in such journals should not be allowed to be cited as references in high-quality original articles, and citing these articles in an investigators' curriculum vitae could be assigned a negative value. However, there is a need for caution and superb judgment because there are journals controlled by industry and also devoted to a single major disease entity that are truly excellent.

7. Journals should preferably be under the supervision and control of scientific and professional societies. Commercial companies that own, control, and publish journals should consider setting up an "independent scientific board of trustees" to control and supervise the scientific part of the publication.

8. Part-time journal editors should have a limited life-span. The terms of full-term journal editors should be renewed after an academic-style peer review every 5 to 10 years.

9. Fraud and plagiarism cannot be totally prevented. Some changes in the methods and style of rewarding investigators and adequate supervision may reduce it to a minimum. Those proven to be guilty should be appropriately punished.

10. We need to devise a fair and appropriate method of dealing with and punishing those guilty of fictitious claims of fraud and plagiarism.

References

1. Comstock GW. Reviews and commentary: Uncontrolled ruminations on modern clinical trials. Am J Epidemiol 1978;108:81–84.
2. Feinstein AR, Horwitz RJ. Double standards, scientific methods, and epidemiological research. N Engl J Med 1982;307:1611–1617.
3. Rahimtoola SH. Coronary bypass surgery for chronic angina—1981: A perspective. Circulation 1982;65:225–241.
4. Feinstein AR. An additional basic science for clinical medicine. II. The limitations of randomized trials. Ann Int Med 1983;99:544–550.
5. Feinstein AR. Current problems and future challenges in randomized clinical trials. Circulation 1984;70:767–774.
6. Rahimtoola SH. A perspective on the three large multicenter randomized clinical trials of coronary bypass surgery for chronic stable angina. Circulation 1985;72(Suppl V):V-123–V-135.

7. Rahimtoola SH. Some unexpected lessons from large multicenter randomized clinical trials. Circulation 1985;72:449–455.
8. Varnauskas E and the European Coronary Surgery Study Group. Survival, myocardial infarction, and employment status in a prospective randomized study of coronary bypass surgery. Circulation 1985;72(Suppl V):V-90–V-101.
9. Moser M. Treating hypertension: A review of clinical trials. Am J Med 1986;81(Suppl 6C):25–32.

44

The Electrocardiogram as a Marker for Future Cardiovascular Events

Charles Fisch

Introduction

Since its introduction by Einthoven in 1903, the electrocardiogram (ECG) has been used as an aid in the diagnosis of suspected heart disease, for confirmation of known heart disease, and less often as an index of functional and anatomical severity. More recently, and largely due to the high prevalence of coronary heart disease (CHD), the ECG has been used to detect asymptomatic ischemic heart disease. ECG changes have also been studied as a potential marker for future events. Since, for all practical purposes, in the western countries, hypertensive cardiovascular (CV) disease and CHD are the most common forms of heart disease, future events are those of angina pectoris, myocardial infarction, and CV death, either sudden or nonsudden.

This brief discussion deals with (1) the role of the ECG as an independent marker for CHD, (2) ECG abnormalities as an independent marker for future CV events, (3) ECG as an independent marker for sudden death, (4) ECG as a prognostic indicator following myocardial infarction, and (5) the significance of clinical setting in which the ECG is recorded.

From: Brugada P, Wellens HJJ. CARDIAC ARRHYTHMIAS: Where To Go From Here? Mount Kisco, NY, Futura Publishing Company, Inc., © 1987.

The ECG as an Independent Marker of CHD and Future CV Events

The prognostic significance of left ventricular hypertrophy (LVH) was studied in 5209 individuals enrolled in the Framingham study.[1] Over a period of 12 years, 3.0% developed a definite and 4.5% developed a possible pattern of LVH. At entry into the study, 76 or 1.5% had a definite and 88 or 1.7% a possible pattern of LVH. In the course of the study, 60% with definite and 20% of those with possible LVH were dead. Forty-four percent of all the 264 CV deaths were preceded by LVH. Importantly, at entry, of the 76 individuals with definite LVH, 54 were free of clinically evident heart failure, valvular disease, or CHD, suggesting that LVH may be an independent marker of heart disease. It was concluded from that study that even in the absence of overt signs of heart disease, LVH pattern carries a "grave prognosis." This is particularly true for the definite form of LVH.

In the Tecumseh study[2] of 4678 persons over the age of 20, 47 individuals had nonspecific T-wave inversion without symptoms or clinical evidence of CV disease. Twelve died; their mean age at the time of death was 70. While 5.0 deaths would be expected, 12 died, a difference significant at 0.5% level.

In the International study[3] of 12,770 men ages 40 to 59, QRS complexes with a Q and QS configuration, most likely due to past myocardial infarction, were associated with a high incidence of CV deaths. Of the 83 individuals with the Q or QS configuration, 18 died within 5 years. Similarly negative T-waves were associated with a high incidence of CV deaths. Furthermore, in individuals free of clinical heart disease at time of entry, flat or diphasic T-waves were often predictors of subsequent clinical CHD. In this study, the prevalence of other ECG abnormalities was low and the associated deaths too few in number to permit a statistical analysis.

One hundred and three asymptomatic men out of a cohort of 1400 professional aircrew and air control officers were found to have minor ST-segment and T-wave changes.[4] When subjected to an exercise study using the Bruce protocol, 19 exhibited positive responses. The study also indicated that three-eighths of those with "significant" CHD presented with minor ST-segment and T-wave changes in the resting ECG.

In the Brusselton study[5] of 2119 males, ages 40–79, presence of a Q or QS pattern, negative, flat or biphasic (<1 mm in depth) T-wave, ST-segment depression of 0.5 to 1.0 mm, and left anterior divisional block were associated with a CV mortality higher than expected. The mortality ratio was 3.7, 3.5, 2.3, 2.1, and 1.6, respectively.

The results of the three Chicago epidemiologic studies[6] of 1893 white men indicate that the CV and especially CHD death rate was significantly higher in individuals with major ECG changes than that in those individuals with a normal resting ECG. The respective mortality ratios were 3.75 and 2.43. This, however, was not true in the group with minor ECG changes where the death rates from CV disease and CHD specifically were 1.46 and 1.05, respectively. Importantly, there was evidence suggesting that the ECG abnormalities had an independent relationship to the three endpoints of the study, namely, all deaths, deaths due to CV and CHD disease.

ECG and Risk of Sudden Death

During a 6-year follow-up study of 2456 individuals in the Tecumseh study, there were seven sudden deaths in individuals with normal ECG.[2] During the same period, 38 deaths were observed in individuals with abnormal ECG. The ECG findings associated with higher incidence of sudden death included bilateral BBB, LBBB, and old myocardial infarction. The number of individuals in each of the above-listed categories was 4, 18, 26 and the number of sudden deaths was 3, 5, 5, respectively. There were only six sudden deaths in a group of 124 individuals with LVH.

In a 16-year study of males ages 45 to 74, there were 234 deaths due to CHD, of which 109 were sudden.[7] The results of this study suggested that CHD can be suspected in asymptomatic patients with LVH and who also exhibit one or more of the conventional risk factors. This group of individuals had an incidence of sudden death 5-fold greater than individuals without LVH.

In a 4-year follow-up study,[8] 17,705 men were divided into three groups: (1) 311 with a previous myocardial infarction (of this group, 40 or 12.9% died suddenly); (2) 9166 who were employed (of this group, 87 or 9.5% died suddenly); (3) 2828 who were asymptomatic (of this group, 50 or 0.62% died suddenly). The ECG abnormalities associated with an increased incidence of sudden death included intraventricular conduction defects, QRS with a Q and QS configuration, abnormal left axis deviation, ST-segment depression, and T-wave abnormality. The vast majority of the abnormal ECGs were recorded in the post-infarction group.

Seventy sudden deaths were recorded in a 30-year follow-up study of 3883 former Air Force pilots, pilots in training, and licensed pilots.[9] Twenty had a normal prior ECG while 50 (71.4%) exhibited ECG abnormalities, including ST-segment and T-wave changes (31.4%), PVC (15%), LVH (12.9%), LBBB (7.1%), and LAFB (5.7%). All of the ECG changes, other than LAFB, were associated with a higher incidence of sudden death.

The ECG After Myocardial Infarction

The Coronary Drug Project[10] enrolled 2035 individuals age 30 to 65. All suffered a myocardial infarction 3 months prior to enrollment and all were followed for 3 years. While the overall mortality was 12.6%, the mortality in the group with normal ECG was 4.1%. In the group with any codeable ECG abnormality, the mortality was 13.1%. The mortality for moderate, minor, and borderline T-wave abnormalities, Minnesota Code 5.2, 5.3, and 5.4 was 19% ($p<.001$), 13.2% ($p<.05$), and 11.6% (N.S.), respectively. Interestingly, when the T-wave abnormality was the only codeable change, the mortality was 8.5%, similar to the group without T-wave changes. Statistically significant ($p<.01$) increase in mortality was also documented in the presence of QRS complexes with Q, QS configuration and intraventricular conduction delays. ECG changes which did not have a statistically significant correlation with mortality included junctional depression, RBBB, and bifascicular blocks. The mortality in patients with LBBB was excessive among all men, but the numbers were too small to reach a statistical significance.

In the above study, the strongest independent predictor of mortality was a horizontal or downsloping ST-segment depression ($p<.001$). Twenty-five percent of individuals had this abnormality on entry and 45% of the 245 deaths occurred in this group. Mortality among men with 1 mm or more depression, or a downsloping ST-segment, was four times that observed in men without ST-segment abnormality. The numbers were 35.4% and 9.1%, respectively. The difference was statistically significant ($p<.01$).

Abnormal ECG and the Clinical Setting

Two studies addressed specifically the issue of importance of the clinical setting in evaluating an ECG abnormality as a potential marker for future events.[8,11]

In a study of 17,705 individuals, the latter were separated into three groups, namely, those with previous infarction, those employed and those who were known to be asymptomatic. The incidence of sudden death in each group was 12.9, 0.95, and 0.62%, respectively,[8] attesting to the importance of the clinical setting in which the ECG is recorded.

In another study involving 18,403 men,[11] there were 277 deaths due to CHD. In the asymptomatic individuals, with the exception of prominent Q waves and atrial fibrillation, no ECG abnormality achieved a 5 year CHD morbidity rate of even 5%. The ECG abnormalities that showed a clear association with CHD included intraventricular conduction delays, ST-segment depression, and T-wave changes including minor T-wave inversion or simply flattening. The prognostic significance of each of these ECG changes depended, however, on the clinical state. For example, while the 1 year mortality rate for those with LBBB complicating acute myocardial infarction was 50% in the ambulatory setting, of the 286 men with LBBB the 5 year mortality rate was only 5%. Similarly, in 103 men with T-wave inversion and symptomatic CHD, the 5 year mortality rate was 21%, while in 88 asymptomatic individuals with the same changes only 3% died. In essence, in men under medical care the mortality in presence of a given ECG abnormality was four times greater than in men not under medical care.

One hundred and sixty deaths were recorded in a prospective study of 554 patients with chronic bifascicular and trifascicular block with an average follow-up period of 42.4 months.[12] There was no significant difference in number of CV deaths or sudden deaths among patients with different ECG patterns. The vast majority had accompanying heart disease manifest by congestive failure or acute myocardial infarction. It appears from that study that the major determinant of mortality in presence of fascicular blocks is the severity of the underlying heart disease rather than the conduction defect per se.[13]

Comments

The ECG is used increasingly for screening of apparently healthy individuals in an effort to identify latent disease when present, and as an assessment of fitness for clearance for employment in sensitive occupations. It is also used increasingly in epidemiological studies designed to study the prevalence of CHD. Unfortunately, the resting ECG is neither a sensitive nor a specific marker for occult heart disease and furthermore the prognosis of many of the abnormalities is unclear.[14] The diagnostic and prognostic value of a given ECG abnormality differs greatly depending on the population studied and the reason for which the ECG is recorded. In keeping with the Bayes Theorum, an abnormal ECG recorded in a population with a low prevalence of cardiac disease is much more likely to be a false positive for presence of clinically significant heart disease. It is also recognized that in this group, the ECG abnormality carries a low risk for future events. However, the same ECG changes when recorded in a population with a high prevalence of heart disease, i.e., ischemic heart disease, is very likely to be a true positive and a significant prognostic sign. It has been suggested that the prognosis of a given ECG abnormality for future events is two to four times worse when discovered during a clinical evaluation than if noted during a screening procedure.[11] In essence, the prognosis of a given ECG abnormality varies depending on whether it is recorded as a screening procedure or in the course of clinical practice. Failure to recognize these facts may result in crippling "aetrogenic" heart disease.

In patients with known heart disease, some of the ECG abnormalities reach statistical significance as an independent prognostic marker. These include ST-segment and T-wave changes, and abnormal Q waves; the latter is usually a sign of a previous infarction. At this point in time there is no data which permits a clearcut differentiation of the significance of ST-segment and T-wave changes in patients with and without signs of heart disease. It has been suggested, however, that these changes may be a marker of latent heart disease. Whatever meager data is available indicate that the prognostic significance of an abnormal ST-segment or T-wave is dependent to a large extent on presence or absence of heart disease. For example, moderate T-wave inversion, Minnesota code 5:2, when associated with a history of heart disease was found to have a 21% 5 year mortality, while the mortality for the same ECG abnormality in the absence of symptoms was 3%.[11]

The strong association of LVH with future events including a high mortality regardless of whether the LVH is associated with clinical finding of heart disease or not, suggested by the Framingham study,[1] is not shared by all investigators. Rose and co-workers[11] state, "For example, in the Framingham study, LVH in men aged 45 to 62 carried an estimated 4 year mortality of 30%, a risk not equalled in this study even for major Q waves." Similarly, in the Brusselton study,[5] LVH was not associated with "significantly increased cardiovascular mortality." It is the impression of this author that LVH is often associated with organic heart disease and the latter is associated with an increased morbidity and mortality from CV causes. This divergence of opinion warrants further study.

In respect to bundle branch blocks not due to acute myocardial infarction, the evidence indicates that incidence of new events including deaths are dependent on the severity of the underlying heart disease and that the ECG changes are not an independent prognostic marker.[10,14] This is understandable in light of the fact that ECG abnormalities rarely reflect myocardial function, often the major determinant of prognosis.

The findings of the Coronary Drug Study[10] strongly suggest that in post-infarction patients, ECG changes may provide prognostic information independent of other clinical and laboratory findings. The changes include ST-segment depression, acquired intraventricular conduction delays, and Q waves. These ECG abnormalities were associated with the highest mortality during the 3 year follow-up period.

The literature dealing specifically with the ECG as a potential marker for sudden death is meager. This is especially true in the groups with an abnormal ECG but without clinically demonstrable heart disease. The few available studies have inherent limitations which include, among others, infrequency with which the ECG are recorded. As a result, conversion of a normal ECG to abnormal may be missed. Similarly, methods of confirming or ruling out clinical heart disease in large cohorts may be unreliable. Although the majority of sudden deaths occur in individuals with an abnormal ECG, thus speaking for a reasonable sensitivity, the specificity of abnormal ECG for sudden death is poor. Many patients with abnormal ECGs die of noncardiac causes or of cardiac causes but do not die suddenly.

The data relating the ECG to other variables such as prognosis for future events including angina, myocardial infarction, CV death and sudden death, presence or absence of clinical heart disease, presence or absence of anatomical heart abnormalities, and severity of myocardial impairment are often divergent. This is exemplified by the fact that although ECG abnormalities are as a rule acquired[15] and thus are probably associated with some form of cardiac pathology, the long-term prognosis of some may be no different than in presence of a normal ECG. Failure of the ECG abnormality as an independent marker is due to the fact that it is the severity of the cardiac pathology and function that are the most sensitive determinants of prognosis, and these are rarely reflected in the ECG.

The potential contribution of the ECG to identification of patients at risk for future events is tied to the fact that these occur largely in individuals with ischemic heart disease.[16] The ECG may contribute to recognition of individuals at risk by aiding in identification of the individual with CHD.

Acknowledgment: This research was supported in part by the Herman C. Krannert Fund; by Grants HL-06308 and HL-07182 from the National Heart, Lung and Blood Institute of the National Institutes of Health, U.S. Public Health Service; and the American Heart Association, Indiana Affiliate, Inc.

References

1. Kannel WB, Gordon T, Offutt D. Left ventricular hypertrophy by electrocardiogram: Prevalence, incidence, and mortality in the Framingham study. Ann Intern Med 1969;71:89–105.

2. Chiang BN, Perlman LV, Fulton M, Ostrander LD, Epstein FH. Predisposing factors in sudden cardiac death in Tecumseh, Michigan: A prospective study. Circulation 1970; 41:31–37.
3. Blackburn H, Taylor HL, Keys A. XVI. The electrocardiogram in prediction of five year coronary heart disease incidence among men aged forty through fifty nine. Circulation 1970;41/42(suppl I):1–154–161.
4. Joy M, Trump DW. Significance of minor ST segment and T wave changes in the resting electrocardiogram of asymptomatic subjects. Br Heart J 1981;45:48–55.
5. Cullen K, Stenhouse NS, Wearne KL, Cumpston GN. Electrocardiograms and 13 year cardiovascular mortality in Busselton study. Br Heart J 1982;47:209–212.
6. Cedres BL, Liu K, Stamler J, Dyer AR, Stamler R, Berkson DM, Paul O, Lepper M, Lindberg HA, Marquardt J, Stevens E, Schoenberger JA, Shekelle RB, Collette P, Garside D. Independent contribution of electrocardiographic abnormalities to risk of death from coronary heart disease, cardiovascular diseases and all causes. Circulation 1982;65:146–153.
7. Kannel WB, Doyle JT, McNamara PM, Quickenton P, Gordon T. Precursors of sudden coronary death. Factors related to the incidence of sudden death. Circulation 1975;51:606–613.
8. Pedoe HDT. Predictability of sudden death from resting electrocardiogram: Effect of previous manifestations of coronary heart disease. Br Heart J 1978;4040:630–635.
9. Rabkin SW, Mathewson FAL, Tate RB. The electrocardiogram in apparently healthy men and the risk of sudden death. Br Heart J 1978;40:636–643.
10. Blackburn H. The prognostic importance of the electrocardiogram after myocardial infarction. Ann Int Med 1972;77:677–689.
11. Rose G, Baxter PJ, Reid DD, McCartney P. Prevalence and prognosis of electrocardiographic findings in middle-aged men. Br Heart J 1978;40:636–643.
12. McAnulty JH, Rahimtoola, SH, Murphy E, DeMots H, Ritzman L, Kanarek, PE, Kauffman S. Natural history of "high-risk" bundle branch block. N Engl J Med 1982; 307:138–143.
13. Fisch GR, Zipes DP, Fisch C. Bundle branch block and sudden death. Prog Cardiovasc Dis 1980;23:187–224.
14. Fisch C. Role of the electrocardiogram in identifying the patient at increased risk for sudden death. JACC 1985;5(6):6B–8B.
15. Fisch C. The electrocardiogram in the aged. Cardiovasc Clin 1981;12:65–74.
16. Spain DM, Bradess VA, Mohr C. Coronary atherosclerosis as a cause of unexpected and unexplained death: An autopsy study from 1949–1959. JAMA 1960;174:384–388.

45

Relations Between University and Industry

Ivan M.G.P. Bourgeois

Introduction

The relations between universities and industry are influenced by the perceived role of both parties, the socio-economic environment, and the culture of that part of the world where both parties are located.

The Role of the University and Industry

The cooperation between university and industry has for several years been a theme of many discussions, especially in Western Europe. Historically the role of the universities in Europe was to be a training center for the elite and to be a focal point for fundamental research for the sake of know-how. With democratization, its role has shifted to that of a contributor to the development of the country through education and research from which industry, as well as the population of the country through job creation, will benefit.

The role of industry is to provide products and service to the population in the most cost effective manner within the social economic environment in which they operate.

Socio-Economic Factors

Education and Communication

For several decades now there has been an explosion in education. Illiteracy has been virtually eliminated in the industrialized countries and is rapidly regressing in the undeveloped countries. During the 20th century, the need for education has led to the phenomenal development of colleges and universities.

Over the centuries this increased general knowledge has transformed the population from agrarian workers to factory workers and recently to collaborators in the service industries. It has also created a need for increased communication resulting in the recent phenomenal development of the travel and communications business. As new products and ideas are rapidly widely distributed, there is a general trend to invest in research and development to maintain a competitive edge with innovative products. This is clearly visible in growth-oriented companies, at industrial and national levels. Recently major research efforts in the field of fundamental physics or space programs has been on a transcontinental level.

Economic Development

In the industrialized nations, the number of people involved in research and development is roughly 2% of the population. The educational budgets in those countries are among the highest. These heavy investments are made to maintain or to develop the relative competitive situation of those countries.

Research and development projects in the high technology area receive a favorable audience at all levels of the population some examples of which are microelectronics, telecommunications, information processing, biotechnology, transportation, aeronautics, and medical electronics.

Governments contribute to the creation of such new fields by investing in university research and fundamental technologies or, as in Japan, creating an overall agency to coordinate technological-oriented research. Also several nations have pooled their research investment in specific fields such as Euratom, CERN, and recently the Eureka project in the hope of major economic spin-offs, such as those which were derived from space and other programs in the recent decades. These nations have been major contributors to the actual development of microelectronics, data processing, and telecommunications. They also have contributed to the creation of new materials.

Private Investments

Many of those major projects are carried out in the research laboratories of leading universities or companies. Some brilliant young researchers have seen the potential of responding to a market need with new products made possible by newly developed technology and have started their own companies. Since the success of Silicon Valley, showing a phrenetic growth of young successful innovative companies, there is an increased recognition for an entrepreneurial attitude. Capital from private investors, i.e., venture capital, became available to help young innovative entrepreneurs to start up a company. This new attitude has spread over the world and is influencing government subsidies to companies in Western Europe. Major corporations have increased their research efforts to exploit fully the opportunity offered by the new technology. They have introduced new products which could hardly be conceivable a quarter of a century ago. Some striking examples are portable calculators, digital watches, computers, composite materials, and video communications.

Cultural Factors

Different countries, ethnic groups, and religions have their own scales of value and are influencing socio-economic values via the political system. The lifestyle and the way of doing business differs from country to country. In undeveloped countries the first priority is adequate nutrition, while in the developed nations it is increased wealth. Here different priorities of how to achieve wealth improvement are present in different nations: health education, capitalization, redistribution. The relative value depends on the political choice.

Organizations and individuals have behavior patterns that have been built up over the centuries and that are part of their cultural heritage. Respect for those patterns and objectives is essential for a successful cooperation. Deviations could lead to communication problems and misunderstandings, which could be the cause of major frustrations.

Conditions for a Successful Relationship

It is an impossible task to give a set of rules that will ensure a successful relationship between university and industry. The university has a broad role of educating, training, and performing fundamental as well as applied research. The interest of industry covers a very large field, which is related to the great diversity of products it manufactures or services it delivers.

In this section, cooperation between universities and industry in Western Europe will be discussed within the framework of medical technology, especially in the field of implantable electronics, where the author has the largest part of his experience.

The Implantable Electronics Industry

The flagship product of the implantable electronics industry is the cardiac pacemaker. From the original concept of maintaining an acceptable heart rate by electrical stimulation of the cardiac muscle, pacemakers became more sophisticated with the development of microelectronics. Microelectronics made programmable and rate variable pacemakers possible. Programmable pacemakers can be attuned by the physician to the clinical condition of the patient by noninvasive telemetry. Rate variable pacemakers adapt their stimulation frequency to the instantaneous need of the patient. Reliability, longevity, size reduction, and electrode improvements have made the implantable pacemaker into one of the most cost-effective therapies. Clinical research on the use of electrical stimulation for the treatment of rapid heart rates is progressing. The devices used are implantable defibrillators and antitachycardia pacemakers.

Other applications of implantable electronics are in the field of pain management, the treatment of deafness, respiratory dysfunctions, and peripheral circulatory insufficiencies. In the field of muscle stimulation by implantable electronics, muscle spinal cord correction (scoliosis management), heart assistance concepts, and functional electrical stimulation are under investigation. Functional stimulation is a sequential stimulation of a series of muscles to restore the muscle function in paralyzed patients.

The field of implantable electronics will further develop as implantable sensors are available and will allow continuous ambulatory monitoring.

Implantable electronic controlled drug delivery devices have recently shown therapeutic benefits in the management of certain types of cancer and spasticity. There are preliminary indications that controlled insulin delivery in carefully selected diabetic patients is promising.

Rationale for Cooperation Between Medical Research and Teaching Centers with the Implantable Electronics Industry

The field of implantable electronics has a predetermined disposition to cooperate with universities. Cooperation with clinical researchers, physiologists, and surgeons is essential to define a clinically acceptable product. When the product is ready, it should be clinically evaluated at different centers to verify current clinical functioning and to demonstrate clinical efficacy. This process is essential in the medical device business to be able to introduce a new concept or a product to the market. Concerns regarding the cost of health care in relation to the gross national product are voiced around the world. Clinical efficacy and cost effectiveness are key determinates to an overall health care of the population, which conditions business success.

The medical faculty of any given university is in an excellent position to contribute to health care improvement. Medical researchers should have a key role in the clinical definition of new concepts and participate in the clinical evaluation of those new devices made by industry. Also as new therapies evolve, medical research and teaching centers can educate their students in the use of those new therapeutic tools.

Key Elements in Establishing a Cooperation Between University and Industry

Before starting to discuss any cooperation, it is of paramount importance that the two following questions are satisfactorily answered:

- Do both parties have a common objective and receive a reward when they achieve the objective?
- Do both parties have the authority to enter into an agreement and do they have the necessary resources to carry out the agreement?

The answers to those questions should be given not only taking into account the input of the individuals but also that of the respective organizations. The socio-economic attitude in the country relative to the type of research to be carried out should also be taken into consideration.

When the decision is made to enter into a research cooperation, the following two actions should take place:

- Write a formal agreement in which the objectives, the duties, and the rewards are clearly defined and documented.
- Ensure formal regular progress reporting versus the objective and the plan.

Some Practical Hints

Definition of the Parties

The cooperation between university and industry has been quoted many times. From the first contacts it should be clear whether the intended relationship is with a representative of the university or an individual working at the university.

Understanding the Nature of the Cooperation

There are three different types of cooperation: (1) consultation; (2) clinical evaluation; and (3) clinical research.

Consultation is an exchange of information from a knowledgeable person to an interested party.

Clinical evaluation is the last phase of a product development cycle, the objective of which is to verify the clinical functioning of the device, related to the design intention. These clinical evaluation studies are scientific in nature and are conducted according a protocol agreed upon by the investigator and the manufacturer. There are guidelines for the clinical evaluation of pacemakers issued by NASPE (North American Society for Pacing and Electrophysiology) and the EWGCP (European Working Group on Cardiac Pacing). Most countries have adopted the declaration of Helsinki 1975, and clinical evaluation should follow those statements. Several countries require preregistration of the device to be evaluated and have introduced clinical evaluation requirements.

Clinical research is orientated toward finding new therapeutic or diagnostic methods that could lead to improvements of currently available devices or results in new devices. As with clinical evaluation, clinical research is governed by the declaration of Helsinki. It is essential that both parties understand the nature, the objectives, and the limitations of such programs. These studies should be done according to protocol and data should be analyzed regularly. The information exchange between both parties should be in depth.

Ownership of Information and Publication Rights

An academic researcher's motivation is influenced by the number of innovative publications that he can present, while a manufacturer could have a more subtle attitude. When a product is marketed, the manufacturer likes to see as many scientific publications as possible related to that product. Manufacturers are more hesitant regarding the publication of preliminary research data to protect their competitive edge or patent protection. Negative clinical experience should be communicated to all investigators involved in such research programs.

Dealings Between Organizations

Cooperation between two organizations who do not have the same basic objective can create much frustration through misunderstandings. The presence of a champion in both organizations will facilitate the process. Both champions should define the joint objective and explain to the sponsors (management) how that joint objective fits the individual organizations' objectives. These champions should ensure that proper agreements are made and that resources will be made available and they should monitor progress relative to those agreements.

They should be aware of regulatory, organizational, and other potential constraints to such agreements, as well as to their implementation.

The champions are vital to the success of the cooperation, and should be able to meet the expectations of the sponsors. To fullfil this complex role, mutual trust of the champions is essential, as is the continuous backing of the sponsors.

Classical Traps to Avoid

Manage Expectation Gaps

Entering into an agreement creates a lot of excitement, usually based on the conviction of achieving the goal of the agreement or further spin-offs of that research. This excitement could be misleading and create expectations that are not covered by the contract, yet those expectations could later prove to be the reason for having signed the contract.

Therefore it is essential that both parties understand the objectives of the agreement and discuss what could happen at the end of the contract. It is also imperative to achieve a clear understanding, by both parties, of what will occur if one of the parties terminates the agreement prior to its expiration. Cultural closeness and open communication between champions are essential in this context. For major agreements, the establishment of a trust relationship is *a must* to avoid expectation gaps.

Cooperation between university and industry also creates a lot of excitement in the community. In Western Europe, governments are the main providers of funds to universities. In recent years there has been a reduced level of government funding, due to the economical crisis. On the other hand, governments are willing to fund significant parts of research if an industrial partner is associated with the university and especially if the industry partly funds the project.

Plan Landmarks in the Agreement

Sometimes people tend to believe that agreements will remain forever. The continuation of agreements is dependent on achievement of objectives and changes in the environment demanding for new resource allocations. Building landmarks, i.e., time limits, resource limits, and measuring points into the plan, will enhance the positive outcome of the agreement and will also put agreed limits to it.

Conclusion

Cooperation between university and industry, if properly agreed upon and implemented, will benefit to all parties involved. The academic researcher will be supported in his scientific work and have access to the advanced technologies which the manufacturers have. The university will benefit from an image of openness and targeted oriented research complementary to their basic research. They will be perceived by doing it to contribute to the society via the industrial spin-off of their research. The manufacturer will benefit from the knowledge that is made available at the university and the assistance he receives complementary to his research efforts.

46

How Everything Started in Clinical Electrophysiology

Richard Langendorf

Introduction

When the organizers of the Maastricht meeting invited me more than a year ago to participate and give a perspective lecture on "How everything started in clinical electrophysiology," I accepted with some hesitation. I did not know exactly what I was expected to present. In my letter of acceptance I stated that I might approach the topic from a very personal standpoint; I hope it is a not-too-personal one. How did clinical, i.e., bedside, electrophysiology start?

A main reason was the endeavor to better understand the mechanisms of arrhythmias observed at the bedside. Some, but not all, of the disturbances of impulse formation and conduction had been studied in the experimental animal and had helped clarify their counterpart in man.

Electrical stimulation of the heart for the study of human arrhythmias has been performed for more than two decades.[1] The combination with intracardiac recordings of electrical activation, notably electrical activity from the bundle of His, greatly increased interpretation of the mechanisms of human arrhythmias. I would like to concentrate on one aspect of the electrophysiology of disturbed impulse formation, that of parasystole, and one aspect of disturbed impulse conduction, that of concealed conduction. They will illustrate how these mechanisms, suspected from simple electrocardiographic tracings, could be confirmed by sophisticated electrophysiologic techniques. They also will illustrate the continuum from noninvasive to invasive arrhythmology.

From: Brugada P, Wellens HJJ. CARDIAC ARRHYTHMIAS: Where To Go From Here? Mount Kisco, NY, Futura Publishing Company, Inc., © 1987.

Parasystole

The manifestations of parasystole, so named by Kaufman and Rothberger in 1920,[2] have become understood only during the last decade. The application to human arrhythmias by Drs. Gordon Moe, Jose Jalife, and co-workers[3] of data obtained from ingenious biological and mathematical models has made it possible to understand the behavior of parasystolic rhythms.

It is clear today that parasystole is a much more frequent mechanism of abnormal impulse formation than previously realized. The recognition of the possibility of electrotonic modulation of the parasystolic pacemaker by the dominant rhythm has changed the traditional concepts in relation to the electrocardiographic diagnosis of parasystole.

Parasystole can occur in any heart structure: the atria, the atrioventricular junction, or the ventricles. Even the sinus node can manifest parasystolic activity, as recently demonstrated by Jalife and Michaels[4] (Fig. 1). The possibility of sinus node extrasystoles had been recognized in the electrocardiogram for a long time.[5] The diagnosis was made using two very simple criteria: (1) an atrial premature beat with a P-wave configuration indicating an origin in the sinus node, and (2) the absence of a compensatory pause after the extrasystole, with a return cycle that equaled the sinus cycle length. The possibility of parasystole in the sinus node reveals fascinating aspects in the diagnosis of sinus node arrhythmias.

Parasystole has been most frequently diagnosed at the ventricular level. The

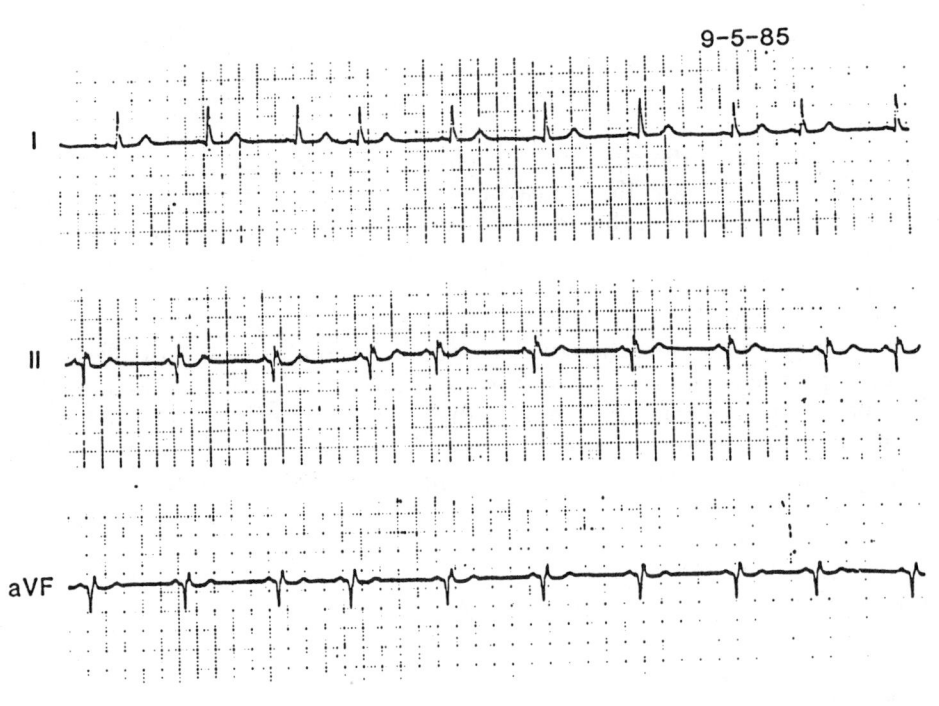

Figure 1: Sinus node parasystole (see text for details).

way the diagnosis was made will have to be adapted after the observations by Moe and Jalife of the possibility of parasystolic modulation. Figure 2 is an example of ventricular ectopic beats showing the same morphology and marked variations in the coupling interval to the preceding sinus beat. However, the long interectopic cycles are not multiples of the short interectopic cycles, a criterion which was used in the diagnosis of parasystole. On the basis of the new observations on parasystolic modulation, we know that the lack of a mathematical relation between short and long interectopic cycles does not rule out parasystole. The parasystolic pacemaker is slowed when sinus impulses occur during the first half of the parasystolic focus cycle and is accelerated when sinus impulses occur during the second half of the parasystolic cycle.

A fixed coupling interval of premature beats does not rule out parasystole. Numerous explanations can be given for the occurrence of a fixed coupling interval during parasystole. One of these explanations is the phenomenon of so-called "reversed coupling" caused by a similar rate of the parasystolic and dominant pacemaker. This phenomenon can be observed in Figure 3, where it was reproduced by pacing the human ventricle with a demand pacemaker and a slower, asynchronous (parasystolic) pacemaker.

Parasystole was a rather well-understood phenomenon from simple electrocardiographic tracings. The whole spectrum of its possible manifestations was opened, however, with the advent of more sophisticated techniques to study, produce, reproduce, and simulate that phenomenon. The same has happened with the interpretation of reentry from electrocardiographic tracings. We know nowadays that a varying coupling interval of reentrant extrasystoles can be the

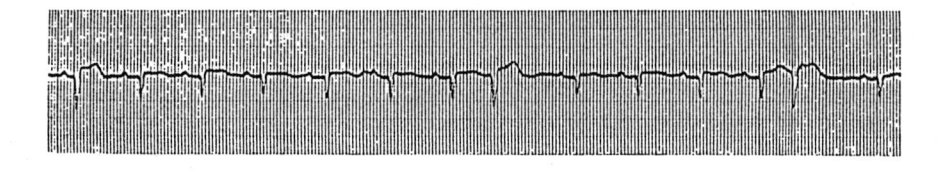

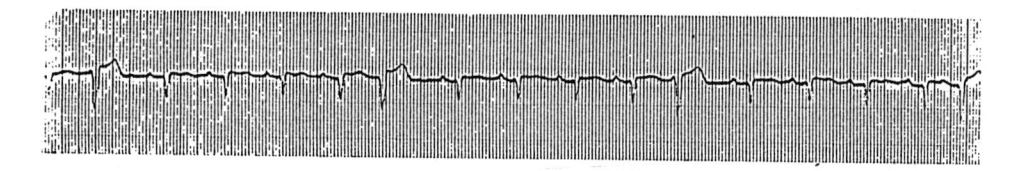

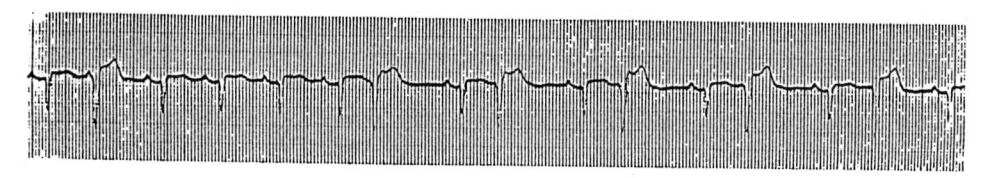

Figure 2: Modulated parasystole (see text for details).

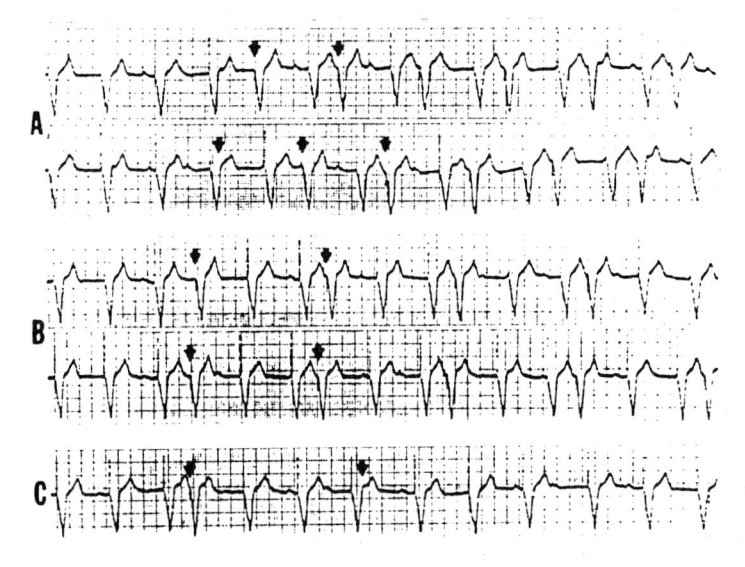

Figure 3: Parasystole with fixed coupling (see text for details).

result of varying degrees of delay in conduction in the reentrant pathways. Figure 4 demonstrates such progressive delay in the coupling interval of premature beats in a case of intermittent bigeminy,[7] a mechanism later confirmed when the refined electrophysiology techniques became available,[8] as shown in Figure 5. Another important observation that was also later confirmed was the variation in the number of spontaneous premature beats in relation to the frequency of the dominant pacemaker. These variations have important implications for the interpretation of the efficacy of antiarrhythmic drugs and are probably not taken sufficiently into account.

With the recognition of modulation of parasystolic pacemakers, electrocardiographic manifestations of parasystole, such as exit block from a parasystolic pacemaker or the concept of intermittent parasystole, require extensive reassessment at the present time.

Concealed Conduction

I introduced the term "concealed conduction" about 40 years ago on the occasion of the Second Inter-American Congress of Cardiology. That Congress has held at the Instituto Nacional de Cardiologia in Mexico, now named after the founder, Dr. Ignacio Chavez. The reality of concealed conduction was clear from electrophysiologic tracings, but definitive proof could only be obtained when the phenomena which were concealed in the surface electrocardiogram became evident from endocavitary recordings. At the same time, new forms of concealed conduction were recognized, which are concealed even when using endocavitary recordings. Electrical stimulation has helped in understanding the phenomenon of concealed conduction. Figure 6 was obtained during atrial stimulation in

History of Clinical Electrophysiology • 719

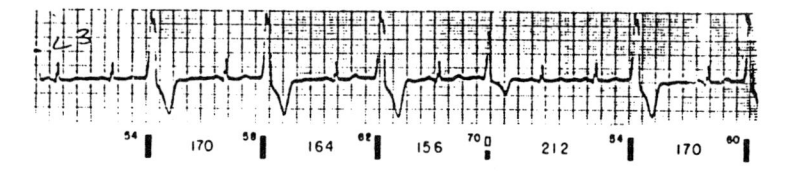

Figure 4: Bigeminy with progressively longer coupling interval (see text).

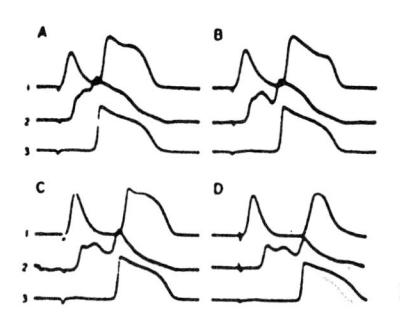

Figure 5: Variable coupling intervals of reentrant impulses due to increasing conduction time in a reentrant pathway (see text). (Reproduced with permission.[8])

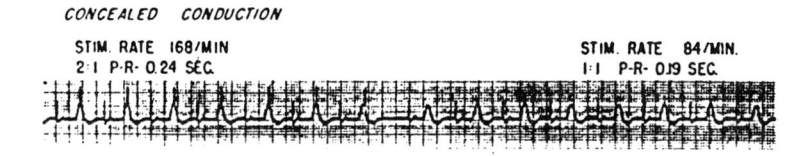

Figure 6: Concealed conduction of apparently blocked impulses (see text).

humans during an experience published[9] and performed at the Michael Reese Hospital in 1925. During that study, the methodology as previously reported by Sir Thomas Lewis and Arthur Master in 1925 in the dog[10] was used by us in humans. Figure 6 gives indirect evidence of concealed conduction of apparently completely blocked impulses. Full evidence for that phenomenon came from the studies by Ling and Gerard 10 years later when electrical stimulation was combined with recordings of electrical activation from different portions of the conduction system of the heart.[12,13] Recordings of electrical activity from the bundle of His were initiated in 1960 by Girard, Puech and co-workers,[14] and introduced as a clinical method by Damato's group in 1969.[15] Programmed electrical stimulation of the heart became a clinical method of study of arrhythmias after the studies by Wellens.[16] By combining electrical stimulation with endocavitary recordings, the site of origin and pathways of human arrhythmias can be very accurately determined. These methods have fully validated many observations which were made from simple electrocardiographic tracings. They have also confirmed many assumptions based on indirect evidence from the electrocardiogram. In relation to

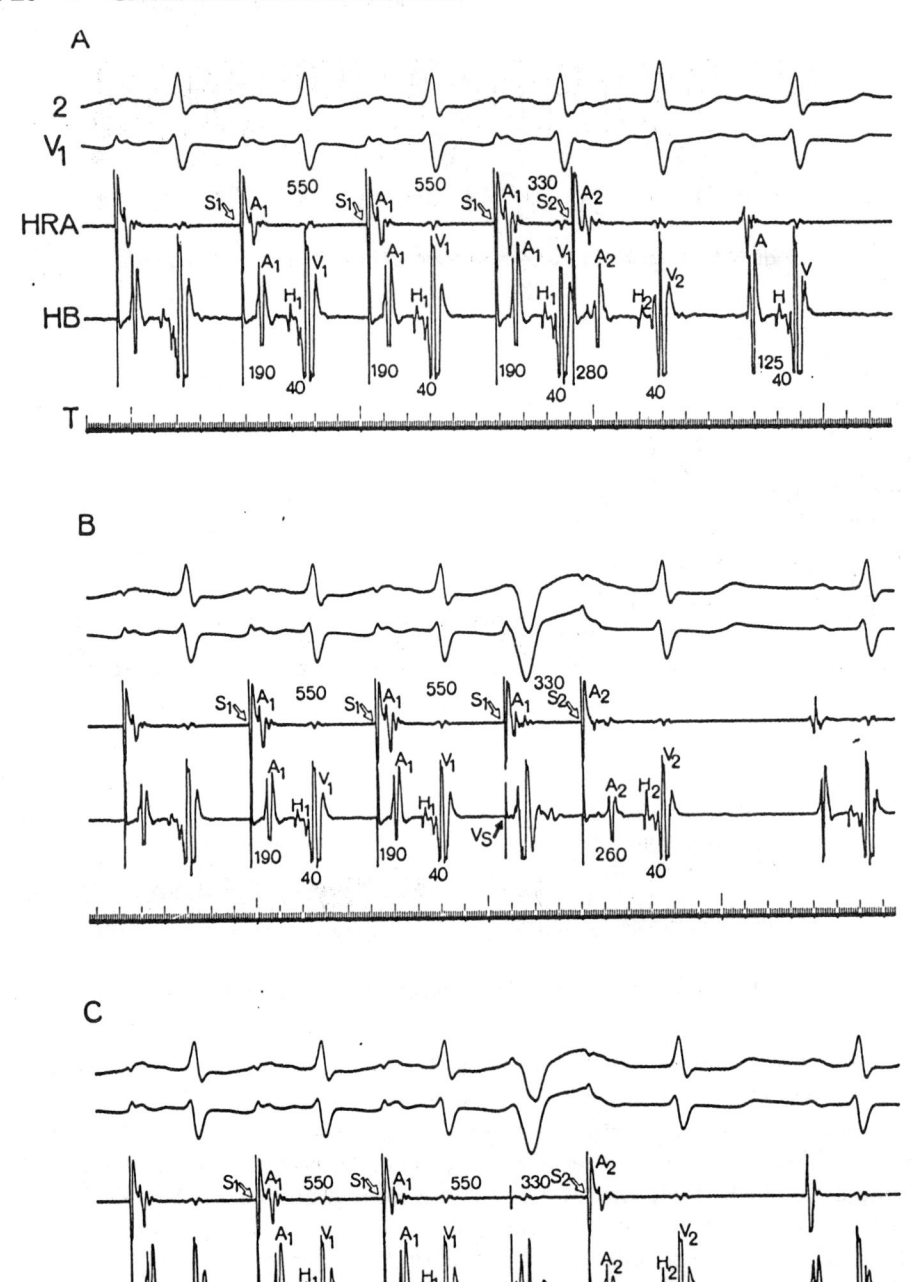

Figure 7: Facilitation of anterograde conduction after retrograde concealed conduction in the AV node (see text). (Reproduced with permission.[17])

concealed conduction, they have taught us many interesting things, among them the possible facilitating effect of concealed conduction upon subsequent conduction[17,18] as shown in Figure 7. This facilitating effect was first described by Wolferth[19] and held responsible for a pseudo-supernormal phase of conduction. The reality of these phenomena would be confirmed by Moore and Spear later on.[20]

Conclusion

The development of clinical electrophysiology was a naturally occurring process based upon the need to better understand the arrhythmias which occurred at the bedside and the growing availability of technology which made these types of studies possible in humans. Both abnormal impulse formation and conduction have been extensively studied by these techniques. It was the continuous flow of information from the electrocardiogram to the experimental laboratory and to the clinical electrophysiology laboratory and back that made possible a better understanding of the mechanisms of human arrhythmias, which was the first step toward better treatment.

References

1. Langendorf R, Pick A. Artificial pacing of the human heart. Its contribution to the understanding of the arrhythmias. Am J Cardiol 1971;28:516–525.
2. Kaufmann R, Rothberger CJ. Beiträge zur Entstehungsweise extrasystolischer Allorhythmien. 4. Mittlg. Über Parasystolie, eine besondere Art extrasystolischer Rhythmusstörungen. Ztschr. f. d. ges. Exp. M. 1920;11:40.
3. Antzelevitch C, Jalife J, Moe GK. Electrotonic modulation of pacemaker activity: Further biological and mathematical observations on the behavior of modulated parasystole. Circulation 1982;66:1225–1232.
4. Jalife J, Michaels DC, Langendorf R. Modulated parasystole originating in the sinoatrial node. Circulation 1986; Vol. 74.
5. Wenckebach KF, Winterberg H. Die unregelmässige Herztätigkeit Leipzig: Engelmann, 1927:196.
6. Langendorf R, Pick A. Parasystole with fixed coupling. Circulation 1967;35:304–315.
7. Mack I, Langendorf R. Factors influencing the time of appearance of premature systoles (including a demonstration of cases with ventricular premature systoles due to reentry but exhibiting variable coupling). Circulation 1950;1:910–921.
8. Cranefield PF, Wit AL, Hoffman BF. Genesis of cardiac arrhythmias. Circulation 1973;47:190–204.
9. Langendorf R, Pick A, Edelist A, Katz LN. Experimental demonstration of concealed AV conduction in the human heart. Circulation 1965;32:386–393.
10. Lewis T, Master AM. Observations upon conduction in the mammalian heart. A-V conduction. Heart 1925;12:209.
11. Ling G, Gerard RW. The normal membrane potential in frog sartorius fibers. J Cell Comp Physiol 1949;343:383.
12. Alanis J, Lopez E, Mandoki J, Pilar G. Propagation of impulses through the atrioventricular node. Am J Physiol 1959;197:1171.
13. Hoffman BF, Paes de Carvalho A, de Mello WC, Cranefield PF. Electrical activity of single fibers of the atrioventricular node. Circ Res 1959;7:11.

14. Giraud G, Puech P, Latour H, Hertault J. Variations de potentiel liées a l'activité du système de conduction auriculoventriculaire chez l'homme (enregistrement electrocardiographique endocavitaire). Arch Mal Coeur 1960;53:757.
15. Scherlag BJ, Lau SH, Helfant RH, Berkowitz WD, Stein E, Damato AN. Catheter technique for recording His bundle activity in man. Circulation 1969;59:13–18.
16. Wellens HJJ. Electrical stimulation of the heart in the study and treatment of tachycardias. Baltimore: University Park Press, 1971.
17. Shenasa M, Denker S, Mahmud R, Lehman M, Gilbert CJ, Akhtar M. Atrioventricular nodal conduction and refractoriness after intranodal collision from antegrade and retrograde impulses. Circulation 1983;67:651–660.
18. Mahmud R, Lehman M, Denker S, Gilbert CJ, Akhtar M. Atrioventricular sequential pacing: differential effect on retrograde conduction related to level of impulse collision. Circulation 1983;68:23–32.
19. Wolferth CC. The so'called supernormal recovery phase of conduction in heart muscle. Am Heart J 1928;3:706.
20. Moore EN, Spear JF. Experimental studies on the facilitation of A-V conduction by ectopic beats in dogs and rabbits. Circ Res 1971;29:29.

XI

New Prospects in Diagnosis and Treatment of Arrhythmias

47

New Forms of Anomalous Conduction in the AV Junction

Benjamin J. Scherlag
Masayuki Sakurai
Raed Sweidan
Ralph Lazzara

Introduction

In the mid 1970s, several basic studies were performed in our laboratories on the effects of ischemia on AV and intraventricular conduction caused by ligation of the anterior septal artery in the dog heart.[1-5] In more than 150 such experiments we have documented various forms of conduction abnormalities including tachy- and bradycardia bundle branch blocks, Mobitz type I and type II AV block, paroxysmal AV block, and intra-His as well as bilateral bundle branch block. However, in one experiment we observed a severe form of intra-His bundle block which was associated with the loss of initial forces in the QRS and the appearance of delta waves. Due to the singularity of these observations, none of our previous reports alluded to these findings, although a previous report used an illustration from this case in the context of describing His bundle dissociation.[6] Prior to anterior septal artery ligation, records of two standard leads, II and aVR were made, as well as a simultaneously recorded His bundle electrogram (Fig. 1). The insets below the His bundle recordings show magnifications of the His bundle deflection. In the control state (panel A) the H-V interval is within the normal

From: Brugada P, Wellens HJJ. CARDIAC ARRHYTHMIAS: Where To Go From Here? Mount Kisco, NY, Futura Publishing Company, Inc., © 1987.

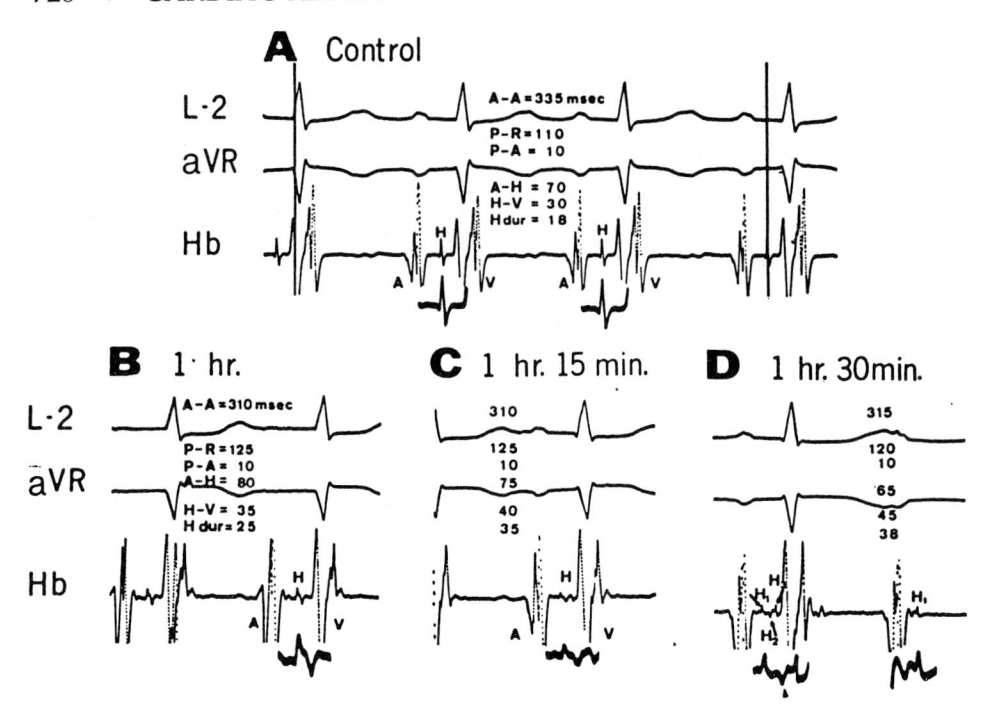

Figure 1: Evolution of intra-His bundle block caused by ischemia after ligation of the anterior septal artery in the dog heart. The three traces from above are: electrocardiographic leads II (L-2) and aVR; His bundle electrogram (Hb). In the control state, panel A, and His potential duration of 18 ms and H-V of 30 ms are in the normal range for the dog heart. The magnified His bundle deflection is shown below the Hb recording. In panels B–D, 1–1.5 hours after anterior septal artery ligation, there is a progressive amplitude reduction and increased duration of the His potential, which fractionates into three portions (H_1, H_2, H_3). The H-V also prolonged to 45 ms prior to block distal to H_1 (panel D). (Reproduced by permission. Arch Inst Cardiol Mex 1980;50:131–140.)

range for the dog heart, 30 ms, and the duration of the His bundle potential has a normal value of 18 ms.

In panels B and C, about 1 hour after ligation of the anterior septal artery, which supplies the basal interventricular septum underlying the His bundle, we observed a marked decrease in the amplitude and an increase in the duration of the His bundle potential to 25 and 35 ms (see insets). The severity of the intra-His bundle block became apparent at 1 hr and 30 min after coronary artery ligation with the development of a tripartite His potential, H_1, H_2, and H_3. The occurrence of second degree intra-His bundle block was indicated by a dropped beat showing only atrial and H_1 potentials. Note that in the control and ischemic states, leads II and aVR exhibit normal initial vectors represented by Q and R waves, respectively.

Within the same time frame, vagal-induced slowing of the heart rate caused a bradycardia-dependent conduction delay (Fig 2). This was manifest as an exacerbation of the intra-His bundle block with H-V intervals reaching 140 ms. Associated with this marked intra-His bundle block was the loss of the initial deflections

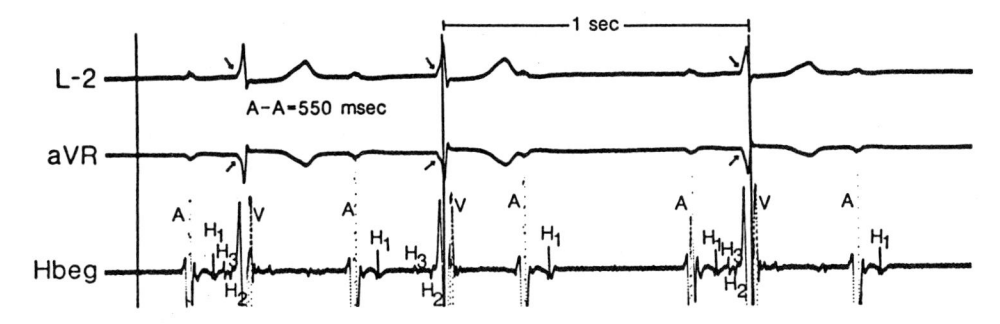

Figure 2: The appearance of delta waves associated with severe intra-His bundle block. The traces are the same as in Figure 1 minutes after the development of second degree AV block. Vagal-induced slowing of the heart rate (A - A = 550 ms) exacerbated the intra-His bundle block by prolonging the H-V interval up to 140 ms. Note the temporal dissociation of conduction within the His bundle as evidenced by the temporal reversal of H_2 and H_3 potentials (compare to Figure 1). These changes are concomitant with loss of initial Q and R waves in the ECG leads and the appearance of delta waves (arrows).

of the QRS complexes in the standard ECG leads which were replaced by delta-like waves, i.e., slurred R and Q waves in leads II and aVR, respectively.

These observations provided the incentive for the studies described below. Our objective was to reproduce conditions of severe intra-His bundle block in order to regularly induce delta wave formation. In this way, a mechanistic hypothesis could be developed to explain the basis of this phenomenon.

Methods

Eighteen adult mongrel dogs were anesthetized with sodium pentobarbital, 30 mg/kg, administered intravenously. After a 12-lead ECG was recorded, the right heart was exposed at the fourth intercostal space, and a pericardiotomy through a thoracotomy. The upper lobe of the right lung was ligated and excised in order to expose the major inflow vessels to the right heart. The azygous vein was ligated and ligatures placed around the superior and inferior vena cavae to be used for temporary inflow restriction later in the study.

Plunge wire electrodes were placed into the atrium near the sinoatrial node and the right ventricular free wall near the apex. The right common carotid sheath was dissected in the neck and wires placed into the intact right vagosympathetic trunk.[7] The right carotid artery was ligated and a bipolar or tripolar pacing catheter was introduced and passed to the noncoronary cusp at the aortic root.[8] By contrast electrographic monitoring, a stable His bundle electrogram was registered.[8]

During normal sinus rhythm, two standard ECG leads, II and aVR or V_2 were monitored on an oscillographic recorder (Honeywell E for M, VR-12) which was interfaced with a Gould electrostatic recorder (ES1000) or a Siemens-Elema ink-jet recorder. In addition to the ECG leads, the following electrograms were displayed: sinoatrial area, His bundle, and right ventricular apex. Right vagosympathetic trunk stimulation, as described previously,[7] was used to slow the sinus rate or to induce sinus arrest and/or AV nodal block, depending on the intensity of stimulation.

Atrial pacing at progressively higher rates was initiated using a Grass S-88 stimulator and stimulus isolation unit. The heart rate at which AV nodal Wenckebach cycles occurred was noted. Ventriculoatrial (VA) conduction was tested by pacing the ventricle from the site of the recorded right ventricular electrogram. The rate at which retrograde Wenckebach cycles occurred was noted in those dogs showing VA conduction. Arterial blood pressure was monitored continuously using a pressure transducer (Statham P24D) attached to a polyethylene cannula inserted into a femoral artery.

All ECG leads were recorded with standard filter settings of DC to 250 Hz while electrogram frequency limits ranged from 30-250 Hz. Recordings were made at paper speeds of 100 to 250 mm/sec with reading errors of 5 and 2.0 ms, respectively.

In order to obtain a detailed characterization of the AV junctional area from the right heart, a fingertip bipolar electrode (2 mm interelectrode distance) was inserted into the right atrium during inflow occlusion of the vena cavae and secured by a pursestring suture. The caval obstruction was removed in order to allow blood flow to resume. Any air trapped was released from the heart around the fingertip by transiently loosening the pursestring suture.

Figure 3 shows, in schematic fashion, the position of the fingertip electrode within the right heart and the characteristic electrograms recorded at three junctional sites (1, 2, and 3) at the proximal atrial, middle His bundle, and distal ventricular locations of the His bundle.

In order to induce various forms of AV block, 0.5 cc (average amount) of a 1% lidocaine solution was injected at the junction of the His bundle and basal ventricular septum (either at site 2 or site 3) (Fig. 3). Site 2 was the interface of the mid-His bundle and ventricular septum, whereas site 3 was the recorded junction of the His and right bundle branch.

Results

In the control state, right atrial pacing showed 1:1 conduction up to an average rate of 310 ± 43/min, whereas with right ventricular pacing, Wenckebach cycles occurred at an average rate of 223 ± 32/min. In nine dogs, no VA conduction was seen at any pacing rate above the sinus rate.

Injection of Lidocaine at the His–Right Bundle Injection

AV block was induced after lidocaine injection into the His bundle region and in 50% of cases (9 of 18) anomalous AV conduction was noted, i.e., 1:1 conduction with delta waves which initiated ventricular depolarization. Two forms of anomalous conduction were seen. In four dogs, delta waves were associated with left bundle branch block pattern during induced heart block. The injection site was the

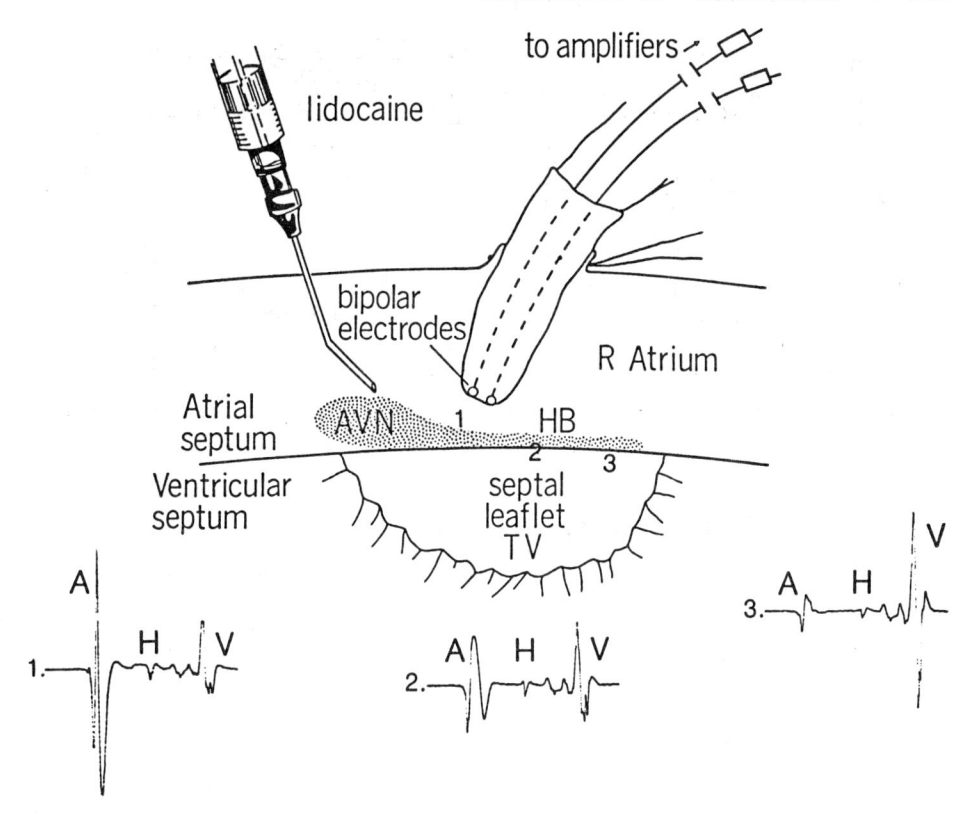

Figure 3: Diagram of the methodology for localized induction of AV block. During a brief interruption of venous inflow to the heart, a fingertip bipolar electrode was inserted through the anterior wall and secured by a pursestring suture. The three electrograms below correspond to the numbered positions at proximal, mid- and distal His bundle sites. In these studies, lidocaine injection from a tuberculin syringe was localized to sites 2 and 3. AVN = atrioventricular node; HB = His bundle; TV = tricuspid valve; R = right; A, V, N = His bundle electrogram consisting of atrial, His bundle, and ventricular deflections.

distal His bundle–right bundle junction. Figure 4 shows the development of complete heart block after the localized injection of lidocaine into the distal His bundle area (at site 3) (Fig. 3). Initially, a complete right bundle branch block pattern with a prolonged H-V interval was observed (H-V = 50 ms) (compare panel B with control panel A). The development of complete heart block ensued, which was localized distal to the His bundle deflection, (panel C). In this and one other case there was a slowing of the heart rate from control (A − A = 370 ms) to the onset of complete heart block (A − A = 630, panel B; A − A = 410, panel C). In the other cases, the heart rate stayed the same or increased slightly at the onset of complete heart block.

Within an average of 8–20 minutes (Fig. 5), conducted beats appeared during high degree heart AV block (panel A) since the P-R intervals were similar. Slowing of the heart rate with right vagosympathetic trunk stimulation confirmed the presence of conducted beats with constant P-R intervals and left bundle branch block patterns. Significantly, the ventricular depolarization was initiated by a

A. CONTROL

R-R=370 msec

L-2

V$_2$

H-V=30 msec

Hbeg

B. RBBB after lidocaine injection

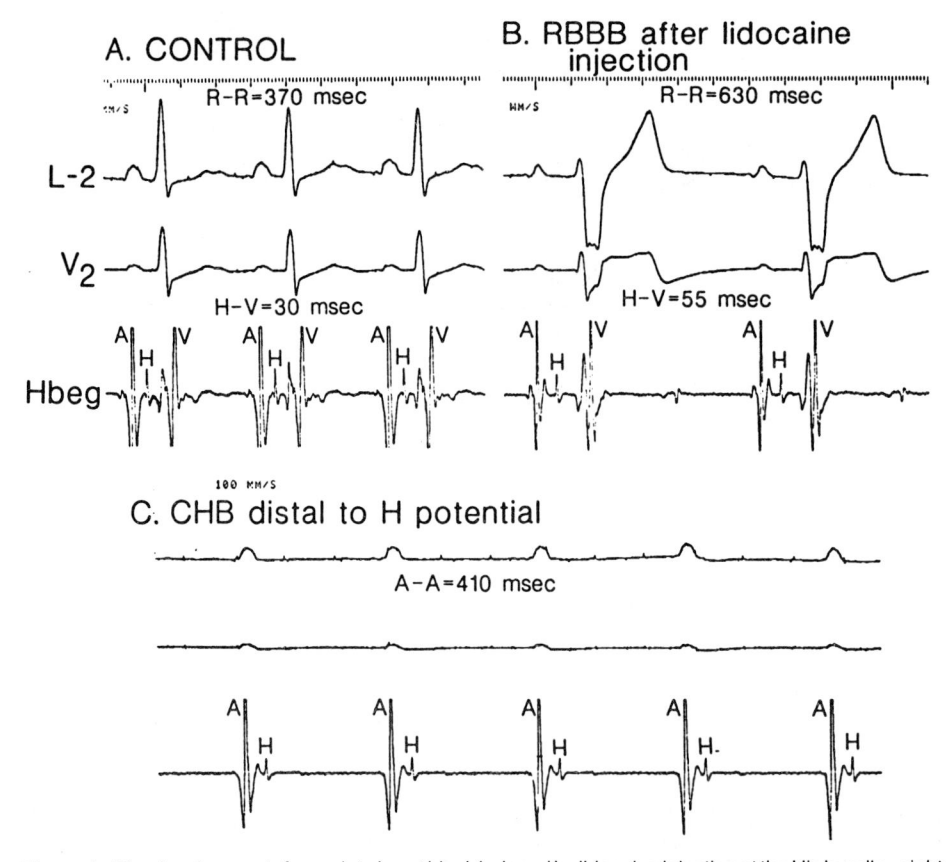

R-R=630 msec

H-V=55 msec

C. CHB distal to H potential

A-A=410 msec

Figure 4: The development of complete heart block induced by lidocaine injection at the His bundle – right bundle junction. Traces from above: ECG leads II (L-2) and V$_2$; His bundle electrogram (Hbeg). In the control state (panel A), the H-V interval measured 30 ms, within the normal range. Injection of lidocaine (panel B) 0.5 cc – 1% solution, caused slowing of the heart rate (A – A = 630 ms) and H-V prolongation to 50 ms with a complete right bundle branch block pattern. Within 2 minutes complete AV block distal to the recorded His bundle potential (panel C) was observed as the atrial rate accelerated, A – A = 410 ms.

delta wave. In leads II and aVR, left bundle branch block in the dog heart is commonly associated with prominent Q and R waves, respectively,[1,4] in contrast to these findings of an initial delta wave.

Injection of Lidocaine at the Mid-His bundle

Induction of complete heart block by localized injection of lidocaine at the mid-His bundle region provided a somewhat different form of QRS abnormality in five dogs. Figure 6 illustrates sinus rhythm after partial recovery of 1:1 AV conduction after induced complete AV block. The first beat has a normal QRS configuration in both leads II and aVR with a prolonged P-R interval. However, an analysis of the proximal and distal His bundle electrograms showed the marked AV delay to be due mostly to a tripartite His deflection (H, H', H'') indicative of

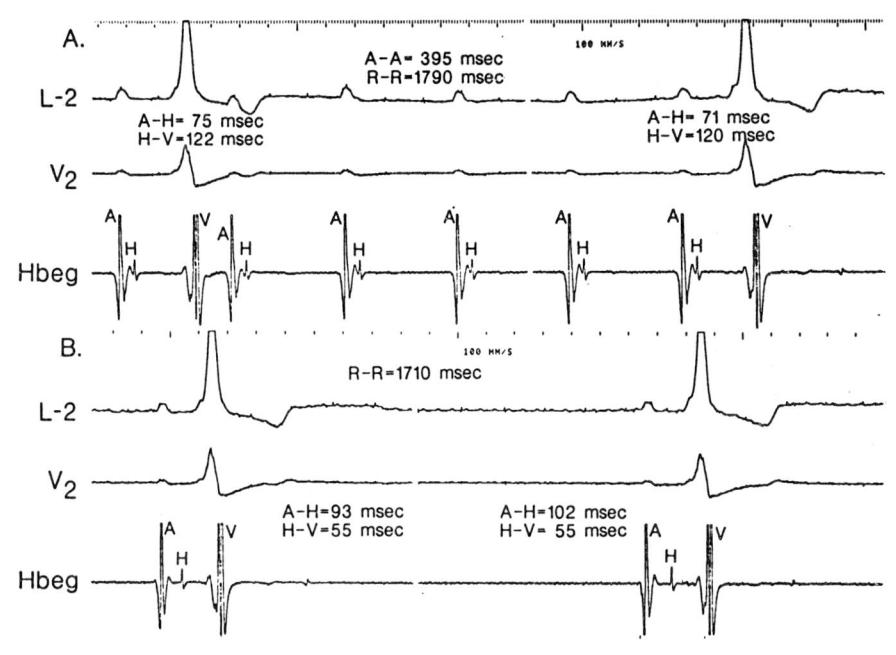

Figure 5: Demonstration of conducted beats with initial delta waves and prolonged ventricular activation time during high grade AV heart block. Panel A, 10–12 minutes after induction of complete AV block, apparent conducted beats, with delta waves and left bundle branch block patterns, were observed. Note similar A-H (75, 71 ms) and H-V intervals (122, 120 ms). Vagal-induced slowing of the heart rate (A − A = 1710 ms) allowed 1:1 AV conduction with the same delta wave and complete left bundle branch block pattern as in A. However, the A-H intervals prolonged (93, 102 ms) due to increased intensity of vagal stimulation whereas the H-V shortened (55 ms) probably due to reduction of repetitive concealed conduction as the atrial rate slowed.

intra-His bundle block. The last deflection, which is evident in the first beat, became partially obscured by the onset of the ventricular depolarization in the subsequent beats. Note that in the proximal His bundle recording, the terminal deflection associated with ventricular activity (so-called septal potential[9]) coincides with the S-wave or R^1 in the ECG leads, leads II and aVR, respectively.

From the second to the fifth beat, the initial left to right mid-septal vector, i.e., Q wave in lead II, is replaced by a prominent delta wave. There were concurrent changes in the proximal His bundle electrogram such that the terminal septal potential is reduced in amplitude. The duration of ventricular depolarization was slightly increased (as a result of the delta wave) from 50 to 70 ms. In addition, there was a concomitant reduction in the amplitude of the S and R' waves in leads II and aVR. The implications of these changes will be discussed below. Delta waves and a duration of ventricular depolarization within normal limits ≤ 75 ms were seen in five dogs in whom the lidocaine injection was made at site 2 (Fig. 3), mid-His bundle. On the other hand, delta waves and a left bundle branch block pattern (average duration of ventricular depolarization = 120 ms) were seen in four experiments. In each case, the injection site was the distal His−right bundle junction (site 3, Fig. 3).

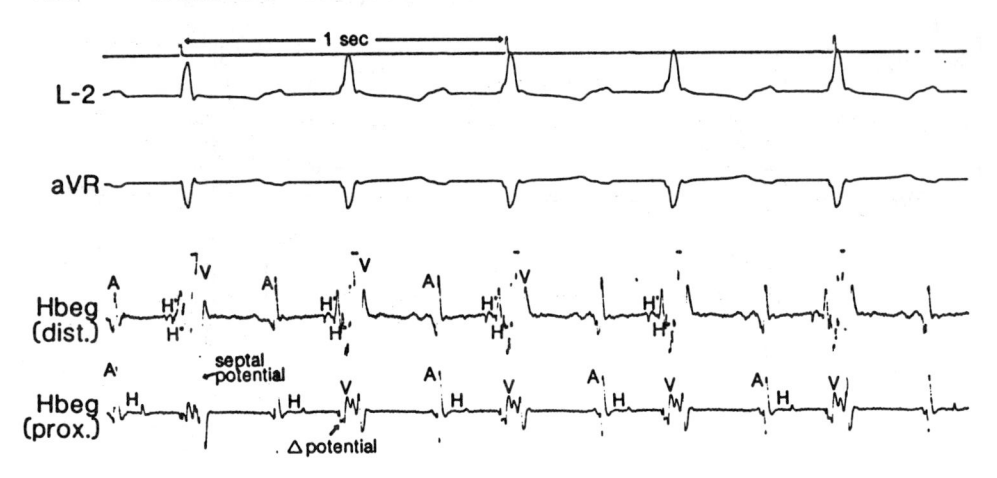

Figure 6: Delta wave formation with a normal duration of ventricular activation caused by mid-His bundle injection of lidocaine. The traces are the same for the ECG leads as in previous figures. Two His bundle electrograms are shown from the electrode catheter in the aorta (Hbeg, distal) and the fingertip electrode at the bottom (Hbeg, proximal). The first beat displays a normal QRS complex but the intra-His bundle block is evidence since there is a tripartite His potential (H, H', H'') with an intra-His delay of 107 ms (H-H'' interval). Note the septal potential in the proximal His bundle electrogram of the first beat. Its amplitude markedly diminished in the subsequent beats in which an initial delta wave was seen. Concomitantly, there appeared a distinct initial deflection in the proximal Hbeg recording (Δ potential) coincident with the delta wave (see text for discussion).

VA Conduction During Induced AV Block

Another aspect of anomalous or ectopic conduction was the observation of unexpected VA conduction that was manifest during lidocaine-induced AV block. Figure 7, panel A, shows a sinus beat with recordings of ECG leads II, aVR, His bundle electrograms from the aortic root (distal His potential, H') and the right heart (proximal His potential, H'), as well as electrograms from the right ventricular (RV) septum and the sinus node (SA) area in the right atrium. Right ventricular pacing (panel B) at 185 beats/minute in the control state, prior to induced AV block, allowed identification of the His potential during retrograde VA conduction. The H-A interval (taken from the proximal His bundle recording) was constant at 98 ms. Note the retrograde activation of the atrium, from the AV node-His bundle area to the sinus node region. The mid-His bundle injection of lidocaine caused a progressive intra-His bundle block, and within 1–2 minutes progressed to complete AV heart block localized distal to the H potential. Right ventricular pacing was used to maintain a normal heart rate.

Within 8–10 minutes, evidence of retrograde VA conduction began to appear although complete AV heart block persisted. In Figure 8, pacing from the same right ventricular site as in the control state (Fig. 7) and at a comparable rate (180 beats/min versus 185/min in the control state) induced VA conduction. The first three beats showed a pattern of low to high right atrial activation consonant with retrograde conduction. Note the progressive prolongation of the pacer impulse (PI)-atrial (A) interval (167, 172, 176 ms) prior to the occurrence of VA block, in the

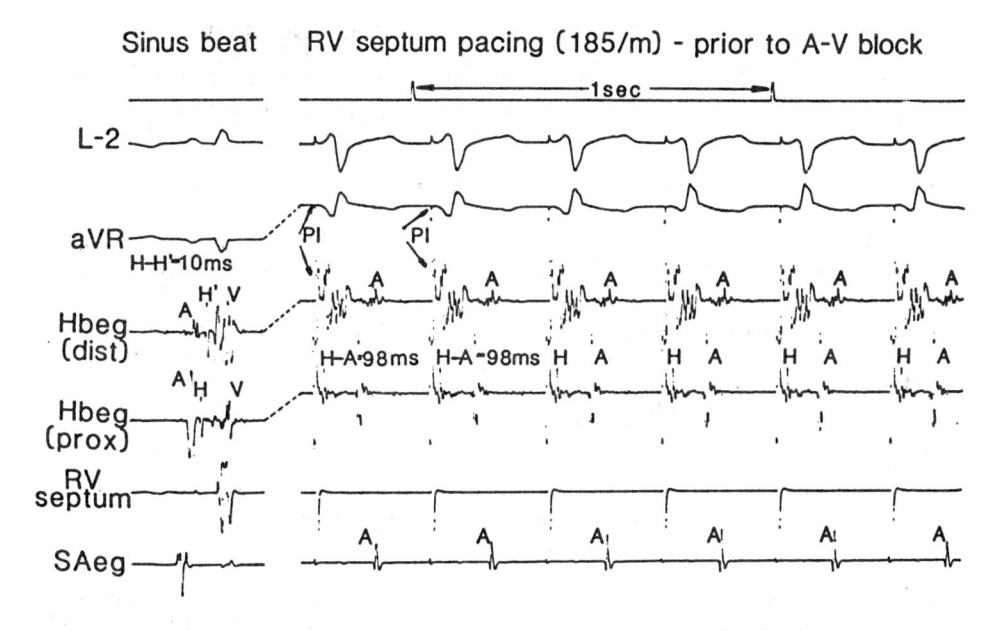

Figure 7: Example of retrograde (VA) conduction during ventricular pacing at 185 beats/min in the control state. Traces from above are: standard ECG lead II (L-2) and aVR; electrograms from the distal and proximal His bundle (Hbeg); right ventricular (RV) septum and sinus node area (SAeg). During the sinus beat (panel A), the intra-His bundle conduction time (H-H′) was 10 ms. During RV septum pacing at 185/min (panel B), the retrograde H-A interval measured 98 ms. Note the retrograde sequence of atrial activation with low atrial activation preceding high atrial recordings. PI = pacer impulse.

fourth beat. The identification of the retrograde His bundle potential (H) was partly determined by its absence during the blocked beat. The next three ventricular paced beats showed a regular but dissociated atrial and ventricular rhythm. The atrial activation sequence suggested a sinus node origin of the supraventricular complex. Each A wave was associated with a proximal H potential indicative of persistent complete AV block distal to recorded H potential. Since the H potential was captured by the sinus impulse, it was absent at the time it would be expected to appear (↓ arrow) during retrograde activation as seen in the first three beats in the tracing. Also note that the apparent retrograde AV nodal conduction time was 57 ms compared to an H-A interval of 98 ms during the control state at a comparable heart rate. Possible explanations of this parodoxical finding will be discussed below.

Another unusual observation during ventricular pacing was noted in two dogs in whom retrograde VA conduction could not be recorded after induced complete AV block. Figure 9, panel A, shows the response to pacing at the right ventricular apex at a rate (63/min), just faster than the sinus rate (61/min). No retrograde (VA) conduction was noted as the sinus impulse (SAeg) activated the low right atrial potential in the His bundle electrogram (Hbeg). Complete AV blockade was evident with the block localized distal to the recorded His bundle potential (H). However, pacing (60/min) from the fingertip bipolar electrode (interelectrode distance, 2 mm) placed on the basal right ventricular septum in the

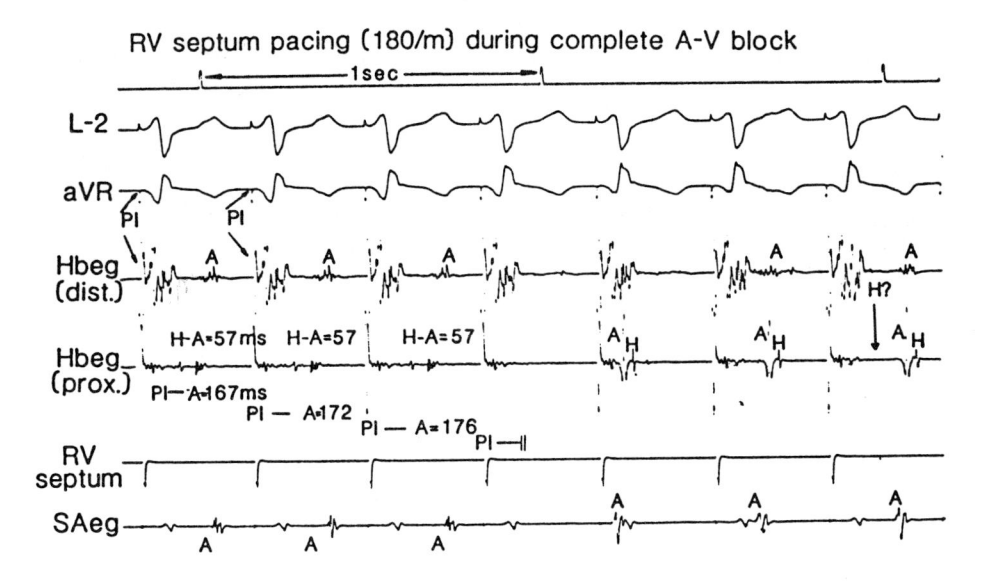

Figure 8: Resumption of VA conduction 10 minutes after the induction of complete AV block; however, the persistence of AV block is evident by the constant-coupled A-H interval each of which is *not* followed by QRS complexes. RV septum pacing at 180 beats/min (approximating the pacing rate in Figure 8, control state) induced retrograde VA conduction with a Wenckebach sequence. The pacer impulse (PI) to A interval progressively increased (167, 172, 176 ms) until retrograde VA block occurred in the fourth beat. Resumption of antegrade A-H conduction in the last three beats "usurped" the His potential so that it is absent during ventricular pacing (H?). Note that during successful VA conduction, the H-A interval is constant (H − A = 57 ms) yet is significantly shorter than the H-A interval measured during VA conduction in the control state (Fig. 8). Possible explanations of these findings are considered in the discussion section.

area of the lidocaine injection, resulted in 1:1 VA conduction with the low right atrium preceding the sinus node area electrogram (see Discussion section for interpretation of these findings).

Discussion

The purpose of the present study was to induce sever intra-His bundle block in an attempt to reproduce the conditions for delta wave formation. Previously, a single case of ischemically induced intra-His bundle block was associated with such an alteration of initial QRS vectors (Figs. 1, 2). We chose the method of localized lidocaine injection into the His bundle area because of extensive experience with this technique in producing varying degrees of AV block.[10-12] Admittedly, injection of lidocaine into conducting tissue raises questions regarding the concentration of the drug at the injection site and the damage of the needle insertion itself. Despite these misgivings, the results provided consistent patterns of anomalous conduction dependent on the site of injection (see below) as well as a 50% success rate in producing delta waves which was the original intention. The use of the fingertip bipolar electrode was particularly helpful in achieving these

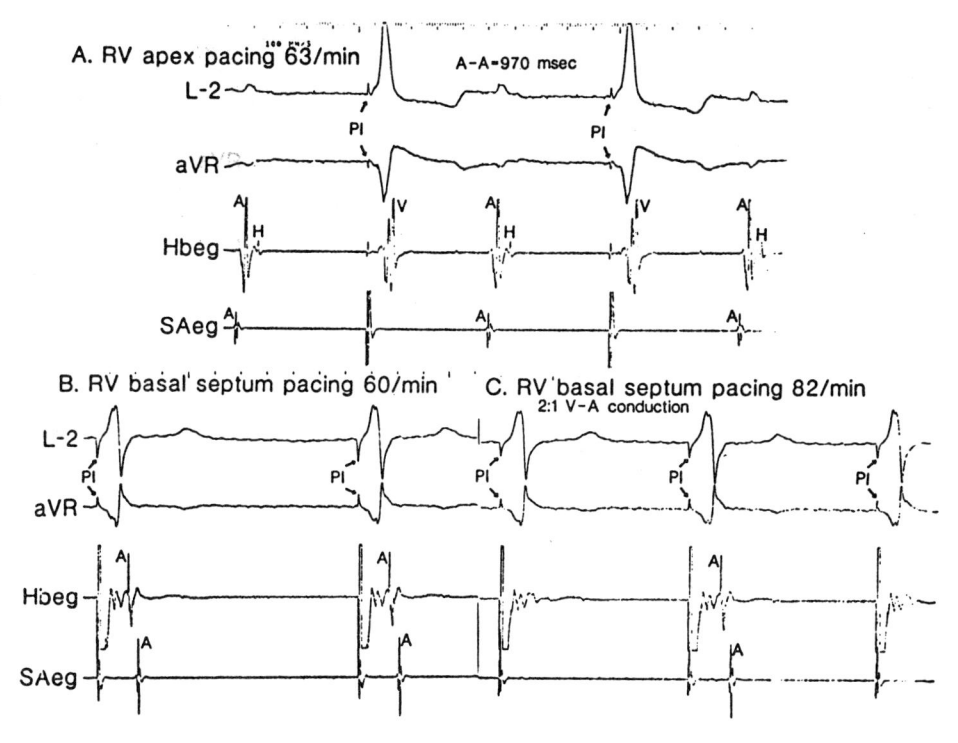

Figure 9: Site-dependent success of VA conduction during complete AV block induced by intra-His bundle injection of lidocaine. In panel A, pacing from the right ventricular apex at 63/min, slightly faster than the sinus rate, failed to induce VA conduction. Atrial activation from high to low occurred regularly (A − A = 970 ms) and complete AV block localized distal to the H potential is evident. Panel B, pacing from the right ventricular base in the area of the lidocaine injection at a rate of 60/min shows 1:1 VA conduction whereas pacing at 82/min from the same site (panel C) results in 2:1 VA conduction. PI = pacer impulse.

results. With it, the AV junction could be explored electrically and also palpation aided in localizing the sites for lidocaine injection.

Injection of Lidocaine at the His–Right Bundle Junction

Four of the nine dogs in whom delta waves were induced showed common features based on a site of lidocaine induced AV block at the His–right bundle junction. In each case, lidocaine injection was guided by the electrical recordings made with the fingertip electrode. Each of the four experiments showed a prolonged ventricular depolarization with a left bundle branch block pattern. Of interest, the conducted beats appeared only after several minutes (average 11 min) of complete AV block, but prior to the return of AV conduction due to dissipation of lidocaine's local anesthetic action. The anomalous conduction pattern was most convincingly detected during slowing of the heart rate with right vagal stimulation (Fig. 5B). The possibility that these beats (Fig. 5) were coincidental escape beats was unlikely because there were long strips in which the P-R intervals were relatively constant. Also, with greater intensity of vagal stimulation, true escape beats could be identified. The question arises regarding the activation sequence by which these conducted beats arose. The delta wave, itself, is indicative of an initial activation vector starting at the base of the heart directed toward the apex rather than the normal left to right vector that starts at the midventricular portion of the interventricular septum in the dog heart.[13] Since there was induced block distal to the recorded His bundle potential, it would appear that the impulse left the His bundle and directly entered the basal septum to produce the delta wave. We have coined the term "ectopic" conduction which is defined as a special form of anomalous conduction whereby the impulse prematurely or unexpectedly exits the conduction system.[14] Spread of the impulse relatively uniformly to the right and left sides of the heart mainly through regular myocardium would produce a wide ventricular depolarization with a diffuse intraventricular conduction pattern. Instead, a left bundle branch block pattern was seen (Fig. 5), indicating an early activation of the right heart and late activation of the left. Such a pattern suggests that the right bundle was entered early by the impulse after the inscription of the delta wave. One could postulate that the area of damage that caused the initial complete right bundle branch block (Fig. 4B) and then complete AV block also served as a bridge for the impulse to leave the His bundle and reenter the right bundle branch.

How could lidocaine accomplish both of these apparently contradicting actions? The initiation of AV block is readily understandable due to the strong local anesthetic action of lidocaine[15] which blocks conduction in excitable tissues. However, in high concentrations, lidocaine may induce a lypolytic action causing dissolution of cell membranes in adjacent tissues, e.g., His bundle or right bundle and nearby ventricular myocardial cells of the basal interventricular septum.

It has been reported that "healing over" of damaged cell membranes[16] and "reconnection" of contiguous cells are associated with construction of new gap junctions[16-18] which can occur in 3–20 minutes.[19] This timing is consonant with the appearance of conducted beats with delta waves 8–20 minutes after lidocaine-induced AV block. The electrical reconnection of cardiac cells with newly formed apposing gap junctions has been shown to have a higher resistance to current flow than normal cell to cell connections, i.e., intercalated discs.[18,20] Evidence of such high resistance connections induced between the right bundle branch and adjacent ventricular myocardium was found after lidocaine was injected at the bundle muscle interface using in vitro preparations.[14] In these previous studies, intracellular recordings at the site of induced Purkinje to muscle connection was characterized by a prominent foot potential which has been used as hallmark of slow conduction.[21] Indeed, it was this site that showed failure of conduction when stressed by high rates of pacing.[14]

Injection of Lidocaine at the Mid-His Bundle Site

In response to lidocaine injection at the mid-His bundle region, similarities and differences were noted compared to more distal injection, discussed above.

Delta wave formation was noted in five dogs in whom this site of injection was used. However, delta waves could not be discerned with certainty during the induced complete AV block. Only during the return of AV conduction were the delta waves readily and reproducible seen (Fig. 6). In each case there was an association with marked intra-His bundle block (49–110 ms). In all cases the fractionated His potential consisted of two fragments (one case) and three fragments (four cases) which was recorded during the delta-initiated ventricular depolarization. This association did not exclude the finding that normal QRS complexes, which occurred in runs or intermittently, also showed marked fractionation (Fig. 6, 1st beat). Still, when the marked intra-His delay returned to control, the delta wave was invariably replaced with normal initial forces in the ventricular depolarization.[14]

In the instances of delta wave induction with normal configuration and duration of ventricular depolarization (Fig. 6), one could postulate that the lidocaine injection caused very slow conduction through the His bundle to the rest of the heart normally and concurrently caused ectopic conduction, i.e., premature leak of the impulse, from the His bundle to the underlying ventricular septum, thus inducing the initial delta wave.

It is interesting to note that the normal activation of the crest of the septum in the proximal His bundle electrogram (Fig. 4, 1st beat septal potential) occurs coincident or just after the S wave in lead II.[9,10,22] With the appearance of the delta wave (2nd–5th beat), there is an abrupt decrease in the amplitude of the septal potential with the similarly abrupt appearance of an initial potential, coincident with the delta waves in the standard ECG leads. One could argue that the early activation of the crest of the septum by ectopic conduction was the cause of the early potential thereby diminishing the amplitude late septal potential. In support of this premise, the S wave in lead II and R' in lead aVR are also diminished in amplitude in the anomalously conducted beats.

VA Conduction During Induced AV Block

Since the focus of the injection site of lidocaine is the His bundle, damage to adjacent ventricular septum is to be expected due to the large area of the latter in regard to the almost microscopic area of former. Since the His bundle is also located within the atrial septum,[23] lidocaine damage to the His bundle–atrial interface would also be expected for the same reasons. If ectopic conduction and delta wave formation is the result of antegrade passage of the impulse from the His bundle to ventricular septum, it would seem reasonable to find conduction from the His bundle directly to the atrium during retrograde or VA conduction. In eight dogs (43%), retrograde conduction could be demonstrated during complete antegrade AV block (Fig. 8). The fact that the ventricular impulse was able to engage the His bundle during AV block could be construed as evidence for direct conduction from ventricle to His without initial use of the bundle branch system. Also in the case illustrated and in two other experiments retrograde H-A time was shorter during complete AV block than in the control state at comparable heart rates. Again, a possible explanation is the ectopic conduction of the impulse directly from the His bundle to the atrium. This type of bypass of the AV node would explain the shortened H-A time even at the same pacing rate. Other evidence implicating the possibility of ectopic conduction was the finding that four of nine dogs who showed no VA conduction prior to the AV block had retrograde conduction after lidocaine-induced AV block.

In two experiments, pacing from the right ventricular apex did not result in VA conduction (Fig. 9A) whereas pacing from the site of lidocaine injection at the base of the interventricular septum (through the fingertip) electrodes did induce 1:1 and 2:1 VA conduction. One might argue that retrograde conduction in site of stimulation was the damaged zone. Even if a bypass tract was utilized for VA conduction in this instance, why would lidocaine-induced damage enhance its conductivity? Moreover, anomalous conduction induced by lidocaine injection at the mid-right bundle–ventricular septum interface could not be explained by latent bypass fibers since these kinds of paraspecific fibers have not been described for the bundle branches.[24,25]

Clinical Implications

Damage to the crest of the interventricular septum in clinical circumstances can occur as the result of myocardial ischemia and infarction or sclero-degenerative disease. There are several reports in the clinical literature describing the appearance of pre-excitation during or soon after acute myocardial infarction.[26,27] Two clinical studies of patients with documented intra-His bundle block[29,30] have both recently reported loss of initial electrical forces in escape beats originating from the damaged His bundle. A careful perusal of these reports clearly shows delta waves in the standard leads similar to those which were induced in our dog experiment after localized lidocaine injections. Berman[29] and Mangiardi et al.[30] suggest that the explanation for these findings is "that impulses from the common bundle may bypass the fibers predestined to activation of the interventricular septum." It would appear from the animal experiments described in this and in other reports[14] that ectopic conduction may be another working hypothesis to explain the unusual clinical findings.

Acknowledgments: This research has been supported by a grant from the Veterans Administration. The authors thank LaVonna Blair for her excellent technical assistance and Pamela Tomey for her dedicated secretarial efforts in our behalf.

References

1. El-Sherif N, Scherlag BJ, Lazzara R, Samet P. Pathophysiology of tachycardia- and bradycardia-dependent block in the canine proximal His-Purkinje system after acute myocardial ischemia. Am J Cardiol 1974;33:529–540.
2. Scherlag BJ, El-Sherif N, Lazzara R. Experimental model for the study of Mobitz type II and paroxysmal A-V block. Am J Cardiol 1974;34:309–316.
3. El-Sherif N, Scherlag BJ, Lazzara R. Conduction disorders in the canine proximal His-Purkinje system following acute myocardial ischemia. I. The pathophysiology of intra-His bundle block. Circulation 1974;49:837–847.

4. El-Sherif N, Scherlag BJ, Lazzara R. Conduction disorders in the canine proximal His-Purkinje system following acute myocardial ischemia. II. The pathophysiology of bilateral bundle branch block. Circulation 1974;49:848–857.
5. El-Sherif N, Scherlag BJ, Lazzara R, Hope RR, Williams DO, Samet P. The pathophysiology of tachycardia-dependent paroxysmal A-V block after acute myocardial ischemia: Experimental and clinical observations. Circulation 1974;50:515–528.
6. Mendoza I, Scherlag BJ, El-Sherif N, Lazzara R, Hope R. Lesiones del haz de His: Correlacion clinica y experimental. Arch Inst Cardiol Mex 1980;50:131–140.
7. Lazzara R, Scherlag BJ, Robinson MJ, Samet P. Selective in situ parasympathetic control of the canine sinoatrial and atrioventricular nodes. Circ Res 1973;32:393–401.
8. Scherlag BJ, Abelleira JL, Samet P. Electrode catheter recordings from the His bundle and left bundle in the intact dog. In Kao FF, Koizumi K, Vassalle M, eds. Research in Physiology, Bologna, Aulo Gaggi, 1771;223–238.
9. El-Sherif N, Scherlag BJ, Lazzara R. Electrode catheter recordings during malignant ventricular arrhythmia following experimental acute myocardial ischemia: Evidence for reentry due to conduction delay and block in ischemic myocardium. Circulation 1975;51:1003–1014.
10. Scherlag BJ, Kosowsky BD, Damato AN. Technique for ventricular pacing from the His bundle of the intact heart. J Appl Physiol 1967;22:584–587.
11. Kosowsky DB, Scherlag BJ, Damato AN. A reevaluation of the atrial contribution to ventricular function: A study using His bundle pacing. Am J Cardiol 1968;21:518–524.
12. Scherlag BJ, Abelliera JL, Narula OS, Samet P. The differential effects of ouabain on sinus, A-V nodal, His bundle and idioventricular rhythms. Am Heart J 1971;81:227–235.
13. Amer NS, Stuckey JH, Hoffman BF, Cappelletti RR, Domingo RT. Activation of the interventricular septal myocardium studied during cardiopulmonary bypass. Am Heart J 1960;70:381–389.
14. Scherlag BJ. Evidence for ectopic conduction in vivo and in vitro. In Barley JJ, ed. Proceedings of the 1986 Engineering Foundation Conference. Computerized Interpretation of the Electrocardiogram XI. New York, 1986;155.
15. Moss AJ, Patton RD. Antiarrhythmic Agents. CC Thomas, Springfield, IL, Chapter 6.
16. DeMelto WC. The healing-over process in cardiac and other muscle fibers. In DeMello WC, ed. Electrical Phenomena in the Heart. New York, Academic Press, 1972; 323–351.
17. Lowenstein WR. Cellular communication by permeable membrane junctions. In Weismann G, Claiborne R, eds. Cell Membranes: Biochemistry, Cell Biology and Pathology. New York, HP Publishing Company, 1975, Chapter 11.
18. Scherlag BJ, Abelleira JL, Samet P. Electrode catheter recordings from the His bundle and left bundle in the intact dog. In Kao FF, Koizumi K, Vassalle M, eds. Research in Physiology. Bologna, Aulo Gaggi, 1971;223–238.
18a. de Mello WC. Intercellular communication in cardiac muscle: Physiological and pathophysiological implications. In Zipes DP, Jalife J, eds. Cardiac Electrophysiology and Arrhythmias. New York, Grune and Stratton, 1985, Chapter 8.
19. de Mello WC, Motto GE, Chopeau M. A study on the healing-over of myocardial cells of toads. Circ Res 1969;24:475–487.
20. Page E, Manjunath CK. Communicating junctions between cardiac cells. In Fazzard HA, ed. Heart and Cardiovascular System, New York, Raven Press, 1986, Chapter 29.
21. Hoffman, BF, Cranefield PF. Electrophysiology of the Heart. New York, McGraw-Hill, 1960, Chapter 5.
22. Hoffman BF, Cranefield PF, Stuckey, Bagdonas AA. Electrical activity during the P-R interval. Circ Res 1960;8:1200–1211.
23. James TN. Morphology of the human A-V node with remarks pertinent to its electrophysiology. Am Heart J 1961;62:756–771.
24. Baird JA, Robb JS. Study, reconstruction, and gross dissection of the atrioventricular conducting system of the dog heart. Anta Rec 1950;108:747–763.
25. James TW, Sherf L, Urthather F. Fine structure of the bundle-branches. Br Heart J 1974;36:1–18.

26. Fabre H. Wolff-Parkinson-White syndrome after infarct: Stability during 15 years; disappearance 2 years ago. Arch Mal Colm 1970;63:301.
27. Mathew G, Raferty E. Accelerated atioventricular conduction after myocardial infarction: A study using His bundle electrograms. Br Heart J 1973;35:985.
28. Goel BG, Han J. Manifestations of the WPW syndrome after myocardial infarction. Am Heart J 1974;87:633.
29. Berman ND. The surface electrocardiogram in complete intra-His heart block. J Electrocardiol 1978;11:151–158.
30. Mangiardi L, Ronzani G, Goita F, Presbitero P, Conte MR, Diheo M, Commodo E, Brusca A. Clinical and elctrocardiographic features and long-term results of electrical therapy in patients with isolated His bundle disease. Am Heart J 1986;112:1183–1191.

48

Manipulation of the Autonomic Nervous System in the Prevention of Sudden Cardiac Death

Peter J. Schwartz

Introduction

A causal relationship between changes in the activity of the autonomic nervous system and sudden cardiac death has been clearly demonstrated and is by now generally accepted.[1-6]

An increase in sympathetic activity can trigger life-threatening arrhythmias even in some individuals with a normal heart;[3,7] however, this chapter will focus on the condition in which the autonomic nervous system plays more frequently a critical arrhythmogenic role, i.e., in ischemic heart disease.

Numerous experimental studies have suggested that a significant degree of protection from sudden cardiac death can be achieved by specific manipulations of the autonomic nervous system. Specifically, ablation of left-sided sympathetic nerves, daily exercise, and vagal stimulation will be briefly discussed here. It is worth noting that all these operations modify the autonomic balance in the same direction, i.e., toward a relative decrease in the sympathetic and a relative increase in the vagal outflow to the heart.

These interventions reflect recent developments in the understanding of the complex relationship existing between acute myocardial ischemia, the autonomic nervous system, and malignant arrhythmias. As they have largely originated from the extensive studies in a specific animal model for sudden death,[8] this will be described first.

From: Brugada P, Wellens HJJ. CARDIAC ARRHYTHMIAS: Where To Go From Here? Mount Kisco, NY, Futura Publishing Company, Inc., © 1987.

An Animal Model for Sudden Death

As discussed elsewhere,[9] there is growing evidence[10-13] suggesting that ventricular fibrillation is often triggered by a transient ischemic episode usually associated with signs of sympathetic hyperactivity and more likely to occur in patients with a healed myocardial infarction (MI). These considerations have guided the design of the experimental protocol.[8]

Dogs are instrumented for the recording of hemodynamic variables, including left ventricular pressure and coronary flow, and a balloon occluder is positioned around the circumflex coronary artery. The left anterior descending coronary artery is ligated, below the origin of the first diagonal branch, in order to produce a myocardial infarction that usually involves approximately 20% of the left ventricular mass.

One month after the production of an anterior myocardial infarction, dogs engage in an exercise stress test on a motor-driven treadmill. At the beginning of the last minute of exercise, a balloon occluder, previously positioned around the circumflex coronary artery, is inflated for 2 minutes to produce acute myocardial ischemia. This short-lasting ischemic episode affects the last minute of exercise and the first minute after exercise. This sequence of events allows separation between arrhythmias dependent on cessation of exercise or on release of occlusion. This model shows what may happen to a patient with a prior myocardial infarction who engages in exercise and has a brief reduction in coronary flow, leading to acute myocardial ischemia, cardiac pain, and arrest of exercise. It is important to note that such a brief coronary occlusion does not induce ventricular arrhythmias at rest, whereas when it is coupled with exercise, it frequently elicits malignant arrhythmias that are particularly frequent within seconds from cessation of exercise. Figure 1 shows a typical example of the event occurring with this protocol.

The incidence of ventricular fibrillation is well defined, given the large number of dogs studied so far. Indeed, as 90 dogs out of 151 developed ventricular fibrillation during the exercise plus ischemia test, this incidence is 60%. A most important characteristic of this model is the reproducibility of the outcome during the test; i.e., if a dog develops ventricular fibrillation (these animals are defined as "susceptible" to sudden death), the same event will repeat itself for several months whenever the exercise and ischemia test are repeated. The same applies to those dogs that survive the test (these animals are defined as "resistant" to sudden death). Reproducibility is important because it allows internal control analysis of the efficacy, or lack of it, of a variety of potentially protective interventions. These animals perform the exercise plus ischemia test having steel paddles strapped to their chest and connected to a defibrillator so that, if ventricular fibrillation occurs, they can be defibrillated within seconds and studied again over time. The lethal arrhythmias in this model depend on the interaction between the following five variables: acute myocardial ischemia, sympathetic and vagal reflexes, level of heart rate, exercise, and its cessation.

A significant insight came from the analysis of the heart rate response to ischemia during exercise. This was stimulated by the unexpected observation that

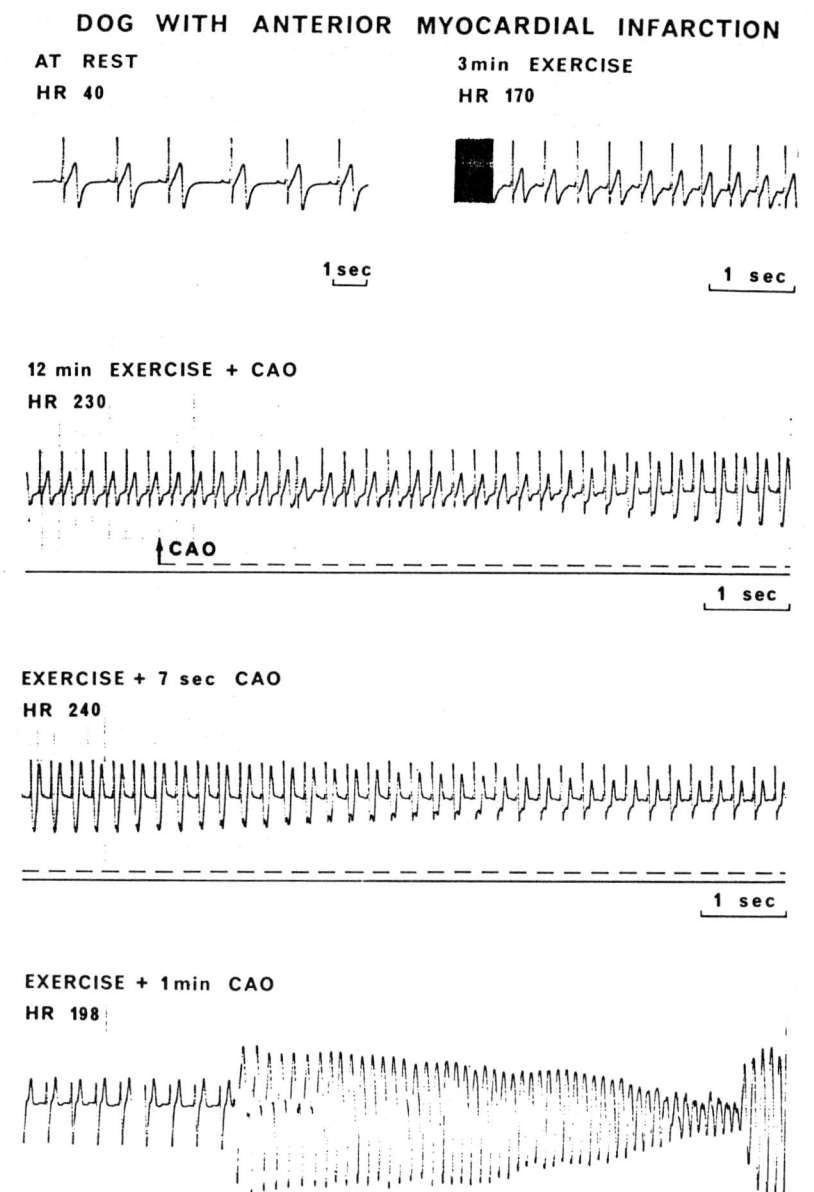

Figure 1: Example of the most frequent sequence of events during the exercise plus ischemia test. This dog had at rest an unusually low heart rate (HR) which increased rapidly with exercise. After 12 min of exercise the heart rate was already 230 beats/min and coronary arterial occlusion (CAO) was produced. Within a few seconds, major ischemic changes appeared but were short-lived, as indicated by the two continuous strips. Exercise ended after 1 min of occlusion, and within 1 sec, ventricular flutter appeared and rapidly deteriorated into VF. Coronary arterial occlusion was immediately released, without benefit. (From ref. 8.)

most "resistant" dogs had a decrease in heart rate during the first minute of coronary occlusion, despite continuation of exercise. As illustrated in Figure 2, this decrease in heart rate was quite marked (up to 60–70 beats/min in some cases) and indicated that very powerful vagal reflexes were operant. By contrast, all susceptible dogs had a marked increase in heart rate, often at the beginning of the coronary occlusion. Among the resistant dogs, those without myocardial infarction had more pronounced heart rate decreases, as if the presence of myocardial infarction had interfered with these reflexes.

The presence of powerful vagal reflexes in the resistant animals raised the question of the possibility of identifying in advance which animals would survive the exercise plus ischemia test. Despite the large body of evidence that indicates that the autonomic nervous system plays a critical role in triggering ventricular fibrillation, there has been no attempt to use autonomic reflexes to discriminate between postmyocardial infarction patients at high and low risk for sudden death.[9] Changes in the heart rate mediated by the baroreceptor reflex can provide a meaningful and feasible way to assess the autonomic neural control of the heart.

Clinical studies had suggested that the baroreflex function may be altered after a myocardial infarction.[14,15] We examined whether there is a relationship between the autonomic reflex control of the heart and the susceptibility to sudden death that would identify subgroups at higher risk.

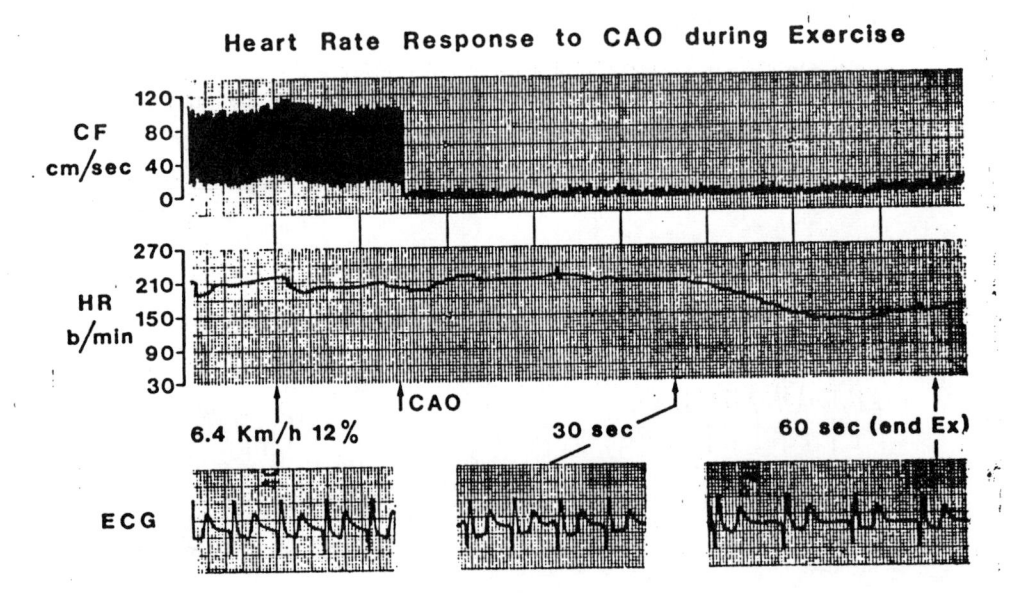

Figure 2: The three panels show the circumflex coronary flow velocity, heart rate, and ECG during the occlusion of the circumflex artery performed during exercise in a dog with a 1-month-old anterior myocardial infarction. The occlusion was initiated after 15 minutes of exercise when the speed reached was 6.4 km/h, and the inclination of the treadmill was 12%. The figure shows, without interruptions, the first minute of occlusion and the moment of cessation of exercise (occlusion is always maintained for an additional minute). For the first 30 seconds, heart rate oscillated around 210 beats/min, and then strikingly decreased to 130 beats/min while the animal continued to run. When the treadmill stopped (end Ex) and occlusion continued, there were no arrhythmias. (From ref. 9.)

One month after an anterior myocardial infarction, the baroreceptor reflex control of the heart rate was assessed by the method of Smyth and colleagues.[16] Phenylephrine, 10 μg/Kg, was used to raise systolic arterial pressure by 30–50 mmHg. Each RR interval was plotted as a function of the preceding systolic pressure. A least-squares-fit linear regression was performed, and the reflex control of the heart rate was expressed as the slope of the linear regression line (an index of the baroreceptor reflex sensitivity). A greater steepness of the slopes reflects mostly the efficiency of the vagal reflexes (Fig. 3). A flatter baroreflex slope indicates a combination of weak vagal reflexes and of strong sympathetic activity; it may also reflect in part an impaired left ventricular function.

The baroreflex slope was determined in dogs with and without an anterior myocardial infarction. Those with myocardial infarction were divided into two groups according to their response to the exercise plus ischemia test.[17] It was evident that the normal dogs had a much steeper baroreflex slope. Twelve dogs were studied in control conditions and 17 were studied 4 weeks after a myocardial infarction (11 were susceptible and six were resistant). The baroreflex slope was significantly greater in control dogs compared to the infarcted dogs (26.1 ± 15.4 vs 9.2 ± 8.4 ms/mmHg) and, more importantly, in resistant compared to susceptible dogs (17.9 ± 8.6 vs 4.4 ± 2.3 ms/mmHg) (Fig. 4).

The relationship between depressed baroreflex sensitivity and increased

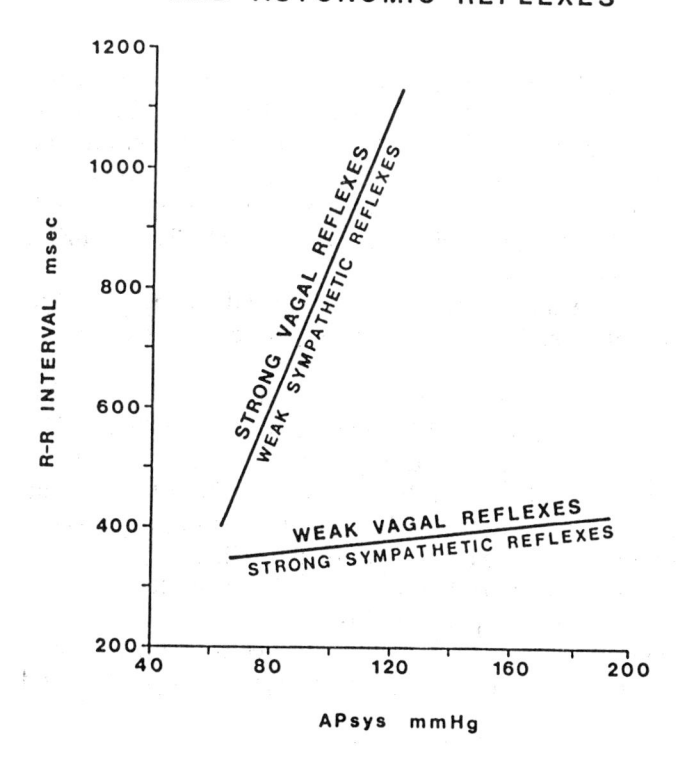

Figure 3: An example of the relationship between R-R interval or heart rate and arterial blood pressure is shown. The upper curve would represent a response primarily characterized by an increase in efferent vagus nerve activity to the SA node. Lower curve would be the opposite. Sympathetic neural activity may be altered in an opposite direction to vagus nerve activity but does not contribute greatly to heart rate control under these conditions. (From ref. 9.)

Response to Phenylephrine 10μg/Kg

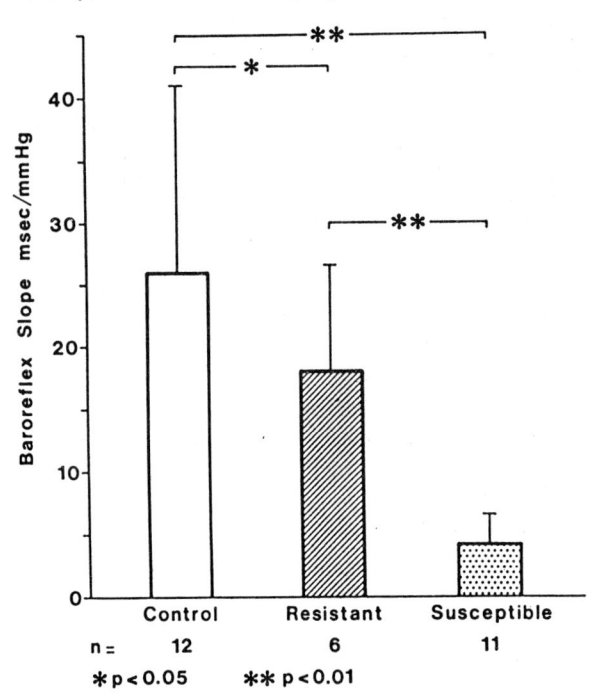

Figure 4: Baroreflex sensitivity of 12 control, 11 resistant, and 11 susceptible dogs. The control animals are without myocardial infarction, the resistant and susceptible ones are tested 4 weeks after the production of an anterior myocardial infarction. All the differences noted are statistically significant. (From ref. 9.)

susceptibility to ventricular fibrillation in this model has been confirmed by the extension of our ongoing study. So far, 151 dogs with a 1-month-old anterior myocardial infarction and with data on baroreflex sensitivity underwent the exercise plus ischemia test. As shown in Figure 5, where the dashed area is an arbitrary gray zone, for a post-MI dog which has a baroreflex slope below 9 ms/mmHg, there is a 95% probability of developing ventricular fibrillation during the exercise plus ischemia test.

These results have, of course, suggested the possibility of their application to post-myocardial infarction patients. Accordingly, two separate prospective studies have been initiated.

The first study compares the baroreflex sensitivity of healthy controls and post-MI patients at 15 days, 3 months, and 12 months after infarction.[18] The baroreflex sensitivity is significantly decreased in patients 15 days after MI and tends to increase over time so that by 3 months post MI, it is back to the same values present in the normal population. It must be noted that baroreflex sensitivity does not change over time among the control population. These data strongly suggest that, at least in some individuals, baroreflex sensitivity is altered after a MI; however, because of the group comparison, this could remain an unproven assumption. The actual demonstration of this phenomenon comes from an experimental study in which baroreflex sensitivity was measured in 34 dogs before and

BAROREFLEX SENSITIVITY AND SUDDEN DEATH

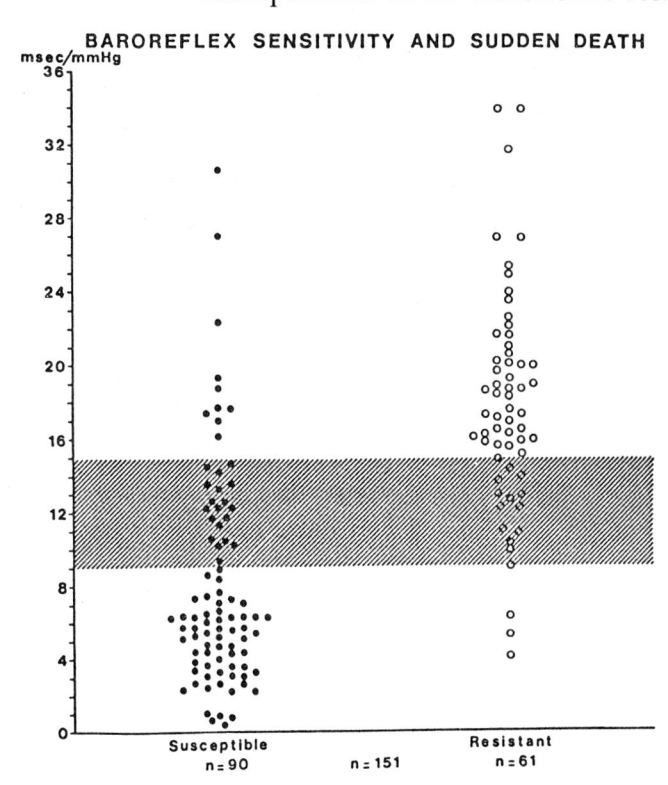

Figure 5: Baroreflex sensitivity in 151 post-infarction dogs and its relationship to susceptibility to sudden death. The darkened area is an arbitrary grey zone. Below the limit of 9 ms/mmHg, 95% of the dogs are susceptible to sudden death, whereas above 15 ms/mmHg, the great majority proves to be resistant to sudden death during the exercise plus ischemia test.

after MI:[19] baroreflex sensitivity was clearly decreased 4 weeks post-myocardial infarction in 79% of these animals. This represents the evidence that indeed baroreflex sensitivity is reduced after MI in the majority of individuals, in comparison to the initial values.

The second study has involved, so far, the evaluation of baroreflex sensitivity in 64 patients[20] with a first MI who also underwent thorough hemodynamic evaluation. This ongoing prospective study already yielded promising information. Indeed, the analysis of these preliminary data shows that the baroreflex sensitivity of the four deceased patients is markedly lower than that of the survivors (3.2 ± 2.2 vs 9.4 ± 4.5 ms/mmHg, $p < 0.01$). Moreover, among the patients with depressed baroreflex sensitivity (> 1 SD below the mean) mortality was 43% (3 out of 7) compared to 1.7% (1 out of 57) among the other patients. A depressed baroreflex sensitivity suggests the presence of a derangement in the autonomic balance due to a reduced vagal activity, probably combined with increased sympathetic activity. This clinical study supports the growing concept that reduced vagal efferent activity may favor cardiac electrical instability.

Taken together, these ongoing studies suggest that the quantitative analysis of autonomic reflexes may contribute to the identification of high risk subgroups of post-MI patients.

Left Stellectomy

The rationale for the clinical use of left cardiac sympathetic denervation has been repeatedly discussed in detail.[21,22] Here, only a brief overview of the experimental data will be made to be followed by the results of this intervention in patients with ischemic heart disease.

The Arrhythmogenic Role of Left Sympathetic Nerves

The different effects of right and left cardiac sympathetic nerves and the importance of sympathetic imbalance in the genesis of cardiac arrhythmias have been recently reviewed in detail.[23] Whereas right-sided sympathetic stimulation induces only sinus tachycardia, stimulation of cardiac nerves that originate from the left stellate ganglion produces a variety of rhythm disorders. Most of these arrhythmias are supraventricular.[24-26] Even if infrequently, however, stimulation of the left stellate ganglion may initiate major arrhythmias such as ventricular tachycardia, even in an intact heart.[27]

Not surprisingly, this arrhythmogenic potential of left-sided sympathetic stimulation becomes much more evident in a myocardium already electrically unstable because of a recent myocardial infarction or an acute myocardial ischemia both in experimental animals as well as in humans.[5,27,28]

Figure 6 shows ventricular premature beats, including a couplet, elicited by touching with a blunt instrument the left stellate ganglion of a patient who suffered an anterior wall myocardial infarction 50 days earlier. This observation was made just prior to performing a high thoracic left sympathectomy. In the experimental laboratory, this phenomenon can be more quantitatively and reproducibly demonstrated. Indeed, these notions have contributed to the development of an experimental animal model in which left-threatening arrhythmias are reproducibly induced by the combination of acute myocardial ischemia and sympathetic hyperactivity, the latter being produced through electrical stimulation of the left stellate ganglion.[29] This model has already proved to be quite useful for testing and comparing different antiarrhythmic drugs.[30,31]

Thus, after removal of the left stellate ganglion, a decreased incidence of cardiac arrhythmias may be expected.

Left Stellectomy and Ventricular Vulnerability

The antiarrhythmic and, more important, the antifibrillatory effect of left stellectomy has been demonstrated in a variety of experimental conditions. This effect becomes more complete with chronic denervation, partly because of the massive neural activation at the moment of surgical section. Indeed, with pharmacological blockade or blockade by cold, the antiarrhythmic effect becomes immediately evident.

Left stellate ganglion blockade by cold was found capable of preventing ventricular tachyarrhythmias elicited by short-lasting coronary artery occlu-

A.B. 50 YEARS - DURING ANESTHESIA

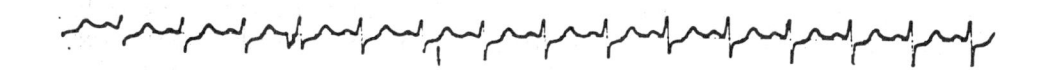

LEFT STELLATE GANGLION STIMULATION

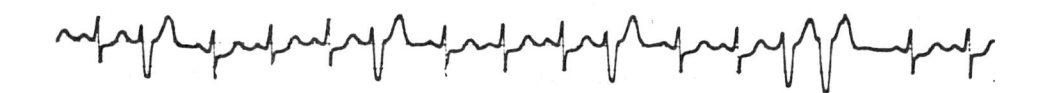

|1 sec|

Figure 6: Electrocardiographic tracing in an anesthetized man 50 days after occurrence of an anterior myocardial infarction complicated by ventricular fibrillation. The patient was in sinus rhythm until the left stellate ganglion was mechanically stimulated, leading to frequent premature ventricular beats and couplets. (From ref. 5.)

sions.[27] Left stellectomy modifies two electrophysiological parameters relevant to arrhythmogenesis: ventricular refractoriness and ventricular fibrillation threshold. Left stellectomy shifted the strength-interval curve, used as an index of ventricular excitability, later in diastole; thus, this lengthening of ventricular refractoriness reflects a decreased excitability.[32] The ventricular fibrillation threshold is increased, by either left stellectomy or cold blockade of the ganglion, by 73% when compared to control conditions indicating a significant decrease in the propensity to ventricular fibrillation.[33] This finding, obtained in 1975, was important in raising the possibility that left stellectomy be considered as one of the ways to reduce, in high risk patients, the likelihood of an episode of ventricular fibrillation.

The antifibrillatory effect of left stellectomy has also been observed in unanesthetized animals. It was first reported that among 32 dogs with a prior anterior myocardial infarction exposed to a 10-minute occlusion of the circumflex coronary artery, the incidence of ventricular fibrillation was reduced from 65% to 33% in the left stellectomized animals compared to the control group.[34] Later on it was found in the animal model for sudden death described above[8] that while the incidence of ventricular fibrillation was 60% among 151 control dogs, it was reduced to zero in 14 dogs which underwent left stellectomy.

A significant aspect of the antifibrillatory action of left stellectomy is that it is not accompanied by negative effects on left ventricular function. Using left ventricular dP/dt max as a reliable index of ventricular contractility, we found that left stellectomy did not affect cardiac performance either at rest or during a submaximal exercise stress test.[35] Even more important, for its clinical implications, was the subsequent finding of a similar lack of negative inotropic action in dogs with a 1-month-old myocardial infarction,[36] both at rest and during exercise. In the same animals, the beta-adrenergic blocking agent, propranolol, while leaving unmodified contractility at rest, severely reduced its increase during exercise. The lack of detrimental effects of left stellectomy is explained by the compensatory action of the right stellate ganglion:[23] a significant advantage of a selective denervation which has profound electrophysiologic effects without entirely depriving the myocardium of the necessary adrenergic support.

Left Stellectomy and Coronary Flow

The relationship between the autonomic nervous system and coronary circulation has been recently reviewed by Feigl[37] who in 1967 had shown that electrical stimulation of the left stellate ganglion could induce coronary vasoconstriction in anesthetized dogs pretreated with beta-blockers.[38]

Despite the great importance of these findings, the significance of the neural mechanisms in physiologic conditions in the unanesthetized state remained elusive.

Myocardial reactive hyperemia is an index of the capability of the coronary bed to dilate, which can be evaluated in chronically instrumented dogs to allow the investigation of the mechanisms of neural control in the conscious state. In this way, we found the left stellectomy greatly increases myocardial reactive hyperemia and that alpha-adrenergic blockade produces qualitatively similar results.[39] It is noteworthy that in the same experiments, right stellectomy had no effect on myocardial reactive hyperemia. This represented the first evidence of a dominant alpha-mediated vasoconstrictor tone present in conscious animals. Subsequently, we have demonstrated that left stellectomy increases coronary flow even when metabolic demands are increased physiologically by exercise.[35] In other words, neural activity can limit coronary flow even during exercise, thus constituting a reserve mechanism.

Does the presence of the left stellate ganglion also affect the degree and the extent of ischemia induced by a coronary artery occlusion? An affirmative answer comes from a study with Janse.[40] In anesthetized dogs, brief coronary occlusions were performed in control conditions and with various autonomic interventions including left stellectomy while recording direct current extracellular electrograms simultaneously from 60 left ventricular epicardial sites. In 10 out of 13 cases, left stellectomy resulted in a reduction of the degree of depression of the QT segment, and thus resulted in a reduction of the ischemia induced by the occlusion of the vessel in the same animal (Fig. 7).

Thus, the absence of the left stellate ganglion reduces the severity of ischemia and the extent of the area affected in the ischemic process or, at least, delays the occurrence of these changes. This may be of particular clinical relevance in the case of transient ischemic episodes.

These findings raised the question of whether coronary artery occlusion in a left stellectomized animal would result in a somewhat smaller infarct area. Ac-

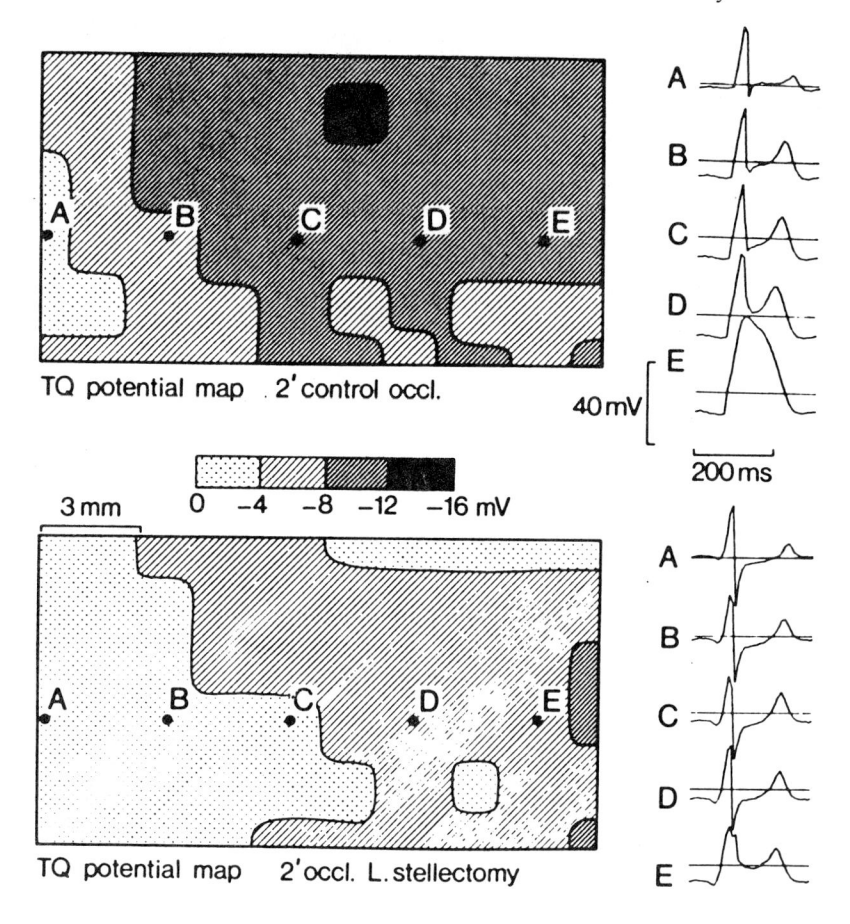

Figure 7: Selected direct-current electrograms recorded 2 min after coronary occlusion from sites A to E. On the left, the area from which 60 electrograms were simultaneously recorded is indicated and isopotentials during the QT segment are shown. The upper panel depicts the situation during the control occlusion and the lower panel shows the situation 2 min after a subsequent occlusion was made when the left stellate ganglion had been removed. Note that the degree of the ischemic changes is less marked after stellectomy. (From ref. 40.)

cordingly, we have evaluated the effect of left stellectomy on the infarct size produced by an 8-hour occlusion of the left descending coronary artery, at its origin, in anesthetized cats.[41] The infarct size was measured directly using the nitro-blue tetrazolium staining technique. In 20 cats compared to 20 controls, left stellectomy significantly reduced the infarcted area by approximately 25% of the total heart weight. As we have used the total heart weight, the salvage of ventricular myocardium is significant also from a biologic point of view and will affect, in all likelihood, long-term ventricular function.

Through alpha-adrenergic mechanisms, left-sided cardiac sympathetic nerves exert a significant role in the control of the coronary circulation. Under pathologic conditions, such as coronary artery stenosis or occlusion, these effects may acquire further importance and determine the extent of myocardium that will undergo irreversible damage, probably by regulating perfusion through collateral vessels. In terms of ischemia-induced arrhythmias, left stellectomy may play a very significant role, when the ischemic episodes are transient and not prolonged, by preventing the development of ischemic changes of such a magnitude that would trigger malignant arrhythmias.

Summary of Experimental Data

Left stellectomy has both antiarrhythmic and antifibrillatory effects, improves the capability of the coronary bed to dilate and reduces both the degree and the extent of myocardial ischemia, and does not interfere with left ventricular function at rest and during exercise even in animals with a prior myocardial infarction. All together, these data make logical the evaluation of the left stellectomy as a potential way to reduce the incidence of sudden cardiac death in high risk subgroups of post-myocardial infarction patients.

Left Stellectomy in Post-MI Patients

A nontraditional intervention such as left stellectomy (high thoracic left sympathectomy in humans) could be performed only in a group of patients at very high risk for sudden cardiac death. One such group was identified by a specifically designed epidemiologic study.[42]

After identification of 70 patients with an anterior myocardial infarction and 55 patients with an inferior myocardial infarction, all complicated in the acute phase by ventricular fibrillation and discharged alive, 125 additional patients who had a myocardial infarction uncomplicated by ventricular fibrillation were selected (control subjects). Cases and controls were matched for the following variables: sex (all males), age (same ± 2 years), coronary care unit (same), epoch of myocardial infarction (same ± 3 months), site of myocardial infarction (same). Left ventricular dysfunction and prior myocardial infarction were present in only a few patients. Patients receiving either acute or long-term treatment with beta-adrenergic blocking agents were not included. The average follow-up was 59 months. The cumulative mortality during the first 5 years for the patients with inferior myocardial infarction without ventricular fibrillation (6%, 11%, 13%, 13%, and 13%) was modest and significantly different from that of inferior myocardial infarction complicated by ventricular fibrillation (6%, 11%, 20%, 20%, and 25%). In contrast, a striking difference (Fig. 8) appeared when the cumulative mortality of patients with anterior myocardial infarction without ventricular fibrillation (9%, 13%, 17%, 27%, and 27%) was compared with that of patients with anterior myocardial infarction complicated by ventricular fibrillation (32%, 40%, 46%, 49%, and 54%) ($p < 0.005$). This group also had a very high incidence of sudden death (71%). This is particularly evident in the first year post myocardial infarction when the incidence of nonsudden cardiac death was almost identical among the patients with anterior myocardial infarction complicated and noncomplicated by

Manipulation of the Autonomic Nervous System

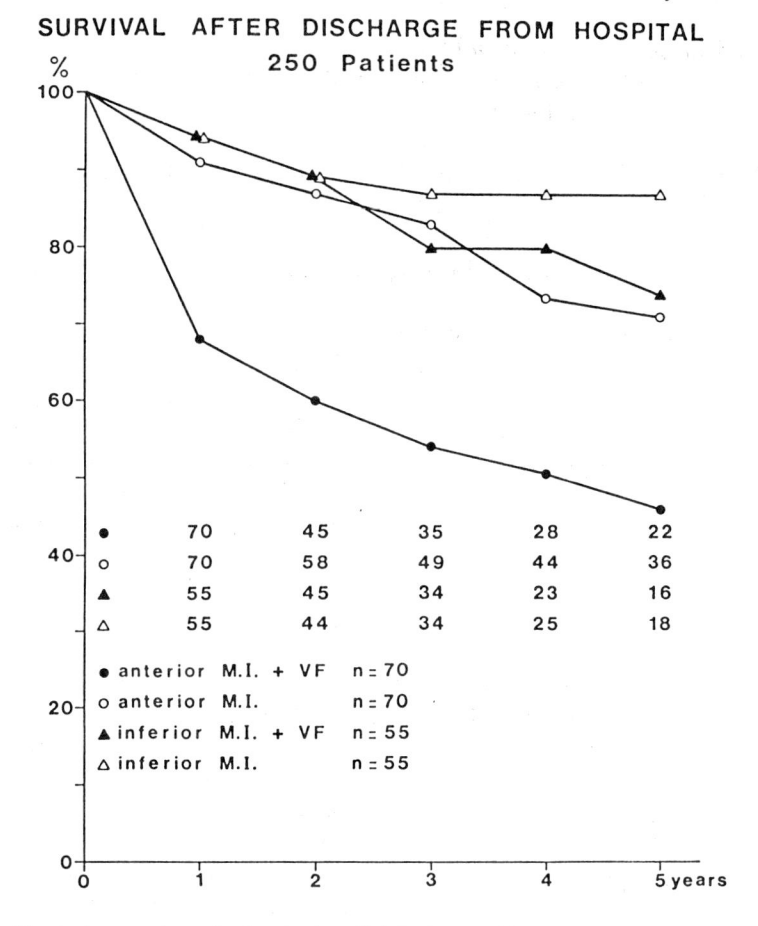

SURVIVAL AFTER DISCHARGE FROM HOSPITAL
250 Patients

		1	2	3	4	5 years
●		70	45	35	28	22
○		70	58	49	44	36
▲		55	45	34	23	16
△		55	44	34	25	18

● anterior M.I. + VF   n = 70
○ anterior M.I.   n = 70
▲ inferior M.I. + VF   n = 55
△ inferior M.I.   n = 55

Figure 8: Survival curves for patients after hospital discharge with anterior acute myocardial infarction (MI) grouped according to age and presence of ventricular fibrillation (VF). The numbers represent the number of patients studied at each interval. Within each age group, survival rates are significantly lower in patients with VF in the 0 to 2-year interval ($\geq$ 65 years: Z = 2.6, $p < 0.01$; > 65 years: Z = 1.59, $p = 0.05$). (From ref. 42.)

ventricular fibrillation (9% vs 6%), so that almost the entire difference depends on the disproportionate number of sudden deaths present in the group of patients with anterior myocardial infarction complicated by ventricular fibrillation. This study showed, in contrast to the currently held view, that patients with an anterior myocardial infarction complicated by ventricular fibrillation represent a subgroup at very high risk of sudden death.

Based on the results of this epidemiologic study, we have proceeded with the design of a randomized, placebo-controlled, multicenter study with the specific goal of assessing the potential efficacy of high thoracic left sympathectomy in reducing sudden cardiac death and of comparing it with that of a beta-adrenergic blocking agent.[43] Accordingly, 144 patients surviving an anterior myocardial infarction complicated by ventricular fibrillation or ventricular tachycardia were randomized to placebo, the beta-blocker oxprenolol (160 mg SR), and to high thoracic left sympathectomy. The study was double blind for the two pharmacological treatments. To add to the homogeneity of the population under study, only patients below 65 years and with a first myocardial infarction were considered. The mean follow-up was 20 months. The mortality in the placebo group, as correctly predicted, was very high (22%) and was dramatically decreased both by oxprenolol (2.7%) and by high thoracic left sympathectomy (3.6%). These results are statistically significant according both to "drug efficacy" and to "intention to treat" analysis.

This multicenter study, unique for the population studied and for the evaluation of high thoracic left sympathectomy, shows that not only beta-adrenergic blockade but also selective cardiac sympathetic denervation can significantly reduce the incidence of sudden cardiac death in post-myocardial infarction patients. The practical implications of this study is that high thoracic left sympathectomy may represent an interesting therapeutical approach for the high risk post-myocardial infarction patients with contraindications to beta-blockade.

Daily Exercise

The relationship found, and discussed above, between baroreflex sensitivity and susceptibility to sudden cardiac death raised the question of the possibility of modifying cardiac vagal efferent activity as a physiological means to prevent ventricular fibrillation. Daily exercise may be one such method.

Endurance exercise training alters the autonomic nervous system, resulting in an apparent increase in vagal efferent activity and in a decrease in sympathetic efferent activity. Specifically, heart rate at submaximal workload is reduced in dogs after 8–10 weeks of exercise training.[44,45] Acetylcholine content[46] and the quantity of acetylcholine transferase[47] obtained from hearts of trained rats were increased when compared to untrained rats. These data suggested that exercise training enhanced cardiac parasympathetic activity. Exercise training has resulted in simular hemodynamic changes in humans.[48]

Using the exercise plus ischemia protocol, we investigated whether daily exercise would alter the propensity to life-threatening arrhythmias, particularly in those dogs with a healed myocardial infarction identified to be at higher risk of sudden death.[49]

Three groups of dogs, all with a 1-month-old anterior myocardial infarction, were studied: one of the resistant dogs and two of the susceptible ones. They were so identified by the outcome of the first exercise plus ischemia test and by the baroreflex slopes, which always matched. The resistant and one group of susceptible dogs were treated with daily exercise for a 6-week period, while the other group of susceptible dogs was rested in a cage for the same length of time. In this way we could rule out time as a potential cause of possible changes in the exercise-treated group. The baroreceptor reflexes were evaluated using the phenylephrine test every 2 weeks, and after 6 weeks the exercise plus ischemia test was repeated.

The dogs were exercised by running on a motor-driven treadmill 5 days/

week. On alternate days, the major portion of each exercise period consisted of either spring or endurance running. The duration of each exercise period increased weekly: during the first week each session lasted a total of 35 minutes, while during the sixth week the period had increased to 60 minutes.

Exercise produced a striking change in the baroreflex slopes. This is shown in Figure 9. Within a few weeks, the almost flat baroreflex slopes of the susceptible dogs became quite similar to those of the resistant animals. Similarly, within 2 weeks of exercise, the heart rate decrease for 30 mmHg among susceptible dogs changed so much (from -14.6 ± 8.7 to -54 ± 15.2 beats/min) that it became undistinguishable from that of the resistant dogs (-50 ± 9 beats/min). This is shown in Figure 10, together with the fact that almost no change occurred over time among the susceptible dogs resting quietly in a cage.

Is there any relationship between the dramatic changes in the baroreceptor reflexes and the susceptibility to sudden death? The exercise plus ischemia test failed to elicit ventricular fibrillation or significant arrhythmias in the animals that completed 6 weeks of exercise. This is true for both the resistant animals, as expected, and more importantly, the susceptible dogs. In contrast, all but one of the susceptible dogs cage-rested for 6 weeks developed ventricular fibrillation during the exercise plus ischemia. The relationship among the baroreflex slopes, exercise or cage rest, and survival is shown in Figure 11. It seems important to

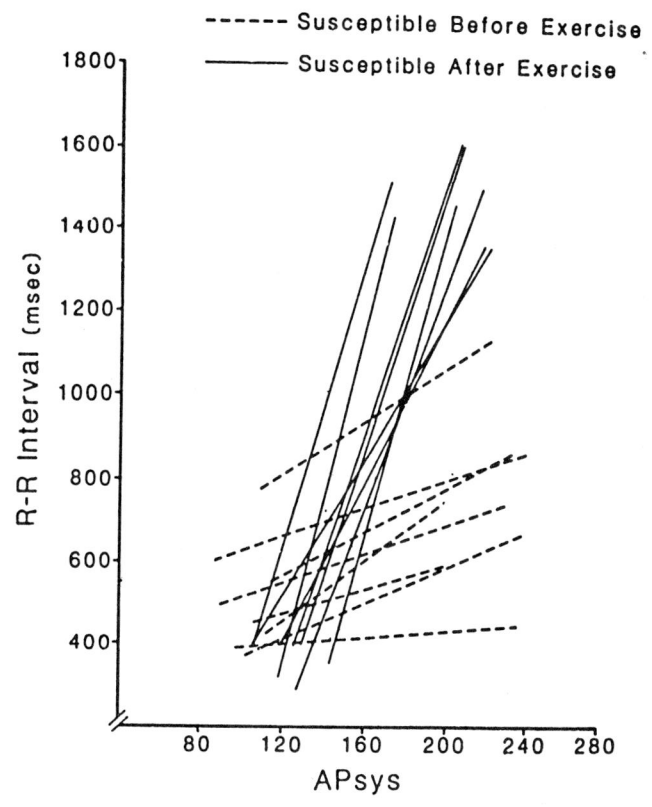

Figure 9: Regression analysis for all susceptible dogs before and after 6 weeks of daily exercise. Modified from Billman GE, Schwartz PJ, Stone HL. The effects of daily exercise on susceptibility to sudden cardiac death. (From ref. 9.)

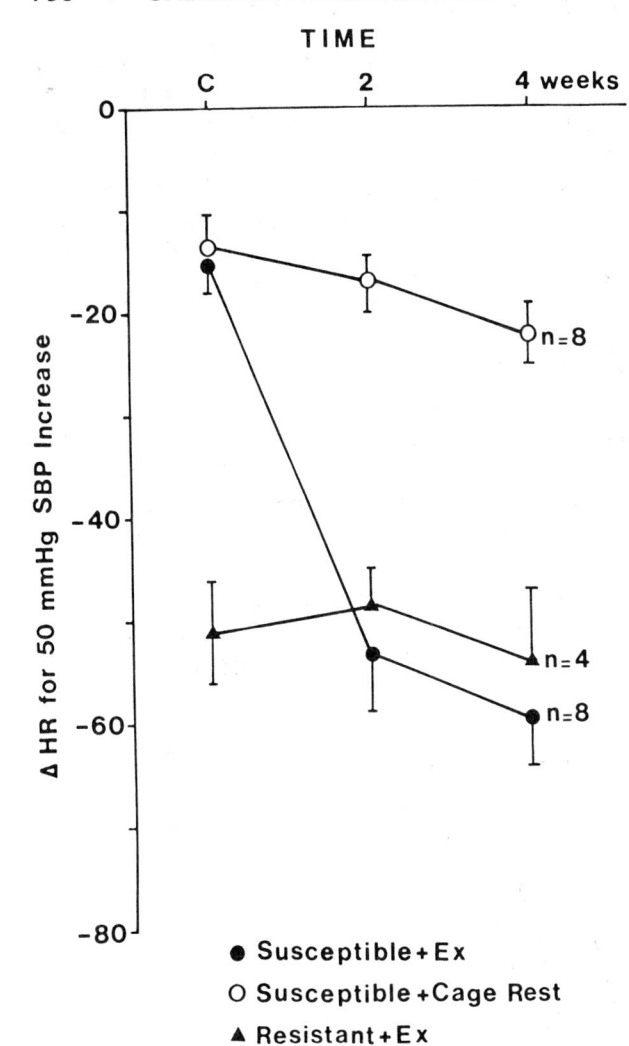

Figure 10: The change in the heart rate from control heart rate to a 50 mmHg elevation of arterial pressure in three groups of animals. Data were taken in each group before, 2 weeks after, and 4 weeks after the susceptible group had entered a 4-week exercise program. The susceptible plus cage rest and the resistant plus exercise showed very little change over this time span. (From ref. 9.)

note that the only susceptible cage-rested dog that survived the exercise plus ischemia test was also the only one that, for unknown reasons, had a baroreflex slope that had increased spontaneously to reach the resistant range (from 4.4 to 16.7 ms/mmHg). Although one must be wary of anecdotes, it is also important in experimental research not to miss biologic messages; this one dogs seems to be telling us something about the relationship between baroreceptor reflexes and susceptibility to sudden death.

The changes induced by exercise are not permanent as shown in Figure 12. When a susceptible dog, with a flat baroreflex slope and ventricular fibrillation during the exercise plus ischemia test, had 6 weeks of exercise, its baroreflex slopes increased markedly and it survived during the repetition of the exercise plus ischemia test. After having been returned to cage rest for an additional 6

EFFECT OF 6WK EXERCISE ON BAROREFLEX SLOPES AND ON SURVIVAL

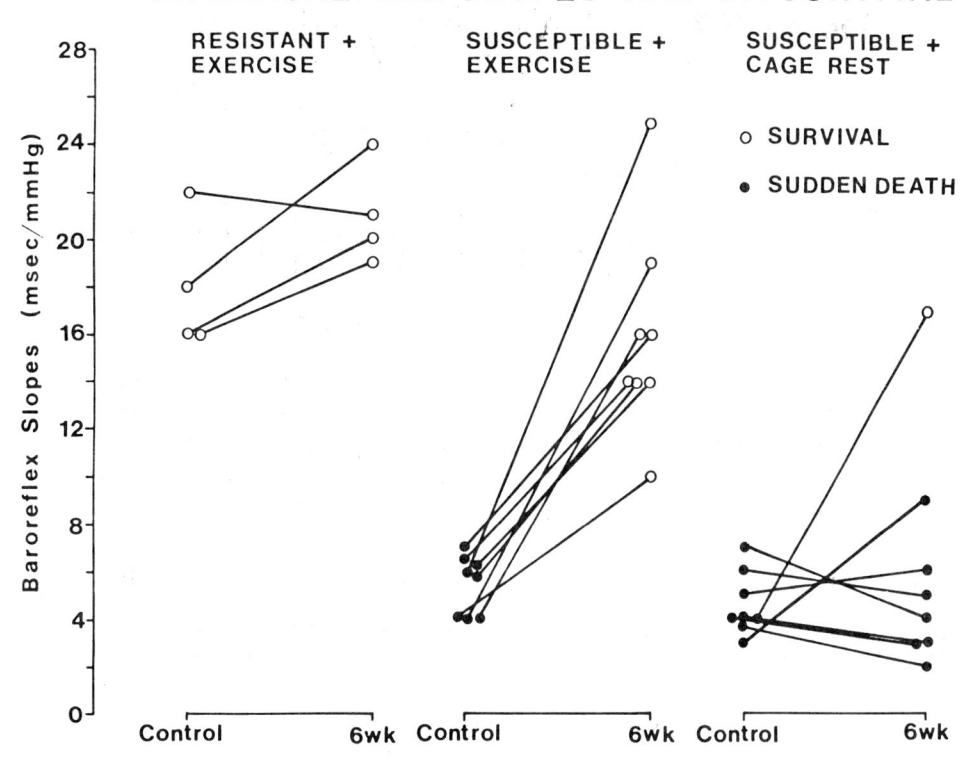

Figure 11: Baroreflex slopes before and after 6 weeks of either daily exercise or cage rest. All animals were tested with exercise plus ischemia at these times. Sudden death on the treadmill is indicated by the closed circles, survival by the open circles. It is evident that while the resistant dogs were unaffected by exercise, the susceptible showed a clear increase in the baroreflex slopes, which was matched by survival during the exercise plus ischemia test. The only susceptible dog in the cage rested group that survived the exercise plus ischemia test is also the only one whose baroreflex slope had returned into the resistant range. (From ref. 49.)

weeks, however, its baroreflex slopes became flat again and, when exposed to the exercise plus ischemia test, it again developed ventricular fibrillation. Therefore, whatever changes are induced by exercise (at least a 6-week period), which reduce susceptibility to sudden death, seem to be reversible.

The mechanisms by which daily exercise modifies the baroreceptor reflexes and cardiac electrical stability require further investigations, which are already under way in our laboratories. In this study, the dogs had not yet reached a trained state. For the dog, 8–10 weeks of exercise are necessary to produce classic training effects, consisting of increased skeletal muscle oxidative enzyme activity and lower heart rate during submaximal exercise. A striking point is represented by the fact that the changes in baroreceptor reflexes occur within 2 weeks. Exercise improves the cardiac function, including ejection fraction and stroke volume.[50-52] A combined effect on autonomic reflexes (increase in vagal

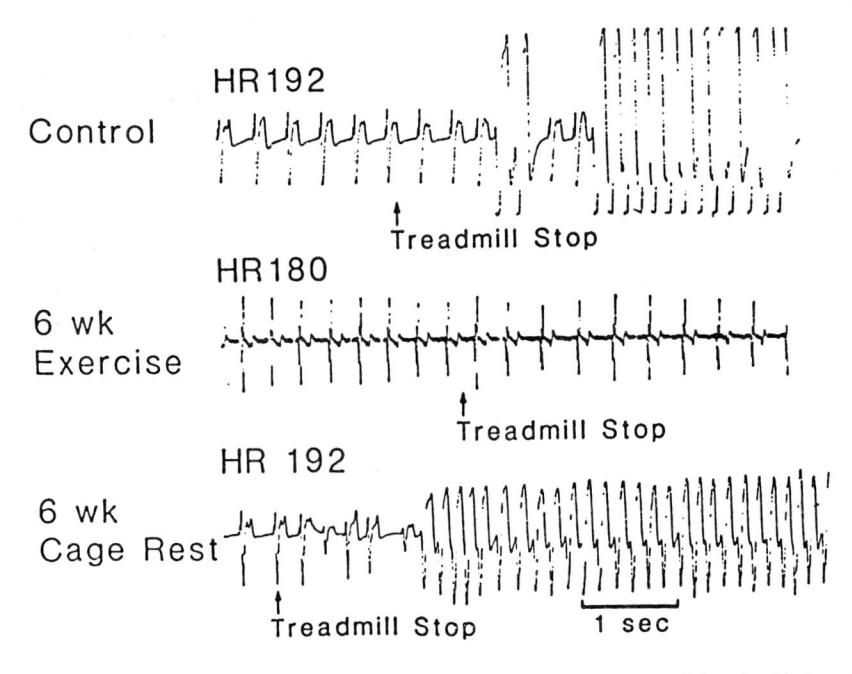

Figure 12: Actual recordings of the exercise plus ischemia test from one susceptible animal before daily exercise (control), at the end of 6 weeks' daily exercise, and after 6 weeks' cage rest that followed the exercise period. The animal developed VF before daily exercise but not after completion of the exercise program. This protection was reversed by 6 weeks' cage rest. (From ref. 49.)

and decrease in sympathetic reflexes) and on left ventricular function may have affected the results.

Clinical studies on the effects of exercise on cardiovascular mortality in patients recovering from myocardial infarction have been inconclusive. Although a recent article,[53] using a questionable cumulative analysis of several studies, suggests a reduction in sudden death among post-myocardial infarction patients participating in an exercise program, no firm conclusion can yet be made. This is largely due to the fact that the exercise programs have mostly involved the already low risk groups and that the enrollment criteria have usually created a considerable bias toward low risk individuals. With a low mortality, it is always difficult to prove a beneficial effect of any intervention. This makes interesting the seemingly favorable trend for the patients involved in the exercise program. What is needed, however, is a carefully controlled study in a medium-high risk subgroup of patients.

Vagal Stimulation

The effect of vagal activity during acute myocardial ischemia has been the issue of an interesting controversy (for details, see ref. 6). Critical work in this area has been performed by Kent, Corr, Verrier, and their associates.

Kent and co-workers[54,55] demonstrated that vagal stimulation increases the threshold for ventricular fibrillation in both the normal and the ischemic canine heart. They also provided the evidence for the cholinergic innervation of the specialized conducting system. The same group[56] showed that vagal stimulation decreases the number of animals developing spontaneous ventricular fibrillation. Corr and Gillis[57,58] reported that the presence of intact vagi protected against ventricular fibrillation, an effect independent of heart rate. Verrier, Lown, and associates have provided, through numerous studies, evidence for the fact that the protective effect of vagal stimulation depends on the level of preexisting cardiac sympathetic tone.[59-62] Others[63,64] were unable to confirm a protective effect of vagal stimulation on the threshold for ventricular fibrillation, an indirect index of ventricular vulnerability to fibrillation.

As to reperfusion arrhythmias, our group[65] has recently shown that in cats, vagal stimulation significantly reduces the incidence of ventricular tachyarrhythmias. This effect is largely but not entirely mediated by the attendant decrease in heart rate.

The data available from these experimental studies and also from clinical observations[66] suggest that, as far as survival is concerned, the results of dominant vagal reflexes at time of acute myocardial ischemia are complex. If vagal dominance is limited and helps to preserve an optimal heart rate,[67] antagonizing also the more deleterious effects of sympathetic hyperactivity, electrical stability increases and survival is more likely. On the other hand, if vagal reflexes are excessive and lead to bradycardia and hypotension, they may facilitate ventricular fibrillation or result in asystole or electromechanic dissociation.

A major limitation of all the studies involving vagal stimulation is represented by the fact that they have been performed in anesthetized animals. We have decided to utilize our post-myocardial infarction model for sudden death and to evaluate in conscious dogs the effects of vagal stimulation performed through chronically implanted electrodes. These experiments are currently performed in our laboratories in Oklahoma City and in Milan.[68] In the first group of experiments, the intensity of vagal stimulation is adjusted so that heart rate decreases by approximately 80-100 beats/min without producing major side effects. So far, this has resulted in a striking protection from ventricular fibrillation (Fig. 13). The exercise plus ischemia tests with and without vagal stimulation are of course performed in the same animals to allow an internal control analysis and maximizing the advantages of chronic preparations (Fig. 14). Experiments in which heart rate is maintained constant by ventricular pacing during vagal stimulation are currently being performed. It would seem from the initial results that the protective effect of vagal stimulation is mostly dependent on the attendant heart rate decrease. From a practical point of view, the fact remains that vagal stimulation, performed through a chronically implanted electrode during acute myocardial ischemia substantially reduces the incidence of ventricular fibrillation.

Conclusions

The availability of an animal model in which life-threatening arrhythmias can be reproducibly generated by the interaction between factors that are clinically

VAGAL STIMULATION AND VENTRICULAR FIBRILLATION

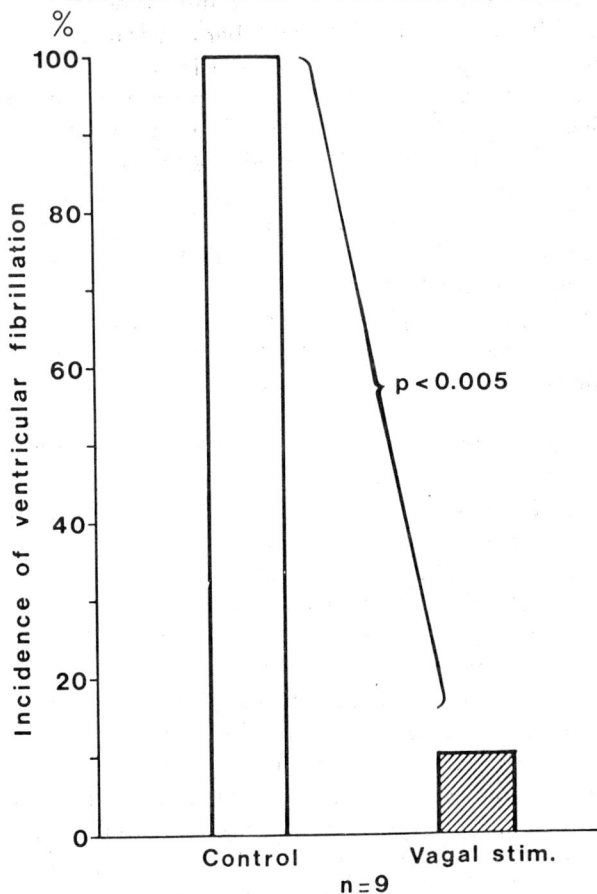

Figure 13: Incidence of ventricular fibrillation in nine dogs susceptible to sudden death in control condition and in a subsequent exercise plus ischemia test during which electrical vagal stimulation was performed. Vagal stimulation results in a striking protection from ventricular fibrillation.

relevant (acute myocardial ischemia, physical exercise) in a clinically relevant setting (conscious animals, healed myocardial infarction) have allowed the acquisition of novel information on the relationship between the autonomic nervous system and sudden death.

Previous data from our own group suggesting an antifibrillatory action of left stellectomy in the absence of significant side effects have been confirmed and have led to a clinical trial unique for the population studied and for the therapy employed. It was found that left cardiac sympathetic denervation dramatically decreases the incidence of sudden cardiac death (but also of total mortality) among a high risk subgroup of post-MI patients.

It was found that the analysis baroreceptor reflexes, employing a technique already applicable to man, allows the identification of subgroups of post-myocardial infarction animals at high risk for ventricular fibrillation. Ongoing

CONTROL

HR 295 b/min

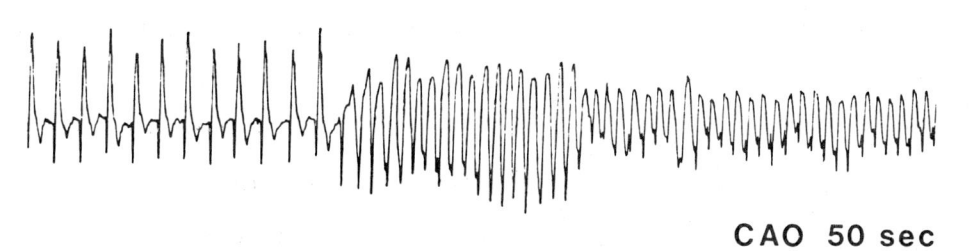

CAO 50 sec

VAGAL STIMULATION

HR 125   HR 80

CAO 45 sec   ↓ end of CAO

1 sec

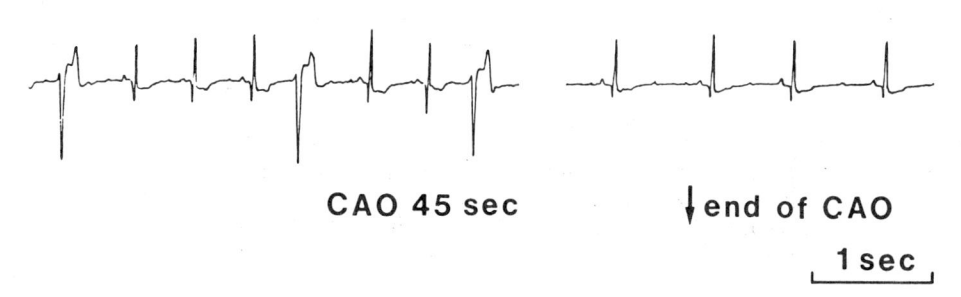

Figure 14: Electrocardiographic recording in a susceptible dog during an exercise plus ischemia test 1 month after myocardial infarction. In the upper tracing, the control test: 50 sec after the coronary artery occlusion (CAO), onset of ventricular tachycardia which deteriorated into ventricular fibrillation. In the lower tracing, the same dog in which electrical stimulation of the right cervical vagus is performed during a subsequent exercise plus ischemia test: only few premature ventricular beats are noted.

studies in post-MI patients seem to confirm the validity of this concept that may contribute to a better and early identification of high risk subgroups. It was also shown that modification of the baroreceptor reflexes by daily exercise is associated with an increased electrical stability and with the shift from high to low risk subgroups.

Finally, an implantable device that allows electrical stimulation of the right vagus in conscious animals has been devised and is currently used in the sudden death animal model. Preliminary results indicate that vagal stimulation, largely through its effect on heart rate, can prevent ventricular fibrillation induced by myocardial ischemia in dogs with a healed myocardial infarction.

It does seem that experimental cardiovascular research is entering a new phase in which we are learning how to manipulate the autonomic nervous system in order to decrease susceptibility to sudden cardiac death. It is exciting to realize that, with all probability, most of this information can be transferred to humans.

References

1. Schwartz PJ, Brown AM, Malliani A, Zanchetti A, eds. Neural Mechanisms in Cardiac Arrhythmias. New York, Raven Press, 1978.
2. Lown B, Verrier RL. Neural activity and ventricular fibrillation. N Engl J Med 1976;294:1165–1170.
3. Lown B. Sudden cardiac death: the major challenge confronting contemporary cardiology. Am J Cardiol 1979;43:313–328.
4. Malliani A, Schwartz PJ, Zanchetti A. Neural mechanisms in life-threatening arrhythmias. Am Heart J 1980;100:705–715.
5. Schwartz PJ, Stone HL. The role of the autonomic nervous system in sudden coronary death. Ann NY Acad Sci 1982;382:162–180.
6. Corr PB, Yamada KA, Witkowski FX. Mechanisms controlling cardiac autonomic function and their relation to arrhythmogenesis. In The Heart and the Cardiovascular System. HA Fozzard, E Haber, RB Jennings, AM Katz, eds. Raven Press, New York 1986, p 1343–1404.
7. Schwartz PJ. Idiopathic long QT syndrome: Progress and questions. Am Heart J 1985;109:399–411.
8. Schwartz PJ, Billman GE, Stone HL. Autonomic mechanisms in ventricular fibrillation induced by myocardial ischemia during exercise in dogs with healed myocardial infarction: An experimental preparation for sudden cardiac death. Circulation 1984;69:790–800.
9. Schwartz PJ, Stone HL. The analysis and modulation of autonomic reflexes in the prediction and prevention of sudden death. In Zipes DP, Jalife J, eds. Cardiac Electrophysiology and Arrhythmias. New York, Grune & Stratton, 1985;165–176.
10. Roelandt J, Klootwijk P, Lubsen J, Janse MJ. Sudden death during longterm ambulatory monitoring. Eur Heart J 1984;5:7–20.
11. Gradman AH, Bell PA, DeBusk RF. Sudden death during ambulatory monitoring. Clinical and electrocardiographic correlations: Report of a case. Circulation 1977;55:210–211.
12. Myerburg RJ, Epstein K, Gaide MS, Wong SS, Castellanos A, Gelband H, Cameron JS, Bassett AL. Cellular electrophysiology in acute and healed experimental myocardial infarction. Ann NY Acad Sci 1982;382:90–115.
13. Adgey AAJ, Devlin JE, Webb SW, Mulholland HC. Initiation of ventricular fibrillation outside hospital in patients with acute ischaemic heart disease. Br Heart J 1982;47:55–61.
14. Bennett T, Wilcox RG, Hampton JR. Cardiovascular reflexes in patients after myocardial infarction: Effect on long term treatment with beta-adrenoceptor antagonists. Br Heart J 1980;44:265–270.
15. Eckberg DL. Parasympathetic cardiovascular control in human disease: A critical review of methods and results. Am J Physiol 1980;239:H581–H593.
16. Smyth HS, Sleight P, Pickering GW. Reflex regulation of arterial pressure during sleep in man. Circ Res 1969;24:109–121.
17. Billman GE, Schwartz PJ, Stone HL. Baroreceptor reflex control of heart rate: A predictor of sudden cardiac death. Circulation 1982;66:874–880.
18. Schwartz PJ, Zaza A, Pala M, Grassi G, Mancia G, Stone HL, Zanchetti A. Transient impairment in baroreceptor reflexes in the first year post myocardial infarction: A prospective study. Circulation 1984;70:(suppl II) 874.
19. Vanoli E, Stramba-Badiale M, De Ferrari GM, Cerati D, Billman G, Schwartz PJ. Baroreflex sensitivity and sudden death in conscious dogs before and after myocardial infarction. J Am Coll Cardiol 1987 (in press).
20. La Rovere MT, Specchia G, Mazzoleni C, Mortara A, Schwartz PJ. Baroreflex sensitivity in post-myocardial infarction patients. Correlation with physical training and prognosis. Circulation 1986;74:(suppl III) 514.
21. Schwartz PJ. The rationale and the role of left stellectomy for the prevention of malignant arrhythmias. In Clinical Aspects of Life-Threatening Arrhythmias. HM

Greenberg, HE Kulbertus, AJ Moss, PJ Schwartz, eds. Ann NY Acad Sci 1984;427: 199–220.
22. Schwartz PJ, Zaza A. The rational basis and the clinical value of selective cardiac sympathetic denervation in the prevention of malignant arrhythmias. Eur Heart J 1986;7:(suppl A) 107–118.
23. Schwartz PJ. Sympathetic imbalance and cardiac arrhythmias. In Randall WC, ed. Nervous Control of Cardiovascular Function. Oxford Univ Press, 1984;225–251.
24. Armour JA, Hageman GR, Randall WC. Arrhythmias induced by local cardiac nerve stimulation. Am J Physiol 1972;223:1068–1075.
25. Hageman GR, Goldberg JM, Armour JA, Randall WC. Cardiac dysrhythmias induced by autonomic nerve stimulation. Am J Cardiol 1973;32:823–830.
26. Kralios FA, Millar CK. Sympathetic neural effects on regional atrial recovery properties and cardiac rhythm. Am J Physiol 1981;240:H590–H596.
27. Schwartz PJ, Stone HL, Brown AM. Effects of unilateral stellate ganglion blockade on the arrhythmias associated with coronary occlusion. Am Heart J 1976;92:589–599.
28. Harris AS, Otero H, Bocage AJ. The induction of arrhythmias by sympathetic activity before and after occlusion of a coronary artery in the canine heart. J Electrocardiol 1971;4:34–43.
29. Schwartz PJ, Vanoli E. A new experimental model for the study of cardiac arrhythmias dependent on the interaction between acute myocardial ischemia and sympathetic hyperactivity. J Cardiovasc Pharmacol 1981;3:1251–1259.
30. Schwartz PJ, Vanoli E, Zaza A, Zuanettti G. The effect of antiarrhythmic drugs on life-threatening arrhythmias induced by the interaction between acute myocardial ischemia and sympathetic hyperactivity. Am Heart J 1985;109:937–948.
31. Schwartz PJ, Priori SG, Vanoli E, Zaza A, Zuanetti G. Efficacy of Diltiazem in two experimental feline models of sudden cardiac death. J Am Coll Cardiol 1986;8: 661–668.
32. Schwartz PJ, Verrier RL, Lown B. Effect of stellectomy and vagotomy on ventricular refractoriness in dogs. Circ Res 1977;40:536–540.
33. Schwartz PJ, Snebold NG, Brown AM. Effects of unilateral cardiac sympathectomy denervation on the ventricular fibrillation threshold. Am J Cardiol 1976;37:1034–1040.
34. Schwartz PJ, Stone HL. Left stellectomy in the prevention of ventricular fibrillation caused by acute myocardial ischemia in conscious dogs with anterior myocardial infarction. Circulation 1980;62:1256–1265.
35. Schwartz PJ, Stone HL. Effects of unilateral stellectomy upon cardiac performance during exercise in dogs. Circ Res 1979;44:637–645.
36. Schwartz PJ, Gwirtz PA, Stone HL. Cardiac performance before and after left stellectomy in dogs with an anterior myocardial infarction. Proc 8th Europ Congr Cardiol, Paris, 1980;121.
37. Feigl EO. Coronary physiology. Physiol Rev 1983;63:1–204.
38. Feigl EO. Sympathetic control of coronary circulation. Circ Res 1967;20:262–271.
39. Schwartz PJ, Stone HL. Tonic influence of the sympathetic nervous system on myocardial reactive hyperemia and on coronary blood flow distribution in dogs. Circ Res 1977;41:51–58.
40. Janse MJ, Schwartz PJ, Wilms-Schopman F, Peters RJG, Durrer D. Effects of unilateral stellate ganglion stimulation and ablation on elctophysiologic changes induced by acute myocardial ischemia in dogs. Circulation 1985;72:585–595.
41. Vanoli E, Zaza A, Zuanetti G, Stramba-Badiale M, Cerati D, Schwartz PJ, Unilateral stellectomy and infarct size. Eur Heart J 1985;6(suppl I):118.
42. Schwartz PJ, Zaza A, Grazi S, Lombardo M, Lotto A, Sbressa C, Zappa P. Effect of ventricular fibrillation complicating acute myocardial infarction on long-term prognosis: importance of the site of infarction. Am J Cardiol 1985;56:384–389.
43. Schwartz PJ, Motolese M, Pallavini G, Malliani A, Bartorelli C, Zanchetti A, and the Sudden Death Italian Prevention Group. Surgical and pharmacological antiadrenergic interventions in the prevention of sudden death after a first myocardial infarction. Circulation 1985;72(suppl II):358.

44. Stone HL. Cardiac function and exercise training in conscious dogs. J Appl Physiol 1977;42:824–832.
45. Wyatt HL, Mitchell JH. Influences of physical training on the heart of dogs. Circ Res 1974;35:883–889.
46. DeSchryver C, Merteno-Stryhagen J. Heart tissue acetylcholine in chronically exercised rats. Experientia 1975;31:316–318.
47. Ekstrom J. Choline acetyltransferase in the heart and salivary glands of the rat after physical training. QL Exp Physiol 1974;59:73–80.
48. Clausen JP. Circulatory adjustments to dynamic exercise and effect of physical training in normal subjects and patients with coronary artery disease. Progr Cardiosvasc Dis 1976;18:459–495.
49. Billman GE, Schwartz PJ, Stone HL. The effects of daily exercise on susceptibility to sudden cardiac death. Circulation 1984;69:1182–1189.
50. Froehicher V, Jensen D, Atwood JE, McKirnan MD, Gerber K, Slutsky R, Batler A, Ashborn W, Ross J. Cardiac rehabilitation: Evidence for improvement in myocardial perfusion and function. Arch Phys Med Rehabil 1980;61:517–522.
51. Hagberg JM, Eksani AA, Holloszy JO. Effect of 12 months of intense exercise training on stroke volume in patients with coronary artery disease. Circulation 1983;67:1194–1199.
52. Verani MS, Hartung GH, Hoepfel-Harris J, Wellon DE, Pratt CM, Miller RR. Effects of exercise training on left ventricular performance and myocardial perfusion in patients with coronary artery disease. Am J Cardiol 1981;47:797–803.
53. Shephard RJ. The value of exercise in ischemic heart disease: A cumulative analysis. J Cardiac Rehab 1983;3:294–298.
54. Kent KM, Smith ER, Redwood DR, Epstein SE. Electrical stability of acutely ischemic myocardium: Influences of heart rate and vagal stimulation. Circulation 1973;47:291–298.
55. Kent KM, Epstein SE, Cooper T, Jacobowitz DM. Cholinergic innervation of the canine and human ventricular conducting system: Anatomic and electrophysiologic correlation. Circulation 1974;50:948–955.
56. Myers RW, Pearlman AS, Hyman RM, Goldstein RA, Kent DM, Goldstein RE, Epstein SE. Beneficial effects of vagal stimulation and bradycardia during experimental acute myocardial ischemia. Circulation 1974;49:943–947.
57. Corr PB, Gillis RA. Role of the vagus in the cardiovascular changes induced by coronary occlusion. Circulation 1974;49:86–97.
58. Corr PB, Pearle DL, Gillis RA. Coronary occlusion site as a determinant of the cardiac rhythm effects of atropine and vagotomy. Am Heart J 1976;93:60–65.
59. Rabinowitz SH, Verrier RL, Lown B. Muscarinic effects of vagosympathetic trunk stimulation on the repetitive extrasystole threshold. Circulation 1976;53:622–627.
60. Kolman BS, Verrier RL, Lown B. The effect of vagus nerve stimulation upon vulnerability of the canine ventricle. Role of sympathetic-parasympathetic interactions. Circulation 1975;52:578–585.
61. De Silva RA, Verrier RL, Lown B. Effect of physiologic stress and sedation with morphine sulfate on ventricular vulnerability. Am Heart J 1978;95:197–203.
62. Verrier RL, Lown B. Behavioural stress and cardiac arrhythmias. Ann Rev Physiol 1984;46:155–176.
63. Yoon MS, Han J, Tse WW, Rogers R. Effects of vagal stimulation, atropine, and propranolol on fibrillation threshold of normal and ischemic ventricles. Am Heart J 1977;93:60–65.
64. James RGG, Arnold JMO, Allen JD, Pantridge JF, Shanks RG. The effects of heart rate, myocardial ischemia and vagal stimulation on the threshold for ventricular fibrillation. Circulation 1977;55:311–317.
65. Zuanetti G, De Ferrari GM, Priori SG, Schwartz PJ. Protective effect of vagal stimulation on reperfusion arrhythmias in cats. Circ Res (In Press).
66. Pantridge JF. Autonomic disturbance at the onset of acute myocardial infarction. In Schwartz PJ, Brown AM, Malliani A, et al, eds. Neural Mechanisms in Cardiac Arrhythmias. New York, Raven Press, 1978;7–17.

67. Chadda KD, Banka VS, Helfant RH. Rate-dependent ventricular ectopia following acute coronary occlusion. Circulation 1974;49:654–658.
68. Schwartz PJ, Vanoli E, De Ferrari G, Stramba-Badiale M. Vagal stimulation prevents ventricular fibrillation due to acute myocardial ischemia in conscious dogs. (Submitted for publication.)

49

Quantitation of Myocardial Ischemic Surface and Volume by NADH And Magnetic Resonance Imaging With Correlation to Ventricular Arrhythmias

Alden H. Harken
Anirban Banerjee
John Sun
Glenn J.R. Whitman

Introduction

Although substantial advances have been made in rendering emergency medical care and cardiac resuscitation, the survivors of "sudden cardiac death" are prone to recurrent episodes of malignant arrhythmias.[1]

The common denominator of both left ventricular scar and ventricular irritability is myocardial ischemia. One does not necessitate the other, but they frequently co-exist. Boineau and Cox[4] first postulated asynchronous electrical activation in acutely ischemic myocardium. This investigation suggested that electrical inhomogeneity in the heart predisposed to reentrant tachyarrhythmias. Recent microelectrode studies[5-7] have confirmed that the electrophysiologic derangements required for the development of reentry do exist in acute and chronically

From: Brugada P, Wellens HJJ. CARDIAC ARRHYTHMIAS: Where To Go From Here? Mount Kisco, NY, Futura Publishing Company, Inc., © 1987.

infarcted myocardium. These electrophysiologic derangements are most noted in the transition or "borderzone" between normal and ischemic/hypoxic myocardium; this borderzone contains adjacent cells with markedly different electrophysiologic properties. It appears that the electrical inhomogeneity, which exists in the borderzone, may play an important role in the increased susceptibility to tachyarrhythmias following myocardial injury. Investigations[8-10] using histologic techniques combined with electrophysiologic studies have correlated anatomically nonuniform (heterogeneous) myocardial injury with increased susceptibility to sustained reentrant ventricular tachyarrhythmias in the canine heart.

Ischemic myocardial damage may lead to recurrent malignant ventricular tachyarrhythmias. The purpose of this manuscript is (1) to explore avenues suggesting that the myocardial infarct anatomy or pattern of myocardial ischemia may influence the degree of susceptibility to sustained reentrant ventricular tachyarrhythmias, and (2) to investigate the possibilities of applying magnetic resonance imaging (MRI) techniques to delineate more precisely the ischemic-perfused perimeter and surface area.

Magnitude of Clinical Problem

Recurrent sustained ventricular tachycardia almost always co-exists with myocardial ischemia. Antiarrhythmic drug and pacemaker therapy are successful in controlling ventricular tachyarrhythmias in a substantial number of patients, but some 40% continue to have recurrent tachyarrhythmias despite these interventions.[1-3] The advent of new electrophysiologically directed surgical techniques has allowed the surgeon to take an increasing role in the therapy of ventricular tachyarrhythmias. At present, the most frequently utilized operation for medically refractory ventricular tachycardia is electrophysiologically directed endocardial resection. In this instance, a 1 to 2 mm thick sheet of endocardium is removed. By experience, we have found that the site of earliest ventricular activation during ventricular tachycardia is typically at the border of left ventricular scar and viable myocardium. Programmed electrical stimulation permits the scanning of electrical diastole with the introduction of programmed electrical extrastimuli in the electrophysiology laboratory. Programmed pacing has proved to be of considerable importance, both in confirming the existence of arrhythmias and in substantiating drug efficacy. Notably, both the morphology and rate of arrhythmias induced by programmed pacing correlate well with those abnormal rhythms occurring spontaneously.

Unfortunately, a substantial number of patients with documented malignant ventricular arrhythmias are refractory to all medical therapy.[11,12] Without successful therapy, these patients might be relegated to an approximate 67% annual mortality.[13] Surgery has resulted in ventricular arrhythmia control in selected patients previously resistant to all medical regimen.[14] With surgical excision of ventricular muscle (or ischemic borderzone), an additional surgical injury necessarily occurs. If indeed the pattern of this ventricular injury is significant, then it behooves us to explore the relationship between scar patterns and tachyarrhythmias.

Delineation of Infarct Pattern: NADH Fluorescence Photography

Myocardial ischemia has previously been displayed and delineated by NADH fluorescence photography in our laboratory.[15,16] A heart is examined either in vivo[16] or on a perfusion apparatus.[15] In the exposed heart, a coronary artery is identified and reversibly noose occluded (Fig. 1). Two 400 joule xenon flash tubes are then directed at the left ventricle filtered through 330–380 nanometer filters. A 350 microsecond flash is then produced. Emitted fluorescence designating reduced NADH is filtered at 440–510 nanometers and a photograph is taken. This technique permits delineation of the oxygen supply/demand ratio over the entire surface of the epicardium or frozen myocardial specimen.

Nicotinamide adenine dinucledotide (NADH) fluorescence photographs are taken of the epicardial and myocardial surfaces. This photographic technique may be used to exhibit the adequacy of myocardial oxygen supply. NADH fluorescence photographs are taken with a Bronica S2A camera. Corning 9788 and Wratten 45 filters are placed over the camera lens to allow transmission of NADH fluorescence in the 430–510 nanometer region. NADH fluorescence excitation is provided by two 400 joule xenon flash tubes (EG and G FX-47C3) covered by Corning 5840 filters to provide 330–380 nanometer excitation.

Correlation of Myocardial Ischemic Pattern With Predisposition to Ventricular Arrhythmias

The coronary artery occlusion/reperfusion model produces a heterogeneous infarct in the dog[16] Fifteen dogs were anesthetized and underwent a left thoraco-

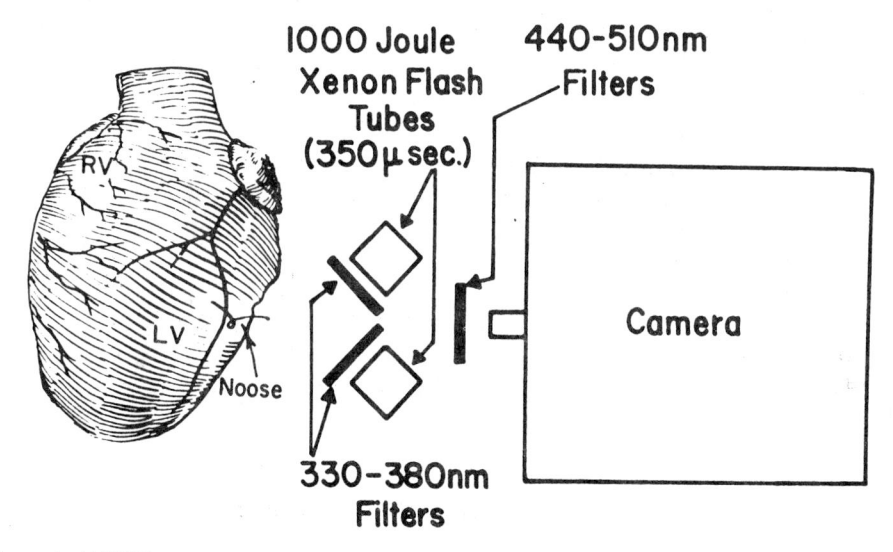

Figure 1: NADH fluorescence photography of an isolated perfused heart undergoing a noose occlusion segmental infarct.

tomy.[17] In five dogs, the pericardium was opened and a pursestring suture was placed in the left atrium (group A). In five dogs, a "closed" endocardial resection was performed via the left atrium (group B). In this group, a biopsy forceps was passed through the pursestring suture in the left atrium through the mitral valve and 10 bites (100 mg each) of apical endocardium was removed. An additional five dogs were subjected to mid-left anterior descending coronary artery occlusion and reperfusion following 2 hours. The dogs were studied electrophysiologically by standard techniques 2 weeks postoperatively. Using programmed unipolar cathodal stimulation with three premature excitations, none of the control operated dogs (group A) exhibited ventricular tachycardia at any site. Similarly, in the dogs that underwent "closed" endocardial resection (group B), ventricular tachycardia was not inducible at any site. Sustained ventricular tachycardia, however, was reproducibly inducible in four of the five dogs with chronic heterogeneous infarctions produced by the occlusion/reperfusion procedure (group C).

In addition, 40 guinea pig hearts were isolated and perfused in the standard Langendorff fashion. The distribution of myocardial ischemia was determined from NADH fluorescence photographs. Negatives were uniformly enlarged and printed. Area and perimeter lengths of ventricular NADH fluorescence were obtained using a desk-top computer/planimeter. A standard clinical stimulation protocol using programmed electrical stimulation was used to assess predisposition to arrhythmias. Hearts not subjected to experimental injury underwent electrophysiologic testing and served as controls. Homogeneous, confluent patterns of myocardial ischemia were created by ligation of a left coronary artery. Heterogeneous mottled patterns of myocardial anoxia were produced by either decreasing perfusate oxygen concentration from 95% to 10% (high-flow hypoxia) or decreasing coronary flow to 40% of baseline (low-flow ischemia).

None of ten control or ten homogeneously ischemic hearts displayed spontaneous or inducible tachyarrhythmias. Conversely, nine of ten heterogeneously hypoxic hearts ($p < 0.001$) and nine of ten heterogeneously ischemic hearts ($p < 0.001$) displayed spontaneous or induced sustained tachyarrhythmias. Mean total perimeter length of the NADH fluorescence (millimeters) was zero for controls, 70 ± 10 for the homogeneously ischemic hearts, 200 ± 10 for the heterogeneously hypoxic hearts, and 170 ± 10 for the heterogeneously ischemic hearts.

We conclude that in both guinea pigs and dogs an anatomically heterogeneous pattern of injury does increase the perimeter length (anoxic-perfused interface) as compared with a homogeneous injury pattern. This perimeter represents borderzone tissue between normal and ischemic/hypoxic myocardium, the area previously shown to contain the necessary electrophysiologic substrates for reentrant arrhythmias. Anatomic heterogeneity does appear to increase the amount of electrically heterogeneous tissue and therefore predisposes to an increased susceptibility to reentrant arrhythmias in animals with experimental myocardial ischemia.

Delineation of Infarct Pattern: Magnetic Resonance Imaging

MRI is currently being employed widely in the study of the cardiovascular system.[18] The high soft tissue contrast allows discrimination among fat, pericardium, and myocardium, while the absence of signal from rapidly flowing blood in the lumen of blood vessels and in the cardiac chambers allows these structures to be clearly visualized without the aid of contrast agents.

Further useful information about pathological conditions of the heart is becoming available by exploiting the differences in T_1 and T_2 relaxation times. Recent investigations[18] have revealed that as early as 30 minutes after induction of ischemia there is prolongation of T_1 and T_2 relaxation times. In the early stages myocardial edema and inflammation are largely responsible for these observations which correlate with increased water content of ischemically damaged myocardium and remain significantly prolonged up to about 28 days post-infarction. Thereafter, T_1 and T_2 times tend towards the normal, but chronic infarcts (older than 56 days) are distinguished by diminished signal intensity and short T_2 times (relative to normal myocardium), presumably due to greater fibrous tissue content in these scars.

At the present, we are focusing on (1) accurate imaging of these scarred areas exploiting only the T_1 and T_2 differences and MRI parameters for maximal contrast, preferably without the use of paramagnetic contrast agents (e.g., gadolinium-DTPA which is taken up by only perfused tissue), and (2) quantitation of perimeter (or surface area) of the scar as well as its enclosed area (or volume). The following discussion deals solely with this latter objective of quantitating the three-dimensional surface area and volume of a selected region of interest (ROI).

Magnetic Resonance Imaging and Quantitation Methods

Images were obtained on a 1.89 T BIOSPEC spectrometer (Bruker Instruments, Billerica, MA). The probe used was a 10 cm diameter slotted-tube resonator tuned to 80.554 MHz for protons (1-H). Images were made with a multislice 2-D FT experiment,[19] using the first echoes acquired with a TE 27 ms and TR of 1.1 sec. All NMR slices of myocardium were 3.2 mm thick and separated by 2 mm. The resolution in the x and y dimensions was 0.4 mm/pixel. The 90° and 180° pulses were sinc-shaped and the total experiment duration to obtain the 16 slices was 8 minutes.

At autopsy, a patient's heart is placed in the probe, positioned within the 28.5 cm bore magnet as described above. Coronal slices at 5 mm intervals are taken of the ventricles from base to apex (16 total). For example, zoomed (2X) photographs of three sequential slices are shown (Figs. 2, 3, and 4). The bright area on the right ventricular wall of Figure 2 (suggestive of infarcted myocardium), is chosen as the region of interest (ROI).

The magnetic resonance image (Fig. 2), containing the ROI is then scanned by a Thunderscan™ image digitizer (Thunderware, Inc., Sunnyvale, CA). This infra-red scanner scans horizontally with nine vertical beams, at 200 dots/inch to digitally transfer the photographic data to the computer (Fig. 5). The scan parameters are magnification (2X), contrast 80%, and brightness 140%. The image is reversed (black and white) (Fig. 6) on the computer, and outlined by placing dots around all positive pixels (Fig. 7). Now, a mouse-controlled cursor is used to isolate a portion of the outlined image which represents the infarct, (the ROI), (Fig. 8, top). The outline of the ROI are pixels computer counted to give *perimeter*

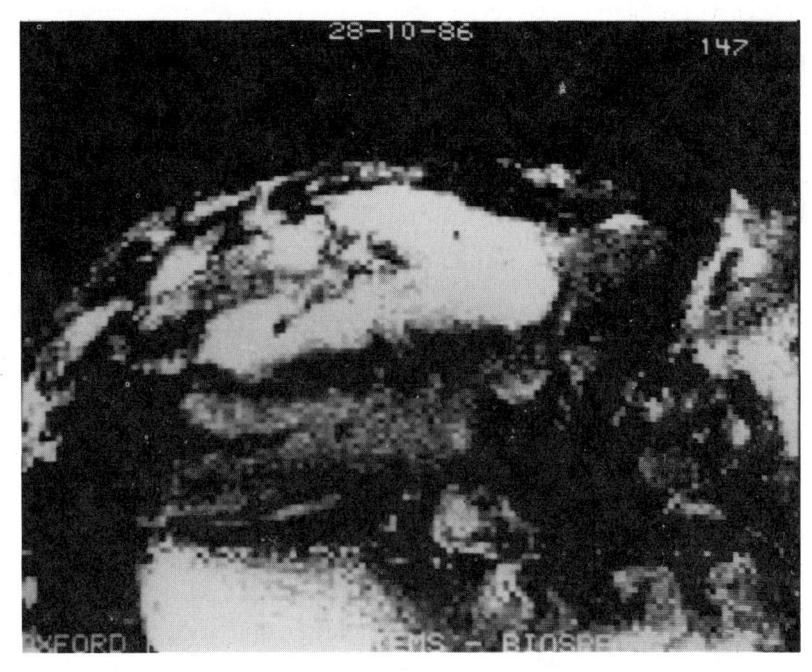

Figure 2: Zoomed portion (2X) of a magnetic resonance image of an isolated human heart. The slice is approximately 12 cm from the apex and 3.2 mm thick. The bright area on the right ventricular wall is nominated as a region of interest.

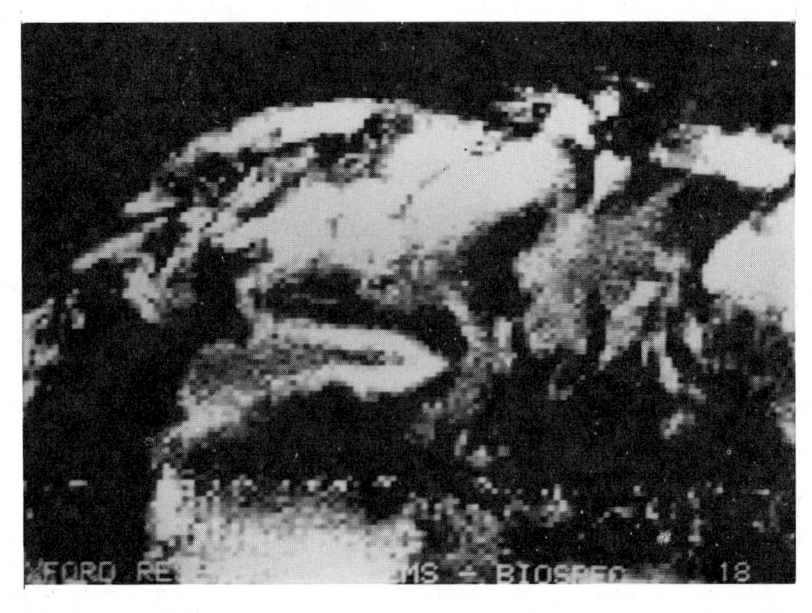

Figure 3: Zoomed portion (2X) of a magnetic resonance image of an isolated human heart. This slice is displaced approximately 2 mm from Figure 2, toward the apex.

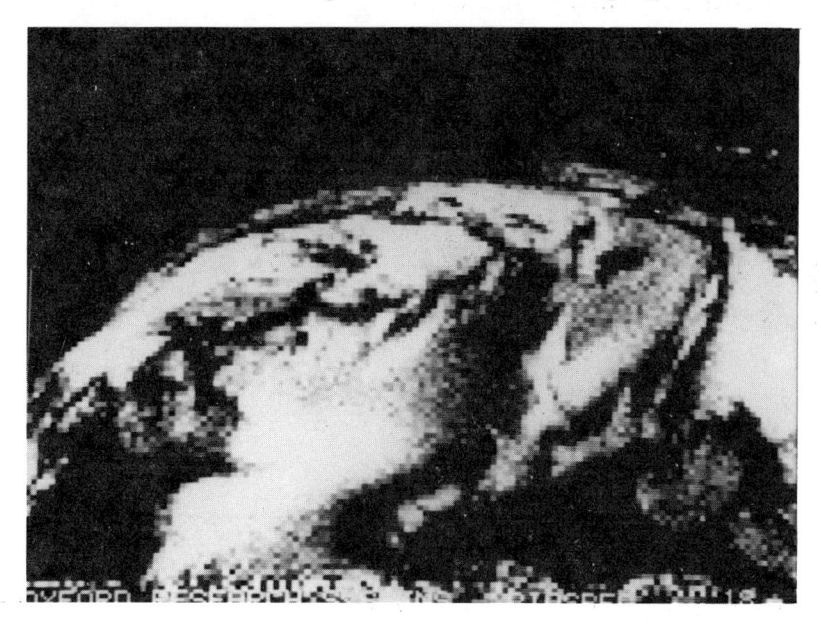

Figure 4: Zoomed portion (2X) of a magnetic resonance image of an isolated human heart. This slice is also displaced approximately 2 mm from Figure 3, toward the apex.

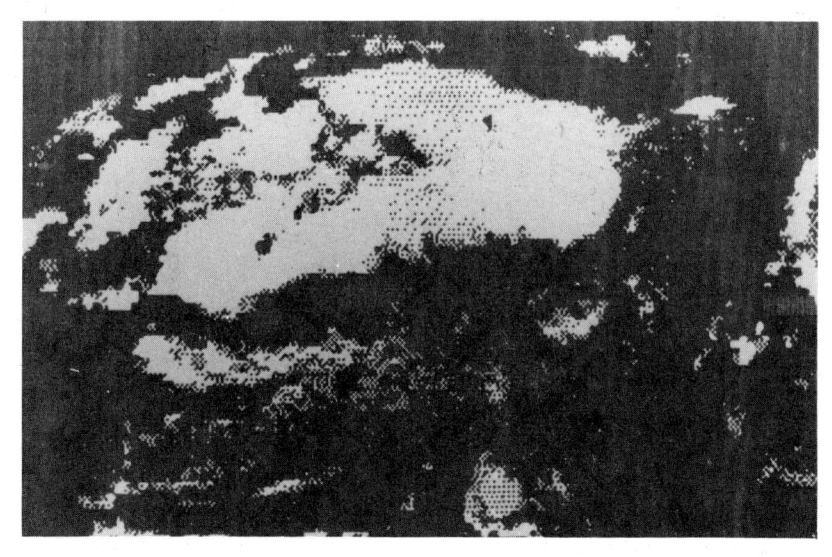

Figure 5: Digitized image of Figure 2. Digitization parameters are magnification (2X), contrast 80% and brightness 140%.

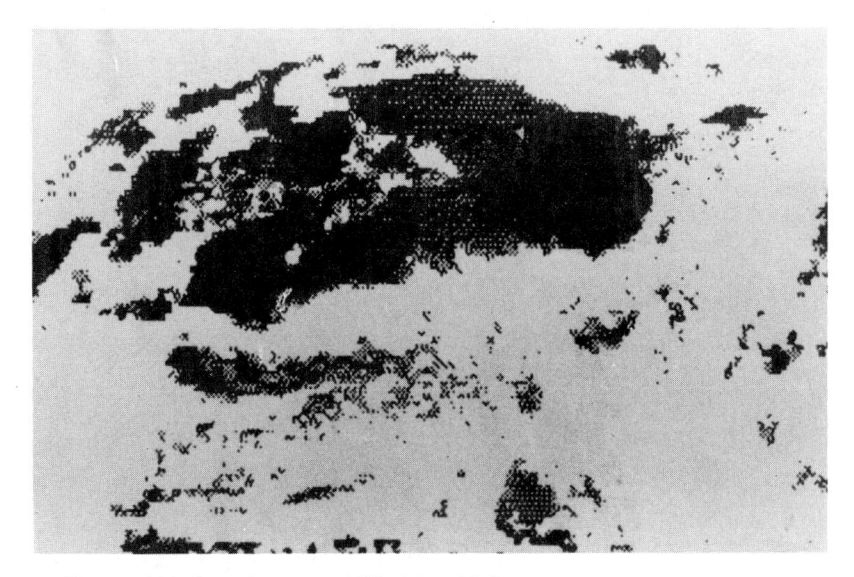

Figure 6: The previous figure is reversed (black to white).

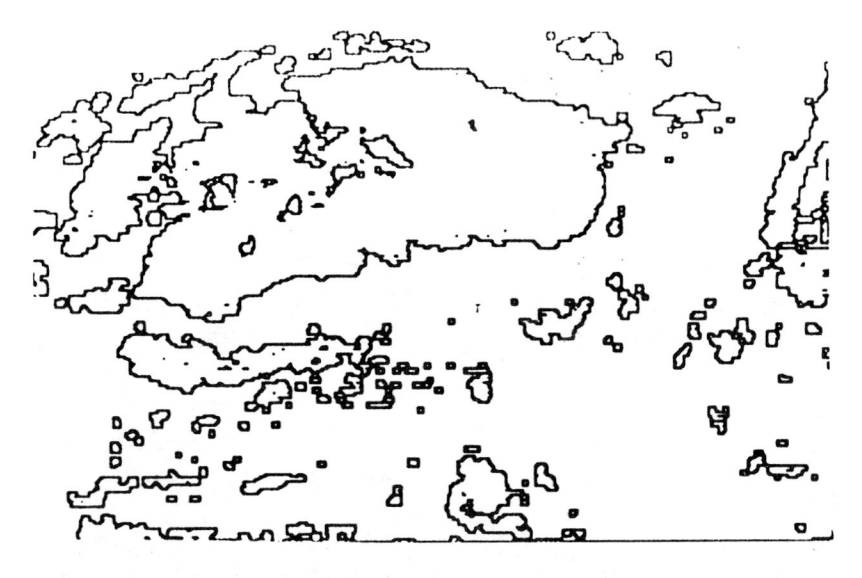

Figure 7: An outlined image, obtained by placing dots around all positive pixels of Figure 6.

lengths. The ROI is then completely filled with a pixel-grid (Fig. 8, bottom) and the number of pixels in the grid computer counted to give the *two-dimensional area* of the ROI. Any nonconfluent "islands" within the ROI have their perimeter lengths and areas computed separately.

Figure 9 shows the isolated ROIs from Figures 2, 3, and 4 as three-dimensional

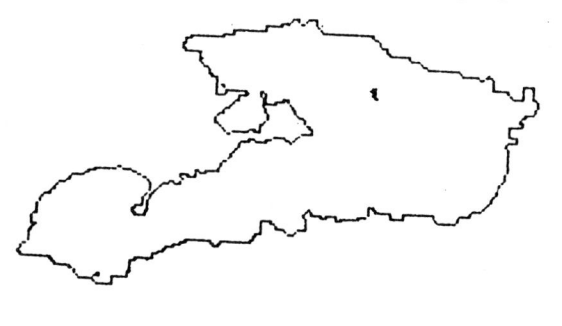

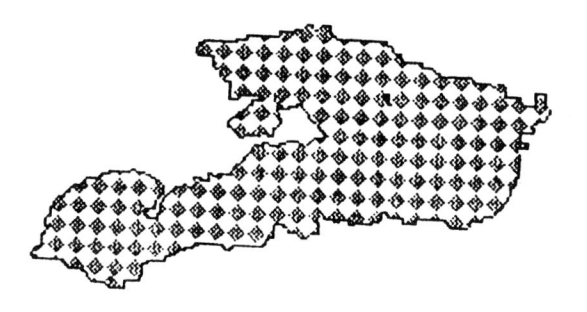

Figure 8: Top: The ROI is isolated. The pixels along the outline are computer counted to give the perimeter length. Bottom: The ROI is filled with a pixel-grid. The total number of pixels within the ROI are computer counted to give the two-dimensional area.

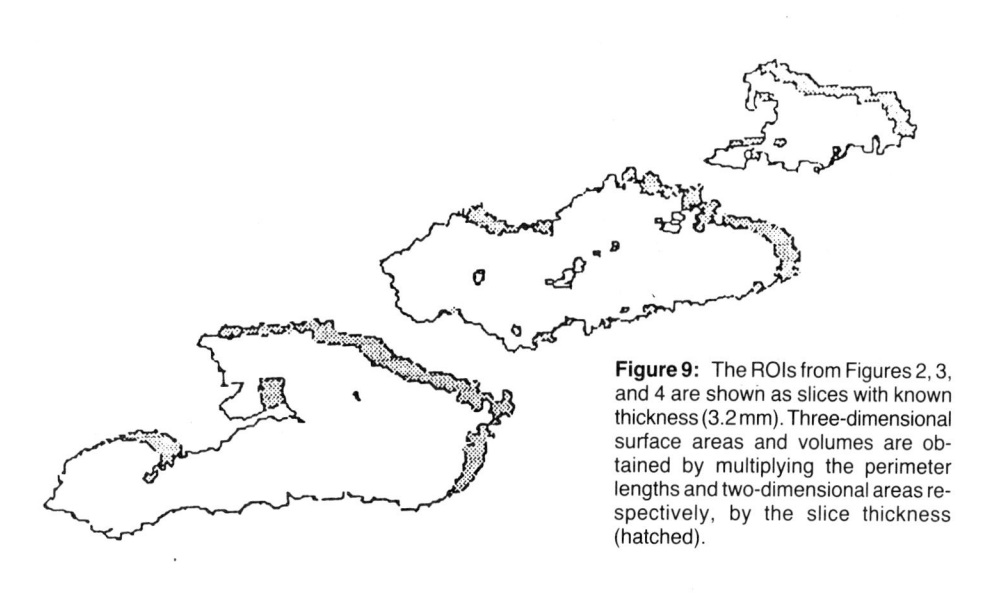

Figure 9: The ROIs from Figures 2, 3, and 4 are shown as slices with known thickness (3.2 mm). Three-dimensional surface areas and volumes are obtained by multiplying the perimeter lengths and two-dimensional areas respectively, by the slice thickness (hatched).

Table I
Three-Dimensional Surface Areas and Volumes for Figures 2, 3, and 4*

Figure	2	3	4
Perimeter (cms)	11.3	7.9	5.0
Two Dimensional Area (cm^2)	2.8	2.7	0.64
Slice Thickness (cm)		0.32	
Three Dimensional Surface Area (cm^2)	3.6	2.5	1.6
Volume (cm^3)	0.88	0.87	0.21

*Obtained by multiplying the perimeter lengths and two dimensional areas respectively, with the slice thickness (3.2 mm).

slices, and Table I lists three-dimensional surface areas and volumes that were obtained by multiplying the perimeters and two-dimensional areas, respectively, by the slice-thickness.

We conclude that animal models of actue myocardial ischemia produced in a heterogeneous pattern predispose to ventricular instability and ventricular tachyarrhythmias. We present a noninvasive method of delineating the perimeter, three-dimensional surface area, and volume of any selected region of interest. We continue our efforts to obtain many more, progressively thinner slices, with high x, y spatial resolution, to obtain better approximations to the true surface area and volume.

References

1. Ruskin JN, DiMarco JP, Garan H. Out-of-hospital cardiac arrest. N Engl J Med 1980; 303:607–613.
2. Grube SM: Instantaneous and sudden deaths: Clinical and pathological differentiation in coronary artery disease. JAMA 1973;225:1319–1328.
3. Mason JW, Winkle RA. Accuracy of the ventricular tachycardia induction study for predicting long-term efficacy and inefficacy of anti-arrhythmic drugs. N Engl M Med 1980;303:1973.
4. Boineau JL, Cox JF. Slow ventricular activation in acute myocardial infarction. Circulation 1973;48:702.
5. Wong SS, Bossett AL, Cameron JS, et al. Dissimilarities in the electrophysiologic abnormalities of lateral border and central infarct zone cells after healing of myocardial infarction in cats. Circ Res 1982;51:486.
6. Bukauskas F. Electrophysiology of the normal-to-hypoxic transition zone. Circ Res 1982;51:321.
7. Janse MJ, Cinca J, Morena H, et al. The "borderzone" in myocardial ischemia. Circ Res 1979;44:576.
8. Karagueuzian HS, Fenoglio JJJ, Weis MB, et al. Protracted ventricular tachycardia induced by premature stimulation of the canine heart after coronary artery occlusion and reperfusion. Circ Res 1979;44:833.
9. Michelson EL, Spear JE, Moore EN. Electrophysiologic and anatomic correlates of sustained ventricular tachyarrhythmias in a model of chronic myocardial infarction. Am J Cardiol 1980;45:583.

10. Wetstein L, Michelson EL, Simson MB, Harken AH. Increased normoxic-to-ischemic tissue borderzone as the cause for re-entrant ventricular tachyarrhythmias. J Surg Res 1982;32:526.
11. Mason JW, Winkle RA. Electrode-catheter arrhythmia induction in the selection and assessment of anti-arrhythmic drug therapy for recurrent ventricular tachycardia. Circulation 1978;58:971.
12. Vandepol CJ, Farshidi A, Spielman SR, Greenspun AM, Horowitz LN, Josephson ME. Incidence and clinical significance of induced ventricular tachycardia. Am J Cardiol 1980;45:725–731.
13. Graboys TB, Lown B, Podrid PJ, DeSilva RA. Survival of patients with malignant ventricular arrhythmia treated with anti-arrhythmic agents (abstr). Circulation 1979; 60:II–255.
14. Harken AH, Horowitz LN, Josephson ME. The surgical treatment of ventricular tachycardia. Ann Thorac Surg 1980;30:499–508.
15. Barlow CH, Harken AH, Chance B. Evaluation of cardiac ischemia by NADH fluorescence of photography. Ann Surg 1977;186:737.
16. Harken AH, Barlow CH, Harden WR III, Chance B. Two and three dimensional display of myocardial ischemic "borderzone" in dogs. Amer J Cardiol 1978;42:954–959.
17. Wetstein L, Michelson E, Euler D, Simson M, Spear J, Nattel S, Josephson M, Moore EN, Harken AH. Mechanism and surgical therapy of re-entrant ventricular tachyarrhythmias. Surg Forum 1981;32:266–268.
18. Higgins CB, and McNamara MT. Magnetic Resonance Imaging of Ischemic Heart Disease. Prog Cardiovascular Diseases 1986;28:257–266.
19. Edelstein WA, Hutchison JMS, Johnson G, Redpath T. Spin-warp imaging. Phys Med Biol 1980;25:751–756.

50

Characterizing Cardiac Ion Channels Using the Bilayer Reconstitution Technique

Joseph A. Hill, Jr.
Harold C. Strauss

Introduction

The advent of single channel recording techniques has extended the purview of cardiac electrophysiology to the level of molecular and atomic events. Using these techniques, investigators are able to observe directly the amplitude and duration of elementary current pulses that occur upon channel opening. From such observations, inferences can be made concerning the molecular mechanisms of channel gating and ionic permeation. These inferences, then, are clues that help define the structure-function relationships of ionic channels. An understanding of channel function can settle controversies not answered by lower resolution macroscopic current measurements. Single channel studies pose new questions and provide agendas for future research. Ultimately, they help us understand the roles channels play in excitable membrane physiology and pathology and provide a substrate for the development of new therapeutic modalities.

Currently there are two techniques at the channel biophysicist's disposal for recording single channel current: patch clamp recording and channel reconstitution.[1] Patch clamping[2] involves electrical isolation of a small patch of native cell membrane and the measurement of transmembrane current at high gain. The experimenter may either excise the patch or leave it in contact with the cell

From: Brugada P, Wellens HJJ. CARDIAC ARRHYTHMIAS: Where To Go From Here? Mount Kisco, NY, Futura Publishing Company, Inc., © 1987.

(cell-attached patch). If the isolated patch is small enough, it will contain only one or several channels. Channel reconstitution, in contrast, involves the biochemical isolation of channel protein and incorporation of the protein into an artificial membrane environment. Under appropriate conditions, one can reconstitute one or several channels and record unitary current. Thus, these two methodologies have obvious similarities. However, their relative strengths and weaknesses dictate the role each plays in the elucidation of different aspects of channel physiology.

In this chapter, we review basic aspects of single channel reconstitution technology. We outline the issues that can be addressed using single channel techniques, particularly as they relate to cardiac tissues. These issues are divided into conduction mechanisms and gating mechanisms. Finally, we summarize the limitations of current reconstitution technology.

The Reconstitution Technique

Langmuir and Waugh[3] were the first to study the formation of lipid membranes. Then, only a few years after the foundations of modern electrophysiology were laid by Hodgkin and Huxley,[4] efforts to reconstruct electrical excitation phenomena in model membranes began. Mueller et al.[5] introduced a system consisting of a septum with a hole in it capable of supporting a planar bilayer separating two aqueous solutions. These investigators demonstrated that the electrical capacitance of the lipid film was consistent with that of a molecular bilayer. In 1969, planar bilayer studies provided the first direct observations of ionic current through single ion channels.[6]

Today, the reconstitution technique has been used to study channels from many different tissues including sarcoplasmic reticulum,[7,8] skeletal muscle transverse tubule,[9] electroplax organ,[10] brain microsomes,[11] and cardiac sarcolemma[12,13] to name a few. The first and most detailed studies to date were directed at a voltage-dependent K channel from skeletal muscle sarcoplasmic reticulum.[7,8] One of the least well-characterized systems presently is the heart. Coronado and Latorre[12] were the first to investigate cardiac membranes; they identified three K channels and one Cl channel, all of which exhibited the complex kinetics of long, silent closed states and "noisy" open states. A monovalent cation channel from cardiac sarcoplasmic reticulum with properties similar to one from skeletal muscle has been described.[13-16] In addition, calcium channels from cardiac membranes have been studied in model membranes systems.[17,18]

The first step in channel reconstitution is the isolation of vesiculated membrane fragments. Cells from the tissue of interest are disrupted, and the cytoplasmic proteins solubilized and discarded. Membrane microsomes are then prepared. In cardiac tissue, the membrane microsomes come from three primary sources: surface sarcolemma, sarcoplasmic reticulum, and mitochondrial membranes. These three types of vesicle are separated on the basis of density using a differential density centrifugation procedure. At the same time, the vesicles are loaded with an osmotic agent (e.g., sucrose).

Artificial bilayers (also referred to as planar lipid bilayers and black lipid films) can be prepared in a number of ways. Probably the most common technique is "painting" Mueller-Rudin type bilayers.[5] In this approach, phospholipid is dispersed in a solvent (usually an n-alkane such as decane) and spread across a small (50–300 μm diameter) aperture. This lipid-decane suspension will spontaneously transform into a heterogeneous system consisting of a planar bimolecular membrane and decane-lipid suspension excluded to a surrounding annulus and to microlenses. A stable Mueller-Rudin bilayer will last several hours. All records illustrated here were made using this technique.

Bilayers for reconstitution can also be prepared using a "folding" technique.[19] Lipid monolayers, formed at the air-water interface of two aqueous solutions, can be apposed across a tiny aperture and coalesced into a "folded," alkane-free bilayer. These planar membranes are typically large (like Mueller-Rudin bilayers) but offer the potential advantage of not requiring decane. In addition, it is possible to form bilayers assymetric in lipid. Protein incorporation, however, involves exposing the protein to a monolayer environment with unknown consequences.

Small bilayers can be formed at the tips of patch-type pipettes ("tip-dip" technique).[20] This strategy offers the distinct advantages of low input capacitance (low noise) and excellent frequency response. However, the probability of a fusion event declines with the decrease in surface area; this technique is difficult to use with a "non-fusogenic" preparation. Finally, spherical bilayers can be prepared and patch recordings made from the vesicle surface.[21] This technique offers frequency response advantages similar to the tip-dip technique. Disadvantages include having to expose the protein to detergent and/or several freeze-thaw steps.

With Mueller-Rudin bilayers, vesicle protein is usually incorporated by vesicle fusion with the bilayer. After preparing the vesicles, they are added to the aqueous solution on one side (termed the *cis* chamber) of the bilayer (Fig. 1). This bath is connected to a voltage-command signal. The bath on the other side of the bilayer (termed *trans*) is connected to a current-to-voltage converter circuit and is thereby held at virtual ground. A vesicle will fuse with the bilayer when all of the following conditions obtain: (1) osmotic gradient across the bilayer such that water moves *trans* to *cis*, (2) osmotic gradient across the vesicle such that the vesicles swell, and (3) the presence of divalent cations in the *cis* chamber.[22,23] Importantly, the orientation of a particular channel protein tends to be uniform between experiments.[24] By measuring transmembrane current at high gain (10^9

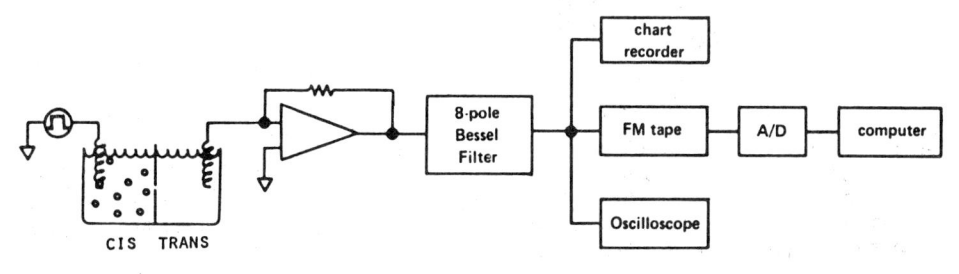

Figure 1: Schematic diagram of the planar bilayer system in our laboratory.

782 • CARDIAC ARRHYTHMIAS

V/A), one observes rectangular current pulses that represent channel openings and closings (Fig. 2). This current signal is low-pass filtered and recorded for subsequent analysis (usually computer-aided).

Properties of Ionic Channels

Channels are enzymes; they function to reduce the energy barrier that separates two chemical species and thereby catalyze the forward and backward rates of a chemical reaction. The reaction is the transmembrane movement of various ionic species; the parameter of interest is reaction rate (i.e., current). In the absence of channels, the rate of transmembrane ionic diffusion (across an area of

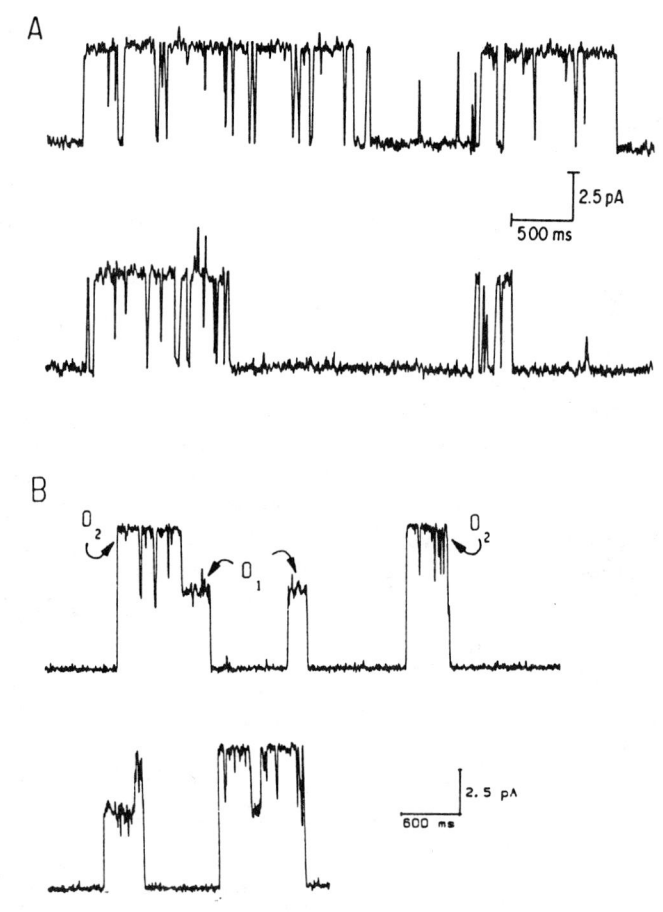

Figure 2: Single channel records of reconstituted cardiac channels. Panel A: cardiac sarcolemmal calcium-activated channel; experimental conditions: *cis* [K] = 73 mM, *trans* [K] = 50 mM, [Ca^{2+}] less than 100 nM; open = up, amplitude = 4.95 pA, bandwidth = 100 Hz (taken from Hill et al.[57]). Panel B: cardiac sarcoplasmic reticulum K channel with two open states (0_1, 0_2) indicated; open = up, amplitudes = 4.1 pA (0_1), 7.6 pA (0_2), bandwidth = 100 Hz.

membrane equivalent to that occupied by a large protein molecule) is on the order of 10^{-4} ions/s or 10^{-11} pA (1 pA = 10^{-12} A). The rate of ionic diffusion through a channel is on the order of tens of picoamps, an increase of 10^{12}. Current as a function of driving force is usually quantified in terms of conductance (inverse resistance) derived as the slope of a current versus voltage (I-V) plot.

Viewed from this perspective, many classic features of enzymatic reactions are manifest in the permeation reaction. For example, permeation exhibits saturation kinetics with substrate (ion) concentration. Permeation can be competitively inhibited by substrate analogues (blockers), and the reaction shows tight substrate specificity (ionic selectivity). Channels undergo rapid conformational changes to nonconducting "off" states; examples of traditional enzymes that undergo similar conformational changes include hemoglobin[1,25] and superoxide dismutase.[26] This "on–off" transition in channels, termed *gating*, can be influenced by a variety of physiologic and nonphysiologic parameters. Membrane potential, chemical ligands (e.g., acetylcholine, Ca^{2+}, amino acids, adenine nucleotides), temperature, and covalent chemical modification can modulate gating kinetics in certain channels.

As with conduction, the analysis of gating is usually couched in terms of a chemical reaction. Here the reactant(s) are closed state(s) and the product(s) are open state(s). For example,

$$C_1 \underset{\beta}{\overset{\alpha}{\rightleftharpoons}} C_2 \underset{\delta}{\overset{\gamma}{\rightleftharpoons}} 0 \qquad \text{(scheme I)}$$

where C_1 and C_2 are closed states 1 and 2, respectively, and 0 represents the open state.

Interesting aspects of the gating reaction include rate (rates of transition between each of the states) and more. These rates, however, are different from the traditional definition; obviously, it no longer makes sense to speak in terms of moles of reactant being converted per unit time. Rather, we wish to quantify a "rate" that is occurring within a single molecule. Therefore, reaction rate is quantified as a probability, or the chance that the molecule under study will undergo a reaction step in any given unit of time. Thus, for example, the rate constant γ for the reaction $C_2 \to 0$ in scheme I is measured in units of time^{-1}. In addition to reaction rate, the numbers of reactants and products (numbers of states), concentrations of reactants [dwell time in the closed state(s)], and products [dwell time in the open state(s)] all reveal important aspects of the underlying molecular processes. In this formulation, the units of concentration are units of time.

Ionic channels have been categorized into four classes.[27] *Ion-selective* channels select for ions of a certain electric charge and exhibit substantial selectivity among ions of that charge. The Na, K, and Cl channels involved in action potential generation in nerve and muscle are familiar examples of these. In general, these channels have conductances on the order of 10 pS in the presence of 0.1 M salt. *Valence-selective* channels are absolutely selective for ions of a given charge but show little discrimination among ions of that charge. Examples from this group include the acetylcholine receptor of the neuromuscular junction and the gramicidin A channel. Channels in the *nonselective* group are highly conductive and relatively nonselective. K-selective channels comprise a fourth group; they are highly conductive channels from animal cell membranes. These *maxi-K* channels greatly favor K permeation over other monovalent cations, yet conduct in the range of 130–200 pS in the presence of 0.1 M K.

Channels can also be categorized according to general features of their conduction and gating mechanisms. Categories based on gating properties include ligand-gated channels and voltage-dependent channels. Alternatively, other schemes divide channels into single-ion, multiple-ion, free diffusion, and multiple-ion single file depending upon the mechanisms of ionic permeation.

Experimental Characterization of Ionic Channels

The Conduction Process

The goals of investigating mechanisms of channel-mediated ion transport are (1) to elucidate the ways in which ions and drugs interact with the channel during ionic permeation, and (2) to elucidate crucial aspects of channel geometry. These goals are achieved by studying the conduction reaction's rate, specificity, concentration-dependence, temperature-dependence, and inhibition by channel blockers.

Single Channel Current

Unitary channel current from two different K-conducting channels reconstituted from canine ventricular microsomes is shown in Figure 2. In panel A, a sarcolemmal channel exhibiting Ca-dependent gating kinetics is shown. Note the bursting pattern of the open state. Channel openings are punctuated by short-lived closures and separated by very long-lived closures. In panel B, a K-conducting channel from cardiac sarcoplasmic reticulum is depicted. The bursting kinetics pattern is absent here. Rather, we see two degrees of "openness," labeled 0_1 and 0_2.

Unitary current through the calcium-activated channel (Fig. 2, panel A) is plotted as a function of holding potential in Figure 3. This I-V relation, recorded under bi-ionic conditions (see below), is linear. A linear I-V relation is that expected of a simple resistor, and is said to be ohmic. A best fit line is shown superimposed on the data whose slope is 120 pS.

Channel Selectivity

A great deal of valuable information can be gleaned from the study of ionic selectivity.[28] First of all, selectivity serves as the most commonly used basis for distinguishing different types of channels (e.g., Na, Ca, and K channels). Second,

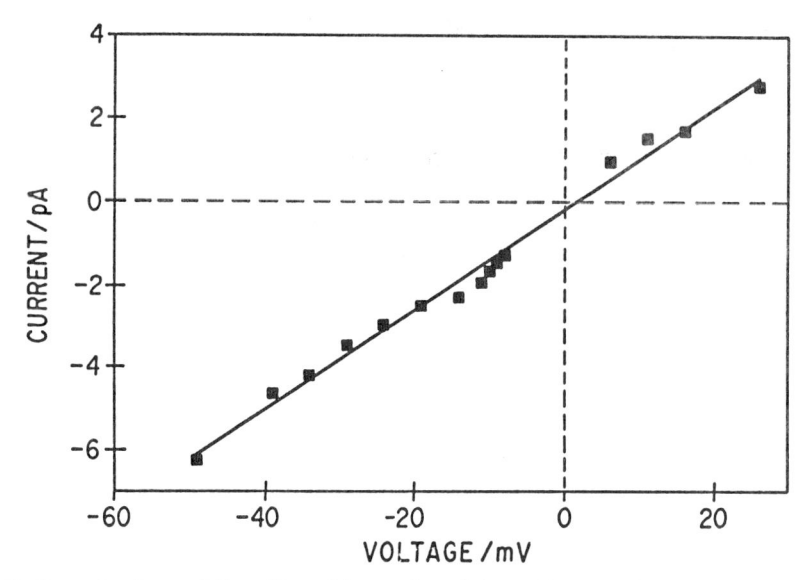

Figure 3: Current-voltage relation of the calcium-activated channel from ventricular muscle; experimental conditions: 100 mM NaOAc *cis*, 100 mM KOAc *trans*. A fitted line is superimposed (slope = 120 pS, x-intercept = +2 mV) (taken from Hill et al.[57]).

selectivity analysis sheds light on the anatomy of the channel protein, both in physical terms (steric interactions between ion and channel) and in functional terms (electrical interactions). The part of the conduction pathway in which selectivity takes place (if regarded as a single discrete location) is operationally termed the selectivity filter. The goal, in summary, is to learn about the selectivity filter's dimensions and structure and its location within the electric field.

There are two general approaches to the study of selectivity, and each method addresses a different aspect of the process.[7,27] Comparing single channel conductances in the presence of a series of ionic species along a column of the periodic table (plus other ions of similar size and hydrated radius) characterizes selectivity under steady state conditions. Measuring ratios of permeabilities addresses selectivity as an equilibrium process.

Permeability ratios are conveniently measured by bathing the membrane with ions of one type (x) on the *cis* side and ions of another type (y) on the *trans* side (termed bi-ionic conditions). The zero-current ("crossover") potential under such asymmetric ionic conditions is determined by interpolation. By assuming ionic independence and involving the Goldman-Hodgkin-Katz equation, the permeability ratio (P_y/P_x) is seen to be a function of the "crossover" potential, V_o:

$$P_y/P_x = (\alpha_x/\alpha_y) \exp(FV_o/RT) \qquad (a)$$

where α_x, (α_y) represents the activity of ion x (y), F is the Faraday constant, R is the gas constant, and T is absolute temperature. This permeability ratio is independent of ion concentration for both free diffusion pores and single-ion pores.

The permeability ratio is, in general, a function of ionic activity for multi-ion pores.

Conduction as a Function of Concentration

For most ionic channels, unitary conductance reaches a maximum value as ion activity increases. For single-ion channels, conductance obeys single saturation kinetics and follows a Michaelis-Menten hyperbola:

$$\gamma_i = \frac{\gamma_i^{max}\, \alpha_i/K_i}{1 + \alpha_i/K_i} \quad (b)$$

where γ_i^{max} represents the maximum conductance of ion (i), α_i is the activity of ion i, and K_i is the apparent dissociation constant. Analogous to conventional enzyme reactions, the initial slope of the saturation curve (γ_i^{max}/K_i) models the biomolecular reaction of an ion entering the channel from aqueous solution. In the limit of very high ion concentration, γ_i^{max} represents the first-order process of the ion leaving the channel. For the case of multiple-ion channels (e.g., gramicidin A),[29] conductance increases linearly at first. At large concentrations, however, conductance may actually decrease as all binding sites become filled, and permeant ions block their own passage through the pore.

The delayed rectifier K channel of the squid giant axon exhibits a biphasic conductance-activity relation.[30] Conductance initially increases steeply with K activity and then gradually reaches a linear phase. Such behavior is characteristic of a special type of multiple-ion pore, the multiple-ion, single file channel.

Temperature Effects

Ionic flux past the selectivity filter requires energy and this energy can be divided into two parts: electrical and nonelectrical terms. Maximal conductance can be taken as a measure of the rate constant of this flux. This rate constant for ion i (k_i) is expressed in terms of absolute rate theory:

$$k_i = v \exp(-\Delta G_i^*/RT) \quad (c)$$

where v is the attempt (vibration) frequency, ΔG_i^* is the activation free energy in the usual RT units. This free energy term has both enthalpic and entropic components:

$$\Delta G^* = \Delta H^* - T\Delta S^* \quad (d)$$

where ΔH^* and ΔS^* are the activation enthalphy and entropy, respectively. Combine these two relations, and plot $\ln k_i$ versus $1/T$ to obtain an Arrhenius plot. The slope of this plot depends on ΔH^* and not on ΔS^*. In other words, the enthalpic contribution to the activation energy for a given transition will determine its temperature dependence. As expected, the activation enthalpy for aqueous conductivity of alkali metal cations is a relatively small 4.3–4.5 kcal/mole.[31]

Lipid Charge Effects

The extent to which lipid charge affects channel behavior is a function of the electrostatic interaction between lipid head groups and the channel protein. This interaction is modulated by screening ions, neutralization of lipid charge by binding substances, and by the physical distance between lipid charge and an active site within the protein. In other words, the interaction is a function of the surface potential set up by the charged lipid components in the bilayer and the extent to which the channel protein senses that surface potential.

It is known that cation concentration at the surface of a negatively charged membrane is much higher than that in the bulk solution.[32] Such variations in concentration affect channel function by effectively shifting the conductance along the conductance-activity curve (these effects are quantified by the Gouy-Chapman-Stern treatment[33] of the electrified interface). In reconstitution experiments, single channel conductance recorded from bilayers composed of negatively charged phospholipid (e.g., phosphatidylserine, phosphatidylglycerol, phosphatidic acid) will be greater than that from neutral membranes (phosphatidylcholines, phosphatidylethanolamines, cholesterol). The magnitude of the increase is a measure of the effective surface potential sensed by the mouth of the channel protein. If the mouth of the channel protrudes out of the plane of the membrane, then some of the surface potential will exert no influence. At the same time, lateral separation of the pore entryway from the negatively charged lipid in the plane of the membrane may partially screen the protein from the profile. This separation, in turn, may be due to the size of the channel protein or the presence of tightly bound native phospholipid that accompanied the channel into the bilayer.

Channel Blockers

There are many substances that when presented to an ionic channel fail to permeate; some of these substances also prevent the permeation of ions through the pore and are called blockers. By analyzing the effects of a number of blockers of widely varying sizes, dimensions, and charge, one can gain insight into the architecture of the selectivity filter and the binding site of the blocker. For instance, what are the dimensions of the filter, and what is its effective charge? Where is the blocker binding site located, and is it the same site at which a permeating ion transiently binds in its journey through the pore? Is the selectivity filter the site at which permeant ions bind in a rate-limiting fashion? Lastly, blockade experiments will serve in the future as a valuable assay for the investigation and development of therapeutic channel blockers.

Analysis of the Site of Blockade

Voltage Dependence: A common feature of ionic blockers is their ability to transform a linear current-voltage relation into a highly nonlinear one. This effect is termed voltage-dependence of block and reflects the interaction of a charge blocker compound with a binding site within the electric field of the diffusion pathway. A quantitative analysis of this phenomenon has been offered by Woodhull.[34] In this analysis it is assumed that there exists a single site S somewhere within the channel that can bind a blocker B.

$$S + B \underset{k_{-1}}{\overset{k_1}{\rightleftharpoons}} SB \qquad \text{(scheme II)}$$

This reaction is taken to be sensitive to voltage according to the following:

$$K_D(V) = k_{-1}/k_1 \qquad (e)$$

where $K_D(V)$ is a voltage-dependent dissociation constant for the reaction. One can then derive an expression relating open channel probability [P(open)] to the dissociation constant at zero voltage $K_D(0)$ such that:

$$P(\text{open}) = \{1 + \{[B]/K_D(0)\} \exp(z\delta FV/RT)\}^{-1} \qquad (f)$$

where S is located the fractional distance δ down the electric field and senses a fraction δV of the total applied potential V. Here z is the valence of the blocking ion.

For the case of single-ion channels, the power dependence of blocker concentration $z\delta$ is less than 1. Some channels, however, have experimentally derived $z\delta$ values greater than 1. The delayed rectifier of squid giant axon, for example, apparently senses a fraction of the total applied potential that is greater than 1.[30] This observation is interpreted to indicate that more than one blocking ion binds to the channel at a time. It is consistent with the notion that this channel is a multiple-ion channel in which the ions are constrained to move in a single file.

Some blockers form blocked states that are short-lived with respect to the frequency response of the amplifier (Fig. 4). In these circumstances, one expects to observe only an average apparent open-state conductance equal to the time average of true open and true blocked conductances.[35] If Cs block (of a K channel, for instance) results from a single-site interaction with the channel, then the inhibition should follow a titration curve of the form:

$$\frac{\gamma}{\gamma_o} = \{1 + Cs/K_D(V)\}^{-1} \qquad (g)$$

where γ signifies channel conductance at a given Cs concentration, γ_o signifies channel conductance in the absence of Cs, and $K_D(V)$ is the dissociation constant of the blocking reaction at a given potential. If one further assumes that voltage

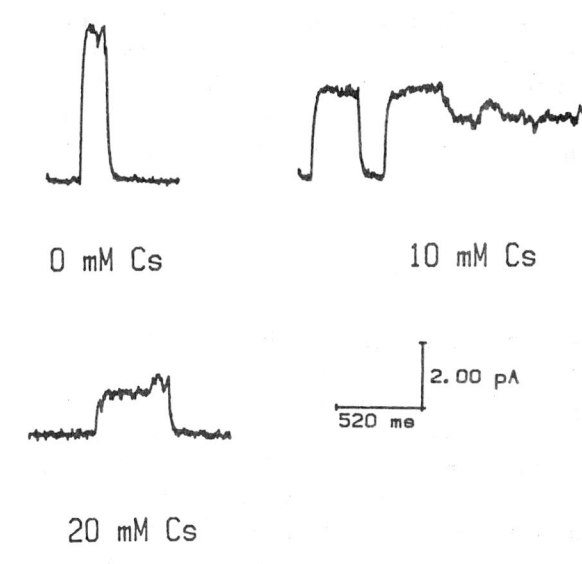

Figure 4: Single channel records of the cardiac sarcoplasmic reticulum K channel; experimental conditions: 100 mM KOAc symmetrical with Cs added as indicated, open = up. Current amplitudes (0_2, 0_1) are 5.44, 3.29 pA (control, 0_1 not shown); 2.65, 1.74 pA (10 mM Cs); 1.71, 1.28 pA (20 mM Cs), bandwidth = 60 Hz.

dependence results from the blocking ion's moving into the transmembrane electric field, then the fraction of channel-mediated conductance not blocked by Cs should be described by the following expression (compare with equation f):

$$\frac{\gamma}{\gamma_o} = \{1 + \{ [Cs]/K_D(0) \} \exp (\delta FV/RT) \}^{-1} \quad \text{(h)}$$

Lastly, if one assumes that both *cis* and *trans* Cs reach the binding site for blockade, then K_D's for both the *cis* and *trans* reactions may be calculated from this analysis.[35,36]

Analysis of the Site of Blockade

Competition of Block: Classical Michaelis-Menten analysis of blockade provides useful information concerning the importance of competitive versus non-competitive mechanisms. Reciprocal single channel conductance is plotted as a function of reciprocal ionic activity. Provided that a linear relation is derived, a dissociation constant for blocker binding may be calculated, and competitive versus noncompetitive aspects of the reaction revealed.

Probing the Structural Features of the Channel

Hille and co-workers[37,38] and Miller and Coronado[39,40] have pioneered the use of ions of a varying size to probe the structural features of the selectivity filter. Using compounds widely varying cross-sectional area, these investigators have measured selectivity filter dimensions in a K channel in nerve[37] and the sarcoplasmic reticulum K channel of skeletal muscle.[39,40] By analyzing conductance as a function of molecular cross-sectional area, they have determined the critical dimension beyond which channel conductance drops sharply. They have interpreted this to represent the dimension beyond which steric hindrance prevents ionic permeation.

Eyring Rate Theory Analysis

A useful approach to the understanding of channel-mediated ion transport is to model the process as the movement of an ion over a series of kinetic barriers within the diffusion pathway. Eyring absolute rate theory focuses on the high energy transition state of ion movement across the energy barriers to derive expressions for the rates of ion movement through the pore. Thus, the conduction pathway is modeled as a corrugated energy profile of energy peaks and wells. This analysis has been extended to the case of single ion channels with an arbitrary number of barriers and wells by Läuger.[41] Often it is useful to impose the simplifying assumption to the "peak energy offset condition" offered by Hille.[42] Here, all of the peak heights, measured relative to the outside solution, for a given ion are assumed to differ from those of a second ion by a constant free energy amount.

This type of analysis synthesizes much of the information gathered in the study of a particular channel's conduction properties. The number of ions allowed in the channel and the effective distance at which voltage-dependent block occurs (δ) are reasonable first guesses at the number of energy wells and their relative positions. There must, of course, be n + 1 energy barriers for the case of n wells.

The Gating Process

The ultimate goal of gating studies is to understand the molecular processes underlying the cellular regulation of ion flow. The fulfillment of this goal requires knowledge of the structural, biochemical, and electrophysiological properties of ionic channels. The channels from animal tissue about which we have detailed information in all three areas are the acetylcholine receptor[43,44] and the Na channel of nerve.[11,45]

Thermodynamics

Most channels exhibit complicated gating reactions; usually there are numerous open and closed states and these are often connected in complicated ways. Some reaction pathways may be voltage-dependent or ligand-dependent. Certain states may be "absorbing" (as the Na channel inactivated state). Some states may be very long-lived, up to tens or hundreds of seconds. Others are very short-lived, with time constants of a few microseconds. In fact, it is almost certainly true that most channels have gating states that are completely unresolvable by current recording technology.

These limitations are not absolute; certain aspects of the gating reaction can still be analyzed and useful information derived. For instance, short-lived open events may be lumped together with a short-lived "flicker" closed state to define a new state termed a "burst." This new "event" can then be treated as a true state and analyzed accordingly; rate constants and lifetimes can be calculated and assigned. This type of simplification is not only necessary, but has some justification for channels that spend a great deal of time in a few states. Simplification of the model to two or three "states" (each of which may comprise more than one physical state) is justified when just a few states are physiologically significant.

The following two-state reaction scheme serves as the starting point for most discussions of gating processes:

$$\text{closed} \underset{\beta(V)}{\overset{\alpha(V)}{\rightleftharpoons}} \text{open} \qquad \text{(scheme III)}$$

where $\alpha(V)$ and $\beta(V)$ are the voltage-dependent opening and closing rate constants, respectively. Such a simple two-state model is well suited to the application of straightforward equilibrium thermodynamic analysis. It may, in fact, represent one of the schemes to which a very complicated gating reaction is simplified. For example, such a scheme might be appropriate for a channel that displays one open and two closed states, one of which is a short-lived flicker closed state (e.g., C_1 and C_2 in scheme I).

As mentioned above, we think of the gating process as a chemical reaction wherein two species of different chemical energy are separated by an activation energy barrier. Applying the Boltzmann equation of these states (scheme III) indicates that:

$$\frac{n_{open}}{n_{closed}} = \exp\{-\Delta G/RT\} \qquad (i)$$

when n_{open} (n_{closed}) represents the number of channels open (closed), and ΔG is the total Gibbs free energy of the opening reaction. Rearrangement results in the familiar expression:

$$P(open) = \{1 + \exp(\Delta G/RT)\}^{-1} \qquad (j)$$

where P(open) denotes the probability of channel opening. If one then assumes that the total Gibbs free energy ΔG is composed of a "chemical" part ΔG_i and an electrical part (the energy difference of the dipole moments of the two protein conformations in the electrical field, zFV), then

$$\Delta G = \Delta G_i + zFV \qquad (k)$$

where z equals the effective gating charge.[46] Rearrangement reveals a linearized expression:

$$\ln\{[1-P(\text{open})]/P(\text{open})\} = \Delta G_i/RT + zFV/RT \qquad (1)$$

A plot of $\ln\{[1-P(\text{open})]/P[\text{open}]\}$ versus V should be linear and will determine both ΔG_i and z.

Opening probability for the calcium-activated channel is plotter versus holding potential in Figure 5. A theoretical relation as described above is superimposed. The fitted parameters indicate an effective gating charge (z) of -2.5 and a chemical energy of channel opening of -2.2 kcal/mole. The gating charge indicates that 2.5 negative charges move from the *trans* chamber to the *cis* chamber on channel opening. Negative Gibbs free energy indicates that the open state is preferred at 0 mV.

Kinetics

Clearly from the above, a kinetic analysis must go hand-in-hand with any thermodynamic analysis of the gating process. Initial analysis involves determining the number of open and closed states within the constraints outlined above. Then it is possible to estimate the rate constants to and from each state and determine which, if any, are voltage-dependent, ligand-dependent, or otherwise subject to metabolic control.

Channel gating is a binomial process in that (1) a channel is either open or closed, on or off, and (2) each gating transition is assumed to be statistically

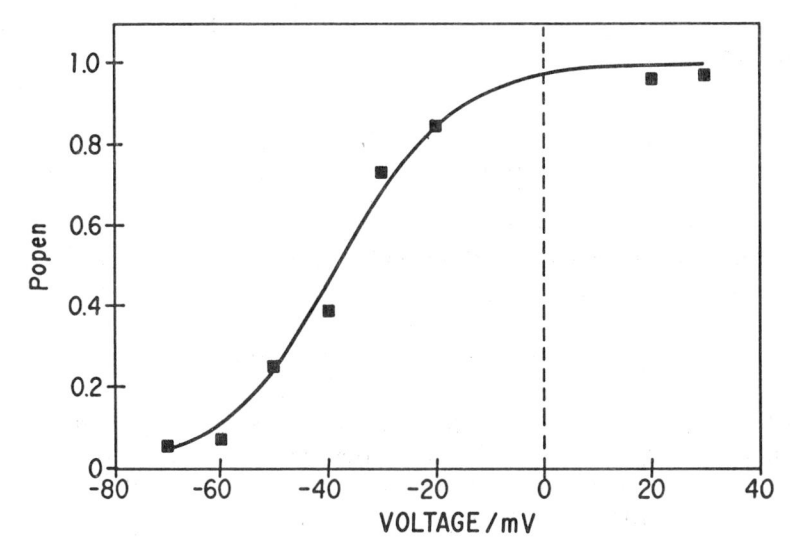

Figure 5: Calcium-activated channel open probability versus holding potential; experimental conditions: *cis* $[Ca^{2+}]$ is less than 100 nM; a curve of the form $P(\text{open}) = \{1 + \exp(\Delta G/RT)\}^{-1}$ (where $\Delta G = \Delta G_i + zFV$) is depicted, $z = -2.5$, $\Delta G_i = -2.2$ kcal/mole (taken from Hill et al.[57]).

independent of all other transitions. Thus, the gating reaction should be binomially distributed. It is known that as the binomial probability p approaches zero, the binomial distribution approaches a Poisson distribution. In fact, it is widely accepted that the Poisson distribution can be applied to the open and closed states of channel gating. It follows that if the gating reaction represents a Poisson process, then the waiting time t for the first occurrence of an opening or a closing transition is exponentially distributed.

Prob (channel stays open throughout the interval [0, t]) =

$$\text{Prob (open lifetime} > t) \text{ and is proportional to } \exp(-\alpha t) \qquad (m)$$

where α is the sum of the rate constants for all routes by which the open channel can be shut. Therefore, it follows that the mean open time equals $1/\alpha$ from

$$\int_0^\infty \alpha \cdot t \cdot \exp\{-\alpha t\} \, dt = 1/\alpha \qquad (n)$$

or equivalently, the mean open time equals the time constant τ of the open time probability distribution ($\tau = 1/\alpha$). This analysis is not unique to the open state but rather can be applied to closed states as well.

For the case of multiple open (or closed) states, the lifetime of each state will be exponentially distributed. Thus the total length of time spent open (closed) will be distributed as the sum of each individual open (closed) state's exponential distribution. This principle outlines, then, the first step in a kinetic analysis of channel gating; one must estimate the number of conducting and nonconducting states. This is accomplished by constructing an open (closed) state duration histogram and fitting the histogram with a probability density function which is the sum of an arbitrary number of exponential functions (Fig. 6). The time constant τ_i of each function i corresponds to the mean open (closed) time of conducting (nonconducting) state i.

It is also possible to estimate the number of events unresolved by the recording system. Assuming all of the missed events arise from the states defined by the event duration distributions, then it is a simple matter to calculate the expected frequency of an event of duration less than the resolution limit ϵ: the number of unresolved events equals

$$1 - P(t > \epsilon) = 1 - \int_\epsilon^\infty \alpha \exp\{-\alpha t\} \, dt = 1 - \exp\{-\alpha \cdot \epsilon\} \qquad (q)$$

Metabolic Regulation

There is a wide range of metabolic regulatory factors that modulate channel function in the heart. Protein phosphorylation is a mechanism of calcium channel regulation.[47] Adenosine triphosphate (ATP) has been shown to be an important

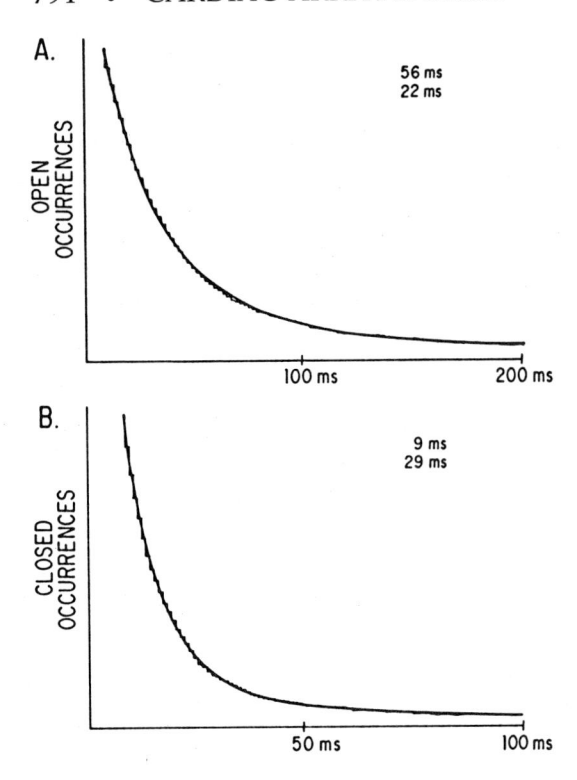

Figure 6: Cumulative event duration probability distributions for the open and closed states, calculated from a record with 1590 open events; experimental conditions: holding potential = −40 mV, same solutions as Figure 1. The sum of two exponential functions is superimposed on each histogram with time constants (ms) as indicated (taken from Hill et al.[57]).

regulatory factor for K channels in ventricular muscle.[48,49] Intracellular calcium ions regulate calcium-activated channels in nerve,[50,51] skeletal muscle,[52,53] smooth muscle,[54] and cardiac muscle.[55–57] Hydrogen ion activity also modulates channel gating. This effect is mediated by the protonation or deprotonation of crucial amino acid moieties on the channel protein and can serve as a tool for identifying important primary structural aspects of the channel. By varying pH and monitoring gating variables, one is able to determine the pKa of any effect observed and deduce from that which amino acids are involved. As before, it is important to impose experimental perturbations that are symmetric about the bilayer; pH must be changed on both sides of the membrane in order to avoid proton-induced asymmetries in surface potential.

Assumptions and Limitations of the Reconstitution Technique

The forte of the reconstitution approach is the high degree of control it affords over experimental variables. Single channel molecules are isolated and characterized in a chemically defined artificial membrane. The aqueous and electrical milieu can be completely controlled, and experimental perturbations can be varied independently. The effects of repeated solution changes on the same channel molecule can be investigated. Nominally identical channels from different tissues can be studied under identical conditions. With the discovery of highly specific, high-affinity ligands, reconstitution assists in the purification of channel proteins and in the elucidation of important structure-function relations (e.g., bungarotoxin, acetylcholine receptor;[43] tetrodotoxin, Na channel;[11,45] charybdotoxin, Ca-activated K channel[58]).

Thus the power of the isolation-reconstitution system is clear. It provides for the detailed characterization of complex mechanisms in a simplified system. Experimental manipulations can be imposed independently and with great precision on both sides of the membrane. In addition, channels that are inaccessible with the patch clamp technique may be studied in detail (e.g., transverse tubular and sarcoplasmic reticulum channels). Finally, the technique provides the important link to functional integrity in the biochemical characterization of transport proteins.

Assumptions

The single channel reconstitution technique invokes a number of assumptions. For example, it is implicitly assumed that the greatly simplified system for study of channel function is at least reminiscent of the physiological milieu of the native channel protein. Much could be learned about channel function even if this assumption were proved invalid, but the scientist must be cognizant of it when comparing reconstitution data with patch clamp experiments or cellular macroscopic currents.

Channels in bilayers are also assumed to incorporate irreversibly and with fixed orientation. Further, channels in bilayers are assumed to function independently of one another. Single channel data are assumed to correspond with ensemble average macroscopic currents in artificial membranes. These assumptions have been established in one system.[8]

Limitations

It is appropriate to question whether channels in bilayers behave as channels in native membranes. The extent to which they do determines how the observations are interpreted; if they behave very differently (for any of the reasons listed below), then extrapolations to native systems are clearly inappropriate.

Deleterious Effects of the Biochemical Fractionation Procedures

This is a serious concern, as channels are exposed to depolarizing conditions and to low ionic strength solutions. In addition, they may be exposed to proteolytic degradation as intracellular proteases are released and activated during cell lysis and membrane vesiculation. For these reasons, membrane isolations are generally performed in the cold (4°C) in order to decrease proteolytic enzyme activity. In addition, protease inhibitors are often included in the solutions.

Deleterious Effects of the Reconstitution Procedure: Some reconstitution procedures involve the use of detergents. Others extract surrounding lipid from the channel proteins and thus remove them from their membrane milieu. These methods are relatively harsh and great care must be exercised to insure that protein denaturation does not occur. Some methods, notably the fusion technique, are relatively mild by contrast; transfer of channels to the planar membrane occurs after native vesicles make contact with monolayers. The transfer is viewed as a "dilution" of the membrane fragment into a vast excess of bilayer phospholipids without involving the extraction of the channel from its native environment. Thus channel proteins never come in contact with detergent, and they do not leave the native membrane until reconstituted.

It is possible that some bilayer lipids or fatty acids may produce deleterious effects. The decane solvent used to suspend the phospholipid is also a potential problem as it may change or damage the channel protein structure; as volatile alkanes are anesthetics, the fear has arisen that solvent-containing bilayers might be anesthetized. Importantly, however, the composition of the bilayer is under experimental control. Further, studies of bilayers have shown that the apposed acyl chains on the lipid molecules tend to interdigitate and to exclude solvent molecules trapped in the film ("demixing") (for a review, see reference 59). Finally, channel studies have shown that such effects are relatively minor.[8]

Limited Bandwidth Considerations

Planar bilayer membranes used for reconstitution typically have 100–400 pF of capacitance. This represents a substantial amount of input capacitance for the current-to-voltage circuitry. Low-pass filtering is required in order to achieve an acceptable signal-to-noise ratio. As discussed above, one expects to miss any channel states of less than some fixed duration (hundreds of μs to a few ms). Large amounts of input capacitance also make the analysis of transient events more difficult to study as large capacitive transients obscure a portion of the experimental record. Many of these difficulties are avoided using bilayers of smaller capacitance as described earlier.

Correspondence Between Electrophysiology of Native Membranes and the Properties of Channels in Bilayers

Even after every attempt has been made to minimize deleterious effects on channels, channels incorporated into bilayers may display some properties not anticipated by studies of native membranes. Two variables that bear on this point are (1) the source of the membranes, and (2) the selection process that determines the type of channel transferred to the bilayer.

Contamination of sarcolemmal preparations with intracellular or peripheral membranes: Purity of plasma membranes is an important concern as contaminants, even if present in small quantities, may donate channels to the bilayer. Cardiac sarcolemma has been extensively characterized in terms of a variety of plasma membrane markers and markers for contaminating membranes.[60-62] For instance, a cardiac sarcolemmal preparation may contain, in addition to surface membrane, cleft and transverse-tubule membranes that have been shown to migrate with light surface membrane fractions from skeletal muscle.[63] A certain amount of sarcoplasmic reticulum and mitochondrial membrane contamination is expected as well.[60-62]

Selective incorporation of channels: There may be 10^6 and 10^7 channels in vesicles that are in contact with the surface of the bilayer. It is possible, however, to manipulate the experimental conditions to limit the number to one or two channels actually transferred. Thus, there is a tremendously selective reaction by which some channels incorporate rather easily while others do not. Studies of phospholipid interactions suggest that some forms of vesicles are "fusogenic," while others do not fuse easily. It is often possible to modulate fusion rate by varying the lipid or solvent composition of the bilayer. However, it follows that the bilayer assay alone does not allow one to infer whether or not the recorded channels are representative of the entire population of channels present in the vesicles or the tissue of origin. At present, there appears to be no simple resolution of this issue.

Perspective

Currently there are three major strategies for the elucidation of basic cardiac electrophysiology: studies at the level of tissues, cells, or molecules. Tissue studies generally involve transmembrane potential measurement and control using microelectrodes. Resolution is at the level of small volumes of tissue and hence thousands of channels, pumps, and carriers. Such experiments measure changes in electrical potential or syncytial currents in response to laboratory perturbation. Cellular measurements also involve voltage and current measurement and/or control. They examine the electrical responses of isolated cells to experimental manipulations. Resolution is at the level of hundreds of molecules. Most recently, single channel methods allow investigation at the most basic of these levels, i.e., single molecules (and single atoms with molecules).

In this chapter, we dealt only with single channel reconstitution. However, equally important insights have been provided by the technologies of single cell isolation, cell dialysis, patch clamping, and pump current measurement in cardiac and other tissues. The nicotinic acetylcholine receptor and the sodium channel have already been cloned and, as such, their primary structures elucidated. Most recently, Numa and co-workers have cloned and expressed the muscarinic acetylcholine receptor.[64] Logothetis et al.,[65] using purified guanine nucleotide binding proteins, recently have elucidated the pathway whereby the atrial muscarinic acetylcholine receptor is coupled to a K channel. Future use of molecular genetics approaches such as cloning and site-specific mutagenesis will no doubt be applied to these and other membrane channels with profound results.

The implications of these molecular studies for the future of cardiology are extremely significant. As alluded to above, single channel studies allow for the development and testing of specific channel blockers. Some of these agents may prove therapeutically more useful in the treatment of arrhythmias than currently available agents which are rather nonspecific in their blocking action. In addition, specific blockers will be useful in the laboratory for the dissection and characterization of complicated membrane currents. The heart is notorious for geometric complexity and overlapping currents (diffusion, pump-mediated, exchanger-mediated); specific, high-affinity blocking compounds are the essential tools of the cardiac electrophysiologist. With them, it is possible to determine the relative contributions of different electrogenic processes to complex membrane events such as repolarization and arrhythmias. Thus, specific blockers will indirectly benefit the cardiac patient, as they facilitate the study of current mechanisms.

The existence of channel subtypes may lead to clinically important developments. For instance, single channel studies have uncovered three different types of calcium channel in a single cell.[66] Further, it is well known that there are significant differences in the pharmacology of sodium channels of nerve and cardiac muscle; the tetrodotoxin affinity of nerve sodium channels is about 100 times greater than cardiac,[67,68] while the efficacy of local anesthetics in heart is much greater. It may be possible to exploit these phenomena to develop tissue-specific blocking agents. As an example, a sodium channel blocker similar to lidocaine but with fewer central nervous system side effects would be very useful clinically.

It is possible that abnormal channel proteins may underlie certain congenital or acquired arrhythmias, although this is entirely speculative at present. Changes in channel protein modulation may underlie abnormal function in cardiac disease states (e.g., energy substrate depletion, calcium overload); we may be able to exploit our understanding of modulation pathways to benefit the cardiac patient.

In summary, studies at the level of single molecules have revolutionized cardiac electophysiology. We are now analyzing the atomic and molecular mechanisms that underlie transmembrane current, investigating old problems with state-of-the-art resolution. It is only a matter of time before we begin to address aspects of abnormal cardiac electrical function. In fact, one reconstitution study dealing with cardiac arrhythmias has already appeared.[57] Certainly, the elucidation of single channel processes will ultimately be relevant at the bedside.

Acknowledgments: We are indebted to Dr. Roberto Coronado for introducing us to single channels and providing help along the way. We are also grateful to Drs. Augustus O. Grant, John W. Moore, and C. Frank Starmer for many helpful discussions.

References

1. Hille B. Ionic channels of excitable membranes. Sunderland, MA, Sinauer, 1984.
2. Hamill OP, Marty A, Neher E, Sakmann B, Sigworth FJ. Improved patch-clamp techniques for high-resolution current recording from cells and cell-free membrane patches. Pflugers Archiv 1981;391:85–100.
3. Langmuir I, Waugh DF. The adsorption of proteins at oil-water interfaces and artificial protein-lipid membranes. J Gen Physiol 1938;21:745–755.
4. Hodgkin AL, Huxley AF. A quantitative description of membrane current and its application to conduction and excitation in nerve. J Physiol (London) 1952;117:500–544.
5. Mueller P, Rudin DO, Tien HT, Westcott WC. Reconstitution of excitable cell membrane structure in vitro. Circulation 1962;26:1167–1171.

6. Bean RC, Shepperd WC, Chan M, Eichner J. Discrete conductance fluctuations in lipid bilayer protein membranes. J Gen Physiol 1969;53:741–757.
7. Coronado R, Rosenberg RL, Miller C. Ionic selectivity, saturation, and block in a K^+-selective channel from sarcoplasmic reticulum. J Gen Physiol 1980;76:425–446.
8. Labarca P, Coronado R, Miller C. Thermodynamic and kinetic studies of the gating behavior of a K^+-selective channel from the sarcoplasmic reticulum membrane. J Gen Physiol 1980;76:397–424.
9. Moczydlowski E, Latorre R. Gating kinetics of Ca^{2+}-activated K^+ channels from rat muscle incorporated into planar lipid bilayers. J Gen Physiol 1983;82:511–542.
10. Miller C. Open-state substructure of single chloride channels from Torpedo electroplax. Phil Trans R Soc Lond B 1982;299:401–411.
11. Hartshorne RP, Keller BU, Talvenheimo JA, Catterall WA, Montal M. Functional reconstitution of the purified brain sodium channel in planar lipid bilayers. Proc Natl Acad Sci USA 1985;82:240–244.
12. Coronado R, Latorre R. Detection of K and Cl channels from calf cardiac sarcolemma in planar lipid bilayer membranes. Nature 1982;298:849–852.
13. Hill JA, Coronado R, Strauss HC. Reconstitution of canine ventricular ion channels in a planar lipid bilayer system. Circulation, Part II, 1985;72:III–36.
14. Tomlins B, Williams AJ, Montgomery RAP. The characterization of a monovalent cation-selective channel of mammalian cardiac muscle sarcoplasmic reticulum. J Membr Biol 1984;80:191–199.
15. Hill JA, Coronado R, Strauss HC. Reconstitution of a highly conductive K channel from canine ventricular sarcolemma. Biophys J 1986;49:346a.
16. Hill JA, Coronado R, Strauss HC. Conduction and selectivity in a K channel from cardiac sarcoplasmic reticulum. Biophys J (in press).
17. Ehrlich BE, Schen CR, Garcia ML, Kaczorowski GJ. Incorporation of calcium channels from cardiac sarcolemmal membrane vesicles into planar lipid bilayers. Proc Natl Acad Sci USA 1986;83:193–197.
18. Rosenberg RL, Hess P, Reeves JP, Smilowitz H, Tsien RW. Calcium channels in planar lipid bilayers: insights into mechanisms of ion permeation and gating. Science 1986;231 (4745):1564–1566.
19. Montal M, Darszon A, Schindler H. Functional reassembly of membrane proteins in planar lipid bilayers. Q Rev Biophys 1981;14:1–79.
20. Coronado R, Latorre R. Phospholipid bilayers made from monolayers on patch-clamp pipettes. Biophys J 1983;43:231–236.
21. Tank DW, Miller C, Webb WW. Isolated-patch recording from liposomes containing functionally reconstituted chloride channels from Torpedo electroplax. Proc Natl Acad Sci USA 1982;79:7749–7753.
22. Miller C, Racker E. Ca^{++}-induced fusion of fragmented sarcoplasmic reticulum with artificial planar bilayer. J Membr Biol 1976;30:283–300.
23. Cohen FS. Fusion of liposomes to planar bilayers. In Miller C, ed. Ion Channel Reconstitution. New York, Plenum Press, 1986;131–138.
24. Miller C. Integral membrane channels: Studies in model membranes. Physiol Rev 1983;63:1209–1242.
25. Perutz M. Regulation of oxygen affinity of hemoglobin: Influences of structure of the globin on the heme ion. Ann Rev Biochem 1979;48:327–386.
26. Getzoff ED, Tainer JA. Superoxide dismutase as a model ion channel. In Miller C, ed. Ion Channel Reconstitution. New York, Plenum Press, 1986;57–74.
27. Latorre R, Miller C. Conduction and selectivity in potassium channels. J Membr Biol 1983;71:11–30.
28. Eisenman G, Horn R. Ionic selectivity revisited: The role of kinetic and equilibrium processes in ion permeability through channels. J Membr Biol 1983;76:197–225.
29. Hladky SB, Haydon DA. Ion transfer across lipid membranes in the presence of gramicidin A. I. Studies on the unit conductance channel. Biochim Biophys Acta 1972;274:294–312.
30. Begenisich T, Smith C. Multi-ion nature of potassium channels in squid axons. Curr Top Membr Transp 1984;22:353–369.

31. Robinson RA, Stokes RH. Electrolyte Solutions. New York, Academic Press, Inc., 1955.
32. McLaughlin S. Electrostatic potentials at membrane-solution interfaces. Curr Top Membr Transp 1977;9:71–144.
33. McLaughlin S, Mulrine GAN, Gresalfi T, Vaio G, McLaughlin A. Adsorption of divalent cations to bilayer membranes containing phosphatidylserine. J Gen Physiol 1981;77:445–473.
34. Woodhull AM. Ionic blockade of sodium channels in nerve. J Gen Physiol 1973;61:687–708.
35. Coronado R, Miller C. Decamethonium and hexamethonium block K^+ channels of sarcoplasmic reticulum. Nature 1980;288(5790):495–497.
36. Coronado R, Miller C. Voltage-dependent caesium blockade of a cation channel from fragmented sarcoplasmic reticulum. Nature 1979;280:807–810.
37. Hille B. Potassium channels in myelinated nerve. Selective permeability to small cations. J Gen Physiol 1973;61:669–686.
38. Dwyer TM, Adams DJ, Hille B. The permeability of the endplate channel to organic cations in frog muscle. J Gen Physiol 1980;75:469–492.
39. Coronado R, Miller C. Conduction and block by organic cations in a K^+-selective channel from sarcoplasmic reticulum incorporated into planar phospholipid bilayers. J Gen Physiol 1982;79:529–547.
40. Miller C. Bis-quaternary ammonium blockers as structural probes of the sarcoplasmic reticulum K^+ channel. J Gen Physiol 1982;79:869–891.
41. Läuger P. Ion transport through pores: a rate-theory analysis. Biochim Biophys Acta 1973;311:423–441.
42. Hille B. Ionic selectivity, saturation, and block in sodium channels. A four-barrier model. J Gen Physiol 1975;66:535–560.
43. Changeux J-P, Devillers-Thiery A, Chemouilli P. Acetylcholine receptor: An allosteric protein. Science 1984;255:1335–1345.
44. Montal M, Anholt R, Labarca P. The reconstituted acetylcholine receptor. In Miller C, ed. Ion Channel Reconstitution. New York, Plenum Press, 1986;157–204.
45. Noda M, Shimizu S, Tanabe T, Takai T, Kayano T, Ikeda T, Takahashi H, Nakayama H, Kanaoka Y, Minamino N, Kangawa K, Matsuo H, Raftery MA, Hirose T, Inayama S, Hayashida H, Miyata T, Numa S. Primary structure of Electrophorus electricus sodium channel deduced from cDNA sequence. Nature 1984;312:121–127.
46. Ehrenstein G, LeCar H. Electrically gated ionic channel in lipid bilayers. Q Rev Biophys 1977;10:1–34.
47. Tsien RW, Bean BP, Hess P, Lansman JB, Nilius B, Nowycky MC. Mechanisms of calcium channel modulation by beta-adrenergic agents and dihydropyridine calcium agonists. J Mol Cell Cardiol 1986;45:691–710.
48. Noma A. ATP-regulated K^+ channels in cardiac muscle. Nature 1983;305(8):147–148.
49. Trube G, Hescheler J. Inward-rectifying channels in isolated patches of the heart cell membrane: ATP-dependence and comparison with cell-attached patches. Pflugers Arch 1984;401:178–184.
50. Yellen G. Single Ca^{2+}-activated non-selective cation channels in neuroblastoma. Nature 1982;296:357–359.
51. Krueger BK, French RJ, Blaustein MB, Worley JF. Incorporation of Ca^{2+}-dependent K^+ channels, from rat brain, into planar bilayers. Biophys J 1982;37:170a.
52. Blatz AI, Magleby KL. Ion conductance and selectivity of single calcium-activated postassium channels in cultured rat muscle. J Gen Physiol 1984;84:1–23.
53. Vergara C, Moczydlowski E, Latorre R. Conduction, blockade and gating in a Ca^{2+}-activated K^+ channel incorporated into planar bilayers. Biophys J 1984;45:73–76.
54. Walsh JV, Singer JJ. Ca^{++}-activated K^+ channels in vertebrate smooth muscle cells. Cell Calcium 1983;4:321–330.
55. Colquhoun D, Neher E, Reuter H, Stevens CF. Inward current channel activated by intracellular Ca in cultured cardiac cells. Nature 1981;294:255–277.

56. Callewaert G, Vereecke J, Carmeliet E. Existence of a calcium-dependent potassium channel in the membrane of cow cardiac Purkinje cells. Pflugers Arch 1986;406:424–426.
57. Hill JA, Coronado R, Strauss HC. Reconstitution of single calcium-activated channels from heart: Toward a molecular understanding of triggered arrhythmias. (submitted for publication).
58. Miller C, Moczydlowsk E, Latorre R, Phillips M. Charybdotoxin, a protein inhibitor of single Ca^{2+} channels from mammalian skeletal muscle. Nature 1985;313:316–318.
59. White SH. The Physical Nature of Planar Bilayer Membranes. In Miller C, ed. Ion Channel Reconstitution. New York, Plenum Press, 1986;3–35.
60. Jones LR, Maddock SW, Besch HR. Unmasking effect of alamethicin on the (Na^+,K^+)-ATPase, β-adrenergic receptor-coupled adenylate cyclase, and cAMP-dependent protein kinase activities of cardiac sarcolemmal vesicles. J Biol Chem 1980;255(20):9971–9980.
61. Jones LR, Besch HR. Isolation of canine cardiac sarcolemmal vesicles. In Schwartz A, ed. Methods of Pharmacology. Plenum Press, 1984;1–12.
62. Jones LR. Rapid preparation of canine cardiac sarcolemmal vesicles by sucrose flotation. In S. Fleisher, ed. Methods in Enzymology (in press).
63. Rosenblatt M, Hidalgo C, Vergara C, Ikemoto N. Immunological and biochemical properties of transverse tubular membranes isolated from rabbit skeletal muscle. J Biol Chem 1981;256:8140–8148.
64. Kubo T, Fukuda K, Mikami A, Maeda A, Takahashi H, Mishina M, Haga T, Haga K, Ichiyama A, Kangawa K, Kojima M, Matsuo H, Hirose T, Naum S. Cloning, sequencing and expression of complementary DNA encoding the muscarinic acetylcholine receptor. Nature 1986;323(6087):411–416.
65. Logothetis DE, Kurachi Y, Galper J, Neer EJ, Clapham DE. The βγ subunits of GTP-binding proteins activate the muscarinic K^+ channel in heart. Nature (in press).
66. McCleskey EW, Fox AP, Feldman D, Tsien RW. Different types of calcium channels. J Exp Biol 1986;124:177–190.
67. Brown AM, Lee KS, Powell T. Sodium current in single rat heart muscle cell. J Physiol (London) 1981;381:479–500.
68. Cohen CJ, Bean BP, Colatsky TJ, Tsien RW. Tetrodotoxin block of sodium channels in rabbit Purkinje fibers. Interaction between toxin binding and channel gating. J Gen Physiol 1981;78:383–411.

51

Laser Ablation for Tachyarrhythmia Control: Current Status and Future Development

Sanjeev Saksena

Introduction

Medical applications of laser energy were developed shortly after the advent of this new technology.[1-4] Early users have included surgical disciplines such as ophthalmology and gynecology. This was followed by endoscopic application in gastroenterology and pulmonary medicine. In this decade, considerable investigative effort has been devoted to examining potential cardiovascular applications.[5-7] Experimental studies suggested the feasibility of myocardial ablation with laser energy.[8-12] Pilot clinical studies have reported on the use of laser ablation techniques in patients with ventricular tachycardia (VT) and supraventricular tachycardias (SVT).[7,13-17] This report will detail the physical and experimental basis of the laser ablation technique and analyze early clinical experiences with particular attention towards future development of the technique.

Physical Considerations for Cardiovascular Laser Energy Sources

The principles of laser action were developed in the early 20th century[18] and the actual technology was developed in the 1950s.[1,2] Laser energy is emitted when excited atoms or molecules fall back to their basal energy level and emit

From: Brugada P, Wellens HJJ. CARDIAC ARRHYTHMIAS: Where To Go From Here? Mount Kisco, NY, Futura Publishing Company, Inc., © 1987.

electromagnetic radiation.[7] This radiation has similar wavelengths (monochromatic), is parallel, and in the same phase. This results in a narrow concentrated energy beam seen as a laser beam emission. Many elements and compounds can undergo laser action and laser beams can have widely varying wavelengths and characteristics, depending on the initiating chemical reaction. Table I enumerates some laser energy sources under evaluation for cardiovascular application and their physical characteristics. Figure 1 shows a prototype argon laser system currently under evaluation at our center. This is a 222 V 15 watt argon laser with a water-cooled laser tube.

Laser beams can be directed with optical systems. Transmission of laser energy to its cardiovascular site of application requires focusing of the laser beam into an optical fiber. In our prototype system, a prism and mirror arrangement directs the beam into an optical coupler which focuses the beam into a 300 micron quartz optical fiber. The development of suitable optical transmission systems is necessary for cardiovascular application of specific laser energy sources. Since there is some energy loss during optical fiber transmission, it is necessary to evaluate delivered energy at the fiber tip for precision and control during cardiac applications. An external power measurement device is usually employed for this purpose. (Fig. 1). Furthermore, laser energy can be dissipated or selectively absorbed by emission into specific media. Thus, the wavelengths present in argon laser beams are selectively absorbed by hemoglobin components present in blood. This can result in experimentally and clinically significant interactions.[7,19,20] Laser fibers are housed within specialized guiding catheter systems.[5,7] This permits transportation of the laser fiber to desired sites of application within the cardiovascular system.[7,8,21,22]

Ablation may be accomplished directly using the laser beam emission or employing the laser beam in conjunction with a metal tip to produce indirect thermal effects. Figure 2 illustrates the tip of an optical fiber within a guiding catheter under investigation in our laboratory. We have employed the optical fiber itself in experimental and clinical studies. A major concern with the use of polished fiber-tip alone is the possibility of fiberoptic tip damage. This is usually seen when the top comes into contact with the myocardial surface which has been heated by the beam.[23,24] It is most frequently observed with the use of continuous wave laser radiation and minimized by the pulsed mode.[24] Alternatively, the fiber tip may be protected by a metallic tip which can protect the tip but qualitatively limits the type of lesion elicited.[25,26]

Table I
Laser Energy Sources*

Element/Compound	Wavelength (nm)	Optical Fiber
Argon	496,514	Yes
Neodymium-yttrium-aluminum garnet	1064	Yes
Carbon dioxide	10,600	Under development
Krypton fluoride excimer	248	Under development

*Physical and optical transmission characteristics of certain laser energy sources which could be suitable for cardiovascular application. Of these, only the argon laser is in the visible light spectrum.

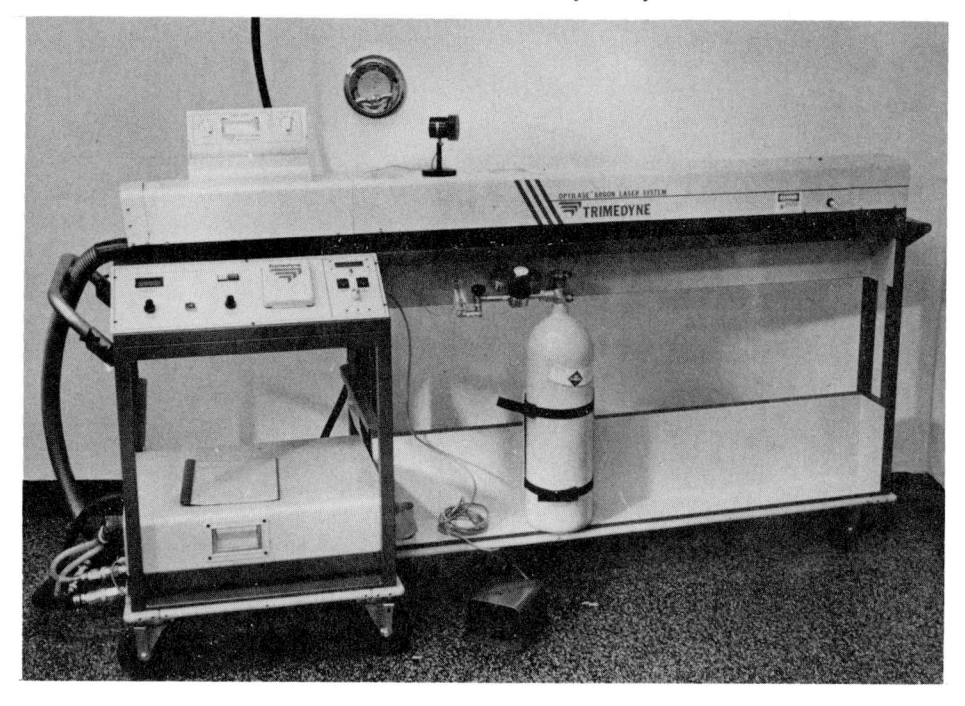

Figure 1: A prototype argon laser system with 15 watt power output. A water-cooled laser tube is employed. The front panel has a pulse modulator and the external power meter is mounted on top of the laser tube. A foot pedal is employed to operate the laser. (Reprinted with permission from Futura Publishing Co., Mt. Kisco, NY.)

Experimental Basis for Laser Ablation

The interaction of laser energy with different myocardial tissues has been studied experimentally in a variety of situations. Fundamental effects of laser radiation in human myocardium relate to thermal injury induced by the beam. Histologic examination of normal and diseased human ventricle has revealed lesions consistent with thermal effects.[7,9,11] Continuous wave argon laser discharges produce a central crater due to tissue vaporization lined by charred carbonized tissue and a zone of coagulation necrosis. Pulsed laser discharges reduce the extent of tissue carbonization and produce vaporization with lesser degrees of coagulation necrosis.[7,24] Direct tissue temperature measurements during in vitro irradiation of canine myocardium with an Nd-YAG laser was performed by Lee and co-workers.[23] They demonstrated a marked rise in tissue temperature at the site of irradiation with a temperature gradient in surrounding tissues. Cessation of irradiation was associated with rapid return to baseline tissue temperature. These thermal effects of laser beams can be modified by the laser delivery mode as well as by the superfusing medium. In saline medium, the dimensions of the induced lesion are significantly smaller, particularly with respect to depth.[9] However, the presence of a warm blood medium may enhance these effects and lesion dimensions are comparable to direct tissue irradiation.[9,19,21]

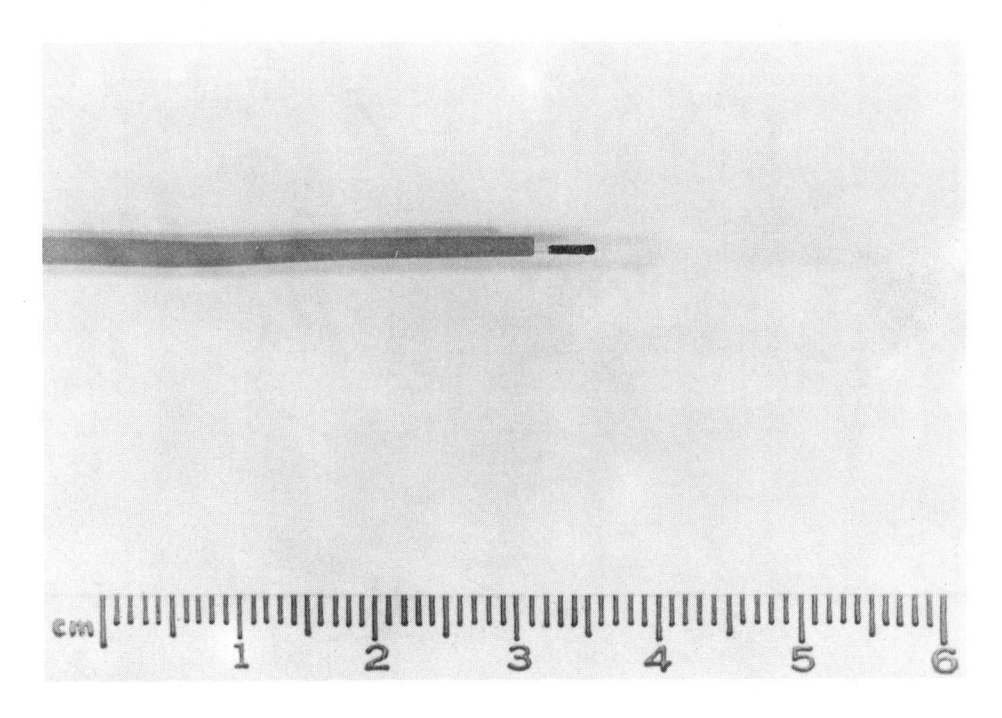

Figure 2: Quartz optical fiber within a guiding catheter system. The fiber tip is polished but unprotected.

Lesions produced by different laser energy sources can show some qualitative variability with respect to the extent of tissue vaporization and coagulation. Laser energy in the infrared spectrum, e.g., Nd-YAG, can produce largely coagulation,[21] while ultraviolet radiation such as a xenon fluoride excimer can exclusively vaporize tissue.[10,12] Argon laser energy produces mixed lesions.[7,11] However, modification of the energy delivery mode and medium can be employed to alter the type of lesion elicited.[7] Figure 3 shows examples of endocardial ablation of ventricular myocardium achieved with continuous wave (panel A) and pulsed (panel B) argon laser discharges. Note the substantial decrease in tissue carbonization and coagulation necrosis with the pulsed mode.

The effects of laser energy can also vary quantitatively on the anatomic substrate for ablation. Normal human ventricular myocardium can be significantly ablated with energies of 100 to 200 J and is often perforated by continuous discharges of > 300 J.[11] In diseased human ventricle from patients with VT, the lesion size is greatly reduced. In this tissue, lesions require 200 to 400 J/cm^2 density to achieve significant endocardial ablation.[11,14,15] Perforation is rarely observed even with energies up to 1000 J.[11] Ablation of human atrium or atrioventricular (AV) junction requires extremely low energies with single bursts of > 25 J, often producing perforation.[27] Figure 4 shows a lesion produced by rapid pulsed discharges with a total delivered energy of 19 J. Note the almost complete penetration of the atrial wall. Pulsed argon laser energy delivery provides control and precision of the extent of ablation within the prescribed dose energy relationships.[7] This prevents perforation and inadvertent injury to adjoin-

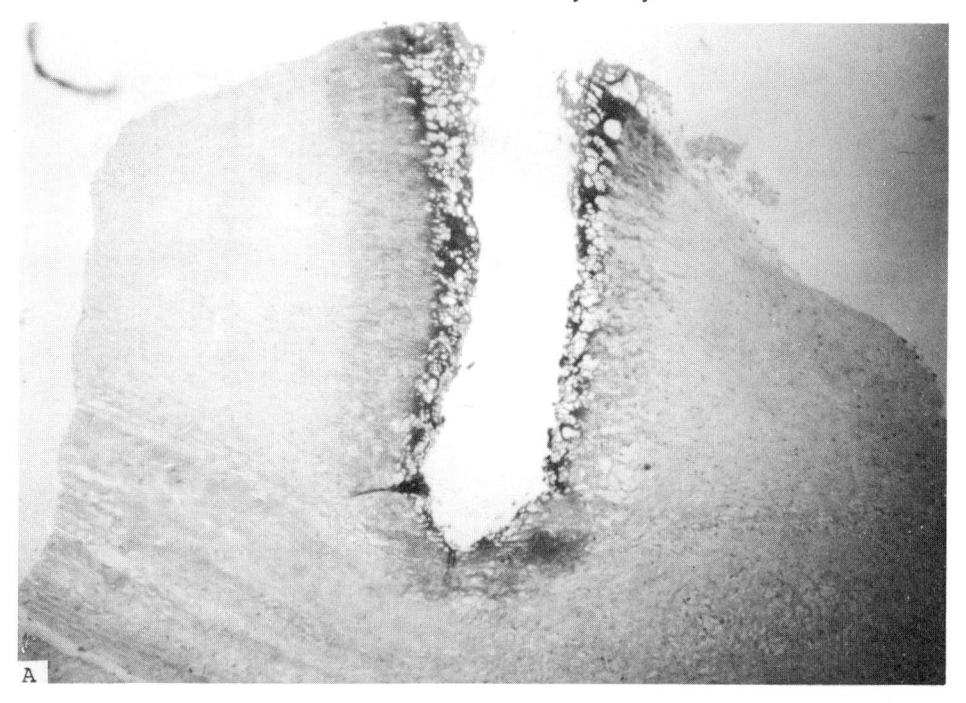

Figure 3A: Myocardial lesion created by a continuous wave argon laser discharge. Note the crater due to tissue vaporization, surrounding carbonization and coagulation necrosis of ventricular myocardium.

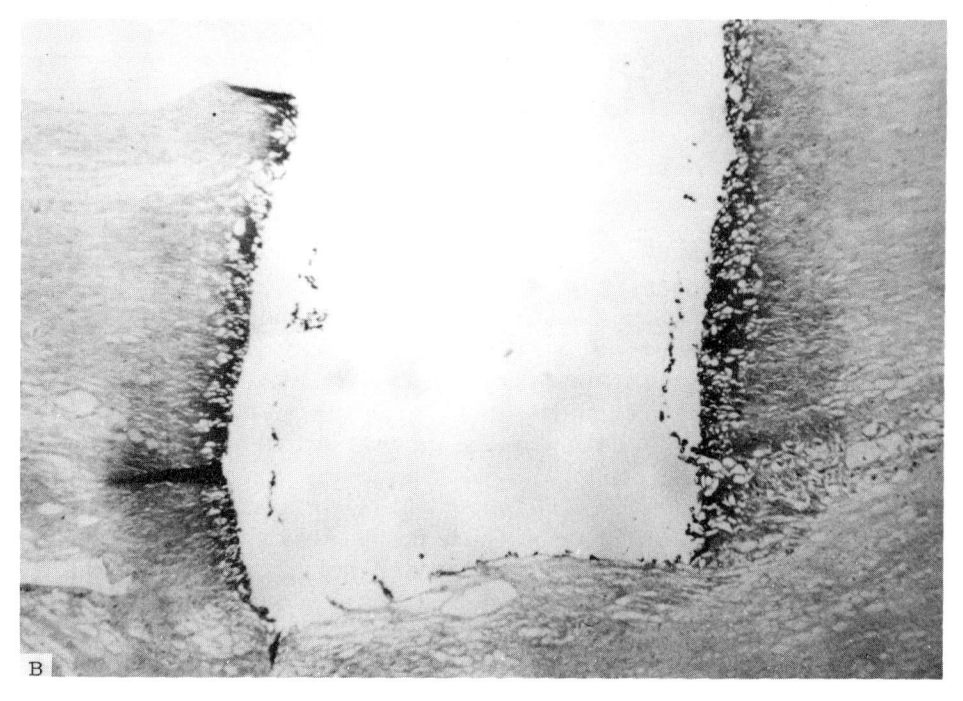

Figure 3B: Myocardial lesion created by pulsed argon laser discharges. Note the crater has minimal carbonization of its margins and limited coagulation necrosis.

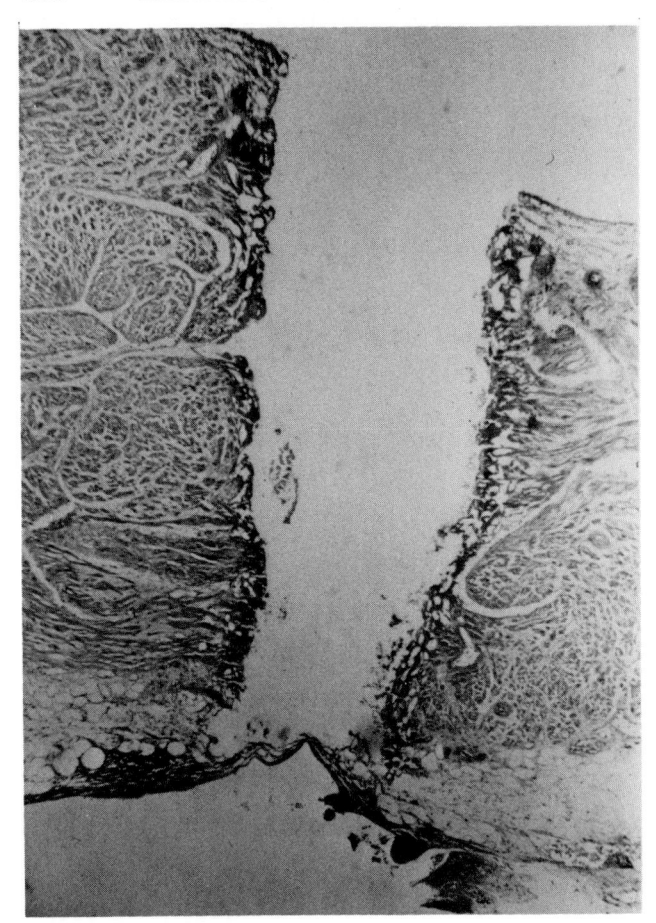

Figure 4: Lesion created by low power pulsed argon laser discharges in human atrium with a total delivered energy of 19 J. Note the penetration of the entire atrial wall with only epicardium remaining intact. There is virtually no carbonization present.

ing or deeper cardiac and vascular structures. Furthermore, modification of conduction rather than ablation may be feasible with controlled pulsed laser energy delivery techniques.[22,27] *High energy continuous wave* laser discharges are extremely undesirable when ablation of SVT is being considered. Figure 5 shows ablation in the AV groove with low power rapid pulsed argon laser discharges. Note the controlled vaporization of tissue in the AV groove.

In summary, experimental data is now available to establish feasibility of laser ablation techniques for ablation in a variety of arrhythmogenic substrates. The ability to control laser energy with pulsed techniques, variable power output, fiberoptic transmission methods, and superfusing media permitted development of the clinical ablation technique. A single flexible laser energy source with a minimum range of power outputs from 2 to 20 W optically coupled to a flexible fiberoptic transmission system with pulse control is suitable for such applications. A number of prototype laser systems can fulfill these requirements and it is highly conceivable that a variety of clinically suitable systems will become available.

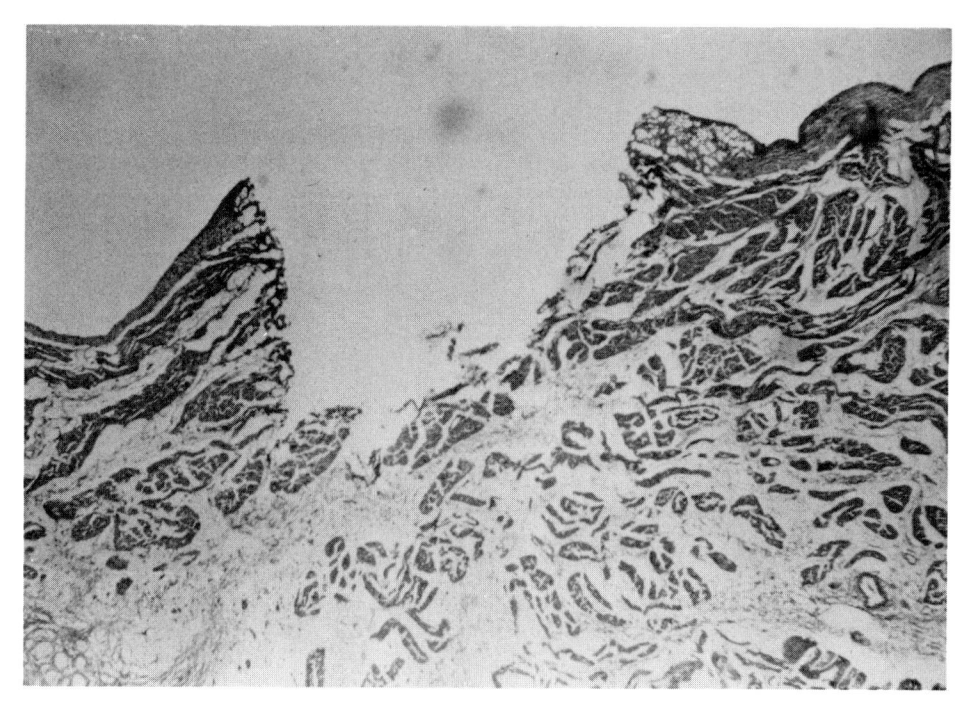

Figure 5: Superficial controlled ablation of the atrioventricular sulcus by low power rapid pulsed argon laser discharges. Note the vaporization of the endocardium and atrial muscle with preservation of deep muscle layers and epicardial fat.

Clinical Experience with Laser Ablation Methods

Early clinical experience is now being acquired with intraoperative use of the laser ablation method. Experimental studies were undertaken by Lee and co-workers in 1981 and in our laboratory since 1983. The first formal studies of the effects of laser energy on canine AV junction were reported by Narula in 1984 and in human diseased ventricle were reported from our laboratory in 1985. Preliminary clinical data with a *nonmap-guided* approach in patients with VT using an Nd-YAG laser were first reported by Mesnildrey and co-workers in 1985.[13] We reported the first experience with a *map-guided* approach in patients with VT using an argon laser in 1986.[7,14,28] Application of argon laser energy for ablation of SVT associated with the Wolff-Parkinson-White (WPW) syndrome was initially reported from our center in 1986.[16,27,28] However, detailed reports of clinical application are scanty[7,15,16] and this field must be considered to be in rapid evolution at this time. Thus, this report will be rapidly updated with increasing clinical experience.

The details of the patient population included in our initial studies is shown in Table II. Nine patients had recurrent and refractory VT and three patients had life-threatening SVT associated with the WPW syndrome. The presenting symp-

Table II
Patient Characteristics*

Pt #	Age	Sex	Dx	Symptom	Prior Antiarrhythmic Drug Trials	LVEF (%)
Ventricular Tachycardia:						
1.	69	M	CAD	syncope	6	37
2.	69	M	CAD	CA	5	45
3.	62	M	CAD	syncope	5	11
4.	67	M	CAD	syncope, CA	7	30
5.	57	M	CAD	syncope, CA	5	30
6.	63	M	CAD	CA	5	39
7.	54	M	CAD	CA	4	23
8.	53	M	CAD	CA	5	34
9.	71	F	CAD	CA	7	22
Supraventricular Tachycardia:						
1.	27	M	WPW	CA	—	> 50
2.	19	M	WPW	syncope	—	> 50
3.	42	F	WPW	syncope, CA	—	> 50

*Clinical characteristics of patients with recurrent supraventricular and ventricular tachycardia undergoing intraoperative laser ablation.
Pt = patient; Dx = diagnosis; LVEF = left ventricular ejection fraction; CAD = coronary artery disease; CA = cardiac arrest; WPW = Wolff-Parkinson-White syndrome.

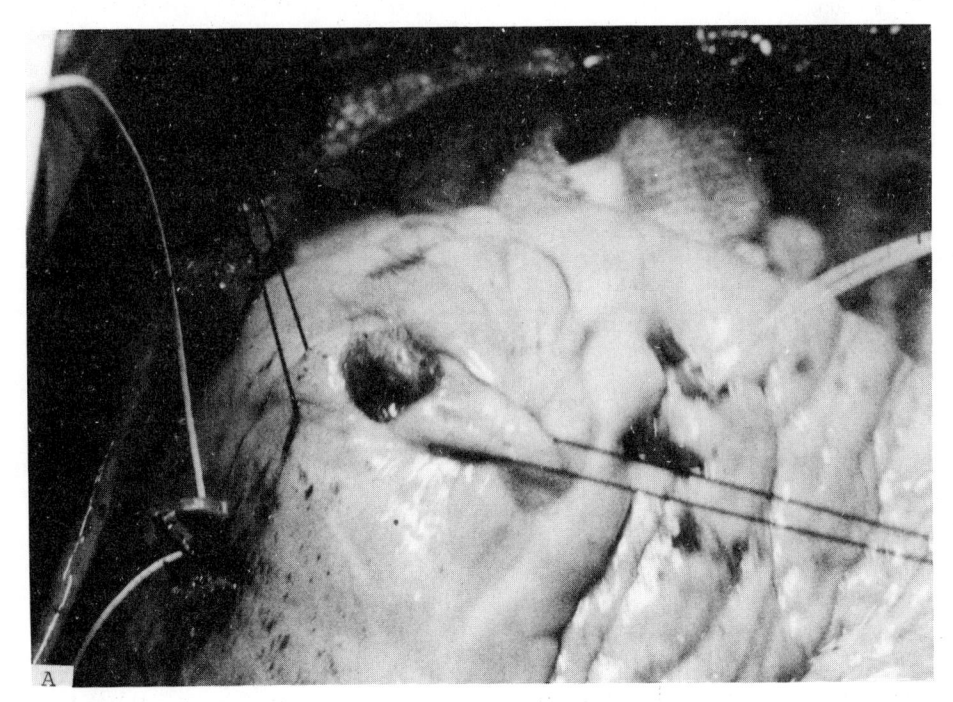

Figure 6A: Argon laser ventriculotomy in a patient with refractory ventricular tachycardia. High power pulsed laser discharges were employed.

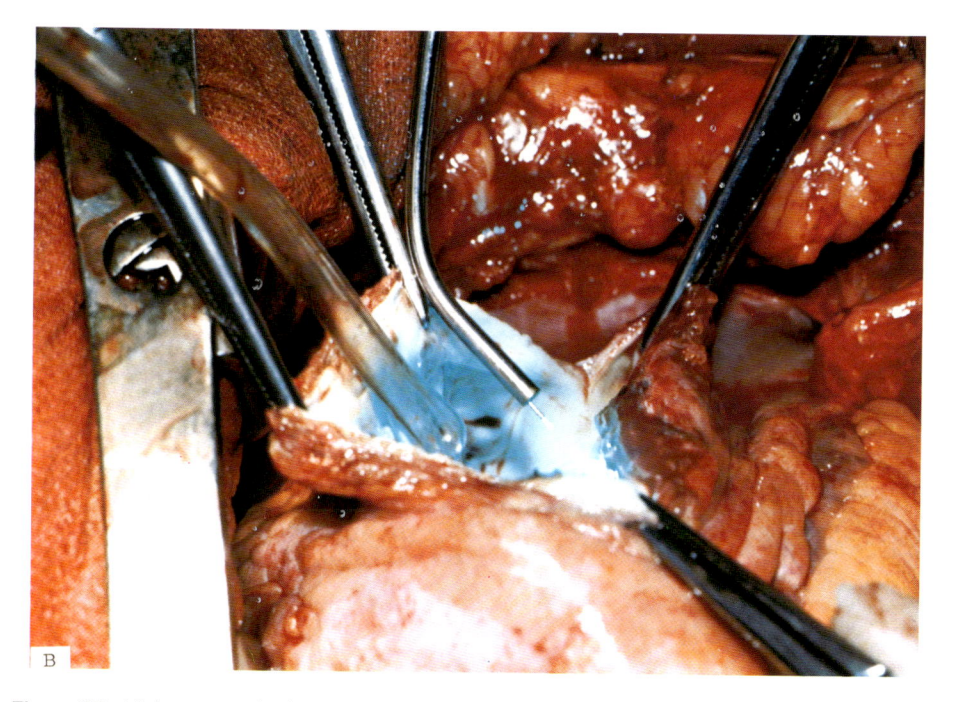

Figure 6B: High power pulsed argon laser endocardial ablation of arrhythmogenic ventricular myocardium in a patient with ventricular tachycardia. An optical fiber/laser catheter system was employed.

toms are shown in the table. Patients with VT had an age range of 54 to 71 years, had failed a mean of 5 ± 1 drug trials, and all patients had coronary artery disease. The extent of coronary artery disease was left main coronary artery obstruction in one patient, single vessel disease in one patient, two-vessel disease in two patients, and three-vessel disease in six patients. The mean left ventricular (LV) ejection fraction was 29 ± 10%. Three patients with SVT had the WPW syndrome. Their presenting symptoms were cardiac arrest (one patient) or syncope (two patients). Their ages ranged from 19 to 43 years and the LV ejection fraction was > 50% in all patients. These patients underwent preoperative and intraoperative cardiac mapping to localize the site of VT origin or the location of the accessory bypass tract. The site of VT origin was defined on the basis of presence of presystolic electrical activity during VT.[15] The location of the accessory tract was determined at the site of earliest retrograde activation during orthodromic SVT.[16,27,28]

In six patients with VT, an intraoperative laser ventriculotomy was performed (Fig. 6A). Endocardial mapping was then completed. Laser endocardial ablation was performed with high power pulsed argon laser discharges (Fig. 6B). Fourteen VT morphologies were mapped in these nine patients, and 12 sites of VT origin were considered surgically unresectable. Endocardial resection was performed alone at the two resectable VT sites. At eight VT sites, only laser endocardial ablation was performed, and in the remaining four VT sites, laser ablation was combined with limited resection. Eleven of 12 laser ablation sites were either in the interventricular septum (n = 8) or posterior papillary (n = 3). The mean area ablated for each VT morphology was 11 ± 7 cm^2, and the mean delivered energy was 232 ± 125 J/cm^2. Electrogram recordings from the ablation site showed preservation of normal myocardial electrical activity in underlying tissues.[15] After laser ablation, postoperative electrophysiologic (EP) studies showed suppression of spontaneous and inducible VT for 13 of the 14 preoperative morphologies. One morphology remained inducible in a patient who received < 90 J/cm^2 of laser energy due to concern regarding disruption of the posterior papillary muscle. In this patient who had continuous incessant VT preoperatively, a single paroxysmal episode of spontaneous VT occurred in the second postoperative week. This was easily supressed by procainamide, to which he had been unresponsive and had inducible VT preoperatively. Postoperatively, all patients had no inducible or spontaneous VT on no drug therapy (eight patients) or procainamide therapy in the remaining patient.

In patients with SVT, a laser atriotomy was performed in the lateral right atrium in two patients to open the chamber for endocardial ablation of a posterior septal accessory tract. A bloodless laser atriotomy was then performed at just above the AV junction in all three patients. Low power (3 to 5 W) rapid pulsed laser discharges were employed to avoid damage to adjoining vascular structures. This was followed by blunt dissection in the AV groove. The mean length of the atriotomy was 33 ± 14 mm and the mean delivered energy for the atriotomy was 53 ±31 J/cm of incision. Energy density ranged from 25 to 50 J/cm^2. Blunt dissection was employed in the AV sulcus to complete the procedure in the epicardial fat pad. The location of the bypass tract was left posterolateral in one patient and posterior septal in two patients. The atriotomy was sutured and significant bleeding was not observed. Transient postoperative heart block was observed in one patient with a posterior septal tract which subsequently resolved. Postoperative cardiac monitoring and EP studies showed no spontaneous or inducible SVT in any patient. All patients were discharged without antiarrhythmic drug therapy or permanent pacemaker implantation. Figure 7A shows a resting 12-lead ECG in a patient who subsequently underwent laser atriotomy and ablation. Postoperatively, disappearance of the preexcitation pattern is noted (Fig. 7B). There were no intraoperative or immediate postoperative hemodynamic or arrhythmic deaths.

Figure 8 illustrates the hemodynamic sequelae of intraoperative argon laser ablation. Hemodynamic parameters measured preoperatively and postoperatively showed no change in mean pulmonary capillary wedge pressure, ejection fraction, or cardiac index. After discharge, 11 of 12 patients were in New York Heart Association class I or II with one patient remaining in New York Heart Association class III.

Clinical experience with the Nd-YAG laser has been reported from two centers.[13,17] Mesnildrey and co-workers employed a nonmap-guided approach and performed a complete encircling thermoablation of the margins of a left ventricular aneurysm or infarction. In their early experience with 12 patients with VT, there were three immediate postoperative deaths due to low cardiac output. Late VT recurrences (incidence 15%) have been reported.[29] An overall arrhythmia-free rate of 71% was noted. This less favorable experience needs to be analyzed with two important variables, viz use of a nonmap-guided approach and the

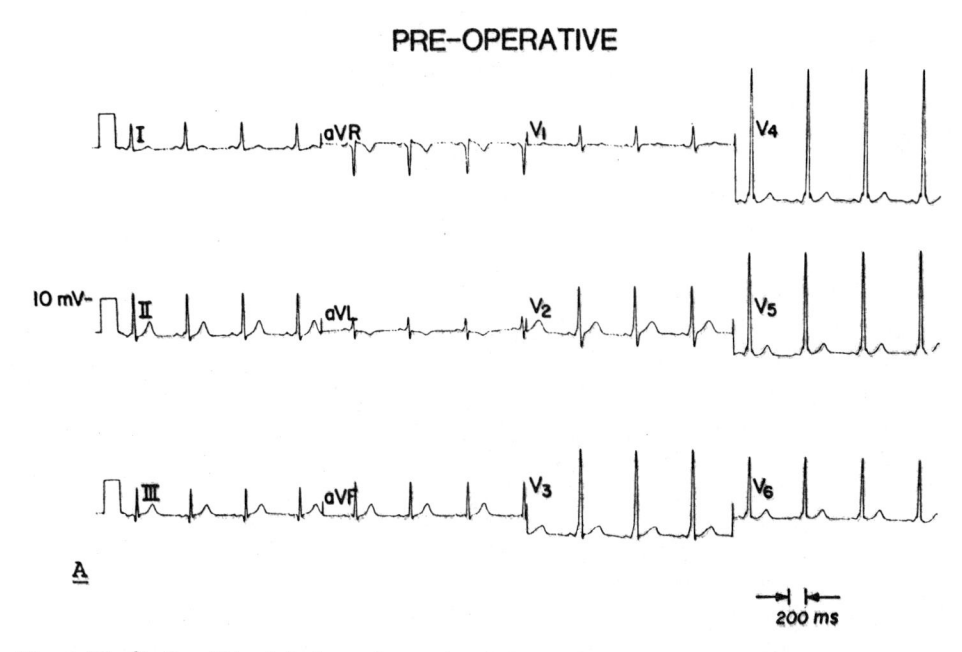

Figure 7A: Resting 12-lead electrocardiogram in a patient with supraventricular tachyarrhythmias and the Wolff-Parkinson-White syndrome prior to laser atriotomy and ablation. Note the typical preexcitation pattern.

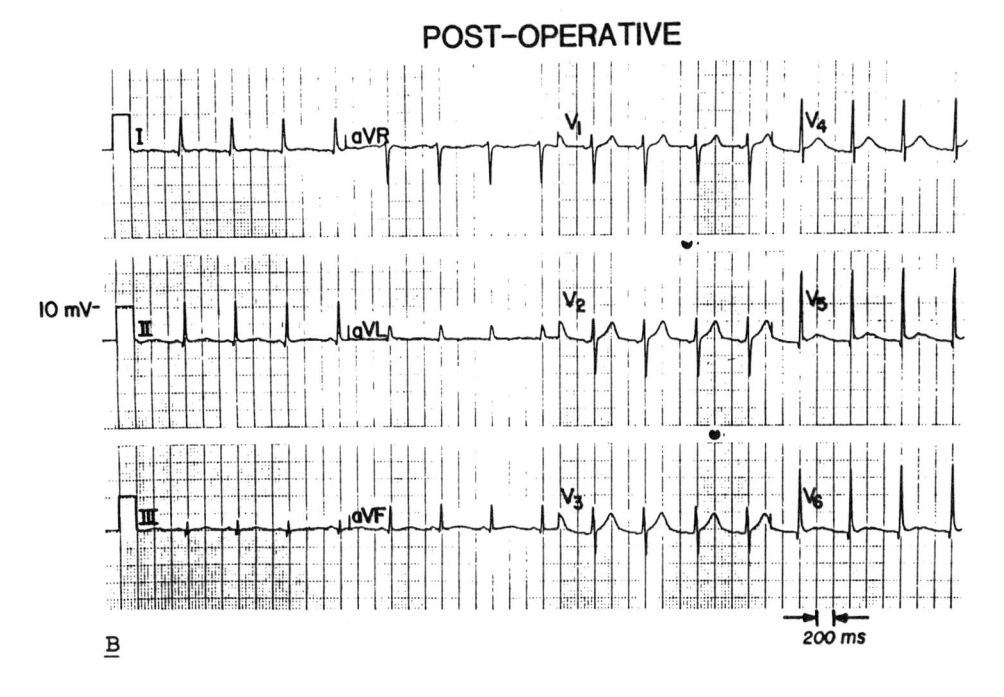

Figure 7B: Resting 12-lead electrocardiogram in the same patient after laser atriotomy. Note the disappearance of the preexcitation pattern. This patient had no spontaneous or inducible supraventricular tachycardia postoperatively.

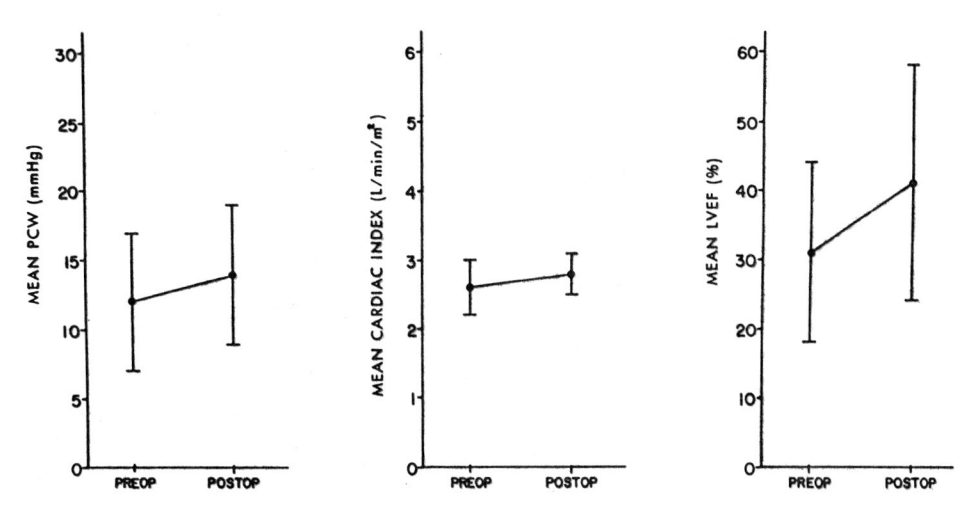

Figure 8: Hemodynamic parameters before and after intraoperative laser ablation in patients with sustained ventricular tachycardia and poor left ventricular function. Note the stable postoperative parameters which are unchanged from preoperative values. PCW = pulmonary capillary wedge pressure; LVEF = left ventricular ejection fraction.

extensive myocardial damage resulting from an encircling thermoablation using a high power laser. A more favorable experience with the Nd-YAG laser has been reported by Svenson and co-workers in 14 patients with recurrent VT using a map-guided approach.[17] The mean energy density employed for ablation in this study was 1006 J/cm^2 with a mean irradiated area of 30 + 3 cm^2. In this report, there was one intraoperative death and one immediate postoperative death, for an overall mortality of 11%. Eighty-four percent of patients were arrhythmia-free during follow-up on no drug therapy.

Future Development of the Laser Ablation Technique

The future applications of the laser ablation technique could potentially include intraoperative and transcatheter ablation of arrhythmogenic tissues. In analyzing feasibility, both general concerns with laser methods and specific issues related to each application need to be considered. The major advantages of the laser technique include precise and rapid ablation in diseased tissues. It produces less myocardial dysfunction than other ablation methods.[21] The healing properties of laser-induced lesions are superior and the healed lesion may be less arrhythmogenic.[30,32] The argon laser-induced lesion vaporizes superficial scar, has focal effects, and appears to leave behind electrically active myocardium.[15,31] The Nd-YAG lesion produces photocoagulation of large myocardial segments producing a dense homogenous scar.

The major concerns with the use of laser ablation techniques include lack of control of the extent of damage, induced myocardial dysfunction, thrombogenicity, and myocardial rupture as well as long-term efficacy and safety. Continuous wave laser energy delivery is inherently associated with limited ability to control extent of damage. Pulsed energy delivery techniques permit control and precision and produce comparable lesions to continuous wave discharges.[24] Thus, pulsed laser energy delivery would potentially provide controlled ablation. The extent of myocardial dysfunction is clearly related to the amount of delivered energy. In general, limited ablation with lower energy densities will minimize this complication. Map-guided approaches are clearly superior in this regard and are essential for ablation of the AV node–His bundle, accessory bypass tracts, and VT foci. We have achieved successful ablation with the argon laser technique with considerably lower energy densities than with the Nd-YAG photocoagulation method. This is particularly important in patients with VT who have severely compromised LV function. Future developments will need to determine the minimum amount of tissue needed for successful ablation of SVT and VT as well as the minimum energy density. Current information would suggest that in patients with VT, the mean area for successful ablation of one VT morphology could be < 12 cm^2, and the minimum energy should exceed 100 J/cm^2 but is probably less than 400 J/cm^2 for argon laser energy. Noninvasive postoperative studies with 2-D echocardiograms have revealed no evidence of mural thrombosis and postoperative embolic events have not been reported. No documented case of myocardial perforation or rupture after laser ablation is currently available. Data on long-term efficacy and safety are available only for mean follow-up periods ranging from 6 to 18 months.

These data suggest that initial efficacy and safety are maintained during this period.

Specific issues for the intraoperative technique remain. The laser technique permits ablation of VT foci in regions hitherto considered to have poor surgical resectability.[32] This issue had limited effectiveness of surgical resection methods.[32] Improved results can be expected with the laser method leading to less stringent patient selection criteria for intraoperative arrhythmia ablation. Furthermore, bloodless incision of atrium and ventricle is feasible. Thus, it has potential as an adjunct to conventional methods and with improvements may even compete with standard mechanical resection. A major limitation currently is the lack of refinement in available prototype equipment, including cumbersome fiberoptics. Significant innovations will be needed to reduce the equipment size and improve delivery techniques yet maintain and even enhance versatility. Issues of personnel safety and training need to be addressed. Rapid mapping techniques with multiple recording electrodes, display, and analysis methods will further enhance the technique. Finally, equipment cost is a significant issue and needs to be examined.

The transcatheter technique remains another potential application of this energy source. Catheter ablation of arrhythmogenic foci has three major elements: (1) issues related to the ablation energy source, (2) a need for satisfactory catheter-based energy delivery systems, and (3) an understanding of the anatomic substrate for ablation. In the instance of laser techniques, considerable work has been focused on the first and last issues.[7-11] There is a lack of information on adequate catheter energy delivery systems. We have used a catheter/laser fiber energy delivery system for intraoperative use.[7] However, specialized guiding catheter systems will be necessary for intracardiac use in vivo. Our recent experience with a prototype fiberoptic angioscopic system for visualization has yielded limited results.[7] Electrically guided active fixation catheter systems housing laser fibers will be essential in this effort.[33] The products of laser ablation have been considered largely soluble and unlikely to produce embolism.

In summary, significant progress has already been made in the use of laser energy for tachycardia ablation. Experimental and initial clincal data support more widespread evaluation of this physical energy for this purpose as well as further development of both intraoperative and catheter applications. In view of the existing widespread industrial and biologic applications of laser energy, there is good reason to expect this "promise" to be realized, providing a fascinating future direction for development of clinical electrophysiology.

Acknowledgments: The author acknowledges the major contribution of Doctors Mansoor Hussain, Isaac Gielchinsky and Arun Gadhoke, and of Mr. Demetris Pantopoulos in the development of the laser technique. The excellent secretarial assistance of Ms. Ruth Harrison in preparation of this manuscript is greatly appreciated.

References

1. Schawlow AL, Townes CH. Infrared and optical lasers. Physiol Rev 1958;112: 1940–1942.
2. Maiman TH. Stimulated optical radiation in ruby. Nature 1960;187:493–494.

3. Zaret MM, Ripps H, Siegel IM, Breinin GM. Laser photocoagulation of the eye. Arch Ophthalmol 1963;69:97−104.
4. Kapany NS, Peppers NA, Zweng HC, Flocks M. Retinal photocoagulation by laser. Nature 1963;199:146−149.
5. Saksena S. Cardiovascular applications of laser technology. Cardiology 1984;1:27−31.
6. Lee G, Ikeda RM, Chan MC, Stobbe D, Kozina J, Jiang MC, Reis RL, Mason DT. Current and potential uses of lasers in the treatment of atherosclerotic disease. Chest 1984;85:429−434.
7. Saksena S, Gadhoke A. Laser therapy for tachyarrhythmias: A new frontier. PACE 1986;9:531−550.
8. Lee G, Ikeda RM, Theis J, Stobbe D, Ogata C, Lui H, Reis RL, Mason DT. Effects of laser irradiation delivered by flexible fiberoptic system on the left ventricular internal myocardium. Am Heart J 1983;106:587−590.
9. Saksena S, Ciccone J, Chandran P, Rothbart ST, Pantopoulos D, Lee B. Laser ablation of normal and diseased human ventricle (abstr). J Am Coll Cardiol 1985;5:473.
10. Isner JM, Donaldson RF, Deckelbaum LI, Clark RH, Laliberte SM, Ucci AA, Salem EN, Konstam MA. The excimer laser: Gross, light microscopic and ultrastrucutural analysis of potential advantages for use in laser therapy of cardiovascular disease. J Am Coll Cardiol 1985;6:1102−1109.
11. Saksena S, Ciccone J, Chandran P, Rothbart ST, Pantopoulos D, Lee B. Laser ablation of normal and diseased human ventricle. Am Heart J 1986;112:52−60.
12. Downar E, Butany J, Jares A, Storcheff BP. Endocardial photoablation by excimer laser. J Am Coll Cardiol 1986;7:546−550.
13. Mesnildrey P, Laborde F, Piwnica A. Encircling thermoexclusion by the Nd-YAG laser without mapping: A new surgical technique for ischemic ventricular tachycardia (abstr). Circulation 1986:72(Suppl III):III−389.
14. Saksena S, Hussain SM, Gielchinsky I, Gadhoke A, Pantopoulos D. Successful mapping-guided argon laser ablation of ventricular tachycardia in man (abstr). Circulation 1986;74(Suppl II):II−186.
15. Saksena S, Hussain SM, Gielchinsky I, Gadhoke A, Pantopoulos D. Intraoperative mapping-guided argon laser ablation of malignant ventricular tachycardia. Am J Cardiol 1987 (in press).
16. Saksena S, Hussain SM, Gielchinsky I, Gadhoke A, Pantopoulos D. Intraoperative mapping-guided argon laser ablation of malignant supraventricular and ventricular tachycardia. In Progress in Clinical Pacing. Santini M, Pistolese M, Alliegro A, eds. Rome, T. F. Begliomini, 1986;564−571.
17. Svenson RH, Gallagher JJ, Selle JG, Zimmern SH, Fedor JM. Intraoperative laser photoablation of venticular tachycardia (abstr). Circulation 1986;74(Suppl II):II−461.
18. Einstein A. On the quantum theory of radiation. Physikalische Zeitschrift 1917;18:121
19. Saksena S, Gadhoke A, Hussain SM. Feasibility of intraoperative laser ablation of ventricular tachycardia: Studies in intact animal ventricle and in diseased human ventricle resected from patients with ventricular tachycardia. New Trends in Arrhythmias 1986;2:285−292.
20. Abela GS, Fenech A, Crea F, Smith W, Conti R. Blood enhances the thermal effects of argon laser energy on the arterial wall (abstr). J Am Coll Cardiol 1985;5:408.
21. Lee B, Gottdiener JS, Fletcher RD, Rodriguez ER, Ferrans VJ. Transcatheter ablation: Comparison between laser photoablation and electrode shock ablation in the dog. Circulation 1985;71:579−586.
22. Narula OS, Bharati S, Chan MC, Embi AA, Lev A. Microsection of the His bundle with laser radiation through a pervenous catheter: Correlation of histologic and electrophysiologic data. Am J Cardiol 1984;54:186−192.
23. Lee B, Rodriguez ER, Notargiocomo A, Ferrans VJ, Chen Y, Fletcher RD. Thermal effects of laser and electrical discharge on cardiovascular tissue: Implications for coronary artery recanlization and endocardial ablation. J Am Coll Cardiol 1986;8: 193−200.

24. Ciccone J, Saksena S, Pantopoulos D. Comparative efficacy of continuous and pulsed argon laser ablation of human diseased ventricle. PACE 1986;9:697–704.
25. Hussein H. A novel fiberoptic laser probe for treatment of occlusive vessel disease: Optical and laser technology in medicine. Optical Laser Technol Med 1986;605:59–62.
26. Sanborn T, Faxon D, Haudenschild C, Ryan T. Experimental angioplasty: Circumferential distribution of laser thermal injury with a laser probe. J Am Coll Cardiol 1985;5:934–938.
27. Saksena S, Hussain SM, Gielchinsky I, Pantopoulos D, Wasty N, Rothbart ST, Alizedah J. Intraoperative mapping-guided argon laser ablation of malignant supraventricular and ventricular tachycardia. J Am Coll Cardiol 1987 (in press).
28. Saksena S. Laser ablation of tachycardias: Experimental basis and preliminary clinical application. Proceedings of International Symposium on Non-Pharmacological Therapy of Tachyarrhythmias. Dusseldorf, 1986 (in press).
29. Mesnildrey P. Unpublished data.
30. Gerrity RG, Loop RD, Goldbert LAR. Arterial response to laser operation for removal of atherosclerotic plaques. J Thorac Cardiovasc Surg 1983;85:409–421.
31. Merillat JE, Levine JH, Waxman HF, Stern MD, Spear JF, Moore EN, Kadish AA, Fonyer J, Guzman R, Guarnieri T. Laser ablation leads to more focal electrophysiologic effects compared to catheter delivered high energy ablation (abstr). J Am Coll Cardiol 1986;7:237A.
32. Saksena S, Hussain SM, Wasty N, Gielchinsky I, Parsonnet V. Long-term efficacy of subendorcardial resection in refractory tachycardia: Relationship to site of arrhythmia origin. Ann Thorac Surg 1986;42:685–689.
33. Saksena S, Tarjan P, Bharati S, Boveja B, Cohen D, Joubert T. A new technique for successful low energy His bundle ablation among a suction electrode catheter (abstr). Circulation 1986;74(Suppl II):II–387.
34. Isner JM, Clarke RH, Donaldson RF, Aharon A. Identification of photoproducts liberated by in vitro argon laser irradiation of atherosclerotic plaque, calcified valves and myocardium. Am J Cardiol 1985;55:1192–1196.

Index

A

Ablation, 477–478, 479–480
  of atrioventricular junction, 530–533
  complications, 532, 535
  electrode catheter, 529–537, 539–565
  equipment, 545–547
  laser, 803–815
  registry, 529–537
  ventricular tachycardia, 533–537, 539–565
Accessory pathways, 243–268
Afterdepolarization
  delayed, 129, 130–137, 139, 157–165
  early, 154–157, 226–227
Ambulatory monitoring. *See* Holter monitoring
Amiodarone, 500–502
Anesthesia, 108
Anisotropy, 24–48, 79, 244–245, 258–263
Antiarrhythmic drugs, 48, 299–309
  arrhythmogenic potentials of, 227–228
  atrioventricular conduction, depressing, 490
  after cardiac arrest, 514
  clinical classification of, 485–493
  efficacy of, measuring, 466
  electrophysiologic changes by, 219–228, 495–503
  extrasystoles, use on, 490
  responses expected, 486–488
  for sustained tachycardias, 488–490
  for ventricular tachycardia or ventricular fibrillation, 462–463
Arrhythmia
  atrial, 67–80, 278–281
  benign to lethal, 411–412
  cardiac arrest, 505–522
  catecholergic, 491
  catheter electrical ablation of, 529–537, 539–563
  digitalis, 491
  after fulguration, 561
  ischemic, 83–102, 105–123, 105–123, 227, 491
  junctional, 273–278
  mechanisms of, 148–150
  morphologic characteristics, 3–25
  pharmacological suppression of, 159–165
  phases, 110–111
  rate dependency vs. adrenergic dependency, 414
  sinus node reentry, 53–63
  sudden death, as determinant of, 356–358
  supraventricular, 271–281
  therapies, 403–418, 421–430, 435–450
  triggered activity, 129–142, 147–165
  ventricular, 421–430, 435–450, 767–776
  See also specific types of arrhythmias
ATP, 94–102
Atrial fibrillation. *See* Fibrillation, atrial
Atrial flutter. *See* Flutter, atrial
Atrial tachycardia. *See* Tachycardia, atrial
Atrioventricular junction
  ablation, 530–533
  conduction in, 725–738
  reentry tachycardia, 595–598, 600–601
Atrioventricular node
  conduction, 209–217, 490, 497–499
  reentry tachycardia, 643–644
Automaticity, 150–154
Autonomic nervous system, 741–761

B

Brechenmacher fiber, 13

C

Calcium, 157–158, 159, 487
Cardiac arrest
  antiarrhythmic drugs for, 514
  causes, 509

hospital care for, 507–508
implantable devices, use of, 517–518
out-of-hospital, 505–522
programmed electrical stimulation after, 515–517
risk of recurrence, 508
survivors of, 506–507, 509–521
Cardiac mapping. See Mapping
Cardiac metabolism, 84–85
Cardiomyopathy
dilated, 447–448
hypertrophic, 353–364, 367–375, 448–449
Catecholamine, 158
Catheter, electrode, 529–537, 539–565
Circus movement, 68–69, 76–78, 148
Conduction
accessory pathways, 243–268
atrioventricular junction, 725–738
atrioventricular node, 209–217, 490, 497–499
concealed, 718–719
His-Purkinje, 499–500
ion channels, 784–790
reentry models, 78–79
sinus node, 58–62
velocity, 114, 175–176, 191–207, 222–224
Coronary artery
disease, 391–398
occlusion, 107

D

Defibrillator, implantable, 478, 480, 517–518, 561–562, 655–660, 663–678, 681–686
availability, 673–674
clinical results, 668–671, 681–686
costs, 676–677
replacement, 672
system components, 666–668
Digitalis, 160–162, 491
Drugs, antiarrhythmic. See Antiarrhythmic drugs
Dysplasia, right ventricular, 433–464

E

Ebstein's anomaly, 17, 19
Echo beat, 55–58, 62–63
Electrocardiogram, 237–239
abnormal, as marker, 702, 703
Fourier transform analysis, 311–326
ischemic heart disease detection, 699–701
after myocardial infarction, 701–702

signal averaging, 299–309, 315–316, 330, 334
sudden death risk, determination of, 701
See also Holter monitoring
Electrode catheter, 529–537, 539–565
Electronics industry, 707–715
Electrophysiology, 86–91, 112–121, 556
antiarrhythmic drugs, 219–228, 495–503
bioelectric amplifiers, 246–247
cardiac ion channels, 779–798
conduction velocity, 114
electrograms, 245–246, 247–250
excitability, 115–117
hypertrophic cardiomyopathy, testing for, 358–361
invasive vs. noninvasive strategies, 403–418
membrane potential, 112–114, 131–134
origins, 715–721
reconstitution technique, 780–782, 794–799
resistance, 112
in supraventricular tachycardia, 233–241
therapeutic considerations, 240–241
ventricular fibrillation, 117–123
waveform analysis, 243–268
Entrainment, 171–172, 174–188, 204–206
Exercise, 440, 754–758

F

Fibrillation, atrial, 67–80, 254, 488, 600, 601, 644
Fibrillation, ventricular
mechanisms of, 117–121
after myocardial infarction, 445–446
therapies for, 457–469, 471–482
Fluorescence photography, NADH, 769–770
Flutter, atrial, 67–80, 488, 642–643
Fourier transform analysis, 311–326
Fulguration. See Ablation
Fulgurator, 545–546

G

Gating, 790–794

H

Heart
metabolism, 84–85
rate, 108–109

See also Arrhythmia; Cardiac arrest
His-Purkinje conduction, 499–500
Holter (ambulatory) monitoring, 331, 335, 421
  classification of data, 408–409
  efficiency of, 465–466
  of exercise-induced arrhythmias, 440
  limitations, 405–408
  methodological considerations, 436–439
  vs. programmed electrical stimulation, 421, 425–426, 427–428, 429, 435–436

I

Infarct, 107–108
  electrocardiogram after, 701–702
  during fulguration, 561
  late death after, 377–387
  magnetic resonance imaging, 770–776
  NADH fluorescence photography, 769–770
  programmed stimulation after, 330, 338, 339–340, 344, 345–346, 442–446
  sudden death after, 329–340, 343–350
Ion channels, 779–798
  mechanism of, 784–794
  properties of, 782–784
Ischemia, 83–102, 105–123
  collaterals, 107
  coronary artery occlusion, 107
  electrocardiogram, detection by, 699–701
  electrophysiological alterations during, 86–91, 112–121
  energy utilization during, 85–86
  experimental models, 106–110
  heart rate, 108–109
  potassium loss during, 91–102
  size of area, 106, 767–776
  sympathetic nervous system, 110
  therapy against, 509–511
  See also Infarct

J

James fiber, 13

L

Laser, 803–815
Lev's disease, 13

M

Magnetic resonance imaging, 770–776
Mahaim fibers, 10, 19–23

Mapping
  computerized intraoperative, 613–636
    multipoint intraoperative systems, 615–619
  pace, 192–202
  percutaneous, 529–537
  single-point intraoperative systems, 614–615
  in supraventricular tachycardia, 629–633
  of ventricular tachycardia, 605–610, 624–626, 633–635
  in Wolff-Parkinson-White syndrome, 191, 621–624, 626–628
Metablolism, cardiac, 84–85
Monitoring. *See* Holter monitoring
Myocardial infarction. *See* Infarct

N

NADH fluorescence photography, 769–770
Nervous system, autonomic, 741–761
Nervous system, sympathetic, 110
Nodoventricular fibers, 599, 601

P

Pacing
  antitachycardia, 285–294, 478, 480
  beat delay, 203–204
  fulguration's effect on, 561–562
  mapping, 192–202
  overdrive, 135–142
  patient experience, 288–293
  tachyarrhythmias, treatment of, 176–179, 204–207
Paladino's tract, 19
Parasystole, 716–718
Potassium
  ATP-sensitive channel, 94–102
  loss during ischemia, 91–102
Preexcitation, ventricular, 3–15
  atrio-fascicular and intranodal bypass tracts, 12–15
  atrioventricular connections, 7–8, 15–19
  morphologic basis, 6–15
  nodoventricular and fasciculo-ventricular connections, 8–11, 19–23
  pathology, 4–6
Programmed, stimulation electrical
  after cardiac arrest, 515–517
  with cardiomyopathy, 376–375, 447–449
  efficiency of, 465–466

vs. Holter monitoring, 421, 425–426, 427–428, 429, 435–436
after infarct, 330, 338, 339–340, 344, 345–346, 442–446
proarrhythmic effects of, 464–465
ventricular, 421–430, 440–449

R

Reentry
  anisotropic, 79
  atrial, 72–76
  atrioventricular junction tachycardia, 595–598, 600–601
  atrioventricular node tachycardia, 643–644
  circuits, 68, 179–188
  models of, 76–80
  rhythms, 141–142, 172–173
  sinus node, 53–63
  slow conduction in, 175–176
  and transient entrainment, 174–175
  ventricular, 27–48
  in ventricular fibrillation, 117–123
  wavelength, role of, 72–76
Refractory period, atrial and ventricular, 209–217, 500
Repolarization
  asynchronous, 222–224
  local differences in, 225–227
Research, control of, 689–697
Rhythms
  automatic, 139–141
  reentrant, 141–142, 172–173

S

Sinus node
  conduction, 58–62
  reentry, 53–63
  spontaneous cycle length, 209–217, 497
Sodium-potassium pump-inhibition, 157, 224–225
Stellectomy, left, 748–754
Sudden death
  arrhythmias as a determinant of, 356–358
  with coronary artery disease, 391–398
  in hypertrophic cardiomyopathy, 353–364
  after myocardial infarction, 329–340, 343–350
  predictions of, 354–355, 701
  prevention of, 122–123, 377–387, 741–761
  in recurrent ventricular tachycardia, 463

Superventricular tachycardia. *See* Tachycardia, superventricular
Surgery
  for atrial fibrillation, 644
  for atrial tachycardia, 644–645
  mapping, 605–610, 613–636
  for supraventricular tachycardia, 591–602, 640–644
  for ventricular tachycardia, 645–649
  for Wolff-Parkinson-White syndrome, 573–587
Sympathetic nerve, stimulation of, 209–217
Sympathetic nervous system, 110

T

Tachyarrhythmias
  entrainment of, 171–188
  laser ablation, 803–815
  pacemaker treatment, 176–179, 204–207
  reentrant rhythm, 172–174
  reentry circuit, 179–184
  See also specific types of tachyarrhythmias
Tachycardia, atrial, 599, 601, 644–645
Tachycardia, atrioventricular junction reentry, 595–598, 600–601
Tachycardia, atrioventricular node reentry, 643–644
Tachycardia, supraventricular
  antiarrhythmic drugs for suppression of, 488–489
  electrophysiological studies, 233–241
  mapping, 629–633
  narrow QRS, 234–235
  pacing mode to terminate, 285–294
  surgical treatment of, 591–602, 640–644
  wide QRS, 235–239
  See also Wolff-Parkinson-White syndrome
Tachycardia, ventricular
  ablation, 533–537, 539–565
  anisotrophy, effect of, 27–48
  antiarrhythmic drugs for, 489–490, 500
  electrocardiogram in management of, 299–309, 311–326
  entrainment of, 171–172, 174–188, 204–206
  idiopathic, drug treatment of, 463–464
  idiopathic, programmed stimulation of, 449
  inducible, 332–333, 534
  mapping, 605–610, 624–626, 633–635
  pacing, effect of, 204–207

during slow conduction, 191–207
sudden death in, 463
surgery for, 645–649
therapies, 457–469, 471–482
Therapies
  ablation, 477–478, 479–480
  cardioverter/defibrillator, implantable, 478, 480
  Holter monitoring, 405, 408–409, 421, 425–426, 427–428, 429, 435–440
  medical, 478, 480
  noninvasive vs. invasive, 403–418, 435–450
  programmed stimulation-guided, 421–430, 440–449
  selection criteria, 471–482
  surgery, antitachycardia, 477, 479
Torsade de pointes, 490–491
Triggered activity
  delayed afterdepolarization-induced, 129, 130–137, 139, 157–165
  early afterdepolarization-induced, 154–157
  initiation of, 134–135
  overdrive pacing, response to, 135–142

V

Vagus nerve, stimulation of, 209–217, 758–759
Ventricular fibrillation. *See* Fibrillation, ventricular
Ventricular tachycardia. *See* Tachycardia, ventricular

W

Waveform analysis, 243–268
Wavelength, role of, 72–76
Wolff-Parkinson-White syndrome
  ablation in, 271
  accessory atrioventricular connections, 7–8, 15–18, 22–23
  atrio-fascicular and intranodal bypass tracts, 12–15
  circus movement tachycardia in, 148
  Mahaim connections, 19–22
  mapping of, 191, 621–624, 626–628
  nodoventricular and fasciculo-ventricular connections, 8–11, 22–23
  surgical treatment, 573–587, 640–642
  ventricular preexcitation, 3–15, 23–25